Potter & Perry's Essentials of Nursing Foundation

SOUTH ASIA EDITION

Patricia A. Potter
Anne Griffin Perry
Patricia A. Stockert
Amy M. Hall

Adaptation Editor
Suresh K. Sharma

Potter & Perry's Essentials of Nursing Foundation

SOUTH ASIA EDITION

Patricia A. Potter, RN, MSN, PhD, FAAN
Formerly, Director of Research
Patient Care Services
Barnes-Jewish Hospital
St. Louis, Missouri

Anne Griffin Perry, RN, MSN, EdD, FAAN
Professor Emerita
School of Nursing
Southern Illinois University—Edwardsville
Edwardsville, Illinois

Patricia A. Stockert, RN, BSN, MS, PhD
President, College of Nursing
Saint Francis Medical Center College of Nursing
Peoria, Illinois

Amy M. Hall, RN, BSN, MS, PhD, CNE
Dean, School of Nursing
Franciscan Missionaries of Our Lady University
Baton Rouge, Louisiana

South Asia Edition Editor
Suresh K. Sharma, PhD, RN, FNRS
Professor and Principal
College of Nursing
All India Institute of Medical Sciences
Jodhpur, Rajasthan, India

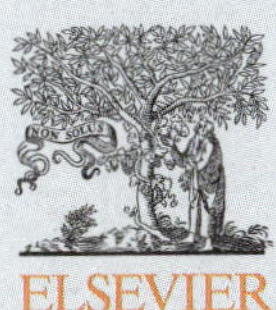

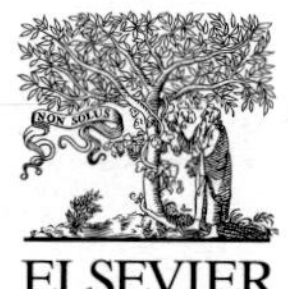

ELSEVIER

RELX India Pvt. Ltd.
Registered Office: 818, Indraprakash Building, 8thFloor, 21, Barakhamba Road, New Delhi-110001
Corporate Office: 14th Floor, Building No. 10B, DLF Cyber City, Phase II, Gurgaon-122 002, Haryana, India

Essentials for Nursing Practice, 9e, Patricia A. Potter, Anne Griffiin Perry, Patricia A. Stockert, Amy M. Hall.

ISBN: 978-0-323-48184-7

Herdman, T.H. & Kamitsuru, S. (Eds.) Nursing Diagnoses—Definitions and Classification 2012-2014

In order to make safe and effective judgments using NANDA-I nursing diagnoses, it is essential that nurses refer to the definitions and defining characteristics of the diagnoses listed in the work.

This adaptation of Essentials for Nursing Practice, 9e, by Patricia A. Potter, Anne Griffiin Perry, Patricia A. Stockert, Amy M. Hall was undertaken by RELX India Private Limited and is published by arrangement with Elsevier Inc.

Potter & Perry's Essentials of Nursing Foundation, South Asia Edition, Patricia A. Potter, Anne Griffiin Perry, Patricia A. Stockert, Amy M. Hall.
Adaptation Editor: Suresh K. Sharma

Adaptation ISBN: 978-81-312-5780-7

First Printed in India 2021, Reprinted 2022

Notice

The adaptation has been undertaken by RELX India Pvt. Ltd. at its sole responsibility. Practitioners and researchers must always rely on their own experience and knowledge in evaluating and using any information, methods, compounds or experiments described herein. Because of rapid advances in the medical sciences, in particular, independent verification of diagnoses and drug dosages should be made. To the fullest extent of the law, no responsibility is assumed by Elsevier, authors, editors or contributors in relation to the adaptation or for any injury and/or damage to persons or property as a matter of products liability, negligence or otherwise, or from any use or operation of any methods, products, instructions, or ideas contained in the material herein.

Although all advertising material is expected to conform to ethical (medical) standards, inclusion in this publication does not constitute a guarantee or endorsement of the quality or value of such product or of the claims made of it by its manufacturer.

This publication is licensed for sale in Bangladesh, Bhutan, India, Maldives, Nepal, Pakistan and Sri Lanka only. Circulation of this version outside these territories is unauthorized and illegal.

Content Strategist: Deepti Damodaran
Head of Content Project Management-APAC: Shabina Nasim
Content Project Manager: Supriya Barua Kumar

Printed in India by Balaji Art, Mumbai.

Adaptation Editor

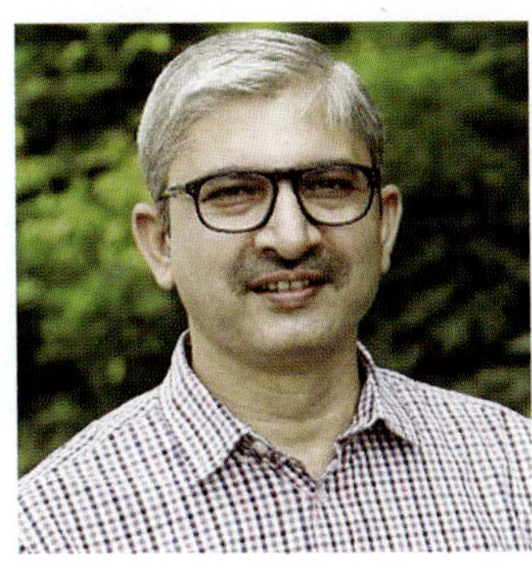

Prof Suresh K. Sharma is currently a Professor-cum-Principal, College of Nursing, All India Institute of Medical Sciences (AIIMS), Jodhpur, Rajasthan, India. He is also ICN-GNLI 2020 Scholar at International Council of Nursing, Global Nursing Leadership Institute, Geneva, Switzerland. He received his Bachelor of Science degree in Nursing from Rajiv Gandhi University of Health Sciences, Bengaluru, his Master of Science degree in Medical-Surgical Nursing from National Institute of Nursing Education, PGIMER, Chandigarh, under Panjab University, Chandigarh, and his Doctoral degree in Nursing Administration from Panjab University, Chandigarh. Prof Sharma is a Post-Doctoral Fellow of Nursing Research Society of India (NRSI) and he obtained observership in Clinical Nursing Research at University of York, Yorkshire, UK.

He received his University Gold Medal for obtaining First Position in the university during his Bachelor and Master degrees. He is also registered as an RN in Board of Registered Nursing, California, USA. He has been conferred with the prestigious Indian nursing award "*Florence Nightingale Award-2001*" from Florence Nightingale Nurses' Welfare Association and Anglo-Indian Unity Center, Bangalore. He is member of 15 different national and international nursing societies and associations including American Association of Critical Care Nursing, Sigma Theta Tau International, and International Network for Doctoral Education in Nursing. He is also the fellow of International Network for Doctoral Education in Nursing and Sigma Theta Tau International USA.

Prof Sharma has taught undergraduate, postgraduate, and doctoral program nursing students, working as a Lecturer, Associate Professor, and Professor of Nursing at College of Nursing Dayanand Medical College & Hospital, Ludhiana, Punjab, and All India Institute of Medical Sciences, Rishikesh and Jodhpur. He is also active internationally through his association with Liverpool John Moores University, Liverpool, UK, as external advisor, and has acted as an invigilator for South African Nursing Council, Acardia, Protoria, South Africa.

He is a prolific writer and has published several text books in nursing; he has also reviewed several books, contributed many chapters in books, and published more than 100 research papers in national and international nursing journals. Prof. Sharma's clinical, educational, and research interest involves the generation and dissemination of empirical evidences in nursing to improve the quality of nursing care, education, and administration. He has special interest for research in the areas of nursing education, Critical Care Nursing, diabetes, and endocrinology nursing, where he has carried out 20 research projects as principle investigator or co-investigator and also guide for 10 doctoral-level students.

Prof Sharma is presently the section editor of *Journal of Medical Evidence*, and peer reviewer of *Nursing and Midwifery Research Journal*. In addition, he is also serving as a member of editorial board of several national and international health sciences journals, namely *Journal of Caring Science, International Journal of Nursing Education, International Journal of Nursing Care*, and *International Journal of Nursing Education & Practice* published from Canada. Prof Sharma is the Founder President of Society of Perioperative Nursing, India, and Society for Critical Care Nursing, India.

Prof Sharma has presented more than 150 research papers/lectures/talks at international- and national-level conferences, seminars, symposiums, and workshops. He has also chaired sessions in more than 30 national- and international-level conferences and participated in more than 200 national- and international-level conferences. Prof Sharma also acted as internal and external examiner for undergraduate-, postgraduate-, and doctoral-level nursing programs in different universities and nursing boards.

He is practicing as a nurse educator, administrator, and researcher with a philosophy: *"preparing clinically competent nurses to offer cost effective quality care."* He is devoted in generating the empirical evidences to provide the quality nursing care at affordable cost and maintaining standard of nursing care, education, and nursing administration par excellence.

Reviewers of First South Asia Edition

1. ***Bimla Kapoor, PhD, RN***
   Former Director,
   School of Health Sciences,
   Indira Gandhi National Open University,
   New Delhi, India

2. ***Manju Vatsa, PhD, RN***
   Former Principal,
   College of Nursing,
   All India Institute of Medical Sciences,
   New Delhi, India

3. ***Latha Venkatesan, PhD, RN***
   Principal,
   College of Nursing,
   All India Institute of Medical Sciences,
   New Delhi, India

4. ***Rathi Balachandran, PhD, RN***
   Assistant Director General (Nursing),
   Ministry of Health & Family Welfare,
   Government of India,
   New Delhi, India

5. ***Sukhpal Kaur, PhD, RN***
   Lecturer,
   National Institute of Nursing Education,
   PGIMER,
   Chandigarh, India

6. ***MJ Kumari, PhD, RN***
   Professor & Principal (Actg),
   College of Nursing,
   JIPMER,
   Puducherry, India

7. ***Anigrace Kalaimathi, PhD, RN***
   Registrar,
   Tamil Nadu Nursing Council,
   Chennai,
   Tamil Nadu, India

8. ***Asha P Shetty, PhD, RN***
   Professor-cum-Principal,
   College of Nursing,
   All India Institute of Medical Sciences,
   Bhubaneshwar, India

9. ***Triza Jeevan, PhD, RN***
   Principal,
   DMCH College of Nursing,
   Dayanand Medical College & Hospitals,
   Ludhiana,
   Punjab, India

10. ***Reena Jerish, PhD, RN***
    Professor & Principal,
    College of Nursing,
    Christian Medical College & Hospitals,
    Ludhiana,
    Punjab, India

11. ***Manju Chuganni, PhD, RN***
    Dean,
    School of Nursing & Allied Health,
    Jamia Hamdard University,
    New Delhi, India

12. ***Jyoti Sarin, PhD, RN***
    Principal & Director,
    MM College of Nursing,
    Maharishi Markandeshwar University,
    Ambala, India

13. ***S Madhavi, PhD, RN***
    Principal & Professor,
    KMCH College of Nursing,
    Coimbatore,
    Tamil Nadu, India

14. ***Mehmooda Regu***
    Former Principal,
    College of Nursing,
    Sher-I-Kashmir Institute of Medical Sciences,
    Srinagar,
    Jammu & Kashmir, India

15. ***Assuma Beevi, PhD, RN***
    Joint Director,
    MIMS Academy,
    Kozhikode,
    Kerala, India

16. ***Ratna Prakash, PhD, RN***
    Professor & Principal,
    Pal College of Nursing,
    Haldwani,
    Uttarakhand, India

17. ***HCL Rawat, MScN, RN***
    Professor & Principal,
    University College of Nursing,
    Baba Farid University of Health Sciences,
    Faridkot,
    Punjab, India

18. ***Rita Lakhani, PhD, RN***
Principal,
School of Nursing,
DY Patil University,
Thane,
Maharashtra, India

19. ***Anil Sharma, PhD, RN***
Professor & Principal,
Manikaka Topawala Institute of Nursing,
Charusat, Changa,
Gujrat, India

20. ***Pragna Dabhi, PhD, RN***
Registrar,
Gujrat Nursing Council,
Ahmedabad,
Gujrat, India

21. ***Shiv K Mudgal, PhD, RN***
Professor & Principal,
Akal College of Nursing,
Baru Sahib,
Himachal Pradesh, India

22. ***Mamta Verma, MScN, RN***
Professor & Principal (Actg),
College of Nursing,
All India Institute of Medical Sciences,
Bhopal, India

23. ***Lily Podder, PhD, RN***
Associate Professor,
College of Nursing,
All India Institute of Medical Sciences,
Bhopal, India

24. ***Smita MV, PhD, RN***
Associate Professor,
College of Nursing,
All India Institute of Medical Sciences,
Bhubaneshwar, India

25. ***Sonali Jadhav, PhD, RN***
Principal
Ramaiah Institute of Nursing Education and Research
Bangalore, India

26. ***Prabhjot Saini, PhD, RN***
Professor & Principal,
SKSS College of Nursing,
Sarabha, Ludhiana,
Punjab, India

27. ***Narinder K Walia, PhD, RN***
Professor & Principal,
Saraswati Education Society Group,
Mohali,
Punjab, India

28. ***Nochovono Tase, MScN, RN***
Lecturer,
College of Nursing,
North Eastern Indira Gandhi Regional Institute of Health & Medical Sciences,
Shillong,
Meghalaya, India

29. ***Mahipal Singh, PhD, RN***
Professor & Principal,
Akhil Bharti Vidyapeeth College of Nursing,
Sikar,
Rajasthan, India

30. ***Elsa Sanatombi Devi, PhD, RN***
Professor,
Manipal College of Nursing,
Manipal Academy of Higher Education,
Manipal,
Karnataka, India

31. ***Rakhi Mishra, MScN, RN***
Assistant Professor,
College of Nursing,
All India Institute of Medical Sciences,
Rishikesh, India

32. ***Rajesh Kumar, PhD, RN***
Assistant Professor,
College of Nursing,
All India Institute of Medical Sciences,
Rishikesh, India

33. ***Medha Verma, MScN, RN,***
Kingsbury Court Care Home,
Bisley England, United Kingdom

34. ***Tarika Sharma, MScN, RN***
Lecturer,
College of Nursing,
Institute of Liver and Biliary Sciences,
New Delhi, India

35. ***Milan Tirwa, MScN, RN***
Associate Professor,
All India Institute of Medical Sciences,
College of Nursing.
New Delhi, India

36. ***Nipin Kalal, MScN, RN***
Assistant Professor
College of Nursing,
All India Institute of Medical Sciences,
Jodhpur, India

Contributors of 9th Edition

Carolyn Wright Boon, MSN, BSN
Assistant Professor
Saint Francis Medical Center College of Nursing
Peoria, Illinois

Linda Cason, DNP, MSN, BSN
Clinical Nurse Specialist
Deaconess Hospital, Inc.
Evansville, Indiana

Lori Catalano, JD, MSN, RN, CCNS, PCCN
Assistant Professor of Clinical Nursing
College of Nursing
University of Cincinnati
Cincinnati, Ohio

Edith Claros, PhD, MSN, RN, APHN-BC
PMHNP Track Coordinator and Associate Professor
School of Nursing
MCPHS University
Worcester, Massachusetts

Janice C. Colwell, RN, MS, CWOCN, FAAN
Advanced Practice Nurse
Surgery
University of Chicago Medicine
Chicago, Illinois

Margaret Ecker, RN, MS
Nurse Consultant
Los Angeles, California;
Director of Nursing Quality, retired
Kaiser Permanente Los Angeles
Los Angeles, California

Jane Fellows, MSN, CWOCN
Wound/Ostomy CNS
Advanced Clinical Practice
Duke University Health System
Durham, North Carolina

Linda Felver, PhD, RN
Associate Professor
School of Nursing
Oregon Health & Science University
Portland, Oregon

Susan Fetzer, BA, BSN, MSN, MBA, PhD, CNL
Professor
College of Health and Human Services
University of New Hampshire
Durham, New Hampshire;
Director of Research
Patient Care Services
Southern New Hampshire Medical Center
Nashua, New Hampshire

Victoria N. Folse, PhD, APN, PMHCNS-BC, LCPC
Director and Professor; Caroline F. Rupert Endowed Chair of Nursing
School of Nursing
Illinois Wesleyan University
Bloomington, Illinois

Lorri A. Graham, DNP, RN
Associate Professor
Saint Francis Medical Center College of Nursing
Peoria, Illinois

Susan Hendricks, EdD, MSN, RN, CNE
Associate Dean for Undergraduate Programs
School of Nursing
Indiana University
Indianapolis, Indiana

Cassandra Horack, MS, PSL, BSN
Vice President Quality and Safety
OSF HealthCare Saint Francis Medical Center
Peoria, Illinois

Noël Marie Kerr, PhD
Assistant Professor
School of Nursing
Illinois Wesleyan University
Bloomington, Illinois

Jerrilee Lamar, PhD, RN, CNE
Associate Professor of Nursing
Dunigan Department of Nursing and Health Sciences
University of Evansville
Evansville, Indiana

Nancy Laplante, PhD, RN, AHN-BC
Associate Professor
School of Nursing
Widener University
Chester, Pennsylvania

Angela McConachie, FNP, DNP
Assistant Professor
Faculty
Goldfarb School of Nursing at Barnes-Jewish College
St. Louis, Missouri

Judith A. McCutchan, ASN, BSN, MSN, PhD
Adjunct Faculty
Nursing
University of Evansville
Evansville, Indiana

Staci McIntosh, MS, RD
Assistant Professor (Lecturer)
Department of Nutrition and Integrative Physiology
University of Utah
Salt Lake City, Utah

Emily McKenna, APN, CNS
INI Neurology
OSF HealthCare Saint Francis Medical Center
Peoria, Illinois

Jill Parsons, PhD, RN
Associate Professor
Nursing
MacMurray College
Jacksonville, Illinois

Theresa Pietsch, PhD, RN, CRRN, CNE
Associate Professor
Division of Nursing & Health Sciences
Neumann University
Aston, Pennsylvania

Sandra L. Richmond, DNP, MS, RN, CSN
Dean, School of Nursing and Health Sciences
Pennsylvania College of Technology
Williamsport, Pennsylvania

Anita Shoup, DNP, RN, CNS-SP, CNOR
Assistant Professor; Coordinator, Simulation/Experiential Learning
Nursing
Heritage University
Toppenish, Washington

Reviewers

Michelle Aebersold, PhD, RN, CHSE, FAAN
Clinical Associate Professor and Director of Simulation
University of Michigan School of Nursing
Ann Arbor, Michigan

Lezley Anderson, MA, MSN, RN
Assistant Professor
Saint Francis Medical Center College of Nursing
Peoria, Illinois

Colleen Andreoni, DNP, MSN, ANP-BC, FNP-BC
Advanced Practice Nurse
Board Certified Nurse Practitioner
Northwestern Medicine Regional Medical Group
Chicago, Illinois

Suzanne L. Bailey, PMHCNS-BC, CNE
Associate Professor of Nursing
University of Evansville
Evansville, Indiana

Leigh Ann Bonney, PhD, RN, CCRN
Associate Professor
Saint Francis Medical Center College of Nursing
Peoria, Illinois

Denise Branchizio, DNP, MSN, RN
Assistant Professor of Nursing
New Jersey City University
Jersey City, New Jersey

Anna M. Bruch, RN, MSN
Nursing Professor
Illinois Valley Community College
Oglesby, Illinois

Sheryl Buckner, PhD, RN, ANEF
Assistant Professor/Lab Director
University of Oklahoma Earl and Frances Ziegler College of Nursing
Oklahoma City, Oklahoma

Pat Callard, DNP, RN, CNL
Associate Professor of Nursing
College of Graduate Nursing
Western University of Health Sciences
Pomona, California

Kim Clevenger, EdD, MSN, RN, BC
Associate Professor of Nursing
Morehead State University
Morehead, Kentucky

Tracy Colburn, RN, MSN, C-EFM
Associate Professor of Nursing
Lewis and Clark Community College
Godfrey, Illinois

Barbara A. Coles, PhD, RN-BC, LHRM
Adjunct Professor
American Public University System
Charles Town, West Virginia

Janice C. Colwell, RN, MS, CWOCN, FAAN
Advanced Practice Nurse
Surgery
University of Chicago Medicine
Chicago, Illinois

Pamela Cook, PhD(c), MSN, RN, CNS
Assistant Professor
Bloomsburg University
Bloomsburg, Pennsylvania

Eileen Costantinou, MSN, RN-BC
Practice Specialist, Senior Coordinator
Barnes-Jewish Hospital
St. Louis, Missouri

Graciela Lopez Cox, MSN, RN
Assistant Professor
Samuel Merritt University
Sacramento, California

Pamela A. Dettenmeier, PhD(c), DNP, ANP-BC
Associate Professor of Medicine
Director CPAP Adherence Clinic
Adult Nurse Practitioner
Division of Pulmonary, Critical Care & Sleep Medicine
Saint Louis University
St. Louis, Missouri

Holly Johanna Diesel, PhD, RN
Associate Professor and Academic Chair of the Accelerated and RN to BSN Program
Goldfarb School of Nursing at Barnes-Jewish College
St. Louis, Missouri

Christine R. Durbin, PhD, JD, RN
Associate Professor and Chair, Primary Care & Health Systems Department
Southern Illinois University School of Nursing
Edwardsville, Illinois

Amber Essman, DNP, MSN, FNP-BC, CNE ARNP
Confluence Health;
Visiting Professor
Chamberlain College of Nursing
Moses Lake, Washington

Kelly L. Fisher, PhD, RN, FNAP
Dean, School of Nursing
Endicott College
Beverly, Massachusetts

Linda R. Garner, PhD, RN, APHN-BC, CHES
Associate Professor
Southeast Missouri State University
Cape Girardeau, Missouri

Linda Hansen-Kyle, PhD, RN, CCM
Chair (Retired) Second Degree Program
Azusa Pacific University
Azusa, California;
University of San Diego
San Diego, California;
University of Phoenix
Tempe, Arizona

Nicole M. Heimgartner, MSN, RN, COI
Vice President
Connect: RN2ED
Dayton, Ohio

Kathleen C. Jones, MSN, RN, CNS
Associate Professor of Nursing
Walters State Community College
Morristown, Tennessee

Shari Kist, PhD, RN, CNE
Associate Professor
Goldfarb School of Nursing at Barnes-Jewish College
St. Louis, Missouri

Kimberly Leppert, MSN, RN, ACNS-BC, CNOR, ONC
Surgery Clinical Supervisor
Swedish Health Services-Ballard
Seattle, Washington

Kathryn A. Lever, RN, MSN, WHNP-BC
Associate Professor of Nursing
Dunigan Family School of Nursing and Health Sciences
University of Evansville
Evansville, Indiana

Mary M. Lopez, PhD, RN
Associate Dean, Research
Western University of Health Sciences
Pomona, California

Angela McConachie, DNP, FNP
Assistant Professor
Goldfarb School of Nursing at Barnes-Jewish Hospital
St. Louis, Missouri

Janis Longfield McMillan, RN, MSN, CNE
Associate Clinical Professor
Northern Arizona University
Flagstaff, Arizona

Pamela Molnar, RN, CEN
Decatur Morgan Hospital
Decatur, Alabama

Katrin Moskowitz, DNP, FNP
Doctor of Nursing Practice
Meriden, Connecticut

Katie Murphy, RN, MSN, PHN
Virtual Nurse Educator
Quintiles/Abbvie
Chicago, Illinois

Wendy R. Ostendorf, RN, MS, EdD, CNE
Professor of Nursing
Neumann University
Aston, Pennsylvania

Veronica (Ronnie) Peterson, BA, BSN, MS
Manager of Clinical Support
UW-Medical Foundation
Madison, Wisconsin

Victoria Plagenz, PhD, MS, BSN
Assistant Professor
University of Great Falls
Great Falls, Montana

Melissa Anne Radecki, MSN, NEd, RN, PCCN
Nursing Instructor
Florida Southern College
Lakeland, Florida

Cherie R. Rebar, PhD, MBA, RN, COI
Affiliate Faculty
Indiana Wesleyan University
Marion, Indiana;
Consultant
Xavier University School of Nursing
Cincinnati, Ohio

Anita K. Reed, MSN, RN
Chair, Community Health Practice
St. Elizabeth School of Nursing
Saint Joseph' s College
Lafayette, Indiana

Jill R. Reed, PhD, APRN-NP
Assistant Professor
University of Nebraska Medical Center, College of Nursing
Kearney, Nebraska

Rhonda J. Reed, MSN, RN, CRRN
Learning Resource Center Director—Technology Coordinator
Indiana State University
Terre Haute, Indiana

Maura C. Schlairet, EdD, MA, MSN, RN, CNL
Professor of Nursing, Bioethicist
College of Nursing and Health Sciences
Valdosta State University
Valdosta, Georgia

Susan Parnell Scholtz, RN, PhD
Associate Professor of Nursing
Moravian College
Bethlehem, Pennsylvania

Elizabeth Sibson-Tuan, MS, RN
Bay Area Preceptor Coordinator
Samuel Merritt University
Oakland, California

Crystal Slaughter, DNP, APN, ACNS-BC
Associate Professor
Saint Francis Medical Center College of Nursing
Peoria, Illinois

Emily G. Smith, DNP, RN, CRRN, CNE, FNAP
Assistant Professor
Endicott College
Beverly, Massachusetts

Mindy Stayner, PhD, MSN, RN
Professor
Northwest State Community College
Chamberlain College of Nursing
Capella University
Archbold, Ohio

Laura M. Streeter, BSN, RN, SCRN, GCPH
Stroke Program Nurse
University of Missouri Health System
Columbia, Missouri

Linda Turchin, RN, MSN, CNE
Associate Professor of Nursing
Fairmont State University
Fairmont, West Virginia

Claudia C. Turner, MSN, RN
Professor of Nursing
Temple College
Temple, Texas

Heidi Tymkew, PT, DPT, MHS, CCS
Clinical Specialist
Barnes-Jewish Hospital
St. Louis, Missouri

Kim Webb, MN, RN
Adjunct Nursing Instructor
Pioneer Technology Center
Ponca City, Oklahoma

Anne M. Welsh, MSN-Ed, RN
Assistant Professor
Lewis and Clark Community College
Godfrey, Illinois

Estella J. Wetzel, MSN, APRN, FNP-C
Family Nurse Practitioner
AANP, OAAPN
Dayton, Ohio

Laura M. Willis, DNP, APRN, FNP-C
Co-President, Connect: RN2ED
Beavercreek, Ohio;
Family Nurse Practitioner
Urbana, Ohio

Paige Wimberley, PhD, APRN, CNS, CNE
Associate Professor of Nursing
Arkansas State University
Jonesboro, Arkansas

Valerie Yancey, PhD, RN
Associate Professor
Southern Illinois University Edwardsville
Edwardsville, Illinois

Jean Yockey, PhD, FNP-BC, CNE
Assistant Professor
University of South Dakota
Vermillion, South Dakota

Contributors of Previous Edition

Jeanette Spain Adams, RN, PhD, CRNI, APRN

Michelle Aebersold, PhD, RN

Elizabeth A. Ayello, RN, BSN, MS, PhD, CS, CETN

Marjorie Baier, RN, PhD

Sylvia Baird, RN, BSN, MM

Brenda A. Battle, MBA, BSN, RN

Lois Bentler-Lampe, RN, MS

Peggy Breckenridge, MSN, FNP

Judith C. Brostron, RN, BA, JD, LLM

Victoria M. Brown, RN, BSN, MSN, PhD, HNC

Jeri Burger, RN, PhD

Gale Carli, MSN, MSHed, BSN, RN

Rhonda Comrie, PhD, RN

Kelly Jo Cone, RN, BSN, MS, PhD

Roslyn Corcoran, RN, BSN

Eileen Costantinou, RN, MSN, BC

Ruth Curchoe, RN, MSN, CIC

Rick Daniels, RN, BSN, MSN, PhD

Carolyn Ruppel D' Avis, RN, BSN, MSN

Christine Durbin, RN, JD, PhD

Sharon J. Edwards, RN, BSN, MSN, PhD

Martha Keene Elkin, RN, MSN, IBCLC

Linda Fasciani, RN, BSN, MSN

Susan J. Fetzer, RN, BA, BSN, MSN, MBA, PhD

Leah Frederick, MS, RN, CIC

Cynthia S. Goodwin, RN, BSN, MSN

Lois C. Hamel, BS, MS

Janis Waite Hayden, RN, EdD

Maureen Huhmann, MS, RD

Tara Hulsey, RN, PhD, CNE, FAAN

Judith Ann Kilpatrick, RN, MSN, DNSc

Carl A. Kirton, RN-C, BSN, MA, ACRN, ANP

Lori Klingman, RN, MSN

Kristine L' Ecuyer, RN, MSN, CCNS

Kathryn A. Lever, RNC, MSN, WHNP-BC

Ruth Ludwick, RN, BSN, MSN, PhD, RN-C

Suzanne Lugerner, RN, MS, LN, CNSC, CNS

Mary Kay Knight Macheca, RN, BSN, MSN(R), CS, CDE

Deborah L. Marshall, RN, MSN

Carol McGinnis, DNP, RN, CNS, CNSC

Rita G. Mertig, RNC, MS, CNS

Mary Dee Miller, RN, BSN, MS, CIC

Elaine Neel, BSN, MSN

Geralyn A. Ochs, RN, ADN, BSN, MSN

Marsha Evans Orr, RN, MS, CS, CNSN

Wendy R. Ostendorf, MS, EdD

Dula F. Pacquiao, EdD, RN, CTN

Nancy Panthofer, RN, BSN, MSN

Elizabeth S. Pratt, RN, MSN, ACNS-BC

Julia Balzer Riley, RN, MN, AHN-C, CET®

Kristine A. Rose, RN, MSN

Janice J. Rumfelt, BSN, MSN, EdD, RNC

Marilyn Schallom, MSN, CCRN, CCNS

Matthew R. Sorenson, RN, PhD

Sharon Souter, RN, BSN, MSN

Elizabeth Speakman, RN, EdD

Rachel E. Spector, BS, MS, PhD, CTN, FAAN

Susan Speraw, RN, PHD, CNP

Donna L. Thompson, MSN, CRNP, FNP-BC, CCCN

Jelena Todic, MSW, LCSW

Riva Touger-Decker, PhD, RD, FADA

Ann Tritak, RN, EdD

Ellen Wathen, PhD, RN, BC

Pamela Becker Weilitz, DNP, APRN, ANP-BC

Joan Domigan Wentz, MSN, RN

Paige Wimberley, PhD, APN, CNS, CNE

Terry L. Wood, PhD, RN, CNE

Rita Wunderlich, PhD, RN, CNE

Valerie Yancey, RN, PhD

Barbara Yoost, RN, BSN, MSN, CNS

I wish to dedicate this edition of Essentials to the many friends who make up my family. Each one contributes in so many ways to support and value the work I am able to do. Special thanks to Ruth, a wonderful listener and advocate; Jim, a valued friend and kind man; Bess, always adding humor and love to my life; and Anne, a consummate writing colleague and lifelong mentor.

Patricia A. Potter

To all nursing faculty and professional nurses who work each day to advance clinical nursing. Your commitment to nursing education and nursing practice inspires us all to be the guardians of the discipline.

I also want to thank my husband Bob for his loving support.

Anne Griffin Perry

I was blessed to have an incredible nursing role model in my life—my mother, Evelyn M. Clark, RN. Your dedication and service to nursing inspired me to pursue my career as a professional nurse. Your unwavering support of my endeavors provided a foundation for me to continue to grow in my nursing role. Your encouragement and pride in my accomplishments was tremendous. Thank you for starting me on my path to a long and satisfying career in nursing and nursing education. I love you and miss you!

Patricia A. Stockert

To my family, especially Greg, Jacob, Isaac, and Mom and Dad. Thank you for your love, support, and patience, without which I would not be able to chase my dreams. Thank you also to the nursing faculty at Franciscan Missionaries of Our Lady University. Your never-ending compassion and commitment to nursing education inspires me every day. And finally, to my Varsity Sports running friends, who keep me grounded and who have helped me integrate into my new community. Despite all those really hot and long runs, y'all haven't killed me yet!

Amy M. Hall

Foreword

Nurses are among the country's most vital and tireless caregivers, which has been proved and witnessed by everyone during the COVID-19 pandemic, more than ever before. In the last few decades, nursing profession in India has grown from hospital-based occupational training to undergraduate-, postgraduate-, and doctoral-level nursing education. Furthermore, nowadays nurses are also trained in specialized nursing and midwifery practitioner programs in the country. Nurse clinicians have independent, collaborative, and facilitating roles in health care including bedside care, patient advocacy, health education, assisting physician and surgeons in diagnostic, and treatment interventions. Bedside nurses are involved in a wide range of activities such as initial assessment; vital signs monitoring; maintaining hygiene, positioning, promotion of rest, comfort. and sleep; infection prevention and control; practicing barrier nursing; feeding; medication administration; wound care; meeting needs of oxygenation, fluid, and electrolyte; elimination; providing perioperative nursing care; discharge teaching; and other nursing interventions to meet patient's basic and advanced health care needs.

It well known that *'Potter and Perry's Essentials of Nursing Practice'* is a widely appreciated textbook among nursing faculty, nurse practitioners, nursing scholars, and undergraduate and postgraduate nursing students. I am delighted to see the comprehensiveness of this textbook, which precisely covers all the fundamental concepts, skills, and techniques of nursing practice. I am sure that this South Asian edition of *Potter and Perry's Essentials of Nursing Foundation* will not only provide the well-established authentic content of international standard but also cater to the specific curricular needs of nursing students and faculty of the region.

I found this textbook reader friendly to the complex topics, which will help the beginners easily grasp the fundamentals of nursing practice. I also found that this textbook is presented in an uncluttered, straightforward manner. This textbook uses many bulleted lists to make the material visually interesting; in addition, figures, images, boxes, and tables have further contributed to this purpose. Thus, this textbook facilitates the readers to grasp the information quickly and to learn more efficiently. Nevertheless, the lucidity of the content will provide ease in reading and learning for students with non-English background. I hope that this textbook will be an excellent ready reference on the subject of *Nursing Foundation* for nursing faculty, nurse clinicians, clinical nurse specialists, nurse practitioners, undergraduate and postgraduate nursing students, and other health care professionals.

Dr Sanjeev Misra
MS, MCh, FRCS (Eng), FRCS (Glasgow), FICS, FACS (USA), FAMS, FNASc, DSc (Hc)
Professor of Surgical Oncology
Director
All India Institute of Medical Sciences
Jodhpur, Rajasthan, India

Preface to the First South Asia Edition

The nursing profession has always responded to dynamic changes and continual challenges. Today's nurses must be prepared to adapt to the continual changes occurring in health care. They play a vital role in the delivery of multidisciplinary health care services. The practice arena is changing—moving more toward the community setting. The focus of care is also changing, with more emphasis being placed on health promotion and restorative care. Even the patients are changing—more cultural diversity exists, and the percentage of older adult patients continues to increase. Patients are far more involved in and informed about health care.

Despite—or perhaps because of—these changes, it is essential that the basics of nursing remain the foundation of practice. Nurses must be knowledgeable and professional. They must be both technically proficient and personally caring. And they must be able to synthesize a broad array of knowledge and experience when providing care for their patients.

We continue to cover all the fundamental nursing concepts, skills, and techniques that students must master before moving on to other areas of study. In addition, we address the changes in practice that affect how and where nurses use the skills and knowledge they acquire.

FEATURES

We have designed this text to welcome the new student to nursing, communicate our own love for the profession, and promote learning and understanding. We know that today's students are busy and, too often, are overwhelmed by all that they must learn and do. They want their texts to focus on the most current, factual, and essential content and skills. We want to ensure that these students are ready to continue with their education and ultimately be prepared for all of the challenges of practice. To this end, we have included the following key features:

- Students will appreciate the **clear, engaging writing style.** The narrative actually addresses the reader, making this textbook more of an active instructional tool than a passive reference. Students will find that even complex technical and theoretical concepts are presented in a language that is easy to understand.
- The **attractive, functional design** will appeal to today's visual learner. The clear, readable type and bold headings make the content easy to read and follow. Each special element is consistently color keyed so that students can readily identify important information.
- Hundreds of **large, clear, full-color photographs and drawings** reinforce and clarify key concepts and techniques.
- The implementation narrative consistently addresses health promotion, acute care, and restorative and continuing care to reflect a focus on **community-based nursing** and **health promotion.**
- Information related to the **Quality and Safety Education for Nurses (QSEN)** initiative is highlighted with activities integrated into each chapter. These activities incorporate one of the six key competencies and relate back to the progressive chapter case study scenarios.
- **More than 35 nursing skills** are presented in a clear, two-column format with steps and rationales. Skills include delegation guidelines and clinical decision points that alert students to steps that require special assessment or specific technique for safe and effective administration.
- **Procedural guidelines** provide streamlined step-by-step instructions for performing very basic skills.
- Care of the **older adult** and **patient teaching** are stressed throughout the narrative and are also highlighted in special boxes.
- **Learning aids** to help students identify, review, and apply important content in each chapter, including Objectives, Key Terms, Key Points.
- **Printed lists** on the inside back cover provide information about locating specific assets in the book, including Skills, Procedural Guidelines, and Patient Teaching boxes.

New to South Asia Edition

- A complete comprehensive coverage of syllabus of nursing foundation prescribed by the **Indian Nursing Council** for undergraduate and postgraduate nursing students has been presented.
- The **historical background** and development of **nursing in India** has been included in the existing content. In addition, a brief highlight of the existing nursing education and nursing cadres in India has also been added.
- **Health care delivery system in India** and the role of nurse in primary health care has also been incorporated in the existing content of community-based care.
- The book has been adapted to include the much needed Indian health care policies and procedures, such as **Indian National Health Policy-2017**, code of ethics for nurses in India, medico-legal issues in health care in India, and Indian hospital waste management guidelines.
- Illustrations and pictorial presentation has been **adapted to the Indian context** and background.
- Nursing procedures and protocols have been **customized to Indian nursing needs** and resources.
- The presentation of content has been made more **comprehensive and lucid to adapt** to the needs of Indian nursing faculty and students.
- Some of the **much-needed content has been added** to existing content, such as admission and discharge of patient, environmental safety of patient, infection control and machinery, equipment and linen management, care of patients in alterations, care of critically ill patients, and first aid.
- **Evidence-based Practice** boxes have been updated with new PICO questions. These boxes provide a summary of

nursing research evidence related to that specific topic and then explain its implications for nursing practice. These boxes have been updated to reflect current research topics and trends.

Thank you for delving into a different learning format; nurses like you, who are open to new ideas and situations, will make positive changes for patients, families, and communities and in the health care systems in India and abroad. We wish you the best of luck in your nursing career.

Suresh K. Sharma

Preface to the Instructor

The nursing profession is always responding to dynamic change and continual challenges. Today's nurses must be prepared to adapt to the continual changes occurring in health care. They play a vital role in the delivery of multidisciplinary health care services. The practice arena is changing—moving more to the community setting. The focus of care is also changing, with more emphasis being placed on health promotion and restorative care. Even the patients are changing—more cultural diversity exists, and the percentage of older adult patients continues to increase. Patients are far more involved in and informed about health care.

Despite—or perhaps because of—these changes, it is essential that the basics of nursing remain the foundation of practice. Nurses must be knowledgeable and professional. They must be both technically proficient and personally caring. And they must be able to synthesize a broad array of knowledge and experience when providing care for their patients.

We continue to cover all of the fundamental nursing concepts, skills, and techniques that students must master before moving on to other areas of study. In addition, we address changes in practice that affect how and where nurses use the skills and knowledge they acquire.

FEATURES

We have designed this text to welcome the new student to nursing, communicate our own love for the profession, and promote learning and understanding. We know that today's students are busy and, too often, are overwhelmed by all that they must learn and do. They want their texts to focus on the most current, factual, and essential content and skills. We want to ensure that these students are ready to continue with their education and will ultimately be prepared for all of the challenges of practice. To this end, we have included the following key features:

- Students will appreciate the **clear, engaging writing style.** The narrative actually addresses the reader, making this textbook more of an active instructional tool than a passive reference. Students will find that even complex technical and theoretical concepts are presented in a language that is easy to understand.
- The **attractive, functional design** will appeal to today's visual learner. The clear, readable type and bold headings make the content easy to read and follow. Each special element is consistently color keyed so students can readily identify important information.
- Hundreds of **large, clear, full-color photographs and drawings** reinforce and clarify key concepts and techniques.
- The **five-step nursing process** serves as the organizing framework for all clinical chapters. This logical, consistent framework for narrative discussions is further enhanced by special boxes that highlight assessment, care plans, and evaluation of outcome achievement.
- **Ongoing case studies** in each chapter introduce "real-world" patients, families, and nurses. The chapter follows the case study through the steps of the nursing process, helping students see how to apply the process, as well as critical thinking, to the care of patients. Cases take place in both acute and community settings and include patients and nurses from a variety of cultural backgrounds.
- **Nursing Care Plans** guide students on how to conduct an assessment and analyze the defining characteristics that indicate nursing diagnoses. The plans include NIC and NOC classifications to familiarize students with this important nomenclature. The evaluation sections of the plans show students how to evaluate and then determine the outcomes of care.
- **Concept Maps** included in clinical chapters show you the associations among multiple nursing diagnoses for a patient with a selected medical diagnosis, as well as their relationship to nursing interventions.
- The implementation narrative consistently addresses health promotion, acute care, and restorative and continuing care to reflect a focus on **community-based nursing** and **health promotion.**
- Information related to the **Quality and Safety Education for Nurses (QSEN)** initiative is highlighted with activities integrated into each chapter. These activities incorporate one of the six key competencies and relate back to the progressive chapter case study scenarios.
- **More than 35 nursing skills** are presented in a clear, two-column format with steps and rationales. Skills include delegation guidelines and clinical decision points that alert students to steps that require special assessment or specific technique for safe and effective administration.
- **Procedural guidelines** provide streamlined step-by-step instructions for performing very basic skills.
- Care of the **older adult** and **patient teaching** are stressed throughout the narrative and are also highlighted in special boxes.
- **Learning aids** to help students identify, review, and apply important content in each chapter include Objectives, Key Terms, Key Points, and Review Questions.
- **Printed lists** on the inside back cover provide information on locating specific assets in the book, including Skills, Procedural Guidelines, Nursing Care Plans, and Patient Teaching boxes.

New to This Edition

- A **new chapter on "Complementary, Alternative, and Integrative Therapies"** addresses content that is now included on the NCLEX® examination.
- A **new Refl ective Learning** section in each chapter helps students better understand and reflect on their

clinical and simulation experiences as they move through their first nursing course.

- **Evidence-Based Practice** boxes have been updated with new PICO questions. These boxes provide a summary of nursing research evidence related to that specific topic and then explain its implications for nursing practice. These boxes have been updated to reflect current research topics and trends.

LEARNING SUPPLEMENTS FOR STUDENTS

- The **Evolve Student Resources** are available online at http://evolve.elsevier.com/Potter/essentials and include the following valuable learning aids organized by chapter:
  - Review Questions with Answers and Rationales
  - Answers to QSEN Activity Scenarios
  - Case Studies with Questions
  - Printable Key Points
  - Video Clips
  - Interactive Skills Performance Checklists
  - Fluids and Electrolytes Tutorial
  - Audio Glossary
  - Concept Map Creator
  - Conceptual Care Map
  - Calculation Tutorial
  - Answers to Student Study Guide
  - Content Updates
- A thorough **Study Guide** by Patricia A. Castaldi provides students with a wide variety of exercises and activities to enhance learning and comprehension. This study guide features case studies with related questions; chapter review sections with matching, fill-in-the-blank, and multiple-choice questions; study group questions; and instructions for creating and using study charts.
- **Virtual Clinical Excursions** is an exciting workbook and CD-ROM experience that brings learning to life in a virtual hospital setting. The workbook guides students as they care for patients, providing ongoing challenges and learning opportunities. Each lesson in *Virtual Clinical Excursions* complements the textbook content and provides an environment for students to practice what they are learning. This CD/workbook is available separately or packaged at a special price with the textbook.

TEACHING SUPPLEMENTS FOR INSTRUCTORS

- The **Evolve Instructor Resources** (available online at http://evolve.elsevier.com/Potter/essentials) are a comprehensive collection of the most important tools instructors need, including the following:
  - **TEACH for Nurses** ties together every chapter resource you need for the most effective class presentations, with sections dedicated to objectives, teaching strategies, nursing curriculum standards (including QSEN/NLN Competencies, BSN Essentials, and Nursing Concepts), instructor chapter resources, student chapter resources, and an in-class case study discussion. Teaching Strategies include relationships between the textbook content and discussion items. Examples of student activities, online activities, and large group activities are provided for more "hands-on" learning.
  - The **Test Bank** contains a revised set of more than 950 questions with answers coded for NCLEX® Client Needs category, nursing process, and cognitive level. The Exam-View software allows instructors to create new tests; edit, add, and delete test questions; sort questions by NCLEX® category, cognitive level, nursing process step, and question type; and administer and grade online tests.
  - **PowerPoint Presentations** include over 1400 slides for use in lectures. Art is included within the slides, and progressive case studies include discussion questions and answers.
  - The **Image Collection** contains hundreds of illustrations from the text for use in lectures.
- **Simulation Learning System** is an online toolkit that helps instructors and facilitators effectively incorporate medium- to high-fidelity simulation into their nursing curriculum. Detailed patient scenarios promote and enhance the clinical decision-making skills of students at all levels. The system provides detailed instructions for preparation and implementation of the simulation experience, debriefing questions that encourage critical thinking, and learning resources to reinforce student comprehension. Each scenario in *Simulation Learning System* complements the textbook content and helps bridge the gap between lectures and clinicals. This system provides the perfect environment for students to practice what they are learning in the text for a true-to-life, hands-on learning experience.

MULTIMEDIA SUPPLEMENTS FOR INSTRUCTORS AND STUDENTS

- **Nursing Skills Online 4.0** contains 19 modules rich with animations, videos, interactive activities, and exercises to help students prepare for their clinical lab experience. The instructionally designed lessons focus on topics that are difficult to master and pose a high risk to the patient if done incorrectly. Lesson quizzes allow students to check their learning curve and review as needed, and the module exams feed out to an instructor grade book. Modules cover Airway Management, Blood Therapy, Bowel Elimination/ Ostomy, Cardiac Care, Closed Chest Drainage Systems, Enteral Nutrition, Infection Control, Maintenance of IV Fluid Therapy, IV Fluid Therapy, Administration of Parenteral Medications: Injections and IV Medications, Nonparenteral Medication Administration, Safe Medication Preparation, Safety, Specimen Collection, Urinary Catheterization, Caring for Central Vascular Access Devices (CVAD), Vital Signs, and Wound Care. Available alone or packaged with the text.
- **Mosby's Nursing Video Skills: Basic, Intermediate, Advanced, 4th edition,** provides 126 skills with overview information covering skill purpose, safety, and delegation guides; equipment lists; preparation procedures; procedure videos with printable step-by-step guidelines; appropriate follow-up care; documentation guidelines; and interactive review questions. Available online, as a student DVD set, or as a networkable DVD set for the institution.

Authors

Acknowledgement of First South Asia Edition

I would like to thank past and present reviewers and contributors and the entire Elsevier team for their contribution to the 'Potter & Perry's Nursing Foundation', South Asian Edition. Also, I would like to thank Patricia A. Potter, Anne Griffin Perry, Patricia A. Stockert, Amy M. Hall and Elsevier for giving me permission and opportunity to adapt this legendary textbook in the South Asian context. **A special thanks to my Dr Shiv Kumar Mudgal**, Tutor (Nursing), Rakhi Mishra, Assistant Professor (Nursing), Priya Sharma, Tutor (Nursing), and Ravin Bishnoi, Nursing Officer for their significant contribution in adaption of this edition. My special thanks to my wife Reena Sharma for tolerating my endless hours with books, journals and computer. Everyone has come to respect the enormity of the task and how each step affects the next. I am proud of this accomplishment.

Suresh K. Sharma

Acknowledgements, 9th Edition

The ninth edition of *Essentials for Nursing Practice* is the result of a continued collaboration among all authors, contributors, and editorial team members. Having professional colleagues to work with, trust, and challenge one another is a gift—one that ensures a timely and accurate text.

This textbook cannot be created without the support, guidance, and creative direction from our editorial team, designer, and production staff. Likewise, no book is successful without the hard work and dedication of its marketing team. We are also very fortunate regarding the manner in which staff from the electronic media division of Elsevier has produced products that complement the text and ensure its success. We wish to make special mention of some important individuals.

Tamara Myers, Director, is a dedicated professional who continually challenges the author team to create a state-ofthe-art revision. Her enthusiasm and knowledge creates an environment for the writing, editorial, and production teams to develop a relevant and creative textbook that reflects contemporary nursing practice.

Tina Kaemmerer, Senior Content Development Specialist, is a dedicated professional whose organizational skills ensure that this project remains on target. She effectively collaborates with all members of the writing team in tracking manuscript through the publication process, in problem solving, and in being an invaluable resource for authors, contributors, and the production team.

Paula Catalano, our Book Designer, has developed a visually distinctive textbook design. Her expertise created a text that is visually appealing yet easy for our readers to use. Paula is also credited for her creativity and vision for the design of the cover art and her direction in implementing the overall design of the text.

Many thanks and gratitude go to members of the Production Team. Jodi Willard, Senior Project Manager, is a tireless and dedicated professional. As an accomplished project manager, she keeps us on deadline while ensuring consistency in formatting, presentation, and style. Her sense of humor and ability to always remain calm under pressure are invaluable attributes. She is one of a kind. Jeff Patterson, Publishing Services Manager, has contributed support throughout the editing and final pages.

A tip of the hat must always go to the sales and marketing team, headed by Julie Burchett and Megan Atencio, who provided us direction early in the planning stage of *Essentials for Nursing Practice*. Their knowledge of market trends and needs helps us to make revisions of high quality.

Many thanks to our contributors, clinicians, and educators, who share their experiences and knowledge about nursing practice in helping to create informative, accurate, and current information. Their knowledge of their own clinical specialties ensures we have a state-of-the-art textbook. We are fortunate to be associated with excellent nurse authors who are able to convey standards of nursing excellence through the printed word.

A heartfelt thanks to our many reviewers for their expertise, candor, knowledge of the literature, and astute comments that assist us in developing a text with high standards that reflect professional nursing practice today.

After many years of collaboration, we find ourselves very fortunate and humble. *Essentials for Nursing Practice* and the other textbooks we have been able to develop have made important contributions to nursing practice. It remains a work of love.

Patricia A. Potter
Anne Griffin Perry
Patricia A. Stockert
Amy M. Hall

Contents

1 Health and Wellness

OBJECTIVES

After reading this chapter, the student should be able to:

- To define health, and discuss the concept and dimensions of health.
- To discuss the Maslow's hierarchy human needs model of health and illness and its relationship to patients' attitudes toward health and health practices.
- To explain illness–wellness continuum with relevant examples.
- To describe the factors influencing health beliefs, health practices, and illness behaviors.
- To explain how different types of causes and risk factors affect a person's health.
- To describe a nurse's role in helping patients modify their health risks and change their health behavior.
- To define concept of illness and illness behavior and describe factors that influence illness behavior.
- To explain how illness affects a patient and his or her family.
- To discuss the nurse's role in caring for people, communities, and populations in various states of health and illness.

KEY TERMS

acute illness, p. 7
chronic illness, p. 7
health, p. 2
illness, p. 7
illness behavior, p. 7
Maslow's hierarchy of needs, p. 3
risk factor, p. 5

INTRODUCTION

Nurses play a key role in helping individuals, families, communities, and populations become or remain healthy. Nurses are considered to be health experts because they are caregivers, advocates, and educators. Nowadays, health information is readily available through electronic and print media. However, people often have difficulty determining which information is accurate and helpful. Because of your expertise in health, your patients, family, and friends will frequently ask you questions about how to use this information to become healthier. If you can help a person remain well, you can reduce the frequency of that person accessing health care, which reduces the health care costs. Thus, it is very important for nurses to help patients make changes to improve their health and wellness.

CONCEPT OF HEALTH AND WELLNESS

The widely accepted definition of health, given by the World Health Organization (WHO), includes three basic dimensions—physical, mental, and social well-being. However, many other aspects of health need to be considered, e.g., spiritual, emotional, vocational, and political dimensions of health. Health is a state of being that people define in relation to their own values, personality, and lifestyle. Each person has a personal concept of health. Pender et al. (2015) define health as the actualization of inherent and acquired human potential through goal-directed behavior, competent self-care, and satisfying relationships with others while adjustments are made as needed to maintain structural integrity and harmony with the environment.

Individuals' views of health vary among different cultural orientations. Pender (1996) explains that "all people free of disease are not equally healthy." Views of health have broadened to include not only physical well-being but also mental, social, and spiritual well-being and a focus on health at the family and community levels.

To help patients identify and reach health goals, nurses discover and use information about their concepts of health. Pender et al. (2015) suggest that for many people, conditions of life rather than pathological states define health. Life conditions can have positive or negative effects on health long before an illness is evident. Life conditions include socioeconomic variables such as environment, diet, lifestyle practices or choices, and many other physiological and psychological variables.

Health and illness are defined according to individual perception. Health often includes conditions previously considered to be illness. For example, a person with epilepsy who has learned to control seizures with medication and who functions at home and work or a person fully recovered from a stroke with limited paralysis and living independently may no longer consider himself or herself ill. A nurse needs to consider the total person and the environment in which the person lives to individualize nursing care and enhance meaningfulness of the patient's future health status.

In a nutshell, health is

- not merely absence of disease but complete physical, mental, social, and spiritual well-being of an individual.
- the ability to maintain normal roles and responsibilities.
- the process of adaptation to physical and social environment in different situations and phases of life.
- striving toward optimal wellness.

Definition of Health

Defining **health** is a difficult task. Therefore, there are many definitions of health offered from time to time but most of them were criticized for one or more reasons. Some of the commonly referred definitions are as follows:

Health is a state of complete physical, mental, and social well-being, not merely the absence of disease or infirmity.

—WHO, 1947

Health is the condition of being sound body, mind, or spirit, especially freedom from physical disease or pain.

—Webster's Dictionary

Health is soundness of body or mind; that condition in which its functions are duly and efficiently discharged.

—Oxford English Dictionary

WHO defines health as a "state of complete physical, mental and social well-being and not merely the absence of disease or infirmity" (1947, 2017). Every person has a different definition of health (Pender et al., 2011). A person who is free from disease is not necessarily healthy (Pender, 1996). **Health** is a state of being influenced by a person's values, personality, and lifestyle. For many people, health is defined by the circumstances surrounding their life rather than their physical condition (Pender et al., 2011). Nurses individualize nursing care by considering the whole person and the environment to help patients reach their health goals. Individual perceptions of health are affected by a person's health beliefs and change as a person ages. For example, the definition of health for older people is often affected by the ability to function independently, the presence of or management of symptoms, acceptance of current health status, being connected to others, and having energy (Song and Kong, 2015).

Dimensions of Health and Wellness

Health and wellness has several dimensions, mentioned as follows (Fig. 1.1).

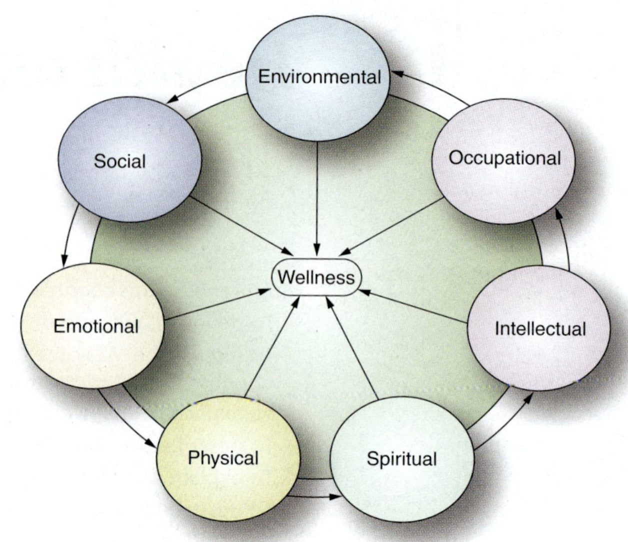

Fig. 1.1 Dimensions of health and wellness.

Physical Dimension

- Ability to carry out daily tasks/self-care abilities
- Ability to achieve fitness
- Ability to maintain nutrition
- Ability to avoid abuses

Social Dimension

- Ability to interact successfully
- Ability to develop and maintain intimacy
- Ability to develop respect and tolerance for others

Emotional Dimension

- Ability to manage stress
- Ability to express emotion

Intellectual Dimension

- Ability to learn
- Ability to use information effectively

Spiritual Dimension

- Belief in some force that serves to unite

Occupational Dimension

- Ability to achieve balance between work and leisure

Environmental Dimension

- Ability to promote health measure that improves
- Standard of living
- Quality of life

Table 1.1 depicts the relationship between human dimensions of health and basic human needs.

Table 1.1 Relationship Between Human Dimensions and Basic Human Needs

Dimension	Basic Human Need	Examples
Physical	Physiologic needs	Breathing circulation, temperature intake of food and fluids, and elimination of waste movement
Environmental	Safety and security needs	Housing community/ neighborhood climate
Sociocultural	Love and belonging needs	Relationships with others, communications with others, support system being part of a community, and feeling loved by others
Emotional	Self-esteem needs	Fear, sadness, loneliness, happiness, and accepting self
Intellectual and spiritual	Self-actualization needs	Thinking, learning, decision-making, values, beliefs, fulfillment, and helping others

MASLOW'S HIERARCHY OF NEEDS

Maslow's hierarchy of needs (Maslow, 1954), also known as "*basic human needs model*," helps you understand an individual's motivation to achieve optimal health. This model explains the basic needs of patients and families, their behaviors, and their readiness to take part in health activities. Maslow's original model describes human needs using a hierarchical pyramid divided into five levels (Fig. 1.2). According to Maslow, individuals have to meet lower level needs before they are able to satisfy higher level needs. As people meet the needs of one level, they move up to the next level. Unmet needs motivate human behavior.

- ***First***, a person needs to meet basic *physiological* needs such as oxygen, water, food, sleep, and shelter before progressing to higher level needs. When basic needs are not met, an affected person feels sick or irritated or experiences pain or discomfort. These feelings motivate an individual to satisfy the need.
- ***The second level*** on the hierarchy of needs consists of *safety and security needs*, which include establishing stability and consistency. These psychological needs include the security of a home and a family. For example, a woman in an abusive relationship is unable to move to the next level of love and belongingness because she is constantly concerned for her safety.
- ***The third level*** on the hierarchy, *love and belongingness*, is a desire to belong to groups. It consists of the need to feel loved and accepted by others.
- ***The fourth level*** deals with the need for *self-esteem*. Self-esteem results from mastery of a task and includes the recognition gained from others.
- ***The highest level*** of needs on the hierarchy is *self-actualization*, which is the desire to become everything that one is capable of becoming. Individuals at this level are concerned with maximizing their potential.

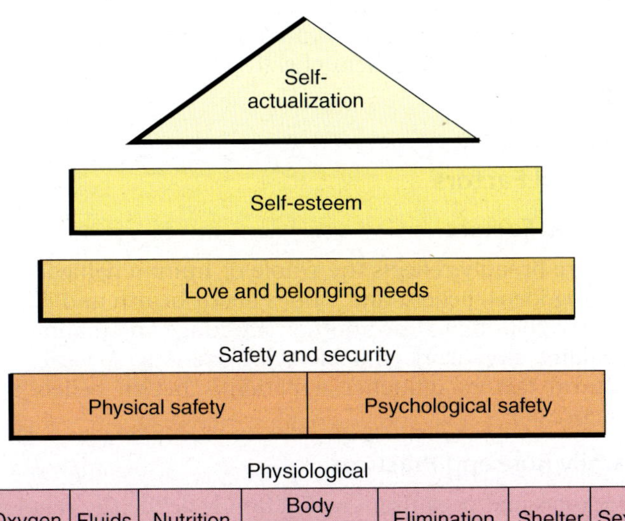

Fig. 1.2 Maslow's hierarchy of needs. (From Maslow AH, Frager RD, Fadiman J: *Motivation and personality*, ed 3. Copyright ©1987. Reprinted by permission of Pearson Education, Inc., New York, New York.)

Maslow (1970) expanded his model to include cognitive, aesthetic, and transcendence needs to incorporate needs that could not be explained by his original model. In the expanded model, cognitive and aesthetic needs come between esteem and self-actualization needs (McLeod, 2016). According to Maslow (1970), cognitive needs are hardwired in all of us and include the needs for knowledge, understanding, meaning, and predictability. Aesthetic needs are universal and include the appreciation and search for beauty and balance. Cognitive and aesthetic needs help explain why patients respond better when they understand their health problems and when they are in attractive surroundings with peaceful colors. Transcendence needs refer to the need to help others achieve self-actualization and are the highest needs.

You can use Maslow's hierarchy as a framework when addressing patient needs and prioritizing patient care. Unless a patient's basic needs are met, higher levels in the pyramid are not relevant. Patients approach life differently.

The requirements to satisfy the needs of each level of the hierarchy vary from person to person. Therefore, you need to thoroughly assess the individual needs of each patient. For example, in caring for patients with psychological issues such as depression or risk for suicide, safety and security needs are a priority. As a nurse, you need to provide all patients with physical and psychological safety.

ILLNESS–WELLNESS CONTINUUM

Travis's illness–wellness continuum model signifies that wellness is a process, never a static state. The illness–wellness continuum was first envisioned by John W. Travis in 1972. Once it was published in 1975, the continuum became an immediate success, an easy way to illustrate what this newly emerging wellness concept was all about (Fig. 1.3).

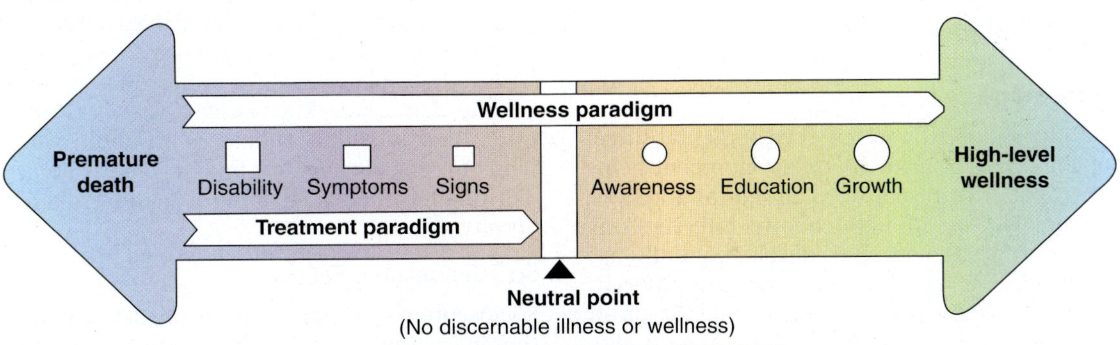

Fig. 1.3 Illness–wellness continuum model.

In this model, the opposite directions are joined at a neutral point. Moving to the right of the neutral point indicates increasing wellness which is achieved by awareness, education, and growth. Moving to the left indicates decreasing wellness due to various disabilities and signs, and symptoms of illness.

There are actually many degrees of wellness, just as there are many degrees of illness. The illness–wellness continuum illustrates the relationship of the treatment paradigm to the wellness paradigm.

The treatment paradigm (drugs, herbs, surgery, psychotherapy, acupuncture, and so on) can bring you up to the neutral point, where the symptoms of disease have been alleviated.

The wellness paradigm, which can be used at any point on the continuum, helps you move toward higher levels of wellness. The wellness paradigm directs you beyond neutral and encourages you to move as far to the right as possible. It is not meant to replace the treatment paradigm on the left side of the continuum, but to work in harmony with it. If you are ill, then treatment is important, but do not stop at the neutral point. Use the wellness paradigm to move toward high-level wellness.

FACTORS INFLUENCING HEALTH

Health is influenced by various external and internal factors. Peoples' beliefs about their own health, their health practices, and the manner in which they care for themselves ultimately influence their health status. Health beliefs are a person's ideas and attitudes about health. These beliefs often directly influence health practices irrespective of whether there is evidence to support them. Health practices are activities that individuals perform to care for themselves. They include activities of daily living such as bathing and brushing teeth and formal activities such as taking medications and visiting the health care provider for routine checkups. Nowadays, health care focuses on the role of patients and their responsibility for self-care. The ability to care for oneself is as important for healthy living as managing a complex medical regimen for a chronic illness. Many factors influence patients' health beliefs, health practices, and self-care. Internal and external factors influence how a person thinks, acts, and will deal with an illness. Consider the effect of these internal and external factors and incorporate appropriate interventions based on a person's unique characteristics when you deliver nursing care. The various internal and external factors which influence the health are discussed as follows.

Internal Factors

Developmental Stage

Our concept of illness depends on our developmental stage. Knowledge of the stages of growth and development helps you predict your patient's response to an actual illness or the threat of future illness. Your educational interventions need to be age appropriate as well as developmentally appropriate to be effective. For example, you use different techniques to teach healthy diet choices to a child versus an adult. You also use different techniques for people whose developmental age differs from their chronological age.

Intellectual Background

A person's beliefs about health are shaped in part by knowledge (or misinformation) about body functions and illnesses, educational background, and past experiences. Cognitive abilities shape the *way* a person thinks, including the ability to understand factors involved in illness and apply knowledge of health and illness to personal health practices.

Emotional Factors

A person's degree of anxiety or stress influences health beliefs and practices. How people handle stress throughout each phase of life influences their personal reaction to illness. A person who generally is very calm may have little emotional response during illness, whereas a person normally unable to cope with stress may overreact to illness or deny the presence of symptoms and does not take therapeutic action (see Chapter 31).

Spiritual Factors

Spirituality is a cultural factor reflected in how a person lives his or her life including the values and beliefs exercised, the relationships established with family and friends, and the ability to find hope and meaning in life. Spiritual health often provides motivation to engage in health-promoting activities and enhances mental and physical health during times of illness. You need to understand patients' spiritual beliefs to incorporate them effectively in nursing care (see Chapter 32).

External Factors

Cultural Factors

Culture broadly reflects the whole of human behavior, including ideas, beliefs, and values about health and illness; ways of relating to one another; language and manners of speaking; and work and lifestyle practices. A variety of cultural factors influence a patient's health beliefs and practices.

Family Role and Practices

The roles and organization of a family define the relationship of insiders and outsiders and include concepts related to family goals and priorities and how each member defines health and illness and values preventive health practices (see Chapter 33). There is usually a person in the family responsible for health-related decisions; for example, parental health beliefs, attitudes, perceptions, and misperceptions have a direct effect on a family's health practices. The family's socioeconomic status, family structure, and parental practices also affect a family's health. A person raised in a family that believes in the importance of preventive care such as dental checkups twice a year is more likely to continue those health practices as an adult, whereas parents who have misconceptions and unhealthy perceptions about diet quality often contribute to eating habits that lead to obesity.

Socioeconomic Factors

Socioeconomic factors are social determinants of health that increase the risk for illness and influence how a person defines and reacts to illness (see Chapter 33). Socioeconomic variables also determine how and where patients access medical care and receive treatment, how they pay for their health care, and the potential reimbursement to the health care agency or patient. Poor access to health care is one social determinant of health that contributes to health disparities. Economic variables affect a patient's level of health by increasing the risk for disease and influencing how or at what point the patient enters the health care system. In addition, economic status affects a person's participation in treatment to maintain or improve health. A person who has high utility bills, a large family, and a low income may give a higher priority to food and shelter than to prescribed drugs or treatment or foods for special diets.

CAUSES AND RISK FACTORS FOR DEVELOPMENT OF ILLNESS

Infections, injuries, faulty genes, and unhealthy lifestyle are the main causes of illness. Infectious diseases and disorders are mainly caused by bacteria, viruses, fungi, and parasites. A **risk factor** is any attribute, quality, trait, or environmental condition that increases vulnerability of an individual, community, or population to an illness or accident. Risk factors do not cause diseases or accidents, but they increase the chance that an individual, community, or population will experience a particular disease or accident. You assess for risk factors to identify a patient's health status. A person's knowledge of risk factors sometimes influences health beliefs and practices. People can modify some risk factors such as dietary choices, whereas other risk factors such as genetics or age are nonmodifiable.

Nonmodifiable Risk Factors

Nonmodifiable risk factors such as age, gender, genetics, and family history cannot be changed. Use your knowledge of nonmodifiable risk factors to provide secondary prevention. Age increases susceptibility to certain illnesses and accidents. For example, children are at risk for accidental deaths due to drowning. The risk for heart disease, diabetes, and many cancers increases with age for both genders.

A person's gender sometimes is a risk factor for diseases or accidents. For example, the risk for asthma is higher in men than women. However, by the age of 20 years, the number of men and women who have asthma is about equal, and by the age of 40 years, more women have asthma. Men have a higher risk for cardiovascular disease (CVD) than premenopausal women. However, after menopause, the risk for CVD is similar between men and women.

An individual's family history and genetics are also risk factors for some illnesses. Breast, ovarian, and colon cancer appear to have a genetic link. A person with a family history of diabetes or CVD has a higher risk of developing these diseases. Sometimes, it is difficult to determine whether the family link to illness is related to genetics, lifestyle choices, or environmental exposure, or a combination of these factors. For example, you are caring for a female patient with obesity who develops high blood pressure. Her parents suffer from high blood pressure, and her husband smokes. It is challenging for you to determine which risk factor—lifestyle, genetics, or environmental toxins—caused her condition, or if all factors were involved. Main modifiable, nonmodifiable, and environmental risk factors of illness have been discussed as follows.

Modifiable Risk Factors

Some risk factors such as lifestyle practices and health-related behaviors can be modified. Although some practices can positively affect health, practices with potential negative effects are risk factors. Examples of modifiable risk factors include overeating or poor nutrition, insufficient rest and sleep, and poor personal hygiene. Other habits that put a person at risk for illness include tobacco use, alcohol or drug abuse, and activities involving a threat of injury such as drinking alcohol or texting while driving. Some habits are risk factors for specific diseases. For example, excessive sunbathing increases the risk for skin cancer, and being overweight increases the risk for CVD. Examples of modifiable behavioral risk factors that are leading causes of mortality are tobacco use, obesity, lack of physical activity, poor control of blood pressure, high cholesterol, and not being immunized for vaccine-preventable diseases. Modifiable risk factors, especially for people who are 10–24 years of age, include behaviors that lead to unintentional injuries (e.g., texting while driving and bullying); use of tobacco, alcohol, and other drugs; sexual behaviors leading to unintended pregnancy and sexually transmitted infections; unhealthy diet choices; and physical inactivity. Current evidence emphasizes the need for preventive care and shows the effect that lifestyle choices have on our health care system, our economy, and our communities.

Lifestyle behavior choices affect people throughout their life. For example, a teenager whose nutritional choices lead to obesity will most likely experience the effects of obesity later in life. Patients of all ages are vulnerable to the influences of unhealthy lifestyle patterns. You can influence the choices your patients make to prevent or change unhealthy behaviors and promote healthy lifestyle patterns. Therefore, you need to understand the relationship between growth and development, lifestyle behaviors, and your patients' health status. Use developmentally appropriate evidence-based interventions when teaching about wellness-promoting lifestyle behaviors (Box 1.1).

Environment

The environment is affected by physical, chemical, biological, social, and psychosocial factors. Our environment includes the physical space in which we live; the air, water, soil, and food that is all around us; and the biological, chemical, and radiological exposures we experience. All of these can increase the likelihood that certain illnesses will occur. Some home environments increase the risk that a person will contract and spread infections, whereas some cancers are more likely to develop when people live near toxic waste disposal sites. Environmental exposure rarely occurs one time, in one location, and from one source because we are constantly interacting with our environment.

Risk Factor Identification

You identify modifiable and nonmodifiable risk factors to help patients understand what they need to modify or eliminate to promote wellness and prevent illness. Health

BOX 1.1 **Evidence-Based Practice**

PICO Question: Are individualized developmentally appropriate health promotion interventions effective in increasing patients' activity levels?

Summary of Evidence

Being physically active is important in preventing many health issues such as obesity, cardiovascular disease, cancer, and type 2 diabetes. Many people of all ages do not participate in regular physical activity. Nurses are in key positions to provide health education to patients, families, and communities to promote physical activity. Walking is an activity that people of all ages can usually do and is effective in helping people lose weight or maintain a healthy weight (Adams et al., 2015; Yan et al., 2015). Current evidence shows that effective health promotion interventions are individualized and take a patient's age and developmental level into consideration. Interventions that are effective with younger people are not typically effective with older adults. When high school–age and college-age patients receive positive, individualized text messages regularly that encourage exercise such as walking and address barriers, goal-setting, motivation, and connection with others, the messages are frequently effective in helping patients increase the number of steps they take every day and engage in regular physical activity (Yan et al., 2015; Thompson et al., 2016). Community-based groups that encourage walking and exercise are often effective in helping middle-aged and elderly patients increase their physical activity (Resnick et al., 2014; Adams et al., 2015). Health promotion interventions that emphasize connections with others are effective in patients of all ages (Resnick et al., 2014; Thompson et al., 2016).

Application to Nursing Practice

- Ensure the health education you provide to your patients is connected to their developmental needs (Yan et al., 2015).
- Include connections with significant others when designing health promotion strategies for patients of all ages (Resnick et al., 2014).
- Encourage patients to set realistic, measurable goals, and encourage them to use pedometers if possible to count their steps daily (Adams et al., 2015).

risk appraisals assess individuals, families, or communities for the presence of factors that increase specific health threats. You will often find risk factors through patient interviews and reading medical records. You need to link the risk factors you identify with educational programs and other community resources to help people make lifestyle changes to reduce their risks.

CHANGING HEALTH BEHAVIORS

Once you identify a patient's risk factors, you implement appropriate and relevant health education and counseling to help a person change a risky health behavior or implement a new behavior to modify the risk for a disease or injury. It is essential to engage and collaborate with patients when determining which changes they perceive they need to make or are willing to make. Patients typically will not change a behavior unless they see a need and are motivated and supported to change. This will also often require family caregiver support.

Aim your attempts to help a patient stop a health-damaging behavior (e.g., tobacco use or alcohol misuse) or adopt a healthy behavior (e.g., make healthy food choices or exercise). Changing health behavior, especially long-term lifestyle habits, is difficult. Adopting healthy behaviors to reduce risk factors requires patients to change. As a nurse, you are challenged to motivate and facilitate health behavior change in working with individuals, families, and communities. Use evidence-based guidelines when helping your patients make health behavior changes.

You will better help your patients make difficult behavioral changes if you apply knowledge about the process of change. Current evidence supports that many people go through a series of five stages of behavior change (Table 1.2), ranging from precontemplation, when a person has no intention to change, to the maintenance stage, when a person maintains a changed behavior. Change typically is not a linear process; most people relapse and recycle through the stages of change frequently. When relapse occurs, a person returns to the contemplation or precontemplation stage before attempting change again. Although patients will often feel like relapse is a failure, you need to help them view it as a learning process. Patients can apply what they learned in their next attempt to change. Health promotion interventions have a greater effect if you time them appropriately to match a patient's specific stage of change. For example, teaching a patient who is in the contemplation stage and does not routinely eat fruits

Table 1.2 Stages of Behavior Change

Stage	Definition
Precontemplation	Does not intend to make changes within the next 6 months. Patient is unaware of the problem or underestimates it. "There is nothing that I really need to change."
Contemplation	Considering a change within the next 6 months. Patient says that he or she is seriously considering a change. "I have a problem, and I really think I need to work on it."
Preparation	Has tried to make changes, but without success. Patient intends to take action in the next month. "I started to exercise regularly, but it didn't last long. I'll probably try again in a few weeks."
Action	Actively engaged in strategies to change behavior. This stage sometimes lasts up to 6 months. It requires commitment of time and energy. "I am really working hard to stop smoking."
Maintenance	Sustained change over time. This stage begins 6 months after action has started and continues indefinitely. It is important to avoid relapse. "I need to avoid people who smoke so I'm not tempted to start smoking again."

Data from Prochaska JO, DiClemente CC: Stages of change in the modification of problem behaviors, *Prog Behav Modif* 28:184, 1992; and Conn VS: A staged-based approach to helping people change health behaviors, *Clin Nurs Spec* 8(4):187, 1994.

and vegetables to immediately begin eating five fruits and vegetables a day is not effective. It is better to encourage this patient to think about the costs and benefits of eating five fruits and vegetables a day to help the patient move into the preparation stage.

Health care professionals design interventions and wellness strategies for people in all stages of behavior change. For example, current evidence shows that initiating tobacco cessation in hospital settings is very successful. However, if there are no resources or programs available or patients are not aware of available programs, they miss the opportunity to make a behavior change to improve their health. Patients maintain changes over time when you help them integrate the changes into their daily routine. True change comes from a patient's desire to change. Maintenance of healthy lifestyles prevents hospitalizations and potentially lowers the cost of health care. Your advice and support may help patients adapt to a healthier lifestyle.

ILLNESS AND ILLNESS BEHAVIOR

Illness is not the same as disease. Disease is a pathophysiological process, whereas **illness** is a state in which a person's physical, emotional, intellectual, social, developmental, or spiritual functioning is diminished or impaired compared with previous experience. A person can feel ill in the presence or absence of disease. For example, cancer is a disease. Some patients with cancer feel ill, whereas others continue to function as usual. Some patients with breast cancer feel well physically but experience spiritual distress. Many patients find health within illness. Sometimes, illness motivates an individual to adopt positive health behaviors. Although you need to be familiar with different types of diseases and their treatments, be concerned more with illness, which includes the effects of disease and treatments on a person's functioning and well-being in all dimensions.

Acute and Chronic Illness

Acute and chronic illnesses affect many dimensions of functioning. An **acute illness** is usually short term. The symptoms appear abruptly, are intense, and often subside after a relatively short period. A **chronic illness** usually lasts longer than 6 months. Patients fluctuate between maximal functioning and serious health relapses that are sometimes life threatening.

Because of advances in public health, medicine, and biomedical technology, acute and infectious diseases are no longer major causes of death, disease, and disability. Chronic illnesses (e.g., diabetes, heart disease, stroke, cancer, arthritis, and obesity) are the most common, costly, and preventable of all health problems (CDC, 2016). You need to learn how to help patients prevent and manage their chronic illness or disabilities to enhance wellness and improve patients' quality of life (tertiary prevention).

Self-management

Programs that teach chronic disease management must use a holistic approach and include family caregivers when appropriate. The Chronic Disease Self-Management Program (CDSMP) is one of the most widely used evidence-based programs for people with a variety of chronic illnesses. CDSMP is community-based and includes self-management education workshops led by people with the chronic illness. It upholds that people with different chronic illnesses have similar self-management needs and problems, that people can learn how to become responsible for the daily management of their diseases, and that people who are confident and knowledgeable about their disease management will have positive health outcomes. Taking responsibility for living well with illness strengthens patients. Therefore, encourage patients to ask questions about their health care and make informed decisions. The process of learning self-management skills is crucial when learning to live with a chronic illness. The management of chronic illnesses promotes health within illness and addresses human comfort and quality of life. You are able to reduce the impact of chronic illness on an individual and society by providing quality, comprehensive, patient-centered care.

Factors Influencing Illness Behavior

People have different attitudes and reactions to illness. Medical sociologists call this reaction **illness behavior**. People who are ill generally adopt illness behaviors (cognitive, affective, and behavioral reactions) that are influenced by sociocultural and social psychological factors. Illness behaviors affect how people monitor their bodies, define and interpret their symptoms, take remedial actions, and use the health care system. Although people react to an illness in a variety of ways, patients often use illness behavior displayed in sickness to manage difficulties in life. People who have more positive coping skills, greater social support, and a good perceived health status tend to report less illness behaviors. Internal and external variables affect illness behavior. The influences of these variables affect how likely a patient is to seek health care and participate in therapy, which ultimately affects health outcomes.

Internal Factors

Internal variables are patients' perceptions of symptoms and the nature of illnesses. If patients believe that the symptoms of their illnesses disrupt their normal routine, they are more likely to seek health care assistance than if they do not perceive the symptoms as disruptive. If they believe that the symptoms are serious or perhaps life threatening, they are also more likely to seek assistance. A person awakened by crushing chest pains in the middle of the night generally views this symptom as potentially serious and life threatening and will probably be motivated to seek assistance. However, some patients fear serious illness and react by denying it and not seeking medical assistance.

External Factors

External variables influencing a patient's illness behavior include the visibility of symptoms, social group, cultural variables, accessibility of the health care system, and social support. The visibility of the symptoms of an illness affects body image and illness behavior. A patient with a visible symptom or a recognizable symptom such as crushing chest pain, intense headache, or a high fever is more likely to seek assistance than a patient who has symptoms that are less visible or recognizable such as the nonspecific symptoms associated with ovarian cancer (e.g., fatigue, bloating, trouble eating, and feeling full quickly).

Patients' social groups help them accept or deny the threat of illness. Families, friends, and coworkers all influence patients' illness behavior. Patients often react positively to social support while practicing positive health behaviors. How patients perceive health and the effects of disease and its interpretation vary according to a patient's culture and family.

Economic variables are social determinants of health that influence the way a patient reacts to illness. Financial difficulty will often lead a patient to delay treatment. This is especially common in patients who are uninsured or underinsured. The health care system is a socioeconomic system that patients enter, interact within, and exit. For many patients, entry into the system is complex or confusing, and some patients seek nonemergency medical care in an emergency department because they do not have access through insurance or do not know how to obtain health services otherwise. The physical proximity of patients to a health care agency often influences how soon they enter the system after deciding to seek care.

IMPACT OF ILLNESS ON PATIENT AND FAMILY

An illness of a family member affects the function of an entire family unit. A patient and family commonly experience behavioral and emotional changes and changes in body image, self-concept, family roles, and family dynamics.

Behavioral and Emotional Changes

Individual behavioral and emotional reactions depend on the nature of an illness, a patient's attitude toward the illness, the reaction of others to the illness, and the variables of illness behavior. Short-term, non–life-threatening illnesses evoke few behavioral changes in the functioning of a patient or family. For example, a parent who has a severe cold lacks the energy and patience to spend time in family activities and prefers not to interact with the family. This is a behavioral change, but it is subtle and does not last long. Some even consider such a change a normal response to illness.

Severe illness, particularly one that is life threatening, leads to more extensive emotional and behavioral changes such as anxiety, shock, denial, anger, and withdrawal. These are common responses to the stress of illness. You develop interventions to help patients and families cope with and adapt to this stress because the stressors usually cannot be changed.

Impact on Body Image

Body image is the subjective concept of physical appearance. Our perception of body image changes as we grow and develop (see Chapter 29). Some illnesses result in changes in physical appearance. Patients and families react differently to these changes. Their reactions depend on the type of changes (e.g., the loss of a limb or an organ), the adaptive capacity of a family, the rate at which changes take place, and the support services available.

When a profound change in body image occurs, such as after a mastectomy or leg amputation, a patient generally adjusts by experiencing phases of the grief process (see Chapter 27). Initially, the change or impending change shocks the patient. As the patient and family recognize the reality of the change, they become anxious and sometimes withdraw. As they acknowledge the change, they gradually move toward accepting their loss. During rehabilitation, the patient is ready to learn how to adapt to the change in body image.

Impact on Self-Concept

Self-concept is your mental self-image of all aspects of your personality. It depends in part on body image and roles but also includes other aspects of psychology and spirituality. Self-concept is important in relationships with other family members. A patient whose self-concept changes because of illness is sometimes no longer able to meet family expectations, leading to tension or conflict. As a result, family members change their interactions with the patient. While providing care, you observe changes in a patient's self-concept (or in the self-concepts of family members) and develop a care plan to help a patient adjust to the changes resulting from the illness (see Chapter 29).

Impact on Family Roles and Family Dynamics

A person has many roles in life such as wage earner, decision maker, professional, and parent. When an illness occurs, the roles of the patient and family change. Patients and their families generally adjust more easily to subtle, short-term changes caused by minor acute illness, such as when a child gets strep throat. However, long-term changes caused by sudden acute and severe health problems (e.g., stroke or head injury from a motor vehicle accident) or the diagnosis of a chronic illness (e.g., type 1 diabetes or cancer) require an adjustment process similar to the grief process (see Chapter 31). A patient and family often need specific counseling and guidance to help them cope with the role changes.

Family dynamics is the process by which the family functions, makes decisions, gives support to individual members, and copes with everyday changes and challenges. Because of the effects of illness, family dynamics often change. Another family member sometimes needs to assume a patient's usual roles and responsibilities. This often creates tension or anxiety in the family. Include the whole family as appropriate while helping patients attain their maximal level of functioning and well-being.

ROLE OF NURSES IN HEALTH AND ILLNESS

Patients receive care related to their health and illness needs in all health care settings. Although nurses are often the key members of the health care team to provide information to patients about health, wellness, and illness, patients' needs are very complex. Thus, as a nurse, you need to collaborate with other members of the health care team to successfully improve the health of individuals, families, and communities. Value, respect, and trust the other members of the health care team as you work together to develop an appropriate plan of care. Ensure that a patient's interests are at the center of the plan. Understand how each team member can contribute to a patient's health or illness care and determine how you can best work together to help your patient. Effective teams communicate with and listen to each other clearly and frequently.

KEY POINTS

- Health and wellness are not merely the absence of disease and illness. A person's state of health, wellness, or illness depends on his or her values, attitudes, personality, and lifestyle.
- Unmet needs motivate human beings. Basic human needs must be met before an individual is able to focus on higher level needs.
- Consider internal and external factors that influence patients' health beliefs and practices when planning nursing care.
- Risk factors threaten health, influence health practices, and are important considerations in illness-prevention activities. Some risk factors are modifiable, whereas others are nonmodifiable.
- Improvement in health often requires a change in health behaviors.
- Illness behavior influences how patients respond to illness. Patients who cope better tend to respond better to illnesses.
- Illness has many effects on the patient and family, including changes in behavior and emotions, family roles and dynamics, body image, and self-concept.

REFERENCES

Adams T, Burns D, Forehand JW, Spurlock A. A community-based walking program to promote physical activity among African American women. Nurs Womens Health 2015;19(1):26.

Ball JW, Dains J, Flynn J, Solomon B, Stewart R. Seidel's guide to physical examination. 9th ed. St. Louis: Elsevier; 2018.

Centers for Disease Control and Prevention (CDC). Chronic disease overview. 2016. Available from: https://www.cdc.gov/chronicdisease/overview/.

Maslow AH. Motivation and personality. New York: Harper & Row; 1954.

Maslow AH. Motivation and personality. 2nd ed. New York: Harper & Row; 1970.

Maslow AH. Motivation and personality. 3rd ed. Upper Saddle River, NJ: Prentice Hall; 1987.

McLeod S. Maslow's hierarchy of needs. 2016. Available from: http://www.simplypsychology.org/maslow.html.

Pender NJ, Health promotion and nursing practice. 3rd ed. Stamford: Appleton & Lange; 1996.

Pender NJ, Murdaugh CL, Parsons MA. Health promotion in nursing practice. 6th ed. Upper Saddle River, NJ: Prentice Hall; 2011.

Pender NJ, Murdaugh, C, Parsons, MA. Health promotion in nursing practice. 7th ed. Boston: Pearson; 2015.

Resnick B, Michael K, Griffith K, Klinedinst J, Galik E. The impact of PRAISEDD on adherence and initiation of heart health behaviors in senior housing. Public Health Nurs 2014;31(4):309.

Song M, Kong E. Older adults' definitions of health: a metasynthesis. Int J Nurs Stud 2015;52(6):1097.

Thompson D, Cantu D, Ramirez B, Cullen KW, Baranowski T, Mendoza J, et al. Texting to increase adolescent physical activity: feasibility assessment. Am J Health Behav 2016;40(4):472.

World Health Organization (WHO) Interim Commission: Chronicle of WHO. Geneva: The Organization; 1947.

World Health Organization (WHO). Constitution of WHO principles. 2017. Available from: http://www.who.int/about/mission/en/.

Yan AF, Stevens P, Wang Y, Weinhardt L, Holt CL, O'Connor C, et al. mHealth text messaging for physical activity promotion in college students: a formative participatory approach. Am J Health Behav 2015; 39(3):395.

2 The Health Care Delivery System

OBJECTIVES

After reading this chapter, the student should be able to:

- To discuss the three levels of prevention.
- To describe the health care delivery system in India.
- To explain the different types of healthcare agencies offering health care.
- To discuss the types of settings in which professionals provide various levels of health care.
- To explain composition of health care team in hospital and role of team members.
- To discuss the role of nurses in various health care settings.
- To explain approaches nurses can use to improve patient satisfaction.
- To describe issues in health care delivery system for nursing in India

KEY TERMS

INTRODUCTION

The health care delivery system has changed significantly in the last 3 decades. Efforts have been made to reduce the costs of health care while improving access to the health care system and ensuring high-quality outcomes. Until recently, however, the costs of health care skyrocketed each year. Millions of Indians had limited access to health care, there were limited incentives for people to engage in healthy behaviors, and participants had no accepted method for measuring and evaluating health care outcomes.

Initiatives of Government of India such as National Rural Health Mission (2005), National Urban Health Mission (2013), and Ayushman Bharat National Health Protection Mission (2018) have been launched to transform primary, secondary, and tertiary health care system in India. In addition, there are several other national health programs functional in India to promote health, prevent illness, and facilitate provisions of care and rehabilitation for different selected diseases and disorders. Presently, India spends 1.4% of GDP on the health expenditure of the country. However, the National Health Policy, 2017, envisages raising government health spending to 2.5% of the GDP by 2025 in a time-bound manner.

Despite the provision of these national health programs and recent health care–related initiatives, India is ranked 130 of 189 countries in the Human Development Index Report, 2018, issued by United Nations Development Programme (UNDP). India is fastest growing economy in the world but the following facts depict the level of ignorance of the health sector in India.

- India spends 1.4% of GDP on the health, which is lowest in the world. Sri Lanka spends 1.8% of its GDP, whereas the figures in China and Thailand are 2.3% and 3.3%, respectively. The corresponding figure for the United States is in excess of 7%, whereas European nations such as the United Kingdom, Spain, Germany, and Italy spend 6.5%–8% of their GDP on health care.
- Seventy percent of overall household expenditure of Indians happened on medicines.
- Large Indian population (estimated >469 million) do not have regular access to essential medicines.
- Significant large number of urban (68%) and rural (58%) population seek their health care services from private health care facilities.
- Huge out-of-pocket expenditure on health care services is pushing about 55 million Indians below poverty every year and 33 million of this is only because of unaffordable cost of medicines.
- Surprisingly, there is no operation theatre in 63% primary health centers (PHCs) and 27% did not have labor rooms, whereas 82% community health centers lack specialties in surgery, pediatrics, obstetrics, and gynecology.

As you begin your career in nursing, you will soon realize that the Indian health care system is quite complex and constantly changing. You will better succeed in your career if you understand the functioning of the health care system and the role nurses play. Nursing is a caring discipline. The profession's values are rooted in helping people to regain, maintain, or improve their health; prevent illness; and find comfort and dignity at the time of death. Nowadays, the health care system overall is trying to move in the same direction.

As a result of global health care transformations, the practice of nursing is changing in every country. The American Nurses Association (ANA) takes this position: "Registered nurses are educated and practice within a holistic framework that views the individual, family, and community as an interconnected system that can keep us well and help us heal. Registered nurses are fundamental to the critical shift needed in health services delivery, with the goal of transforming the current 'sick care' system into a true 'health care' system."

Challenges to health care leaders nowadays include reducing health care costs while ensuring high-quality care for patients, improving access and coverage for more people, and encouraging healthy behaviors. Health care providers are discharging patients sooner from hospitals, resulting in more patients needing nursing homes or home care. Often families provide care for their loved ones in the home setting. Nurses face major challenges to prevent gaps in health care across health care settings so that individuals remain healthy and well within their own homes and communities.

HEALTH PROMOTION, WELLNESS, AND ILLNESS PREVENTION

Health promotion, health education, and illness prevention are closely related and sometimes overlap. All are focused on the future; the differences between them involve motivations and goals.

- **Health promotion** is a key component of public health and uses a variety of strategies, such as health education, legislation, and policy to help individuals, groups, and communities increase control over and improve their health. It also focuses on:
  - Improving quality of life by motivating people to reach stable level of health and decrease the incidence of illness.
  - Reducing effect of disability, premature death, and costs of medical treatment.

  Strategies for health promotion
    - Engage or adopt specific healthy behaviors, such as smoking-cessation programs by actively involving the individual.
    - Routine exercise and good nutrition to sustain present levels of health and prevent the risk of disease.
    - Strict policies or legislation in country, such as bars should ban smoking and reduce exposure to secondhand smoke.
- **Health education** teaches people how to care for themselves in a healthy way. It helps patients to achieve new understanding and control of their lives. It includes:
  - Physical awareness of self and environment.
  - Prevention of stress and its management.
- **Illness prevention** protects patients from actual or potential threats to health, such as obtaining immunizations. These activities help people avoid declines in health or functional level.

Illnesses, particularly chronic illnesses increase the cost of health care. Improving self-management and providing preventive services reduce health care need and cost. Therefore, you need to educate your patients about improving their ability to improve and manage their health. You do this by helping them recognize the effects their choices have on their health.

LEVELS OF ILLNESS PREVENTION

There are three levels of prevention in public health and health promotion. As a nurse, you will provide care in all four levels.

- **Primordial prevention:** It includes actions and measures that inhibit the emergence of risk factors in the form of environmental, social, cultural, behavioral and economic milieu, which can have adverse health consequences in the long terms.
  - Relatively new concept and catching good attention for prevention of chronic illness such as obesity, hypertension, coronary artery diseases, and diabetes.
  - Focus on early age because this is the time when lifestyle is formed, for example, eating patterns, physical activities, sleeping habits, smoking, and alcohol consumption, which can have significant impact on health during adulthood.
  - This can be achieved through individual and mass health education to promote healthy lifestyle among children and distancing them from harmful lifestyle practices.
- **Primary prevention** is true prevention. Its goal is to reduce the incidence of disease. Many primary prevention activities (e.g., federally funded immunization programs, water treatment) are supported by the government. It includes intervention such as
  - health education to reduce the risk of developing type 2 diabetes.
  - ensuring communities have safe water sources, implementing blood-borne pathogen regulations, and inspecting restaurants to ensure safe food handling.
- **Secondary prevention** focuses on preventing the spread of disease, illness, or infection once it occurs. Nurses who practice secondary prevention identify and treat people who have new cases of a disease or identify people who have been exposed to a disease but do not have the disease yet. For example:
  - Health screenings and contacting health care employees after exposure to a patient with an unknown diagnosis of tuberculosis.
  - Screening activities may lead to primary prevention interventions such as providing health teaching.
- **Tertiary prevention** focuses on reducing complications of long-term disease and disabilities through treatment and rehabilitation. It involves
  - Preventing further disability or reduced functioning.
  - Helping patients to achieve as high a level of functioning as possible, despite limitations caused by illness or impairment.

For example, you provide tertiary prevention when you help patients who have had a stroke adapt to their impaired mobility so that they can walk and prepare meals again.

LEVELS OF HEALTH CARE

Three-tier health care delivery system exists in India—primary, secondary, and tertiary level of health care. Levels of care describe the scope of services and settings delivered by health care providers to patients in all stages of health and illness. A fundamental and necessary function of health care system is to provide sound *referral system*.

- It must be a two-way exchange of information and returning patient to those who referred them for follow-up care.
- It will ensure continuity of care and inspire confidence of the patients and family in the system. However, unfortunately in developing countries like India, health care system remains weak and ideally there is no true referral system.

Each level of care has different requirements and opportunities for a nurse. For example, in your role within a primary care setting, you will be involved in patient assessment.

- You will identify changes in chronic conditions or the development of new acute conditions.
- You will teach new mothers how to care for their babies or young adults how to use an inhaler.
- In a continuing care setting, you will apply gerontology nursing principles to help patients adapt to permanent health changes so that they can remain active and engaged.

Levels of care are not the same as levels of prevention. Levels of prevention describe the focus of health-related activities in a care setting.

- These include timely containment of risk factors (primordial prevention), health promotion and disease prevention (primary prevention), curing of disease (secondary prevention), and reducing complications (tertiary prevention).
- At every level of care, nurses and other health care providers offer a variety of prevention services. For example, a nurse working in a specialized **acute care** (secondary/tertiary) hospital setting monitors the recovery of a patient following open heart surgery while also providing health promotion information to the family caregiver concerning diet and exercise.
- Health care reform has led to changes unique to each level of care. For example, the health care system now places greater emphasis on wellness.
- Wellness care focuses on the health of populations and communities rather than simply curing an individual's disease. In wellness care, nurses help lead communities and health care systems in coordinating resources to better serve their populations.

Thus, the current national health policies emphasis more resources toward primary care. Finding strategies to better address patient needs at all levels of care is critical to improving the health care system (Box 2.1).

Primary Health Care

It is the first level of contact of individuals, the family, and community with the national health system, where primary health care is provided. As a level of care, it is close to the people, where most of their health problems can be dealt with and resolved. In India, primary health care is delivered through PHCs and subcenters (Table 2.1).

- Primary health care team, auxiliary nurse midwives (ANMs), multipurpose health workers through and village health care team, trained dais, village health guide, Anganwadi workers, accredited social health activist (ASHA) not only provide primary health care but also

BOX 2.1 Examples of Health Care Services

Preventive Care

- Adult screenings for blood pressure, cholesterol, tobacco use, and cancer
- Pediatric screenings for hearing, vision, autism, and developmental disorders
- Human immunodeficiency virus (HIV) screening for adults at higher risk
- Wellness visits
- Immunizations
- Diet counseling
- Mental health counseling and crisis prevention
- Community legislation (seat belts, air bags, bike helmets)

Primary Care (Health Promotion)

- Diagnosis and treatment of common illnesses
- Ongoing management of chronic health problems
- Prenatal care
- Well-baby care
- Family planning
- Patient-centered medical home

Secondary (Acute Care)

- Urgent or emergency care
- Acute medical–surgical care: ambulatory, hospital
- Radiological procedures

Tertiary Care

- Highly specialized: intensive care, inpatient psychiatric facilities
- Specialty care (e.g., neurology, cardiology, rheumatology, dermatology, oncology)

Restorative Care

- Rehabilitation programs (e.g., cardiovascular, pulmonary, orthopedic)
- Sports medicine
- Spinal cord injury programs
- Home care

Continuing Care

- Long-term care: assisted living, nursing centers
- Psychiatric and older-adult day care

Table 2.1 Health Promotion in Preventive and Primary Care Settings

Type of Service	Purpose	Available Programs/Services
School health	Comprehensive programs integrate health promotion principles into a school curriculum. Services emphasize program management, interdisciplinary collaboration, and community health principles. Research shows a link between the health outcomes of young people and their academic success (CDC, 2015b).	Health education Physical education and physical activity Nutrition environment and services Health services Physical environment Social and emotional climate Counseling, psychological, and social services Employee wellness Family engagement Community involvement
Occupational health	The workplace is an important setting for delivering comprehensive health protection, health promotion, and disease-/accident-prevention programs. Americans working full time spend an average of more than one-third of their day, 5 days per week at the workplace (CDC, 2015a). The goal is to increase worker productivity, reduce absenteeism, reduce health risks, and reduce use of expensive medical care.	Environmental surveillance Create company policies that promote healthy behaviors such as a tobacco-free campus policy Work environment: offer healthy foods through vending machines or cafeterias Physical assessment and health screening Health education classes Communicable disease control Counseling
Physicians' offices	Physicians' offices provide primary health care and diagnose and treat acute and chronic illnesses. Practitioners are beginning to focus more on health promotion practices. Advanced nurse practitioners often partner with a physician in managing a patient population.	Routine physical examination Health screening Diagnostics Disease management
Nurse-managed clinics	Nurse-managed clinics or centers deliver nursing services with a focus on health promotion and health education, chronic disease assessment and management, and support for self-care and caregivers. Clinics often are associated with a school, college, department of nursing, federally qualified health center, or independent nonprofit health care agency (AACN, 2014).	Day care Clinical education site for other health care providers in school Physical examinations, cardiovascular checks Prevention services: diabetes and osteoporosis screenings, smoking-cessation programs, and immunizations. Health risk appraisal Wellness counseling Employment readiness Acute and long-term care management
Block and parish nursing	Nurses deliver health care services to patients (e.g., older adults or those unable to leave their home) within their own religious communities. Nurses provide services that are unavailable in traditional health care systems.	Running errands/transportation Respite care Counseling Spiritual health: balancing body and mind health to achieve overall wellness
Community centers	Centers provide comprehensive and cost-effective primary care and supportive services that promote access to health care. Services are often provided to a specific patient population (e.g., well-baby care, mental health care, diabetes care) within underserved communities. Centers are sometimes affiliated with a hospital, medical school, church, or other community organization. Care offered by community centers is culturally appropriate and delivered in languages that many people in the community speak (Center for American Progress, 2010).	Physical assessment and health screening Nutrition education Translation services Dental care Mental health services Care coordination and case management Specialty care (e.g., orthopedic, cardiac, or podiatric care) Disease management Health education

bridge the cultural and communication gap between the rural people and health care system.

- India being signatory in "Health for All" by CE 2000, the primary health care system has been reorganized and strengthened to make the primary health care delivery system more efficient.
- Health promotion is a key to quality health care. Effective health promotion programs help patients develop healthier lifestyles.

The Centers for Disease Control and Prevention (CDC, 2015a) notes that employees who adopt healthy behaviors through health promotion programs not only reduce their risk for developing disabling or life-threatening diseases and their associated costs but also improve their everyday quality of life including their physical, mental, and emotional health. The focus of health promotion is to

- keep people healthy through personal hygiene, good nutrition, clean living environment, regular exercise, rest, and the adoption of positive health attitudes.
- reduce the costs of health care by reducing the incidence of disease and minimizing complications, thereby reducing the need to use expensive health care resources.

In contrast, preventive care is more disease oriented and focuses on reducing and controlling risk factors for disease through activities such as immunization and diet counseling.

At the primary care level, health care providers deliver interventions that improve health outcome for an entire population. Community-based primary health care programs consider societal and environmental factors when addressing the health needs of communities.

The primary level of health care includes:

- Medical health care services
- Health education
- Nutritional counseling
- Maternal/child health care
- Family planning
- Control of diseases

Secondary Health Care

The next higher level of care is the secondary health care level. The traditional reason people use health care services such as a hospital is to diagnose and treat illness. When the nature or severity of a condition makes primary care insufficient, secondary and tertiary care often become necessary. In India, this kind of care is generally provided in district hospitals and community health centers, which also serve as the first referral level.

- Presently, total 4823 community health centers have been established by upgrading the PHCs, each community health center covering a population of 80,000 to 1.20 lakh with 30 beds and specialists in surgery, medicine, obstetrics, and gynecology and pediatrics with X-ray and laboratory facilities.
- The difference between secondary and tertiary care arises from the complexity of a patient's medical needs.
- **Secondary health care** is provided by a specialist or agency on referral by a primary health care provider. It requires more specialized knowledge, skill, or equipment than the primary care physician or nurse practitioner can provide.

Tertiary Health Care

The tertiary level is a more specialized level than secondary care level and requires specific facilities and attention of highly specialized health workers.

- Tertiary health care is specialized consultative care, usually provided on referral from secondary medical personnel.
- This level of care is provided by the regional or central level institutes, such as medical college hospitals, all India institutes, regional hospitals, specialized hospitals, and other apex institutes of the country.
- Tertiary care, also called *acute care*, typically is expensive, especially if a patient has waited to seek care until after symptoms have developed (Fig. 2.1).

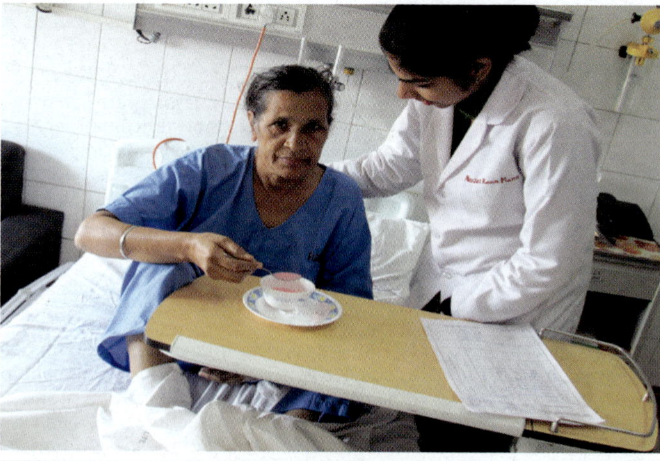

Fig. 2.1 Delivering nursing services in assisted-living facilities promotes physical and psychosocial health. (Copyright © Sharma SK.)

TYPES OF HEALTH CARE AGENCIES

The health care system is intended to deliver the health care services. In India, health care system is represented by six major sectors or agencies that differ from each other by health technology applied and by source of funding for operation. These are

I. **Public health sector**
   - Primary health care
     - PHCs
     - Subcenters
   - Hospitals/health centers
     - Community health centers
     - Rural hospitals
     - District hospitals
     - Specialty hospitals (mental health hospitals, maternal and child hospitals, etc.)
     - Teaching hospitals
   - Health insurance scheme
     - Employees' State Insurance
     - Central Government Health Scheme
   - Other agencies
     - Defense services
     - Railway hospitals

II. **Private sector**
   - Private hospitals, polyclinics, nursing homes, and dispensaries

III. **Indigenous System of Medicine (AYUSH)**
   - Ayurveda
   - Yoga
   - Unani
   - Siddha
   - Homeopathy

IV. **Voluntary health agencies**

V. **National health programs**

VI. **Faith healers and unregistered practitioner**

Primary Health Care in India

In 1977, the Government of India launched a rural health scheme based on the principle of planning "placing people's health in people's hands." It is a three-tier system of health care delivered in rural area based on the recommendations of the Shrivastav Committee in 1975. Close on the heels of these recommendations, an international conference at Alma-Ata in 1978 set the goal of an acceptable level of health for all the people of the world by the year 2000 through primary health care approach. As a signatory to the Alma-Ata Declaration, the Government of India was committed to achieving the goal of health for all through primary health care approach, which seeks to provide universal comprehensive health care at a cost that is affordable.

Keeping in view the World Health Organization (WHO) goal of **Health for All** by CE 2000 , the Government of India evolved a National Health Policy based on the

BOX 2.2 Role of Nurse in Primary Health Care

- Providing antenatal, natal, and postnatal care to pregnant women.
- Offering the immunization services to the eligible mothers and children.
- Educating the couples about temporary and permanent family planning methods and facilitating them to avail the desired method.
- Identifying and managing the nutrition-related problems of mother and children in the community through screening, education, and offering the dietary supplements.
- Promoting health and preventing diseases in the community through active participation in national health programs.
- Recording and reporting the vital statistics including birth, death, expecting mothers, infants, and children to relevant health authorities.
- Nurse working in primary health care facilities also offers the treatment for the minor ailments in case the physician is not available.
- Assisting the medical officer in medical termination of pregnancy, whenever it is required.
- Providing training to dais, village health guide, ASHA, and so on.

primary health care approach. It laid down a plan of action for reorienting and shaping the existing rural health infrastructure with specific goals to be achieved by 1985, 1990, and 1995 within the framework of the Sixth (1980–1985) and Seventh (1985–1990) Five Year Plans and the new 20-Point Programme. Steps were taken to implement the National Health Policy objectives toward achieving health for all by the year 2000. During the last decade, further development of rural health infrastructure took place in view to implement National Health Policy 2000, National Population Policy 2002, and more recently National Rural Health Mission with formulation of Indian Public Health Standards. Nurses play a vital role in the primary health care as depicted in Box 2.2.

Village Level

One of the basic tenets of primary health care is universal coverage and equitable distribution of health resources, that is, health care must penetrate into the farthest reaches of rural area, and that everyone should have access to it. To implement this policy at the village level, the following schemes are operational:

- National Village Health Guide Scheme
- Training of local dais
- Integrated Child Development Scheme
- ASHA

Subcenter Level

The subcenters are the peripheral outposts of the existing health delivery system in the rural area. They are being established on the basis of one subcenter for every 5000 population in general and one for every 3000 population in hilly, tribal, and backward areas. Presently, total 148,366 subcenters are established in India. The subcenters provide infrastructure with the community at the grassroots level, providing all the primary health care services. Of particular importance are the packages of services such as immunization; antenatal, natal, postnatal care; prevention of malnutrition and common childhood diseases; family planning services and counselling. They also provide elementary drugs for minor ailments such as acute respiratory infections (ARIs), diarrhea, fever, and worm infestation, and carry out community needs assessment. Besides the above, the government implements several national health and family welfare programs through these frontline workers.

BOX 2.3 Functions of Primary Health Center

The functions of the primary health center in India cover all the eight *essential* elements of primary health care as outlined in the Alma-Ata Declaration. They are as follows:

- Medical care
- Maternal and child health care including family planning
- Safe water supply and basic sanitation
- Prevention and control of locally endemic diseases
- Collection and reporting of vital statistics
- Education about health
- National health programs, as relevant
- Referral services
- Training of health guides, health care workers, local dais, and health assistants
- Basic laboratory services

Primary Health Centre Level

The concept of PHC is not new in India. The Bhore Committee in 1946 gave the concept of PHC as a basic health unit, to provide as close to the people as possible, an integrated curative and preventive health care to the rural population with emphasis on preventive and promotive aspects of health care. The Bhore Committee aimed at having a health center to serve a population of 10,000–20,000 with six medical officers, six public health nurses, and other supportive staff. But in view of the limited resources, the Bhore Committee's recommendations could not be fully implemented, even after a lapse of 60 years.

The health planners in India have visualized the primary health care services and their subcenter as the proper infrastructure to provide health services in rural areas. The Central Council of Health at its first meeting held in January 1953 had recommended the establishment of PHC in community development blocks to provide comprehensive health care to rural population. The Alma-Ata Declaration in 1978 setting the goals of health for all by CE 2000 has ushered in a new philosophy of equity and a new approach, the primary health care approach. The National Health Plan (1983) proposed recognition of PHCs on the basis of one PHC for every 30,000 rural population in the plain and one PHC for every 20,000 population in hilly, tribal, and backward areas for more effective coverage. Presently, total 24,049 PHCs have been established in India. The basic functions of PHC are depicted in Box 2.3.

Secondary and tertiary health care services in India are provided through public or private hospital and health centers. The discussion about hospitals is given in the subsequent section.

HOSPITALS IN INDIA

The word *hospital* is derived from the Latin word *hospice*. In fact, the words hospital, hostel, and hotel all are derived

BOX 2.4 Basic Functions of the Hospital

Diagnostic: Hospitals provide the diagnostic services for the early and prompt diagnosis of illnesses.
Therapeutic: Hospitals provide the curative services to the sick people.
Emergency care: Hospitals provide the emergency to the patients' acute illnesses.
Critical care services: Hospitals provide the advanced tertiary care for the patients suffering from life-threatening illnesses.
Rehabilitation: Hospitals also provide the facilities for physical therapy and rehabilitation.
Preventive services: Hospitals also provide the preventive services such as antenatal care, immunization, communicable disease prevention, and baby clinic.
Health promotion: Hospitals also actively participate in health promotion activities such as health education and family welfare clinics.
Education and training: Hospitals also provide platform to offer the education for medical, nursing, and paramedical students.
Research: Hospitals are places where research is carried out to expand body of knowledge in the field of health sciences.

from the common Latin root *hospice*. Meaning of *hospice* is "host" or "an establishment where a guest is received and cared." WHO defines the hospital as an "integral part of the social and medical organization, the function of which is to provide for the population, complete health care, both curative and preventive and whose outpatient services reach out to the families and its environment; the hospital is also a center for the training of health workers and biosocial research." Nowadays, hospital means an institution in which sick or injured persons are treated and healthy persons are helped to promote and maintain an optimum level of well-being. A modern hospital is an institution that possesses adequate accommodation and well-qualified and experienced personnel to provide services of curative, restorative, preventive, and promotive characteristics of the highest quality possible to all people, regardless of race, color, creed, or economic status. It conducts educational and training programs for the health personnel particularly required for patient care and hospital services. It also conducts research in assisting the advancement of medical services and hospital services, and conducts programs of health education (for details about function of hospitals, refer to Box 2.4).

Types of Hospitals

Hospitals can be classified per ownership/control, clinical basis, patients' LOS, and teaching or nonteaching status. Per ownership basis, the hospitals can be public, voluntary, private, and corporate. The public hospitals can be further classified as central government hospitals and state government hospitals. Private hospitals can be missionary or charitable trust hospitals (see details in Table 2.2).

History of Hospitals In India

Early Indian rulers considered the provision of institutional care to the sick as their spiritual and temporal responsibility. The forerunners of the present hospitals can be traced to the times of Buddha, followed by Ashoka. India could boast of a very well organized hospital and health care system even in the ancient times. The writings of Sushruta (6th century BCE) and Charaka (CE 200), the famous surgeon and physician, respectively, were considered for their standard work for many centuries with instructions (in Charaka Samhita) for the creation of hospitals for provisions of lying in; children rooms, maintenance, and sterilization of bed linen with steam and fumigation; and use of syringes and other medical appliances. Medicine based on

Table 2.2 Types/Classification of Hospitals

BASED ON OWNERSHIP OF HOSPITAL	
Public hospitals	These hospitals are run by the central or state government or municipal bodies/corporations with a service motive. These hospitals may be general hospitals or specialized hospitals.
Charitable hospitals	These hospitals are established under Societies Registration Act and run for service motive. These are generally funded by donations, grants, and aids from philanthropic organizations.
Private hospitals	These hospitals are generally owned by an individual or a group of individuals, which are generally self-funded and run for commercial purpose.
Corporate hospitals	These hospitals are established by registered companies and generally run for the commercial purposes.
BASED ON CLINICAL SPECIALTIES	
General hospitals	These hospitals are run to provide only general medical, surgical, maternity, and pediatrics care for the community.
Specialized hospitals	These hospitals are run to provide specialized care such as cardiology, neurosciences, nephrology, oncology, ophthalmology, mental health, and maternal health services.
BASED ON LENGTH OF STAY	
Long-term hospitals	These hospitals provide care to the people who require long-term services for chronic diseases such as Alzheimer disease.
Short-term hospitals	These hospitals provide care to the people with short acute illness such as cardiac hospitals.
Day care hospitals	These hospitals offer care only during daytime. Patients are admitted on the same day, procedure is performed, and then discharged on the same day. For example, eye care hospitals.
BASED ON DIVERSITY IN AIM OF HOSPITALS	
Teaching hospitals	These hospitals are run for the dual purpose—teaching the medical, nursing, and other health care students and providing the care to the people.
Nonteaching hospitals	These hospitals are run to offer only health care services to the people, without any purpose of providing the teaching to the health science students.

the Indian system was taught in the ancient university of Taxila. Charaka Samhita, a treatise of surgical knowledge, was compiled during CE 400 .

The most notable of the early hospitals were those built by king Ashoka (273–232 BCE). There were rituals laid down for the nurses and the physicians who were enjoined to wear white clothes and promised to keep the confidence of the patients. However, the age of Indian medicine started declining from Mohammedan invasions during the 10th century. The Mohammedans brought with them their Hakims who followed the Greek system of medicine, which came to be known as *Unani*. The system and its physicians started to prosper at the expense of Ayurveda and its Vaidyas. However, the influence of Ayurveda continued in the south.

The modern system of medicine in India was introduced in the 17th century with the arrival of European Christian missionary in South India. In the 17th century, the East India Company, the forerunner of the British Empire in India, established its first hospital in 1664 at Chennai for its soldiers and in 1668 for civil population. European doctors started getting popular and during the later part of the 18th and the 19th century, there was a steady growth of modern system of medical practice and hospitals, pushing the indigenous system to the background. Organized medical training started with the first medical college opening in Calcutta in 1835, followed by Mumbai in 1845, and Chennai in 1850. Thereafter, these services swelled up and in 1885, there were 1250 hospitals and dispensaries in British India. After independence, from time to time various committees were constituted to study the health services; these committees have recommended increasing need of hospitals and health centers. Nowadays, we have more than 20,000 secondary and tertiary care providing hospitals in India. However, 70% of the country's health care infrastructure is under the private sector. The basic traditional organization of a hospital is presented in Fig. 2.2.

HEALTH CARE TEAM

No single agency can deliver the entire range of medical care and health care. Achievement of health and medical care can be best if many professional groups of workers such as physicians, nurses, paramedical workers, health educators, health visitors, public health engineers, and many others share a common unifying goal. This joint effort materializes through team work.

In health care, teamwork has been defined as a dynamic process involving two or more health care professionals with complementary backgrounds and skills, sharing common health goals and exercising concerted physical and mental effort in assessing, planning, or evaluating patient care.

Teamwork is increasingly advocated by health care policy makers as a means of assuring quality and safety in the delivery of services. The functional classification of teams concerned with group health and personal health is as follows:

- The **health care team,** which consists of all those who are involved in improving health in a community setting without necessarily being in active contact with the patients.
- The **medical care team,** which consists of those professional and paraprofessionals who provide service for the patient generally in a hospital setting but without any direct or personal contact with the patient.
- The **patient care team,** which comprises any group of professionals and semiprofessionals in a hospital setting who jointly provide service that brings them into direct contact with the patient.

Therefore, health and medical services cannot be delivered through any one agency. As discussed earlier, all the responsibility devolves on the three health sectors—environmental health, public health, and personal health sector. In addition, the two other service systems indirectly connected with

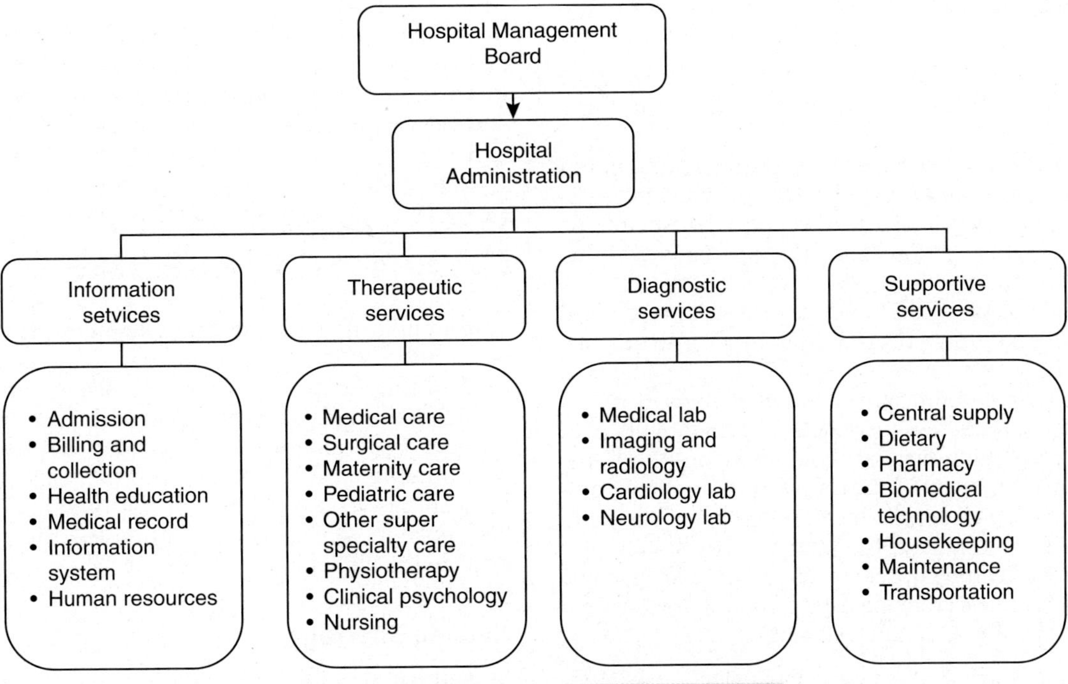

Fig. 2.2 Traditional organization chart of a hospital.

Table 2.3 Bombay Nursing Homes Registration Act (June 2006) Recommendation for Ward Staff

Category of Staff	Staff to Bed Ratio Round the Clock
Resident medical officer	1 for every 10 beds
Registered nurse	1 for every 5 beds
General duty assistant	1 for every 3 beds
Sweeper	1 for every 5 beds

health are the social welfare services and the educational services.

A general hospital includes variety of people involved directly and indirectly for the care of patients such as physicians, nurses, technicians, paramedical staff, general duty assistants, and sweepers. Bombay Nursing Homes Registration Act, 2006, has provided recommendations of ward staff in a general hospital, which is presented in Table 2.3. It was recommended that there should be one Resident Medical Officer for 10 beds, one registered nurse for 5 beds, one general duty assistant for 3 beds, and one sweeper for 5 beds round the clock.

PATIENT SATISFACTION

Patient satisfaction is the responsibility of all health care providers. This is more important than ever because patient satisfaction measures are linked to quality of health care services provided to them. Patient perceptions of the quality of their health care are incorporated into quality assessment. As a result, health care organizations have made patient-centered care a major component of their health care missions. Hospitals now report patient satisfaction scores for patient care units monthly. All health care staff members help identify satisfaction trends and determine ways to improve quality of care. Hospitals and other health care agencies use a variety of instruments to measure patient satisfaction, such as:

- Instruments provided by private vendors. These usually are not published, and their reliability and validity are unclear.
- Public and standardized instruments such as patient satisfaction questionnaires: PSQ-18 and consumer assessment health plans (e.g., HCAHPS). Such instruments have the advantage of good reliability and validity; however, they have a limited scope of survey questions.
- Internally developed instruments. These are derived mainly from questions extracted from other instruments. The HCAHPS survey has 32 questions that ask patients to respond about communication with physicians, communication with nurses, responsiveness of hospital staff, pain management, communication about medicines, discharge information, cleanliness of the hospital environment, quietness of the hospital environment, transition of care, and willingness to recommend the hospital. The survey also includes four screening questions and seven demographic items, which are used for adjusting the mix of patients across hospitals and for analytical purposes.

Recently, the factors that affect patient satisfaction, including relational communication techniques, hourly rounding (Box 2.5), and bedside shift report, have been the focus of many research studies. Common factors that positively affected patient satisfaction in these studies included interpersonal skills, especially the courtesy and respect of health care providers, as well as the communication skills of explanation and clear information. These factors were more influential than other technical skills such as clinical competency and hospital equipment.

BOX 2.5 Evidence-Based Practice

PICOT Question: In acute care hospitals, does the use of hourly rounding by registered nurses influence patient satisfaction?

Summary of Evidence

Patient satisfaction is a key measurement that affects both hospital quality ratings and reimbursement. Nurses spend a great deal of time with patients and thus have a large influence on patients' perceptions of their experiences and level of satisfaction. A systematic review of studies examining the effects of hourly rounding shows that evidence supporting the use of hourly rounding in inpatient care is of low-to-moderate strength because the studies were not conducted in a consistent manner (Mitchell et al., 2014). However, evidence from this study suggests that purposeful, hourly rounding improves patients' perceptions of nursing staff responsiveness in units where this may have been a problem. Hourly rounding can reduce patient falls and use of nurse call system and improves patient satisfaction scores. Hourly nurse rounding is possibly also a cost-effective intervention because it reduces injuries related to patient falls and pressure injuries, both of which often extend hospital length of stays (Brosey and March, 2014).

Application to Nursing Practice

- Proactive and regular checks of hospitalized patients during hourly rounds may reduce patient anxiety and minimize uncertainty that a nurse will be available to assist with basic needs.
- The use of a script or structure of tasks to be performed during rounding may be beneficial. Those tasks correspond to the "four Ps": bathroom ("potty"), positioning, pain control, and proximity of personal items (Meade et al., 2006).
- The approach to rounding may differ by patient care setting (e.g., hourly rounding, rounding every 30 min [emergency department], or involvement of RN or nursing assistive personnel).

ISSUES IN HEALTH CARE DELIVERY FOR NURSING

Your familiarity with the issues facing health care will help you understand the expectations, programs, and policies used in the institution where you begin your nursing career. For example, controlling health care costs has been a major issue for the last 2 decades and has affected the way nursing care is provided and the staffing models used in hospitals. These issues will not only affect the choices you make in your career but also affect the quality of care provided to all patients.

Nursing Shortage

India is training highest number of nurses in the world and it is also one of the top five exporters of nurses across the globe. However, this exporting country is in crippling shortage of nurses because of rapid migration of nurses to other countries for the better pay and working conditions. WHO recommends 2.5 nurses per 1000 population; however, India has only 1.7 nurses per 1000 population, which means that India is currently short of about 2.5 million nurses.

In past two decades, there had been steep growth in number of nursing institutes. In 2004, there were 165 BSc Nursing Colleges, which increased nearly ten folds to 1507 in 2012. Similarly, institutes offering General Nursing and Midwifery and Auxiliary Nurse Midwifery program also increased from 659 and 485 in 1997 to 2487 and 1307 in 2012, respectively. However, situation is more worrisome because of declining enrolment of students in nursing education and a very poor quality of education facilities in the country.

The poor quality of academic infrastructure in nursing institutes of the country may be because of rapid mushrooming of institutes, weak accreditation system by central and state nursing councils, political interference, and corruption in accreditation process of statutory bodies. Consequently, India is producing nurses with poor clinical acumen and emotional intelligence. The scarcity of nurses in the country is leading the private health sector to fill its demand by employing untrained nurses or undertaking nurse poaching from other health institutions. Only 40% of the total nursing workforce in the country is said to be active because of low recruitment, migration, attrition and dropouts due to poor working conditions.

Patient-Centered Care

Patient-centered care is much more than simply "individualizing" patient care. A critical component of patient-centered care is the nurse, patient, and family caregiver partnering to identify the patient's health care needs within the context of the patient's lifestyle. Patient-centered care also requires the entire health care team to collaborate so that the patient and family caregiver are engaged in the care process and associated decisions. This is a major shift in how care is delivered, empowering the patient and family caregiver to participate in the plan of care. Following are the eight principles of patient-centered care based on input from patients, families, and health care experts:

1. **Respect for patients' values, preferences, and expressed needs.** Engage patients in decision-making, recognizing that they are individuals with their own unique values and preferences. Treat patients with dignity, respect, and sensitivity to their cultural values and autonomy.
2. **Coordination and integration of care.** Coordinate care to reduce patients' feelings of vulnerability:
   - Coordinate clinical care
   - Coordinate ancillary and support services
   - Coordinate frontline patient care
3. **Information and education.** Improve communication with patients and families:
   - Provide information about clinical status, progress, and prognosis
   - Provide information about processes of care
   - Provide information to facilitate autonomy, self-care, and health promotion
4. **Physical comfort.** Provide physical comfort throughout the care experience including pain management, assistance with activities and daily living needs, and provide comforting hospital surroundings and environment.
5. **Emotional support and alleviation of fear and anxiety.** Professional caregivers need to pay attention to patients' fear and anxiety:
   - Anxiety over physical status, treatment, and prognosis
   - Anxiety over the effect of the illness on themselves and family
   - Anxiety over the financial impact of illness
6. **Involvement of family and friends.** Support family and friends in taking a role in a patient's experience. Family dimensions of patient-centered care include:
   - Providing accommodations for family and friends
   - Involving family and close friends in decision-making
   - Supporting family members as caregivers
   - Recognizing the needs of family and friends
7. **Continuity and transition.** Offer support and resources so that patients can care for themselves after discharge or receive the assistance they need:
   - Provide understandable, detailed information about topics such as medications, physical limitations, and dietary needs
   - Coordinate and plan treatment and services to continue after discharge
   - Provide information about access to clinical, social, physical, and financial support continually
8. **Access to care.** Patients need to know they can access care when it is needed, especially ambulatory care:
   - Access to hospitals, clinics, and physician offices
   - Availability of transportation
   - Ease in scheduling appointments
   - Availability of appointments when needed
   - Accessibility of specialists or specialty services when a referral is made
   - Clear instructions provided on when and how to get referrals

Technology in Health Care

- Technological advances continually affect health care organizations and change the ways nurses deliver evidence-based care to patients. Emerging technologies that will change nursing practice include genetics and genomics, less invasive and more accurate tools for diagnosis and treatment, three-dimensional printing, robotics, biometrics, EHRs, and computerized physician/provider order entry and clinical decision support. Technology makes your work easier in many ways, but it does not replace your judgment. For example, when you manage an i.v. infusion smart pump, you monitor the device to ensure that it infuses on schedule and without complications despite its numerous automatic settings. An infusion device infuses at a constant rate, but you must confirm that the rate is calculated correctly. An infusion device sets off an alarm if the infusion slows, making it important for you to respond to the alarm and fix the problem. Technology does not replace a nurse's astute, critical eye, and clinical judgment.
- Robotics is a form of emerging technology that will greatly affect how nursing is practiced in the future. Experts estimate that robotic use will grow because of

workforce shortages, a growing elderly population, and a call for higher quality care not subject to human limitations. Robotic applications include food service, medication distribution, infection control, surgery, and diagnosing patients. Another area with great potential for impacting nursing is the use of robots as direct care providers reports that there are daily care robots designed to support older patients and people with disabilities in activities such as preparing and serving meals and daily care tasks. In addition, exoskeleton-powered robots can help patients with paraplegia stand with the goal of reducing morbidity and augmenting physical therapy. The implications for nursing are significant. Nurses must be on the frontline in deciding how robotics is used to advocate for patients and families as well as ensuring that professional standards of care are delivered.

- Telemedicine is a technology that relies on interactive video and uses medical information gathered and reviewed at one site (e.g., a hospital, home, clinic, or urgent care center) and transmits treatment recommendations to another site to improve a patient's clinical health status. A variety of applications and services use two-way video, smartphones, wireless tools, and other forms of telecommunications technology. However, varying state policies on telemedicine use and reimbursement pose an obstacle to wider adoption of this emerging practice. Research shows that specific telemedicine applications (e.g., the Hospital at Home model and management of chronic illness) save patients, providers, and payers money compared with traditional approaches.

Health Care Disparities

Health care services are more concentrated in urban areas, and rural areas are seriously deprived. There were clear inequalities in the distribution of these training institutions among states. Although the Empowered Action Group states account for almost half of the country's population, they house only approximately one,Äëfifth of the medical colleges and a quarter of the dental and nursing institutes.

The distribution of nurses in India presents a picture of imbalance across states. The state with low-mortality rates reported higher availability of nurses as compared with the states experiencing low-health status. The rural–urban distribution of nurses showed that more nurses preferred working in the urban areas. However, the need for nursing services is more in the rural than the urban areas because of lower health status and higher mortality rates experienced by rural population. The nurses working in urban areas were nearly three times more in number than the nurses employed in the rural areas.

KEY POINTS

- Levels of health care describe the scope of services and settings in which health care is delivered to patients in all stages of health and illness.
- The primary level of health care includes medical health care services, health education, nutritional care, maternal/child health care, family planning, and control of diseases.
- Nurses and other health care providers offer preventive services at every level of health care.
- Hospitals deliver health care to patients who are acutely ill and need comprehensive specialized secondary and tertiary health care.
- Access of rural Indians to health care is affected by economic factors (rural Indians are more likely to live below the poverty level), cultural and social differences, educational shortcomings, lack of recognition of the problem by legislators, and the isolation of living in remote rural areas.
- The holistic model of care is used within integrated health care systems and delivers a coordinated continuum of services that supports patients with chronic conditions and improves the health of specific populations.
- Expertise in assessment is a critical competency of home health nurses.
- Preventive services are health-related activities delivered in a care setting and include promoting health and preventing disease (primary prevention), curing disease (secondary prevention), and reducing complications (tertiary prevention).
- Barriers to effective discharge planning include ineffective communication, lack of role clarity among health care team members, and lack of resources.
- In restorative care settings, nurses know that success depends on their effective and early partnering with patients and their families.
- As a nurse, you can promote patient satisfaction through interpersonal skills including courtesy, respect, and good communication skills.
- The nursing shortage opens vast opportunities to nurses. If you pursue further education and follow trends in health care, many professional options will be available to you.

REFERENCES

American Association of Colleges of Nursing (AACN). Policy brief: nurse-managed health clinics: increasing access to primary care and educating the healthcare workforce. 2014. Available from: https://www.aacnnursing.org/Policy-Advocacy/Government-Affairs.

Brosey L, March KS. Effectiveness of structured hourly nurse rounding on patient satisfaction and clinical outcomes, J Nurs Care Qual 2014;30(2). Available from: https://www.researchgate.net/publication/265863446_Effectiveness_of_Structured_Hourly_Nurse_Rounding_on_Patient_Satisfaction_and_Clinical_Outcomes.

Center for American Progress. The importance of community health centers: engines of economic activity and job creation. 2010. Available from: https://www.americanprogress.org/issues/healthcare/report/2010/08/09/8195/the-importance-of-community-health-centers/.

Centers for Disease Control and Prevention (CDC). Workplace health promotion: health outcome measures. 2015a. Available from: http://www.cdc.gov/workplacehealthpromotion/model/evaluation/outcomes.html.

Centers for Disease Control and Prevention (CDC). Whole school, whole community, whole child (WSCC): a collaborative approach to learning and health. 2015b. Available from: http://www.cdc.gov/healthyschools/wscc/index.htm.

Meade CM, Bursell AL, Ketelsen L. Effects of nursing rounds: on patients' call light use, satisfaction, and safety. Am J Nurs 2006;106(9):58-70.

Mitchell MD, Lavenberg JG, Trotta RL, Umscheid CA. Hourly rounding to improve nursing responsiveness: a systematic review. J Nurs Adm 2014;44:462-72.

3 History of Nursing and Nursing as a Profession

OBJECTIVES

After reading this chapter, the student should be able to:

- To discuss the history of nursing in India.
- To explain contribution of Florence Nightingale in Indian nursing.
- To define nursing and discuss the concept of nursing.
- To discuss philosophy, aims, and objectives of nursing.
- To explain characteristics, nature, and scope of nursing.
- To discuss the qualities of a nurse.
- To enlist categories of nursing personnel.
- To define profession and describe characteristics of professionalism in nursing.
- To discuss the importance of education in professional nursing practice.
- To describe the purpose of professional standards of nursing practice.
- To describe the roles and career opportunities for nurses.
- To discuss the influence of social, political, and economic changes on nursing practices.
- To explain importance of values in nursing profession.

KEY TERMS

Auxiliary nurse midwife, p. 31
advanced practice registered nurse (APRN), p. 32
American Nurses Association (ANA), p. 27
caregiver, p. 29
certified nurse-midwife (CNM), p. 32
certified registered nurse anesthetist (CRNA), p. 32
Chief nursing officer, p. 31
clinical nurse specialist (CNS), p. 29
code of ethics, p. 33
Indian Nursing Council, p. 25
International Council of Nurses (ICN), p. 27
nurse administrator, p. 31
nurse educator, p. 31
nurse practitioner (NP), p. 31
nurse researcher, p. 32
nursing, p. 27
patient advocate, p. 30
Quality and Safety Education for Nurses (QSEN), p. 35
registered nurse (RN), p. 31

INTRODUCTION

Nursing is an art and a science. As a professional nurse, you learn to deliver care artfully with compassion, care, and respect for each patient's dignity and personhood. As a science, nursing practice is based on a body of knowledge that is continually changing with new discoveries and innovations. When you integrate the science and art of nursing into your practice, the quality of care you provide to your patients is at a level of excellence that benefits patients and their families. Your patients' health care needs are multidimensional. Thus, your care reflects patients' needs as well as the needs and values of society and professional standards of care. In addition, your care should integrate evidence-based practices to provide the highest level of care.

The patient is the center of your practice. The patient includes the individual, family, and/or community. Patients have a wide variety of health care needs, experiences, vulnerabilities, and expectations; this is what makes nursing both challenging and rewarding. Making a difference in your patients' lives is fulfilling. For example, you help a dying patient find relief from pain, help a young mother learn parenting skills, or find ways for older adults to remain independent in their homes. Nursing offers personal and professional rewards every day.

As a nurse, you can choose a variety of career paths including clinical practice, education, research, management, administration, and entrepreneurship. As a student, it is important for you to understand the scope of nursing practice and how nursing influences the lives of your patients. You are required to provide nursing care according to standards of practice and follow a code of ethics. Professional practice includes knowledge from social and behavioral sciences, biological and physiological sciences, and nursing theories. In addition, nursing practice incorporates ethical and social values, professional autonomy, and a sense of commitment and community.

Expert clinical nursing practice is a commitment to the application of knowledge, ethics, standards of practice, and clinical experience. Your ability to interpret clinical situations and make complex decisions is the foundation for your nursing care and the basis for the advancement of nursing practice and the development of nursing science. Clinical expertise takes time and commitment. Critical thinking skills are essential to nursing (see Chapter 18). When providing nursing care, you need to make clinical judgments and decisions about your patients' health care needs on the basis of knowledge, experience, and standards of care. Critical thinking and reflection help you gain and interpret scientific knowledge, integrate knowledge from clinical experiences, and become a lifelong learner. This includes integrating knowledge from basic science and nursing knowledge bases, applying knowledge from past and present experiences, applying critical thinking attitudes to a clinical situation, and implementing intellectual and professional standards (see Chapter 18). When you provide well-thought-out care with compassion and care, you provide each of your patients the best of the science and art of nursing care.

HISTORY OF NURSING IN INDIA

History of nursing is as ancient as existence of human being. Throughout the ages, the sick, the disabled, and the helpless have needed the protective, tender, and loving care, which is nursing. Nursing as a science of healing, caring, and allaying of physical suffering of men and women and as a noble and humane profession was known to many ancient people and civilizations including those of India, but as a systematic science and organized profession, its history may not be very old.

Since the beginning of the profession, nurses have studied and tested new and better ways to help patients. Patients are most vulnerable when they are injured, sick, or dying. Nowadays, nurses are active in determining the best practices for patient care related to problems such as skin care management, pain control, nutritional management, and care of older adults. Nurse researchers are leaders in expanding knowledge in nursing and other health care disciplines. Their work provides evidence for practice to ensure that we have the best available evidence to support our practices.

Nurses are also active in social policy and political arenas. With their professional organizations, they lobby for health care legislation. For example, nurses have lobbied for laws promoting smoke-free environments and stronger antitobacco laws, setting up antigang coalitions, establishing safer environments for walking and physical fitness in their communities, and advocating for breastfeeding.

Knowledge of the history of the nursing profession increases your ability to understand the social and intellectual origins of the discipline. Although it is not practical to describe all the historical aspects of professional nursing, some of the more significant milestones are described in the following paragraphs.

Nursing in Ancient India

History indicates that nursing education and practices are ancient in India. It is documented that world's first nursing school was started in India during 250 BCE, where only men were trained as nurses. The status of ancient Indian nursing as well as medicine far exceeded that of the west, to an extent that streets and roads near hospitals were lined specifically with trees that had medicinal properties. In ancient India, only men were considered pure to be trained as nurse; however, it was evident from old photographs and painting arts (Fig. 3.1) that older experienced women were offering help in childbirth to other women. These traditional birth attendants or "*dais*" were believed to have indigenous knowledge of herbs, diet, and skills of massage techniques to ease the pains of pregnancy and delivery, which was passed from one generation to another to practice.

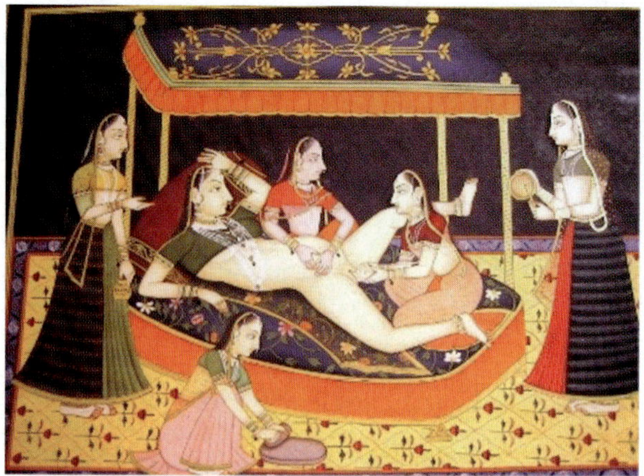

Fig. 3.1 Women helping in childbirth in ancient India.

- Roots of nursing can be traced in the Vedic period during which Ayurveda had mentioned nurse as one of the four important wings of treatment. In India, the Ayurvedic system of medicine has been practiced since 3000 BCE, which stressed on hygiene and prevention of illness. This was strongly promoted by the kings of various times and was also mostly practiced by great sages. Atreya was the first great physician and teacher of Ayurveda. Nurses in this era worked primarily as assistants to the Ayurvedic physicians in the preparation of medicines and application of topical medicines and care of wounds.
- In 1500 BCE, it was thought that diseases are attributed to demons and the treatment given was primarily to exorcize the demons. Role of nurses was not very clear during this period.
- About 700 BCE, the practice of medicine had passed into the hands of Brahmins, who were scholars and members of the priestly class. Banaras became the center of medical education.
- As early as 700–600 BCE, there are evidence of practice of surgery and medicine. The preparation of various drugs and compounding for administration is well explained by the great physician Charaka in his book "*Charaka Samhita*" or Compendium of Charaka, which was believed to be compiled between 100 BCE and 200 BCE. It also describes that nurses must be knowledgeable, skilled at preparing formulations and dosage, sympathetic toward everyone, and clean. Code of ethics for physicians and nurses was also found in this book.
- In the 4th century BCE, *Sutrasthanam* gave the description of nurse as the "man" to be..."*that person alone who*

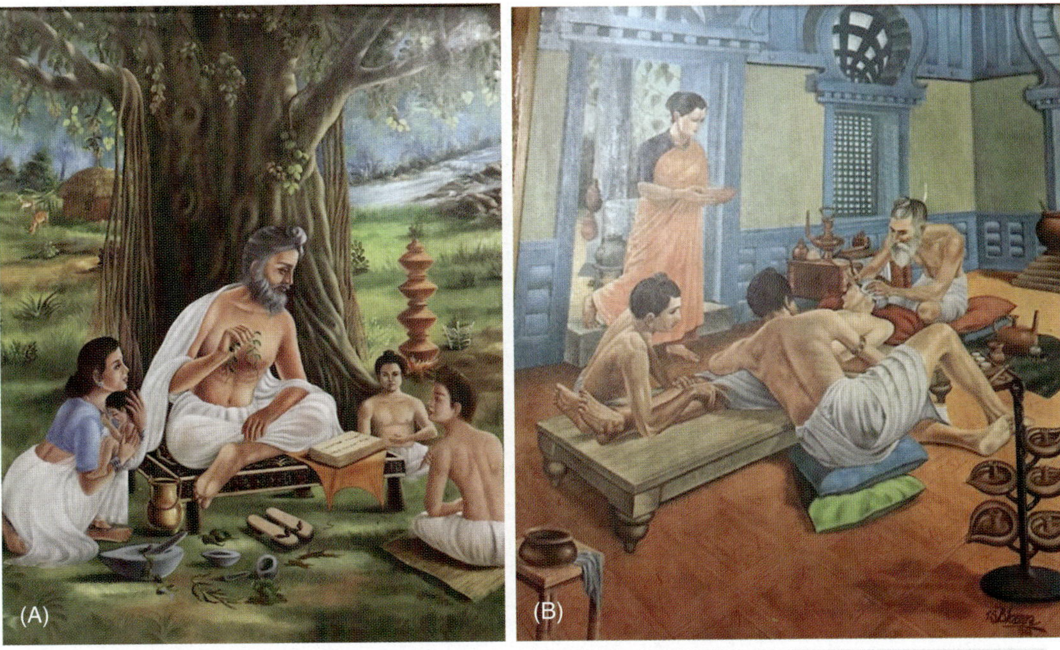

Fig. 3.2 Men as nurses with ancient Indian physician Charka (A) and assisting ancient Indian surgeon Sushruta (B).

is fit to nurse or to attend the bedside of a patient, whom is coolheaded and pleasant in his demeanor, does not speak ill of anybody, is strong and attentive to the requirements of the sick, and strictly and indefatigably follows the instructions of the physician." Fig. 3.2 depicts male nurses assisting ancient Indian physician Charka (Fig. 3.2A) and assisting ancient Indian surgeon Sushruta (Fig. 3.2B).

- Medical education was introduced in ancient universities of "Nalanda" and "Thakshashila" between 600 BCE and CE 600. In 264 BCE, King Ashoka was greatly moved by the human sufferings after the war of Kalinga. He founded a large number of hospitals and monastery universities, which later became famous for their medical schools. The nursing of patients seems to have been devoted primarily to men, a great deal of unrewarded work. The qualities expected of nurses were good behavior, purity, cleverness, kindness, and skill.
- Preaching of *Buddha* in the spirit of compassion to others, the development of scientific medicine grew espousing the benefits to humanity. However, there are distinct texts that refer specifically to nursing practice and care during this time. For example, it was the *Charaka Samhita* and *Sushruta Samhita*, 4th century BCE Indian medical (healer) texts, through which nursing came to be recognized for what it was—an art defined by the "*four feet*" (tetrad desiderata) as possessing skill, knowledge, cleanliness, and affection for the patient.
- "Unani" system of medicine developed during the Arab civilization. It was practiced in Indo-Pakistan subcontinent. The role of nurses in this system is unknown because it was not discussed anywhere.

Nursing in pre-Christian times was mostly driven by the belief that one should render services of love to humanity without any reward. It was equal to one's sincere love to God. Although these ancient 4th century BCE Indian texts provide some early insight and affirmation to the role of the nurse and especially that of the male nurse, it must be remembered that the practice of "medicine," or healing as it should be ideally referred to, and nursing was an integral part of this system of medicine. Thus, prior to the 20th century, Indian nurses were usually young men and older women with women acting only as midwives for assisting with childbirth.

Nursing During British Rule in India

- Portuguese first brought modern medicine including nursing to India but the French and British later established and consolidated modern medical and nursing services in India.
- The first European hospital was built by the Portuguese, in 1510 by Albuquerque in Goa. The East India Company required hospitals to take care of the white settlers working in trade or living in the settlements around trading ports and factories. The company set up hospitals in the three centers in the 17th and the 18th centuries—Bombay, Madras, and Calcutta. Early time image of Government general hospital, Madras has been presented in Fig 3.3.
- The development of nursing in India was curtailed by the low state of women, the caste system, illiteracy, and political unrest.
- As the East India Company set its root in India, a small hospital for soldiers was started in 1664 in a house at Fort St. George, Madras. It was documented that these hospitals were not open to native Indians for a significant period of time.
- Madras General Hospital is the first hospital built by the British for native Indians in 1772. The Presidency General Hospital, Calcutta, was established in 1796 and

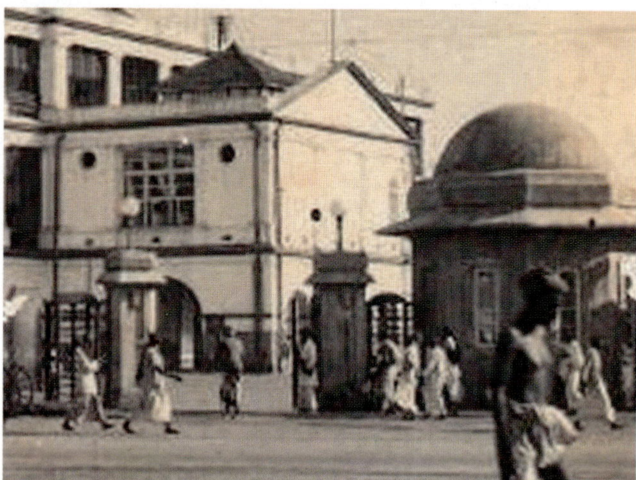

Fig. 3.3 Government General Hospital in 1930s. (Courtesy: TOI)

during 1800–1820 about four hospitals were built in Madras.

- By 1772, the Madras General Hospital was training native Indians along with European and Eurasians in western methods of diagnosis, treatment, and preparation of medicines. These trained persons were posted in various places of the then Madras Presidency to assist the qualified doctors. However, these assistants were not designated as nurses despite of their roles being similar to those of nurses.
- In 1859, scheme for training of nurses was sanctioned by the Government of Bengal and a nursing training center was opened at Calcutta.
- In the succeeding years, nursing schools were established all over the country in collaboration with government and private hospitals.
- In 1843, one of the earliest hospitals in Bombay, the JJ Group of Hospitals was started. Later, this hospital played an important role in the development of nursing in the country.
- The first training school for midwives in Madras was sanctioned in 1854 by the government with the aim of improvising the system of nursing in India; Florence Nightingale made some detailed suggestions and in 1865 sent out graduates from the Nightingale School of Nursing at St. Thomas Hospital, London, to India. As a result, in 1867, the first training school for the Indian girls was established at St. Stephens Hospital in Delhi.
- In 1871, another school of nursing was started in Government General Hospital, Madras, with 6-month diploma midwives program with four students. Four lady superintendents and four trained nurses from England were posted to Government General Hospital, Madras, Madras.
- By this time, the health service was established as a general rule, with the help of nurses from western countries. Government hospital nurses were recruited directly from Britain or religious order of nurses to organize hospitals services. Mission hospital nurses were recruited from Europe and North America.

Contribution of Florence Nightingale in Indian Nursing

In *Notes on Nursing: What It Is and What It Is Not*, Florence Nightingale established the first nursing philosophy based on health maintenance and restoration (Nightingale, 1860). She saw the role of nursing as having "charge of somebody's health" based on the knowledge of "how to put the body in such a state to be free of disease or to recover from disease" (Nightingale, 1860). She developed the first organized training program for nurses in 1860, the Nightingale Training School for Nurses at St. Thomas' Hospital in London. Nightingale volunteered during the Crimean War in 1853 and visited the injured at the battlefield hospitals even at night, carrying her lamp; thus, she was known as "the lady with the lamp." As a result of Nightingale's organization and improvement of the sanitation facilities at the battlefield hospitals, the mortality rate at the Barracks Hospital in Scutari, Turkey, was reduced from 42.7% to 2.2% in 6 months (Donahue, 2011). Perhaps one of Nightingale's greatest contributions was the maintenance of statistics to show the efficacy of her strategies.

Florence Nightingale has a significant influence over nursing in India, and was the first lady to have such an influence on this discipline in the country. She came to India with prioritized interests in welfare of the British army in India. However, later she also contributed in the improvement of sanitation and health care services for the civil population of India by starting formal training in nursing for Indian women. Some of the key historical milestone contributions by Miss Florence Nightingale in India are as follows:

- In 1850s, the high mortality rate of British soldiers from illness in India drew the attention of Miss Florence Nightingale.
- In 1860, Miss Florence Nightingale conducted a survey in India to collect as much information as possible about conditions of the army stations in India. A questionnaire titled "Circular of Enquiry" was send to every military station in India.
- In 1862, she submitted her report titled "Observation." It reported the death rate in the British Army as 69 per 1000. The main cause being poor sanitation, unpotable drinking water, overcrowding, and a hot climate. Surprisingly, living conditions of native soldiers in British army was far worse.
- On December 4, 1863, Sir John Lawrence on request of Lord Stanley spoke to Miss Nightingale about sanitary reforms in India. A week later, she left to visit India for the first time on this request.
- In January 1864, along with Dr Sutherland, Dr Farr, and Sir Robert Rawlinson, she prepared draft of "Sanitary Code of India" for reforms for sanitation in India consisting of details of water supply, drainage, sanitation, hospital, and so on. Subsequently, sanitary reforms took place and hospitals were built for the care of British army people.
- In 1865, she prepared detailed suggestions on the system of nursing for hospitals in India. Under directions of Lady Napier, then Governor of Madras, Miss Nightingale

could gradually bring female nurses into Indian hospitals because no formal training for nurses existed in India at the time.

- In 1867, some of the nursing graduates were moved from Nightingale School of Nurses at St. Thomas Hospital, England, to start a similar school in India at St. Stephen Hospital, Delhi, for Indian women. Later, more nursing training institutes were started in India under the guidance of Miss Florence Nightingale.
- In 1870, she was selected as an honorary member of the Bengal Social Science Association.
- In January 1884, with the cooperation of Lord Roberts, she obtained an official sanction for the employment of Indian female nurses in military hospitals in India, at Ambala and Rawalpindi (which is in Pakistan now).
- In 1891, when she was 71 years old, she fought for better sanitation, water supply, and reduced taxation for Indian people. She succeeded in 1894. This was her final active work in India, but she still continued in an advisory capacity.

Establishment of Military Nursing Services

- The history of Military Nursing Services (MNS) dates back to March 28, 1888, when 10 qualified British nurses arrived to Bombay and set up nursing services in Indian military hospitals.
- The first lady superintendent Miss Locke trained in London was appointed with her second-in-command Miss Foxley at the military hospital. Orderlies however, were appointed to look after the patients.
- In 1893, the training for orderlies who looked after the bedside nursing care, such as bathing the patients, feeding the patients, making the beds of the patients, was started. In the same year, nursing services in the British Army were designated as Indian Army Nursing Services (IANS).
- In 1896, the service was gradually increased and the permanent cadre of British Army Nursing established and thereafter those trained nurses were granted Commission in British Army.
- In 1902, the British Army Nursing Service had been formulated and Queen Alexandra became the first President of the British Army Nursing Services in the United Kingdom and soon it had been redesignated as Queen Alexandra's Military Nursing Services for Indians (QAMNS).
- In 1914, Temporary Indian Nursing Service (TINS) was started for the nursing care of the Indian Soldiers and after a decade permanent nursing service was formed, which was designated as Indian Military Nursing Services (IMNS) in 1927.
- During the World War II, many nurses from permanent nursing services were sent to different places of Middle East, Africa, Europe, and the Far East, where they worked in base and field hospitals, casualty clearing stations, and hospital ships. Their work in these most tiring conditions was universally acclaimed and raised the status and prestige of the service. In recognition of their enormous service, IMNS was made to be a part of the Indian Army and the status of its members was made equivalent to the commissioned officers.
- In 1947, the IMNS was renamed as MNS, which exists till today and Colonel DG Howard was appointed as Chief Principal Matron, which was earlier headed by QAMNS Officer.
- Since then, quite a lot of changes happened in MNS in terms of upgradation of ranks and establishment of nursing colleges in MNS. Presently, the highest rank in the MNS is Major General.
- Presently, there are six colleges functioning under MNS, namely College of Nursing AFMC, Pune; College of Nursing, Command Hospital, Calcutta; College of Nursing, INHS, Asvini; College of Nursing, Army Hospital Research and Referral, New Delhi; School of Nursing, Command Hospital, Lucknow; and School of Nursing, Command Hospital, Air Force, Bangalore, which offers diploma in General Nursing and Midwifery, BSc Nursing, and MSc Nursing degrees.

Significant Milestones of Nursing in Independent India

- After the independence in 1947, the community development program of the government and the expansion of hospital service created a large demand for nurses, auxiliary nurse midwives (ANMs), health visitors, midwives, nursing tutors, and nursing administrators.
- The Indian Nursing Council (INC) was constituted in 1949 under the Indian Nursing Council Act, 1947.
- In 1956, Miss Adrenwala was appointed as the first nursing advisor to the Government of India. The development of nursing in India was greatly influenced by the Christian missionaries and the international agencies such as the World Health Organization (WHO), UNICEF, Red Cross, and UNSAID.
- In 1959, the first master's degree course, a two-year postgraduate program, began at the Rajkumari Amrit Kaur College of Nursing, Delhi.
- Christian Medical College, Vellore, started with College of Nursing in 1909 with 15 Indian women. The graduate course, however, began in 1946. It now has postgraduate and doctoral programs.
- Other significant institutes of nursing training were started. The Christian Medical College, Ludhiana, was established in 1894 by two Scottish sisters, one of them a nurse. She simply started by opening a dispensary in Chaura Bazaar and gave "simple advice" to women in need. The school of nursing was established in 1889 and basics of primary health care were taught to the students. Year 1973 saw the start of the 4-year nursing program and MSc Nursing was started in 1987 with affiliation to Panjab University, Chandigarh.
- In 1963, the School of Nursing in Trivandrum instituted the first 2-year postcertificate bachelor's degree program.
- In 1964, College of Nursing, Post Graduate Institute of Medical Education and Research, Chandigarh, was started with aim of improving nursing education in the region. Initially, they started with three students for post basic BSc Nursing, slowly increased their seats to accommodate more students. In 2003, this institute is upgraded as National Institute of Nursing Education and nowadays running full-fledged state of the art nursing

institute with undergraduate and postgraduate nursing education.

- Efforts were made by the Government of India to make significant development in the field of nursing by framing number of committees from time to time for rendering advice on different health problems. Bhore Committee (1946), Shetty Committee (1954), Mudaliar Committee (1962), Chadha Committee (1963), Mukherjee Committee (1965), Mukherjee Committee (1966), Jungalwalla Committee (1967), Kartar Singh Committee (1974), Shrivastav Committee (1975), Rural Health Scheme (1977), and High Power Committee on Nursing and Nursing Profession (1987–1989) have significantly contributed to the growth and development of nursing in India.
- Nursing is progressively transforming in India through liberal availability of higher education for nurses, opportunities of international migration in developed countries, and improved pay for nurses in government sectors. However, there is a long way to go.
- A significant brain drain has been observed in Indian nurses; it may be because of poor social status of nursing, pathetic working conditions, and very low pay. Nurses trained in India started migrating to western world for their green pasture, especially to the United States, Canada, the United Kingdom, Australia, New Zealand, Ireland, and gulf countries.

Revolutionary Era of Nursing Education in India

- In 1867, first formal nursing training for the Indian women was started at St. Stevens Hospital at Delhi.
- In 1871, the Government General Hospital at Madras started with the first school of nursing for midwives with four students.
- During 18th and 19th centuries, many nursing schools started in different parts of India to train Indian women, predominantly by mission hospitals. However, there was lack of uniform educational standards in these nursing schools.
- Dr BC Roy in 1897 put a tremendous effort to raise the standards of nursing in India for both male and female nurses.
- To formulate nursing training standards and rules, conduct examinations, and give diplomas for the mission hospital, United Board of Examiners was established in North India (in 1907–1970), South India (1913), and Mid India (1926).
- In 1908, the Trained Nurses' Association of India (TNAI) was formed to uphold the dignity and the honor of nursing profession.
- In 1918, first school for health visitors was started at Lady Reading Health School, Delhi. Two English nurses, Miss Griffin and Miss Graham, were appointed to give training to and to supervise the nurses.
- During the 1920s and 1930s, there was a rapid development in medical technology, which caused a shift in the techniques used by the nurses. Technical methods gained more importance.
- In 1926, Madras state formed the first registration council to provide basic standards in nursing education and training. This was the beginning of the practice of licensed nurses in India.
- Seven health centers were set up in the cities of Delhi, Madras, Bangalore, Lucknow, Trivandrum, Pune, and Calcutta from 1931 to 1939, with the help of the Rockefeller Foundation.
- After World War II in 1945, the value of medical care gained more importance as compared with nursing care.
- Because of the advancement of technology in the field of medicine, the role of a nurse has changed from obeying and carrying out doctors' orders to carrying out knowledgeable, prompt observation and taking decisions and helping the patients to become self-sufficient.
- In 1946, the first 4-year basic bachelor's degree program was established at the Rajkumari Amrit Kaur College of Nursing in Delhi and College of Nursing, CMCH, Vellore, Tamil Nadu.
- In 1949, INC was established to maintain a uniform standard of training for nurses, midwives, and health visitors and regulate the standards of nursing in India. INC Act was passed in 1947 that was amended in 1950 and 1957.
- In 1951, a two-year ANM course was established in St. Mary's Hospital at Punjab.
- In 1960, MSc program was established in Rajkumari Amrit Kaur College of Nursing, Delhi.
- In 1964, BSc Nursing (post basic) program in administration and education was started at College of Nursing, PGIMER, Chandigarh, with assistance from WHO under Post Basic Education Project; later on, 4-year basic BSc Nursing course was started. In 1977, MSc Nursing course in medical–surgical nursing was started, and later other specialties were added.
- Nursing education has seen rapid expansion during 1995–2015, where a number of nursing educational institutes expanded in multiple folds to meet the requirement of trained nurses in the country. However, this rapid mushrooming of nursing educational institutes has seen the declining standards of nursing education in the country.
- In 2003, College of Nursing, PGIMER, Chandigarh, and College of Nursing, CMC, Vellore, were designated as WHO collaborating centers for nursing and midwifery.
- In 2006, College of Nursing, AIIMS, New Delhi, has started superspecialization in Master's in Nursing program, and later INC has adapted the same curriculum and also started post basic diploma courses in superspecialty nursing.
- Nursing education is predominately imparted through private institutes; however, recently Government of India has invested significant amount of funds to open nursing schools and colleges in government sector. In addition, central government has also opened nursing colleges in each new AIIMS institute, which will give a significant impetus in providing cost-effective quality nursing education for Indian nurses.
- In 2017, INC also launched Nurse Practitioner in Critical Care (NPCC) nursing program.
- Initially, nurses obtained their doctorates in allied fields such as psychology, education, administration, and sociology. However, recently PhD in nursing is also available in the country through PhD consortium of WHO, INC, and Rajiv Gandhi University of Health Sciences, Bengaluru, and expanding over the time.

- Government of India is also in the process to enact National Nursing and Midwifery Commission (NNMC) Act, 2020, on the lines of National Medical Commission Bill to improve quality of nursing education and practices in the country.

CONCEPT AND DEFINITIONS OF NURSING

The word *nurse* originated from the Latin word "*nurtix*," which means "to nourish." The nurse is defined as a person who nourishes, fosters, protects, and who is prepared to take care of sick, injured, and aged people. With the expanding role and functions of the nurse in society these days, however, any one definition is too limited to define nursing.

Nursing is an art and science. It may be defined as service to the individual which helps him/her to obtain or maintain a healthy state of mind or body and the relief of pain and discomfort.

—Hemmer and Henderson

Nursing is a unique function of the nurse, i.e. to assist the individual, sick or well, in the performance of those activities contributing to health or recovery (or to a peaceful death) that he/she would perform unaided if he/she had the necessary strength, will or knowledge, and to do so in such a way as to help him/her to gain independence as rapidly as possible.

—Virginia Henderson

The **American Nurses Association (ANA)** defines **nursing** as *the protection, promotion, and optimization of health and abilities; prevention of illness and injury; alleviation of suffering through the diagnosis and treatment of human response; and advocacy in the care of individuals, families, communities, and populations* (ANA, 2010b).

The International Council of Nurses (ICN, 2010) has another definition: *Nursing encompasses autonomous and collaborative care of individuals of all ages, families, groups and communities, sick or well and in all settings. Nursing includes the promotion of health; prevention of illness; and the care of ill, disabled, and dying people. Advocacy, promotion of a safe environment, research, participation in shaping health policy and in patient and health systems management, and education are also key nursing roles.*

Both of these definitions support the prominence and importance that nursing holds in providing safe, patient-centered health care to the global community.

When giving care, it is essential to provide a specified service according to standards of practice and to follow a code of ethics. Professional practice includes knowledge from social and behavioral sciences, biological and physiological sciences, and nursing theories. In addition, nursing practice incorporates ethical and social values, professional autonomy, and a sense of commitment and community. Expert clinical nursing practice is a commitment to the application of knowledge, ethics, aesthetics, and clinical experience. Your ability to interpret clinical situations and make complex decisions is the foundation for your nursing care and the basis for the advancement of nursing practice and the development of nursing science. Critical thinking skills are essential to nursing.

The term *nurse* may be elaborated as follows:

N—Noble
U—Understanding
R—Responsible
S—Sincere
E—Empathetic

PHILOSOPHY OF NURSING

Philosophy of nursing states our thoughts on what we believe to be true about the nature of the profession of nursing and provide a basis for nursing activities. It endorses ethical values we hold as basic and bases our beliefs in theory.

ICN states the philosophy of nursing as follows:

- We work as a collaborative team to continuously improve the health and well-being of ourselves and the community.
- We accept and respect our patients' unique view of self and their world.
- We believe in the involvement of the professional nurse in shared governance, and we incorporate research and evidence-based practice in the development of standards of care.
- Nurses are responsible for lifelong learning, accountability for their practice, and participation in interdisciplinary activities.

INC believes in the concept of health as laid down by WHO: "Health is a state of complete physical, mental and social well-being and not merely the absence of disease or infirmity." INC recognized that basic nursing education is a formally recognized program of study providing a broad and sound foundation in the behavioral, life, and nursing sciences for the general practice of nursing, for a leadership role, and for the post basic education in specialties for advanced nursing practice.

- The council believes that this basic course in nursing should prepare nurses for occupying first-level positions in nursing in all kinds of health care settings.
- The council recognizes that nursing is a profession that is influenced by advances in science and technology.
- It believes that skills in all aspects of communication are also essential for learning and for the practice of nursing.
- The council also recognizes that the nature of nursing is such that a substantial portion of learning of the students is acquired in the clinical field(s) of practice.
- It further recognizes the interdependence of nursing and allied professions and occupations in promoting, maintaining, and restoring health and prevention of diseases.
- The council believes that it has a responsibility in helping the students to develop pride in their profession besides keeping them abreast with current knowledge and professional trends for a successful career ahead.

AIMS AND OBJECTIVES OF NURSING

The aim of nursing practice can broadly be described as to promote health, to prevent illness, to restore health, and last but not the least, to facilitate coping with disability or death.

Promoting Health

Health promotion is a framework for nursing activities. Nurse considers patient's self-awareness, health awareness, and use of resources while providing care through knowledge and skill. A nurse performs the following to promote health:

- Facilitating decision about enhancement of quality of life and encouraging acceptance of responsibility for one's own health.
- Increasing health awareness by teaching certain behaviors and factors that can prevent deterioration in health.
- Encouraging health promotion by providing information and referrals.
- Teaching self-care activity to maximize achievement of goal.

Preventing Illness

- Nurse prevents illness primarily by teaching, which include educational programs and community programs for promoting healthy habits, such as smoking-cessation programs, stress-reduction seminars, and physical fitness programs.
- Education through literatures, television, radio, and internet.

Restoring Health

The steps involved in restoring health are as follows:

- Focusing on early detection of disease for rehabilitation and teaching during recovery.
- Promoting diagnostic measurements for early detection of disease, such as promotion of annual health checkups.
- Providing direct care to person who is ill.
- Collaborating with other health care providers.

Facilitating Coping with Disability and Death

Altered function decreases an individual's ability to carry out activities of daily living and the expected role. Nurse can facilitate an optimum level of function by maximizing the patient's strengths and potentials through teaching and referring both the patient and his or her family to community resources during the last phase of life. Nurse prepares the patient's family for death and living as comfortably as possible until death occurs.

Nursing Practice

Nursing is a dynamic and supportive profession guided by its code of ethics and is rooted in caring, a concept evident throughout its four fields of activity: practice, education, administration, and research.

CHARACTERISTICS OF NURSING

The key characteristics of nursing are as follows:

- Nursing is an art and science of caring.
- Nursing involves close personal contact with the recipient of care.
- Nursing is concerned with services that take humans into account as physiological, psychological, and sociological organisms.
- Nursing is committed to promoting the health goals of individuals, families, communities, and nation in its best manner possible.
- Nursing is committed to personalized services for all persons without regard to color, creed, and social or economic status.
- Nursing is committed to involvement in ethical, legal, and political issues in the delivery of health care.

NATURE OF NURSING

- Nursing is caring.
- Nursing is science and art.
- Nursing is holistic.
- Nursing is adaptive.
- Nursing is patient centered.

RECIPIENTS OF NURSING

- *Consumer:* He or she is an individual, a group of people, or a community that uses a service.
- *Patient:* He or she is a person who is waiting for or undergoing medical treatment and care.
- *Client:* He or she is a person who engages the advice or services of another who is qualified to provide this service.

FUNCTIONS OF A NURSE

Following are some essential functions of nursing:

- *Caregiver*: Assists patient physically and psychologically; provides direct care and shows concern for patient welfare and accepts the patient as a person.
- *Counselor:* Helps patient to recognize and cope with stressful psychological or social problems, to develop and improve interpersonal relationships, and to promote personal growth; provides emotional, intellectual, and psychological support.
- *Clinical and ethical decision maker*: As an advocate of the patient and family, makes the clinical and ethical decisions for the ultimate benefit of the patient and the family; in several instances, nurse acts on behalf of the patient and secures patient's health care rights and stands up for them.
- *Protector and clinical advocate:* Protects patient's rights; involves concern for and actions on behalf of the patient to bring about a change.
- *Change agent:* Initiates changes or assists patients to make modifications in themselves or in the system of care.
- *Case manager:* Makes decisions, coordinates activities of others, and allocates resources; plans, gives direction, develops staff, monitors operations, gives the rewards fairly, and represents both staff and administrations as needed.
- *Rehabilitator:* Plays an important role in restoration of health of the patient; the nurse works with patient to regain the health status as close as possible to the premorbidity state.

- *Comforter:* Helps in promoting the comfort of patient and family during the period of care.
- *Communicator:* Supports the patient through health care team and supports people in community.
- *Teacher:* Provides information and helps the patient to learn or acquire new knowledge and technical skills; interprets information to the patient.
- *Leader:* As a leader, coordinates the activities of members of the nursing staff in delivering nursing care, and has personnel, policy, and budgetary responsibilities for a specific nursing unit or agency.
- *Researcher:* Participates in identifying significant researchable problems and scientific investigation.

QUALITIES OF A NURSE

To become a good nurse, a person should be:

- Self-confident
- Humble and honest
- Loyal
- Cooperative
- Good listener
- Keen observer
- Good administrator
- Good supervisor
- Impartial
- Capable
- Good workman
- Responsible
- Accountable
- Competent
- Advocate

CATEGORIES OF NURSING PERSONNEL

Following are the different categories of nursing personnel:

- *Bedside nurse:* A nurse working in an institution with patients to provide direct bedside nursing care.
- *Public health nurse/community health nurse:* Usually deals with families and communities for health promotion, disease prevention, and health restoration activities.
- *Industrial/occupational nurse:* A nurse working in factories, offices, and companies for promotion and restoration of health and prevention of diseases/injuries.
- *Military nurse:* A nurse working in a military base.
- *Private duty nurse:* Privately hired nurse to take care of someone in need.
- *Independent nurse practitioner:* A nurse who has completed an advanced-level specialized nursing program and is certified to practice as independent nurse practitioner.
- *Clinical nurse specialist (CNS):* A nurse who has completed a master's degree in a specialty and has considerable clinical expertise in that specialty. Such a nurse provides expert care to individuals. They may belong to specialties such as psychiatric nurse, pediatric nurse, critical care nurse, cardiothoracic nurse, stoma nurse, and diabetes specialist nurse.
- *Nurse midwife:* A nurse who has completed a program in midwifery, provides prenatal and postnatal care, and delivers babies to women with uncomplicated pregnancies.
- *Nurse anesthetist:* A nurse who has completed the course of study in an anesthesia school and carries out assessment of the preoperative status of patients. They ensure the anesthesia and monitor during surgical procedures.
- *Nurse educator:* A nurse usually with advanced degree, who teaches in clinical or educational settings, teaches theoretical knowledge and clinical skills, and conducts research.
- *Nurse researcher:* A nurse who is involved in planning, conducting, and disseminating the research among nurses to promote the evidence-based nursing practice.
- *Nurse administrator:* A nurse who functions at various levels of management in health care settings and is responsible for the management and administration of resources and personnel involved in giving patient care.
- *Nurse entrepreneur:* A nurse who has an advanced degree and manages health care–related business.

ROLES AND RESPONSIBILITIES OF NURSE

As a nurse you are responsible for obtaining and maintaining specific knowledge and skills for a variety of professional roles and responsibilities. Nurses provide care and comfort to patients in all health care settings. Their concern for meeting patients' needs remains the same whether care focuses on health promotion and illness prevention, disease and symptom management, family support, or end-of-life care.

Caregiver

As **caregiver**, you help patients maintain and regain health, manage disease and symptoms, and attain a maximal level function and independence through the healing process. You provide evidence-based nursing care to promote healing through both physical and interpersonal skills. Healing involves more than achieving improved physical well-being. You need to meet all health care needs of a patient by providing measures that restore the patient's emotional, spiritual, and social well-being. As a caregiver, you help the patient and family set goals and assist them with meeting these goals with minimal financial cost, time, and energy.

Most nurses provide direct patient care in an acute care setting, whereas some pursue a specific area of specialty practice such as pediatrics, critical care, or emergency care. Many specialty care areas require some experience as a medical–surgical nurse and certification in advanced cardiac life support and critical care, emergency nursing, or trauma nursing.

As health care returns to the home care setting, there are increased opportunities for you to provide direct care in a patient's home or community. Use the nursing process and critical thinking skills to provide care that is restorative, curative, and evidence-based. Educate your patients and their families to promote health maintenance and self-care.

In collaboration with other health care team members, focus your care on returning patients to their home at an optimal functional status.

Advocate

As a **patient advocate**, you protect your patient's human and legal rights and provide assistance in asserting these rights if the need arises. As an advocate, you act on behalf of your patient, securing and standing up for your patient's health care rights. For example, you provide information to help a patient decide whether or not to accept a treatment, or you find an interpreter to help family caregivers communicate their concerns. You sometimes need to defend patients' rights in a general way by speaking out against policies or actions that put patients in danger or conflict with their rights.

Educator

As an **educator**, you explain concepts and facts about health, describe the reason for routine care activities, demonstrate procedures such as self-care activities, reinforce learning or patient behavior, and evaluate patients' progress in learning. Sometimes, patient teaching is unplanned and informal. For example, during a casual conversation, you respond to questions about the reason for an intravenous infusion, a health issue such as smoking cessation, or necessary lifestyle changes. Other teaching activities are planned and more formal such as when you teach your patient to self-administer insulin injections. Always use teaching methods that match your patient's capabilities and needs, and incorporate other resources such as family members or caregivers in teaching plans.

Communicator

Your effectiveness as a **communicator** is central to the nurse—patient relationship. It allows you to know your patients, including their strengths and weaknesses and their needs, and when possible, to know the family's concerns and needs. Communication is essential for all nursing roles and activities. You routinely communicate with patients and families, other nurses and health care professionals, resource persons, and the community. Without clear communication, it is impossible to give comfort and emotional support, give care effectively, make decisions with patients and families, protect patients from threats to well-being, coordinate and manage patient care, assist patients in rehabilitation, or provide patient education. The quality of communication is a critical factor in meeting the needs of individuals, families, and communities (see Chapter 4).

Leader

Leaders are found in all areas of nursing and at all levels, functioning in both formal and informal settings. As a leader, you will work with others to create a vision and then make decisions and take action to achieve this vision. You will assess the situation, identify strategies using the best evidence, and guide others toward the vision. Your behaviors and attitudes will impact those that you lead. As a leader, you must inspire others. A good leader should have the skills of self-awareness, self-management, social awareness, and relationship management. Effective leadership requires you to grow through ongoing personal development and good communication skills. One strategy to develop your leadership skills is to select a mentor who models effective leadership. Your mentor can be your role model, coach, and teacher.

Manager

Health care environment these days is fast paced and complex. Nurse managers need to establish an environment for collaborative patient-centered care to provide safe, quality care with positive patient outcomes. A manager coordinates the activities of members of the nursing staff in delivering nursing care and has personnel, policy, and budgetary responsibilities for a specific nursing unit or agency. The manager uses appropriate leadership styles to create a nursing environment for the patients and staff, which reflects the mission and values of the health care organization. Ensuring adequate nurse staffing, which is essential for the good patient outcome (Box 3.1).

BOX 3.1 Evidence-Based Practice

PICO Question: Are patient outcomes improved in hospitals with adequate nursing staffing versus hospitals with lower nursing staffing?

Summary of Evidence

There is a growing body of research that shows that nurse staffing does impact patient outcomes, patient survival, and the occurrence of adverse events. A secondary data analysis from 661 hospitals showed that there was a significantly lower 30-day readmission rate for patients with heart failure in hospitals that had high nurse staffing, thus reducing health care costs (Giuliano et al., 2016). Higher nurse staffing was also found to significantly increase the survival of patients in an intensive care unit (West et al., 2014). Patients experiencing an in-hospital cardiac arrest were more likely to survive when there was a decreased patient to nurse ratio (McHugh et al., 2016). Cho et al. (2016) found that larger numbers of patients assigned to a nurse increased the occurrence of medication errors, pressure injury formation, and falls with injuries. Studies demonstrating the positive impact that nurse to patient ratios have on outcomes provide nursing administrators with evidence to support hiring of qualified professional nurses.

Application to Nursing Practice

- Consider the nurse to patient ratio when looking at a hospital or unit for employment.
- Adequate nursing levels help to improve the nursing work environment (Cho et al., 2016).
- Improved working conditions increase the likelihood of patient survival in emergency events (McHugh et al., 2016).
- Continuing research needs to be conducted to study the economic impact of nurse staffing and improved patient outcomes (Giuliano et al., 2016).

SCOPE OF NURSING PRACTICES

Innovations in health care, expanding health care systems and practice settings, and the increasing needs of patients have created new nursing roles. Nowadays, most nurses practice in hospital settings, community-based care, ambulatory care, and nursing homes or extended care settings.

Nursing allows you to commit to lifelong learning and career development to provide patients the state-of-the-art care they need. Career roles are specific employment positions or paths. Because of increasing educational opportunities for nurses, the growth of nursing as a profession, and a greater concern for job enrichment, the nursing profession offers expanded roles and different kinds of career opportunities. You will probably switch career roles more than once. Take advantage of the different clinical practice and professional opportunities. These career opportunities include auxiliary nurse midwives, registered nurse and midwives, nurse educators, nurse administrators, and nurse researchers.

Auxiliary Nurse Midwives

An ANM is trained for a period of 1.5 years at a recognized nursing school or training center. Traditionally, ANMs were trained in the nursing school run by the government. However, recently in last few years, more and more ANM training schools opened in the private sector. ANMs are mainly deployed in the primary health centers or community health centers for the community health nursing services.

Registered Nurses and Registered Midwives

As a profession, nursing requires that its members possess a significant amount of education. A 3-year diploma in General Nursing and Midwifery (GNM) or 4-year degree in nursing, that is, BSc Nursing/BSc (Hons) Nursing leads a nurse to become registered nurse (RN) and registered midwife (RM) in India. They are ideally employed in secondary and tertiary care hospitals. However, RN and RM are also employed in PHCs and CHCs in some of the states based on the requirement of the particular state.

Nurse Practitioner

The role of nurse practitioners (NPs) is recently developed in India and first batch of NPs in critical care is passed in year 2019. Unfortunately, there is no Nursing Practice Act in country to define scope of practices for the NPs in India and neither any of the state nursing council has any provision of registration title for the NPs. However, nurses are hopeful that Nursing Practice Act and defined scope of practice and separate registration title for the NPs in India will be established in near future. The Ministry of Health and Family Welfare, Government of India, is planning to enact NNMC Act, 2020, to sort out these issues and regulate nursing practices in the country.

In developed world, the **NP** is an advanced practice registered nurse (APRN) who provides health care to a group of patients, usually in an outpatient, ambulatory care, or community-based setting. The major NP categories are acute care, adult, family, pediatric, women's, psychiatric mental health, and geriatric. The NP provides comprehensive care, directly managing the medical care of patients who are healthy or have chronic conditions, and establishes a collaborative provider–patient relationship, working with a specific group of patients or with patients of all ages and health care needs.

Nurse Educator

A **nurse educator** works primarily in nursing institute or in the staff development department to teach working nurses. A faculty member in a school of nursing or college of nursing is responsible for teaching current nursing practice, trends, theory, and necessary skills in laboratories and clinical settings to educate students to become professional nurses. Nurse educators in educational programs of nursing usually have postgraduate degrees in nursing and additional education such as a doctorate or an advanced degree in nursing, education, or administration.

Nurse educators in staff development departments of health care institutions provide educational programs for nurses within their institutions. These programs include orientation of new personnel, critical care nursing courses, assisting with clinical skill competency, safety training, instruction about new equipment or procedures, and participation in developing nursing policies and procedures.

The primary focus of the nurse educator in a patient education department of an agency is to teach patients and their families how to self-manage their illness or disability. These nurse educators are usually specialized and certified, such as a certified diabetes educator (CDE) or an ostomy care nurse and see only a specific population of patients. However, the roles of nurse educator in staff development departments and patient nurse educators are limited to only few corporate hospitals in India.

Nurse Administrator

A **nurse administrator** manages patient care and the delivery of specific nursing services within a health care facility. Nursing administration often begins with positions such as the senior nursing officer, nursing supervisor, or assistant nursing superintendent. Experience and additional education lead to a higher management position such as deputy nursing superintendent of a specific unit or area or an upper management position such as nursing superintendent, chief nursing officer (CNO), or director of nursing services.

Now initial nursing administration positions usually require at least a baccalaureate degree in nursing, and CNO or director of nursing positions generally require a master's degree. However, in government hospitals, nurses through promotional avenues may be promoted to these higher positions without master's degree in nursing. In western world, nurse administrators compulsorily need master's nursing degree for these higher nursing administrative positions and they frequently too have advanced degrees such as Master of Nursing Administration, MBA, Master of Hospital Administration (MHA),

Master of Public Health (MPH), or Master of Health Service Administration.

In health care organizations these days, CNO and director of nursing often have responsibilities for all clinical functions within a hospital. This may include all ancillary personnel who provide and support patient care services. The nurse administrator needs to be skilled in business and management and understand all aspects of nursing and patient care. Functions of administrators include budgeting, staffing, strategic planning of programs and services, employee evaluation, and employee development.

Nurse Researcher

The **nurse researcher** investigates problems to improve nursing care and further define and expand the scope of nursing practice. The nurse researcher in western countries often works in an academic setting, hospital, or independent professional or community service agency. The preferred educational requirement is a doctoral degree, with at least a master's degree in nursing. However, in India, the position of nurse researchers has not yet well established, except if isolated position in some of educational institutes and in the universities.

The scope discussed in the subsequent section does not exist in India; however, it is given for the purpose that nursing students' could understand that the following scope of nursing exists in the western world and it may be implemented in India on the basis of needs and feasibility in the country.

Advanced Practice Registered Nurse

APRN is the most independently functioning nurse. An APRN has a master's degree or Doctor of Nursing Practice (DNP) degree in nursing; advanced education in pathophysiology, pharmacology, and physical assessment; and certification and expertise in a specialized area of practice. In 2008, the APRN Consensus Work Group and the National Council of State Boards of Nursing APRN Advisory Committee developed the Consensus Model for APRN Regulation: Licensure, Accreditation, Certification, and Education. The Consensus Model identified that the title of APRN is for nurses with advanced graduate–level knowledge prepared in one of four roles: CNS, NP, certified nurse-midwife (CNM), and certified registered nurse anesthetist (CRNA). The educational preparation for the four roles is in at least one of the following six populations: adult-gerontology, pediatrics, neonatology, women's health/gender related, family/individual across life span, and psychiatric mental health. APRNs function within their area of practice to plan or improve the quality of nursing care for patients and their families.

Clinical Nurse Specialist

A **CNS** is an APRN who is an expert clinician in a specialized area of practice. The specialty may be identified by a population (e.g., geriatrics), setting (e.g., critical care), disease specialty (e.g., diabetes), type of care (e.g., rehabilitation), or type of problem (e.g., pain). A CNS practices in all health care settings.

Certified Nurse-Midwife

A **CNM** is an APRN who is educated in midwifery and is certified by the American College of Nurse-Midwives. The practice of nurse-midwifery involves providing independent care for women during normal pregnancy, labor, and delivery and care for the newborn. It includes providing some gynecological services such as routine Papanicolaou (Pap) tests, family planning, and treatment for minor vaginal infections.

Certified Registered Nurse Anesthetist

A **CRNA** is an APRN with advanced education earned in a nurse anesthesia accredited program. Nurse anesthetists provide surgical anesthesia under the guidance and supervision of an anesthesiologist, who is a physician with advanced knowledge of surgical anesthesia.

NURSING AS A PROFESSION

Nursing is not simply a collection of specific skills, and you are not simply a person trained to perform specific nursing tasks. Nursing is a profession. No one factor absolutely differentiates a job from a profession, but the difference is important in terms of how you practice. To act professionally, you administer quality patient-centered care in a safe, conscientious, and knowledgeable manner. You are responsible and accountable to yourself and your patients and peers. A profession has the following primary characteristics:

- It requires a basic liberal foundation and an extended education of its members.
- It has a theoretical body of knowledge leading to defined skills, abilities, and norms.
- It provides a specific service.
- Members of a profession have autonomy in decision-making and practice.
- The profession as a whole has a code of ethics for practice. A profession is an occupation that requires extensive education, special knowledge, skill, and preparation.

Characteristics and Criteria of a Profession

Specialized education. Specialized education is an important aspect of professional status. There are four means of entry into registered nursing: general nursing and midwifery diploma, baccalaureate degree, master's degree, and doctoral degree in nursing.

Body of knowledge. As a profession, the nursing is establishing a well-defined body of knowledge and expertise. A number of nursing conceptual frameworks contribute to the knowledge base of nursing and give direction to the nursing practice, education, and ongoing research.

Service orientation. A service orientation differentiates nursing from an occupation pursued primarily for profit. Nursing has a tradition of service to others. This service, however, must be guided by certain rules, policies, or codes of ethics.

Ongoing research. Increasing research in nursing is contributing to nursing practice. Most early research was directed to the study of nursing education. In 1960s, studies were often related to the nature of knowledge base underlying nursing practice. Since 1970s, nursing research has focused on practice-related issues.

Code of ethics. The nursing profession requires integrity of its members, that is, a member is expected to do what is right regardless of the personal cost. Ethical codes change as the needs and values of the society change. Nursing has developed its own codes of ethics and in most instances has set up means to monitor the professional behavior of its members. Code of ethics for nurses in India is developed by INC and is published in 2006 as a document titled "The Code of Ethics for Nurses in India."

Autonomy. A profession is autonomous if it regulates itself and sets standards for its members. To practitioners of nursing, autonomy means independence at work, responsibility, and accountability for one's actions. Nursing is significantly autonomous in western world; however, in India, it is still struggling to be autonomous in real sense. However, proposed enactment of National Nursing and Midwifery Commission Bill, 2020, by Indian Government has significant hope to provide good level of autonomy to the nursing discipline in the country.

Professional organization. Operation under the umbrella of a professional organization differentiates a profession from an occupation. The national professional organizations in nursing are TNAI, Indian Society of Psychiatric Nursing (ISPN), and Society for Critical Care Nursing (SCCN), India, Society of Perioperative Nursing (SPN), India; some of the prominent international professional organizations in nursing are ICN, ANA, Canadian Nurses Association (CAN), National League for Nursing (NLN), and so on.

PROFESSIONAL NURSING CODE OF ETHICS

A **code of ethics** is a set of guiding principles that all members of a profession accept. It is a collective statement about the group's expectations and standards of behavior. ANA established the first code of nursing ethics decades ago. ANA reviews and revises the code periodically, but principles of responsibility, accountability, advocacy, and confidentiality remain constant (ANA, 2015b).

Advocacy

Advocacy refers to the support of a particular cause. As a nurse you advocate for the health, safety, and rights of patients, including their right to privacy and their right to refuse treatment. Your special relationship with patients provides you with knowledge that is specific to your role as a registered nurse and as such with the opportunity to make a unique contribution to understanding a patient's point of view.

Responsibility

The word **responsibility** refers to a willingness to respect one's professional obligations and to follow through. An example is following an agency's policies and procedures. As a nurse, you are responsible for your actions and the actions of those to whom you delegate tasks. You agree to take responsibility to remain competent to practice so you can follow through on your responsibilities reliably.

Accountability

Accountability refers to the ability to answer for one's actions. You ensure that your professional actions are explainable to your patients and your employer. Health care institutions also exercise accountability by monitoring individual and institutional compliance with national standards established by agencies such as National Accreditation Board for Hospitals & Healthcare (NABH) in India and The Joint Commission (TJC) in the United States. TJC establishes national patient safety guidelines to ensure patient and workplace safety through consistent, effective nursing practices.

Confidentiality

In practice, you cannot share information about a patient's medical condition or personal information to anyone not involved in the care of the patient. There are legislations that define the rights and privileges of patients for protection of privacy. The Medical Council of India's Code of Ethics Regulations protects patient confidentiality by stating that the physicians "shall not disclose the secrets of a patient that have been learnt in the exercise of his/her profession except in a court of law under orders of the Presiding Judge; in circumstances where there is a serious and identified risk to a specific person and/or community; [or in case of] notifiable diseases." The INC's Code of Ethics protects patient confidentiality by stating that the nurse respects individual's right to privacy, maintains confidentiality, and shares information judiciously.

a) Respects the individuals' rights to privacy of their personal information.
b) Maintains confidentiality of privileged information, except in life-threatening situations and uses discretion in sharing information.
c) Takes informed consent and maintains anonymity when information is required for quality assurance/academic/legal reasons.
d) Limits the access to all personal records written and computerized to authorized persons only.

Code of Ethics for Nurses in India

INC has published the Code of Ethics for Nurses in India in 2006 (Box 3.2). The code of ethics for nurses is critical for building professionalism and accountability. Ethical considerations are vital in any area dealing with human beings including nursing research because they represent values, rights, and relationships. Therefore, same code of ethics may imply for a nurse dealing with human subject during a research study.

BOX 3.2 Code of Ethics for Nurses in India (2006)

1. The nurse respects the uniqueness of an individual in provision of care
   Nurse
   1.1. Provides care for individuals without consideration of cast, creed, religion, culture, ethnicity, gender, socioeconomic and political status, personal attributes, or any other grounds
   1.2. Individualizes the care considering the beliefs, values, and cultural sensitivities
   1.3. Appreciates the place of individual in the family and community and facilitates participation of significant others in the care
   1.4. Develops and promotes trustful relationship with individual(s)
   1.5. Recognizes uniqueness of response of individuals to interventions and adapts accordingly
2. The nurse respects the rights of individuals as partners in care and help in making informed choices
   Nurse
   2.1. Respects individuals' rights to make decisions about their care and therefore gives adequate and accurate information for enabling them to make informed choices
   2.2. Respects the decisions made by individual(s) regarding their care
   2.3. Protects public from misinformation and misinterpretations
   2.4. Advocates special provisions to protect vulnerable individuals/groups
3. The nurse respects individual's right to privacy, maintains confidentiality, and shares information judiciously
   Nurse
   3.1. Respects the individuals' rights to privacy of their personal information
   3.2. Maintains confidentiality of privileged information, except in life-threatening situations and uses discretion in sharing information
   3.3. Takes informed consent and maintains anonymity when information is required for quality assurance/academic/legal reasons
   3.4. Limits the access to all personal records written and computerized to authorized persons only
4. The nurse maintains competence to render quality nursing care
   4.1. Nursing care must be provided only by registered nurse
   4.2. Nurse strives to maintain quality nursing care and upholds the standards of care
   4.3. Nurse values continuing education, and initiates and utilizes all opportunities for self-development
   4.4. Nurse values research as a means of development of nursing profession and participates in nursing research adhering to ethical principles
5. The nurse is obliged to practice within the framework of ethical, professional, and legal boundaries
   Nurse
   5.1. Adheres to code of ethics and code of professional conduct for nurses in India developed by Indian Nursing Council
   5.2. Familiarizes with relevant laws and practices in accordance with the law of the state
6. Nurse is obliged to work harmoniously with members of the health care team
   Nurse
   6.1. Appreciates the team efforts in rendering care
   6.2. Cooperates, coordinates, and collaborates with members of the health care team to meet the needs of people
7. Nurse commits to reciprocate the trust invested in nursing profession by society
   Nurse
   7.1. Demonstrates personal etiquettes in all dealings
   7.2. Demonstrates professional attributes in all dealings

VALUES

Values are the social standards, principles, or ideals held by an individual, class, or group that give meaning and direction to life. A value is an abstract representation of what is right, worthwhile, or desirable. Values reflect what people consider desirable and consist of the subjective assignment of worth to behavior.

Nursing is a work of intimacy. Nursing practice requires you to be in contact with patients physically, emotionally, psychologically, and spiritually. In most other intimate relationships, you choose to enter the relationship precisely because you anticipate that your values will be shared with the other person. But as a nurse, you agree to provide care to your patients solely on the basis of their need for your services. The ethical principles of beneficence and fidelity shape the practice of health care and distinguish it from other common human relationships such as friendship, marriage, and employer—employee. But by its very nature, relationships in health care sometimes can occur in the presence of conflicting values.

A **value** is a personal belief about the worth of a given idea, attitude, custom, or object that sets standards that influence behavior. Inevitably you will work with patients and colleagues whose values differ from yours. To negotiate differences of value, it is important to be clear about your own values: what you value, why, and how you respect your own values even as you try to respect those of others whose values differ from yours. The values that an individual holds reflect cultural and social influences, and these values vary among people and develop over time. For example, in some cultures, decisions about health care flow from group or family-based discussion rather than independent decisions by one person. Such a practice may challenge your commitment to respect patient autonomy. Your effort to resolve differing opinions and maintain your cultural competence becomes the hallmark of your commitment to ethical practice.

Values could be classified as (i) personal values and (ii) professional values. Personal values are driven from their society. Examples of personal values are honesty, fairness, sense of humor, self-worth, and love. Although professional values are also the refection of personal values, these are acquired during socialization in the nursing. Some of the key values of nursing discipline are autonomy, dignity and worth of each individual, commitment to service, and education.

Values Clarification

Ethical dilemmas almost always occur in the presence of conflicting values. To resolve ethical dilemmas, one needs to distinguish among value, fact, and opinion. Sometimes, people have such strong values that they consider them to be facts, not just opinions. Sometimes, people are so passionate about their values that they become judgmental in a way that intensifies conflict. Clarifying values—your own, your patients', your coworkers'—is an important and effective part of ethical discourse. In the process of values clarification, you learn to tolerate differences in a way that often (although not always) becomes the key to the resolution of ethical dilemmas.

For some people, it is important to remain silent and stoic in the presence of great pain, and for others it is important to talk about it to understand and control it. Identifying values as something separate from facts can help you find tolerance for others, even when differences among you seem worlds apart.

QUALITY AND SAFETY EDUCATION FOR NURSES

The Robert Wood Johnson Foundation sponsored the **Quality and Safety Education for Nurses (QSEN)** initiative to respond to reports about safety and quality patient care by the Institute of Medicine (IOM). QSEN addresses the challenge to prepare nurses with the competencies needed to continuously improve the quality of care in their work environments (Table 3.1). The QSEN initiative encompasses the competencies of patient-centered care, teamwork and collaboration, evidence-based practice, quality improvement, safety, and informatics. For each competency, there are targeted knowledge, skills, and attitudes (KSAs). Different KSAs apply for nursing students in prelicensure as well as graduate nursing programs.

As you gain experience in clinical practice, you encounter situations in which your education helps you to make a difference in improving patient care. Whether that difference in care is to provide evidence for implementing care at the bedside, identify a safety issue, or study patient data to identify trends in outcomes, each of these situations requires competence in patient-centered care, safety, or informatics.

KEY POINTS

- A profession possesses the characteristics of extended education, theory, service, autonomy, and a code of ethics.
- The essential components of professional nursing are care, cure, and coordination.
- During your education, begin to develop professionalism through an ongoing understanding of what denotes appropriate appearance and behaviors, ethical practices (including those associated with social media), and standards of practice.
- Nursing standards of care offer evidence-based guidelines for nurses to provide and evaluate care.
- State nursing councils regulate the registration of nurses and protect the public health, safety, and welfare with their established State Nursing Council Acts, which primarily regulate education and registration of nurses in the particular state but not the scope of their practice and in absence of Nurse Practice Act in the states and country.
- Nursing responds to the health care needs of society, which are influenced by economic, social, and cultural variables of a specific era.
- Changes in society such as increased technology, new demographic patterns, consumerism, health promotion, and the women's and human rights movements lead to changes in nursing.
- Nursing definitions reflect the practice of nursing by identifying the domain of nursing practice and guiding research, practice, and education.

Table 3.1 Quality and Safety Education for Nurses

Competency	Definition with Examples
Patient-centered care	Recognize the patient or designee as the source of control and full partner in providing compassionate and coordinated care based on respect for patient's preferences, values, and needs. *Examples: Involve family and friends in care. Elicit patient's values and preferences. Provide care with respect for diversity of the human experience.*
Teamwork and collaboration	Function effectively within nursing and interprofessional teams, fostering open communication, mutual respect, and shared decision-making to achieve quality patient care. *Examples: Recognize the contributions of other health team members and patient's family members. Discuss effective strategies for communicating and resolving conflict. Participate in designing methods to support effective teamwork.*
Evidence-based practice	Integrate best current evidence with clinical expertise and patient and/or family preferences and values for delivery of optimal health care. *Examples: Demonstrate knowledge of basic scientific methods. Appreciate strengths and weaknesses of scientific bases for practice. Appreciate the importance of regularly reading relevant journals.*
Quality improvement	Use data to monitor the outcomes of care processes, and use improvement methods to design and test changes to continuously improve the quality and safety of health care systems. *Examples: Use tools such as flowcharts and diagrams to make process of care explicit. Appreciate how unwanted variation in outcomes affects care. Identify gaps between local and best practices.*
Safety	Minimize risk of harm to patients and providers through both system effectiveness and individual performance. *Examples: Examine human factors, basic safety design principles, and commonly used unsafe practices. Value own role in preventing errors.*
Informatics	Use information and technology to communicate, manage knowledge, mitigate error, and support decision-making. *Examples: Navigate an electronic health record. Protect confidentiality of protected health information in electronic health records.*

Adapted from Cronenwett, L., Sherwood, G., Barnsteiner J., Disch, J., Johnson, J., Mitchell, P., Sullivan, D., Warren, J. (2007). Quality and safety education for nurses. *Nursing Outlook*, 55(3)122–131.

REFERENCES

American Nurses Association. (2010b). Nursing's social policy statement: The essence of the profession. ANA Publishing: Silver Spring, MD.

American Nurses Association (ANA). Code of ethics for nurses with interpretive statements. Silver Spring, MD: The Association; 2015b.

Cho E, Chin DL, Kim S, Hong O. The relationships of nurse staffing level and work environment with patient adverse events. J Nurs Scholarsh 2016;48(1):74.

Donahue MP. Nursing: the finest art—an illustrated history. 3rd ed. St. Louis: Mosby; 2011.

Giuliano KK, Danesh V, Funk M. The relationship between nurse staffing and 30-day readmission for adults with heart failure. J Nurs Adm 2016;46(1):25.

International Council of Nursing (ICN). Nursing definitions (2010). Available at: https://www.icn.ch/nursing-policy/nursing-definitions.

McHugh MD, Rochman MF, Sloane DM, Berg RA, Mancini ME, Nadkarni VM, et al. Better nurse staffing and nurse work environments associated with increased survival of in-hospital cardiac arrest patients. Med Care 2016;54(1):74.

Nightingale F. Notes on nursing: what it is and what it is not. London: Harrison & Sons; 1860.

West E, Barron DN, Harrison D, Rafferty AM, Rowan K, Sanderson C. Nurse staffing, medical staffing and mortality in intensive care: an observational study. Int J Nurs Stud 2014;51:781.

4 Communication and Nurse–Patient Relationship

OBJECTIVES

After reading this chapter, the student should be able to:

- Define the concept of communication and understand the meaning of communication.
- Identify the levels, elements, types, methods, and process of communication and its applications.
- Appreciate factors influencing communication.
- Use the methods of effective communication and techniques of therapeutic communication with patients and family.
- Discuss the features of helping relationship when interacting with patients and family.
- Describe phases involved in building and enhancing the nurse–patient helping relationship.
- Explain barriers of effective communication.
- Describe the methods and techniques of effective communication with patient, family, and health care team members.
- Demonstrate effective human relations and communication with vulnerable groups in health care settings.

KEY TERMS

active listening, p. 43
assertiveness, p. 47
autonomy, p. 47
channels, p. 39
circular transactional communication process, p. 38
circular transactional model, p. 38
communication, p. 37
electronic communication, p. 38
empathy, p. 43
environment, p. 39
feedback, p. 39
interpersonal communication, p. 38
interpersonal variables, p. 39
intrapersonal communication, p. 38
message, p. 39
nonverbal communication, p. 40
public communication, p. 38
receiver, p. 39
referent, p. 39
sender, p. 39
small-group communication, p. 38
symmetrical, p. 39
therapeutic communication, p. 43
verbal communication, p. 40

INTRODUCTION

Communication is essential to achieve positive patient outcomes and is a deliberate nursing intervention for engaging patients and families in their own nursing care. Therapeutic communication conveys caring and facilitates positive change through the nursing process. Effective communication with all members of the health care team supports quality and safety initiatives and enhances patient satisfaction. Effective communication among the health care team strengthens nurses' engagement within their work units and organizations and improves nurse retention.

CONCEPT AND DEFINITION OF COMMUNICATION

The term *communication* is derived from the Latin word *communis*, meaning common. In general, communication refers to the reciprocal exchange of information, ideas, facts, opinions, beliefs, feelings, and attitudes through verbal or nonverbal means between two people or within a group of people. It can be defined as a two-way process of exchanging or sharing ideas, feelings, and information.

Communication is a process by which information is exchanged between individuals through a common system of symbols, signs, or behavior.

—**Webster's Dictionary**

Communication is interchange of thoughts, opinions, or information by speech, writing, or signs.

—**Robert Anderson**

Communication is the transmission and interchange of facts, ideas, feelings, or course of action.

—**Leland Brown**

LEVELS OF COMMUNICATION

As a nurse, you communicate at different levels. You communicate with yourself, other individuals, and groups. Each level of communication is important and affects your nursing practice. Even though you have been communicating all your life, effective nursing communication is a complex skill that improves with practice and feedback through reflection and the responses of others.

Intrapersonal communication, also called *self-talk*, is a powerful form of communication that occurs within an individual. Both you and your patients engage in self-talk by forming thoughts internally. These thoughts strongly influence perceptions, feelings, behavior, self-concept, and performance. Self-talk is a mental rehearsal for difficult tasks or situations so that individuals deal with them more effectively. An example is reflection, which you can use to think back on previous patient care situations so that you consider effective and ineffective approaches that you used previously (see Chapter 18). Be aware of the nature and content of your own thinking, and seek to replace negative, self-defeating thoughts with realistic and positive ones. Your intrapersonal "self-talk" affects the way others perceive you in your professional role. Use positive self-talk to boost your confidence as a nurse.

Interpersonal communication is interaction that occurs between two people or within a small group. It refers to nonverbal and verbal behavior within a social context and includes the use of symbols and cues to give and receive meaning. Because the message received is sometimes different from the intended message, validate or mutually negotiate the meaning for all involved. Effective interpersonal communication includes idea and information sharing, problem-solving, expressing feelings, making decisions, accomplishing goals, team building, and personal growth.

Small-group communication is the interaction that occurs when a small number of people meet. This type of communication is usually goal directed and requires an understanding of group dynamics. When nurses work on committees with nurses or other disciplines and participate in patient care conferences, they use a small-group communication process. Communication in these situations should be organized, concise, and complete. All participating disciplines are encouraged to contribute and provide feedback. Good communication skills help each participant better meet a patient's needs and promote a safer care environment.

Public communication is the interaction of one individual with large groups of people. As a nurse, you may have opportunities to speak with groups of patients or consumers about health-related topics. You make special adaptations in eye contact, posture, gestures, voice inflection, and use of media materials to communicate messages effectively.

Electronic communication is the use of technology to create ongoing relationships with patients and their health care team. Secure messaging provides an opportunity for frequent and timely communication with a patient's physician or nurse via a patient portal. An electronic portal enables patients to stay engaged and informed and build a therapeutic relationship with the health care team.

ELEMENTS OF THE COMMUNICATION PROCESS

Communication is an ongoing and continuously changing process. You are changing, the people with whom you are communicating are changing, and your environment is also continually changing. Fig. 4.1 shows an example of a **circular transactional communication process** model. The model shows the situational contextual inputs, channels of communication, interpersonal contextual concepts, and factors affecting the sender and receiver. Nursing situations have many unique aspects that influence the nature of communication and interpersonal relationships. As a professional, you will use critical thinking to focus on each aspect of communication, so that your interactions are purposeful and effective.

Circular Transactional Model

The **circular transactional model** includes several elements: the referent, sender and receiver, message, channels, context or environment in which the communication process occurs, feedback, and interpersonal variables (see Fig. 4.1). In this model, each person in the communication interaction is both a speaker and a listener and can be

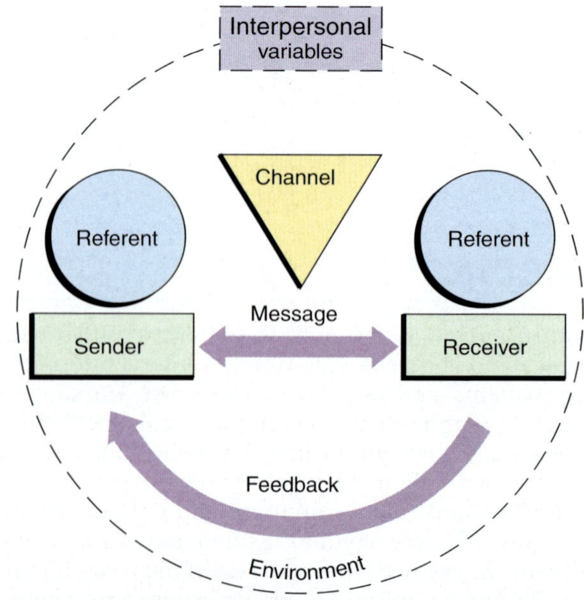

Fig. 4.1 Circular transactional model of communication.

simultaneously sending and receiving messages. Both parties view the perceptions, attitudes, and potential reactions to a sent message. Communication becomes a continuous and interactive activity. Feedback from the receiver or environment enables the communicators to correct or validate the communication. This model also describes the role relationship of the communicators as **complementary** and **symmetrical**. Complementary role relationships function with one person holding an elevated position over the other person. Symmetrical relationships are more equal. For example, a nurse provides education to a patient about a new medication. This would be a complementary role. A group of patients discussing their plans after discharge would be a symmetrical role relationship.

Referent

The **referent** motivates one person to communicate with another. In a health care setting, sights, sounds, sensations, perceptions, and ideas are examples of cues that initiate the communication process. Knowing a stimulus or referent that initiates communication allows you to develop and organize messages more efficiently. For example, a patient request for help prompted by his or her difficulty in breathing causes a different response than a patient request resulting from hunger.

Sender and Receiver

The **sender** is the person who encodes and delivers a message, and the **receiver** is the person who receives and decodes the message. The sender puts the message into verbal and nonverbal symbols that the receiver can understand. The sender's message acts as a referent for the receiver. Transactional communication involves the role of sender and receiver switching back and forth between nurse and patient. A decoding process includes the receiver interpreting the meaning of the word symbols. Active listening is important to accurately decode and understand a message. The more the sender and receiver have in common and the closer the relationship, the more likely they will accurately perceive one another's meaning and respond accordingly. Establishing a rapport with a patient ensures more effective communication.

Message

The **message** is the content of the communication. It contains verbal and nonverbal expressions of thoughts and feelings. Effective messages are clear, direct, and in understandable language. Individuals with communication barriers may need assistance via clarification devices such as hearing aids, interpreters, or pictures to ensure that messages sent and received are understandable. Personal perceptions may also distort the receiver's interpretation of a message. As a nurse, you send effective messages by expressing clearly, directly, and in a manner familiar to a patient. You determine the need for clarification by watching the patient; listen for nonverbal cues that suggest confusion or misunderstanding. Communication is difficult when participants have different levels of education and experience. For example, statements such as "Your incision is well approximated without purulent drainage" means the same as "Your wound edges are close together, and there are no signs of infection"; but the latter is easier to understand. You can also send messages in writing, but make sure that patients are able to read.

Channels

Communication **channels** are means of sending and receiving messages through visual, auditory, and tactile senses. Facial expressions send visual messages; spoken words travel through auditory channels. Touch uses tactile channels. Individuals usually understand a message more clearly when the sender uses more channels to send it.

Feedback

Feedback is the message a receiver receives from the sender. It indicates whether the receiver understood the meaning of the sender's message. Feedback occurs continuously between a sender and receiver. A sender seeks verbal and nonverbal feedback to evaluate the receiver's response and effectiveness of a communicated message. The type of feedback a sender or receiver gives depends on factors such as their background, prior experiences, attitudes, cultural beliefs, and self-esteem. A sender and receiver need to be sensitive and open to one another's messages, to clarify the messages, and to modify behavior accordingly for successful communication.

Interpersonal Variables

Interpersonal variables are factors within both the sender and receiver that influence communication. Perception provides a uniquely personal view of reality formed by an individual's culture, expectations, and experiences. Each person senses, interprets, and understands events differently. A nurse says, "You haven't been talking very much since your family left. Is there something on your mind?" One patient may perceive the nurse's question as caring and concerned; another may perceive the nurse as invading privacy and is less willing to talk. Cultural sensitivity enables you to explore the interpersonal variables such as educational and developmental level, sociocultural background, values and beliefs, emotions, gender, physical health status, and roles and relationships that affect how a patient communicates. Interpersonal variables associated with illness such as pain, anxiety, and medication effects also affect nurse–patient communication.

Environment

The **environment** is the setting for sender–receiver interaction. An effective communication setting provides participants with physical and emotional comfort and safety. Noise, temperature extremes, distractions, and lack of privacy or space create confusion, tension, and discomfort. Environmental distractions are common in health care settings and interfere with messages sent between people. You control the environment as much as possible to create favorable conditions for effective communication.

TYPE AND MODES OF COMMUNICATION

You send messages in many ways: verbally, nonverbally, concretely, and symbolically. People express themselves through language, movements, gestures, voice inflection, facial expressions, and use of space. Many forms of communication combine to create meaning in a sender's message.

Verbal Communication

Verbal communication involves the spoken or written word. Verbal language conveys specific meaning as you combine words. The following sections discuss the most important aspects of verbal communication.

Vocabulary

Communication is unsuccessful if a receiver cannot translate a sender's words and phrases. You will work with people of various cultures who speak different languages. Even people who speak the same language use subcultural variations of words. For example, *dinner* means a midday meal for some, whereas others use *dinner* to mean the last meal of the day. Because medical terms are often misunderstood, you need to use plain language when communicating with people outside the health care field. This means avoiding jargon, using the active voice (e.g., "When you get up ..."), and keeping your sentences and explanations brief.

For many individuals with limited English proficiency (LEP), the inability to communicate in English is the primary barrier to accessing health information and services. These patients require you to use professional interpreters who are able to speak the person's primary language. Health information for people with LEP needs to be communicated plainly in their primary language, using words and examples that make the information understandable.

Denotative and Connotative Meaning

A word sometimes has several meanings. Individuals who use a common language share the **denotative meaning** of a word. The word *baseball* has the same meaning for all individuals who speak English, but the word *code* denotes cardiac arrest primarily to health care providers. The **connotative meaning** is the shade or interpretation of the meaning of a word, which is influenced by the thoughts, feelings, or ideas that people have about the word. Families who are told that a loved one is in serious condition might believe that death is near, but to nurses the term *serious* may simply describe the nature of the illness and not the prognosis.

Pacing

Talking rapidly, using awkward pauses, or speaking extremely slowly and deliberately conveys an unintended message. Consider the following exchange:

Patient: "Do you know if the doctor found anything wrong with me?"

Nurse: "No ... but I'm sure if he did ... he would have come to explain things to you." (Then very rapidly) "Now let's get back to what we were doing."

Long pauses and a rapid shift to another subject may give the impression that you are hiding the truth. Speak slowly, enunciate clearly, and use pauses to stress a particular point or give the listener time to understand.

Intonation and Volume

Tone of voice and volume dramatically affect the meaning of a message, and emotions directly influence tone of voice. A simple question or statement can express enthusiasm, anger, or concern. Be aware of your intonation and volume to avoid sending unintended patronizing or critical messages. If a patient interprets your message as uncaring or condescending, communication is blocked. Pay attention to a patient's intonation and volume for information about his or her emotional state or energy level.

Clarity and Brevity

Effective communication is simple, short, and to the point to minimize confusion. Avoid phrases such as "you know," "right," or "OK?" at the end of every sentence. Give examples to clarify messages for the receiver. Use short sentences and words that express an idea simply and directly.

Timing and Relevance

Timing is critical in communication. Even if a message is clear, poor timing prevents it from being effective. Do not begin routine teaching when a patient is in severe pain, short of breath, or in emotional distress. The best time for interaction is when a patient expresses an interest in communicating because relevant messages are more effective. When a patient is facing emergency surgery, discussing the risks of smoking is less relevant than discussing what the staff will do to prepare the patient for surgery.

Nonverbal Communication

Nonverbal communication includes messages sent through body language without using words. Nonverbal forms of communication include facial expressions; vocal cues; eye contact; and cues such as gestures, posture, touch, odor, physical appearance, dress, silence, and the use of time. Nonverbal communication often reveals true feelings because you may be less censored about nonverbal reactions. A patient who says he or she feels fine but frowns while moving and holds his or her body rigidly is probably in pain. Nonverbal cues add meaning to verbal communication and help you judge the reliability of verbal messages. Nonverbal behaviors vary in different cultures, so gestures or expressions that are acceptable in one culture may have a different meaning and be considered rude in another culture. When communicating with a person from an unfamiliar culture, you need to clarify the meaning of gestures or other nonverbal cues.

Because you communicate using nonverbal messages often without awareness, you need to be aware of your own nonverbal behavior. Be sure that your nonverbal and verbal messages match and convey care and concern. If you say that a patient is getting better but demonstrate an expression of doubt, you do not relieve a patient's anxiety.

Personal Appearance

Physical characteristics, manner of dress and grooming, and jewelry are indicators of well-being, personality, social status, occupation, religion, culture, and self-concept. First impressions are largely based on appearance. Your physical appearance influences a patient's perception of you as a professional and the care you will deliver. You wear uniforms, scrubs, laboratory coats, business suits, or street clothes, depending on your role. Although your dress may not reflect your abilities, it takes longer to establish trust if your clothing detracts from a professional image. Tattoos and body piercings are becoming common in society. However, both can affect the perceptions patients have about your professionalism; they are examples of interpersonal variables, and patients will respond to them. In a study of hospitalized patients, patient care providers with visible tattoos and/or body piercings were not perceived as caring, confident, reliable, attentive, cooperative, professional, efficient, or approachable as providers without tattoos and/or body piercings. Female providers with tattoos were perceived as less professional than male providers with similar tattoos. In many health care settings, any tattoos must be covered by a uniform.

Posture and Gait

The way people sit, stand, and move is a form of self-expression. Posture and gait reflect emotions, self-concept, and health status. An erect posture and a quick, purposeful gait communicate a sense of well-being and confidence. A slumped posture and slow, shuffling gait may indicate depression or fatigue. Leaning forward conveys attention. Leaning backward in a more relaxed manner shows less interest or indicates caution.

Facial Expression

A sender's facial expressions often become the basis for judgments by the receiver. However, because of the diversity in facial expressions, meanings may be misunderstood. Facial expressions reveal, contradict, or suppress true emotions. People are often unaware of the messages their expressions send. When facial expressions are unclear, seek verbal feedback about the sender's intent. A patient who frowns after receiving information may be confused, angry, disapproving, or simply unable to hear you clearly or concentrating on a reply. In this case say, "I notice you're frowning," and have the patient clarify his or her response.

Patients watch nurses closely. Consider the effect that your facial expression has on a patient who asks, "Am I going to die?" The slightest change in the eyes, lips, or face reveals your true feelings. Practice avoidance of showing overt shock, disgust, dismay, or other distressing reactions in a patient's presence.

Eye Contact

Many individuals, regardless of sociocultural differences, maintain eye contact during conversation. By maintaining eye contact, you communicate respect and a willingness to listen. Lack of eye contact may indicate deference, anxiety, defensiveness, discomfort, or a lack of confidence in communicating. You may find that some individuals respond to eye contact by looking away, looking down, or becoming uncomfortable; this may be a cultural difference or may be related to a personal characteristic. Adjust your eye contact to promote an interaction that is comfortable for the patient. If you are in doubt, you may ask the patient about his or her preferences.

Eye movements communicate feelings and emotions. Wide eyes express frankness, terror, and innocence. Downward glances show avoidance or modesty. Raised upper eyelids reveal displeasure, and a constant stare may be associated with hatred or coldness. Avoid significant nurse–patient conversation that involves you looking down on a person; take time to sit down and make eye contact at the same level with a patient. This conveys equality and caring in your nurse–patient relationship. Equalizing the eye level with an angry person can diffuse a situation.

Gestures

A salute, thumbs up, fist bump, and tapping foot are types of gestures. Hands, shoulders, and feet emphasize, punctuate, and clarify the spoken word. Gestures alone carry specific meanings, or they may create messages with other communication cues. A finger pointed toward a person may communicate several different meanings; however, if for example you frown and have a stern tone of voice, the gesture becomes a sign of accusation or threat.

Territoriality and Space

Territoriality is the need to gain, maintain, and defend one's exclusive right to space. *Territory* can be separated and made visible to others such as by a fence around a yard. *Personal space* is invisible, is individual, and travels with a person. During interpersonal interaction, people maintain varying distances between themselves, depending on the nature of the relationship and situation. When personal space is threatened, people respond defensively and communicate less effectively. Examples of nursing actions within the four zones of personal space are listed in Box 4.1.

Because of the nature of caregiving, you must frequently move into a patient's territory and personal space. Convey confidence, gentleness, and respect for privacy, especially when actions require intimate contact. Knock before you enter a room. As you leave, ask if the patient wants the door open or closed. Ask if you can reposition the bed table and clarify which items the patient wants within reach.

FACTORS INFLUENCING COMMUNICATION

Contextual factors influence the nature of communication and interpersonal relationships (Box 4.2). Awareness of these factors helps you to make sound decisions during the communication process.

METHODS OF EFFECTIVE COMMUNICATION

The important strategies to enhance the communication are described in the following sections.

Attention Skills

The sender needs to pay attention to what he or she is trying to communicate, and choose the best words and body language to communicate with; the receiver needs to pay attention to what is being communicated by listening and watching. Attention is primarily governed by the type of attitude sender or receiver has toward each other during communication. *Attitude* is most essential in improving the communication; both sender and receiver need to have a positive and respectful attitude. They should want to communicate, and be willing to work to see that whether communication can take place. Using negative or

BOX 4.1 Nursing Actions within the Zones of Personal Space and Touch

Zones of Personal Space

Intimate Zone (0–18 Inches)

- Holding a crying infant
- Performing physical assessment
- Bathing, grooming, dressing, feeding, and toileting a patient
- Changing a patient's dressing

Personal Zone (18 Inches to 4 Feet)

- Sitting at patient's bedside
- Taking patient's nursing history
- Teaching an individual patient
- Exchanging hand-off communication at change of shift

Social Zone (4–12 Feet)

- Making rounds with a health care provider
- Sitting at the head of a conference table
- Teaching a class for patients with diabetes
- Conducting a family support group

Public Zone (12 Feet and More)

- Speaking at a community forum
- Testifying at a legislative hearing
- Lecturing to a class of students

Zones of Touch

Social Zone (Permission Not Needed)

- Hands
- Arms
- Shoulders
- Back

Consent Zone (Permission Needed)

- Mouth
- Wrists
- Feet

Vulnerable Zone (Special Care Needed)

- Face
- Neck
- Front of body

Intimate Zone (Great Sensitivity Needed)

- Genitalia
- Rectum

BOX 4.2 Factors Influencing Communication

Psychophysiological Context—Internal Factors Influencing Communication

- Physical health (e.g., pain, hunger, weakness, and dyspnea)
- Emotional status (e.g., anxiety, anger, depression, and fear)
- Growth and development status (e.g., age and developmental stage)
- Unmet needs (e.g., safety/security; love/belongingness; and grief resolution)
- Attitudes, values, and beliefs (e.g., confidence in health care providers; meaning of illness)
- Perceptions and personality (e.g., optimistic/pessimistic; trusting/nontrusting)
- Self-concept and self-esteem (e.g., positive/negative)

Relational Context—Nature of Relationship Between Participants

- Social, helping, or working relationship
- Level of trust and self-disclosure between participants
- Degree of sharing among participants
- Shared history of participants
- Balance of power and control

Situational Context—Reason for Communication

- Information exchange
- Goal achievement
- Problem resolution
- Expression of feelings

Environmental Context—Physical Surroundings in which Communication Occurs

- Degree of privacy
- Comfort and safety level
- Noise level
- Presence of distractions

Cultural Context—Sociocultural Elements that Affect Interaction

- Educational level of participants
- Language and self-expression patterns
- Customs and expectations

blaming words shows a poor attitude, using "I" messages and trying to understand the other's point shows a good attitude. Communication can be affected by a poor attitude toward the other person or toward the subject, or just because the sender or receiver is having a bad day. Fear and mistrust can impede communication, as can boredom or lack of interest in the subject. For best communication, try to keep the emotions out of the way until you understand what is being communicated. Therefore, it can be inferred that effective attitude training is essential for efficient communication.

Rapport Building

Rapport building is important in both our professional and personal lives; employers are more likely to employ somebody who they believe will get on well with their current staff. The first task in successful interpersonal relationships is an attempt to build rapport. Building rapport is all about matching ourselves with another person. For many, starting a conversation with a stranger is a stressful event; we can be lost for words, and awkward with our body language and mannerisms. Creating rapport at the beginning of a conversation with somebody new will often make the outcome of the conversation more positive. However stressful and/or nervous you may feel, the first thing you need to do is try to relax and remain calm. By decreasing the tension in the situation, communication becomes easier and rapport grows. Following strategies are quite effective in establishing the rapport in communication:

- Use nonthreatening and "safe topics" for initial small talk. Talk about established shared experiences, the weather, how you travelled to where you are, and so on. Avoid talking too much about yourself and avoid asking direct questions about the other person.

- Listen to what the other person is saying and look for shared experiences or circumstances—this will give you more to talk about in the initial stages of communication.
- Try to inject an element of humor. Laughing together creates harmony; make a joke about yourself or the situation/circumstances you are in but avoid making jokes about them.
- Be conscious of your body language and other nonverbal signals you are sending. Try to maintain eye contact for approximately 60% of the time. Relax and lean slightly toward them to indicate listening, mirror their body language if appropriate.
- Show some empathy. Demonstrate that you can see the other person's point of view. Remember that rapport is all about finding similarities and "being on the same wavelength" as somebody else, so being empathic will help to achieve this.

Empathy Skills

Empathy skills are vitally important in good communication. Empathy is the ability to see the world as another person, and to share and understand another person's feelings, needs, concerns, and/or emotional state. Being empathetic requires two basic components: *effective communication* and *strong imagination*; shared experiences can also help you to empathize. Empathy is a skill that can be developed and, as with most interpersonal skills, empathizing (at some level) comes naturally to most people. You can probably think of examples when you have felt empathy for others or when others have been empathetic toward you. Imagine a colleague becomes stressed at work due to an unfortunate situation in their personal life; their productivity falls and deadlines are missed. If you were empathetic, you might try to relieve their work pressure and offer to help in the best way possible. You could try to imagine how it must feel to be that person and understand why their work commitments were not being met. Thus, thinking empathetically improves the communication.

THERAPEUTIC COMMUNICATION TECHNIQUES

Therapeutic communication techniques are specific responses that encourage the expression of feelings and ideas and convey acceptance and respect. These techniques offer a variety of responses for you to appropriately use in different situations. Although some of the techniques may seem artificial or unnatural at first, your skill and comfort increase with practice and experience.

Conveying Empathy

Empathy is the ability to understand and accept another person's perspective. You can never totally know another's experiences because you are not in that person's situation, but you can try to understand and acknowledge what the person is experiencing. Empathic statements reflect an understanding of what a patient communicated and inform the patient that you heard both the feeling and the factual content of the communication. This allows a patient to validate or clarify feelings and perceptions.

Empathic responses are neutral and nonjudgmental and foster shared respect. Use them to establish trust in very difficult situations. *In the case study, Bud stated that he did not want to come to rely on narcotics because he had worked very hard to turn his life around after he became addicted to narcotic pain relievers. An empathic response from Tim is, "It sounds like you feel very strongly that regardless of your pain, you do not want to use narcotic pain relievers."*

Active Listening

Active listening means being attentive to what a patient is saying both verbally and nonverbally. It facilitates patient communication. Inexperienced nurses sometimes feel the need to talk to prove that they know what they are doing or to decrease anxiety. It is often difficult at first to be quiet and really listen. Active listening enhances trust because you communicate acceptance and respect for a patient. Several nonverbal skills facilitate attentive listening, using the acronym SOLER (Townsend, 2012):

S—*Sit* facing the patient. This posture conveys the message that you are there to listen and are interested in what the patient is saying.

O—*Open* position (i.e., keep arms and legs uncrossed). This position suggests that you are "open" to what the patient says. A "closed" position such as crossing arms conveys a defensive attitude, possibly provoking a similar response in the patient.

L—*Lean* toward the patient. This position conveys that you are involved and interested in the interaction.

E—*Eye* contact. Establish and maintain intermittent eye contact to convey your involvement in and willingness to listen to what the patient is saying. Absence of eye contact or shifting the eyes gives the message that you are not interested in what the patient is saying.

R—*Relax*. It is important to communicate a sense of being relaxed and comfortable with the patient. Restlessness communicates a lack of interest and a feeling of discomfort to the patient.

Sharing Observations

Nurses make observations by commenting on a patient's appearance and how he or she sounds or acts. Stating observations often helps a patient communicate without the need for extensive questioning, focusing, or clarification. This technique helps start a conversation with quiet or withdrawn persons. Do not state observations that will embarrass or anger a patient such as telling someone, "You're a mess!" Even if such an observation is made with humor, a patient can misinterpret the intent.

Sharing observations differs from making assumptions, which means drawing unnecessary conclusions about the other person without validating them. Making assumptions puts a patient in the position of having to contradict you. Examples include your interpretation of a patient's fatigue as depression and assuming that untouched food indicates lack of interest in meeting nutritional goals. Making observations is a gentler and safer technique: "I see you didn't eat any breakfast," "You are clenching your jaw," or a positive observation such as, "I see you've been organizing your papers."

Using Silence

It takes time and experience to become comfortable with silence. Most people have a natural tendency to fill empty spaces with words, but sometimes silence is useful when decisions that require much thought need to be made. Practice remaining mindfully present, but stay silent and listen when interacting with a patient. Silence is especially therapeutic during times of sadness or grief.

Providing Information

Providing relevant information helps your patients make informed decisions, experience less anxiety, and feel safe and secure. Speak in simple language and translate medical terms. When offering options, stress that the patient has the right to make decisions. Provide information that enables others to understand what is happening and what to expect.

Clarifying

Clarifying validates whether a person interpreted a message correctly. Any time a message is unclear or ambiguous, try to restate it or ask the other person to restate it, explain further, or give an example of what he or she means.

Focusing

Focusing directs conversation to a specific topic or issue when a discussion becomes unclear. It limits the area to which the sender can respond. Use it when the sender rambles or introduces many unrelated topics in the same conversation.

Paraphrasing

Paraphrasing is restating the sender's message in the receiver's own words to make sure that the receiver has received information accurately. Be careful not to change the meaning when you paraphrase. Confirm the meaning with the patient.

Summarizing

Summarizing is a concise review of main ideas from a discussion. It brings a sense of satisfaction and closure to an individual conversation or during the termination phase of a nurse–patient relationship. By reviewing a conversation, you focus on key issues and obtain additional relevant information as needed.

Self-Disclosure

You may use self-disclosure during the working phase of a helping relationship. Self-disclosures are personal statements intentionally revealed to the other person to assist the patient. The purpose is to model and educate, foster a therapeutic alliance, validate reality, and encourage autonomy. Keep self-disclosures brief, relevant, and appropriate, and do not introduce your *current* personal concerns or problems into the conversation because this may turn the conversation to focus on your problem. Make these statements to benefit the patient, not you, and use them sparingly so that the patient remains the focus of the interaction.

Instilling Hope

Nurses recognize that hope is essential for healing and learn to communicate a "sense of possibility" to others (see Chapter 32). You give hope by commenting on the positive aspects of the other person's behavior, performance, or response. Sharing a realistic vision of the future and reminding others of their resources and strengths also strengthen hope. You can reassure patients that there are many kinds of hope and that meaning and personal growth can come from illness experiences.

BARRIERS OF COMMUNICATION

Communication is not an easy process and can be hindered by several factors including personal, physiological, physical, environmental, psychological, social, cultural, semantic, and organizational and communication process–related barriers (Fig. 4.2). The barriers of communication are discussed in detail in the subsequent section (Table 4.1).

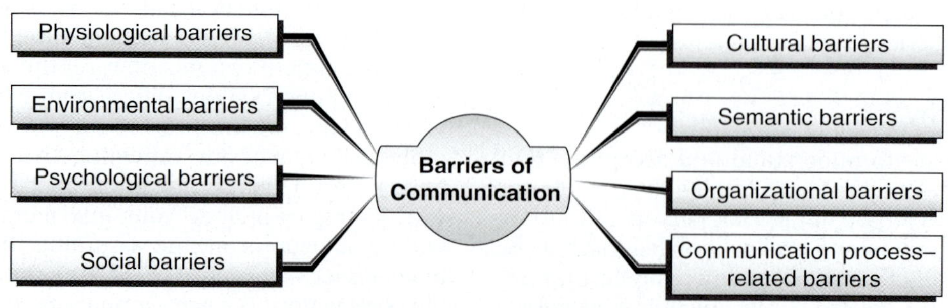

Fig. 4.2 Barriers of communication.

Table 4.1 Barriers of Communication and Methods of Overcoming the Barriers

Categories of Barriers	Description of Barriers of Communication	Methods to Overcome the Barriers of Communication
1. Physiological barriers	Poor retention due to memory problems Lack of attention Discomfort due to illness Poor sensory perception Hearing problems Poor listening skills Information overload Gender physiological differences	Sender and recipient must keep in mind each other's retention and memory abilities Sender and recipient must have each other's complete attention Before initiating communication, the sender and the recipient must ensure each other's comfort Intactness of sensory perception between the sender and the recipient must be considered Limitations of hearing ability must be kept in mind In addition to hearing, the sender and the recipient must ensure active listening between each other Information overload must be avoided Gender differences must be kept in mind
2. Environmental barriers	Loud background noise Poor lighting Uncomfortable setting Unhygienic surroundings and bad odor Very hot or cold room Distance	Background noise must be kept at lowest possible level Good lighting must be ensured to facilitate nonverbal communication Comfortable seating arrangement must be provided for effective communication Hygienic and odor-free environment must be ensured Optimal environmental temperature must be maintained
3. Psychological barriers	Misperception and misunderstanding Distrust and unhappy emotions Emotional disturbance such as anger, jealousy, and suspicion Prejudice, resentment, and antagonism Psychotic or neurotic illness Worry and emotional disturbance Fear, anxiety, and confused thinking	Communication must be carried out in a happy and trustworthy manner The sender and the recipient must refrain from negative emotions such as anger, jealousy, and suspicion The sender and the recipient must avoid feelings of prejudice, resentment, and antagonism The sender and the recipient must be free from fear, anxiety, and confused thinking
4. Social barriers	Diffidence in social norms, values, and behavior Social taboos Different social strata	Diffidence in social norms, values, and behavior must be given due consideration Social beliefs of the sender and the recipient must be kept in mind while communicating
5. Cultural barriers	Ethnic, religious, and cultural differences Cultural traditions, values, and behavior	Cultural difference must be given due consideration Cultural traditions, values, and behavior must be kept in mind

Other Barriers

I. **Semantic barriers**
- Language barriers
- Language jargons
- Faulty language translations
- Individual differences in expression and perception
- Past experiences of an individual
- Failure to listen

II. **Organizational barriers**
- Organizational policy, rules, and regulations
- Technical failure
- Time pressure
- Complexity of organizational structure due to hierarchy
- Size of the organization

III. **Communication process–related barriers**
- Unclear and conflicting messages
- Stereotypical approach
- Inappropriate channels
- Lack of or poor feedback

NONTHERAPEUTIC COMMUNICATION TECHNIQUES

Certain communication techniques hinder or damage professional relationships. These specific techniques are nontherapeutic and often cause recipients to use defenses to avoid being hurt or negatively affected. Nontherapeutic techniques discourage further expression of feelings and ideas and often result in negative responses or behaviors in others.

Inattentive Listening

Behaviors and nonverbal expressions such as fidgeting, breaking eye contact, daydreaming during conversation, and pretending to listen convey the message that what the sender has to say is not important. These behaviors discourage conversation and damage trust. Further examples are looking at your watch, tapping your foot impatiently, and documenting at the computer with your back to the patient.

Overusing Medical Vocabulary

Health care professionals have their own culture and language. Using technical words in discussions with patients can cause confusion and anxiety. Avoid excessive use of such terms or translate them into lay terms (e.g., medicine instead of medication, what you eat or drink instead of intake, get worse or better instead of progressive).

Prying or Asking Personal Questions

Asking irrelevant personal questions simply to satisfy your curiosity is inappropriate and invasive. Limit questions to health-related information.

Giving Approval or Disapproval

Do not impose your own attitudes, values, beliefs, and moral standards on others while in the professional helping role. People have the right to be themselves and make their own decisions. Avoid using terms such as *should, ought, good, bad, right,* or *wrong.* Agreeing, disagreeing, or sharing your opinion sends the subtle message that you are making value judgments about patient decisions. Instead offer options and help the other person anticipate the consequences of decisions. The problem and its solution belong to the patient, not you.

Giving approval or disapproval should be differentiated carefully from providing health care information and education, which are important nursing functions.

Changing the Subject

Changing the subject is a common problem when you are uncomfortable with a topic, but it is insensitive and tends to block further communication.

Automatic Responses

Clichés or stereotypical remarks such as, "You're never given more than you can handle," tend to belittle a patient's feelings and minimize the importance of his or her message. These automatic phrases communicate that you are not taking concerns seriously or responding thoughtfully.

False Reassurance

When a patient is seriously ill or distressed, you may be tempted to offer hope with statements such as, "I'm sure everything will be okay." Although you may be trying to be kind, false reassurance discounts the patient's concerns or situation and tends to block communication.

Asking for Explanations

Sometimes, asking "why" implies an accusation and results in resentment, insecurity, and mistrust. Try to phrase questions without using "why." You could say, "Tell me about the problems you're having with your medicines," rather than, "Why aren't you taking the medicines the doctor prescribed?"

Arguing

Challenging or arguing with someone's perception of a situation denies that his or her perceptions are real. It implies that they are lying, misinformed, or uneducated. Instead, be open and listen to the other person's views and opinion.

Being Defensive

When patients express criticism, listen to what they have to say. Listening does not imply agreement. To discover reasons for a patient's anger or dissatisfaction, you need to listen with a nonjudgmental approach. By avoiding defensiveness, you are able to defuse anger and uncover deeper concerns. Rather than saying, "None of the nurses would intentionally ignore you," you respond, "You feel the nurses are ignoring you."

Sympathy

Sympathy is the concern, sorrow, or pity that you feel for a patient when you personally identify with his or her needs. In contrast to empathy, which tries to understand a patient's experience, sympathy takes a subjective look at the patient's world. Sharing sympathy with another feels good, creates a bond, and minimizes differences; however, it can prevent effective problem solving and impair good judgment. When you share a patient's needs, you are assuming that his or her feelings are similar to your own, and you are unable to help the patient select realistic solutions for problems.

PROFESSIONAL COMMUNICATION

Professional appearance, demeanor, and behavior are important in establishing trustworthiness and competence. A professional is expected to be clean, neat, well groomed, conservatively dressed, and odor-free. Visible tattoos and piercings may not be considered acceptable in some professional settings. Professional behavior reflects warmth, friendliness, confidence, and competence. Professionals speak in a clear, well-modulated voice; use good grammar; listen to others; help and support colleagues; and communicate effectively. Being on time, organized, well prepared, and equipped for the responsibilities of the nursing role also communicate professionalism.

Courtesy

Common courtesy is part of professional communication. To practice courtesy, say hello and goodbye to patients and knock on doors before entering. State your purpose, address people by name, and say "please" and "thank you" to team members. Introduce yourself and state your title. When a nurse is discourteous, others perceive him or her as rude or insensitive. It sets up barriers to forming helping relationships between nurse and patient and causes friction among team members.

Use of Names

Always introduce yourself. Failure to give your name and status (e.g., nursing student, RN, or licensed practical nurse) or acknowledge a patient creates uncertainty about an interaction and conveys an impersonal lack of commitment or caring. Making eye contact and smiling recognize others. Addressing people by name conveys respect for human dignity and uniqueness. Because using last names is respectful in most cultures, nurses usually use a patient's last name in an initial interaction and then use the first name if the patient requests it. Ask how your patients and coworkers prefer to be addressed and honor their personal preferences. Using first names is appropriate for infants, young children, patients who are confused or unconscious, and close team members. Avoid terms of endearment such as "honey," "dear," "grandma," or "sweetheart." Even the closest nurse–patient relationships rarely progress to identities outside of first names. Avoid referring to patients by diagnosis, room number, or other attribute, which is demeaning and sends the message that you do not care enough to know the person as an individual.

Trustworthiness

Trust is relying on someone without doubt or question. Being trustworthy means helping others without hesitation. To foster trust, communicate warmth and demonstrate consistency, reliability, honesty, competence, and respect. Sometimes, it is not easy for a patient to ask for help. Trusting another person involves risk and vulnerability, but it also fosters open, therapeutic communication and enhances the expression of feelings, thoughts, and needs. Without trust, a nurse–patient relationship rarely progresses beyond social interaction and superficial care. Avoid dishonesty at all costs. Withholding key information, lying, or distorting the truth violates both legal and ethical standards of practice. Sharing personal information or gossiping about others sends the message that you cannot be trusted and damages interpersonal relationships.

Autonomy and Responsibility

Autonomy is being self-directed and independent in accomplishing goals and advocating for others. Professional nurses make choices and accept responsibility for the outcomes of their actions. They take initiative in problem-solving and communicate in a way that reflects the importance and purpose of a therapeutic conversation. Professional nurses also recognize their patients' autonomy.

Assertiveness

Assertiveness allows you to express feelings and ideas without judging or hurting others. Assertive behavior includes intermittent eye contact; nonverbal communication that reflects interest, honesty, and active listening; spontaneous verbal responses with a confident voice; and culturally sensitive use of touch and space. An assertive nurse communicates self-assurance; communicates feelings; takes responsibility for choices; and is respectful of others' feelings, ideas, and choices. Assertive behavior increases self-esteem and self-confidence, increases the ability to develop satisfying interpersonal relationships, and increases goal attainment. Assertive individuals make decisions and control their lives more effectively than nonassertive individuals. They deal with criticism and manipulation by others and learn to say no, set limits, and resist intentionally imposed guilt. Assertive responses contain "I" messages such as "I want," "I need," "I think," or "I feel." Nurses may experience ethical issues that make it difficult to use their assertiveness skills for fear of retaliation (e.g., identifying an error made by another health care provider). In such a situation, the individual would need to take steps to resolve this ethical dilemma.

AIDET® is a technique developed by the Studer Group to enable health care workers to provide accurate and timely communication to patients and families while focusing on excellent patient service. It is a technique commonly used in hospitals nowadays. The acronym stands for *A*cknowledge, *I*ntroduce, *D*uration, *E*xplain, and *T*hank you. When using AIDET, a health care worker first acknowledges the person standing in front of him or her with a positive attitude and makes the person feel comfortable. The worker introduces himself or herself and lets the person know what his or her role is in the department and the person's care. It is important to always wear a name badge when working in a health care setting. When possible, the worker gives the patient or family an idea of how long a procedure may take. This keeps the patient informed of any delays that may occur. It is also helpful to let a patient know how long it will take to get results if they are related to testing. When explaining procedures, describe what the patient will experience with the treatment, procedure, or test. Inform him or her of any safety precautions. The worker using AIDET thanks the patient for coming to this organization for care and lets the patient know how much he or she enjoyed working with him or her.

NURSE–PATIENT RELATIONSHIPS

A nurse's application of knowledge, understanding of human behavior and communication, and commitment to ethical behavior create professional relationships. Having a philosophy based on caring and respect for others helps you to be more successful in establishing relationships of this nature.

Phases of Helping Nurse–Patient Relationship

Hildegard Peplau (1952) gave the interpersonal relationship model described in Fig. 4.3. Her model describes the

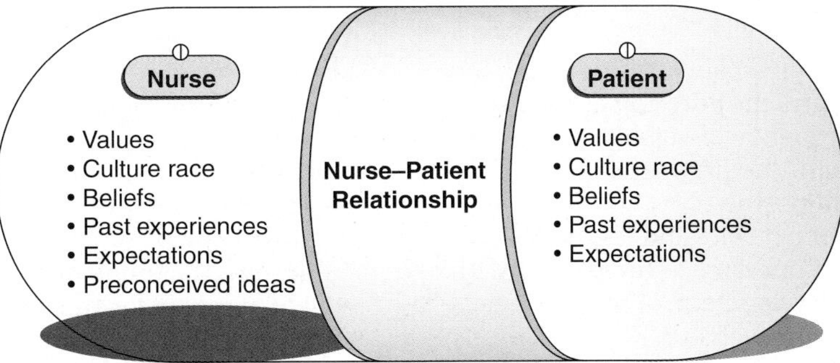

Fig. 4.3 Factors influencing the orientation phase.

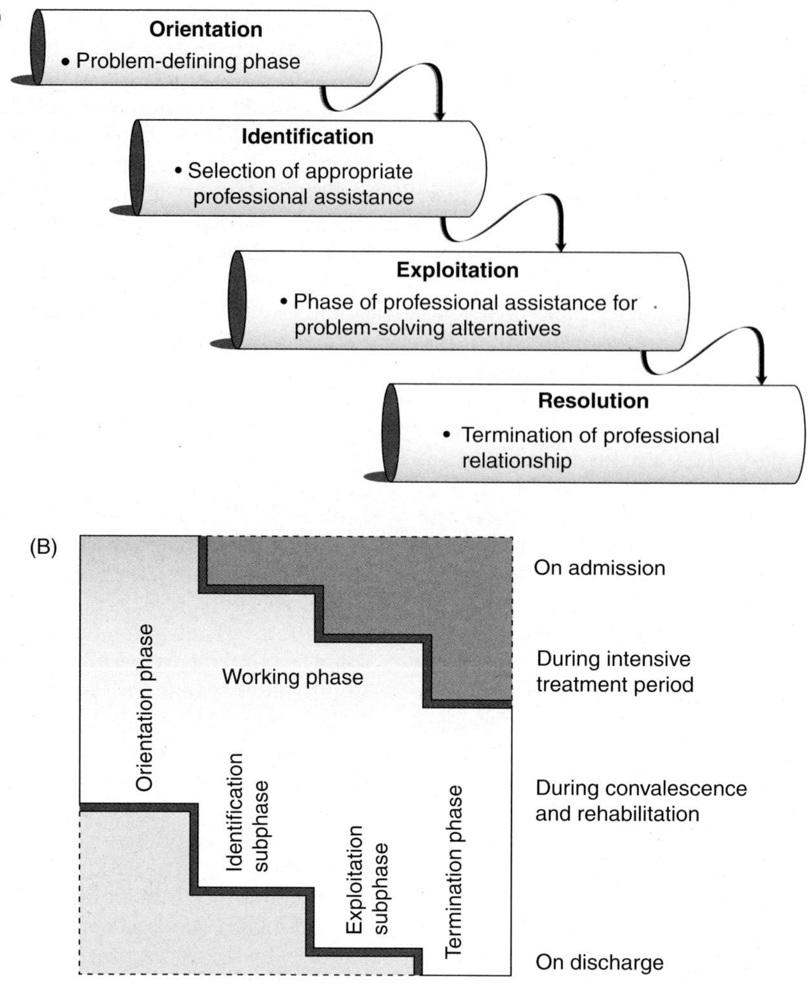

Fig. 4.4 (A) Phases of interpersonal relationships. (B) Phases of an interpersonal relationship with stages of hospitalization.

phases in a nurse–patient relationship in terms of the interpersonal process used in psychodynamic nursing. Peplau's model comprehensively described the four major phases of a nurse–patient relationship, which is discussed in detail next (Fig. 4.4A and B).

Fig. 4.5 illustrates the major concepts in Peplau's framework and their relationships in a nurse–patient relationship.

I. Orientation phase
  - The phase starts with an initial encounter between a nurse as a stranger and the patient having problems.
  - The pact formulation begins between the nurse and the patient. The pact states the duration of the therapeutic relationship, frequency of sessions to be conducted by the nurse with the patient, and details of termination of the relationship.
  - The nurse clarifies his or her roles and responsibilities within the therapeutic boundary to the patient with a view to avoid the development of psychological bonding or dependence on each other.
  - The nurse identifies the patient's problems, defines the problems after understanding them and settles on the type of nursing services needed.
  - After developing a trustworthy relationship, the patients start clarifying doubts, share preconceptions, and convey their needs and expectations to the nurse.
  - There are several factors that may affect the orientation phase in a nurse–patient relationship (values, cultural background, beliefs, past experiences, expectations, and preconceived ideas of both the nurse and the patient). These are presented in Fig. 4.3.

II. Identification phase
  - In this phase, the nurse must approach the patient with empathic understanding to accurately perceive the patient's current feelings.
  - While communicating with patients about their problems, the nurse must avoid vagueness and ambiguity by using specific terminology rather than abstractions. This will help foster understanding between the nurse and the patients.
  - The nurse helps the patients identify their problems in their own context and use the available resources to solve the problems.
  - The nurse helps the patients select the best available professional assistance to solve their problems.
  - The patient's self-esteem will be boosted by having feelings of belongingness and the ability to solve problems.

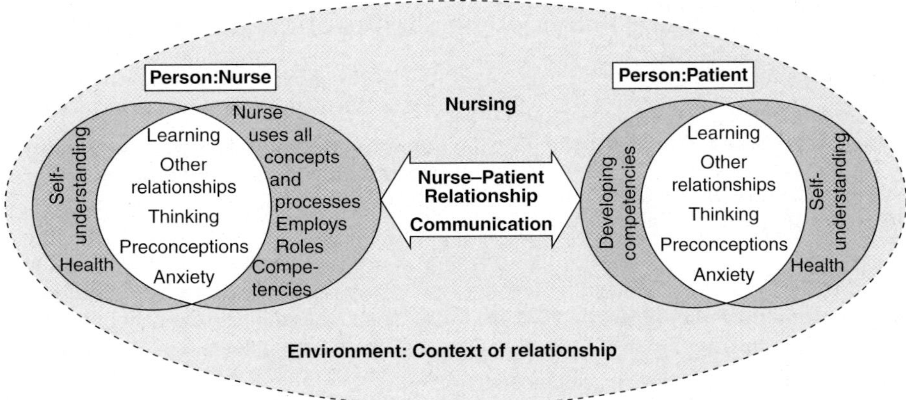

Fig. 4.5 Peplau's framework: major concepts and their relationships.

III. Exploitation phase

- The dictionary meaning of *exploitation* is the process of making use of something to gain as much as possible from it. But during the problematic phase, one feels that there are no resources available that can help the person solve the problem.
- In this phase, the patients are made to understand the problems by exploring all available avenues to solve the problems.
- The nurse can help the patient by extending minimal professional assistance to learn how to explore and exploit the available avenues that can help to solve the problem.
- The patient starts exploiting all the available resources in spite of making requests to others to extend help. Finally, the patient is able to deal adequately with his or her problems.

IV. Resolution phase

- This is the termination of the professional relationship that begins with convalesce and rehabilitation stage of hospitalization and ends with the discharge of the patient.
- As the pact has already formulated in the first phase, the patient is well versed with the termination phase of the therapeutic relationship.
- The patient's needs have already been met by the collaborative efforts of the patient and the nurse in previous phases, so this is the phase to depart from each other therapeutically.
- If psychological dependence persists between both of them, it becomes difficult to resolve the transference or countertransference. A nurse must be aware of the techniques to resolve it.
- The relationship must be terminated by maintaining a healthier emotional balance by both the parties involved and no one should remain dependent on each other.

COMMUNICATING EFFECTIVELY WITH PATIENT, FAMILIES, AND TEAM MEMBERS

Communicating Effectively With Patients

The health of many of the millions of patients we care for may be at risk because of the challenges in understanding and acting on health information. According to national data, there are large percentages of people who cannot read and write. The language that health care providers choose to use when communicating with patients, when speaking and writing significantly impacts whether they understand basic health information and the services needed to make appropriate health decisions. Follow these tips when communicating with patients:

- Organize what you want to say so that the most important points come first. For example, when teaching about a medication, start with its purpose, the dose a patient is to take, and the time to take the medicine. Follow with information about side effects and what to report to a health care provider.
- Break complex information into understandable chunks. For example, say, "This medicine is for your heart. We want you to take a dose once a day. The best time is in the morning about an hour after you usually have breakfast."
- Plan multiple short teaching sessions instead of one long session.
- Use simple language, avoiding jargon and defining technical terms (e.g., use the term *tablets* instead of medication).
- Use the teach-back method (see Chapter 15) to gather important information about patient understanding.
- Use the active voice. An example of active voice is "One of the nurses will give you a prescription before you go home." An example of passive voice is "The prescription for your medicines is being prepared by one of the nurses."

Nurse–Family Communication

Many nursing situations, especially those in community and home care settings, require you to form caring relationships with entire families. The same principles that guide one-on-one communication also apply when the patient is a family unit, although communication within families requires additional understanding of the complexities of family dynamics, needs, and relationships (see Chapter 5).

Nurse–Health Care Team Communication

Communication with other members of the health care team affects patient safety and the work environment. Breakdown in communication, lack of patient education,

BOX 4.3 Nursing Interventions During Phases of the Therapeutic Relationship

Preinteraction Phase—Before Meeting the Patient

- Review available data including medical and nursing histories.
- Talk to other caregivers who may have information about the patient.
- Anticipate health concerns or issues that may arise.
- Identify a location and setting that fosters comfortable, private interaction.
- Plan enough time for initial interaction.

Orientation Phase—When you and the Patient Meet and Get to Know one Another

- Set the tone for the relationship by adopting a warm, empathetic, caring manner.
- Recognize that the initial relationship may be casual, uncertain, and tentative.
- Expect the patient to test your competence and commitment.
- Closely observe and expect to be closely observed by the patient.
- Begin to make inferences and form judgments about the patient's messages and behavior.
- Assess the patient's health status.
- Prioritize patient problems and identify patient goals.
- Clarify the patient's role and your role.
- Form contracts with the patient to specify roles.
- Let the patient know when the relationship will end.

Working Phase—When you and the Patient Work Together to Solve Problems and Accomplish Goals

- Encourage and help the patient express feelings about his or her health.
- Encourage and help the patient with self-exploration.
- Provide information needed to understand and change behavior.
- Encourage and help the patient to set goals.
- Take actions to meet the goals set with the patient.
- Use therapeutic communication skills to facilitate successful interactions.
- Use appropriate self-disclosure and confrontation.

Termination Phase—During the Ending of the Relationship

- Remind the patient that termination is near.
- Evaluate goal achievement with the patient.
- Reminisce about the relationship with the patient.
- Separate from the patient by relinquishing responsibility for his or her care.
- Achieve a smooth transition for the patient to other caregivers as needed.

and poor health care provider accountability are frequent causes of serious injuries in health care settings. When patients move from one nursing unit to another or from one provider to another, there is a risk for miscommunication. To address this risk, health care providers provide detailed hand-off reports at end of shifts or when patients transfer off care units to ensure that patients have a safe and smooth transition in care. TJC Resources recommend that the entire health care team collaborate and coordinate during patient transition. Standardized discharge or transfer procedures and forms reduce the risk of errors during patient transitions. Timely follow-up after discharge or transfer is also encouraged.

Use of a common language such as the SBAR technique for communicating critical information improves perception of communication and information about patients between health care providers. The SBAR technique is a popular communication tool that standardizes communication. SBAR is the acronym for Situation, Background, Assessment, and Recommendation (see Chapter 31). The use of this easy-to-remember, orderly technique is to relay relevant information in a structured and timely manner. Evidence identifies nursing actions that increase effectiveness of nurse-to-nurse interaction and interprofessional communication (Box 4.3).

COMMUNICATING WITH PATIENTS WITH SPECIAL NEEDS

Many health-related and developmental issues contribute to impaired communication. Promoting effective communication in nonvocal patients includes thoroughly assessing communication needs, identifying alternative communication strategies, and creating an individualized plan of care. This includes a patient who is ventilator dependent and cannot speak or an infant who is limited to crying, body movement, and facial expression. Patients who are deaf or hard of hearing or who have LEP require individualized communication approaches. In addition, patients who are unresponsive or heavily sedated are sometimes unable to send or receive verbal messages.

A patient who cannot communicate effectively has difficulty expressing needs and responding appropriately to the environment. Such patients benefit greatly when you adapt communication techniques to their circumstances (Box 4.4). When caring for a patient with the nursing diagnosis of *impaired verbal communication related to a language barrier*, the priority is to have a professional interpreter available. If this cannot be achieved, provide the patient a list with pictures of simple words in the patient's language. The patient's use of these key images enables him or her to communicate basic needs such as food, water, toileting, rest, and need for pain relief. Collaborate with team members and family members when appropriate to design the best communication strategies.

Effective communication improves the quality of your patient's interpersonal relationships and well-being. If a patient uses ineffective communication techniques that interfere with coping or interpersonal relationships, intervene to help him or her send, receive, and interpret messages more effectively. Be a communication role model and teacher to help patients express needs, feelings, and concerns. Help patients develop social interaction skills and communicate thoughts and feelings clearly. This helps them interpret messages sent from others, increasing their autonomy and assertiveness. Methods such as role-playing allow patients to practice situations in which they have difficulty communicating.

Providing Alternative Communication Methods

Patients with physical communication barriers (e.g., patients with a laryngectomy or endotracheal tube) may be

BOX 4.4 Communicating With Patients Who Have Special Needs

Patients who are Hearing Impaired

- Ensure that patient has access to working hearing aids and glasses.
- Reduce environmental noise and distractions.
- Speak at a normal volume and avoid shouting.
- Rephrase instead of repeat if misunderstood.
- Punctuate speech with facial expression and gestures.
- Provide a sign language interpreter if needed.

Patients who are Visually Impaired

- Ensure that patient has access to glasses—corrective lenses and/or magnifying lenses.
- Communicate verbally before touching the patient.
- Orient the patient to sounds in the environment.
- Ensure that lighting is adequate for patient to see the speaker.
- Identify yourself when entering the room and notify the patient when leaving the room.
- Modify written handouts to accommodate degree of visual impairment.
- Offer audiotapes for instructional information.

Patients who are Mute, Unable to Speak, or cannot Speak Clearly

- Answer nurse call system in person.
- Listen attentively, be patient, and do not interrupt or finish patient's sentences.
- Ask simple questions that require "yes" or "no" answers.
- Allow time for understanding and responses.
- Use visual cues (e.g., words, pictures, and objects) when possible.
- Allow only one person to speak at a time.
- Use normal volume and do not shout or speak too loudly.
- Let patient know if you do not understand.
- Use communication aids as needed:
  - Pad and felt-tipped pen or Magic Slate
  - Flash cards
  - Communication board with words, letters, or pictures denoting basic needs
  - Computer toy ("speak and spell" type) for children
  - Call bells or alarms
  - Sign language
  - Use of eye blinks or movement of fingers for simple responses ("yes" or "no")
- Be attentive and responsive to restless physical movements.

Patients who are Cognitively Impaired

- Reduce environmental distractions while conversing.
- Prioritize communication over other tasks.
- Get patient's attention before speaking.
- Use simple sentences and avoid long explanations.
- Avoid shifting from subject to subject.
- Ask one question at a time.
- Allow time for patient to respond.
- Include family and friends in conversations when appropriate.

Patients who are Unresponsive

- Call patient by name during interactions.
- Communicate both verbally and by touch.
- Speak to patient as though he or she could hear.
- Explain all procedures and sensations.
- Provide orientation to person, place, and time as needed.

Patients who do not Speak English

- Speak to patient in a normal tone of voice (shouting may be interpreted as anger).
- Establish a method for patient to signal desire to communicate (nurse call system or bell).
- Avoid using family members, especially children, as interpreters.
- Provide professional interpreter/translator as needed:
  - Use a person familiar with patient's culture and with health care if possible.
  - Allow plenty of time for interpreter to transmit messages.
  - Communicate directly to patient and family rather than to interpreter.
  - Ask one question at a time.
  - Avoid making comments to interpreter about the patient or family (they may understand some English).
- Develop a communication board, pictures, or cards using words translated into English for patient to make basic requests (e.g., pain medication, water, and elimination).
- Have a dictionary (e.g., English/Spanish) available if patient can read.
- Provide written materials in English and in patient's primary language.

unable to speak, or the clarity of speech may be so poor that they need alternative methods of communication (see Box 4.4). To decrease frustration, provide simple communication methods and allow the patient time to respond. The patient must be physically able to use the method you provide (e.g., electronic or physical communication boards or pencil and pad). Patients who are unable to speak are at risk for injury unless they are able to communicate personal needs quickly.

Communicating With Children

Communication with a child requires knowledge of developmental tasks and milestones as well as special considerations to develop a working relationship with the child and family. Confirm that information communicated by the parents is consistent with other reports, including from the child. Offer the child toys or materials so that the parent gives full attention to your information gathering. Give periodic attention to infants and younger children as they play to include them. An older child can be actively involved in communication. Consider the influence of development on language and thought processes.

Children, particularly young children, are especially responsive to nonverbal messages. Sudden movements or gestures can be frightening. Remain calm and gentle and, if possible, let a child make the first move. Use a quiet, friendly, confident tone of voice. A child feels helpless in most situations involving health care personnel, which makes it particularly important to facilitate the presence of parents. When giving explanations or directions, use simple, direct language and be honest. To minimize fear and anxiety, prepare a child by explaining what to expect and seeking input from parents when appropriate. Avoid overly lengthy or involved explanations, and, similar to adults, meet a child at eye level.

BOX 4.5 Care of the Older Adult

Improving Communication

When communicating with older adults, the primary goal is to establish a reliable communication system that all health care team members easily understand. Ideally an interprofessional model delivers effective care for older adults. Communication with older adults requires special attention. Be aware of the physical, psychological, and social changes of aging. Use the following interventions to assist with impaired communication with older adults:

- During conversation, maintain a quiet environment that is free from background noise.
- Avoid shifting from subject to subject; allow time for conversation.
- Be an attentive listener. Use explorative questions to facilitate conversation.
- Avoid long sentences to explain the subject. Try to keep it short, simple, and to the point.
- Allow older adults the opportunity to reminisce. Reminiscing has therapeutic properties that increase the sense of well-being.
- If you are experiencing problems understanding a patient, let the patient know, and facilitate methods that help him or her speak more clearly. Consult with a speech therapist if necessary.
- Include a patient's family and friends in conversations, particularly in subjects known to the patient.
- Be aware of cultural differences among patients.

Drawing and playing with young children allow them to communicate nonverbally (making the drawing) and verbally (explaining the picture). Use a child's drawing as a basis for beginning a conversation.

Communicating With Older Adults

When you are communicating with older adults, avoid use of language that implies that the older adult is feeble; for example, do not speak in a singsong, high-pitched or overly loud voice, and do not use terms that imply the older adult is cute or childlike. Although some older adults experience some loss of sensory function that interferes with sending or receiving messages clearly, each patient is an individual. Many older adults who have some sensory losses adapt to sensory losses and learn to communicate effectively. Other older adults require moderate adaptation. When obvious deficits exist, maximize existing motor and sensory function to help patients communicate more effectively (see Box 4.4). You can make some simple modifications in your approach and the environment to improve communication with older adults (Box 4.5). Identify these challenges and work with patients to enhance effective communication.

KEY POINTS

- Communication is a powerful therapeutic tool and an essential nursing skill used to influence others and achieve positive health outcomes.
- Nurses consider many contexts and factors influencing communication when making decisions about what, when, where, how, why, and with whom to communicate.
- Communication is most effective when the receiver and sender accurately perceive the meaning of one another's messages.
- Effective verbal communication requires appropriate intonation, clear and concise phrasing, proper pacing of statements, and proper timing and relevance of a message.
- Effective nonverbal communication complements and strengthens the message conveyed by verbal communication.
- Strengthen helping relationships by establishing trust, empathy, autonomy, confidentiality, and professional competence.
- Effective communication techniques are facilitative and tend to encourage the other person to openly express ideas, feelings, or concerns.
- Ineffective communication techniques inhibit or block the other person's willingness to openly express ideas, feelings, or concerns.
- Nurses who are experiencing compassion fatigue often have difficulty relating with patients and coworkers.
- A nurse blends social and informational interactions with therapeutic communication techniques so that others explore feelings and manage health issues.
- The language that health care providers choose to use when communicating with patients can significantly impact whether patients understand basic health information.
- When using therapeutic humor, consider timing, receptivity, and content of the humorous intervention.
- When responding to an angry or aggressive patient, remain calm and unhurried, approach the patient slowly and in view, and seek the patient's approval before coming close.
- Older adults with sensory, motor, or cognitive impairments require adaptation of communication techniques to make up for their loss of function and special needs.

REFERENCES

Hildegard P (1952). American Journal of Nursing;52(6):765.

Townsend, MC. (2012). Psychiatric mental health nursing: concepts of care. 8th ed. Philadelphia, 2012, FA Davis.

5 Documentation and Reporting

OBJECTIVES

After reading this chapter, the student should be able to:

- Identify concept and purpose of a health care record.
- Discuss guidelines that fulfill standards of legal and ethical documentation.
- Identify ways to maintain confidentiality of electronic and written records.
- Describe five quality guidelines for documentation.
- Discuss the relationship between documentation and financial reimbursement for health care.
- Describe the different methods and forms used in record keeping.
- Discuss the advantages of standardized documentation forms.
- Identify elements to include when documenting a patient's discharge plan.
- Identify important aspects of home care and long-term care documentation.

KEY TERMS

accreditation, p. 61
acuity ratings, p. 56
case management, p. 59
change-of-shift report, p. 66
charting by exception (CBE), p. 59
clinical decision support system (CDSS), p. 64
clinical information system (CIS), p. 64
computerized provider order entry (CPOE), p. 64
confidentiality, p. 60
critical pathways, p. 59
diagnosis-related groups (DRGs), p. 55
documentation, p. 53
electronic health record (EHR), p. 56
firewall, p. 60
flow sheets, p. 55
focus charting, p. 59
graphic records, p. 55
hand-off report, p. 65
health care information system (HIS), p. 63
incident report (occurrence report), p. 66
interprofessional plan of care, p. 60
medical record, p. 53
nursing informatics, p. 64
password, p. 60
patient care summary, p. 56
problem-oriented medical record (POMR), p. 57
protected health information (PHI), p. 60
SOAP note, p. 58
reports, p. 65
standardized care plans, p. 56
telephone orders (TOs), p. 67
telephone report, p. 67
transfer report, p. 66
variances, p. 59
verbal orders (VOs), p. 67

INTRODUCTION

Documentation is a key communication strategy between health care professionals and a vital element of nursing practice. Health care documentation consists of all information entered into a **medical record,** which may be electronic, paper, or a combination of both formats. The information you enter into the medical record communicates the type and frequency of patient care provided, and provides accountability for the care provided by each member of the health care team. It is necessary to document all the nursing care you provide for each patient including assessment data, interventions, and patient responses in the medical record.

CONCEPT AND DEFINITION OF DOCUMENTATION

Documentation in a patient's medical record is a vital aspect of nursing practice. Nursing documentation needs to be accurate and comprehensive. Nursing documentation systems need to be flexible enough to retrieve clinical data, facilitate continuity of care, track patient outcomes, and reflect current standards of nursing practice. Information in a patient's record provides a detailed account of the level of quality of care delivered. Effective documentation helps ensure continuity of care, saves time, and minimizes the risk of errors. The quality of care, the standards of regulatory agencies and nursing practice, the reimbursement structure in the health care system, and legal guidelines make documentation and reporting an extremely important nursing responsibility. **Documentation** is a nursing action that produces a written account of pertinent patient data, nursing clinical decisions and interventions, and patient responses in a health record.

PURPOSES OF RECORDS

The health care record is a valuable source of data for all members of the health care team. Data entered into the health care record serve many purposes, including communication, legal documentation, reimbursement, education, and research. Health care record data are used for auditing, monitoring, and evaluating care provided to support the process needed for quality and performance improvement. Health care records also serve as sources of research data and as learning resources for nursing and health care education.

Communication

A patient's medical record provides information to all members of the health care team, communicates patient needs and progress toward meeting desired patient outcomes, and maintains continuity of care. The record includes a patient's assessment and responses to interventions and changes made in the plan of care. It is the most current and accurate source of information about a patient's health care status. This information prepares you to know a patient thoroughly so that you can make timely and appropriate care decisions.

Legal Record of Patient Care

Accurate documentation is one of the best defenses for legal claims associated with nursing care. Documentation is an important professional responsibility. To limit liability, your documentation needs to follow organizational standards, which include a clear description of individualized and goal-directed nursing care you provide based on your nursing assessment. You need to document in a timely manner. When documenting, follow agency standards. Documenting all aspects of the nursing process is a critical nursing responsibility that limits nursing liability by providing evidence that you maintained and exceeded practice standards while taking care of patients.

Mistakes in documentation that commonly result in malpractice include (1) failing to record pertinent health or drug information, (2) failing to record nursing actions, (3) failing to record medication administration, (4) failing to record drug reactions or changes in patients' conditions, (5) incomplete or illegible records, and (6) failing to document discontinued medications. Table 5.1 provides guidelines for avoiding these mistakes and gives some examples of basic criteria for legally sound documentation in a medical record.

Table 5.1 Legal Guidelines for Documentation

Guidelines for Electronic and Written Documentation	Rationale	Correct Action
Do not document retaliatory or critical comments about a patient or care provided by another health care professional. Do not enter personal opinions.	Statements can be used as evidence for nonprofessional behavior or poor quality of care.	Enter only objective and factual observations of a patient's behavior or the actions of another health care professional. Quote all patient statements.
Correct all errors promptly.	Errors in recording can lead to errors in treatment or may imply an attempt to mislead or hide evidence.	Avoid rushing to complete documentation; be sure that information is accurate and complete.
Record all facts.	Record must be accurate, factual, and objective.	Be certain that each entry is factual and thorough. A person reading your documentation needs to be able to determine that a patient received adequate care.
Document discussions with providers that you initiate to seek clarification regarding an order that is questioned.	If you carry out an order that is written incorrectly, you are just as liable for prosecution as the health care provider.	Do not record "physician made error." Instead document that "Dr Smith was called to clarify order for analgesic." Include the date and time of the phone call, with whom you spoke, and the outcome.
Document only for yourself.	You are accountable for information that you enter into a patient's record.	Never enter documentation for someone else (exception: if caregiver has left unit for the day and calls with information that needs to be documented; include date and time of entry and reference specific date and time to which you are referring and name of source of information in entry; include that information was provided via telephone).
Avoid using generalized, empty phrases such as "status unchanged" or "had good day."	This type of documentation is subjective and does not reflect patient assessment.	Use complete, concise descriptions of assessments and care provided so documentation is objective and factual.
Begin each entry with date and time and end with your signature and credentials.	Ensures that the correct sequence of events is recorded; signature documents who is accountable for care delivered.	Do not wait until the end of shift to record important changes that occurred several hours earlier; sign each entry according to agency policy (e.g., M. Marcus, RN).
Protect the security of your password for computer documentation.	Maintains security and confidentiality of patient medical records.	Once logged into a computer, do not leave computer screen unattended. Log out when you leave the computer. Make sure that a computer screen is not accessible for public viewing.

Table 5.1 Legal Guidelines for Documentation—cont'd

Guidelines Specific to Written Documentation	Rationale	Correct Action
Do not erase, apply correction fluid, or scratch out errors made while recording.	Charting becomes illegible: it appears as if you were attempting to hide information or deface a written record.	Draw single line through error, write word error above it, and sign your name or initials and date it. Then record note correctly.
Do not leave blank spaces or lines in a written nurses' progress note.	Allows another person to add incorrect information in open space.	Chart consecutively, line by line; if space is left, draw a line horizontally through it and place your signature and credentials at the end.
Record all written entries legibly and in black ink. Do not use felt-tip pens or erasable ink.	Illegible entries are easily misinterpreted, causing errors and lawsuits; ink from felt-tip pen can smudge or run when wet and may destroy documentation; erasures are not permitted in clinical documentation; black ink is more legible when records are photocopied or scanned.	Never use pencil to document in a written clinical record. Never erase entries, use correction fluid, or use pencil. To indicate an error in written documentation, place a single line through the inaccurate information and write your signature with credentials at the end of the text that has been crossed out.

Health Care Reimbursement

Documentation by all members of the health care team is used to determine the severity of illness, the intensity of services received, and the quality of care provided during an episode of care. Insurance companies use this information to determine payment or reimbursement for health care services. **Diagnosis-related groups (DRGs)** are classifications based on a hospitalized patient's primary and secondary medical diagnoses that are used as the basis for establishing Medicare reimbursement for patient care. Hospitals are reimbursed a predetermined dollar amount by Medicare for each DRG. Private insurance carriers and auditors from federal agencies review records to determine the reimbursement that a patient or a health care agency receives. Accurate documentation of nursing services provided as well as supplies and equipment used in a patient's care clarifies the type of treatment a patient received and supports accurate and timely reimbursement to a health care agency and/or patient.

Quality Improvement

Hospitals are required to establish quality improvement programs to conduct objective, ongoing reviews of patient care and to establish standards for quality care. Health care record audits help to determine whether standards of care were met and to identify areas for improvement and staff development. For example, a quality improvement nurse may monitor a unit's records to determine whether the nurses consistently and accurately documented implementation of fall precautions or evaluation of pain measures. Any deficiencies identified are then shared with all members of the nursing staff so that changes in policy or practice can occur.

Research

Some nurses use data in patient records for statistical analysis (e.g., frequency of clinical disorders, complications, use of specific medical and nursing therapies, clinical outcomes achieved during care for specific illnesses, and patient mortality). After obtaining appropriate agency approvals, a nurse researcher reviews patients' records in a research study to collect information about a particular health problem. Analysis of the data contributes to evidence-based nursing practice and quality health care. For example, if a nurse researcher suspects that early ambulation decreases the complication rate in postoperative patients, the researcher reviews the records of select surgical patients to compare the rates of postoperative complications with early versus late ambulation.

Nursing Education

A patient's record contains a variety of information (e.g., medical and nursing diagnoses, signs and symptoms of disease, successful and unsuccessful treatments, diagnostic findings, and patient behaviors). Reading a patient care record is an effective way to learn the nature of a condition and a patient's response to it. Review of patients with similar medical problems allows you to identify patterns and trends. Such information builds your clinical knowledge. As you identify patterns associated with specific diseases and conditions, you are able to anticipate the type of care your patients require and how patients respond to treatment.

TYPES AND FORMS OF COMMON RECORD-KEEPING

Nurses use a variety of electronic or paper documentation forms. The categories or data fields within a form are usually derived from institutional standards of practice or guidelines established by accrediting agencies.

Nursing Admission History

A nurse completes a nursing admission history form when a patient is admitted to a nursing unit. The fields in the form guide you through a comprehensive assessment to identify relevant nursing diagnoses or problems. Completion of this form provides baseline data that are used for comparison when a patient's condition changes.

Flow Sheets and Graphic Records

Acute care and critical care units commonly use flow sheets and graphic records to document physiological data and provision of routine care. Within a computerized documentation system, these forms allow you to quickly and easily enter patient assessment data, such as vital signs, admission and/or daily weights, and percentage of meals eaten. They also facilitate documentation of routine care such as hygiene measures, ambulation, and safety and restraint checks. These documents provide current patient information that is accessible to all members of the health care team so that patient trends can be easily identified. If you document an unusual occurrence or significant change in patient condition on a flow sheet, you should also describe the details of that occurrence or change in a progress note. For example, if a patient's blood pressure becomes dangerously high, you first complete and record a focused assessment on the flow sheet, and then you document the action taken and the patient's response in a progress note.

Patient Care Summary

Many computerized documentation systems generate a **patient care summary** document that you review and sometimes print for each patient at the beginning and/or end of each shift to use as a worksheet for organizing care and in giving hand-off report. The document automatically updates and provides the most current information that was entered into the electronic health record (EHR) and usually includes the following information:

- Basic demographic data (e.g., age, religion)
- Health care provider's name
- Primary medical diagnosis
- Medical and surgical history
- Current orders from the health care provider (e.g., dressing changes, ambulation, glucose monitoring)
- Nursing care plan
- Nursing orders (e.g., education needed, symptom relief measures, counseling)
- Scheduled tests and procedures
- Safety precautions used in a patient's care
- Factors that affect patient independence with activities of daily living
- Nearest relative/guardian or person designated as a patient's health care power of attorney to contact in an emergency
- Emergency code status (e.g., indication of do not resuscitate order)
- Allergies

Standardized Care Plans

Many computerized documentation systems include **standardized care plans** that facilitate the creation and documentation of a nursing and/or interprofessional plan of care. Each standardized plan facilitates safe and consistent care for an identified problem by describing or listing institutional standards and evidence-based guidelines that are easily accessed and included in a patient's EHR. After completing a nursing assessment, the nurse identifies and selects the standardized plans that are appropriate for the patient and are to be included in an individualized plan of care within the EHR. Most computer documentation systems allow these care plans to be modified by creating individualized interventions, goals, and outcomes for each patient.

Standardized care plans are useful when conducting quality improvement audits. They also improve continuity of care among professional nurses. When they are used, the nurse remains responsible for providing individualized care to each patient. Standardized care plans cannot replace a nurse's professional judgment and decision-making. You update care plans on a regular basis to ensure that the documents are appropriate and evidence-based.

Discharge Summary Forms

Nurses help ensure cost-effective care and appropriate reimbursement by preparing patients for a safe, effective, and timely discharge from a health care institution. Developing a comprehensive plan for a safe discharge relies on interprofessional discharge planning. This process includes identification of key clinical outcomes and appropriate timelines for reaching them, the appropriate level of care for discharge, and all necessary resources.

Ideally discharge planning begins at admission. By identifying discharge needs early, nursing and other health care professionals begin planning for discharge to the appropriate level of care, which sometimes includes support services such as home care and any equipment needs. Involve the patient and family in the discharge planning process so they have the necessary information and resources to return home or move to the next level of care. Discharge documentation includes medications, diet, community resources, follow-up care, and the name of a person to contact for questions or in case of an emergency. All this information is included in a discharge summary document that is printed out and given to the patient on discharge (Box 5.1).

Acuity Rating Systems

Nurses use **acuity ratings** to determine the hours of care and number of staff required for a given group of patients every shift or every 24 hours. A patient's acuity level, usually determined by assessment data a reregistered nurse (RN) enters into a computer program, is based on the type and number of nursing interventions (e.g., i.v. therapy, wound care, or ambulation assistance) required by that patient over

BOX 5.1 Guidelines for Information to Include on a Discharge Summary

- Use clear, concise descriptions in the patient's own language.
- Provide step-by-step instructions for how to perform any procedure that the patient or family will be doing independently (e.g., emptying a urinary catheter drainage bag or self-administration of an injectable medication).
- Identify precautions to follow when performing self-care or administering medications.
- List signs and symptoms of complications that a patient needs to report to a health care provider.
- List names and phone numbers of health care providers and community resources that the patient can contact.
- Identify any unresolved problems, including plans for follow-up and continuous treatment.
- List actual time of discharge, mode of transportation, and who accompanied the patient.

a 24-hour period. Although acuity ratings are not part of a patient's health care record, nursing documentation within the health care record provides evidence that supports the assessment of an acuity rating for an individual patient.

The acuity level is a classification used to compare one or more patients with another group of patients. An acuity system classifies patients from 1 (independent in all but one or two aspects of care; almost ready for discharge) to 5 (totally dependent in all aspects of care; requiring intensive care). Using this system, a patient returning from surgery requiring frequent monitoring and extensive care has an acuity level of 3 compared with another patient awaiting discharge after a successful recovery from surgery who has an acuity level of 1. Accurate acuity ratings justify the number and qualifications of staff needed to safely care for patients. The patient to staff ratios established for a unit depend on a composite gathering of 24-hour acuity data for all patients receiving care.

DOCUMENTATION IN HOME CARE SETTINGS

Documentation in the home care setting is different from other areas of nursing. The use of laptop and tablet computers makes it possible for home health care records to be available in multiple locations (i.e., the patient's home and the home care agency), improving accessibility to information and facilitating interprofessional collaboration. Medicare has specific guidelines to establish eligibility for home care reimbursement. Information used for reimbursement is gathered from documentation of care provided in the home care setting. Documentation is both the quality control and the justification for reimbursement from Medicare, Medicaid, or private insurance companies. Information in the home care health care record includes patient assessment, referral and intake forms, the interprofessional plan of care, a list of medications, and reports to third-party payers. Nurses must document all their services for payment (e.g., direct skilled care, patient teaching, skilled observation, and evaluation visits).

Nurses use two different data sets to document the clinical assessments and care provided in the home care setting. Assessment using the Outcome and Assessment Information Set (OASIS) is required for all patients aged 18 years and older (with the exception of prenatal or postnatal patients) who are receiving skilled care through a home health agency that is reimbursed by Medicare or Medicaid. OASIS includes a comprehensive admission assessment and calculates clinical, functional, and service scores to provide justification for reimbursement of services. The Omaha System consists of three components—Problem Classification Scheme, Intervention Scheme, and Problem Rating Scale for Outcomes—and provides a useful model for comprehensive evaluation of nursing care and evaluates the quality of nursing care provided in the home care setting.

DOCUMENTATION IN LONG-TERM CARE SETTINGS

Long-term health care settings include skilled nursing facilities (SNFs), in which patients receive 24-hour-a-day care including housing, meals, specialized (skilled) nursing care, and treatment services, and long-term care facilities, in which patients with chronic conditions receive 24-hour-a-day care including housing, meals, personal care, and basic nursing care. Requirements for documentation in these facilities are governed by individual state regulations, TJC, and CMS. CMS mandates use of the Resident Assessment Instrument (RAI), which includes the Minimum Data Set (MDS) and the Care Area Assessment (CAA) to document data in long-term care facilities. MDS assessment forms are completed on admission and then periodically within specific guidelines and time frames for all residents in certified nursing homes.

MDS data also determine the reimbursement level under the prospective payment system for Medicare Part A residents in an SNF. Communication among nurses; social workers; dietitians; and recreational, speech, physical, and occupational therapists is essential. Documentation in the long-term care setting supports an interprofessional approach to the assessment and planning process for all patients. Compliance with state and federal requirements as well as reimbursement for care provided in a long-term care facility is dependent on accurate completion of the required documentation to justify the care provided.

METHODS OF DOCUMENTATION

There are several documentation methods for recording patient assessment data and progress notes (Box 5.2). Regardless of whether documentation is entered electronically or on paper, each health care agency selects a documentation system that reflects its philosophy of nursing. The same system is used throughout a specific agency and is sometimes used throughout a health care system as well.

Narrative Documentation

Narrative documentation is the method traditionally used to record patient assessment and nursing care provided. It is simply the use of a storylike format to document information. In an electronic nursing information system, this is accomplished through use of free text entry or menu selections. Narrative documentation tends to be time-consuming and repetitious. It requires the reader to sort through a lot of information to locate desired data. However, some nurses believe that in certain situations, use of this method provides better detail of individual patient assessment findings and/or complex patient situations. Physicians and other health care providers review nursing documentation for details about changes in a patient's condition. One of the limitations of electronic documentation is the limited use of narrative documentation. Some areas of the EMR are designed to use multiple checkboxes or drop-down lists, which some believe may not adequately convey the details of significant events that result in a change in patient condition. EMRs that incorporate options for narrative descriptions in a format that is easily retrieved and reviewed may enhance clinician communication and interdisciplinary understanding for patient care.

Problem-Oriented Medical Record

The **problem-oriented medical record (POMR)** is a system of organizing documentation to place the primary

BOX 5.2 Examples of a Nursing Progress Note Written in Different Formats

Narrative Note

Patient stated, "I'm worried about the surgery. Last time I had a lot of pain when I got out of bed." Discussed importance of postoperative ambulation and demonstrated turning, coughing, deep-breathing (TCDB) exercises. Patient set postoperative pain-rating goal at 4 on a scale of 0210. Discussed analgesic plan of care and reassured that analgesics will be offered around the clock as ordered. Encouraged to tell nursing staff as soon as possible if pain is not relieved. Provided with teaching booklet on postoperative care. Stated, "I feel less anxious about my pain now." Verbalized understanding of the importance of postoperative ambulation and confidence in the plan of care.

SOAP (Subjective—Objective—Assessment—Plan) Note

S: "I'm worried about the surgery. Last time I had a lot of pain when I got out of bed."
O: Asking multiple questions about how postoperative pain will be addressed.
A: *Anxiety related to perceived threat of postoperative pain* as evidenced by statement of prior experience with uncontrolled postoperative pain.
P: Explain routine postoperative analgesic plan of care. Encourage to inform nursing staff as soon as possible if pain is not relieved. Explain rationale for early postoperative ambulation and demonstrate TCDB exercises. Provide teaching booklet on postoperative nursing care.

PIE (Problem—Intervention—Evaluation) Note

P: *Anxiety related to perceived threat of postoperative pain* as evidenced by statement of prior experience with uncontrolled postoperative pain.
I: Explained importance of postoperative ambulation and demonstrated TCDB exercises. Described analgesic plan of care. Encouraged to inform nursing staff as soon as possible if pain is not relieved. Provided teaching booklet on postoperative nursing care.
E: Stated, "I feel less anxious about postoperative pain now" and performed return demonstration of TCDB exercises correctly. Needs review of postoperative nursing care.

Focus Charting (Data—Action—Response) Note

D: Patient stated, "I'm worried about the surgery. Last time I had a lot of pain when I got out of bed." Asking frequent questions about postoperative pain management.
A: Discussed importance of postoperative ambulation and demonstrated TCDB exercises. Described postoperative analgesic plan of care that is in place. Provided teaching booklet on postoperative nursing care.
R: Demonstrated TCDB exercises correctly. Needs review of postoperative nursing care. States, "I feel better knowing how my pain will be treated."

focus on patients' individual problems. Data are organized by problem or diagnosis. Ideally, each member of the health care team contributes to a single list of identified patient problems, which coordinates a common plan of care. The POMR has the following major sections: database, problem list, care plan, and progress notes.

Database

The database section contains all available assessment information pertaining to a patient (e.g., history and physical examination, nursing admission history and ongoing assessment, physical therapy assessment, laboratory reports, and radiological test results). The database provides the foundation for identifying patient problems and planning care. As new data become available, the database is revised. It accompanies patients through successive hospitalizations or clinic visits.

Problem List

After analyzing data, health care team members identify problems and make a single problem list. The problem list includes a patient's physiological, psychological, social, cultural, spiritual, developmental, and environmental needs. Team members list the problems in chronological order and file the list in the patient's record to serve as an organizing guide for patient care. Team members add and date new problems as they arise. When a problem is resolved, the text of that problem is highlighted, or lined out, and the date is recorded.

Care Plan

Disciplines involved in a patient's care develop a care plan or plan of care for each problem (see Chapter 19). Nurses document the plan of care in a variety of formats; generally, all of these formats include nursing diagnoses, expected outcomes, and interventions.

Progress Notes

Health care team members monitor and record the progress made toward resolving a patient's problems in progress notes. Health care providers write progress notes in one of several formats or structured notes within a POMR (see Box 5.2).

The SOAP Record

One method is the SOAP note. The acronym **SOAP** stands for—*S*, Subjective data (verbalizations of the patient); *O*, Objective data (that which is measured and observed); *A*, Assessment (diagnosis based on the data); and *P*, Plan (what the caregiver plans to do). An "I" and an "E" are added (i.e., **SOAPIE**) in some institutions. The *I* stands for intervention, and the *E* represents evaluation. The logic of the SOAPIE note format is similar to that of the nursing process. You collect data about a patient's problems, draw conclusions, develop a plan of care, and then evaluate the outcome(s). Each SOAP note is numbered and titled according to the problem on the list that it addresses.

A second progress note used in the POMR is the **PIE** format. It is similar to SOAP charting in its problem-oriented nature. However, a PIE note differs from a SOAP note in that it has a nursing origin. *P* identifies a nursing diagnosis, *I* describes the interventions that will be used to address the problem, and *E* is the evaluation. The format simplifies documentation by unifying the care plan and progress notes. PIE notes also differ from SOAP notes because the narrative does not include assessment information. A nurse's daily assessment data appear on flow sheets, preventing duplication of data. PIE notes are also numbered or labeled according to the patient's problems. Problems that are resolved are dropped from daily documentation after a nurse's review. Nurses document about continuing problems daily with a PIE note for each problem.

The third format used for notes within a POMR is **focus charting**. It involves the use of **DAR** notes, which include

- *D:* Data (both subjective and objective)
- *A:* Action or nursing intervention
- *R:* Response of the patient (i.e., evaluation of effectiveness)

A DAR note addresses patient concerns: a sign or symptom, condition, nursing diagnosis, behavior, significant event, or change in a patient's condition (see Box 5.2). Documentation in this format also follows the nursing process. This format allows nurses to broaden their thinking to include any patient concerns, not just problem areas. Focus charting incorporates all aspects of the nursing process, highlights a patient's concerns, and can be integrated into any clinical setting.

Charting by Exception

The philosophy behind **charting by exception (CBE)** is that a patient meets all standards unless otherwise documented. The method was introduced in the early 1980s, and although the philosophy behind the method has consistently raised professional concern, many computerized nursing documentation systems use a CBE design. Exception-based documentation systems incorporate standards of care, evidence-based interventions, and clearly defined criteria for nursing assessment and documentation of "normal" findings. The predefined statements used to document nursing assessment of body systems are called *within defined limits (WDL)* or *within normal limits (WNL)* definitions. They consist of written criteria for a "normal" assessment for each body system. Automated documentation within a computerized documentation system allows nurses to select a WDL statement or to choose other statements from a drop-down menu that allow description of any assessment findings that deviate from the WDL definition or that are unexpected. You only write a progress note when a patient's assessment does not meet the standardized criteria for "normal" in one or more body systems. When changes in a patient's condition develop, you need to include a thorough and precise description of the effects of the change(s) on the patient and the actions taken to address the change(s) in the progress note.

Case Management and Use of Critical Pathways

The **case management** model of delivering care (see Chapter 2) incorporates an interprofessional approach to documenting patient care. **Critical pathways** (also known as clinical pathways, practice guidelines, critical pathways, or CareMap® tools) are interprofessional care plans that identify patient problems, key interventions, and expected outcomes within an established time frame. The document facilitates the integration of care because all health care team members use the same critical pathway to monitor a patient's progress during each shift or, in the case of home care, every visit. Many organizations summarize the standardized plan of care into critical pathways for a specific disease or condition. For example, in cancer care, some pathways focus on malignancies that have a higher incidence such as breast, colon, prostate, and lung cancers and certain types of blood cancers. Evidence-based critical pathways improve patient outcomes. For example, one critical pathway to manage pain caused by vascular-occlusive crisis in patients with sickle cell disease significantly improved the time interval between patient triage and administration of first analgesic dose and the likelihood of ketorolac administration in a pediatric emergency department.

A critical pathway eliminates nurses' notes, flow sheets, and nursing care plans because the document integrates all relevant information. Unexpected outcomes, unmet goals, and interventions not specified within the critical pathway are called **variances**. A variance occurs when the activities on the critical pathway are not completed as predicted or a patient does not meet the expected outcomes. A positive variance occurs when a patient progresses more rapidly than expected (e.g., use of a Foley catheter is discontinued a day early). An example of a negative variance is when a patient develops pulmonary complications after surgery, requiring oxygen therapy and monitoring with pulse oximetry. You document all variances on the critical pathway (Box 5.3). Analysis of variances identifies trends and provides data to develop an effective action plan to respond to identified patient problems. Variances sometimes result from changes in a patient's health or because of other health complications not associated with the primary reason for which a patient requires care. Once you identify a variance, you modify the patient's care to meet the needs associated with the variance. Over time, health care teams revise critical pathways when similar variances recur.

BOX 5.3 Example of Variance Documentation

You are using a critical pathway for "Routine Postoperative Care" for a 56-year-old man who had abdominal surgery yesterday. One of the expected outcomes for postoperative day 1 on the critical pathway document is "Afebrile with lungs clear bilaterally." This patient has an elevated temperature, his breath sounds are decreased bilaterally in the bases of both lobes of the lungs, and he is slightly confused.

The following is an example of how you document this variance on the pathway:

"Breath sounds diminished bilaterally at the bases. T—100.4; P—92; R—28/min; pulse oximetry 84% on room air. Daughter states he is 'confused' and did not recognize her when she arrived a few minutes ago. Oxygen 2-L nasal cannula started per standing orders. Oxygen saturation improved to 92% after 5 minutes. Dr Lopez notified of change in status. Daughter remains at bedside."

CONFIDENTIALITY OF MEDICAL RECORD AND PATIENT INFORMATION

Nurses are legally and ethically obligated to keep information about patients confidential. Only members of the health care team who are directly involved in a patient's care have legitimate access to the medical record. You discuss a patient's diagnosis, treatment, assessment, and any personal conversations only with members of the health care team who are specifically involved in the patient's care. Do not share information with other patients or with health care team members who are not caring for the patient. Patients have the right to request copies of their medical records and read the information. Each institution has policies that describe how medical records are shared with patients or other people who request them. In most situations, patients are required to give written permission for release of their medical information.

In the United States, the Health Insurance Portability and Accountability Act (HIPAA) of 1996 was the first federal legislation to provide protection for patient records; it governs all areas of patient information and management of that information. To eliminate barriers that potentially delay access to care, HIPAA requires providers to notify patients of privacy policies and to obtain written acknowledgment from patients indicating they received this information. Under HIPAA, the Privacy Rule requires that disclosure or requests regarding health information are limited to the specific information required for a particular purpose. For example, if you need a patient's home telephone number to reschedule an appointment, access to the medical records is limited solely to telephone information. Of equal importance under HIPAA is the Security Rule, which specifies administrative, physical, and technical safeguards for 18 specific elements of protected health information (PHI) in electronic form.

Sometimes, nurses use health care records for data gathering, research, or continuing education. This is permitted as long as you use a record as specified and permission is granted.

- When you are a student learning in a clinical setting, maintaining patient **confidentiality** and compliance with HIPAA are required as part of professional practice.
- You can review patient medical records only for information needed to provide safe and effective patient care. For example, when you are assigned to care for a patient, you need to review the patient's medical record and the **interprofessional plan of care.**
- You *do not* share this information with classmates (except for clinical conferences) and *do not* access the medical records of other patients on the unit.
- Access to an **EHR** is traceable through user log-in information. It is unethical to view medical records of other patients, and breaches of confidentiality will lead to disciplinary action by employers and potentially dismissal from work or nursing school.
- To protect patient confidentiality, you must ensure that any electronic or written materials you use in your student clinical practice *do not* include patient identifiers (e.g., name, room number, date of birth, and demographic information).
- *Never* print material from an EHR for personal use; any information printed must be for professional use only and should not include identifiable information.

Security Mechanisms for Privacy and Confidentiality

There are legal implications associated with the use of electronic documentation. It is possible for anyone to access a computer within a health care agency and gain information about almost any patient. Under HIPAA, ensuring appropriate access to and confidentiality of PHI is the responsibility of all persons working in health care. Therefore, protection of information and computer systems is one of your top priorities. PHI includes health information that identifies the individual, such as demographic data; facts that relate to an individual's past, present, or future physical or mental health condition; provision of care; and payment for the provision of care.

Most computer information system security mechanisms use a combination of logical and physical restrictions to protect information. For example, an automatic sign-off is a safety mechanism that logs a user off a computer system after a specified period of inactivity. Other security measures include firewalls and the installation of antivirus and spyware-detection software. A **firewall** is a combination of hardware and software that protects private network resources (e.g., the information system of the hospital) from outside hackers, network damage, and theft or misuse of information.

Physical security measures include placing computers or file servers in restricted areas or using privacy filters for computer screens that are visible to visitors or other people without access. This form of security has limited benefit, especially if an organization uses mobile wireless devices such as notebooks, tablets, personal computers (PCs), and smartphones. These devices are easily misplaced or lost, falling into the wrong hands. Some organizations use motion detectors or alarms with these devices to help prevent theft.

Access or log-in codes along with passwords are frequently used for authenticating authorized access to electronic records. A **password** is a collection of alphanumeric characters and symbols that a user types into a computer sign-on screen before accessing a program after the entry and acceptance of an access code or user name. Strong passwords use combinations of letters, numbers, and symbols that are difficult to guess. When using a health care agency computer system, it is essential that you do not share your computer password with anyone under any circumstances. A good system requires frequent changes in personal passwords to prevent unauthorized persons from tampering with records. A password does not appear on the computer screen when it is typed, and it should not be known to anyone but the user and information system administrators. Most health care personnel are given access only to patients in their work area. Some staff (e.g., administrators or risk managers) have authority to access all patient records. To protect patient privacy, health care agencies track who accesses patient records and when they access them. Failure to comply with HIPAA can result in civil and criminal penalties for health care agencies and providers. Depending on the nature of a violation, civil penalties can result in minimal fines of $100 to $50,000 per violation and maximum fines of $50,000 per violation with an annual maximum of $1.5 million. Thus, employers have policies for disciplinary action, including loss of employment, that are implemented when nurses or other health care personnel inappropriately access patient information.

HANDLING AND DISPOSAL OF HEALTH CARE INFORMATION

Maintaining the confidentiality of medical records is a fundamental responsibility of all members of the health care team. It is essential to safeguard any information that is printed from the record or extracted for report purposes. For example, you print a copy of a nursing activities work list to use in planning while providing patient care. You refer to information on the list and write notes to record into the computer and share later during hand-off report. Information on the list is PHI; you do not leave it out for view by unauthorized persons. Destroy (e.g., shred) anything that is printed when the information is no longer needed. Nursing students should not print information from the medical record to take away from the hospital to complete written clinical assignments. Instead, patient information needed for clinical assignments should be transcribed to academic forms or notebooks directly from viewing the medical record on the computer screen or the physical chart. All patient data must be de-identified when transcribed onto forms or used for academic papers for clinical courses in nursing school. Any information that is transcribed and must be removed from the clinical setting and any documents that must be printed out must be kept secure and destroyed through shredding or disposal in a locked receptacle as soon as possible.

Historically, information printed from a patient record and/or faxed to other health care providers has been the primary source for accidental, unauthorized disclosure of PHI. All papers containing PHI (e.g., Social Security number, date of birth or age, patient's name or address) must be destroyed after use or after being faxed. Most agencies have shredders or locked receptacles for shredding and later incineration. Nurses also work in settings where they may be responsible for erasing files from a computer hard drive that contain calendars, schedules for surgery or diagnostic procedures, or other daily records that contain PHI. You are responsible to know and follow the record disposal policies in the agency where you work.

Health care facilities and departments have policies for the use of fax machines that specify the kinds of information that can be faxed, who can receive faxed information, where information can be sent, and the process used to verify that information was sent to and received by the appropriate person or persons. Information sent by fax should not exceed what was requested or required for immediate clinical needs. Following are some steps to take to enhance fax security:

- Confirm fax numbers are correct before sending a fax to be sure that you direct information to the proper individual or agency.
- Use a cover sheet for all faxes containing health care information. This eliminates the need for the recipient to read the information to determine to whom a fax needs to be delivered. This is especially important if a fax machine serves a number of different users.
- Authenticate at both ends before transmitting data to verify that source and destination are correct. Use the cover sheet to list intended recipients, the sender, and the phone and fax numbers. Verify the fax number on the transmittal confirmation sheet.
- Use preprogrammed speed-dial keys to eliminate the chance of a dialing error and misdirected information.
- Use the encryption feature on the fax machine. Encoding transmissions makes it impossible to read confidential information without the encryption key.
- Place fax machines in a secure area, and limit machine access to designated individuals.
- Log fax transmissions. This feature is often available electronically on the machine.

GUIDELINES AND STANDARDS FOR QUALITY NURSING DOCUMENTATION

Whether the transfer of patient information occurs through verbal reports or electronic or written documents, you need to follow basic guidelines and standards for nursing documentation. Every health care organization has standards that govern the type of information nurses document and for which they are held accountable. Agency standards or policies often dictate the frequency of documentation such as how often you record a nursing assessment or a patient's level of pain. You are responsible for knowing the standards of your health care organization to ensure that you provide complete and accurate documentation. Nurses are expected to meet the standard of care for every nursing task they perform. Information in patient health care records can be used as evidence in a court of law to demonstrate whether nursing standards of practice were, or were not, met.

In addition, your documentation needs to conform to the standards of the National Committee for Quality Assurance (NCQA) and accrediting bodies such as TJC to maintain institutional **accreditation** and to minimize liability. Health care organizations usually incorporate accreditation standards into policies and revise documentation systems and forms to suit these standards. Current documentation standards require that all patients admitted to a health care agency be assessed for physical, psychosocial, environmental, self-care, spiritual, cultural, knowledge level, and discharge planning needs. Your documentation needs to demonstrate application of the nursing process, describe clinical decision-making, and include evidence of patient and family teaching and discharge planning. In addition to HIPAA standards, health care documentation is affected by standards from state and federal regulatory agencies, the Department of Justice, and CMS.

Quality nursing documentation is necessary to enhance efficient, individualized patient care and has five important characteristics: factual, accurate, current, organized, and complete. According to Beach and Oates (2014), it is easier to maintain these characteristics in your documentation if you continually seek to express ideas clearly and succinctly by doing the following:

- Stick to the facts.
- Write in short sentences.
- Use simple, short words.
- Avoid the use of jargon or abbreviations.

Factual

A factual record contains descriptive, objective information about what a nurse observes, hears, palpates, and smells. Avoid vague terms such as *appears, seems,* or *apparently.* These words suggest you are stating an opinion; they do not accurately communicate facts and do not inform other caregivers about the details regarding the behaviors exhibited by a patient. Objective data are obtained through direct observation and measurement and include description of a patient's behaviors, for example, *"BP 90/50, heart rate 115 and regular, patient diaphoretic and holding both hands over abdominal dressing."* The only subjective data included in the record are statements made by a patient. When recording subjective data, you document a patient's exact words within quotation marks whenever possible. Include objective data to support subjective data so that your documentation is as descriptive as possible. For example, instead of documenting *"the patient seems anxious,"* provide objective signs of anxiety and document the patient's statement about the feelings experienced: *"the patient's heart rate is 110 beats/min, respiratory rate is slightly labored at 22 breaths/min, and the patient states "I feel very nervous."*

Accurate

Using exact measurements establishes accuracy and helps you determine whether a patient's condition has changed in a positive or negative way. For example, a description such as *"Intake, 360 mL of water"* is more accurate than *"Patient drank an adequate amount of fluid."* Documenting that an abdominal incision is *"Approximated, 5 cm in length without redness, drainage, or edema"* is more descriptive than *"large abdominal incision healing well."* Documentation of concise data is clear and easy to understand. Avoid using unnecessary words and irrelevant detail. For example, the fact that the patient is watching television is necessary only when this activity is significant to the patient's status and plan of care.

Use abbreviations carefully to avoid misinterpretation and promote patient safety. TJC (2015) developed a list of "do not use" abbreviations that is used by all health care providers to promote patient safety. In addition, TJC requires that health care institutions develop a list of standard abbreviations, symbols, and acronyms to be used by all members of the health care team when documenting or communicating patient care and treatment. To minimize errors, spell out abbreviations in their entirety when they become confusing.

Correct spelling demonstrates a level of competency and attention to detail. Many terms are easily misinterpreted (e.g., *dysphagia* or *dysphasia*). Some spelling errors result in serious treatment errors (e.g., the names of medications such as lamotrigine and terbinafine or hydromorphone and hydrocodone are similar). Transcribe medication information carefully to ensure a patient receives the correct medication.

All health care record entries should be dated and timed, and the author of each entry must be able to be identified (TJC, 2017). Each entry in a patient's record must end with the caregiver's full name or initials and credentials/title/role such as "Jane Woods, RN." If initials are used in a signature, the full name and credentials/title/role of the individual need to be documented at least once in the health care record to allow others to readily identify that individual. As a nursing student, enter your full name and nursing student abbreviation, such as "David Jones, NS" or "David Jones, SN." The abbreviation for *nursing student* varies between *NS* for *nursing student* and *SN* for *student nurse.* Include information about your educational institution at the end of your signature when required by agency policy.

Current

Timely entries are essential in a patient's ongoing care because delays in documentation can lead to unsafe patient care. Many health care agencies keep records or computers near a patient's bedside to facilitate immediate documentation of information. Document the following activities or findings at the time of occurrence:

- Vital signs
- Pain assessment
- Administration of medications and treatments
- Preparation for diagnostic tests or surgery including preoperative checklist
- Change in patient's status and who was notified (e.g., health care provider, manager, patient's family)
- Admission, transfer, discharge, or death of a patient
- Treatment for sudden change in a patient's status
- Patient's response to treatment or intervention

Most health care agencies use military time, a 24-hour system that avoids misinterpretation of a.m. and p.m. times (Fig. 5.1). Instead of two 12-hour cycles in standard time, the military clock is one 24-hour time cycle. The military clock ends with midnight at 2400 and begins at 1 minute after midnight as 0001. For example, 10:22 a.m. is 1022 military time, and 10:22 p.m. is 2222 military time.

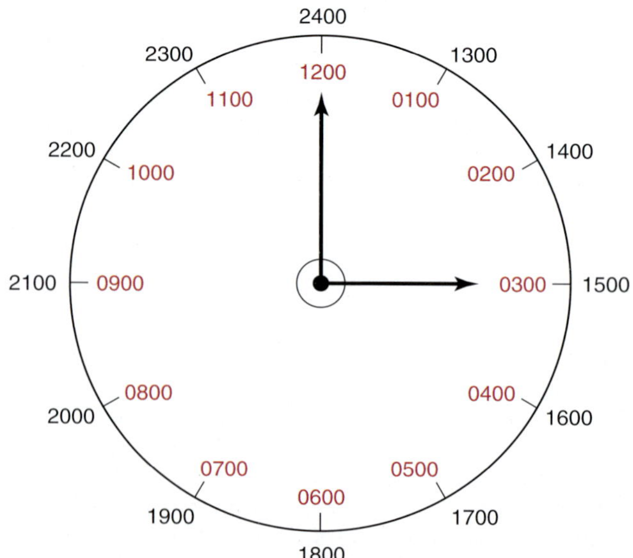

Fig. 5.1 Comparison of 24 hours of military time with the hourly positions for civilian time on the clock face.

Table 5.2 Examples of Criteria for Documentation and Reporting

Topic	Criteria to Report or Record
Subjective assessment data	Patient's description of episode in quotation marks (e.g., *"I feel like an elephant is sitting on my chest, and I can't catch my breath."*) Describe in patient's own words the onset, location, description of condition (severity, duration, frequency, precipitating, aggravating, and relieving factors) (e.g., *"The pain in my left knee started last week after I knelt on the ground. Every time I bend my knee, I have a shooting pain on the inside of the knee."*).
Objective assessment data (e.g., rash, tenderness, breath sounds, or descriptions of patient behavior [e.g., anxiety, confusion, hostility])	Onset, location, description of condition (e.g., 1100: 2-cm raised pale, red area noted on back of left hand). Onset, precipitating factors, behaviors exhibited (e.g., pacing in room, avoiding eye contact with nurse), patient statements (e.g., repeatedly stating, *"I have to go home now."*)
Nursing interventions, treatments, and evaluation (e.g., enema, bath, dressing change)	Time administered, equipment used, patient's response (subjective and objective response) compared with previous treatment (e.g., denied incisional pain during abdominal dressing change, ambulated 300 feet in hallway without assistance)
Medication administration	At time of administration when using a computerized bar-code medication administration program (or immediately after administration), document: time medication given, medication name, dose, route, preliminary assessment (e.g., pain level, vital signs), patient response, or effect of medication (e.g., 1500: Reports *"throbbing headache all over my head."* Rates pain at 6 (scale: 0210). Tylenol 650 mg given p.o. 1530: Patient reports pain level 2 (scale: 0210) and states, *"the throbbing has stopped."*
Patient and/or family teaching	Information presented; method of instruction (e.g., discussion, demonstration, videotape, booklet); and patient response, including questions and evidence of understanding such as teach back, return demonstration, or change in behavior
Discharge planning	Measurable patient goals or expected outcomes, progress toward goals, need for referrals.

Organized

Information entered in a health care record facilitates communication when it is documented in a logical order. Documentation is also more effective when notes are concise, clear, and to the point. To document notes about complex situations in an organized fashion, first think about the situation, and then make decisions about what information and words you need to include before beginning to enter data in the health care record. Application of your critical thinking skills and the nursing process will help you document clearly and comprehensively in a logical order. For example, an organized entry would describe a patient's pain, your assessment and interventions, and the patient's response to treatment.

Complete

You need to ensure the information within a recorded entry or a report is complete, containing appropriate and essential information. Follow established criteria and standards for thorough communication within the health care record or when reporting certain health problems or nursing activities (Table 5.2). Your written entries in a patient's health care record describe the nursing care you administer and the patient's response.

INFORMATICS AND INFORMATION MANAGEMENT IN HEALTH CARE

Information technology (IT) refers to the management and processing of information, generally with the assistance of computers. **Health informatics** is the "application of computer and information science in all basic and biomedical sciences to facilitate the acquisition, processing, interpretation, optimal use, and communication of health-related data. The focus is the patient and the process of care, and the goal is to enhance the quality and efficiency of care provided." A health care information system (HIS) is a group of systems used within a health care organization to support and enhance health care. A HIS consists of two major types of information systems: clinical information systems (CISs) and administrative information systems. Together the two systems operate to make the entry and communication of data and information more efficient. You will find that any single health care agency uses one or several of these systems.

Nursing competence in health care informatics is becoming a priority as health care providers and facilities across the United States implement electronic documentation. You need informatics competencies to deliver safer and more efficient care, to add to the nursing professional knowledge base, and to facilitate the growth of evidence-based practice. Professional organizations such as the Institute of Medicine, The Robert Wood Johnson Foundation, and the National League for Nursing recommend that all nurses acquire a minimal level of awareness and competence in informatics and use of IT. The American Association of Colleges of Nursing established a framework that outlines curricular goals and outcomes in informatics for baccalaureate, masters, and doctoral programs of nursing.

The Technology Informatics Guiding Education Reform (TIGER) Initiative began as a grassroots program in 2006 and was supported by over 70 contributing organizations, two grants from the Robert Wood Johnson Foundation, and one personal endowment. TIGER is focused on better preparing the clinical workforce to use technology and informatics to improve the delivery of patient care. On September 22, 2014, TIGER transitioned to the Healthcare Information and Management Systems Society (HIMSS). Under the direction of HIMSS, the momentum of the grassroots initiative will benefit from the robust volunteer structure that HIMSS can provide so strategies for the recruitment, retention, and training of current and future workforces for informatics education, practice, and research can be advanced.

Competence in informatics is not the same as computer competency. To become competent in informatics you need to be able to use evolving methods of discovering, retrieving, and using information in practice. This means that you learn to recognize when information is needed and have the skills to find, evaluate, and use that information effectively. As a nurse you also need to know how to use clinical databases within your institution and apply the information so you can deliver high-quality, appropriate patient care.

Nursing Informatics

Nursing informatics is broadly defined as the "use of information and computer technology to support all aspects of nursing practice, including direct delivery of care, administration, education, and research." All nurses deal with data, information, and knowledge. It is important that you know how to record, interpret, and report data and critically think and apply that knowledge when providing patient care. Data include numbers, characters, or facts that you collect according to a perceived need for analysis and possible action. You gain knowledge from gathering and using information from several sources. An example is a nurse's review of several, consecutive assessments of a wound documented within the EHR. Reviewing changes in the descriptions of the edges of the wound, color of drainage, and measurements over several days allows the nurse to evaluate and identify a pattern that indicates that the wound is not healing (information). On the basis of evidence available in the scientific literature, the nurse applies knowledge of wound care principles and intervenes to manage the patient's wound to promote healing.

Nursing informatics is also recognized as a specialty area of nursing practice. Informatics nurses have advanced preparation in information management and demonstrate proficiency with informatics to support all areas of nursing practice, including quality improvement, research, project management, and system design. Through the application of nursing informatics, technology is put to practical use to enhance bedside care and education. The application of nursing informatics results in an efficient and effective nursing information system that facilitates the integration of data, information, and knowledge to support patients, nurses, and other providers in decision-making in all roles and settings.

Clinical Information Systems

All members of the interprofessional health care team, including nurses, physicians, pharmacists, social workers, and therapists, use programs available on a **CIS**. These programs include monitoring systems; order entry systems; and laboratory, radiology, and pharmacy systems. A monitoring system includes devices that automatically monitor and record biometric measurements (e.g., vital signs, oxygen saturation, cardiac index, and stroke volume) in acute care, critical care, and specialty areas. The devices electronically send measurements directly to the nursing documentation system.

Order-entry systems allow nurses to order supplies and services from another department. An example is a computer program that provides the ability to order sterile supplies from the central supply department. This eliminates the use of written order forms and expedites the delivery of needed supplies to a nursing unit. Computerized provider order entry (CPOE) systems allow health care providers to directly enter orders for patient care into hospital information system. In advanced systems, CPOE has built-in reminders and alerts that help a health care provider select the most appropriate medication or diagnostic test. The direct entry of orders eliminates issues related to illegible handwriting and transcription errors. In addition, a CPOE system potentially speeds the implementation of ordered diagnostic tests and treatments, which improves staff productivity and saves money because the unit secretary no longer transcribes a written order onto a nursing order form. Orders made through CPOE are integrated within the record and sent to the appropriate departments (e.g., pharmacy or radiology).

Clinical decision support systems (CDSSs) are computerized programs used within the health care setting to aid and support clinical decision-making. When used to support nursing decisions, it is called a nursing CDSS (Fig. 5.2). The knowledge base within a CDSS contains rules and logic statements that link information required for clinical decisions to generate tailored recommendations for individual patients, which are presented to nurses as alerts, warnings, or other information for consideration. For example, an effective CDSS notifies health care providers of patient allergies before ordering a medication, which enhances patient safety during the medication ordering process. CDSSs also improve nursing care. When patient assessment data are combined with patient care guidelines, nurses are better able to implement evidence-based nursing care, resulting in improved patient outcomes.

Nursing Clinical Information Systems

A well-designed **nursing clinical information system (NCIS)** incorporates the principles of nursing informatics

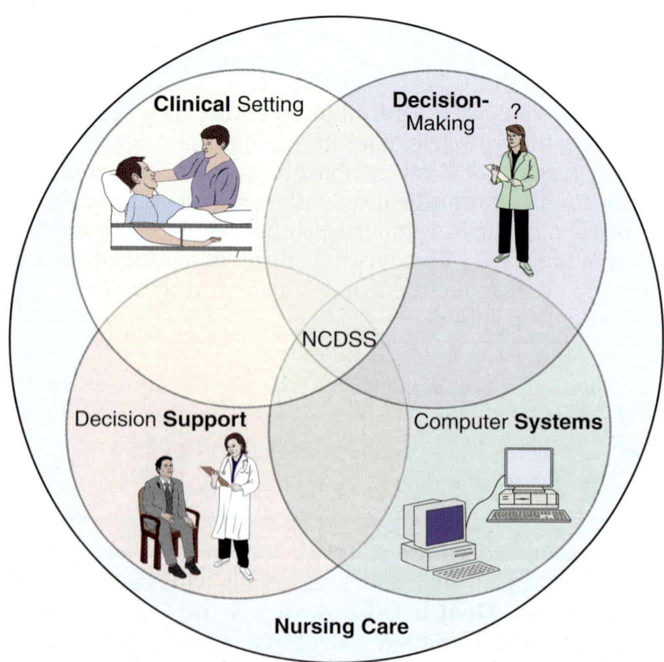

Fig. 5.2 Model of a nursing clinical decision support system (CDSS).

to support the work that nurses do by facilitating documentation of nursing process activities and offering resources for managing nursing care delivery. As a nurse, you need to access a computer program easily, review a patient's medical history and health care provider orders, and then go to the patient's bedside to conduct a comprehensive assessment. Once you complete an assessment, enter data into the computer terminal at the patient's bedside and develop a plan of care from the information gathered. This allows you to quickly share the plan of care with your patient. Periodically return to the computer to check on laboratory test results and document the care you deliver. The computer screens and optional pop-up windows make it easy to locate information, enter and compare data, and make changes.

NCISs have two designs. The nursing process design is the most traditional. It organizes documentation within well-established formats such as admission and postoperative assessment problem lists, care plans, intervention lists or notes, and discharge planning instructions. The nursing process design facilitates the following:

- Generation of a nursing work list that outlines routine scheduled activities related to the care of each patient.
- Documentation of routine aspects of patient care such as hygiene, positioning, fluid intake and output, wound care measures, and blood glucose measurements.
- Progress note entries using narrative notes, CBE, and/or flow sheets.
- Documentation of medication administration (see Chapter 32).

More advanced systems incorporate standardized nursing languages such as the North American Nursing Diagnosis Association-International (NANDA-I) nursing diagnoses, the Nursing Interventions Classification (NIC), and the Nursing Outcomes Classification (NOC) into the software.

The other model for an NCIS is the protocol or critical pathway design. This design facilitates interdisciplinary management of information because all health care providers use evidence-based protocols or critical pathways to document the care they provide. The information system allows a user to select one or more appropriate protocols for a patient. An advanced system merges multiple protocols, using a master protocol or path to direct patient care activities. Standard health care provider order sets are included in the protocols and automatically processed. The system integrates appropriate information into the medication delivery process to enhance patient safety. In addition, the system identifies variances of the anticipated outcomes on the protocols as documentation is entered. This provides all caregivers the ability to analyze variances and offer an accurate clinical picture of a patient's progress.

Advantages of a Nursing Clinical Information System

Anecdotal reports and descriptive studies suggest that NCISs offer important advantages to nurses in practice. According to Hebda and Czar (2013), some specific advantages include:

- Better access to information.
- Enhanced quality of documentation through prompts.
- Reduced errors of omission.
- Reduced hospital costs.
- Increased nurse job satisfaction.
- Compliance with requirements of accrediting agencies (e.g., TJC).
- Development of a common clinical database.
- Enhanced ability to track records.

Many NCISs include content-importing technologies that allow the use of templates, macros, automated data points, and the ability to copy forward either parts of or entire nursing shift assessments that enable nurses to quickly document their assessment or the care they provided. These features have benefits and risks associated with their use. When allergy and current medication lists are automatically imported into nursing admission documentation from a previous hospital encounter, you need to meticulously review this information for accuracy and update it as needed to avoid documentation errors and patient safety concerns. When nursing shift assessment data are copied forward from a previous shift or day, these must be updated so these accurately reflect a patient's current clinical status.

REPORTING

Reports are oral, written, or audiotaped exchanges of information between members of the health care team. A report reflects a summary of activities or observations seen, performed, or heard by the health care provider. Common reports given by nurses include hand-off reports, change-of-shift reports, and transfer reports.

Hand-Off Report

A **hand-off report** occurs any time one health care provider transfers care of a patient to another health care provider. The purpose of hand-off reports is to provide better continuity and individualized care for patients. A hand-off is the process of transferring responsibility for patient care from one provider to another. For example, if you find that a patient breathes better in a certain position, you relay that information to the next nurse caring for the patient.

Standardizing communication during hand-off reports helps ensure patient safety. Face-to-face hand-off communication includes up-to-date information about a patient's condition, required care, treatments, medications, services, and any recent or anticipated changes. In addition, these reports reduce patient care errors.

When a hand-off report is given, it is essential for staff to have an opportunity for last-minute updates to clarify information or to receive information about care events or changes in a patient's condition. Properly performed, a hand-off report provides for patient safety and continuity of care.

An effective hand-off report is quick and efficient. A good report provides a baseline for comparisons and indicates the kind of care anticipated for the next nurse who will be caring for the patient. An organized and concise approach helps you set goals and anticipate patient needs and lessens the chance of overlooking important information.

A sample format frequently includes background information (name, age, and medical diagnosis); primary health problem; unusual occurrences; discharge planning issues; identification of significant changes in measurable terms (e.g., pain scale); observations; findings; times when new, STAT, or prn medications were given; care required such as medications that need to be started, when to assess the effectiveness of STAT or prn medications, or when a dressing needs to be changed next; progress with teaching interventions; and family involvement. It is especially important to report any recent changes or priority situations concerning the patient's condition. Do not include normal findings or routine information retrievable from other sources or derogatory or inappropriate comments about a patient or family.

Change-of-Shift Report

The **change-of-shift report** is a type of hand-off report that occurs at the end of each shift. This report provides the transfer of relevant information from nurses who have completed a shift of care to nurses about to begin a shift of care. Shift reports occur in a variety of ways.

Sometimes, nurses walk with each other from one patient's room to the next. This is called *walking rounds*. Walking reports given in person or during rounds allow you to obtain immediate feedback when questions arise about a patient's care. When you make rounds, the patient and family members can participate in any discussions and care decisions. However, be careful about mentioning information that the patient should not hear (e.g., new laboratory or diagnostic reports not yet explained by the health care provider).

Nurses also give reports orally. Oral reports occur in person with staff members from both shifts participating. Reports can be audiotaped before the end of the shift by the nurse going off duty; the incoming staff listen to the report before assuming patient care. Audiotaped reports often enhance efficiency and minimize social interactions. However, the audiotaped report does not provide the opportunity to raise questions or obtain feedback about the patient's nursing care needs.

Transfer Reports

Patients frequently transfer from one unit to another or to another agency to receive different levels of care. For example, they transfer from intensive care units to general nursing units when the level of care no longer requires intense monitoring. A **transfer report** is another type of hand-off report that involves the nurse on the sending unit communicating information about a patient to the nurse on the receiving unit. Nurses usually give transfer reports by phone or in person. When giving a transfer report, include the following information:

1. Patient's name, age, date of birth, health care provider(s), and medical diagnosis
2. Summary of medical progress up to the time of transfer
3. Current health status (physical and psychosocial)
4. Allergies
5. Emergency code status
6. Family support
7. Current nursing diagnoses or problems and care plan
8. Any critical assessments or interventions to be completed shortly after transfer (helps receiving nurse establish priorities of care)
9. Up-to-date reconciled medication list
10. Need for any special equipment such as isolation equipment, suction equipment, or traction

At the completion of the transfer report, the receiving nurse clarifies information by asking questions about the patient's status. Some institutions require a written transfer report sheet that includes information communicated in the transfer report.

Incident or Occurrence Reports

An incident or occurrence is any event that is not consistent with the routine, expected care of a patient, or the standard procedures in place on a health care unit or within an agency. Examples include patient falls, needlestick injuries, medication administration errors, accidental omission of ordered therapies, a visitor losing consciousness, and any circumstances that lead to injury or pose a risk for patient injury such as a "near miss." A near miss is an incident in which no property was damaged and no patient or personnel were injured, but with a slight shift in time or position, damage or injury could have occurred.

An **incident report (occurrence report)** is completed whenever an incident occurs. Incident reports are an important part of the quality improvement program of a unit or agency; however, they are not part of the health care record. Incident reports contain confidential information; distribution of the report is limited to the individuals responsible for reviewing the forms. Follow agency policy when completing an incident report, and file the report with your agency's risk-management department. Analysis of incident or occurrence reports helps identify system and/or individual human issues in which educational or in-service programs or changes in policies and procedures are needed to reduce the risk of future occurrences.

When an incident occurs, document an objective description of what happened, what you observed, and the follow-up actions taken including notification of the patient's health care provider in the patient's health care record. Remember to evaluate and document the patient's response to the incident in the health care record as well. Do not label this as an "incident," "near miss," or "sentinel event" in the health care record, and do not make any reference to these types of documents. A notation about an incident, near miss, or sentinel event report in a patient's health care record makes it easier for a lawyer to argue that the reference makes the incident report part of the health care record and therefore admissible for attorney review.

DOCUMENTATION OF TELEPHONE REPORTS, TELEPHONE ORDERS, AND VERBAL ORDERS

Document every phone call you make to a health care provider. Your documentation needs to include when the call

BOX 5.4 Guidelines for Telephone and Verbal Orders

- Clearly determine the patient's name, room number, and diagnosis.
- Use clarification questions to avoid misunderstandings.
- Write TO (telephone order) or VO (verbal order), including date and time, name of patient, the complete order; sign the name of the physician or health care provider and nurse.
- Read back any prescribed orders to the physician or health care provider.
- Follow agency policies; some institutions require telephone (and verbal) orders to be reviewed and signed by two nurses.

was made, the number called, who made the call (if you did not make the call), who was called, to whom information was given, what information was given, and what information was received.

Telephone Reports

A **telephone report** needs to include clear, accurate, and concise information. TJC reported that in 2011 verbal and written communication among staff and with patients were listed as one of the 10 most frequently identified root causes of medical errors, also called *sentinel events*. To improve communication, some institutions use SBAR (Situation, Background, Assessment, Recommendation), a communication strategy designed to improve patient safety (see Chapter 11). SBAR standardizes telephone communication of significant events or changes in the patient's condition.

Telephone Orders and Verbal Orders

Telephone orders (TOs) occur when a health care provider gives therapeutic orders over the phone to an RN. **Verbal orders (VOs)** occur when a health care provider gives therapeutic orders to an RN while they are standing in proximity to one another. Use of VOs is discouraged except in urgent or emergent situations. TOs and VOs usually occur at night or during emergencies; they should be used only when absolutely necessary and not for the sake of convenience. In some situations, it is wise to have a second person listen to TOs; some agency policies require it. Check your agency's policy. Box 5.4 provides guidelines that promote accuracy when receiving TOs or VOs.

A nurse receiving a TO or VO enters the complete order into the computer using the CPOE software or writes it out on a physician's order sheet for entry in the computer as soon as possible. After a nurse transcribes an order, the nurse uses the read-back process and documents the process to provide evidence that the information received (e.g., call back instructions and/or therapeutic orders) was verified with the provider.

KEY POINTS

- In response to federal regulations, documentation of health care information continues to shift to electronic rather than paper-based documentation systems.
- Computerized health care records improve continuity of care by providing the ability to compare data from various health care encounters.
- Computerized health care information systems provide patient data in an accessible and organized manner.
- The security of health care computer systems and protection of the confidentiality of patients' health information must remain a top priority.
- The health care record is a confidential, legal, and continuing account of a patient's health care status. It is available to all members of the health care team involved in the patient's care to facilitate communication.
- The health care record provides a legal and financial record of care, aids in clinical education and research, and guides professional and organizational performance improvement.
- Nursing informatics facilitates the integration of data, information, knowledge, and wisdom to support patients, nurses, and other providers in decision-making in all roles and settings.
- Accurate and timely record keeping requires objective documentation of data with precise measurements, correct spelling, and proper use of abbreviations.
- Effective nursing documentation limits liability through objective description of what happened to a patient and clearly indicates that individualized, goal-directed nursing care was provided based on nursing assessment.
- Nursing documentation supports reimbursement to health care agencies through accurate accounting of the use of services and equipment and medications administered.
- Documentation standards for nurses who work in home health care settings are set by Medicare guidelines that establish reimbursement for home health care.
- Documentation in long-term health care settings is interprofessional and closely linked with financial requirements of outside agencies.
- The major purposes of hand-off reports are patient safety, enhanced communication between health care professionals, and continuity of care.
- When information relevant to care is communicated by telephone, verification of information through use of a read-back process should be documented in the health care record.
- Incident (occurrence/event) reports objectively describe any event not consistent with the routine care of a patient. These reports are confidential and are used for quality improvement within an agency. Information about an incident report should never be documented in a patient's health care record.

RESEARCH REFERENCES

Beach J, Oates J. Maintaining best practices in record-keeping and documentation. Nurs Stand. 2014;28(36):45-50.

Hebda TL, Czar P. Handbook of informatics for nurses and healthcare professionals. 5th ed. Boston: Pearson, 2013.

The Joint Commission (2015). Hospital: National patient safety goals. Available at: https://www.jointcommission.org/-/media/deprecated-unorganized/imported-assets/tjc/system-folders/assetmanager/2015_hap_npsg_erpdf.pdf?db=web&hash=5EDBAF733CA6B7679B0B6DEA8165AD00.

The Joint Commission (2017). Hospital: National patient safety goals. Available at: https://www.jointcommission.org/-/media/tjc/documents/standards/national-patient-safety-goals/historical/2017_npsg_hap_erpdf.pdf?db=web&hash=08B0E173E6DB13140B6F719E5FB069FE.

6 Vital Signs

OBJECTIVES

After reading this chapter, the student should be able to:

- Explain the importance of vital signs and guidelines for measuring vital signs.
- Describe the principles and mechanisms of thermoregulation in human body.
- Discuss the factors affecting body temperature.
- Identify the common alterations in body temperature such as pyrexia, hyperthermia, and hypothermia.
- Accurately assess body temperature and understand the use of different types of thermometers.
- Explain the physiology of normal regulation of pulse and assessment of pulse.
- Discuss the use of stethoscope and character of pulse including rate, rhythm, strength, and equality.
- Describe the physiology of respiration and mechanism of breathing.
- Explain physiology of blood pressure and factors that cause variations/alteration in blood pressure.
- Describe the benefits and precautions in measurement of blood pressure.
- Identify acceptable ranges of vital sign values for an infant, a child, and an adult.
- Explain variations in technique used to assess an infant's, a child's, and an adult's vital signs.
- Accurately record and report vital sign measurements.

KEY TERMS

afebrile, p. 72
apnea, p. 82
auscultatory gap, p. 88
antipyretic, p. 73
basal metabolic rate (BMR), p. 70
blood pressure (BP), p. 83
body temperature, p. 69
bradycardia, p. 80
bradypnea, p. 82
capnography, p. 82
cardiac output, p. 78
chemical thermometers, p. 76
conduction, p. 70
convection, p. 70
core temperature, p. 69
diaphoresis, p. 71
diastolic pressure, p. 83
diffusion, p. 81
digital thermometer, p. 76
dysrhythmia, p. 80
electronic thermometers, p. 75
eupnea, p. 81
evaporation, p. 70
febrile, p. 72
fever, p. 72
frostbite, p. 74
heat exhaustion, p. 73
heat stroke, p. 73
hypertension, p. 84
hyperthermia, p. 73
hypotension, p. 85
hypothermia, p. 73
hypoxemia, p. 81
infrared thermometer, p. 75
korotkoff sound, p. 87
nonshivering thermogenesis, p. 70
orthostatic hypotension, p. 85
perfusion, p. 81
pulse, p. 77
pulse deficit, p. 80
pulse pressure, p. 84
pyrexia, p. 72
shivering, p. 70
sphygmomanometer, p. 86
stethoscope, p. 78
systolic pressure, p. 83
tachycardia, p. 80
tachynea, p. 82
vasoconstriction, p. 70
vasodilation, p. 70
ventilation, p. 81

INTRODUCTION

The most frequent and routine measurements obtained by health care providers are those of temperature, pulse, blood pressure (BP), respiratory rate, and oxygen saturation. As indicators of health status, these measures indicate the effectiveness of circulatory, respiratory, neural, and endocrine body functions. Because of their importance, they are referred to as **vital signs.** Pain, a subjective symptom, is often called another vital sign and is frequently measured with the others (see Chapter 11).

Measurement of vital signs provides data to determine a patient's usual state of health (baseline data). Many factors such as the temperature of the environment, the patient's physical exertion, and the effects of illness cause vital signs to change, sometimes outside an acceptable range. Assessment of vital signs provides data to identify nursing diagnoses, implement planned interventions, and evaluate outcomes of care. An alteration in vital signs signals a change in physiological function and the need for medical or nursing intervention.

Vital signs are a quick and efficient way of monitoring a patient's condition or identifying problems and evaluating his or her response to intervention. When you learn the physiological variables influencing vital signs and recognize the relationship of their changes to one another and to other physical assessment findings, you can make precise determinations about a patient's health problems. Vital signs and other physiological measurements are the basis for clinical decision-making and problem-solving. Many facilities adopt early warning scores determined by vital sign data entered into the electronic medical record to alert nurses to potential changes in their patients' conditions.

GUIDELINES FOR MEASURING VITAL SIGNS

A complete set of vital signs is included in a complete physical examination (see Chapter 7). Sometimes, you take vital signs individually to assess a patient's condition. Likewise, a patient's needs and conditions determine when, where, how, and by whom vital signs are measured. Correctly obtaining vital signs, interpreting values, implementing interventions, communicating findings to health care team members appropriately, and recognizing the need for reevaluation are essential nursing skills. Use the following guidelines to help incorporate vital sign measurements into your nursing practice:

1. Measuring vital signs is your responsibility. You may delegate this task in certain situations (e.g., stable patients) to nursing assistive personnel (NAP) (Box 6.1). However, it is your responsibility as the nurse to review vital sign data, interpret their significance, and critically think through decisions regarding implementing appropriate nursing interventions.
2. Assess equipment to ensure that it is working correctly and provides accurate findings.
3. Select equipment based on a patient's condition and physical characteristics (e.g., for a patient who is overweight, use an extra-large size BP cuff rather than an adult size).
4. Vital sign measurements can require removing clothing or exposing areas. Provide patient privacy while being sensitive to cultural norms when measuring vital signs.
5. Know your patient's normal vital sign range. A patient's usual values sometimes differ from the standard range because of age, illness, or physical state. Use a patient's usual values as a baseline comparison.
6. Know a patient's medical history, prescribed medications, therapies, and treatments; these factors can significantly cause vital sign changes.
7. Control or minimize environmental factors that affect vital signs. A patient's respiratory rate taken immediately after exercising does not provide accurate data or a true picture of the patient's condition. Likewise, a patient's temperature taken directly after bathing does not represent an accurate picture of thermoregulation.
8. Use an organized, systematic approach when measuring vital signs.
9. Based on a patient's condition, collaborate with the health care provider to decide the frequency of vital sign assessment. In the hospital, the health care provider orders a minimum frequency of vital sign measurements for each patient. After surgery, treatment intervention, or invasive diagnostic procedures, you obtain vital signs frequently to detect complications. If a patient's physical condition worsens, it is often necessary oto monitor vital signs every 5–10 minutes. You also measure vital signs before, during, and after medication administration. For example, a health care provider may order to hold a cardiac medication for a heart rate (HR) less than 50 beats/min or a systolic blood pressure (SBP) less than 100 mm Hg. Vital sign assessment is also performed when a patient seeks care from a health care provider in the community. Wherever vital signs are measured, you are responsible for judging whether a patient needs more frequent assessments (Box 6.1).
10. Analyze the results of vital sign measurement based on a patient's condition and past medical history (PMH).
11. Verify and communicate significant changes in vital signs. Baseline measurements provide a starting point for identifying and accurately interpreting possible changes. When vital signs appear abnormal, have another nurse repeat the measurement. Inform the charge nurse or health care provider of abnormal vital signs immediately, document findings in your patient's record, and report vital sign changes to nurses during hand-off communications.

BOX 6.1 When to Measure Vital Signs

- On admission to a health care agency
- When assessing patients during home care visits
- In a hospital on a routine schedule according to a health care provider's order or standards of practice
- Before, during, and after a surgical procedure or invasive diagnostic procedure
- Before, during, and after transfusion of blood products
- Before, during, and after administration of medications or applications of therapies that affect cardiovascular, respiratory, or temperature-control functions
- When a patient's general physical condition changes (e.g., loss of consciousness or increased intensity of pain)
- Before, during, and after nursing interventions influencing a vital sign (e.g., before and after a patient currently on bed rest ambulates, before and after a patient performs range-of-motion exercises)
- When a patient reports nonspecific symptoms of physical distress (e.g., feeling "funny" or "different")

BODY TEMPERATURE

Body temperature is the difference between the amount of heat produced by body processes and the amount of heat lost to the external environment.

$$\text{Heat produced} - \text{Heat lost} = \text{Body temperature}$$

Despite environmental temperature extremes and physical activity, temperature-control mechanisms of human beings keep body **core temperature,** or temperature of deep tissues, relatively constant during sleep, exposure to cold, and strenuous exercise. However, surface temperature fluctuates, depending on blood flow to the skin and the amount of heat lost to the external environment. Bodily tissues and cells function efficiently within a relatively narrow temperature range, from 36°C to 38°C (96.8°F to 100.4°F), but no single temperature is normal for all people. For healthy young adults, the average oral temperature is 37°C (98.6°F). In older adults, the average core temperature ranges from 35°C to 36.1°C (95°F to 97°F) as a result of decreased immunity. The circadian rhythm also affects body temperature, with the lowest body temperature at 6 a.m. and the highest at 4 p.m. in healthy people. The circadian rhythm alters body temperature about 0.5°C (0.9°F) throughout each day. An acceptable temperature range for adults depends on age, sex, range of physical activity, and state of health.

Temperatures vary depending on the measurement site. Sites reflecting core temperature such as the pulmonary artery are more reliable indicators of body temperature than sites reflecting surface temperature such as the armpit or axilla. Pulmonary artery temperature monitoring, used in critically ill patients, offers accurate readings because of the blood mix from all regions of the body.

PHYSIOLOGY AND REGULATION OF BODY TEMPERATURE

Physiological and behavioral mechanisms precisely regulate and control body temperature mechanisms (**thermoregulation**). For the body temperature to stay constant and within an acceptable range, the body needs to maintain the relationship between heat production and heat loss.

Neural and Vascular Control

The hypothalamus, located between the cerebral hemispheres of the brain and below the thalamus, controls body temperature by attempting to maintain a comfortable temperature or set point. When the hypothalamus senses an increase in body temperature, it sends out impulses for the release of hormones to reduce body temperature by sweating and **vasodilation** (widening of blood vessels). Vasodilation increases blood flow to the skin, which enables heat loss through radiation. If the hypothalamus senses that body temperature is lower than the set point, it triggers hormone release to increase heat production by muscle shivering or heat conservation by **vasoconstriction** (narrowing of surface blood vessels). Disease or trauma to the hypothalamus or spinal cord, which carries hypothalamic messages, decreases the ability of the body to control body temperature.

Heat Production

Temperature regulation depends on normal heat production processes. Heat produced by the body is a by-product of metabolism, which is the chemical reaction in all body cells. Food is the primary fuel source for metabolism. Activities requiring additional chemical reactions increase the metabolic rate. As metabolism increases, additional heat is produced. When metabolism decreases, less heat is produced. Heat production occurs during rest, voluntary movements, involuntary shivering, and nonshivering thermogenesis.

- Basal metabolism accounts for the heat produced by the body at absolute rest. The average **basal metabolic rate (BMR)** depends on the body surface area. Thyroid hormones also affect the BMR. By promoting the breakdown of body glucose and fat, thyroid hormones increase the rate of chemical reactions in almost all cells of the body. When large amounts of thyroid hormones are secreted, the BMR can increase 100% above normal. The absence of thyroid hormones reduces the BMR by half, causing a decrease in heat production. The male sex hormone testosterone increases BMR. Men have a higher BMR than women.
- Voluntary movements such as muscular activity during exercise require additional energy. The metabolic rate increases during activity, sometimes causing heat production to increase up to 50 times normal.
- **Shivering** is an involuntary body response to temperature differences in the body. The skeletal muscle movement during shivering requires significant energy. Shivering sometimes increases heat production four to five times more than normal. The heat that is produced helps equalize the body temperature, and the shivering ceases. In vulnerable patients, shivering seriously drains energy sources, resulting in further physiological deterioration.
- **Nonshivering thermogenesis** occurs primarily in neonates. Because neonates cannot shiver, a limited amount of vascular brown tissue, present at birth, is metabolized for heat production.

Heat Loss

Heat loss and production occur at the same time. The exposure of the skin to the environment results in constant, normal heat loss through radiation, conduction, convection, and evaporation. Infants and young children have a greater ratio of surface area to body weight; thus, they lose more heat to the environment than adults.

- **Radiation:** Radiation is the transfer of heat between two objects without physical contact. Heat radiates from the skin to any surrounding cooler object.
  - Up to 85% of the surface area of the human body radiate heat to the environment.
  - During surgery, patients often lose excessive amounts of heat in the cool environment of the operating room; thus, you need to closely monitor your patient's temperature during and after surgery.
- **Conduction:** A small amount of heat loss occurs through conduction, which is the transfer of heat from one object to another with direct contact.
  - When warm skin touches a cooler object, heat transfers from the skin to the object until temperatures equalize.
  - In patients with fevers, heat loss increases with the application of ice packs or bathing with tepid water. Applying several layers of clothing reduces conductive loss.
  - The body gains heat by conduction when it contacts materials warmer than skin temperature such as prewarmed blankets.
- **Convection:** Convection is the transfer of heat away from the body by air movement.
  - Fans promote heat loss through convection. The rate of heat loss increases when moist skin comes into contact with slightly moving air.
- **Evaporation:** Heat energy transfers from a liquid to a gas state by evaporation.
  - The body continuously loses heat by evaporation; approximately 600–900 mL of water evaporates daily from the skin and lungs.

- The body promotes additional evaporative heat loss through perspiration or sweating. **Diaphoresis** (i.e., excessive sweating) drastically lowers body temperature and typically manifests on the forehead, upper chest, and arms.

Role of Skin in Temperature Regulation

Skin, subcutaneous tissue, and fat help to maintain body temperature through insulation. Therefore, people with more body fat have more natural insulation than slim or muscular individuals. The skin, or integumentary system (along with neural control), regulates body temperature similar to the way a car radiator controls engine temperature. The car engine generates a great deal of heat. Water pumps through the engine to collect the heat and carry it to the radiator, where a fan transfers the heat from the water to the outside air. The internal organs of the body produce heat, and during exercise or increased sympathetic stimulation the amount of heat produced is more than the usual core temperature. Blood flows from the internal organs, carrying heat to the body surface. At the surface, blood passing through the vascular areas of the hands and feet varies from minimal flow to 30% of the blood pumped from the heart. Heat transfers from the blood through vessel walls to the surface of the skin and is lost to the environment through heat-loss mechanisms.

Behavioral Control

When the environmental temperature falls, a person adds clothing, moves to a warmer place, raises the thermostat setting on a furnace, increases muscular activity by running in place, or sits with arms and legs tightly wrapped together. In contrast, when the temperature becomes hot, a person removes clothing, stops activity, turns on a fan or lowers the thermostat setting on an air conditioner, seeks a cooler place, or takes a cool shower.

FACTORS AFFECTING BODY TEMPERATURE

Many factors affect body temperature. Changes in body temperature within an acceptable range occur when physiological or behavioral mechanisms alter the relationship between heat production and heat loss. Be aware of these factors when assessing temperature variations and evaluating deviations from normal.

Age

At birth, the newborn leaves a warm, relatively constant environment and enters one in which temperatures fluctuate widely. Temperature-control mechanisms are immature. An infant's temperature responds drastically to changes in the environment. Take extra care to protect newborns from environmental temperatures. Provide adequate clothing and avoid exposing infants to temperature extremes. A newborn loses up to 30% of body heat through the head and therefore needs to wear a cap to prevent heat loss. When protected from environmental extremes, the newborn's body temperature is usually within 35.5–37.5°C (95.9–99.5°F).

Temperature regulation is unstable until children reach puberty. The usual temperature range gradually drops as individuals approach older adulthood. The older adult has a narrower range of body temperatures than the younger adult. Oral temperatures of 35°C (95°F) are sometimes found in older adults in cold weather. However, the average body temperature of older adults is approximately 35–36.1°C (95–97°F). Older adults are particularly sensitive to temperature extremes because of deterioration in control mechanisms, particularly poor vasomotor control (control of vasoconstriction and vasodilation), reduced amounts of subcutaneous tissue, reduced sweat gland activity, and reduced metabolism.

Exercise

Muscle activity requires an increased blood supply and carbohydrate and fat breakdown. Any form of exercise increases metabolism and heat production and thus body temperature. Prolonged strenuous exercise such as long-distance running temporarily raises body temperature.

Hormone Level

Women generally experience greater fluctuations in body temperature than men. Hormonal variations during the menstrual cycle cause body temperature fluctuations. Progesterone levels rise and fall cyclically during the menstrual cycle. When progesterone levels are low, the body temperature is a few tenths of a degree below the baseline level. The lower temperature persists until ovulation occurs. During ovulation, greater amounts of progesterone enter the circulatory system and raise the body temperature to previous baseline levels or higher. These temperature variations help to predict a woman's most fertile time to achieve pregnancy.

Body temperature changes also occur in women during menopause (cessation of menstruation). Women who have stopped menstruating often experience periods of intense body heat and sweating lasting from 30 seconds to 5 minutes. During these periods, often intermittent skin temperature increases up to 4°C (7.2°F), referred to as hot flashes. This is caused by the instability of the vasomotor controls for vasodilation and vasoconstriction.

Circadian Rhythm

Body temperature normally changes 0.5–1°C (0.9–1.8°F) during a 24-hour period. However, temperature is one of the most stable rhythms in humans. The temperature is usually lowest between 1:00 and 4:00 a.m.(Fig. 6.1). During the day, body temperature rises steadily to a maximum temperature value at about 4:00 p.m. and then declines to early-morning levels. Temperature patterns are not automatically reversed in people who work at night and sleep during the day. It takes 1–3 weeks for the cycle to reverse. In general, the circadian temperature rhythm does not change with age.

Stress

Physical and emotional stress increase body temperature through hormonal and neural stimulation. These physiological changes increase metabolism, which increases heat production. A patient who is anxious about entering a

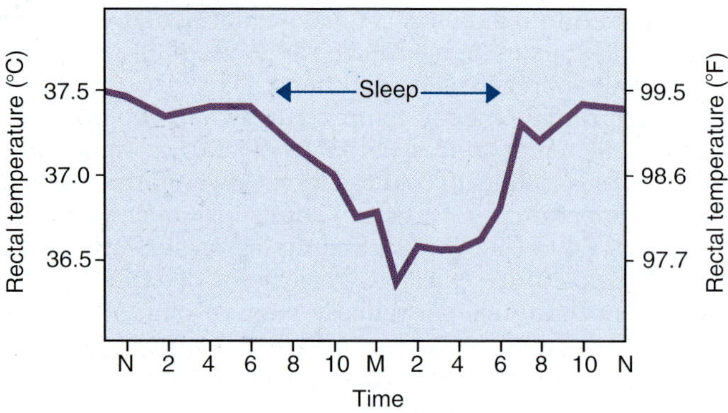

Fig. 6.1 Temperature cycle for 24 hours.

hospital or a health care provider's office often has a higher normal temperature.

Environment

Environment influences body temperature. When placed in a warm room, a patient may be unable to regulate body temperature by heat-loss mechanisms, and the body temperature may elevate. If the patient is outside in the cold without warm clothing, body temperature may be low as a result of extensive radiant and conductive heat loss. Environmental temperatures affect infants and older adults more often because their temperature-regulating mechanisms are less efficient.

TEMPERATURE ALTERATIONS

Body temperature changes are related to excess heat production, heat loss, too little heat production, or any combination of these alterations. The nature of the change affects the type of clinical problems experienced by a patient.

Fever

The condition of **pyrexia** or **fever** occurs because heat-loss mechanisms are unable to keep pace with excess heat production, resulting in an abnormal rise in body temperature. A fever is usually not harmful if it stays below 39°C (102.2°F) in adults or 40°C (104°F) in children. A single temperature reading does not always indicate a fever and often results from outside influences such as a recent increase in physical activity or environmental changes. You determine your patient's fever by taking several temperature readings at different times during the day and comparing them with the patient's usual values.

A true fever results from an alteration in the hypothalamic set point. Substances that trigger the immune system such as bacteria or viruses stimulate the release of hormones in an effort to promote bodily defense against infection. These hormones also trigger the hypothalamus to raise the set point, inducing a **febrile** episode. To reach the new set point, the body produces and conserves heat. The patient experiences chills, shivers, and feels cold, even though the body temperature is rising. If the set point has been "overshot" or if the immune triggers are removed, the skin becomes warm and flushed because of vasodilation. Diaphoresis results in evaporative heat loss. When a fever "breaks," the temperature returns to an acceptable range, and the patient becomes **afebrile.** A fever pattern is present when a febrile episode recurs (Table 6.1).

Table 6.1 Patterns of Fever

Sustained	Constant body temperature continuously more than 38°C (100.4°F) that demonstrates little fluctuation
Intermittent	Fever spikes mixed with usual temperature levels; temperature returns to acceptable value at least once in 24 h
Remittent	Fever spikes and falls without a return to acceptable temperature levels
Relapsing	Periods of febrile episodes mixed with acceptable temperature values; febrile episodes and periods of normothermia sometimes last longer than 24 h

Fever serves as an important defense mechanism. Health care providers are unlikely to treat an adult's fever until it is more than 39°C (102.2°F). Mild temperature elevations enhance the immune system of the body by stimulating white blood cell production. Increased temperature reduces the concentration of iron in the blood plasma, causing bacterial growth to slow. Fever also fights viral infections by stimulating interferon, the natural virus-fighting substance of the body.

Fevers also serve a diagnostic purpose. Fever patterns differ, depending on the causative pyrogen (i.e., the substance such as bacteria that cause the fever). The duration and degree of fever depend on the strength of the pyrogen and the ability of the individual to respond. The term *fever of unknown origin (FUO)* refers to a fever for which the cause cannot be determined.

Treatment for a fever depends on its cause; adverse effects; and strength, intensity, and duration of the elevated temperature. You play a key role in assessing fever and implementing temperature-reducing strategies (Box 6.2). The goal is a "safe" rather than a "low" temperature. Health care providers determine the cause of fever by isolating the causative bacterium or virus by obtaining culture specimens such as urine, blood, sputum, and wound drainage for laboratory analysis. If the culture is bacterial in origin, the health care provider orders antibiotics to be given to effectively destroy bacteria and eliminate the stimulus for fever.

Most fevers in children are of viral origin, last only briefly, and have limited effects. However, children have immature temperature-control mechanisms; therefore, temperatures sometimes rise rapidly. Dehydration and febrile seizures occur during rising temperatures in children between the age of 6 months and 3 years. Febrile seizures are unusual in children older than 5 years. The extent of the temperature change, often exceeding 38.8°C (102°F), seems to be a more important factor than the rapidity of the temperature increase. Interventions for children's fevers are based on their response to the illness and not on the temperature level itself.

Sometimes, a fever results from a hypersensitivity response to a medication, especially when the medication is taken for the first time. These fevers are often accompanied by other allergy symptoms such as rash, hives, or itching. Treatment involves stopping the medication responsible for the reaction.

The objective of fever therapy is to increase heat loss, reduce heat production, and prevent complications. Nondrug therapies (see Box 6.2) for fever increase heat loss by

BOX 6.2 Nursing Management of Patients With Fever

Assessment

- Obtain frequent temperature readings (i.e., tympanic, oral, rectal) during a fever.
- Assess for contributing factors such as dehydration, infection, or environmental temperature.
- Obtain all vital signs.
- Identify physiological response to fever (e.g., diaphoresis, tachycardia, hypotension).
- Assess skin color and temperature and presence of thirst, anorexia, and malaise; observe for shivering and diaphoresis.
- Assess patient comfort and well-being.

Interventions (Unless Contraindicated)

- Before antibiotic therapy, obtain blood cultures when ordered (see Chapter 9). Obtain blood specimens at the same time as a temperature spike, when the causative organism is most prevalent.
- Minimize heat production: reduce frequency of activities that increase oxygen demand such as excessive turning and ambulation; allow rest periods; limit physical activity.
- Maximize heat loss: reduce external covering on patient's body without causing shivering; keep clothing and bed linen dry.
- Satisfy requirements for increased metabolic rate: provide supplemental oxygen therapy as ordered to improve oxygen delivery to body cells; provide measures to stimulate appetite, and offer well-balanced meals; provide fluids (at least 3 L/day for a patient with normal cardiac and renal function) to replace fluids lost through insensible water loss and sweating.
- Promote patient comfort: encourage oral hygiene because oral mucous membranes dry easily from dehydration and have increased potential for bacterial invasion; control temperature of environment without inducing shivering; apply cool, damp cloth to patient's forehead.
- Identify onset and duration of febrile episode phases: examine previous temperature measurements for trends.
- Initiate health teaching as indicated.
- Maintain environmental temperature at 21−27°C (70−80°F).

evaporation, conduction, convection, or radiation. Use caution when implementing nursing interventions and think about heat production and heat-loss mechanisms. For example, when using nursing interventions to enhance body cooling, make sure to avoid stimulating shivering. Shivering is counterproductive because of the heat produced by muscle activity. Physical cooling, including regulating room temperature and using fans (as appropriate) and water-cooled blankets, is appropriate when a patient's own thermoregulation fails or in patients with neurological damage (e.g., spinal cord injury).

An **antipyretic** is a medication that reduces fever. Nonsteroidal drugs such as acetaminophen, salicylates, indomethacin, ibuprofen, and ketorolac reduce fever by increasing heat loss. Health care providers order antipyretics if a fever is more than 39°C (102.2°F). Although not used to treat fever, corticosteroids reduce heat production by interfering with the hypothalamic response. It is important to note that these drugs mask signs of infection by suppressing the immune system. Therefore, patients on steroids need to be observed closely, especially if they are at risk for infection.

Hyperthermia

Hyperthermia is an elevated body temperature related to the inability of the body to promote heat loss or reduce heat production. Fever is an upward shift in the set point, whereas hyperthermia is caused by an overload on the temperature release mechanisms. Any injury to the hypothalamus impairs heat-loss mechanisms. Educate patients at risk for hyperthermia to:

- Avoid strenuous exercise in hot, humid weather.
- Avoid exercising in areas with poor ventilation.
- Drink fluids such as water and clear fruit juices before, during, and after exercise.
- Wear light, loose-fitting, light-colored clothing.
- Wear a protective covering over the head when outdoors.
- Expose themselves to hot climates gradually.

Prolonged exposure to the sun or high environmental temperatures overwhelms the heat-loss mechanisms of the body. Heat also depresses hypothalamic function. These conditions cause **heat stroke,** which is a dangerous heat emergency defined as a body temperature of 40.2°C (104.4°F) or more. Exertional heat stroke is a common cause of death in competitive athletes. Signs and symptoms of heat stroke include giddiness, confusion, delirium, excess thirst, nausea, muscle cramps, visual disturbances, and incontinence. The most important sign of heat stroke is hot, dry skin. Heat stroke can be fatal. Call for emergency assistance as you begin cooling the person using the following methods:

- Move the person out of the sun to the shade or a shelter.
- Cool water immersion is the most rapid means. Ways to cool include placing wet towels over the skin, spraying the person with cool water from a garden hose, and placing oscillating fans in the room.
- If the person can drink, give cool nonalcoholic liquids.
- Continue to take the temperature until it drops to 38.3−38.8°C (101−102°F).

Emergency medical treatment includes applying hypothermia blankets, giving i.v. fluids, and irrigating the stomach and lower bowel with cool solutions.

Heat Exhaustion

Heat exhaustion occurs when profuse diaphoresis results in excess water and electrolyte loss. Caused by environmental heat exposure, a patient exhibits signs and symptoms of deficient fluid volume. First aid includes transporting him or her to a cooler environment and restoring fluid and electrolyte balance.

Hypothermia

Heat loss during prolonged exposure to cold overwhelms the ability of the body to produce heat, causing **hypothermia.** Hypothermia is classified by core temperature measurements as mild, moderate, or severe (Table 6.2). Accidental hypothermia occurs when a person is exposed to a cold environment without protective clothing. Accidental hypothermia usually develops gradually and may go unnoticed for several hours.

Table 6.2 Classification of Hypothermia

Hypothermia	°C	°F
Mild	34–36	93.2–96.8
Moderate	30–34	86–93.2
Severe	Less than 30	Less than 86

The patient experiences uncontrolled shivering, loss of memory, depression, and poor judgment. As the body temperature falls below 34°C (93.2°F), heart and respiratory rates and BP decrease. Intentional hypothermia is a therapeutic approach that reduces the body's need for oxygenated blood. Intentional hypothermia can preserve vital organs during prolonged neurological or cardiac surgery and following a cardiac arrest.

Frostbite occurs when the body is exposed to subnormal temperatures. Ice crystals form inside the cells, and permanent circulatory and tissue damage occurs. Areas particularly susceptible to frostbite are the earlobes, tip of the nose, and fingers and toes. The injured area becomes white, waxy, and firm to the touch. The patient loses sensation in the affected area. Interventions include gradual warming measures, analgesia, and protection of the injured tissue.

The priority treatment for intentional or accidental hypothermia is prevention of a further decrease in body temperature. Removing wet clothes, replacing them with dry ones, and wrapping the patient in blankets are key nursing interventions. In emergencies, when a patient is not in a health care setting, place the patient under blankets next to a warm person, usually skin to skin, for heat conduction. A conscious patient benefits from drinking hot liquids such as soup while avoiding alcohol and caffeinated fluids. Interventions include keeping the head covered, increasing room temperature, or using forced-air warming systems. The cause and severity of the hypothermia dictate the treatments implemented.

Prevention is the key for patients at risk for hypothermia. Provide education to patients, family caregivers, and friends. People at high risk include the very young; the very old; and people debilitated by trauma, stroke, diabetes, drug or alcohol intoxication, and sepsis. Patients with mental illness or handicaps and older adults are at risk for developing hypothermia because they are unaware of the dangers of cold conditions. People without adequate home heating, shelter, diet, or clothing are also at risk.

ASSESSMENT OF BODY TEMPERATURE

Assessment of body temperature regulation requires you to make judgments about the site for temperature measurement, type of device, and frequency of measurement.

Sites

Measure body temperature by using core or body surface sites. The core temperatures of the pulmonary artery, esophagus, and urinary bladder are often used in critical care settings and require continuous invasive monitoring devices placed in arteries or internal organs. The most common sites for intermittent temperature measurements are surface sites such as the tympanic membrane, temporal artery, mouth, rectum, and axilla. Skin temperature obtained by applying noninvasive, chemically prepared thermometer patches to the skin are used for screening a patient's temperature. Core temperature measurement sites are more reliable than surface or skin temperature measurement sites.

To ensure accurate temperature readings, measure each site correctly (see Skill 6.1). Depending on the site used, temperatures normally vary between 36°C (96.8°F) and 38°C (100.4°F). Rectal temperatures are usually 0.5°C (0.9°F) higher than oral temperatures, whereas tympanic and axillary temperatures are usually 0.5°C (0.9°F) lower than oral temperatures. Each temperature measurement site has advantages and disadvantages (Table 6.3). Choose

Table 6.3 Advantages and Limitations of Select Temperature Measurement Sites

Site Advantages	Site Limitations
ORAL	
Easily accessible—requires no position change	Causes delay in measurement if patient recently ingested hot/cold fluids or foods, smoked, or chewed gum
Comfortable for patient	Not used with patients who have had oral surgery, trauma, shaking or chills, or history of seizures
Provides accurate surface temperature reading	Not used with infants; small children; or confused, unconscious, or uncooperative patients
Reflects rapid change in core temperature	Risk for body fluid exposure
Reliable route to measure temperature for intubated patients	
TYMPANIC MEMBRANE	
Easily accessible site	Susceptible to user error
Obtained without disturbing, waking, or repositioning patient	Has low sensitivity for detecting fever compared with standard core temperature measurement methods (i.e., rectal, bladder)
Used for patients with tachypnea without affecting breathing	Requires removal of hearing aids before measurement
Rapid measurement (2−5 s)	Requires disposable sensor cover with only one size available
Unaffected by oral intake of food or fluids or by smoking	Otitis media and cerumen impaction distort readings
Shown to have high precision, sensitivity and specificity (accuracy) in measuring body temperature and a high correlation with nasopharyngeal temperature (Asadian et al., 2016)	Not used with patients who have had surgery of the ear or tympanic membrane
	Does not accurately measure core temperature changes during and after exercise
	Affected by ambient temperature devices such as incubators, radiant warmers, and facial fans
	Anatomy of ear canal makes it difficult to position correctly in neonates, infants, and children younger than 3 years

Table 6.3 Advantages and Limitations of Select Temperature Measurement Sites—cont'd

Advantages	Limitations
RECTAL	
Considered gold standard for estimating core temperature Argued to be more reliable than alternative sites when oral temperature is difficult or impossible to obtain	Lags behind core temperature during rapid temperature changes Not used for patients with diarrhea or patients who have had rectal surgery, rectal disorders, bleeding tendencies, or neutropenia Requires positioning and is a source of patient embarrassment and anxiety Risk for body fluid exposure; thermometer can serve as reservoir for *Clostridium difficile* (CDC, 2015). Requires lubrication Not used for routine vital signs in newborns Readings sometimes influenced by impacted stool
AXILLA	
Safe and inexpensive Recommended only for screening Reliable in stable and preterm infants (Charafeddine et al., 2014)	Long measurement time Requires continuous positioning Poorly reflects core temperature (Reynolds et al., 2014) Measurement lags behind core temperature during rapid temperature changes Not recommended to detect fever in infants and young children Requires exposure of thorax, which results in temperature loss, especially in newborns
SKIN	
Inexpensive Provides continuous reading Safe and noninvasive Used for neonates	Lags behind measurements obtained at other sites during temperature changes, especially during hyperthermia Diaphoresis or sweat impairs adhesion Affected by environmental temperature Cannot be used on patients with adhesive allergy
TEMPORAL ARTERY	
Easy to access without position change Useful for screening body temperature Very rapid measurement No risk for injury to patient or nurse Eliminates need to disrobe or unbundle Comfortable for patient Can be used in premature infants, newborns, and children (Reynolds et al., 2014) Reflects rapid change in core temperature Sensor cover not required	Inaccurate with head covering or hair on forehead Affected by skin moisture such as diaphoresis or sweating Underestimates temperature in patients with fever (Furlong et al., 2015)

the safest and most accurate site for each patient. Use the same site when repeating measurements.

Thermometers

Four types of thermometers are commonly available for measuring body temperature: electronic, infrared, digital, and disposable chemical dot. Mercury-in-glass thermometers are obsolete in the health care setting because of the environmental hazards of mercury. However, some patients may still use mercury-in-glass thermometers at ome. If you find a mercury-in-glass thermometer in the home, teach the patient about safer temperature devices and encourage appropriate disposal of the hazardous device.

Each device measures temperature in either the Celsius or the Fahrenheit scale. Electronic thermometers allow you to convert scales by activating a switch. Use the following formulas for manual conversion:

To convert Fahrenheit to Celsius, subtract 32 from the Fahrenheit reading and multiply the result by 5/9.

$$\text{Example: } (104° - 32°\text{F}) \times \tfrac{5}{9} = 40°\text{C}$$

To convert Celsius to Fahrenheit, multiply the Celsius reading by 9/5 and add 32 to the product.

Electronic Thermometers

Electronic thermometers have a rechargeable battery-powered display unit, a thin wire cord, and a temperature-processing probe or sensor covered by a disposable probe cover (Fig. 6.2). Separate probes are available for oral (blue tip) and rectal (red tip) use. You obtain axillary temperatures with the oral probe. Electronic thermometers provide two modes of operation, 4-second predictive temperatures and 3-minute standard temperatures. In daily clinical situations, the 4-second predictive is more commonly used.

Infrared Thermometer

An **infrared thermometer** relies on thermal radiation to measure body temperature. The tympanic membrane thermometer has an otoscope-like speculum with an infrared sensor tip that detects heat radiated from the tympanic membrane of the ear (Fig. 6.3). Within seconds after placement in the ear canal and pressing the scan button, a sound signals when the peak temperature has been measured, and a reading appears on the display unit. The temporal artery thermometer measures blood flow through the superficial temporal artery. Proper technique involves sweeping an infrared handheld scanner across the forehead then

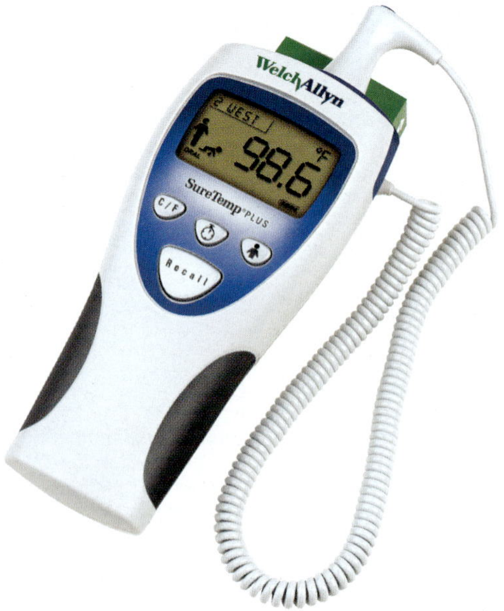

Fig. 6.2 Electronic thermometer with disposable plastic probe cover. (Courtesy Welch Allyn.)

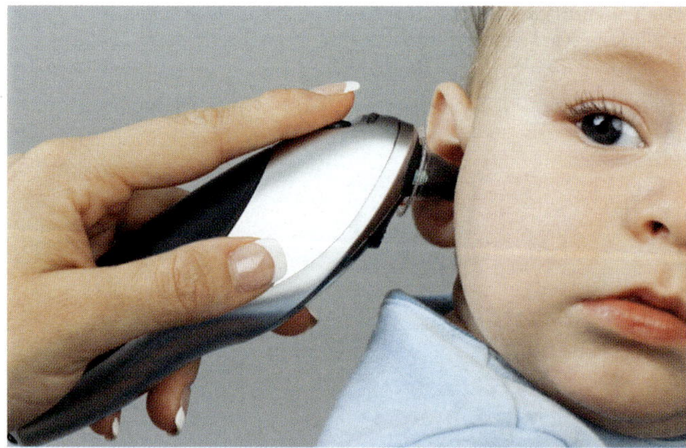

Fig. 6.3 Tympanic membrane thermometer. (Courtesy Welch Allyn.)

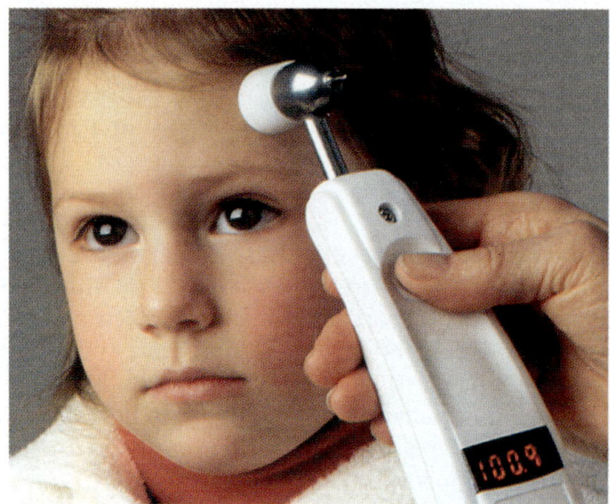

Fig. 6.4 Temporal artery thermometer scanning forehead.

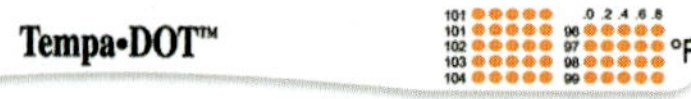

Fig. 6.5 Disposable, single-use thermometer strip. (© Medical Indicators, Inc.)

just behind the ear (Fig. 6.4). After scanning is complete, a reading appears on the display unit.

Digital Thermometer

A **digital thermometer** contains a probe connected to a microprocessor chip, which translates signals into degrees and sends a temperature measurement to a digital display. You use a digital thermometer for oral, rectal, and axillary measurements. The rectal temperature is still the gold standard for estimating core body temperature, but the thermometer is difficult to use in older adults.

Chemical Thermometers

Single-use or reusable **chemical thermometers** are thin strips of plastic with a temperature sensor on one end (Fig. 6.5). The sensor consists of chemically impregnated dots that change color at different temperatures. The Celsius version has 50 dots, each representing temperature increments of 0.1°C over a range of 35.5−40.4°C. The Fahrenheit version has 45 dots with increments of 0.2°F over a range of 96−104.8°F. Chemicals on the thermometer change color to reflect temperature reading, 3 minutes for axilla and 1 minute for oral. Single-use chemical thermometers are useful in caring for patients in emergency departments or in protective isolation and screening temperatures, especially in infants and young children. You need to confirm readings with electronic thermometers when making treatment decisions.

Another form of disposable chemical thermometer is a temperature-sensitive patch or tape. Applied to the forehead or abdomen, temperature-sensitive areas of the patch change color at different temperatures. Home disposable thermometers are useful for temperature screening but are not as accurate as nondisposable electronic thermometers.

Thermal Scanners

New viral diseases caused by coronavirus including COVID-19 are highly contagious in nature and therefore requires temperature measurement with a device without touching the patients' body to prevent the infection transmission, which can be accomplished by use of thermal scanners. The infrared thermal scanners are noninvasive, speedy, cost-effective, and fairly accurate device for individual and mass temperature screening for coronavirus-infected individuals.

In addition, the mass screening device infrared thermography provides a digital image showing temperature patterns. This device was originally used for the identification of inflammation and nerve abnormalities. The accuracy in temperature measurement by this device may be affected by human, environmental, and equipment factors.

Furthermore, it is fact that these thermal scanners measure only skin temperature but not the core body temperature. Therefore, if an individual is exposed to the extreme temperature before taking temperature, these scanners may provide inaccurate readings. The raised body temperature is a common clinical manifestation in many diseases including infectious diseases and thermal scanners can be used as important devices for mass screening of body temperature during infectious disease outbreaks in public.

PULSE

The **pulse** represents the number of cardiac cycles per minute and is the palpable rhythm of blood flow in a peripheral artery. The ejection of blood from the left ventricle during systole enters the aorta after passing through the aortic valve. The ejected blood moves through the major and peripheral arteries (e.g., in the wrist); thus, it feels like a tap when you lightly palpate the artery against underlying bone or muscle. The number of pulsing sensations occurring in 1 minute is the pulse rate. An adult's normal HR ranges from 60 to 100 beats/min. In children, the average HR is significantly increased and varies by age.

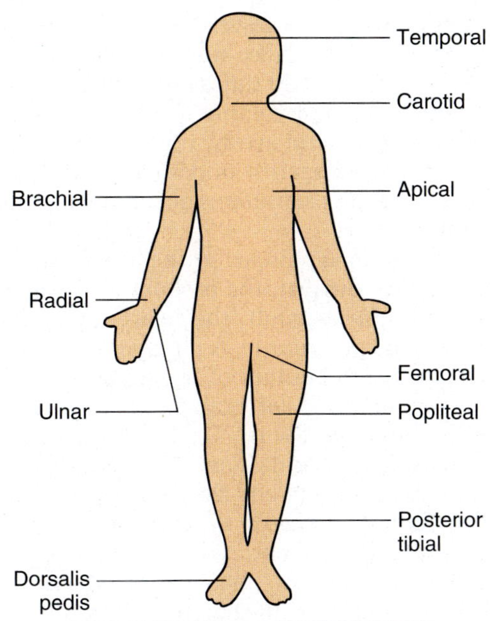

Fig. 6.6 Location of peripheral pulses.

Locating a Peripheral Pulse

You assess any accessible artery for pulse rate (Fig. 6.6); however, the radial and apical locations are the most common sites for pulse rate assessment because each is easy to locate and palpate. When a patient's condition deteriorates suddenly, use the carotid site to quickly locate a pulse. Use the radial or carotid pulse when teaching patients how to monitor their own HRs (e.g., athletes or patients using heart medications). If the radial pulse is abnormal, difficult to palpate, or inaccessible because of a dressing or cast, assess the apical pulse for 1 minute. When a patient takes medication that affects the HR, the apical pulse provides a more accurate assessment. Table 6.4 summarizes pulse sites and criteria for measurement. See Skill 6.2, which outlines radial and apical pulse rate assessment.

PHYSIOLOGY AND REGULATION OF PULSE

Electrical impulses originating from the sinoatrial (SA) node travel through heart muscle to stimulate cardiac contraction. Approximately 60–70 mL of blood enters the aorta with each ventricular contraction (stroke volume [SV]). With each SV ejection, the walls of the aorta distend,

Table 6.4 Pulse Sites

Site	Location	Assessment Criteria
Temporal	Over temporal bone of head, above and lateral to eye	Easily accessible site used to assess pulse in children
Carotid	Along medial edge of sternocleidomastoid muscle in neck	Easily accessible site used in patients with physiological shock or during adult CPR when other sites are not palpable
Apical	Fifth intercostal space at left midclavicular line	Site used to auscultate for apical pulse
Brachial	Groove between biceps and triceps muscles at antecubital fossa	Site used to assess upper extremity blood pressure; used during infant CPR
Radial	Radial or thumb side of forearm at wrist	Common site used to assess character of pulse peripherally; assesses status of circulation to hand
Ulnar	Ulnar side of forearm at wrist	Site used to assess status of circulation to ulnar side of hand; used to perform Allen test
Femoral	Below inguinal ligament, midway between symphysis pubis and anterior superior iliac spine	Site used to assess character of pulse in patients with physiological shock or during CPR when other pulses are not palpable; assesses status of circulation to leg
Popliteal	Behind knee in popliteal fossa	Site used to auscultate lower extremity blood pressure; assesses status of circulation to lower leg
Posterior tibial	Inner side of ankle, below medial malleolus	Site used to assess status of circulation to foot
Dorsalis pedis	Along top of foot, between extension tendons of great and first toe	Site used to assess status of circulation to foot

CPR, cardiopulmonary resuscitation.

creating a pulse wave that travels rapidly toward the distal ends of the arteries. The pulse wave moves 15 times faster through the aorta and 100 times faster through the small arteries than the ejected volume of blood. When a pulse wave reaches a peripheral artery, you can feel it by palpating the artery lightly against underlying bone or muscle. The number of pulsing sensations occurring in 1 minute is the pulse rate.

The volume of blood pumped by the heart during 1 minute is the **cardiac output**, the product of HR and the SV of the ventricle. In an adult, the heart normally pumps 5000 mL of blood per minute. A change in HR or SV does not always change the output of the heart or the amount of blood in the arteries. For example, if a person's HR is 70 beats/min and the SV is 70 mL, the cardiac output is 4900 mL/min (70 beats/min × 70 mL/beat). If the HR drops to 60 beats/min and the SV rises to 85 mL/beat, the cardiac output increases to 5100 mL or 5.1 L/min (60 beats/min × 85 mL/beat).

Mechanical, neural, and chemical factors regulate the strength of ventricular contraction and its SV. But when these factors are unable to alter SV, a change in HR causes a change in cardiac output, which affects BP. As HR increases, there is less time for the ventricular chambers of the heart to fill. As HR increases without a change in SV, BP decreases. As HR slows, filling time is increased, and BP increases. The inability of BP to respond to increases or decreases in HR indicates a possible health problem. Report this to the health care provider.

An abnormally slow, rapid, or irregular pulse alters cardiac output. Assess the ability of the heart to meet the demands of body tissue for nutrients by palpating a peripheral pulse or using a stethoscope to listen to heart sounds (apical rate).

FACTORS AFFECTING PULSE AND ITS ALTERATIONS

Rate, rhythm, strength, and equality of pulse may be affected by variety of factors. Some of the common factors affecting pulse are discussed as follows:

Biological variability
- Individual with different age, race, body built, occupation and time of day and days of week may have different pulse rate.
- Young children, sedentary workers have higher pulse rate than older people and athletes.

Gender
- Females have higher pulse rate than their male counterparts because of smaller cardiovascular system and lower SV.

Exercise, sleep and rest
- During exercise and physical activity, pulse rate increases to meet the increased oxygen demand of the body and for same person it will be less during rest and sleep.
- Long-term sleep deprivation leads to increased pulse rate.

Environment
- Pulse rate may go up during cold weather to keep body warm and pulse rate may also increase during activity at high altitude.

Illness
- Selected cardiovascular, respiratory, and infectious illnesses contribute toward increased pulse rate and pulse rate may be low in some of diseases such as hypothyroidism, typhoid fever, myocarditis, hypokalemia, hypocalcemia, and some of drugs such as lignocaine and antihypertensive drugs.
- Pulse could be rapid and feeble in shock and it could be bounding in case of fluid and electrolyte overload.

Fever
- Fever leads to increased temperature and pulse rate in clients, which generally associated with infectious disorders.

Acute pain and fatigue
- Acute pain and chronic fatigue may cause increased pulse rate.

Emotions
- Anxiety, feeling of nervousness, and a stressful day at work may lead to increased pulse rate.

Music, yoga, and meditation
- Music, yoga, and meditation activate parasympathetic nervous system and thereby help in reducing the pulse rate.

Body position
- Pulse rate in a healthy individual could be lowest while laying down compared with while progressively seating, standing, and moving.

ASSESSMENT OF PULSE

You can assess any artery for pulse rate, but you typically use the radial artery because it is easy to palpate. When a patient's condition suddenly worsens, the carotid site is recommended for quickly finding and assessing the pulse. The heart continues delivering blood through the carotid artery to the brain as long as possible. When cardiac output declines significantly, peripheral pulses weaken and are difficult to palpate.

The radial and apical locations are the most common sites for pulse rate assessment. Use the radial pulse to teach patients how to monitor their own HRs (e.g., athletes, people taking heart medications, and patients starting a prescribed exercise regimen). If the radial pulse is abnormal or intermittent resulting from dysrhythmias or if it is inaccessible because of a dressing or cast, assess the apical pulse. When a patient takes medication that affects the HR, the apical pulse provides a more accurate assessment of heart function. The brachial or apical pulse is the best site for assessing an infant's or a young child's pulse because other peripheral pulses are deep and difficult to palpate accurately.

Assessment of other peripheral pulse sites such as the brachial or femoral artery is unnecessary when routinely obtaining vital signs. You assess other peripheral pulses when conducting a complete physical examination, when surgery or treatment has impaired blood flow to a body part, or when there are clinical indications of impaired peripheral blood flow.

Use of a Stethoscope

You use a **stethoscope** to auscultate the sound waves created by an apical pulse (Fig. 6.7). The four parts of the

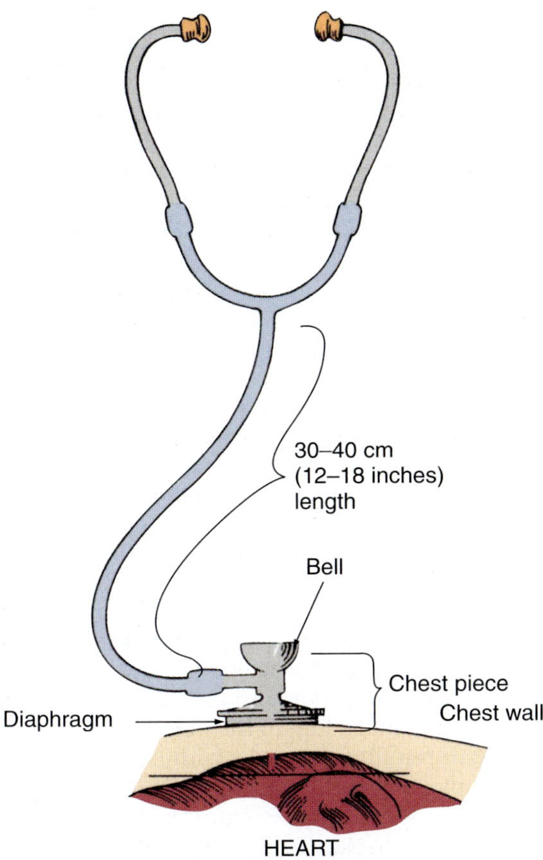

Fig. 6.7 Acoustic stethoscope.

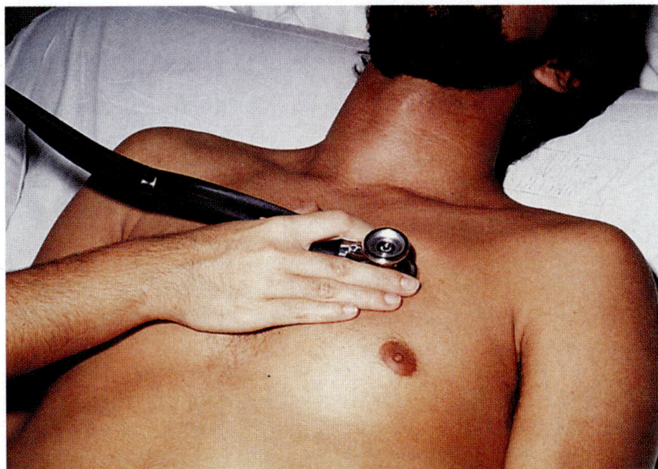

Fig. 6.8 Positioning diaphragm of stethoscope.

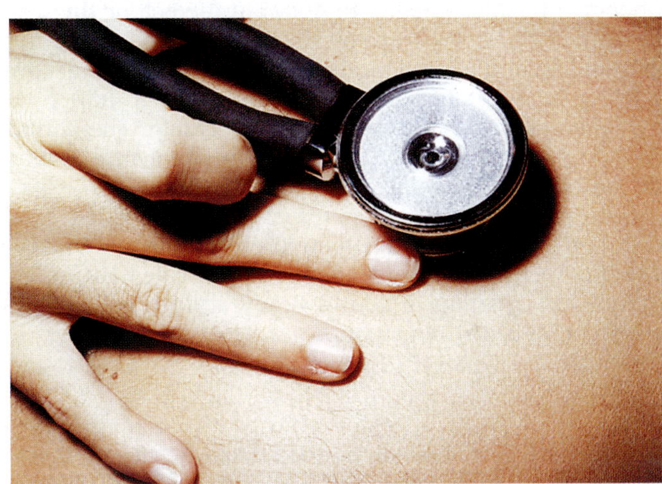

Fig. 6.9 Positioning bell of stethoscope.

stethoscope are the earpieces, binaurals, tubing, and chest piece.

Make sure that the plastic or rubber earpieces fit snugly in the ear canal and that the binaurals are angled and strong enough so that the earpieces stay firmly in place without causing discomfort. The binaurals follow the contour of the ear canal, pointing toward the face when the stethoscope is in place.

The polyvinyl tubing is flexible and 30−45 cm (12−18 inches) in length. Longer tubing decreases sound wave transmission. The tubing is thick walled and moderately rigid to eliminate transmission of environmental noise and prevent kinking, which distorts the sound. Stethoscopes have one or two tubes.

The chest piece consists of a bell and diaphragm that rotates into position. Lightly tap each surface to determine which side is functioning. The diaphragm is the circular, flat-surfaced portion of the chest piece covered with a thin plastic disk. It transmits high-pitched sounds created by the high-velocity movement of air and blood. Use the diaphragm to auscultate bowel, lung, and heart sounds. Position the diaphragm of the stethoscope firmly and directly on the patient's skin because clothing can distort the sound (Fig. 6.8).

The bell is the cone-shaped chest piece usually surrounded by a rubber ring to avoid chilling the patient. It transmits low-pitched sounds created by the low-velocity movement of blood. Use it to auscultate heart and vascular sounds. Apply the bell lightly, resting the chest piece on the skin (Fig. 6.9). Compressing the bell against the skin distorts low-pitched sounds.

One type of stethoscope has one chest piece that combines the bell and diaphragm together. When you use light pressure, the chest piece becomes the bell; when you press the chest piece slightly harder, the bell converts to a diaphragm. The size of the stethoscope chest piece varies from small (used for infants and young children) to large. Determine the appropriate chest piece to use by assessing the surface area being auscultated. Either the diaphragm or the bell can be used for BP measurement (Liu et al., 2016).

The stethoscope is a delicate instrument and requires proper care for optimal function. Remove the earpieces regularly and clean them of cerumen (earwax). Inspect the bell and diaphragm for dust, lint, and body oils. Clean with either alcohol or mild soap and water between patients to reduce bacterial contamination and avoid hospital-acquired infections (Longtin et al., 2016). Do not use fabric stethoscope covers. Covers cannot be washed between patients and can be contaminated with bacteria.

CHARACTERISTICS OF THE PULSE

Assessment of the radial pulse includes measuring the rate, rhythm, strength, and equality. When auscultating an apical pulse, assess rate and rhythm only.

Rate

Before you measure a pulse, review a patient's medical record to obtain a baseline rate. Remember, pulse rates vary with a patient's age. Compare your patient's actual pulse rate with the expected usual values (Table 6.5). When assessing the pulse, consider the variety of factors influencing pulse rate (Table 6.6). A combination of these factors often causes significant changes. If you detect an abnormal rate or rhythm while palpating a peripheral pulse, the next step is to auscultate the apical pulse for 1 minute to obtain a more accurate assessment of cardiac function.

Assess the **apical pulse** by listening for heart sounds (see Chapter 7). After properly positioning the bell or the diaphragm of the stethoscope on the chest, try to identify the first and second heart sounds (S_1 and S_2). At normal slow rates, S_1 is low pitched and dull, sounding like a "lub." S_2 is a higher pitched, shorter sound and creates the sound "dub." Count each set of "lub-dub" as one heartbeat. Count the number of "lub-dubs" occurring in 1 minute.

Pulse rate assessment often reveals variations in HR. Two common abnormalities in HR are **tachycardia** and **bradycardia.** Tachycardia is an abnormally elevated HR, more than 100 beats/min in adults. Bradycardia is a slow HR, less than 60 beats/min in adults.

Table 6.5 Acceptable Ranges of Heart Rate for Age

Age Group	Heart Rate (beats/min)
Infant	120–160
Toddler	90–140
Preschool child	80–110
School-aged child	75–100
Adolescent	60–90
Adult	60–100

Rhythm

Normally, a regular interval of time occurs between each pulse or heartbeat. A regular interval interrupted by an early beat, late beat, or missed beat indicates an irregular rhythm or **dysrhythmia.** A dysrhythmia alters cardiac function, particularly if it occurs repetitively. If your patient has a dysrhythmia, assess how often it is occurring. Dysrhythmias are regularly irregular or irregularly irregular. The health care provider sometimes orders additional tests to evaluate the occurrence of dysrhythmias.

An inefficient contraction of the heart that fails to transmit a pulse wave to the peripheral pulse site creates a **pulse deficit.** To assess a pulse deficit, ask another nurse to assess the radial pulse rate while you assess the apical rate. If you discover a difference between the apical and radial pulse rates, a pulse deficit exists. Pulse deficits are frequently associated with dysrhythmias.

Strength

The strength or amplitude of a pulse reflects the volume and pressure of the blood ejected against the arterial wall with each heart contraction and the condition of the arterial vascular system leading to the pulse site. Normally, the pulse strength remains the same with each heartbeat. Assess both radial pulses at the same time to compare the characteristics of each. Pulse strength or amplitude is assigned a number grade and described as bounding (+4), full or increased (+3), expected and easily palpable (+2), diminished and barely palpable (+1), or absent (0). Evaluate pulse strength and equality during assessment of the vascular system (see Chapter 7).

Equality

Assess radial pulses on both sides of the peripheral vascular system, comparing the characteristics of each. A pulse in one extremity is sometimes unequal in strength or absent in many disease states (e.g., thrombus [clot] formation, aberrant blood vessels, cervical rib syndrome, or aortic dissection). Assess all symmetrical pulses simultaneously except for the carotid pulse. Never measure the carotid pulses simultaneously because excessive pressure occludes blood supply to the brain.

Table 6.6 Factors Influencing Heart Rates

Factor	Increase HR	Decrease HR
Exercise	Short-term exercise	Well-conditioned patient may have a slower than usual resting HR that returns more quickly to resting rate after exercise
Temperature	Fever, heat, hyperthermia	Hypothermia
Emotions	Emotional stress, anxiety, or fear stimulates sympathetic nervous system	Unrelieved severe pain increases parasympathetic stimulation, affecting HR
Medications	Positive chronotropic medications such as epinephrine; stimulants such as caffeine	Antidysrhythmics and cardiotonics affect rate and rhythm of pulse; large doses of narcotic analgesics; general anesthetics
Hemorrhage	Loss of blood increases sympathetic stimulation	
Postural changes	Standing or sitting	Lying down
Pulmonary conditions	Diseases causing poor oxygenation such as asthma and COPD	

COPD, chronic obstructive pulmonary disease; *HR*, heart rate.

ALTERATION OF PULSE

1. **Tachycardia:** Tachycardia is defined as increased pulse rate above the normal baseline highest threshold. For example, in an adult, pulse rate more than 100 is termed as tachycardia. The upper limit of baseline threshold is different for the young children and athletes.
2. **Bradycardia:** Bradycardia is defined as decreased pulse rate below the normal baseline lowest threshold. For example, in an adult, pulse rate less than 60 is termed as bradycardia. The lower limit of baseline threshold is different for the young children and athletes.
3. **Feeble pulse:** Feeble or weak pulse is defined as a very low strength pulse, which is difficult to feel at peripheral pulse assessment sites. It is an indication of low circulatory blood volume and poor cardiac activity signaling for an acute medical emergency and needs immediate medical attention.
4. **Bounding pulse:** Bounding or hyperkinetic pulse is defined as a strong throbbing pulse felt, which is generally associated with circulatory fluid volume overload and forced cardiac activity. It is commonly seen in anemia, anxiety, chronic renal failure, heavy exercise, fever, pregnancy, and hyperthyroidism, and so on.

RESPIRATION

Respiration is the mechanism the body uses to exchange gases between the atmosphere, blood, and cells. It involves three processes: **ventilation** (the mechanical movement of gases into and out of the lungs), **diffusion** (the movement of oxygen [O_2] and carbon dioxide [CO_2] between the alveoli and the red blood cells), and **perfusion** (the distribution of red blood cells to and from the pulmonary capillaries). Analyzing a patient's respiratory status requires integrating assessment data from all three processes. Assess ventilation by determining respiratory rate, depth, and rhythm. You assess diffusion and perfusion by evaluating oxygen saturation.

PHYSIOLOGY AND REGULATION OF RESPIRATION

Breathing generally is a passive process. Normally, a person thinks little about it. The respiratory center in the brain stem regulates the involuntary control of respirations. Adults normally breathe in a smooth, uninterrupted pattern 12–20 times a minute.

The body regulates ventilation using levels of CO_2, O_2, and hydrogen ion concentration (pH) in the arterial blood. The most important factor in the control of ventilation is the level of CO_2 in the arterial blood. An elevation in the CO_2 level causes the respiratory control system in the brain to increase the rate and depth of breathing. The increased ventilatory effort removes excess CO_2 (hypercarbia) by increasing exhalation. However, patients with chronic lung disease have ongoing hypercarbia. For these patients, chemoreceptors in the carotid artery and aorta become sensitive to **hypoxemia,** or low levels of arterial O_2. If arterial oxygen levels fall, these receptors signal the brain to increase the rate and depth of ventilation. Hypoxemia helps to control ventilation in patients with chronic lung disease. Because low levels of arterial O_2 provide the stimulus that allows a patient to breathe, administration of high oxygen levels is fatal for patients with chronic lung disease.

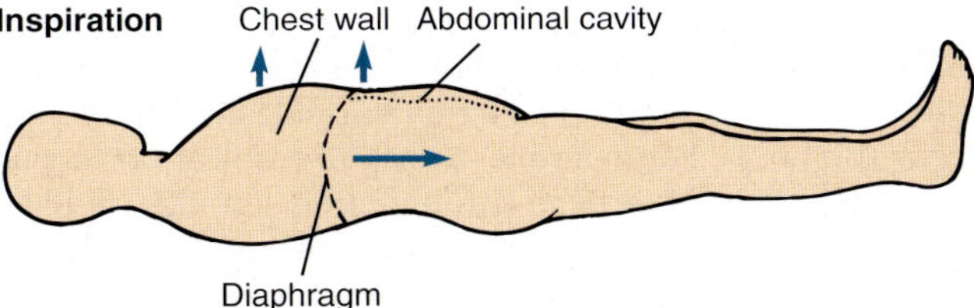

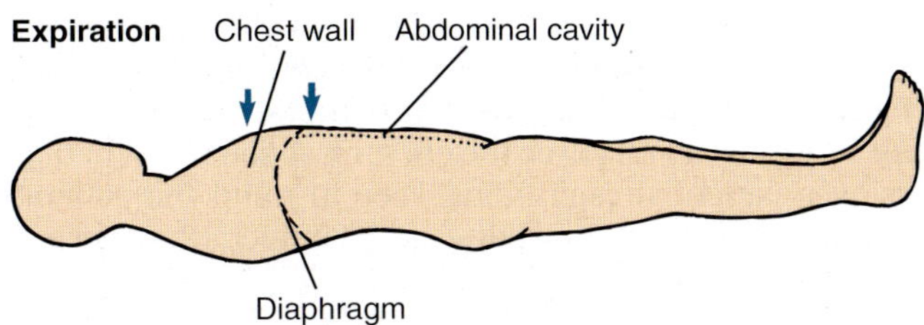

Fig. 6.10 Illustration of diaphragmatic and chest wall movement during inspiration and expiration.

MECHANICS OF BREATHING

Although breathing is normally passive, muscular work is involved in moving the lungs and chest wall. Inspiration is an active process. During inspiration, the respiratory center sends impulses along the phrenic nerve, causing the diaphragm to contract. Abdominal organs move downward and forward, increasing the length of the chest cavity to move air into the lungs. The diaphragm moves approximately 1 cm (4/10 inch), and the ribs retract upward from the midline of the body approximately 1.2–2.5 cm (1/2–1 inch). During a normal, relaxed breath, a person inhales 500 mL of air. This amount is referred to as the tidal volume. During expiration, the diaphragm relaxes, and the abdominal organs return to their original positions. The lung and chest wall return to a relaxed position (Fig. 6.10). Expiration is a passive process. Sighing interrupts the normal rate and depth of ventilation, **eupnea.** The sigh, a prolonged deeper breath, is a protective physiological mechanism for expanding small airways and alveoli not ventilated during a normal breath.

The accurate assessment of respirations depends on the recognition of normal thoracic and abdominal movements. During quiet breathing, the chest wall gently rises and falls. Contraction of the intercostal muscles between the ribs or contraction of the muscles in the neck and shoulders (the accessory muscles of breathing) is not visible. During normal quiet breathing, diaphragmatic movement causes the abdominal cavity to rise and fall slowly.

CHARACTERISTICS OF BREATHING

Respirations are the easiest of all vital signs to assess, but they are often the most haphazardly measured. Do not estimate respirations. Accurate measurement requires observation and palpation of chest wall movement.

A sudden change in the character of respirations is important. Because respiration is tied to the function of numerous body systems, consider all variables when changes occur (Box 6.3). For example, a drop in respirations occurring in a patient after head trauma often signifies injury to the brain stem. Abdominal trauma injures the phrenic nerve, which is responsible for diaphragmatic contraction.

Do not let a patient know that you are assessing respirations. A patient aware of the assessment can alter the rate and depth of breathing. Assess respirations immediately after measuring pulse rate, with your hand still on the patient's wrist as it rests over the chest or abdomen. When assessing a patient's respirations, keep in mind the patient's usual ventilatory rate and pattern, the influence any disease or illness has on respiratory function, the relationship between respiratory and cardiovascular function, and the influence of therapies on respirations. The objective measurements of respiratory status include the rate and depth of breathing and the rhythm of ventilatory movements (see Skill 6.3 on pp. 102–105).

Capnography is the measurement of exhaled carbon dioxide throughout exhalation. At the end of exhalation, the end-tidal carbon dioxide ($ETCO_2$) measurement approximates the $PaCO_2$ in a healthy patient, normally 35–45 mm Hg. In nonintubated patients, $ETCO_2$ can be obtained from a special nasal cannula connected to a monitor that detects the percentage of carbon dioxide exhaled at the end of respiratory cycle. The $ETCO_2$ can be used to evaluate respiratory and cardiac status, whereas interpretation of a continuous recording, or capnogram, can detect changes in ventilation.

BOX 6.3 Factors Influencing the Respirations

Exercise

- Exercise increases respiratory rate and depth to meet the need of the body for additional oxygen and to rid the body of carbon dioxide.

Acute Pain

- Pain alters rate and rhythm of respirations; breathing becomes shallow.
- Patient inhibits or splints chest wall movement when pain is in area of chest or abdomen.

Anxiety

- Anxiety increases respiratory rate and depth as a result of sympathetic stimulation.

Smoking

- Chronic smoking changes pulmonary airways, resulting in increased respiratory rate at rest when not smoking.

Body Position

- Standing or sitting erect promotes full ventilatory movement and lung expansion; stooped or slumped position impairs ventilatory movement; lying flat prevents full chest expansion.

Medications

- General anesthetics, sedative-hypnotics, and excessive doses of opioid analgesics depress respiratory rate and depth.
- Amphetamines and cocaine may increase rate and depth; bronchodilators cause airway dilation that can ultimately slow respiratory rate.

Neurological Injury

- Damage to brain stem impairs the respiratory center and inhibits respiratory rate and rhythm.

Hemoglobin Function

- Decreased hemoglobin levels (anemia) reduce oxygen-carrying capacity of blood, which increases respiratory rate.
- Increased altitude lowers the amount of saturated hemoglobin, which increases respiratory rate and depth.
- Abnormal blood cell function (e.g., sickle cell disease) reduces ability of hemoglobin to carry oxygen, which increases respiratory rate and depth.

Chest Wall Movement

- Constrictive chest or abdominal dressings limit chest wall movement.
- Presence of abdominal incisions limits chest wall movement.

Respiratory Rate

Observe a full inspiration and expiration before counting respirations. The respiratory rate varies with age (Table 6.7). **Bradypnea** is a respiratory rate less than 12 per minute or lower than acceptable limits, whereas **tachypnea** is a rate more than 20 or greater than the acceptable limits. **Apnea** is the lack of respiratory movements. The apnea monitor is a respiratory monitoring device that helps assess respiratory rate. This noninvasive device uses electrodes attached to a patient's chest wall to sense movement. An absence of chest wall movement triggers the apnea alarm. Apnea monitoring is used frequently in the hospital and home to observe for prolonged apneic events in infants.

Ventilatory Depth

Assess the depth of respirations by observing the degree of movement in the chest wall. Ventilatory movements are deep, normal, or shallow. A deep respiration involves a full expansion of the lungs with obvious movement of the rib cage and full exhalation. A normal respiration is relaxed, automatic, and silent. Respirations are shallow when only a small quantity of air passes through the lungs and ventilatory movement is difficult to see. When chest wall movement is unusually shallow or not symmetrical, other techniques may be needed (see Chapter 7). Table 6.8 summarizes types of breathing patterns.

Ventilatory Rhythm

Respiratory rhythm or breathing pattern is either regular or irregular. While assessing respiration, observe the interval between each respiratory cycle. With normal breathing,

Table 6.7 Acceptable Range of Respiratory Rates for Age

Age Group	Rate (breaths/min)
Newborn	35–40
Infant (6 months)	30–50
Toddler (2 years)	25–32
Child	20–30
Adolescent	16–20
Adult	12–20

Table 6.8 Alterations in Breathing Pattern

Alteration	Description
Bradypnea	Rate of breathing is regular but abnormally slow (less than 12 breaths/min).
Tachypnea	Rate of breathing is regular but abnormally rapid (more than 20 breaths/min).
Hyperpnea	Respirations are labored, increased in depth, and increased in rate (more than 20 breaths/min) (occurs normally during exercise).
Apnea	Respirations cease for several seconds. Persistent cessation results in respiratory arrest.
Hyperventilation	Rate and depth of respirations increase. Hypocarbia sometimes occurs.
Hypoventilation	Respiratory rate is abnormally low, and depth of ventilation is depressed. Hypercarbia sometimes occurs.
Cheyne–Stokes respiration	Respiratory rate and depth are irregular, characterized by alternating periods of apnea and hyperventilation. Respiratory cycle begins with slow, shallow breaths that gradually increase to abnormal rate and depth. The pattern reverses; breathing slows and becomes shallow, concluding as apnea before respiration resumes.
Kussmaul respiration	Respirations are abnormally deep, regular, and increased in rate.
Biot respiration	Respirations are abnormally shallow for two to three breaths, followed by irregular period of apnea.

a regular interval occurs between each respiratory cycle. In the presence of irregular breathing pattern such as periods of apnea with shallow or deep breathing, a more detailed physical assessment is imperative (see Chapters 7 and 24). Infants tend to breathe less regularly. Young children sometimes breathe slowly for a few seconds and suddenly breathe more rapidly.

Measurement of Oxygen Saturation (Pulse Oximetry)

Pulse oximetry is the indirect measurement of **oxygen saturation** and is the fifth vital sign (see Skill 6.4). The pulse oximeter contains a photoelectric sensor with two light-emitting diodes (LEDs) of differing wavelengths that measures the SpO_2 level. SpO_2 stands for peripheral **capillary oxygen saturation**, an estimate of the amount of oxygen in the blood. More specifically, it is the percentage of oxygenated hemoglobin (hemoglobin containing oxygen) compared with the total amount of hemoglobin in the blood (Fig. 6.11). Normally, SpO_2 is between 95% and 100%; however, in patients with extensive respiratory disease such as chronic obstructive pulmonary disease (COPD), SpO_2 more than 90% may be an acceptable baseline.

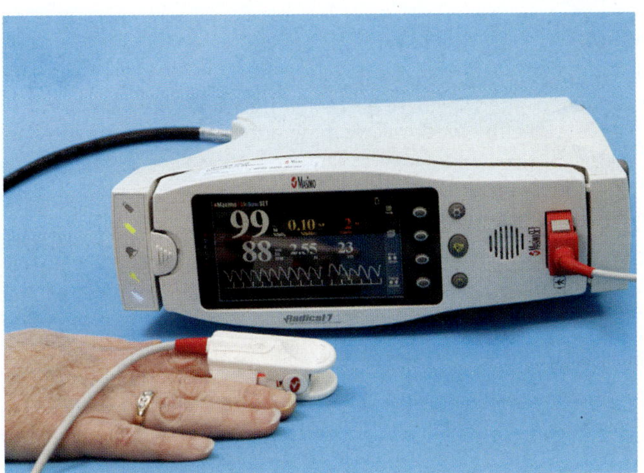

Fig. 6.11 Pulse oximeter connected to finger sensor.

The measurement of SpO_2 is simple and painless and carries fewer risks than invasive measurements of oxygen saturation using arterial blood gas sampling. However, the placement of an oximeter forehead sensor can cause a pressure injury, and therefore it requires frequent monitoring of skin condition. A dry, vascular, pulsatile area (e.g., fingertip, earlobe, forehead) is needed to detect the degree of change in the transmitted light from the oximeter. Factors that affect light transmission such as outside light sources or patient motion also affect the measurement of oxygen saturation. Carbon monoxide in the blood, jaundice, and intravascular dyes can influence the light reflected from hemoglobin molecules. An awareness of these factors allows for accurate interpretation of abnormal SpO_2 measurements. Measuring SpO_2 can be conducted intermittently or continuously to assess ongoing therapies.

Measurement of End-Tidal Carbon Dioxide

$ETCO_2$ values are important to assess when monitoring lung ventilation and perfusion. The noninvasive $ETCO_2$ monitor attaches directly to the ventilator system and measures the exhaled carbon dioxide through sensors. **$ETCO_2$ monitoring** benefits a patient because it is noninvasive and painless and provides an accurate assessment of arterial carbon dioxide retention values. Commonly used in patients on mechanical ventilators, $ETCO_2$ monitoring can also be implemented with patients who are not intubated using a specially designed nasal cannula that can also deliver oxygen (see Chapter 24).

BLOOD PRESSURE

Blood pressure (BP) is the force exerted on the walls of an artery created by the pulsing blood under pressure from the heart. Blood flows throughout the circulatory system because of pressure changes, moving from an area of high pressure to an area of low pressure. Under high pressure, the left ventricle ejects blood into the aorta; the peak pressure is known as **systolic pressure.** When the ventricles relax, the blood remaining in the arteries exerts a minimum or **diastolic pressure.** Diastolic pressure is the minimal pressure exerted against the arterial wall at all times.

The standard unit for measuring BP is millimeters of mercury (mm Hg). The measurement indicates the height to which the BP raises a column of mercury. You record BPs as a ratio with the systolic reading before the diastolic (e.g., 120/80 mm Hg). The difference between systolic and diastolic pressure is the **pulse pressure.** For a BP of 120/80 mm Hg, the pulse pressure is 40.

PHYSIOLOGY OF ARTERIAL BLOOD PRESSURE

BP depends on the interrelationships of cardiac output, peripheral vascular resistance, blood volume, blood viscosity, and artery elasticity. An increase in cardiac output is usually the result of greater heart muscle contractility, an increase in HR, or an increase in blood volume. An increase in cardiac output increases BP. When peripheral arteries constrict such as during periods of stress, peripheral vascular resistance increases, which results in increased BP. As vessels dilate and resistance falls, BP drops. When blood is forced through the rigid arteries, BP rises. If the blood volume decreases, such as during dehydration or hemorrhage, less pressure is exerted against arterial walls, and BP falls. When the percentage of red blood cells increases, the blood viscosity increases, causing the heart to contract more forcefully to move the blood through the circulatory system, resulting in an increased BP.

FACTORS INFLUENCING BLOOD PRESSURE

Many factors continually influence BP. A single measurement does not adequately reflect a patient's BP. BP trends, not individual measurements, guide nursing and medical interventions. Understanding the factors that cause alterations in BP helps to accurately interpret BP measurements (Box 6.4).

ALTERATIONS IN BLOOD PRESSURE

Hypertension

The most common alteration in BP is **hypertension,** an often asymptomatic disorder characterized by persistently elevated BP. Hypertension is defined as SBP more than 140 mm Hg and

BOX 6.4 Factors Influencing Blood Pressure

Age

- BP tends to rise with advancing age:

Age	Average Arterial Pressure (mm Hg)
Newborn (3000 g [6.6 lb])	65/41
1 month	85/54
1 year	86/40
6 years	94/56
10–13 years	103/62
14–17 years	110/65
Adult	<120/80[a]

- Assess the level of BP in a child or adolescent with respect to sex, body size, and age. Larger children have higher BPs than smaller children of the same age (Hockenberry and Wilson, 2015).

Gender

- There is no clinically significant difference in BP levels between boys and girls before puberty.
- After puberty, males have higher BPs.
- During and after menopause, women have higher BPs than men of the same age.

Ethnicity

- The incidence of hypertension is higher in African Americans than in European Americans.
- African Americans tend to develop more severe hypertension at an earlier age and have twice the risk for complications of hypertension such as stroke and heart attack. Hypertension-related deaths are also higher among African Americans.

Sympathetic Stimulation

- Pain, anxiety, and fear stimulate the sympathetic nervous system, causing BP to rise. A full bladder can increase sympathetic stimulation, elevating BP.

Daily Variation

- BP varies throughout the day with lower BP during sleep, increasing during the day.
- BP can drop 10%–20% during nighttime sleep.

Medication and Treatment

- Some medications directly or indirectly affect BP. Opioids, sedatives, general anesthetics, antihypertensives, and vasodilators lower BP, whereas vasoconstrictors, blood, and i.v. fluid infusion raise BP.

Activity

- Older adults often experience a 5- to 10-mm Hg fall in BP about 1 h after eating.
- BP falls as a person moves from lying to sitting or standing position; normal postural variations are minimal.
- Increase in oxygen demand by the body during activity increases BP.

Weight

- Obesity is a risk factor for hypertension.
- In school-aged children, the higher their body mass index, the greater the risk for developing hypertension at an early age.

Diet

- A diet low in sodium and high in potassium can reduce BP. Vegetarian diets and limited alcohol consumption (fewer than two drinks per day for men and one per day for women) are associated with low BP. BP reductions are greater among older adults implementing dietary modifications.

Smoking

- Smoking results in vasoconstriction, a narrowing of blood vessels.

[a]American Heart Association: What is High Blood Pressure, 2016, https://www.heart.org/idc/groups/heart-public/@wcm/@hcm/documents/downloadable/ucm_300310.pdf.

Table 6.9 Classification of Blood Pressure for Adults Aged 18 Years and Older

Category	Systolic (mm Hg)[a]		Diastolic (mm Hg)[a]
Normal	<120		<80
Prehypertension[b]	120–139	Or	80–89
Stage 1 hypertension	≥140	Or	≥90
Stage 2 hypertension	≥160	Or	≥90

Data from James PA, et al: 2014 evidence-based guideline for the management of high blood pressure in adults: report by the panel appointed to the Eighth Joint National Committee (JNC 8), *JAMA* 31:507, 2014.

[a]Treatment based on highest category.

[b]Based on the average of two or more readings taken at each of two or more visits after an initial screening. Patient should not be taking antihypertensive drugs or be acutely ill. When systolic and diastolic blood pressures fall into different categories, select the higher category to classify the individual's blood pressure status. For example, classify 160/92 mm Hg as stage 2 hypertension.

diastolic blood pressure (DBP) more than 90 mm Hg. Patients on antihypertensive medication with acceptable BP measurements are considered to have hypertension. The Joint National Committee on Prevention, Detection, Evaluation, and Treatment of High Blood Pressure (JNC 8) (James et al., 2014) published criteria for categories of hypertension (Table 6.9). Hypertension is a known risk factor for cardiovascular morbidity and mortality. Obesity, cigarette smoking, excessive alcohol intake, elevated blood cholesterol, and continued exposure to stress are risk factors for hypertension. The American Heart Association (AHA) recommends maintaining a BP less than 130/80 mm Hg for high-risk groups, and the treatment goal for persons with cardiac dysfunction is BP less than 120/80 mm Hg (James et al., 2014). Normal BP is considered to be less than 120/80 (AHA, 2016).

A diagnosis of hypertension is based on the average of two or more seated BP measurements, properly measured with well-maintained equipment, at each of two or more visits to an office or clinic after an initial screening (James et al., 2014). Thus, one BP recording revealing a high SBP or DBP does not qualify as a diagnosis of hypertension. However, if a high reading is obtained (e.g., 150/90 mm Hg), encourage the patient to return for another checkup within 2 months.

Hypotension

Hypotension is an SBP less than 90 mm Hg. Although some adults have low BP normally, for most individuals' hypotension is an abnormal finding associated with an illness (e.g., hemorrhage or myocardial infarction). Hypotension occurs when arteries dilate, the peripheral vascular resistance decreases, the circulating blood volume decreases, or the heart fails to provide adequate cardiac output. Hypotension is usually life-threatening and needs to be reported immediately to the patient's health care provider.

Signs and symptoms associated with hypotension include:

- Pallor
- Skin mottling
- Clamminess
- Confusion
- Dizziness
- Chest pain
- Increased HR
- Decreased urine output

Orthostatic hypotension, also referred to as postural hypotension, is a reduction of SBP of at least 20 mm Hg or a reduction of DBP of at least 10 mm Hg within 3 minutes of quiet standing. It occurs when patients experience a drop in BP on rising to an upright position and is associated with symptoms of light-headedness or dizziness. In severe cases, loss of consciousness occurs. Orthostatic hypotension is a risk factor for falls, especially among older adults with hypertension (Angelousi et al., 2014). When a healthy person changes from a lying to sitting to standing position, the peripheral blood vessels in the legs constrict, preventing the pooling of blood in the legs caused by gravity. Orthostatic hypotension occurs when the peripheral blood vessels in the legs are already constricted or are unable to constrict in response to a change in position. Fluid volume deficit from decreased blood volume, dehydration, or recent blood loss; prolonged bed rest; anemia; and antihypertensive medications place patients at risk for orthostatic hypotension. Assess for orthostatic hypotension by obtaining pulse and BP readings with the patient supine, sitting, and standing (Box 6.5).

BOX 6.5 Procedural Guidelines for Measuring Orthostatic Blood Pressure

Equipment

Sphygmomanometer, stethoscope

Steps

1. Identify the patient by using at least two identifiers (e.g., name and birthday or name and medical record number) according to agency policy.
2. Determine whether it is appropriate to measure patient's orthostatic BP. Orthostatic vital signs are not indicated in patients who:
   - Have supine hypotension.
   - Have a sitting BP 90/60 mm Hg or less.
   - Have acute deep vein thrombosis.
   - Exhibit the clinical syndrome of shock.
   - Have severely altered mental status.
   - Have possible spinal injuries.
   - Have lower extremity or pelvic fractures.
   - Are not mobile enough to get out of bed.
3. Perform hand hygiene.
4. Have the patient lie in bed with head of bed flat for a minimum of 3 min, preferably 5 min. With the patient supine, take BP reading in each arm. Select arm with highest systolic reading for subsequent measurements.
5. Leaving BP cuff in place, help the patient to sitting position. Take BP at 1 min. If orthostatic signs or symptoms occur, such as dizziness, weakness, light-headedness, feeling faint, sudden pallor, or sitting BP 90/60 mm Hg or less, put the patient back to bed in the supine position.
6. Leaving BP cuff in place, help the patient to standing position. Take BP at 1 min and 3 min with the patient in standing position. If orthostatic signs or symptoms occur (as previously noted), stop BP measurement, return the patient to bed (if possible), and help the patient to supine position. In most cases, you detect orthostatic hypotension within 1 min of standing.

Continued

BOX 6.5 Procedural Guidelines for Measuring Orthostatic Blood Pressure—cont'd

7. If the patient is unable to stand, take second reading by having the patient sit upright with legs dangling over the edge of the bed.
8. Record the patient's BP in each position (e.g., "140/80 supine, 132/72 sitting, 108/60 standing"). Note any additional symptoms or complaints. A drop in systolic BP of 20 mm Hg or more, a drop in diastolic BP of 10 mm Hg or more, or an experience of light-headedness or dizziness is considered abnormal.
9. Report findings of orthostatic hypotension or orthostatic signs or symptoms to nurse in charge or health care provider. Instruct patient to move slowly when changing from one position to another and to ask for assistance when getting out of bed if orthostatic hypotension is present or orthostatic signs or symptoms occur.
10. Perform hand hygiene.

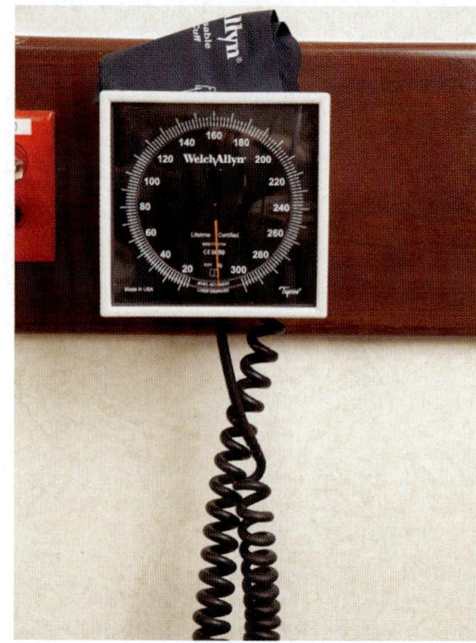

Fig. 6.12 Wall-mounted aneroid sphygmomanometer.

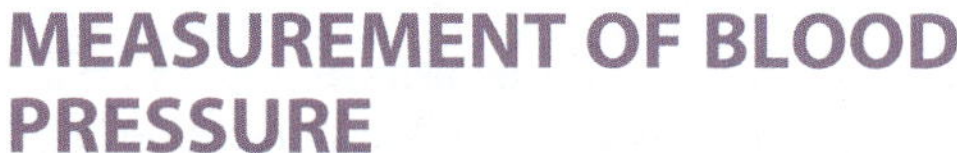

MEASUREMENT OF BLOOD PRESSURE

Measure arterial BP either directly (invasively) or indirectly (noninvasively). The direct method requires the insertion of a thin catheter into an artery by a health care provider. Risks, such as sepsis, associated with continuous invasive BP monitoring require the use of an intensive care setting. The more common noninvasive method requires use of the **sphygmomanometer** and stethoscope. Measure BP indirectly by palpation or auscultation (see Skill 6.5 on pp. 108–112).

Blood Pressure Equipment

Before assessing BP, you need to become comfortable using a sphygmomanometer and stethoscope. A sphygmomanometer includes a pressure manometer, an occlusive cloth or disposable vinyl cuff that encloses an inflatable rubber bladder, and a pressure bulb with a release valve that inflates the bladder. The aneroid manometer has a glass-enclosed circular gauge containing a needle that registers millimeter calibrations (Fig. 6.12). Aneroid manometers are safe, lightweight, portable, and compact. Before using a manometer, be sure that the needle points to zero. Metal parts in the aneroid manometer are subject to temperature variations and need to be checked every 6 months to verify their accuracy.

The release valves of the sphygmomanometer must be clean and freely movable in either direction. The valve, when closed, should hold the pressure constant. Frequent calibration is necessary to ensure accuracy. A sticky valve makes pressure cuff deflation hard to regulate. The pressure bulb and tubing should be airtight.

Cloth or disposable vinyl compression cuffs contain an inflatable bladder and come in several different sizes. The size selected is proportional to the circumference of the limb being assessed. Select a cuff that is at least 40% greater than the arm circumference (or 20% wider than the diameter) of the midpoint of the limb being used to obtain measurements (Fig. 6.13). The bladder, enclosed by the cuff, encircles at least 80% of the arm of an adult and the entire arm of a child. The lower edge of the cuff is above the antecubital fossa if the arm is being used, allowing room for placement of the stethoscope. An improperly placed or fitted cuff causes inaccurate BP measurements (Table 6.10).

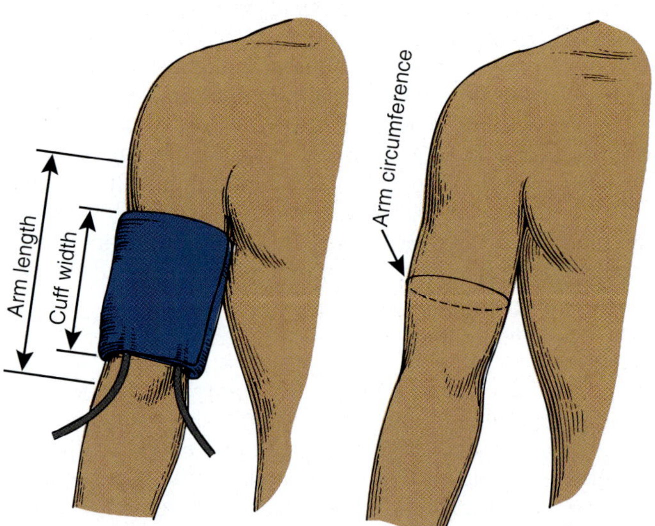

Fig. 6.13 Guidelines for proper blood pressure cuff size. Cuff width equals 20% more than upper arm diameter or 40% of circumference around upper arm and two-thirds of upper arm length.

Auscultation

The best environment to auscultate BP sounds is a quiet room at a comfortable temperature. Although a patient is able to lie or stand, sitting is the best position. It is also best to have a patient assume the same position during each BP measurement to permit a meaningful comparison of values. Before assessment, control factors responsible for artificially high readings such as pain, anxiety, or exertion. *For example, in the case study, Ms Coburn was anxious when first*

Table 6.10 Common Errors in Blood Pressure Assessment

Error	Effect
Bladder or cuff too wide	False-low reading
Bladder or cuff too narrow or too short	False-high reading
Cuff wrapped too loosely or unevenly	False-high reading
Deflating cuff too slowly	False-high diastolic reading
Deflating cuff too quickly	False-low systolic and false-high diastolic reading
Arm below heart level	False-high reading
Arm above heart level	False-low reading
Arm not supported	False-high reading
Stethoscope that fits poorly or impairment of examiner's hearing, causing sounds to be muffled	False-low systolic and false-high diastolic reading
Stethoscope applied too firmly against antecubital fossa	False-low diastolic reading
Inflating too slowly	False-high diastolic reading
Repeating assessments too quickly	False-high systolic reading
Inadequate inflation level	False-low systolic reading
Multiple examiners using different sounds for diastolic readings	False-high systolic and false-low diastolic reading

entering the examination room. After she sees the nurse practitioner, Miguel retakes her blood pressure. Her blood pressure this time is 146/94 mm Hg (first reading was 164/98 mm Hg).

A patient's perception that the physical or interpersonal environment is stressful affects BP. Measurements taken at home are sometimes different from measurements taken at a patient's place of employment or health care provider's office. Home BP devices measuring BP at the wrist lead to falsely elevated values (Casiglia et al., 2016).

During the initial assessment, you obtain and record BPs in both arms. Normally, there is a difference of 5–10 mm Hg between the right and left arms. In subsequent assessments, measure the BP in the arm with the higher pressure. Pressure differences between extremities more than 20 mm Hg indicate vascular problems and need to be reported to the charge nurse or health care provider.

Indirect measurement of arterial BP works on a basic principle of pressure. Blood flows freely through an artery until an inflated cuff applies pressure to tissues and causes the artery to collapse. When the cuff slowly deflates, the point at which blood flow returns and sound appears through auscultation is the SBP.

In 1905, Nikolai Korotkoff, a Russian surgeon, first described the sounds heard over an artery during cuff deflation. The first **Korotkoff sound** is a clear, rhythmic tapping series that corresponds to the pulse rate and gradually increases in intensity. Onset of the sound corresponds to the systolic pressure. A murmur or swishing sound appears as the cuff continues to deflate, which is the second Korotkoff sound. As the artery distends, blood flow becomes turbulent. The third Korotkoff sound is a crisper and more intense tapping. The fourth Korotkoff sound becomes muffled and low pitched as the cuff is further deflated. The onset of the fourth Korotkoff sound is the diastolic pressure in infants and children (Basile and Bloch, 2016), pregnant women, and patients with elevated cardiac output or peripheral vasodilation. The fifth Korotkoff sound is the disappearance of sound; in adolescents and most adults, this sound corresponds with the DBP (Fig. 6.14) (Basile and Bloch, 2016). In some patients, the sounds are clear and distinct, whereas in others only the beginning and the ending sounds are heard.

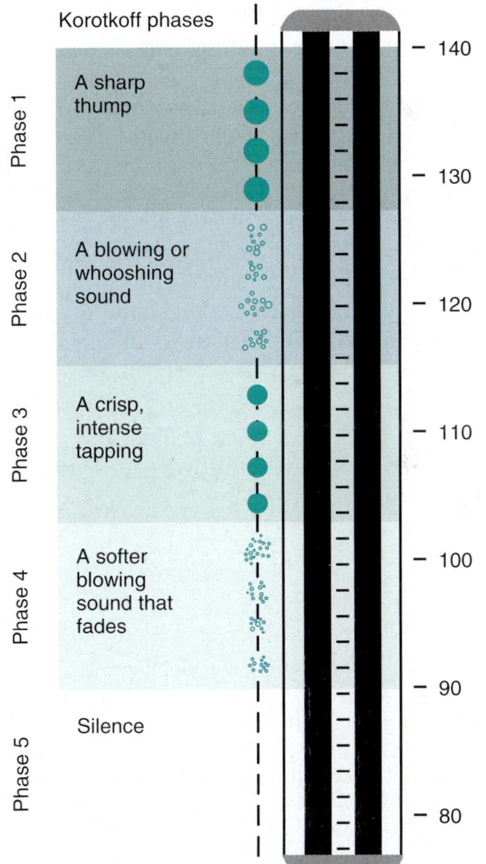

Fig. 6.14 Sounds auscultated during blood pressure measurement can be differentiated into five Korotkoff phases. The blood pressure is 140/90 in this example.

The AHA recommends recording two numbers for a BP measurement: the point on the manometer when the first sound is heard for SBP and the point on the manometer when the fifth sound (disappearance of sound) is heard for DBP (James et al., 2014). Some institutions recommend recording the point when you hear the fourth sound, especially for patients with hypertension. You divide the numbers by slashed lines (e.g., 120/80, 120/100/80), note the arm used to measure the BP, and record the patient's position (e.g., LA 158/78, sitting).

Decisions about patient care and implementing nursing interventions are based on the BP measurements in combination with other findings. Obtaining an accurate BP measurement is critical. There are several possibilities for error if the auscultation procedure is not followed correctly (see Table 6.10). If you are unsure of a reading, ask another nurse to reassess the BP.

Palpation

Indirect measurement of BP by palpation is useful for patients whose arterial pulsations are too weak to create Korotkoff sounds or when there is excessive environmental noise that cannot be controlled. Severe blood loss and weakened heart contractility are examples of conditions that result in BPs too low to auscultate accurately. In this case, you assess the SBP by palpation (Box 6.6). DBP is difficult to determine by palpation. When using the palpation technique, you record the systolic value only and the location and manner in which it was measured (e.g., RA 78/–, palpated).

Sometimes, you use palpation techniques with auscultation. In some patients with hypertension, the sounds heard over the brachial artery when the cuff pressure is high disappear as pressure is reduced and then reappear at a lower level. This temporary disappearance of sound is the **auscultatory gap.** It typically occurs between the first and second Korotkoff sounds. The gap in sound can cover a range of 40 mm Hg, possibly causing an underestimation of SBP or an overestimation of DBP. Be certain to inflate the cuff high enough to hear the true SBP before the auscultatory gap.

BOX 6.6 Procedural Guidelines for Palpating Systolic Blood Pressure

Equipment

Sphygmomanometer

Steps

1. Identify the patient by using two identifiers (e.g., name and birth date or name and medical record number) according to agency policy (TJC, 2016).
2. Perform hand hygiene.
3. Apply BP cuff to extremity selected for measurement.
4. Continually palpate pulse of brachial, radial, or popliteal artery with fingertips of one hand.
5. Inflate BP cuff 30 mm Hg above point at which you no longer can palpate the pulse.
6. Slowly release valve and deflate cuff, allowing manometer needle mercury to fall 2 mm Hg/s.
7. Note point on manometer when pulse is again palpable; this is the systolic BP.
8. Deflate cuff rapidly and completely. Remove cuff from patient extremity unless you need to repeat the measurement.
9. Perform hand hygiene.
10. Record BP as systolic/–, palpated (e.g., BP 108/–, palpated, location) on vital sign flow sheet, in nurses' notes, or electronic medical record. Report abnormal findings to nurse in charge or health care provider.

Palpation of the radial artery helps to determine how high to inflate the cuff. Inflate the cuff 30 mm Hg above the pressure at which the palpated radial pulse disappears and slowly release the cuff until the radial pulse returns. The return of the pulse correlates with the systolic pressure. Document the BP reading with an auscultatory gap (e.g., "BP RA 180/94 with an auscultatory gap from 180 to 160").

Ultrasonic Stethoscope

If you are unable to auscultate Korotkoff sounds because of a weak arterial pulse, use an ultrasonic stethoscope (see Chapter 7). This stethoscope allows you to hear low-frequency systolic sounds and is commonly used in infants and children and for measuring low BP in adults.

Electronic Blood Pressure Devices

Many different styles of electronic BP machines are available to determine BP automatically (Fig. 6.15). Electronic BP machines rely on an electronic sensor to detect the vibrations or sounds caused by the rush of blood through an artery (Box 6.7). When the cuff deflates, one style of BP machine determines the initial burst of oscillations and translates the information to a systolic pressure reading. The machine records a diastolic measurement when the oscillations are lowest, just before they stop. Use electronic devices when frequent BP assessment is necessary such as in patients who are critically ill or unstable, during or after invasive procedures, or when therapies require frequent monitoring (e.g., i.v. heart and BP medications). Box 6.8 lists conditions that are not appropriate for automatic BP devices.

Although electronic BP machines are fast and free up the care provider for other activities, it is necessary to consider their advantages and limitations (Table 6.11). Use the devices when frequent assessment is necessary, during or after invasive procedures, or when therapies require frequent monitoring (Box 6.9).

Lower Extremity Blood Pressure

If your patient has dressings, casts, i.v. catheters, or an arteriovenous fistula or shunt in one arm, select the other

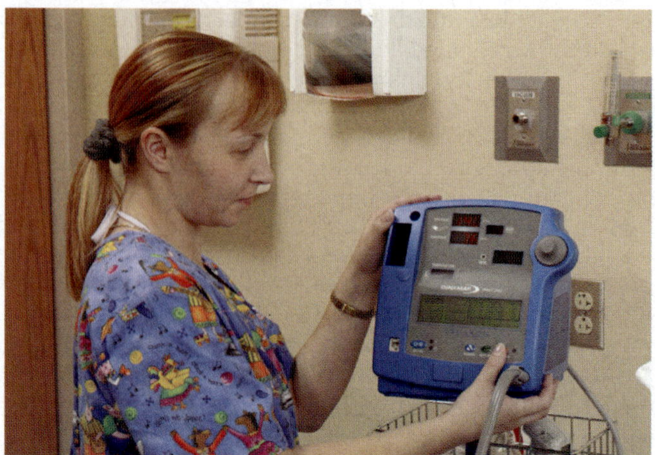

Fig. 6.15 Electronic blood pressure machines vary in appearance.

BOX 6.7 Procedural Guidelines for Electronic Blood Pressure Measurement

Equipment

Electronic BP machine, BP cuff of appropriate size as recommended by manufacturer

Steps

1. Identify the patient by using two identifiers (e.g., name and birth date or name and medical record number) according to agency policy (TJC, 2016).
2. Determine appropriateness of using electronic BP measurement. Patients with irregular heart rate, peripheral vascular disease, seizures, tremors, and shivering are not candidates for this device (Suokhrie et al., 2013).
3. Determine best site for cuff placement (see Skill 6.5).
4. Perform hand hygiene. Help the patient to comfortable position, either lying or sitting. Plug in device and place it near the patient, ensuring that connector hose between cuff and machine will reach.
5. Locate on/off switch and turn machine on to enable device to self-test computer systems.
6. Select appropriate cuff size for the patient extremity and appropriate cuff for machine. Electronic BP cuff and machine are matched by the manufacturer and are not interchangeable.
7. Prepare BP cuff by manually squeezing all the air out of cuff and attaching cuff to connector hose.
8. Remove any constricting clothing to ensure proper cuff application. BP cuff may be placed over a light shirt sleeve (Pinar et al., 2010).
9. Wrap flattened cuff snugly around extremity, verifying that only one finger fits between cuff and patient's skin. Make sure that "artery" arrow marked on outside of cuff is placed correctly (see illustration for Skill 6.5, Step 4).
10. Verify that connector hose between cuff and machine is not kinked. Kinking prevents proper inflation and deflation of cuff.
11. Following manufacturer directions, set frequency control of automatic or manual and press start button. The first BP measurement pumps cuff to pressure of approximately 180 mm Hg. After this pressure is reached, the machine begins a deflation sequence that determines BP. The first reading determines peak pressure inflation for additional measurements.
    Clinical decision point: If unable to obtain BP with electronic device, verify machine connections (e.g., plugged into working electrical outlet, hose–cuff connections tight, machine on, correct cuff). Wait at least 1 min but not more than 2 min to repeat electronic BP; if unable to obtain, use auscultatory technique (see Skill 6.5).
12. When deflation is complete, digital display provides most recent values and flashes time in minutes that have elapsed since measurement occurred.
13. Set frequency of BP measurements and upper and lower alarm limits for systolic, diastolic, and mean BP readings. Intervals between BP measurements are set from 1 to 90 min.
14. Determine measurement frequency and alarm limits on the basis of patient's acceptable range of BP, nursing judgment, and health care provider order.
15. Obtain additional readings at any time by pressing start button. (Sometimes, you need additional readings for unstable patients.) Pressing cancel button immediately deflates cuff.
16. If frequent BP determinations are necessary, leave cuff in place. Remove cuff at least every 2 h to assess underlying skin integrity and, if possible, alternate BP sites. Patients with abnormal bleeding tendencies are at risk for microvascular rupture from repeated inflations. When you are finished using the electronic BP machine, clean BP cuff according to agency policy to reduce transmission of microorganisms.
17. Compare electronic BP readings with auscultatory BP to verify accuracy of electronic BP measurement.
18. Record BP and site assessed on vital sign flow sheet, in nurses' notes, or electronic medical record (per agency policy). Record any signs of BP alterations in nurses' notes.
19. Report abnormal findings to nurse in charge or health care provider.

BOX 6.8 Patient Conditions not Appropriate for Electronic Blood Pressure Measurement

- Irregular heart rate
- Peripheral vascular obstruction (e.g., clots, narrowed vessels)
- Shivering
- Seizures
- Excessive tremors
- Inability to cooperate
- Blood pressure less than 90 mm Hg systolic

arm for BP assessment. When neither upper extremity is appropriate nor available, measure BP in a lower extremity. Comparing upper extremity BP with the BP in the legs is also necessary for patients with certain cardiac and BP abnormalities. The popliteal artery, palpable behind the knee in the popliteal space, is the site for auscultation. Position the cuff with the bladder over the posterior aspect of the midthigh, 2.5 cm (1 inch) above the popliteal artery. Make sure that the cuff is wide enough and long enough to allow for the larger girth of the thigh. For most measurements, place the patient in a prone position. If such a position is impossible, flex the knee slightly for easier access to the artery (Fig. 6.16). The procedure is identical to brachial artery auscultation. SBP in the legs is usually higher by 10–40 mm Hg than in the brachial artery, with the DBP lower (Halm, 2014).

Self-Measurement of Blood Pressure

Improved technology in electronic monitoring devices allows individuals to measure their own BPs in their home with the push of a button. The portable home devices include the aneroid sphygmomanometer and electronic digital readout devices that do not require use of a stethoscope. The electronic devices are easier to manipulate but require frequent recalibration, more than once a year. Because of their sensitivity, improper cuff placement or movement of the arm causes electronic devices to give incorrect readings.

Stationary automatic BP devices are often found in public places such as grocery stores, fitness clubs, airports, or work sites. Users simply rest their arms within the inflatable cuff of the machine, which contains a pressure sensor. A visual display tells users their BP within 60–90 seconds. The reliability of the stationary machines is limited. BP values vary by 5–10 mm Hg or more (for both systolic and diastolic

Table 6.11 Advantages and Limitations of Assessing Blood Pressure Electronically

Advantages	Limitations
▪ Ease of use ▪ Efficient when frequent repeated blood pressure (BP) measurements are indicated ▪ Stethoscope not required ▪ Allows BP to be recorded more frequently, as often as every 15 s, with accuracy	▪ Expensive ▪ Requires source of electricity ▪ Requires space to position machine ▪ Sensitive to outside motion interference; not used in patients with seizures, tremors, or shivers or patients unable to cooperate ▪ Not accurate for hypotensive patients, hypertensive patients, or patients with cardiac dysrhythmias (AACN Practice Alert, 2016) ▪ Should not be used in patients with rapidly changing BPs (McLean, 2015) ▪ May cause low BP in older adults with arteriosclerosis ▪ Systolic readings by automated wrist manometers are the most unreliable, and automated arm monitors tend to provide higher measures than the mercury standard on average (Casiglia et al., 2016) ▪ Adherence to accuracy standards for electronic BP machine manufacturers is voluntary ▪ Vulnerable to error in patients with irregular heart rate and obese extremities ▪ Systolic BP possibly overestimated ▪ Multiple readings are essential to provide clinicians and patients with accurate information on which to base diagnostic and treatment decisions (AACN Practice Alert, 2016)

BOX 6.9 Procedural Guidelines for Automatic Blood Pressure Measurement

Equipment

Electronic BP machine, BP cuff of appropriate size as recommended by manufacturer, pen and vital sign flow sheet in chart or EHR

Steps

1. Identify the patient by using at least two identifiers (e.g., name and birthday or name and medical record number) according to agency policy.
2. Assess need to measure BP and determine patient's baseline BP.
3. Determine appropriateness of using electronic BP measurement.
4. Perform hand hygiene. Inspect condition of extremities to determine best site for cuff placement.
5. Collect and bring appropriate equipment to the patient's bedside. Select appropriate cuff size for patient extremity and appropriate cuff for machine. Electronic BP cuff and machine must be matched by manufacturer and are not interchangeable.
6. Assist the patient to comfortable position, either lying or sitting. Plug device into electric outlet and place it near the patient, ensuring that connector hose between cuff and machine reaches.
7. Locate on/off switch and turn on machine to enable device to self-test computer systems.
8. Remove constricting clothing to ensure proper cuff application.
9. Prepare BP cuff by manually squeezing all the air out of the cuff and connecting it to connector hose.
10. Wrap flattened cuff snugly around extremity, verifying that only one finger can fit between cuff and patient's skin. Make sure that "artery" arrow marked on outside of cuff is placed correctly (see illustration).

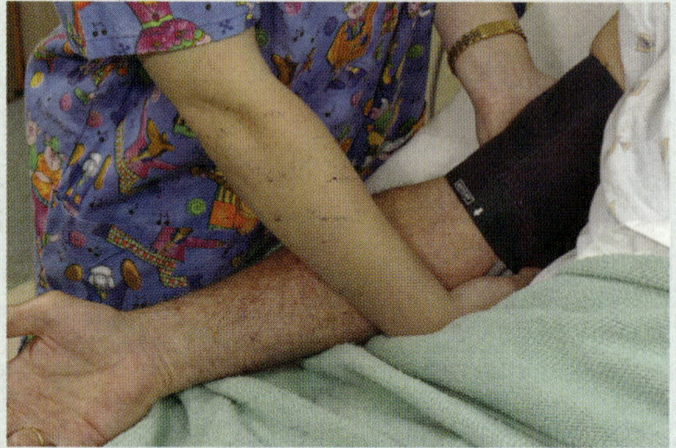

Step 10 Aligning blood pressure cuff arrow with brachial artery.

11. Verify that connector hose between cuff and machine is not kinked. Kinking prevents proper inflation and deflation of cuff.
12. Following manufacturer directions, set frequency control for automatic or manual, and press start button. The first BP measurement pumps cuff to a peak pressure of approximately 180 mm Hg. After this pressure is reached, the machine begins a deflation sequence that determines the BP. The first reading determines peak pressure inflation for additional measurements.
13. When deflation is complete, digital display provides most recent values and flash time in minutes that has elapsed since the measurement occurred (see illustration).

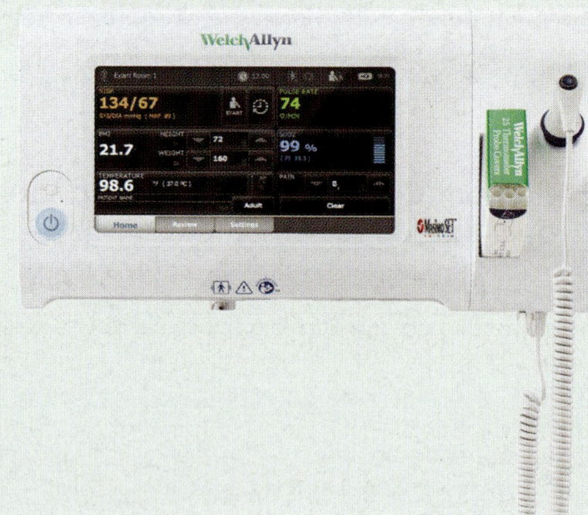

Step 13 Digital electronic blood pressure display. (Image courtesy Welch Allyn.)

Clinical decision point: If unable to obtain BP with electronic device, verify machine connections (e.g., plugged into working electrical outlet, hose–cuff connections tight, machine on, correct cuff). Repeat electronic BP measurement; if unable to obtain, use auscultatory technique.

14. Set frequency of measurements and upper and lower alarm limits for systolic, diastolic, and mean BP readings. Intervals between measurements can be set from 1 to 90 min. A nurse

BOX 6.9 Procedural Guidelines for Automatic Blood Pressure Measurement—cont'd

determines frequency and alarm limits based on patient's acceptable range of BP, nursing judgment, and health care provider order.

15. Obtain additional readings at any time by pressing the start button. Pressing the cancel button immediately deflates the cuff.
16. If frequent measurements are required, the cuff may be left in place. Remove it at least every 2 h to assess underlying skin integrity and if possible alternate measurement sites. Patients with abnormal bleeding tendencies are at risk for microvascular rupture from repeated inflations. When patient no longer requires frequent BP monitoring, remove and clean cuff according to agency policy to reduce transmission of microorganisms.
17. Discuss findings with the patient. Perform hand hygiene.
18. Compare electronic BP readings with auscultatory measurements to verify accuracy of electronic device.
19. Record BP and site assessed on vital sign flow sheet or nurses' notes in chart or EHR; record any signs or symptoms of BP alterations in narrative form in nurses' notes; report abnormal findings to nurse in charge or health care provider.
20. **Use teach back:** "I want to be sure I explained why you need to keep your arm straight while the machine is taking your BP. Tell me why it is important to remain still." Revise your instructions now or develop a plan for revised patient teaching if the patient is unable to teach back correctly.

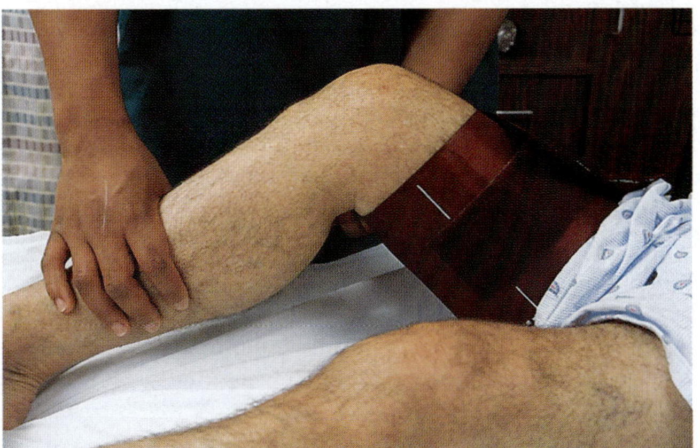

Fig. 6.16 Lower extremity blood pressure cuff positioned above popliteal artery at midthigh with knee flexed.

values) compared with pressures taken with a manual sphygmomanometer.

Self-measurement of BP has several benefits. Sometimes, elevated BP is detected in people previously unaware of a problem. People with prehypertension provide information about the pattern of BP values to their health care provider. Patients with hypertension benefit from participating actively in their treatment through self-monitoring, which helps adherence with treatment. The disadvantages of self-measurement include improper use of the device and risk of inaccurate readings. Some patients are needlessly alarmed with one elevated reading. Some patients with hypertension become overly conscious of their BP and inappropriately self-adjust medications.

Consumers can learn to use self-measurement devices if they have the information needed to perform the procedure correctly and if they know when to seek medical attention. Advise patients of possible inaccuracies in the BP devices, help them understand the meaning and implications of readings, and teach them proper measurement techniques. Encourage them to record the date of their BP readings to assess BP over time and share findings with their health care provider.

Assessment of Blood Pressure in Children

All children 3 years of age through adolescence should have BP checked at least annually. BP values in children change with growth and development. Educate parents about the importance of this routine screening to detect hypertension in children. Measuring BP in infants and children is difficult for several reasons:

1. Smaller cuff size is required.
2. Readings are difficult to obtain in restless or anxious infants and children.
3. Placing stethoscope too firmly on the antecubital fossa causes errors in auscultation.
4. Korotkoff sounds are difficult to hear in children because of low frequency and amplitude; a pediatric stethoscope bell is helpful.

The same auscultation method used with adults is appropriate for children. An infant or child younger than 5 years lies supine with the arm supported at heart level. Have older children sit like adults with arm supported at the heart level. It is important for the child to be relaxed and calm. Allow at least 15 minutes for children to recover from recent activity or excitement before taking a reading. It helps to have a parent nearby. Prepare the child for the unusual sensation of the BP cuff during inflation. Most children understand the analogy of a "tight hug on your arm" and will be more cooperative. Do not choose a cuff based on the name of the cuff (e.g., "infant"); rather base it on actual cuff bladder size. Average width of a cuff bladder for an infant is 2½–3¼ inches; average width of a cuff bladder for a child is 4¾–5½ inches.

SPECIAL CONSIDERATIONS

Physiological changes caused by aging influence the measurement and interpretation of vital signs in older adults (Box 6.10). You often provide patient teaching to patients of all ages related to vital sign results. For example, patients with hypertension require education on risk-factor modification. Teach patients taking cardiac medications that they affect pulse rate and how to check their own pulse.

BOX 6.10 Care of the Older Adult: Considerations When Obtaining Vital Sign Measurements

Temperature

- The normal temperature of older adults is 36°C (96.8°F), which is at the lower end of the acceptable temperature range. Therefore, temperatures considered normal for adults may represent fever in older adults.
- Older adults are very sensitive to slight changes in environmental temperature because their thermoregulatory systems are not as efficient (Touhy and Jett, 2014).
- Decreased sweat gland reactivity in older adults results in a higher threshold for sweating at high temperatures, which leads to hyperthermia and heatstroke.
- With aging, loss of subcutaneous fat reduces the insulating capacity of the skin; older men are at especially high risk for hypothermia.

Pulse Rate

- It is often difficult to palpate the pulse of older adults. A Doppler device provides a more accurate reading.
- Older adults typically have a decreased heart rate at rest (Touhy and Jett, 2014).
- It takes longer for the heart rate to rise in older adults to meet sudden increased demands that result from stress, illness, or excitement. Once elevated, the pulse rate of older adults takes longer to return to normal resting rate.
- When assessing apical rate in older women, lift the breast tissue gently and place the stethoscope at the fifth intercostal space (ICS) or the lower edge of the breast.
- Heart sounds are sometimes muffled or difficult to hear in older adults because of an increase in air space in the lungs.

Blood Pressure

- Older adults often have decreased upper arm mass, which requires special attention to selection of blood pressure (BP) cuff size.
- Skin of older adults is more fragile and susceptible to cuff pressure injury when BP measurements are frequent.
- Older adults sometimes have an increase in systolic BP related to decrease in vessel elasticity, whereas diastolic BP remains the same, resulting in a wider pulse pressure.
- Instruct older adults to change positions slowly and wait after each change to avoid orthostatic hypotension and prevent injuries.

Respiration

- Aging causes ossification of costal cartilage and downward slant of ribs, resulting in a more rigid rib cage, which reduces chest wall expansion. Kyphosis and scoliosis, which may occur in older adults, also restrict chest expansion and decrease tidal volume.
- The respiratory system matures by the time a person reaches the age of 20 years and begins to decline in healthy people after the age of 25 years. Despite this decline, older adults are able to breathe effortlessly as long as they are healthy. However, sudden events that require an increased demand for oxygen (e.g., exercise, stress, illness) can create shortness of breath in older adults (Touhy and Jett, 2014).
- Identifying an acceptable pulse oximeter sensor site is difficult with older adults because of the likelihood of peripheral vascular disease, decreased cardiac output, cold-induced vasoconstriction, and anemia, all of which decrease pulsatile flow.

DOCUMENTING VITAL SIGNS

Enter vital sign data on graphic flow sheets or directly into the electronic health record (EHR) (see Chapter 5). Record any patient teaching regarding vital signs. When a vital sign is above or below the expected value, enter a note in the patient's record regarding the finding, any interventions taken, and the patient's response.

SAFETY GUIDELINES FOR NURSING SKILLS

Ensuring patient safety is an essential role of the professional nurse. To ensure patient safety, communicate clearly with members of the health care team, assess and incorporate the patient's priorities of care and preferences, and use the best evidence when making decisions about your patient's care. When performing the skills of vital sign measurement, remember the following points to ensure safe, individualized patient care:

- Vital sign measurement devices are often shared among patients. Clean each device carefully between patients to decrease the risk for infection.
- BP cuffs and pulse oximetry sensors can apply excessive pressure on fragile skin. Rotating sites during repeated measurements decreases risk for skin breakdown and subsequent pressure injuries.
- Analyze trends of vital sign measurement and report abnormal findings to the health care provider.
- Determine vital sign frequency based on the patient's condition.

SKILL 6.1 Assessing Body Temperature

Equipment

- Thermometer (selected based on the site used)
- Soft tissue or wipe
- Alcohol swab
- Water-soluble lubricant (only for rectal measurements)
- Pen and vital sign flow sheet, record form, or EHR
- Clean gloves (optional), plastic thermometer sleeve, disposable probe or sensor cover
- Towel

STEP	RATIONALE
Assessment	
1. Identify the patient by using at least two identifiers (e.g., name and birthday or name and medical record number) according to agency policy.	Ensures correct patient. Complies with The Joint Commission standards and improves patient safety (TJC, 2018).
2. Determine need to measure patient's body temperature:	Clinical judgment determines need for assessment.
a. Note patient's risks for temperature alterations: ▪ Expected or diagnosed infection ▪ Open wounds or burns ▪ White blood cell count less than 5000/mm^3 or more than 12,000/mm^3 ▪ Immunosuppressive drug therapy ▪ Injury to hypothalamus ▪ Exposure to temperature extremes ▪ Blood product infusion ▪ Hypothermia or hyperthermia therapy ▪ Postoperative status	Certain conditions place patients at risk for temperature alterations and require more frequent temperature measurement and nursing assessment.
b. Assess for other signs and symptoms that accompany temperature alteration: ▪ *Hyperthermia:* Decreased skin turgor, dry mucous membranes; tachycardia; hypotension; decreased venous filling; concentrated urine ▪ *Heat stroke:* Body temperature 40°C (104°F) or more (Goforth and Kazman, 2015); hot, dry skin; tachycardia; hypotension; excessive thirst; muscle cramps; visual disturbances; confusion or delirium ▪ *Hypothermia:* Pale skin; skin cool or cold to touch; bradycardia and dysrhythmias; uncontrollable shivering; reduced level of consciousness; shallow respirations	Physical signs and symptoms alert you to alterations in body temperature.
c. Assess for factors that normally influence temperature:	Allows you to accurately assess for presence and significance of temperature alteration.
▪ Age	Older adults have a narrower range of temperature than younger adults.
Clinical decision point: No single temperature is normal for all people. A temperature within an acceptable range in an adult may reflect a fever in an older adult. Undeveloped temperature-control mechanisms in infants and children cause temperature to rise and fall rapidly.	
▪ Exercise	Muscle activity increases metabolism, which increases heat production and raises temperature.
▪ Hormones	Women have wider temperature fluctuations than men because of menstrual cycle hormonal changes, because body temperature varies during menopause, and because women have a thicker layer of subcutaneous fat.
▪ Stress	Stress elevates temperature by stimulating release of epinephrine.
▪ Environmental temperature	Infants and older adults are more sensitive to environmental temperature changes.
▪ Medications	Some drugs impair or promote sweating, vasoconstriction, or vasodilation or interfere with ability of hypothalamus to regulate temperature.
▪ Daily fluctuations	Body temperature normally changes 0.5–1°C (0.9–1.8°F) during a 24-h period. Temperature is lowest during early morning. Most patients have maximum temperature elevation between 5 p.m. and 7 p.m.; temperature falls gradually during night.
3. Determine appropriate measurement site and device for patient. Use disposable thermometer for patient on isolation precautions.	Determines whether the patient's status contraindicates selection of a specific method or site. Eliminates risk of transferring infection to other patients.
4. Determine previous baseline temperature and measurement site (if available) from patient's record.	Allows you to assess for change in the patient's condition and provides comparison with future temperature measurements.
5. Assess patient's knowledge of procedure.	Encourages cooperation, minimizes risks and anxiety, and identifies teaching needs.
Planning	
1. Provide privacy and prepare bedside environment for patient safety.	Maintains patient comfort and removes barriers that may interfere with procedure.

STEP	RATIONALE
2. Collect and bring appropriate supplies to patient's bedside.	Ensures an organized approach for body temperature measurement.
3. Verify that patient has not had anything to eat or drink and not has chewed gum or smoked within the past 20 min (if having oral temperature measured).	Oral food and fluids, smoking, and gum can alter oral temperature measurement.
4. Explain to patient the way you will measure temperature and the importance of maintaining proper position until reading is complete.	Promotes patient cooperation and increases compliance. Patients are often curious about their temperatures and should be cautioned against prematurely removing thermometer to read results.
Implementation	
1. Perform hand hygiene.	Reduces transmission of microorganisms.
2. Assist patient to comfortable position that provides easy access to temperature measurement site.	Ensures patient's comfort and accuracy of temperature reading.
3. Obtain temperature reading.	
a. **Oral temperature (electronic):**	
(1) *Optional:* Apply clean gloves when there is risk for exposure to respiratory secretions or facial or mouth wound drainage.	An oral probe cover is removable without physical contact and thus does not require gloves.
(2) Remove thermometer pack from charging unit. Attach oral thermometer probe stem (blue tip) to thermometer unit. Grasp top of probe stem, being careful not to apply pressure on ejection button.	Charging provides battery power. Ejection button releases plastic cover from probe stem.
(3) Slide disposable plastic probe cover over the thermometer probe stem until cover locks in place (see illustration).	Soft plastic cover will not break in patient's mouth and prevents transmission of microorganisms between patients.
(4) Ask the patient to open mouth; gently place thermometer probe under tongue in posterior sublingual pocket lateral to center of lower jaw (see illustration).	Heat from superficial blood vessels in sublingual pocket produces temperature reading. With electronic thermometer, temperatures in right and left posterior sublingual pocket are significantly higher than in area under front of tongue.
(5) Ask the patient to hold thermometer probe with lips closed.	Maintains proper position of thermometer during recording.
(6) Leave thermometer probe in place until audible signal indicates completion and patient's temperature appears on digital display; remove thermometer probe from under patient's tongue.	Probe must stay in place until signal occurs to ensure accurate reading.
(7) Push ejection button on the thermometer probe stem to discard plastic probe cover into appropriate receptacle.	Reduces transmission of microorganisms.
(8) If wearing gloves, remove and dispose of in appropriate receptacle and perform hand hygiene.	Reduces transmission of microorganisms.
(9) Return thermometer probe stem to storage position of thermometer unit.	Protects probe stem from damage. Returning thermometer probe stem automatically causes digital reading to disappear.
b. **Rectal temperature (electronic):**	
(1) Draw curtain around bed and/or close room door. Assist patient to side-lying or Sims position with upper leg flexed. Move aside bed linen to expose only anal area. Keep patient's upper body and lower extremities covered with sheet or blanket.	Maintains patient's privacy, minimizes embarrassment, and promotes comfort.
(2) Apply clean gloves. Cleanse anal region when feces and/or secretions are present. Remove soiled gloves, perform hand hygiene, and reapply clean gloves.	Maintains standard precautions when exposed to items soiled with body fluids (e.g., feces).
(3) Remove thermometer pack from charging unit. Attach rectal thermometer probe stem (red tip) to thermometer unit. Grasp top of probe stem, being careful not to apply pressure on ejection button.	Ejection button releases plastic cover from probe stem.
(4) Slide disposable plastic probe cover over thermometer probe stem until cover locks in place.	Soft plastic probe cover prevents transmission of microorganisms between patients.

STEP	RATIONALE
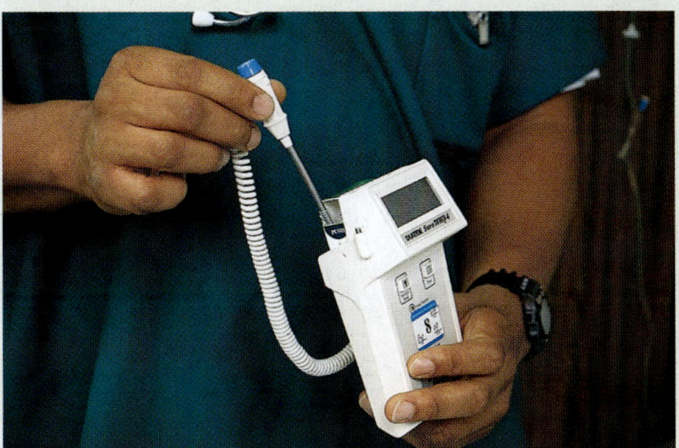 **Step 3a(3)** Nurse inserts electronic thermometer probe stem into probe cover. Cover snaps in place.	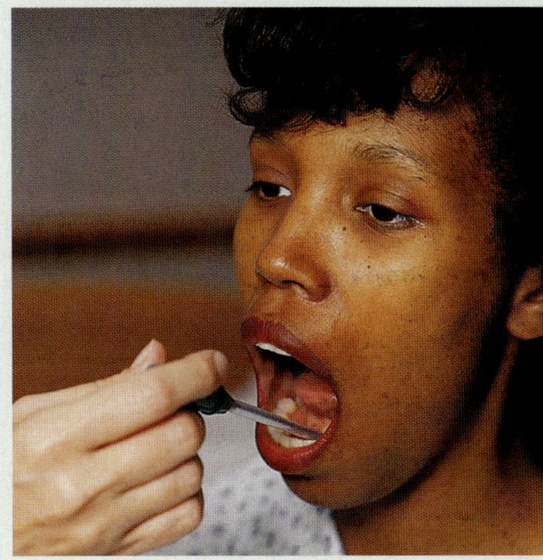 **Step 3a(4)** Probe placed under tongue in posterior sublingual pocket.
(5) Using a single-use package, squeeze a liberal amount of lubricant on tissue. Dip tip of probe cover of thermometer into lubricant, covering 2.5–3.5 cm (1–1½ inches) for adult.	Lubrication minimizes trauma to rectal mucosa during insertion. Using tissue avoids contamination of remaining lubricant in container.
(6) With nondominant hand, separate patient's buttocks to expose anus. Ask the patient to breathe slowly and relax.	Fully exposes anus and relaxes anal sphincter for easier thermometer insertion.
(7) Gently insert thermometer into anus in the direction of umbilicus 3.5 cm (1½ inches) for adult. Do not force thermometer.	Ensures adequate exposure of probe tip against blood vessels in rectal wall.
(8) If you feel resistance during insertion, withdraw immediately. Never force thermometer.	Prevents trauma to mucosa.

Clinical decision point: If you cannot adequately insert thermometer into rectum or resistance is felt during insertion, remove thermometer and consider an alternative method for obtaining temperature.

STEP	RATIONALE
(9) Once positioned, hold thermometer probe in place (see illustration) until audible signal indicates completion and patient's temperature appears on digital display; remove thermometer probe from anus.	Keeps probe in place until signal occurs to ensure accurate reading.
(10) Push ejection button on thermometer stem to discard plastic probe cover into appropriate receptacle. Wipe probe stem with alcohol swab, paying particular attention to ridges where probe stem connects to probe.	Reduces transmission of microorganisms. *Clostridium difficile* has been found to reside on thermometer probes if not cleaned properly.
(11) Return thermometer stem to storage position of recording unit.	Protects probe stem from damage. Returning thermometer stem automatically causes digital reading to disappear.
(12) Wipe patient's anal area with soft tissue to remove lubricant or feces and discard tissue. Assist patient in assuming a comfortable position.	Provides for comfort and hygiene.
(13) Remove and dispose of gloves in appropriate receptacle. Perform hand hygiene.	Reduces transmission of microorganisms.
c. **Axillary temperature (electronic):**	
(1) Draw curtain around bed and/or close room door. Assist patient to supine or sitting position. Move clothing or gown away from shoulder and arm.	Maintains patient's privacy, minimizes embarrassment, and promotes comfort. Exposes axilla for correct thermometer probe placement.
(2) Remove thermometer pack from charging unit. Attach oral thermometer probe stem (blue tip) to thermometer unit. Grasp top of thermometer probe stem, being careful not to apply pressure on ejection button.	Charging provides battery power. Ejection button releases plastic cover from probe stem.
(3) Slide disposable plastic probe cover over thermometer stem until cover locks in place.	Soft plastic probe cover prevents transmission of microorganisms between patients.

STEP	RATIONALE

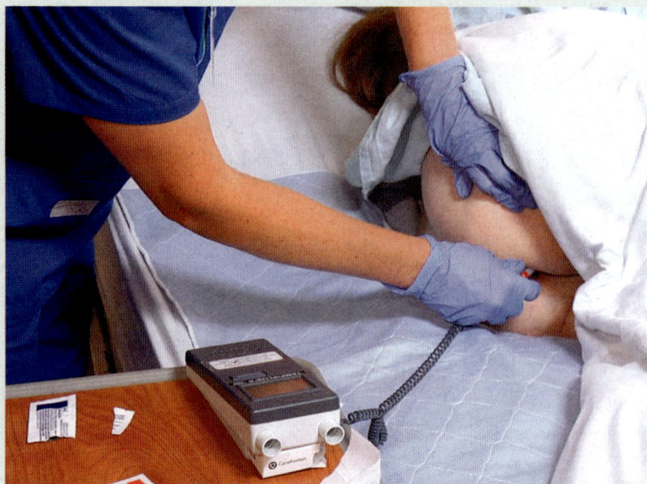

Step 3b(9) Hold rectal thermometer probe in place in anus until audible signal indicates completion. (Copyright © Mosby's Clinical Skills: Essentials Collection.)

STEP	RATIONALE
(4) Raise patient's arm away from torso. Inspect for skin lesions and excessive perspiration; if needed, dry axilla or select alternative site. Insert thermometer probe into center of axilla (see illustration), lower arm over probe, and place arm across patient's chest.	Maintains proper position of thermometer against blood vessels in axilla.

Clinical decision point: Do not use axilla if skin lesions are present because local temperature is sometimes altered and area may be painful to touch.

STEP	RATIONALE
(5) Once thermometer probe is positioned, hold it in place until audible signal indicates completion and patient's temperature appears on digital display; remove thermometer probe from axilla.	Thermometer probe must stay in place until signal occurs to ensure accurate reading.
(6) Push ejection button on thermometer stem to discard plastic probe cover into appropriate receptacle.	Reduces transmission of microorganisms.
(7) Return thermometer stem to storage position of recording unit.	Returning thermometer stem to storage position automatically causes digital reading to disappear and protects stem from damage.
(8) Assist patient in assuming comfortable position, replacing linen or gown.	Restores comfort and a sense of well-being.
(9) Perform hand hygiene.	Reduces transmission of microorganisms.
d. **Tympanic membrane temperature:**	
(1) Assist patient in assuming comfortable position with head turned toward side, away from you. If patient has been lying on one side, use upper ear. Obtain temperature from patient's right ear if you are right-handed. Obtain temperature from patient's left ear if you are left-handed.	Ensures comfort and facilitates exposure of auditory canal for accurate temperature measurement. Heat trapped in ear facing down causes false-high temperature reading. The less acute the angle of approach, the better the probe seal.
(2) Note whether there is obvious cerumen (earwax) in patient's ear canal.	Cerumen impedes the lens cover of speculum. Switch to other ear, or select alternative measurement site.
(3) Remove thermometer handheld unit from charging base, being careful not to apply pressure to ejection button.	Charging base provides battery power. Removal of handheld unit from base prepares it to measure temperature. Ejection button releases plastic probe cover from thermometer tip.
(4) Slide disposable speculum cover over the otoscope-like lens tip until it locks in place. Be careful not to touch lens cover.	Soft plastic probe cover prevents transmission of microorganisms between patients. Lens cover should not have dust, fingerprints, or cerumen obstructing optical pathway.
(5) Insert speculum into ear canal following manufacturer instructions for tympanic probe positioning (see illustration).	Correct positioning of probe with respect to ear canal allows maximal exposure of tympanic membrane.

STEP	RATIONALE

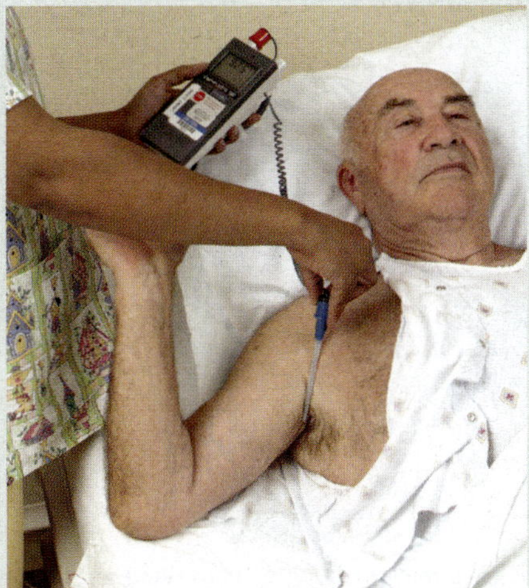

Step 3c(4) Insert thermometer probe into center of axilla.

STEP	RATIONALE
(a) Pull ear pinna backward, up, and out for an adult. For children younger than 3 years, pull pinna down and back, and point covered probe toward midpoint between eyebrow and sideburns. For children older than 3 years, pull pinna up and back (Hockenberry and Wilson, 2015).	The ear tug straightens the external auditory canal, allowing maximum exposure of tympanic membrane and therefore correctly positioning speculum (Hockenberry and Wilson, 2015).
(b) Move thermometer in a figure-eight pattern.	Some manufacturers recommend movement of speculum tip in a figure-eight pattern, which allows sensor to detect maximum tympanic membrane heat radiation.
(c) Fit speculum tip snug in canal, pointing toward the nose.	Gentle pressure seals ear canal from ambient air temperature, which can alter readings 2.8°C (5°F).
(6) Once positioned, press scan button on handheld unit. Leave speculum in place until audible signal indicates completion and patient's temperature appears on digital display.	Pressing scan button causes detection of infrared energy. The speculum probe tip must stay in place until device has detected infrared energy noted by audible signal.
(7) Carefully remove speculum from auditory meatus. Push ejection button on handheld unit to discard speculum cover into appropriate receptacle.	Reduces transmission of microorganisms. Automatically causes digital reading to disappear.
(8) If temperature is abnormal or second reading is necessary, replace probe cover and wait 2 min before repeating in the same ear, or repeat measurement in the other ear. Consider an alternative temperature site or instrument.	Lens cover must be free of cerumen to maintain optical path. Time allows ear canal to regain usual temperature.
(9) Return handheld unit to thermometer base.	Protects sensor tip from damage.
(10) Help patient assume a comfortable position.	Restores comfort and sense of well-being.
(11) Perform hand hygiene.	Reduces transmission of microorganisms.
e. **Temporal artery temperature:**	
(1) Ensure that forehead is dry; dry with a towel if needed.	Moisture interferes with thermometer sensor.
(2) Place sensor firmly on the patient's forehead.	Flush contact avoids measurement of ambient temperature.
(3) Press red scan button with your thumb. Slowly slide thermometer straight across forehead while keeping sensor flat and firmly on skin. Keeping scan button depressed, lift sensor after sweeping forehead and touch sensor on neck just behind earlobe. Read temperature when clicking sound during scanning stops. Release scan button.	Thermometer continuously scans for highest temperature when scan button is depressed. Area behind earlobe is less affected by diaphoresis and verifies temperature.
(4) Gently clean sensor with alcohol swab, return to storage unit, and perform hand hygiene.	Prevents transmission of microorganisms.

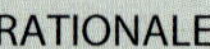

STEP	RATIONALE
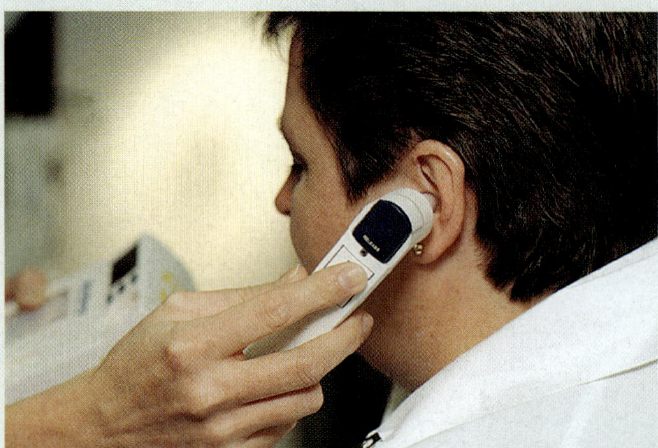 **Step 3d(5)** Tympanic membrane thermometer with probe cover placed in patient's ear.	
4. Inform patient of temperature reading, determine whether the patient has questions, and record measurement.	Promotes participation in care and understanding of health status.
5. Return thermometer to charger.	Maintains battery charge of thermometer unit.
Evaluation	
1. If you are assessing temperature for the first time, establish it as baseline if it is within acceptable range.	Used to compare future temperature measurements.
2. Compare temperature reading with patient's previous baseline and acceptable temperature range for patient's age group.	Body temperature fluctuates within narrow range; comparison reveals the presence of abnormality. Improper placement or movement of thermometer can cause inaccuracies. Second measurement confirms initial findings of abnormal body temperature.
3. If patient has fever, take temperature approximately 30 min after administering antipyretics and every 4 h until temperature stabilizes.	Determines whether temperature begins to fall in response to therapy.
4. **Use teach back:** "I want to be sure I explained how to check your child's temperature at home. Show me how to swipe his forehead using the thermometer." Revise your instruction now or develop a plan for revised patient/family caregiver teaching if patient/family caregiver is unable to teach back correctly.	Evaluates what the patient is able to demonstrate and explain.

Recording and Reporting

- Record temperature and route on vital sign flow sheet or nurses' notes in EHR or chart.
- Record patient's knowledge following evaluation of teach back in nurses' notes.
- Report abnormal findings to nurse in charge or health care provider.

Unexpected Outcomes and Related Interventions

- Patient has temperature 1°C (1.8°F) or more above usual range.
  - Initiate measures to lower body temperature.
    - Cool room environment.
    - Reduce external covering on patient's body to promote heat loss, but do not induce shivering.
    - Keep clothing and bed linen dry.
    - Limit physical activity and sources of emotional stress.
    - Administer antipyretics as ordered.
    - Increase fluid intake to at least 3 L daily (unless contraindicated).
- Patient has temperature 1°C (1.8°F) or more below the usual range.
  - Initiate measures to raise body temperature.
    - Apply warm blankets and, unless contraindicated, offer warm liquids.
    - Apply hyperthermia blankets if ordered.
    - Remove wet clothing or linen.
- Unable to obtain temperature.
  - Reassess correct placement of temperature probe or sensor.
  - Choose alternative temperature measurement site.
  - Obtain alternative temperature measurement device.

SKILL 6.2 Assessing Radial and Apical Pulses

Equipment

- Wristwatch with second hand or digital display
- Stethoscope
- Alcohol swab
- Pen and vital sign flow sheet in chart or EHR

STEP	RATIONALE
Assessment	
1. Identify the patient by using at least two identifiers (e.g., name and birthday or name and medical record number) according to agency policy.	Ensures correct patient. Complies with The Joint Commission standards and improves patient safety (TJC, 2018).
2. Determine need to assess radial or apical pulse rate:	Clinical judgment determines need for assessment.
a. Assess for risk factors for pulse alterations such as history of heart disease, cardiac dysrhythmia, onset of sudden chest pain or acute pain from any site, surgery, sudden infusion of large volume of i.v. fluid, hemorrhage, and medications that alter cardiac function.	Certain conditions place patients at risk for pulse alterations. A history of peripheral vascular disease often alters pulse rate and quality.
b. Assess for signs and symptoms of altered cardiac function such as presence of dyspnea, fatigue, chest pain, orthopnea, syncope, palpitations, edema of dependent body parts, cyanosis, or pallor of skin.	Physical signs and symptoms often indicate alteration in cardiac function, which affects radial pulse rate and rhythm.
c. Assess for signs and symptoms of peripheral vascular disease such as pale, cool extremities; thin, shiny skin with decreased hair growth; and thickened nails.	Physical signs and symptoms indicate alteration in local arterial blood flow.
d. Assess for factors that influence pulse rate and rhythm (see Table 6.6).	Allows you to anticipate factors that alter apical pulse rate, ensuring an accurate interpretation.
3. Determine patient's previous baseline pulse rate (if available) from patient's record.	Allows you to assess for change in condition and provides comparison with future pulse measurements.
4. Determine any report of latex allergy. If patient has latex allergy, ensure that stethoscope is latex-free.	Reduces risk of allergic reaction to stethoscope.
5. If you anticipate need for patient or family caregiver to monitor HR at home, assess their knowledge of the procedure and rationale for measurement.	Determines need for patient or family caregiver instruction.
Planning	
1. Provide privacy for patient; if necessary, draw curtain around bed and/or close door.	Maintains privacy and minimizes embarrassment, helping patient relax.
2. Collect appropriate equipment and bring to patient's bedside.	Ensures an organized approach for assessing a radial pulse.
3. Explain to patient that you will assess radial pulse rate or apical pulse rate (HR). Encourage patient to relax as much as possible. If patient has been active, wait 5–10 min before assessing pulse. If patient has been smoking or ingesting caffeine, wait 15 min before assessing pulse.	Anxiety, activity, caffeine, and smoking elevate HR.
Implementation	
1. Perform hand hygiene.	Reduces transmission of microorganisms.
2. Assist patient with assuming a supine or sitting position.	Provides easy access to pulse sites and chest wall.
a. **Radial pulse:**	
(1) If the patient is supine, place his or her forearm straight alongside or across lower chest or upper abdomen (see illustration A). If sitting, bend patient's elbow 90° and support lower arm on chair or on your arm. Place tips of first two or middle three fingers of hand over groove along radial or thumb side of patient's inner wrist (see illustration B). Slightly extend or flex wrist with palm down until you note strongest pulse.	Fingertips are most sensitive parts of hand to palpate arterial pulsation. Your thumb has pulsation that interferes with accuracy.
(2) Lightly compress pulse against radius, losing the pulse initially, and then relax pressure so that pulse becomes easily palpable.	Pulse assessment is more accurate when using moderate pressure. Too much pressure occludes pulse and impairs blood flow.

STEP	RATIONALE
(3) Determine strength of pulse. Note whether thrust of vessel against fingertips is bounding (4+); full increased, strong (3+); expected (2+); barely palpable, diminished (1+); or absent, not palpable (0).	Accurate description of strength improves communication among nurses and other health care providers and ensures appropriate treatment.
(4) After palpating a regular pulse, look at watch second hand and begin to count rate. Count the first beat after the second hand hits the number on the dial; count as one, then two, and so on.	Rate is determined accurately only after pulse has been palpated. Timing begins with zero. Count of one is first beat palpated after timing begins.
(5) If pulse is regular, count rate for 30 s and multiply total by 2.	A 30-s count is accurate for rapid, slow, or regular pulse rates.
(6) If pulse is irregular, count rate for a full 60 s. Assess frequency and pattern of irregularity.	Inefficient contraction of heart fails to transmit pulse wave, resulting in irregular pulse. Longer time ensures accurate count.
(7) When pulse is irregular, compare radial pulses bilaterally.	A marked difference between pulses indicates that arterial flow is compromised to one extremity, and as a nurse you need to take action.
b. **Apical pulse:**	
(1) Draw curtain around bed and/or close door. Assist patient to supine or sitting position. Move aside bed linen and gown to expose sternum and left side of chest.	Maintains privacy. Exposes portion of chest wall for selection of auscultatory site. Stethoscope diaphragm must touch skin for best sounds.
(2) Locate anatomical landmarks to identify point of maximal impulse (PMI), also called apical *impulse*. The heart is located behind and to the left of sternum with base at top and apex at bottom. Find angle of Louis just below suprasternal notch between the sternal body and manubrium; it feels like a bony prominence (see illustration A). Slip fingers down each side of angle to find second intercostal space (ICS) (see illustration B). Carefully move fingers down left side of sternum to fifth ICS and laterally to left midclavicular line (MCL) (see illustration C). A light tap felt within area 1−2.5 cm (1/2−1 inch) of PMI is reflected from apex of heart (see illustration D).	Use of anatomical landmarks allows correct placement of stethoscope over apex of heart. This position enhances ability to hear heart sounds clearly. If unable to palpate PMI, reposition patient on left side. In the presence of serious heart disease, you may locate PMI to the left of the MCL or at the sixth ICS. The PMI may not be palpated in obese adults or patients with severe pulmonary disease that has changed the shape of the thorax.
(3) Place diaphragm of stethoscope in palm of hand for 5−10 s.	Warming of metal or plastic diaphragm prevents patient from being startled and promotes comfort.
(4) Place diaphragm of stethoscope over PMI at fifth ICS, at left MCL, and auscultate for normal S_1 and S_2 heart sounds (heard as "lub-dub") (see illustrations).	Allow stethoscope tubing to extend straight without kinks that would distort sound transmission. Normal sounds S_1 and S_2 are high-pitched and best heard with diaphragm.
(5) When you hear S_1 and S_2 with regularity, use second hand of watch and begin to count rate: when sweep hand hits number on dial; start counting with zero, then one, two, and so on.	Apical rate is determined accurately only after you are able to auscultate sounds clearly. Timing begins with zero. Count of one is first sound auscultated after timing begins.
(6) If apical rate is regular, count for 30 s and multiply by 2.	The first time the apical rate is measured, it should be counted for 60 s. If the rate is regular, subsequent measurements will be accurate for 30 s.

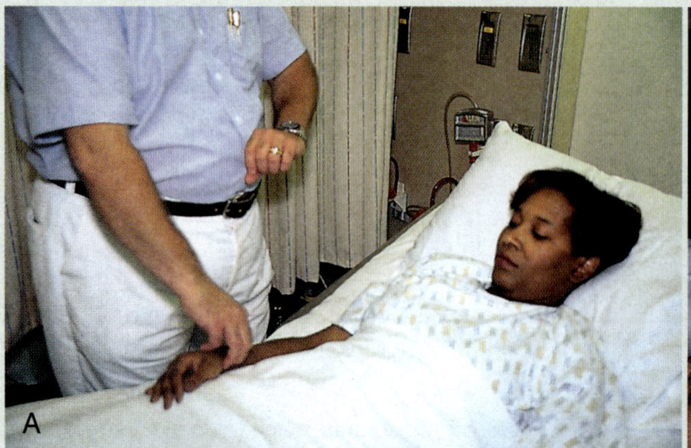

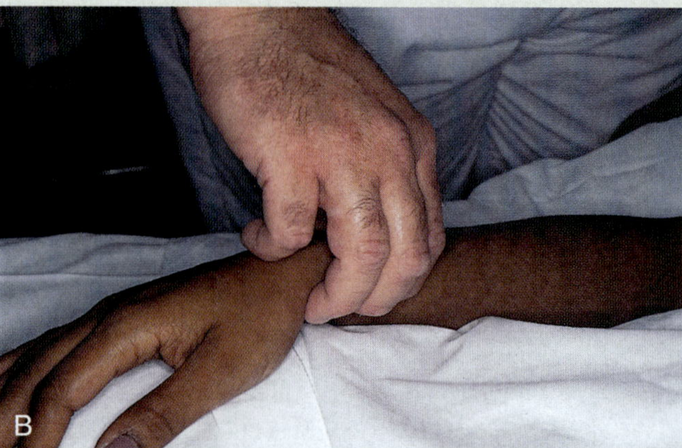

Step 2a(1) A, Pulse check with patient's forearm at side with wrist extended. **B,** Hand placement for pulse check.

STEP	RATIONALE

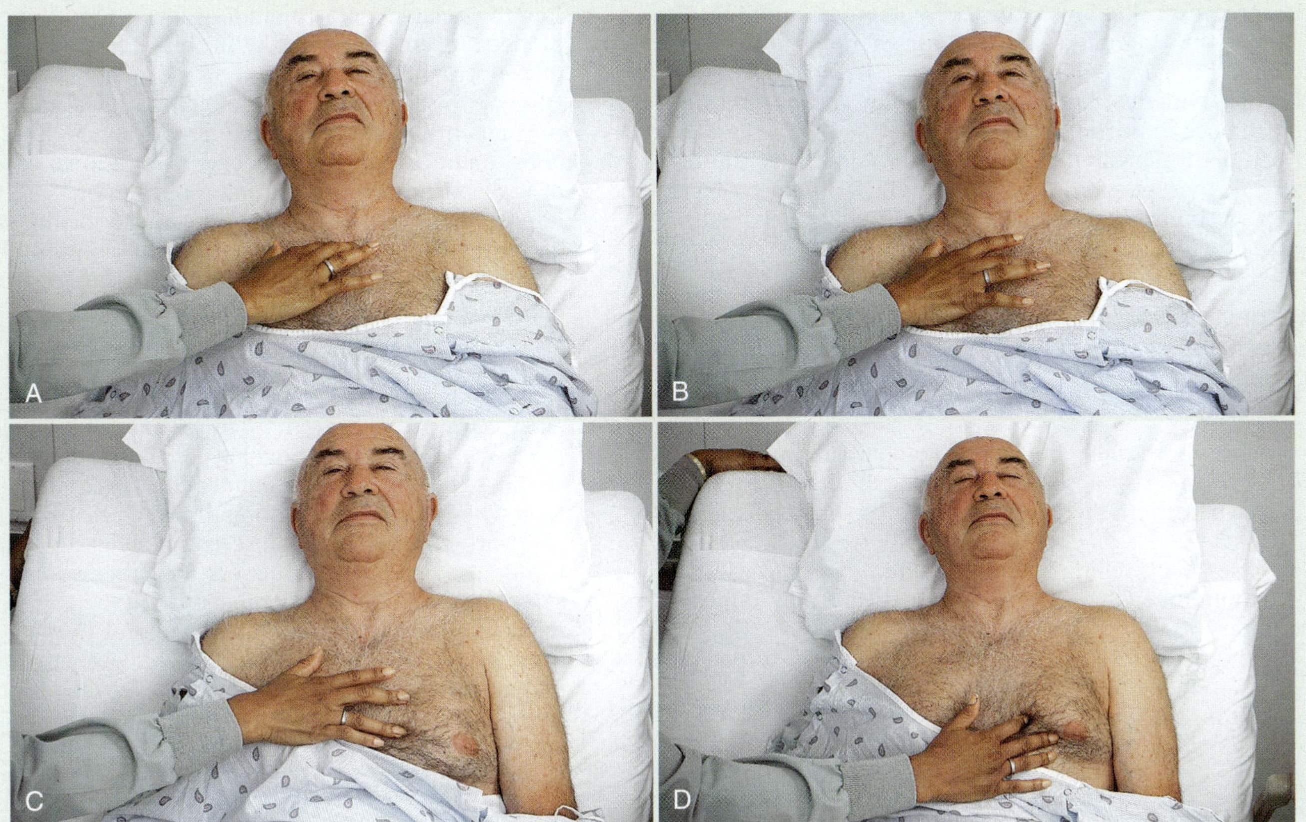

Step 2b(2) **A,** Nurse locates sternal notch. **B,** Nurse locates second intercostal space. **C,** Nurse locates fifth intercostal space. **D,** Nurse locates point of maximal impulse at fifth intercostal space at left midclavicular line.

STEP	RATIONALE
(7) If HR is irregular or patient is receiving cardiovascular medication, count for a full 1 min (60 s).	Irregular rate is more accurately assessed when measured over longer interval.
(8) Note regularity of any dysrhythmia (S_1 and S_2 occurring early or late after previous sequence of sounds) (e.g., every third or every fourth beat is skipped).	Regular occurrence of dysrhythmia within 1 min indicates inefficient contraction of heart and potential alteration in cardiac output.

Clinical decision point: If apical rate is abnormal or irregular, repeat measurement or have another nurse conduct measurement. Original measurement may be incorrect. Second measurement confirms initial findings of an abnormal HR.

STEP	RATIONALE
3. Replace patient's gown and bed linen; assist patient to return to comfortable position.	Restores comfort and promotes sense of well-being.
4. Discuss findings with the patient.	Promotes patient's participation in care and understanding of health status.
5. Perform hand hygiene.	Reduces transmission of microorganisms.

Evaluation

STEP	RATIONALE
1. If assessing pulse for the first time, establish baseline if it is within acceptable range.	Used to compare future HR assessments.
2. Compare HR and pulse character with patient's previous baseline and acceptable range for patient's age.	Allows for assessment of change in patient's condition and presence of cardiac alteration.
3. **Use teach back:** "I want to be sure I explained why it is important to check your pulse at home. Tell me what medication you are taking that would decrease your heart rate." Revise your instruction now or develop a plan for revised patient/family caregiver teaching if patient/family caregiver is unable to teach back correctly.	Evaluates what the patient understands and is able to explain.

Recording and Reporting

- Record pulse site, pulse rate, pulse strength, and apical rate on vital sign flow sheet or nurses' notes in EHR or chart.
- Record patient's knowledge following evaluation of teach back in nurses' notes.
- Document measurement of HR after administration of specific therapies in nurses' notes in EHR or chart.
- Report abnormal findings to nurse in charge or health care provider.

Unexpected Outcomes and Related Interventions

- Patient has weak, thready, or difficult-to-palpate radial pulse.
  - Assess both radial pulses and compare findings.
  - Observe for symptoms associated with ineffective tissue perfusion, including pallor and cool skin distal to weak pulse.
  - Assess for swelling in surrounding tissues or any encumbrance (e.g., dressing or cast) that may impede blood flow.
  - Obtain Doppler or ultrasound stethoscope to detect low-velocity blood flow.
  - Obtain apical pulse.
- An adult patient's HR is less than 60 beats/min (bradycardia) or more than 100 beats/min (tachycardia).
  - Identify related data, including fever, pain, fear or anxiety, recent exercise, low BP, blood loss, or inadequate oxygenation.
  - Observe for signs and symptoms associated with abnormal cardiac function including dyspnea, fatigue, chest pain, orthopnea, syncope, palpitations, edema of body parts, cyanosis, or pallor of the skin.
  - Report findings to nurse in charge and/or health care provider. It may be necessary to withhold prescribed medications that alter HR until health care provider can evaluate need to alter dosage.
  - Be prepared to order and/or obtain an electrocardiogram.
- Patient has an irregular HR.
  - **Assess for pulse deficit:** (a) nurse auscultates apical pulse while a second provider palpates radial pulse; (b) nurse begins 60-second pulse count by calling out loud when to begin counting pulses; (c) the two pulse rates are compared. If pulse count differs by more than 2, a deficit exists; assess for other signs and symptoms of decreased cardiac output.
  - Report findings to nurse in charge and/or health care provider, who may order an electrocardiogram to detect cardiac conduction alteration.

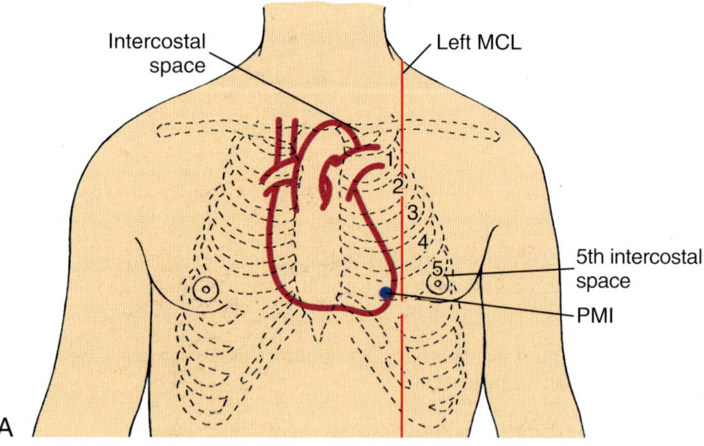

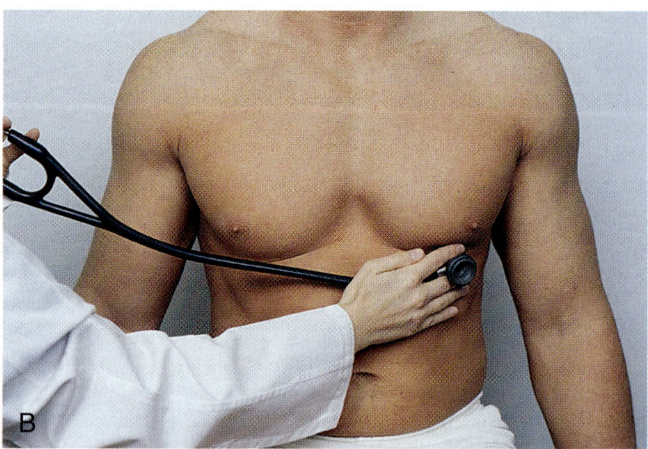

Step 2b(4) **A,** Location of point of maximal impulse *(PMI)* in adult. **B,** Listening to PMI in an adult. *MCL,* midclavicular line.

SKILL 6.3 Assessing Respiration

Equipment

- Wristwatch with second hand or digital display
- Pen and vital sign flow sheet in chart or EHR

STEP	RATIONALE
Assessment	
1. Identify the patient by using at least two identifiers (e.g., name and birthday or name and medical record number) according to agency policy.	Ensures correct patient. Complies with The Joint Commission standards and improves patient safety (TJC, 2018).

STEP	RATIONALE
2. Determine need to assess patient's respirations:	Clinical judgment determines need for assessment.
a. Assess for risk factors of respiratory alterations: ■ Fever ■ Pain and anxiety ■ Diseases of chest wall or muscles ■ Constrictive chest or abdominal dressings ■ Presence of abdominal incisions ■ Gastric distention ■ Chronic pulmonary disease (emphysema, bronchitis, asthma) ■ Traumatic injury to chest wall with or without collapse of underlying lung tissue ■ Presence of a chest tube ■ Respiratory infection (pneumonia, acute bronchitis) ■ Pulmonary edema and emboli ■ Head injury with damage to brain stem ■ Anemia	Certain conditions place patients at risk for ventilatory alterations detected by changes in respiratory rate, depth, and rhythm.
b. Assess for signs and symptoms of respiratory alterations: ■ Bluish or cyanotic appearance of nail beds, lips, mucous membranes, and skin ■ Restlessness, irritability, confusion, reduced level of consciousness ■ Pain during inspiration ■ Labored or difficult breathing ■ Orthopnea ■ Use of accessory muscles ■ Adventitious breath sounds ■ Inability to breathe spontaneously ■ Thick, frothy, blood-tinged, or copious sputum production	Physical signs and symptoms indicate alterations in respiratory status.
c. Assess for factors that influence the character of respirations:	Allows you to anticipate factors that influence respirations, ensuring a more accurate interpretation.
■ Exercise	Respirations increase in rate and depth to meet need for additional oxygen and rid body of carbon dioxide.
■ Anxiety	Anxiety causes increase in respiration rate and depth because of sympathetic nervous system stimulation.
■ Acute pain	Pain alters rate and rhythm of respirations; breathing becomes shallow. Patient inhibits or splints chest wall movement when pain is in area of chest or abdomen.
■ Smoking	Chronic smoking changes pulmonary airways, resulting in increased respiratory rate at rest when not smoking.
■ Medications	Narcotic analgesics, general anesthetics, and sedative-hypnotics depress rate and depth; amphetamines and cocaine increase rate and depth; bronchodilators cause dilation of airways, which ultimately slows respiratory rate.
■ Body position	Standing or sitting erect promotes full ventilatory movement and lung expansion; stooped or slumped posture impairs ventilatory movement; lying flat prevents full chest expansion.
■ Neurological injury	Damage to brain stem impairs the respiratory center and inhibits rate and rhythm.
■ Hemoglobin function	Decreased hemoglobin levels lower the amount of oxygen carried in blood, which results in increased respiratory rate to increase oxygen delivery. An increase in altitude lowers the amount of saturated hemoglobin, which increases respiratory rate and depth.
3. Assess pertinent laboratory/clinical values:	
a. *Arterial blood gases (ABGs):* Normal ranges (values vary slightly among agencies): ■ pH, 7.35–7.45 ■ $PaCO_2$, 35–45 mm Hg ■ HCO_3, 22–28 mEq/L ■ PaO_2, 80–100 mm Hg ■ SaO_2, 95%–100%	Measure arterial blood pH, partial pressure of oxygen and carbon dioxide, and arterial oxygen saturation, which reflect patient's ventilation and oxygenation status.

STEP	RATIONALE
b. *Pulse oximetry (SpO_2):* Normal SpO_2 95%–100% or greater; less than 90% is a clinical emergency (WHO, 2011).	SpO_2 less than 90% is often accompanied by changes in respiratory rate, depth, and rhythm.
c. *Complete blood count (CBC):* Normal CBC for adults (values vary within agencies): ▪ Hemoglobin: 14–18 g/100 mL, male patients; 12–16 g/100 mL, female patients ▪ Hematocrit: 42%–52%, male patients; 37%–47%, female patients ▪ Red blood cell count: 4.7–6.1 million/mm^3, male patients; 4.2–5.4 million/mm^3, female patients	Measures red blood cell count; volume of red blood cells; and concentration of hemoglobin, which reflects patient's capacity to carry oxygen.
4. Determine previous baseline respiratory rate (if available) from patient's record.	Assesses for change in condition and provides comparison with future respiratory measurements.
5. Assess patient's knowledge of procedure and any respiratory alteration that exists.	Encourages cooperation, minimizes risks and anxiety, and identifies teaching needs.

Planning

STEP	RATIONALE
1. Provide privacy.	
2. If the patient has been active, wait 5–10 min before assessing respirations.	Exercise increases respiratory rate and depth. Assessing respirations while patient is at rest allows for objective comparison of values.
3. Assess respirations after pulse measurement in an adult.	Inconspicuous assessment of respirations immediately after pulse assessment prevents patient from consciously or unintentionally altering rate and depth of breathing.
4. Be sure that patient is in comfortable position, preferably sitting or lying with the head of the bed elevated 45–60°.	Sitting erect promotes full ventilatory movement. A position of discomfort causes patient to breathe more rapidly.
5. Explain to patient that you will assess respirations or rate of breathing.	Helps to decrease patient anxiety during measurement.

Clinical decision point: Assess patients with difficulty breathing (dyspnea) such as patients with heart failure or abdominal ascites or in late stages of pregnancy in the position of greatest comfort. Repositioning may increase the work of breathing, which increases respiratory rate.

Implementation

STEP	RATIONALE
1. Perform hand hygiene.	Prevents transmission of microorganisms.
2. Draw curtain around bed and/or close door.	Maintains privacy.
3. Be sure that patient's chest is visible. If necessary, move bed linen or gown.	Ensures clear view of chest wall and abdominal movements.
4. Place patient's arm in relaxed position across abdomen or lower chest, or place your hand directly over patient's upper abdomen.	A similar position used during pulse assessment allows respiratory rate assessment to be inconspicuous. Patient's hand or your hand rises and falls during respiratory cycle.
5. Observe complete respiratory cycle (one inspiration and one expiration) (see illustration).	On inspiration, the diaphragm normally contracts, and the abdominal organs move down to increase the size of the chest cavity. At the same time the ribs and sternum lift outward. On expiration, the diaphragm relaxes upward, and the ribs and sternum return to their relaxed position (see illustration). Rate is accurately determined only after viewing a complete respiratory cycle.
6. After observing a cycle, look at second hand of watch and begin to count rate: when sweep hand hits number on dial, begin time frame, counting one with first full respiratory cycle.	Timing begins with count of one. Respirations occur more slowly than pulse; thus, timing does not begin with zero.

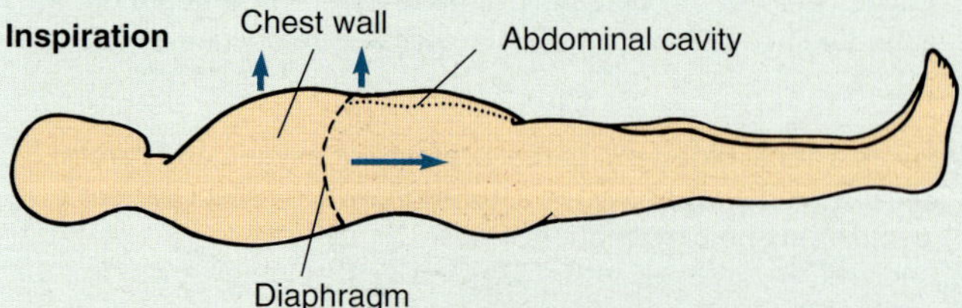

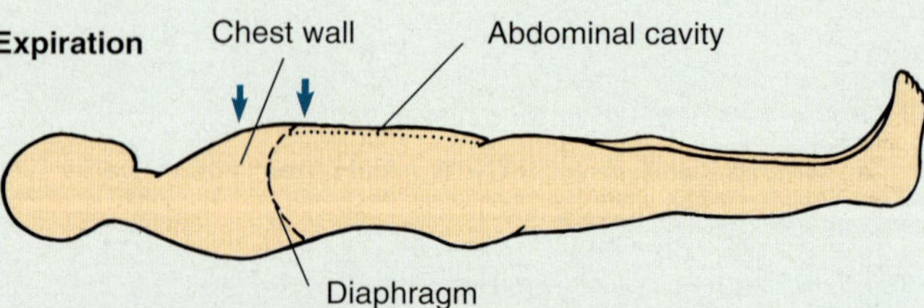

Step 5 Diaphragmatic and chest wall movement during inspiration and expiration.

STEP	RATIONALE
7. If rhythm is regular, count number of respirations in 30 s and multiply by 2. If rhythm is irregular, less than 12, or more than 20, count for 1 full min.	Respiratory rate is equivalent to number of respirations per minute. Suspected irregularities require assessment for at least 1 min.
8. Note depth of respirations by observing degree of chest wall movement while counting rate. Assess depth by palpating chest wall excursion or auscultating posterior thorax after you have counted rate. Describe depth as shallow, normal, or deep.	Character of ventilatory movement reveals specific disease states restricting volume of air from moving into and out of lungs.
9. Note rhythm of ventilatory cycle. Normal breathing is regular and uninterrupted. Do not confuse sighing with abnormal rhythm.	Character of ventilations reveals specific types of alterations. Periodically people unconsciously take single deep breaths or sighs to expand small airways prone to collapse.
Clinical decision point: Any irregular respiratory pattern or periods of apnea (cessation of respiration for several seconds) are symptoms of underlying disease in an adult patient, and you need to report this to the health care provider or nurse in charge. Further assessment and immediate intervention are often necessary.	
10. Replace bed linen and patient's gown.	Restores comfort and promotes a sense of well-being.
11. Discuss findings with patient.	Promotes participation in care and understanding of health status.
12. Perform hand hygiene.	Reduces transmission of microorganisms.
Evaluation	
1. If assessing respirations for the first time, establish rate, rhythm, and depth as baseline if within acceptable range.	Used to compare future respiratory assessment.
2. Compare respirations with patient's previous baseline and usual rate, rhythm, and depth.	Allows you to assess for changes in patient's condition and presence of respiratory alterations.
3. Correlate respiratory rate, depth, and rhythm with data obtained from pulse oximetry and ABG measurements if available.	Evaluation of ventilation, perfusion, and diffusion is interrelated.
4. **Use teach back:** "I want to be sure I explained why you will be reminded to take deep breaths after surgery. Tell me why deep breathing is important." Revise your instruction now or develop a plan for revised patient/family caregiver teaching if patient/family caregiver is unable to teach back correctly.	Evaluates what the patient is able to explain.

Recording and Reporting

- Record respiratory rate, depth, and rhythm on vital sign flow sheet or nurses' notes in EHR or chart.
- Record patient knowledge following evaluation of teach back in nurses' notes.
- Document measurement of respiratory rate after administration of specific therapies in nurses' notes in EHR or chart.
- Record type and amount of oxygen therapy, if used, in nurses' notes.
- Report abnormal findings to nurse in charge or health care provider.

Unexpected Outcomes and Related Interventions

- Adult patient's respiratory rate is less than 12 breaths/min (bradypnea) or more than 20 breaths/min (tachypnea). Breathing pattern is sometimes irregular. Depth of respirations is increased or decreased. Patient complains of dyspnea.
  - Assess for related factors including obstructed airway, abnormal breath sounds, productive cough, restlessness, anxiety, and confusion.
  - Assist patient to supported sitting position (semi-Fowler or high-Fowler) unless contraindicated.
  - Provide oxygen as ordered.
  - Assess for environmental factors that influence patient's respiratory rate such as secondhand smoke, poor ventilation, or gas fumes.
  - Notify health care provider or nurse in charge if alteration continues.
- Patient demonstrates Kussmaul, Cheyne–Stokes, or Biot respirations.
  - Notify health care provider for additional evaluation and possible medical intervention.

SKILL 6.4 Measuring Oxygen Saturation (Pulse Oximetry)

Equipment

- Oximeter
- Oximeter probe appropriate for patient and recommended by manufacturer (single use or reusable are available)
- Acetone or nail polish remover if needed for fingertip sensor
- Pen, vital sign flow sheet or record form, or EHR

STEP	RATIONALE
Assessment	
1. Identify the patient by using at least two identifiers (e.g., name and birthday or name and medical record number) according to agency policy.	Ensures correct patient. Complies with The Joint Commission standards and improves patient safety (TJC, 2018).
2. Determine need to assess patient's oxygen saturation:	Clinical judgment determines need for assessment.
a. Identify risk factors of decreased oxygen saturation including acute or chronic compromised respiratory function, recovery from general anesthesia or conscious sedation, traumatic injury to chest wall with or without collapse of underlying lung tissue, ventilator dependence, and changes in supplemental oxygen therapy.	Certain conditions place patients at risk for decreased oxygen saturation.
b. Assess for signs and symptoms of alterations in oxygen saturation such as altered respiratory rate, depth, or rhythm; adventitious breath sounds (see Chapter 7); cyanotic appearance of nail beds, lips, mucous membranes, and skin; restlessness, irritability, confusion; reduced level of consciousness; and labored or difficult breathing.	Physical signs and symptoms often indicate abnormal oxygen saturation.
3. Assess for factors that normally influence measurement of SpO_2 in addition to oxygen therapy, hemoglobin level, body temperature, and medications such as bronchodilators.	Allows you to accurately assess oxygen saturation variations.
4. Determine previous baseline SpO_2 (if available) from patient's record.	Baseline information provides basis for comparison and assists in assessment of current status and evaluation of interventions.
5. Determine most appropriate patient-specific site (e.g., finger, toe, earlobe, forehead, nose) for sensor probe placement by measuring capillary refill (see Chapter 7). If capillary refill is more than 2 s, select alternative site other than digit.	Sensor requires pulsating vascular bed to identify hemoglobin molecules that absorb emitted light. Changes in SpO_2 are reflected in circulation of finger capillary bed within 30 s and capillary bed of earlobe within 5−10 s. Forehead sensors are preferred for critically ill patients requiring vasopressors.
a. Site must have adequate local circulation and be free of moisture and skin breakdown.	Moisture prevents sensor from detecting SpO_2 levels.
b. Place probe on finger free of polish or artificial nail.	Black or brown nail polish colors alter readings.
c. If tremors are present, use earlobe as site.	Motion artifact is the most common cause of inaccurate readings.
d. If the patient is obese, clip-on probe may not fit properly; obtain a single-use (tape-on) probe.	
6. Determine whether the patient has a latex allergy.	Do not use adhesive sensors if the patient has a latex allergy.
7. Assess patient's knowledge of measurement of oxygen saturation and pulse oximetry.	Encourages cooperation, minimizes risks and anxiety, and identifies teaching needs.
Planning	
1. Provide privacy and prepare environment for patient safety.	Providing privacy and preparing the environment helps you to think about the steps needed and removes clutter from overbed or bedside table.
2. Prepare and organize pulse oximetry equipment.	Ensures organized procedure.
3. Explain purpose of procedure and how you measure oxygen saturation to patient. Instruct patient to breathe normally.	Promotes patient cooperation and increases compliance. Prevents large fluctuations in minute ventilation and possible error in SpO_2 readings.
Implementation	
1. Perform hand hygiene.	Reduces transmission of microorganisms.
2. Position patient comfortably. When using finger as monitoring site, support lower arm.	Ensures probe positioning and decreases motion artifact that interferes with SpO_2 determination.
3. Instruct patient to breathe normally and relax.	Prevents large fluctuations in respiratory rate and depth and possible changes in SpO_2.
4. When using finger as monitoring site, consider removing any fingernail polish with acetone or polish remover. Acrylic nails without polish do not interfere with SpO_2 determination.	Ensures accurate readings. Nail polish may falsely alter saturation.
5. Attach transmittance sensor probe following manufacturer directions. In most sensors involving finger, toe, or ear, the LEDs and the photodetector must be aligned directly across from one another.	Ensures transmission of light between emitter and detector through the digit or ear across the arteriolar bed (Nellcor, n.d.).

STEP	RATIONALE
a. Instruct patient that clip-on probe feels like a clothespin but will not hurt.	Pressure spring tension of sensor probe on peripheral digit or earlobe is unexpected.
6. Attach reflectance sensor to forehead following manufacturer's directions. LEDs are already aligned as part of sensor design. Remove cover over adhesive to apply to forehead or use a Velcro band/device to apply.	Reflects light from the emitter/detector across the skin surface. Forehead site is preferred if patient has poor circulation (Nellcor, n.d.).

Clinical decision point: Do not attach sensor to finger, ear, forehead, or bridge of nose if area is edematous or skin integrity is compromised. Do not attach sensor to fingers that are hypothermic. Select forehead, ear, or bridge of nose if adult patient has history of peripheral vascular disease. Do not use earlobe and bridge of nose sensors for infants and toddlers because of skin fragility. Do not use disposable adhesive sensors if patient has latex allergy. Do not place sensor on same extremity as electronic BP cuff because blood flow to finger is temporarily interrupted when cuff inflates and causes inaccurate readings that trigger alarms.

STEP	RATIONALE
7. Once sensor is in place, turn on oximeter by activating power. Observe pulse waveform/intensity display and audible beep. Correlate oximeter pulse rate with patient's radial pulse. Differences require reevaluation of oximeter sensor placement and may require reassessment of pulse rates.	Pulse waveform/intensity display enables detection of valid pulse or presence of interfering signal. Pitch of audible beep is proportional to SpO_2 value. Double-checking pulse rate ensures oximeter accuracy. Oximeter pulse rate, patient's radial pulse, and apical pulse rate should be the same. Any difference requires reevaluation of oximeter sensor placement and reassessment of pulse rates.
8. Leave sensor in place until oximeter readout reaches constant value and pulse display reaches full strength during each cardiac cycle. Inform patient that oximeter alarm will sound if sensor falls off or patient moves sensor. Read SpO_2 on digital display.	Reading takes 10–30 s, depending on site selected.
9. If continuous SpO_2 monitoring is necessary, verify SpO_2 alarm limits and volume, which are preset by the manufacturer at a low of 85% and a high of 100%. Determine limits for SpO_2 and pulse rate alarms based on each patient's condition. Verify that alarms are on.	Alarms are set at appropriate limits and volumes to avoid frightening patients and visitors.
10. Assess skin integrity every 2 h under sensor. Routinely relocate sensor at least every 24 h or more frequently (see manufacturer's recommendations). This is especially important if skin integrity is altered or tissue perfusion is compromised. Use care during removal to avoid damage to skin.	Sensor tension and sensitivity to disposable sensor adhesive cause skin irritation and lead to disruption of skin integrity. There have been reports of forehead and nasal pressure injuries (Schallom et al., 2016).
11. Help patient return to comfortable position.	Restores comfort and promotes a sense of well-being.
12. Clean the surface of a reusable sensor between patients with 70% isopropyl alcohol solution or solution recommended by manufacturer.	Reduces transmission of infection.
13. Discuss findings with patient as needed.	Promotes participation in care and understanding of health status.
14. Perform hand hygiene.	Reduces transmission of microorganisms.
15. If planning intermittent or spot-checking SpO_2 measurements, remove sensor and turn oximeter power off. Store reusable sensor in appropriate location.	Batteries will run out if oximeter is left on. Sensor probes are expensive and vulnerable to damage.
Evaluation	
1. If you are assessing SpO_2 for the first time, establish it as baseline if it is within acceptable range.	Used to compare future SpO_2 measurements.
2. Compare SpO_2 readings with patient's previous baseline and acceptable values. Note use of oxygen therapy, which can affect SpO_2.	Comparison reveals presence of abnormality.
3. Correlate SpO_2 with SaO_2 obtained from arterial blood gas measurements (see Chapter 24) if available.	Documents reliability of noninvasive assessment.
4. Correlate SpO_2 reading with data obtained from respiratory rate, depth, and rhythm assessment (see Skill 6.3).	Measurements assessing ventilation, perfusion, and diffusion are interrelated.
5. During continuous monitoring, assess skin integrity underneath probe at least every 2 h.	Prevents tissue ischemia.
6. **Use teach back:** "I want to be sure I explained why you need to keep the sensor on your finger. Tell me why this measurement is important and how moving your finger affects the reading." Revise your instruction now or develop a plan for revised patient teaching if patient/family caregiver is unable to teach back correctly.	Evaluates what the patient is able to demonstrate and explain.

Recording and Reporting

- Record SpO_2 on vital sign flow sheet or nurses' notes in EHR or chart.
- Indicate type and amount of oxygen therapy used by patient during assessment.
- Record signs and symptoms of oxygen desaturation in nurses' notes.
- Document oxygen saturation after administration of specific therapies in narrative form in nurses' notes.
- Record patient's knowledge following evaluation of teach back in nurses' notes.
- Record in nurses' notes patient's use of continuous or intermittent pulse oximetry. Document use of equipment for third-party payers.
- Report abnormal findings to nurse in charge or health care provider.

Unexpected Outcomes and Related Interventions

- SpO_2 is less than 90%.
  - Verify that oximeter sensor is intact and properly applied.
  - Observe for signs and symptoms of decreased oxygenation such as anxiety, restlessness, tachycardia, and cyanosis.
  - Verify that supplemental oxygen is delivered as ordered and system is functioning properly.
  - Observe for and minimize factors that decrease SpO_2 such as lung secretions, increased activity, and hyperthermia.
  - Assist patient to a position that maximizes ventilatory effort (e.g., place an obese patient in a high-Fowler position).
- Pulse rate indicated on the oximeter is less than the patient's radial or apical pulse.
  - Reposition sensor probe to an alternative site with increased blood flow.
  - Assess patient for signs of altered cardiac output (e.g., decreased BP, cool skin, confusion).
- Pressure injury develops under sensor site.
  - Remove and relocate sensor.
  - Provide appropriate skin care (see Chapter 16).
  - Inform health care provider.

SKILL 6.5 Blood Pressure Measurement

Equipment

- Aneroid sphygmomanometer
- Cloth or disposable vinyl BP cuff of appropriate size for patient's extremity
- Stethoscope
- Alcohol swab
- Pen and vital sign flow sheet in chart or EHR

STEP	RATIONALE
Assessment	
1. Identify the patient by using at least two identifiers (e.g., name and birthday or name and medical record number) according to agency policy.	Ensures correct patient. Complies with The Joint Commission standards and improves patient safety (TJC, 2018).
2. Determine need to assess patient's BP:	Clinical judgment determines need for assessment.
a. Assess risk factors for BP alterations: ▪ History of cardiovascular disease ▪ Renal disease ▪ Diabetes mellitus ▪ Circulatory shock (hypovolemic, septic, cardiogenic, or neurogenic) ▪ Acute or chronic pain ▪ Rapid i.v. infusion of fluids or blood products ▪ Increased intracranial pressure ▪ Postoperative status ▪ Toxemia of pregnancy	Certain conditions place patients at risk for BP alteration.
b. Assess for signs and symptoms of BP alterations. In patients at risk for hypertension, assess for headache (usually occipital), flushing of face, nosebleed, and fatigue in older adults. In patients at risk for hypotension, assess for dizziness; mental confusion; restlessness; pale, dusky, or cyanotic skin and mucous membranes; and cool, mottled skin over extremities.	Physical signs and symptoms indicate alterations in BP. Hypertension is often asymptomatic until BP is very high.
c. Assess for factors that influence BP:	Allows you to anticipate factors that influence BP, ensuring a more accurate interpretation.
▪ Age	Acceptable values for BP vary throughout life.
▪ Gender	During and after menopause, women often have higher BP values than men of the same age.

STEP	RATIONALE
▪ Daily (diurnal) variation	BP varies throughout day; BP is highest during the day between 10:00 a.m. and 6:00 p.m. and lowest in early morning.
▪ Position	BP falls as person moves from lying to sitting or standing position; normally postural variations are minimal.
▪ Exercise	Increases in oxygen demand by the body during activity increase BP.
▪ Weight	Obesity is an independent predictor of hypertension.
▪ Sympathetic stimulation	Pain, anxiety, or fear stimulates the sympathetic nervous system, causing BP to rise.
▪ Medications	Antihypertensives, diuretics, beta-adrenergic blockers, vasodilators, calcium channel blockers, angiotensin-converting enzyme (ACE) inhibitors, angiotensin receptor blockers (ARBs), and antidysrhythmics lower BP; opioids and general anesthetics also cause a drop in BP.
▪ Smoking	Smoking results in vasoconstriction, a narrowing of blood vessels. BP rises acutely and returns to baseline approximately 30 min after stopping smoking (James et al., 2014).
▪ Ethnicity	Incidence of hypertension is higher in African Americans than in European Americans. African Americans tend to develop more severe hypertension at an earlier age and have twice the risk for complications of hypertension (i.e., stroke, heart attack). Hypertension-related deaths are also higher among African Americans.
3. Determine best site for BP assessment. Avoid applying cuff to extremity when i.v. fluids are infusing, an arteriovenous shunt or fistula is present, or breast or axillary surgery has been performed on that side. Also, avoid applying cuff to traumatized or diseased extremity or one that has a cast or bulky bandage. Use lower extremities when brachial arteries are inaccessible.	Inappropriate site selection may result in poor amplification of sounds, causing inaccurate readings. Application of pressure from inflated bladder temporarily impairs blood flow and can further compromise circulation in extremity that already has impaired blood flow.
4. Determine previous baseline BP and site (if available) from patient's record. Determine any report of latex allergy.	Assesses for change in condition and provides comparison with future BP measurements. If the patient has latex allergy, verify that stethoscope and BP cuff are latex-free.
5. Assess patient's knowledge of procedure and any BP alteration that exists.	Encourages cooperation, minimizes risks and anxiety, and identifies teaching needs.
Planning	
1. Provide privacy and prepare bedside environment for patient safety.	Providing privacy and preparing the environment early help you to think about the steps in the procedure and remove clutter from the over-bed or bedside table.
2. Select appropriate cuff size and ensure that other equipment is in the patient's room.	Use of improper-size cuff causes false-low or false-high reading (Gunes and Efteli, 2016).
3. Explain to the patient that you will assess BP. Have patient rest at least 5 min before measuring lying or sitting BP and 1 min before measuring standing BP. Ask the patient not to speak while you are measuring BP.	Reduces anxiety that falsely elevates readings. Exercise causes false elevations in BP. Deep breathing lowers SBP and DBP up to 5 mm Hg (Zheng et al., 2014). Talking with a patient during assessment increases BP (AACN Practice Alert, 2016).
4. Be sure that the patient has not exercised, ingested caffeine, or smoked for 30 min before assessment of BP.	Smoking increases BP immediately, and increase lasts up to 15 min. The effects of coffee or caffeine increase BP for up to 3 h (James et al., 2014).
Implementation	
1. Perform hand hygiene.	Reduces transmission of microorganisms.
2. Have the patient assume sitting or lying position. Be sure that room is warm, quiet, and relaxing.	Maintains patient's comfort during measurement. Patient's perceptions that the physical or interpersonal environment is stressful affect BP.
3. Assess BP by auscultation:	
a. *Upper extremity:* With the patient sitting or lying, position the patient's forearm at heart level with palm turned up (see illustration). If sitting, instruct the patient to keep feet flat on floor without legs crossed. If supine, the patient should not have legs crossed. If the patient cannot be placed in the prone position, position the patient supine with knee slightly bent. *Lower extremity:* With the patient prone, position the patient so that knee is slightly flexed.	If arm is extended and not supported, the patient will perform isometric exercise that can increase SBP (Gunes and Efteli, 2016). Placement of arm above the level of heart causes false-low reading, 2 mm Hg for each 1 inch above the heart level. Leg crossing can falsely increase BP.

STEP	RATIONALE

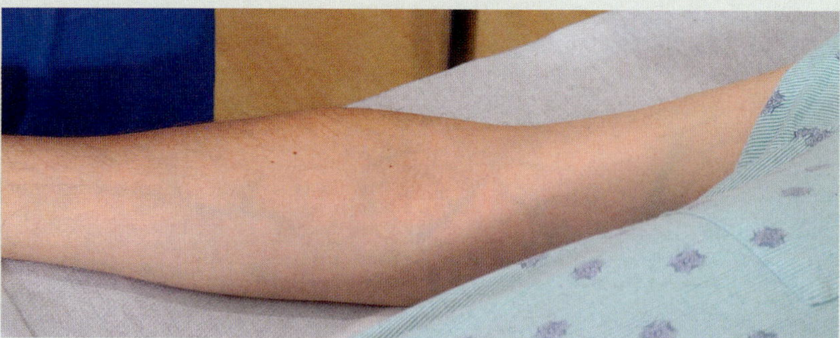

Step 3a Patient's forearm supported on bed. (Copyright © Mosby's Clinical Skills: Essentials Collection.)

STEP	RATIONALE
b. Expose extremity (arm or leg) fully by removing constricting clothing. Cuff may be placed over a sleeve of thin clothing as long as stethoscope rests on the skin.	Ensures proper cuff application. Placing a cuff over rolled-up or thick clothing, especially in older adults, can increase BP (Ozone et al., 2016)
c. Palpate brachial artery (arm; see illustration A) or popliteal artery (leg). With cuff fully deflated, apply bladder of cuff above artery by centering arrows marked on cuff over artery (see illustration B). If cuff does not have any center arrows, estimate center of bladder and place this center over artery. Position cuff 2.5 cm (1 inch) above site of pulsation (antecubital or popliteal space). With cuff fully deflated, wrap it evenly and snugly around the upper arm (see illustration C) or leg (see illustration D).	Brachial artery is along the groove between biceps and triceps muscles above elbow at antecubital fossa. Popliteal artery is just below the patient's thigh, behind knee. Placing bladder directly over artery ensures that you apply proper pressure during inflation. Loose-fitting cuff causes false-high readings.

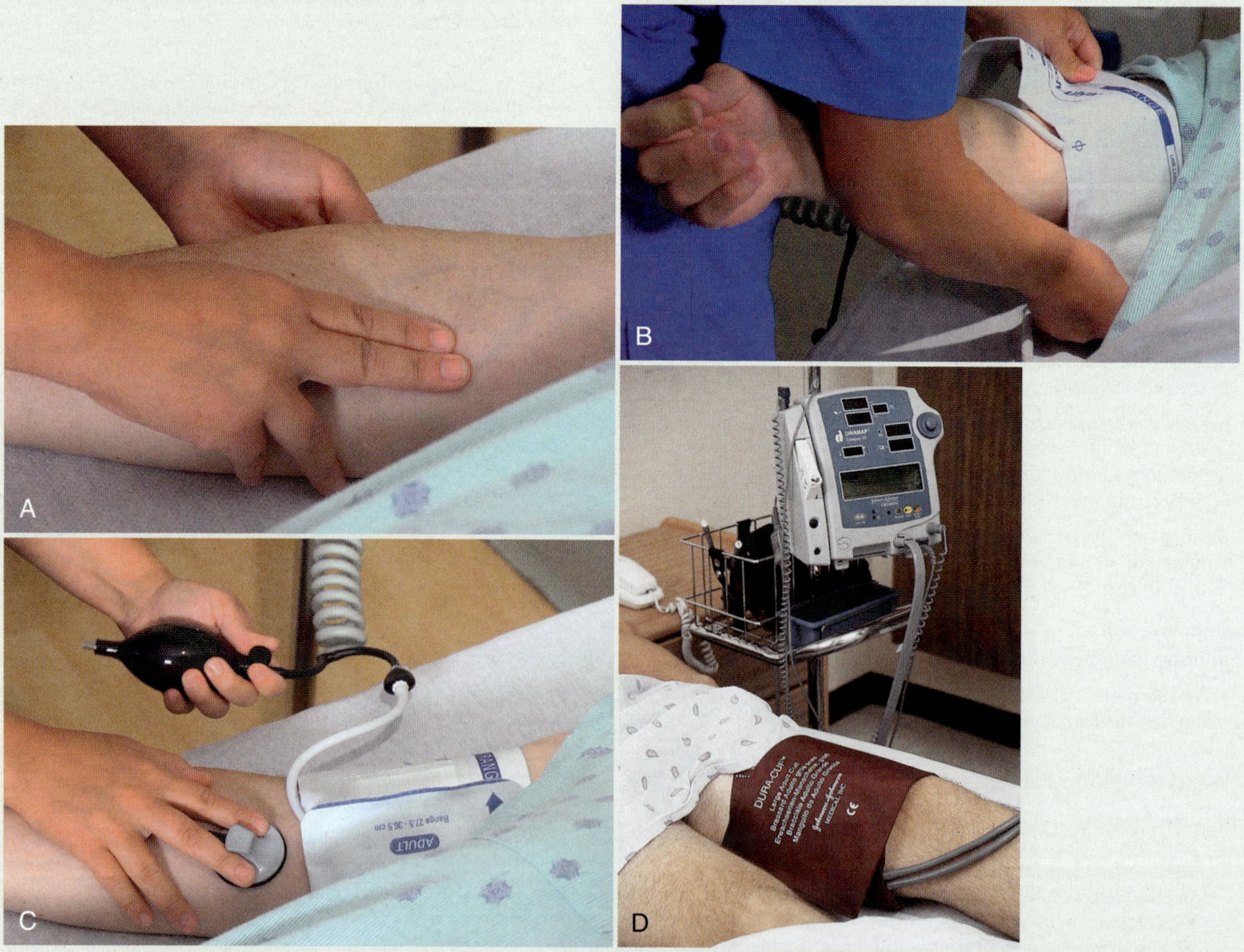

A

B

C

D

Step 3c **A,** Palpating brachial artery. **B,** Aligning blood pressure cuff arrow with brachial artery. **C,** Blood pressure cuff wrapped around upper arm. **D,** Blood pressure cuff applied around thigh. (**A**–**C** copyright © Mosby's Clinical Skills: Essentials Collection.)

STEP	RATIONALE
d. Position manometer gauge vertically at eye level. You should be no farther than 1 m (approximately 1 yard) away.	Looking up or down at scale can result in distorted readings.
e. **Measure BP using two-step method:**	
(1) Palpate brachial or popliteal pulse. Palpate artery distal to cuff with fingertips of nondominant hand while inflating cuff rapidly to pressure 30 mm Hg above point at which pulse disappears. Slowly deflate cuff and note point when pulse reappears. Deflate cuff fully and wait for 30 s.	Estimating prevents false-low readings. Determine maximal inflation point for accurate reading by palpation. If unable to palpate artery because of weakened pulse, use an ultrasonic stethoscope. Completely deflating cuff prevents venous congestion and false-high readings.
(2) Place stethoscope earpieces in ears and be sure that sounds are clear, not muffled.	Ensure that each earpiece follows angle of ear canal to facilitate hearing.
(3) Palpate artery and place bell or diaphragm chest piece of stethoscope over it. Do not allow chest piece to touch cuff or clothing.	Proper stethoscope placement ensures best sound reception. Stethoscope improperly positioned causes muffled sounds that often result in false-low systolic and false-high diastolic readings. The bell provides better sound reproduction, whereas the diaphragm is easier to secure with fingers and covers a larger area.
(4) Close valve of pressure bulb clockwise until tight. Quickly inflate cuff to 30 mm Hg above the patient's estimated SBP.	Tightening valve prevents air leak during inflation. Rapid inflation ensures accurate measurement of SBP.
(5) Slowly release pressure bulb valve and allow manometer needle to fall at rate of 2–3 mm Hg/s.	Too rapid or too slow decline causes inaccurate readings (Gunes and Efteli, 2016).
(6) Note point on manometer when you hear first clear sound. The sound will slowly increase in intensity.	First sound reflects SBP.
(7) Continue to deflate cuff gradually, noting point at which sound disappears in adults. Note pressure to nearest 2 mm Hg. Listen for 20–30 mm Hg after last sound and allow remaining air to escape quickly.	Beginning of the last or fifth sound is indication of DBP in adults (Basile and Bloch, 2016). In children, the distinct muffling of sounds indicates DBP (Basile and Bloch, 2016).
f. **Measure BP using one-step method:**	
(1) Place stethoscope earpieces in ears and be sure that sounds are clear, not muffled.	Earpieces should follow angle of ear canal to facilitate hearing.
(2) Palpate brachial or popliteal artery and place bell or diaphragm chest piece of stethoscope over it. Do not allow chest piece to touch cuff or clothing.	Proper stethoscope placement ensures optimal sound reception. Improperly positioned stethoscope causes muffled sounds that often result in false readings. Bell provides better sound reproduction, whereas diaphragm is easier to secure with fingers and covers larger area.
(3) Close valve of pressure bulb clockwise until tight. Quickly inflate cuff to 30 mm Hg above the patient's usual SBP.	Tightening valve prevents air leak during inflation. Inflation above systolic level ensures accurate measurement of systolic pressure.
(4) Slowly release pressure bulb valve and allow manometer needle to fall at a rate of 2–3 mm Hg/s. Note point on manometer when you hear first clear sound. Sound will slowly increase in intensity.	Too rapid or too slow a decline in mercury level causes inaccurate readings (Gunes and Efteli, 2016). First sound reflects SBP.
(5) Continue to deflate cuff gradually, noting point at which sound disappears in adults. Note pressure to nearest 2 mm Hg. Listen for 10–20 mm Hg after last sound and allow remaining air to escape quickly.	Beginning of fifth sound is indication of DBP in adults (Basile and Bloch, 2016). In children, the distinct muffling of sounds indicates DBP (Basile and Bloch, 2016).
4. AHA recommends average of two sets of BP measurement, 2 min apart. Use second set of BP measurements as baseline. If readings are different by more than 5 mm Hg, additional readings are necessary.	Prevents false-positive readings based on patient's sympathetic response (alert reaction). Repeating measurements too soon creates venous congestion, which makes sounds difficult to hear (Dokoohaki et al., 2015). Averaging minimizes effect of anxiety, which often causes first reading to be higher than subsequent measures (Basile and Bloch, 2016).
5. Remove cuff from patient's arm/leg unless you need to repeat measurement.	Continuous cuff inflation causes arterial occlusion, resulting in numbness and tingling of patient's arm/leg.
6. If this is first assessment of patient, repeat procedure on other arm/leg.	Comparison of BP in both arms/legs detects circulatory problems. (Normal difference of 5–10 mm Hg exists between arms.) Use arm with the higher pressure for subsequent measurements (AACN Practice Alert, 2016).

STEP	RATIONALE

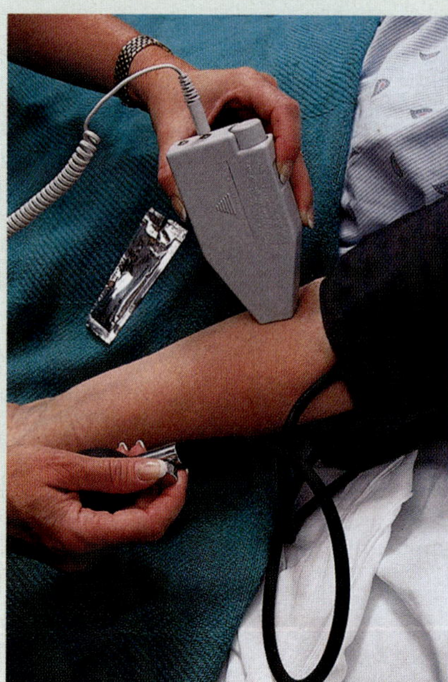

Fig. 6.17 Doppler ultrasonic stethoscope over brachial artery to measure blood pressure.

STEP	RATIONALE
7. Assess SBP by palpation:	
a. Follow Steps 3a through 3d of auscultation method.	
b. Locate and then continually palpate brachial, radial, or popliteal artery with fingertips of one hand. Inflate cuff to pressure 30 mm Hg above point at which you can no longer palpate pulse.	Ensures accurate detection of true SBP once pressure valve is released.

Clinical decision point: If unable to palpate artery because of weakened pulse, use a Doppler device (Fig. 6.17).

STEP	RATIONALE
c. Slowly release valve and deflate cuff, allowing manometer needle to fall at rate of 2 mm Hg/s. Note point on manometer when pulse is again palpable. First palpable pulse reflects SBP.	Too rapid or too slow a decline results in inaccurate readings (Gunes and Efteli, 2016). Palpation helps identify only SBP.
d. Deflate cuff rapidly and completely. Remove cuff from the patient's extremity unless you need to repeat measurement.	Continuous cuff inflation causes arterial occlusion, resulting in numbness and tingling of extremity.
8. Help the patient return to comfortable position and cover upper arm/leg if previously clothed.	Restores comfort and provides a sense of well-being.
9. Discuss findings with the patient.	Promotes participation in care and understanding of health status and makes patient accountable for follow-up assessment. SBP in leg is 10–40 mm Hg higher.
10. Clean earpieces and diaphragm of stethoscope with alcohol swab as needed. Wipe cuff with agency-approved disinfectant if used between patients. Perform hand hygiene.	Reduces transmission of microorganisms. Controls transmission of microorganisms when nurses share stethoscope.

Evaluation

STEP	RATIONALE
1. If assessing BP for the first time, establish baseline BP if it is within acceptable range.	Used to compare future BP measurements.
2. Compare BP reading with the patient's previous baseline and usual BP for the patient's age.	Allows you to assess for change in condition and provides comparison with future BP measurements.
3. **Use teach back:** "I want to be sure I explained why it is important to stand up slowly since you have a high BP. Tell me which of your medications might make you dizzy if you stand up too fast, and tell me what should you do if you suddenly feel dizzy." Revise your instruction now or develop a plan for revised patient/family caregiver teaching if patient/family caregiver is unable to teach back correctly.	Evaluates what the patient is able to explain.

Recording and Reporting

- Record BP and site assessed on vital sign flow sheet or nurses' notes in EHR or chart.
- Record the patient's knowledge following evaluation of teach back in nurses' notes.
- Document measurement of BP and any signs or symptoms of BP alterations after administration of specific therapies in nurses' notes in EHR or chart.
- Report abnormal findings to nurse in charge or health care provider.

Unexpected Outcomes and Related Interventions

- Patient's BP is above acceptable range.
  - Repeat measurement in other extremity and compare findings.
  - Verify correct size and placement of BP cuff.
  - Have another nurse repeat measurement in 1–2 minutes.
  - Observe for related symptoms that are not apparent unless BP is extremely high including headache, facial flushing, nosebleed, and fatigue in older patient.
  - Report BP to nurse in charge or health care provider to initiate appropriate evaluation and treatment.
  - Administer antihypertensive medications as ordered.
- Patient's BP is not sufficient for adequate perfusion and oxygenation of tissues.
  - Compare BP value with baseline.
  - Position patient in supine position to enhance circulation and restrict activity that decreases BP further.
  - Assess for signs and symptoms associated with hypotension including tachycardia; diminished, barely palpable pulse; weakness; dizziness; confusion; and cool, pale, dusky, or cyanotic skin.
  - Assess for factors that contribute to low BP including hemorrhage, dilation of blood vessels resulting from hyperthermia, anesthesia, or medication side effects.
  - Report BP to nurse in charge or health care provider to initiate appropriate evaluation and treatment.
  - Increase rate of i.v. infusion or administer vasoconstriction drugs if ordered.
- Unable to obtain BP reading.
  - Determine that no immediate crisis is present by obtaining pulse and respiratory rates.
  - Assess for signs and symptoms of decreased cardiac output; if present, notify nurse in charge or health care provider immediately.
  - Use alternative sites or procedures to obtain BP: use Doppler or ultrasonic stethoscope; palpate SBP.
- Patient experiences orthostatic hypotension.
  - Maintain patient safety.
  - Return the patient to safe position in bed or chair.

KEY POINTS

- Vital sign measurement includes the physiological measurements of temperature, pulse, BP, respiration, and oxygen saturation.
- You measure vital signs as part of a complete physical examination or in an episodic review of a patient's condition.
- Measure vital signs when your patient is at rest and the environment is controlled for comfort.
- Evaluate vital sign changes with other physical assessment findings using clinical judgment to determine measurement frequency.
- Knowledge of the factors influencing vital signs helps to determine and evaluate abnormal values.
- Changes related to aging influence vital sign measurement and nursing interventions for older adults.
- Vital signs provide a basis for evaluating response to nursing interventions.
- Changes in one vital sign often influence characteristics of the other vital signs.
- Maintain a patient's body temperature by initiating interventions that promote heat loss, production, or conservation.
- Respiratory assessment includes determining the effectiveness of ventilation, perfusion, and diffusion.
- Assessment of respiration involves observing ventilatory movements throughout the respiratory cycle.
- Hypertension is diagnosed only after an average of readings made during two or more subsequent visits reveals an elevated BP.
- Selecting and applying the BP measurement cuff improperly result in errors in BP measurement.
- Routinely assess the condition of the skin underlying an oximeter sensor.

REFERENCES

AACN Practice Alert. Obtaining accurate noninvasive blood pressure measurements in adults. Crit Care Nurse 2016;36(3):e12.

American Heart Association. What is high blood pressure. 2016. Available from: https://www.heart.org/en/health-topics/high-blood-pressure

Angelousi A, Girerd N, Benetos A, Frimat L, Gautier S, Weryha G, et al. Association between orthostatic hypotension and cardiovascular risk, cerebrovascular risk, cognitive decline and falls as well as overall mortality: a systematic review and meta-analysis. J Hypertens 2014; 32:1562.

Asadian S, Khatony A, Moradi G, Abdi A, Rezaei M. Accuracy and precision of four common peripheral temperature measurement methods in intensive care patients. Med Devices (Auckl) 2016;9:301–8.

Basile J, Bloch MJ: Overview of hypertension in adults. UpToDate; 2016. Available from: http://www.uptodate.com/contents/overview-of-hypertension-in-adults.

Casiglia E, Tikhonoff V, Albertini F, Palatini P. Poor reliability of wrist blood pressure self-measurement at home: a population-based study. Hypertension 2016;68:896.

Centers for Disease Control and Prevention (CDC). Healthcare-associated infections: Clostridium difficile infection information for patients. 2015. Available from: https://www.cdc.gov/hai/organisms/cdiff/cdiff_infect.html.html.

Charafeddine L, Tamim H, Hassouna H, Akel R, Nabulsi M. Axillary and rectal thermometry in the newborn: do they agree? BMC Res Notes 2014;31(7):584.

Dokoohaki R, Raeiskarimian F, Rahgosha A, Sharifi M. Frequency of errors of blood pressure measurement among nurses. Int Cardiovasc Res J 2015;9(1):41.

Furlong D, Carroll DL, Finn C, Gay D, Gryglik C, Donahue V. Comparison of temporal to pulmonary artery temperature in febrile patients. Dimens Crit Care Nurs 2015;34(1):47.

Goforth CW, Kazman JB. Exertional heat stroke in Navy and Marine personnel. Crit Care Nurse 2015;35(1):52.

Gunes UY, Efteli EU. Does errors made during indirect blood pressure measurement affect the results? Int J Caring Sci 2016;9(2):520.

Halm MA. Arm circumference, shape and length: how interplaying variables affect blood pressure measurement in obese persons. Am J Crit Care 2014;23(2):166.

Hockenberry MJ, Wilson D. Wong's nursing care of infants and children. 10th ed. St. Louis: Mosby; 2015.

James PA, Oparil S, Carter BL, Cushman WC, Dennison-Himmelfarb C, Handler J, et al. 2014 evidence-based guideline for the management of high blood pressure in adults: report from the panel members appointed to the Eighth Joint National Committee (JNC 8). JAMA 2014;311:507.

Liu C, Griffiths C, Murray A, Zheng D. Comparison of stethoscope bell and diaphragm, and of stethoscope tube length, for clinical blood pressure measurement. Blood Press Monit 2016;21(3):178.

Longtin Y, Schneider A, Tschopp C, Renzi G, Gayet-Ageron A, Schrenzel J, et al. Contamination of stethoscopes and physicians' hands after a physical examination. Mayo Clin Proc 2016;89(3):291.

McLean B. Comparing blood pressure measures: does one measurement equal another? Crit Care Nurse 2015;35(1):75.

Nellcor. Clinicians' guide to Nellcor sensors. n.d. Available from: http://nbninfusions.com/wp-content/uploads/nbnmanuals/Ventilator%20Manuals/Nellcor%20Sensors%20Clinician%27s%20Manual.pdf.

Ozone S, Shaku F, Sato M, Takayashiki A, Tsutsumi M, Maeno T. Comparison of blood pressure measurements on the bare arm, over a sleeve and over a rolled-up sleeve in the elderly. Fam Pract 2016;33(5):517.

Pinar R, et al: The effect of clothes on sphygmomanometric blood pressure measurement in hypertensive patients, J ClinNurs 19: 1861, 2010.

Reynolds M, Bonham L, Gueck M, Hammond K, Lowery J, Redel C, et al. Are temporal artery temperatures accurate enough to replace rectal temperature measurement in pediatric ED patients? J Emerg Nurs 2014;40:46.

Schallom M, Prentice D, Sona C, Mazuski J. Comparison of nasal and forehead oximetry accuracy and pressure injury in critically ill patients, Crit Care Med 2016;44(12):121.

Suokhrie L, et al: Differences in automated and manual blood pressure measurement in hospitalized psychiatric patients, J PsychosocNurs 51(3): 32, 2013.

The Joint Commission (TJC): 2016 National Patient Safety Goals, Oakbrook Terrace, IL, 2016, The Commission. Available at https://www.jointcommission.org/standards/national-patient-safety-goals/. Accessed November 2019.

The Joint Commission (TJC). 2018 National Patient Safety Goals. Oakbrook Terrace, IL: The Joint Commission; 2018. Available from: https://www.jointcommission.org/assets/1/6/NPSG_Chapter_HAP_Jan2017.pdf.

Touhy TA, Jett KF. Ebersole and Hess' gerontological nursing & healthy aging. 4th ed. St. Louis: Mosby; 2014.

World Health Organization (WHO). Pulse Oximetry Training Manual. 2011. Available from: http://www.who.int/patientsafety/safesurgery/pulse_oximetry/who_ps_pulse_oxymetry_training_manual_en.pdf.

Zheng D, Di Marco LY, Murray A. Effect of respiration on Korotkoff sounds and oscillometric cuff pressure pulses during blood pressure measurement. Med Biol Eng Comput 2014;52:467.

7 Health Assessment and Physical Examination

OBJECTIVES

- To describe the component of history collection.
- To discuss the purposes of health assessment.
- To discuss the interview and observation techniques as method of health assessment.
- To describe the techniques used with each physical assessment skill.
- To discuss how cultural awareness influences health assessment.
- To describe proper patient positioning during each phase of the examination.
- To list techniques to promote a patient's physical and psychological comfort during an examination.
- To demonstrate preparation of a therapeutic environment before the physical examination.
- To identify data to collect from the nursing history before an examination.
- To discuss ways to incorporate health promotion and health teaching into an assessment.
- To discuss normal physical findings for patients across the life span.
- To identify self-screening assessments commonly performed by patients.
- To use physical assessment techniques and skills during routine nursing care.
- To document assessment findings on appropriate forms.
- To communicate abnormal findings to appropriate personnel.

KEY TERMS

adventitious sounds, p. 144
arcus senilis, p. 135
atrophy, p. 161
auscultation, p. 121
back channeling p. 117
bruit, p. 149
cerumen, p. 146
concomitant symptoms p. 119
costovertebral angle, p. 157
crackles, p. 145
cyanosis, p. 128
dorsum, p. 129
dyspnea, p. 143
dysrhythmia, p. 148
edema, p. 128
erythema, p. 129
indurated, p. 129
inspection, p. 120
integument, p. 127
intercostal spaces, p. 142
jaundice, p. 128
olfaction, p. 121
orthopnea, p. 143
pallor, p. 128
palpation, p. 120
percussion, p. 121
petechiae, p. 129
phlebitis, p. 152
thrill, p. 149
turgor, p. 129

INTRODUCTION

The health assessment and physical examination are important steps toward providing safe and competent nursing care. As a nurse, you are in a unique position to determine each patient's current health status, distinguish variations from the norm, and recognize improvements or deterioration in his or her condition. As a nurse, you must be able to recognize and interpret each patient's physical and behavioral presentation. By performing health assessments and physical examinations, you identify health patterns and evaluate each patient's response to treatments and therapies.

Nurses gather assessment data about patients' past and current health conditions in a variety of ways, using a comprehensive or focused approach, depending on the patient situation. Assessments are performed at health fairs, at screening clinics, in a health provider's office, in acute care agencies, or in patients' homes. Depending on the outcome of an assessment, a nurse considers evidence-based recommendations for care on the basis of a patient's values, the health provider's clinical expertise, or own personal experience.

A complete health assessment involves a nursing history and physical examination. Through the health history interview, you gather subjective data about a patient's condition. You obtain objective data while observing a patient's behavior and overall presentation. You identify additional objective data through a head-to-toe body system review during the physical examination. With accurate data you create a patient-centered care plan, identifying the nursing diagnoses, desired patient outcomes, and nursing interventions.

INTERVIEW AND OBSERVATION TECHNIQUES

As a nurse, you use the patient interview as the tool to assess a patient's health history. Once you have collected data, you proceed to a physical examination.

Patient-Centered Interview

The first step in establishing a patient-centered database is to collect subjective information by interviewing a patient. An interview is an organized conversation with a patient. The interview focuses on a patient's health history and obtaining information about the current illness (Ball et al., 2015). During the initial interview, you have the opportunity to:

1. Introduce yourself to the patient, explain your role, and explain the roles of others in team who will provide care.
2. Establish a caring patient-centered relationship.
3. Explain how you will conduct the interview (e.g., first you will ask about the patient's current concerns and then collecting other information).
4. Gain insight about the patient's concerns and worries.
5. Determine the patient's goals and expectations of the health care delivery system.
6. Obtain cues to identify topics requiring further investigation and data collection.

Later interviews allow you to further assess a patient's situation and focus on specific problem areas. The interview also helps patients explain their own interpretations and understandings of their conditions and patient and the interviewers are the partners during the whole process.

Always prepare well for the interview. Collect all available information about the patient and create a comfortable environment for the interview. For example, review the information you learn during the hand-off report, and plan to interview the patient during rounds and before you begin to deliver patient care. In a hospital, you often need to relieve a patient's symptoms before the patient can talk comfortably with you. In a patient's home, choose a location that is as quiet and private as possible.

Phases of Interview

The interview consists of three phases: orientation, working, and termination.

Orientation Phase Including Setting an Agenda

During the orientation phase, you establish trust and confidence with a patient. Begin by introducing yourself and explain the purpose of the interview. Assure the patient that all the information will remain confidential and be used only by health care professionals who provide the patient's care (see Chapter 5). HIPAA regulations require patients to sign an authorization before you collect personal health data. The patient usually signs this form in the admitting or screening areas before you meet the patient.

One important goal of the initial interview is to explain to the patient the reason you want to understand the patient's needs.

Another goal of the interview is to begin developing a relationship that enables the patient to become an active partner in care decisions. As the orientation phase proceeds, the patient usually becomes more comfortable in speaking with you.

You first gather demographic data (e.g., date of birth, gender, address, and family members' names and addresses) as specified by the institution. Because this information is the least personal topic, it helps initiate the therapeutic relationship and eases the transition into the working phase of the interview.

Working Phase—Collecting Assessment or Nursing Health History

Start an assessment or nursing health history with open-ended questions rather than yes/no questions. Open-ended questions encourage patients to tell their story in detail. During the working phase, you gather information about the patient's health status. Stay focused, orderly, and unhurried. Obtain the patient's health history using a variety of communication techniques to promote a clear interaction and construct a thorough database (Box 7.1). Techniques you can use include active listening, paraphrasing, and summarizing.

BOX 7.1 Basic Components for a Nursing Health History

- *Biographical information:* Age, address, occupation and working status, marital status, family members, source of health care, and insurance.
- *Reasons for seeking health care:* Goals of care, expectation of the services and care delivered, and expectations of the health care team and system.
- *Present illness or health concern:* Onset, symptoms, nature of symptoms (e.g., sudden or gradual), duration, precipitating factors, relief measures, and weight loss or gain.
- *Health history:* Prior illnesses throughout development, injuries, and hospitalizations; surgeries; blood transfusions; allergies; immunizations; habits (e.g., smoking, caffeine intake, alcohol intake, and alcohol or drug abuse); prescribed and self-prescribed medications; over-the-counter medications; work habits; relaxation activities; and sleep, exercise, and eating or nutritional patterns.
- *Family history:* Health status of immediate family and living relatives; cause of death of relatives; and risk factor analyses for cancer, heart disease, diabetes mellitus, kidney disease, hypertension, and mental disorders.
- *Environmental history:* Hazards, pollutants, and physical safety.
- *Psychosocial and cultural history:* Primary language, cultural group, community resources, mood, attention span, and developmental stage.
- *Review of systems:* Head-to-toe review of all major body systems and patient's knowledge of and compliance with health care (e.g., frequency of breast or testicular self-examination or last visual acuity examination). (Another option for an approach is to use *functional health patterns* as the method for organizing assessment data.)

Termination Phase—Ending the Interview

As in the other phases of the interview, the termination phase requires skill on the part of the interviewer. Give your patient a clue that the interview is coming to an end. For example, you might say, "There are just two more questions" or "We'll be finished in 5 to 6 minutes." This helps a patient maintain direct attention without being distracted by wondering when the interview will end. This approach also gives the patient a chance to ask questions. When ending the interview, summarize the important points and ask your patient whether the summary is accurate. End the interview in a friendly manner, telling the patient when you will return to provide care.

Interview Techniques

How you conduct an interview is just as important as the questions you ask. During an interview, you are responsible for directing the flow of the discussion so patients have the opportunity to freely contribute stories about their health problems to enable you to get as much detailed information as possible. Because a patient's report includes subjective information, validate data from the interview later with objective data. For example, if a patient reports difficulty breathing, this will lead you to further assess respiratory rate and lung sounds during the physical examination.

Observation

Observation is powerful. Observe a patient's nonverbal communication such as use of eye contact, body language, or tone of voice. While observing nonverbal behavior, appearance, and interaction with the environment, you determine whether the data you obtained are consistent with what the patient states verbally. Your observations lead you to pursue further objective information to form accurate conclusions. If you establish a trusting nurse–patient relationship, the patient feels comfortable asking you questions about the health care environment, planned treatments, diagnostic testing, and available resources.

Open-Ended Questions

In a patient-centered interview, you try to find out, in the patient's own words, his or her health goals and any concerns or problems that exist and their probable cause. Patients are the best resources for talking about their symptoms or relating their health history. Begin by asking a patient an *open-ended question* to elicit his or her story. An open-ended question gives a patient discretion about the extent of his or her answer (Ball et al., 2015). For example, "So, tell me more about ...." or "What are your concerns about this?" or "Tell me how you're feeling." The use of **open-ended questions** prompts patients to describe a situation in more than one or two words.

Leading Question

These questions are the most risky because of possibly limiting the information provided to what a patient thinks you want to know (Ball et al., 2015). Examples include, "It seems to me this is bothering you quite a bit. Is that true?" or "Now, that wasn't very hard to do, was it?"

Back Channeling

Reinforce your interest in what a patient has to say through the use of good eye contact and listening skills. Also use **back channeling**, which includes active listening prompts such as "all right," "go on," or "uh-huh." These indicate that you have heard what a patient says, are interested in hearing the full story, and are encouraging the patient to give more details.

Probing

As a patient tells his or her story, encourage a full description without trying to control the direction the story takes. This requires you to probe with further open-ended statements such as "Is there anything else you can tell me?" or "What else is bothering you?" Each time a patient offers more detail, probe again until the patient has nothing else to say and has told the full story. Always stay observant. If a patient becomes fatigued or uncomfortable, know that it is time to postpone an interview.

Direct Closed-Ended Questions

As you learn information from a patient, you will ask direct questions to seek specific information. This approach takes the information provided in a patient's story and more fully describes and identifies specific problem areas. For example, a patient reports experiencing indigestion over the course of several days and acknowledges having some diarrhea and loss of appetite. The patient's explanation for the cause relates to a recent series of trips that changed his eating habits. The nurse focuses on the symptoms the patient identifies and the general indigestion problem by asking **closed-ended questions** that limit answers to one or two words such as "yes" or "no" or a number or frequency of a symptom. For example, ask, "How often does the diarrhea occur?" or "Do you have pain or cramping?" The technique allows you to acquire specific information about health problems such as symptoms, precipitating factors, or relief measures.

A good interviewer leaves with a complete story that contains enough details for understanding a patient's perceptions of his or her health status and the information needed to help identify nursing diagnoses and/or collaborative health problems (see Chapter 19). Always clarify or validate any information about which you are unclear. Make no assumptions.

PURPOSES OF HEALTH ASSESSMENT AND PHYSICAL EXAMINATION

A health assessment and physical examination are conducted as an initial evaluation in triage for emergency care; for routine health screening; to determine eligibility for health insurance, military service, or a new job; or to admit a patient to a hospital or other health care setting. As a nurse, you may focus an initial assessment on a patient's chief concern—the reason the patient is seeking health care. Use a health assessment and physical examination to:

1. Gather baseline information about a patient's health status.
2. Supplement, confirm, or refute information learned during the health history.
3. Identify or confirm actual or at-risk nursing diagnoses.

4. Make clinical judgments about a patient's current or changing health status and ability to manage it.
5. Evaluate the outcomes of care.

NURSING HEALTH HISTORY

You gather a **nursing health history** during an initial or early contact with a patient. The history is a key component of a comprehensive assessment. Most health history forms (manual and electronic) are structured. However, on the basis of information you gain as you conduct the patient-centered interview, you learn which components of the history to explore fully and which require less detail. A good assessor learns to refine and broaden questions as needed to correctly assess a patient's unique needs by determining patient's priorities. A comprehensive history covers all health dimensions (Fig. 7.1), allowing you to develop a complete plan of care.

Cultural Considerations

Obtaining a nursing health history requires cultural competence. This involves self-awareness, reflective practice, and knowledge of a patient's core cultural issues (Ball et al., 2015). Adapt each assessment to the unique needs of patients of backgrounds and cultures different from your own. Be respectful; understand these differences; and do not impose your own attitudes, biases, and beliefs (e.g., attitudes toward aging, obesity, or lifestyle). Having a genuine curiosity about a patient's beliefs and values lays a foundation for a trusting patient–nurse relationship (Ball et al., 2015). Avoid making stereotypes; the assumptions tied to stereotypes (e.g., obese patients do not exercise regularly) can lead you to collect inaccurate information. Draw on knowledge from your assessment and ask questions in a constructive and probing way to allow you to truly know who a patient is (Box 7.2). If you are unsure about what a patient is saying, clarify to prevent making the wrong diagnostic conclusion.

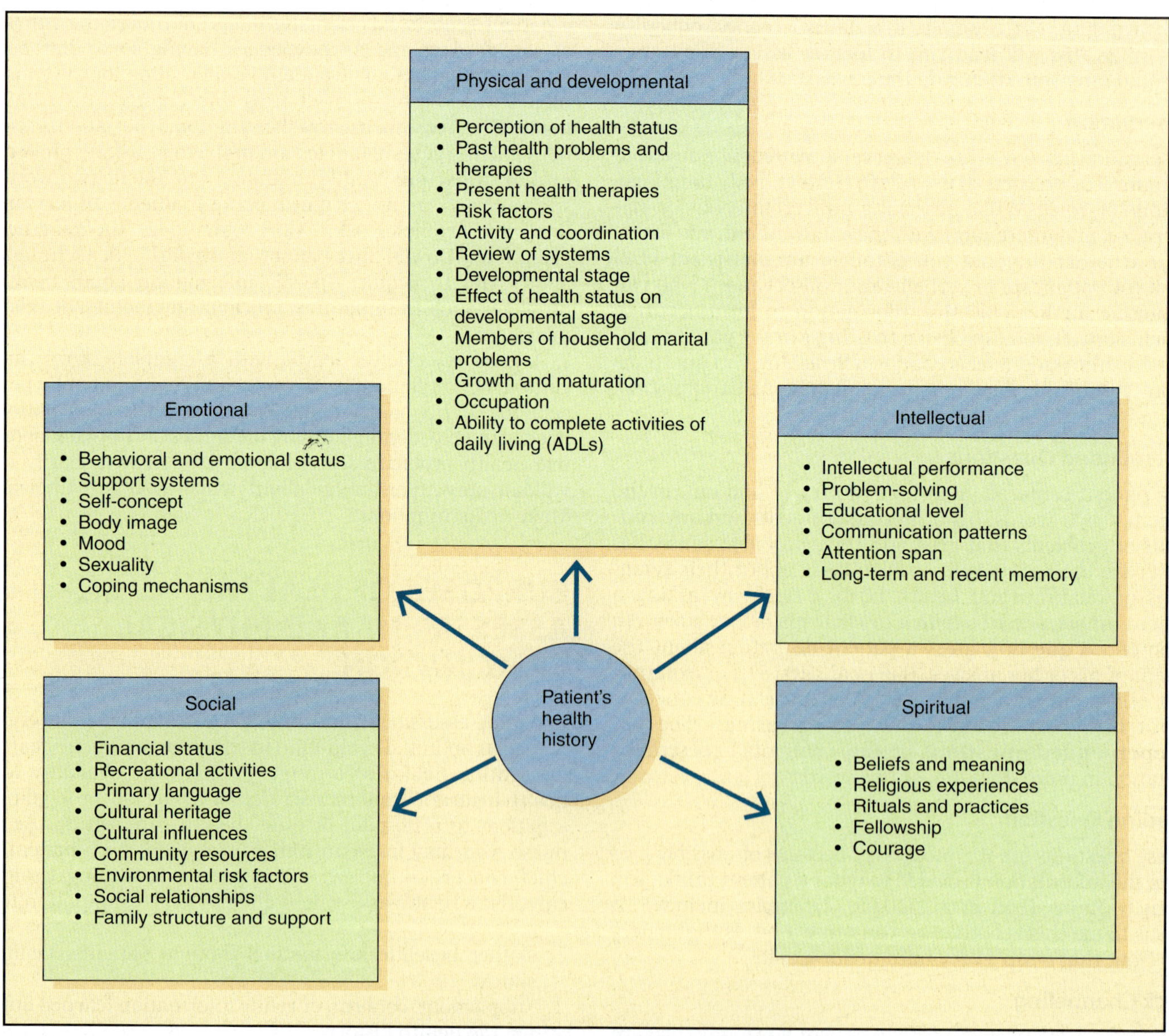

Fig. 7.1 Dimensions for gathering data for a health history.

BOX 7.2 Cultural Aspects of Care

To successfully explore a patient's illness or health care problems, use a patient-centered approach. Elicit patient values, preferences, and expressed needs as part of your clinical interview. Ensure the interview is inclusive. Remove barriers to having families present on the basis of patient preferences.

Implications for Patient-Centered Care

- When talking about a patient's illness, try to understand it "through the patient's eyes."
- What do you think is wrong with you?
- What worries you most about your illness?
- When talking about treatments, value a patient's expertise with own health and symptoms.
- What should we do to eliminate your problem?
- Which types of treatment do you use?
- What benefit do you expect from the treatment?

If there is a cross-cultural difference between you and your patient, ask yourself these questions:

- What is unique to your patient's culture and its impact on the treatment plan?
- What potential is there to have a cultural misunderstanding? If one exists, try to correct it.
- Which types of treatments or health practices do you use?

Components of the Nursing Health History

Most health histories contain the same components. Do not let a history form shape your assessment entirely. Decide what information you need on the basis of your patient's needs, responses to your questions, and changing status during the interview.

Biographical Information

Biographical information is factual demographic data that include a patient's age, address, occupation, and working status; marital status; source of health care; and types of insurance. The staff in an admitting office usually collects this information.

Chief Concern or Reason for Seeking Health Care

This is the information you gather when you initially set an agenda during a patient-centered interview. Compare what you learn from the patient with the "chief complaint," which is often typed on the patient's admission sheet. Ask a patient why he or she is seeking health care (e.g., "Tell me, Mr Lynn, what brought you to the clinic today"). You record the patient's response in quotations to indicate the subjective response. As you explore a patient's reason for seeking health care, you will learn the chronological and sequential history of his or her health problems (Ball et al., 2015). Clarification of a patient's perception identifies potential needs for symptom management, education, counseling, or referral to community resources.

Patient Expectations

It is important to assess a patient's expectations of health care providers (e.g., being diagnosed correctly, receiving comfort measures, or being treated successfully for a disease). Patient satisfaction, a standard measure of quality for all hospitals throughout the country, can be perceived by patients as poor if their expectations are unmet. Patients typically have expectations of receiving information about their treatments and prognosis and a plan of care for returning home. During the initial interview, a patient expresses expectations when entering the health care setting. Later, as a patient interacts with health care providers, assess whether these expectations have changed or been met.

Present Illness or Health Concerns

If a patient presents with an illness, collect essential and relevant data about the symptoms and their effects on the patient's health. Apply critical thinking intellectual standards (See Chapter 18) and use the acronym PQRST to guide an assessment:

- **P—Provokes** (e.g., precipitating and relieving factors): What causes symptom? What makes it better or worse? Are there activities (e.g., exercise) that affect it?
- **Q—Quality:** What does the symptom feel like? If the patient cannot describe, offer probes such as "Is it sharp? Dull? Burning?"
- **R—Radiate:** Where is the symptom located? Is it in one place? Does it go anywhere else? Have patient be as precise as possible.
- **S—Severity:** Ask a patient to rate the severity of a symptom on a scale of 0−10. This gives you a baseline with which to compare in follow-up assessments.
- **T—Time:** Assesses onset and duration of symptom. When did it start? Does it come and go? If so, how often and for how long? What time of day or day of the week?

Also, assess whether the patient has **concomitant symptoms**. Does he or she experience other symptoms along with the primary symptom? For example, does nausea accompany pain?

Past Health History

A health history provides a holistic view of a patient's health care experiences and current health habits (see Fig. 7.1). Assess whether a patient has ever been hospitalized or injured or has had surgery. Include a complete medication history (including herbal and over-the-counter [OTC] drugs). Also essential are descriptions of allergies, including allergic reactions to food, latex, drugs, or contact agents (e.g., soap). If the patient has an allergy, note the specific reaction and treatment on the assessment form and special arm band provided. Assessing for the use of alcohol, tobacco, caffeine, or recreational drugs (e.g., methamphetamine or cocaine) determines a patient's risk for diseases involving the liver, lungs, heart, or nervous system.

It is essential to gather information about the type of habit and the frequency and duration of use. Assessing patterns of sleep (see Chapter 10), exercise (see Chapter 14), and nutrition (see Chapter 20) are also important when planning nursing care. Ultimately your aim is to match a patient's lifestyle patterns with approaches in the plan of care as much as possible.

Family History

The family history includes data about immediate and blood relatives. Your objective is to determine whether a patient is at risk for illnesses of a genetic or familial nature and to identify areas of health promotion and illness prevention.

The family history also reveals information about family structure; interaction, support, and function that often are useful in planning care. If a patient's family is not supportive, it is better not to involve the family in care. Stressful family relationships are sometimes a significant barrier when you try to help patients with problems involving loss, self-concept, spiritual health, and personal relationships.

Psychosocial History

A psychosocial history provides information about a patient's support system, which often includes a spouse or partner, children, other family members, and close friends. The history also includes information about ways that a patient and family typically cope with stress (see Chapter 31). Behaviors that patients use at home to cope with stress such as walking, reading, or talking with a friend can also be used as nursing interventions if the patient experiences stress while receiving health care. In addition, you need to learn whether the patient has experienced any recent losses that create a sense of grief (see Chapter 28).

Spiritual Health

Life experiences and events shape a person's spirituality. The spiritual dimension represents the totality of one's being and is difficult to assess quickly (see Chapter 32). Review with patients their beliefs about life, their source for guidance in acting on beliefs, and the relationship they have with family in exercising their faith. Also assess rituals and religious practices that patients use to express their spirituality. Patients may request availability of these practices while in a health care setting.

METHODS OF PHYSICAL EXAMINATION

A comprehensive physical examination involves the use of five skills: inspection, palpation, percussion, auscultation, and olfaction.

Inspection

Inspection is the use of vision to distinguish normal from abnormal findings. It is important to know what to consider normal for patients of different age, gender, or cultural group. With experience, you are better able to recognize normal variations among patients. Inspection is a simple technique, and the quality of an inspection depends on your willingness to be thorough and systematic. To inspect body parts accurately follow these principles:

1. Make sure that adequate lighting is available.
2. Position and expose body parts so that you can view all surfaces.
3. Inspect each area for size, shape, color, symmetry, position, and abnormalities.
4. When possible, compare each area inspected with the same area on the opposite side of the body.
5. Use additional light (e.g., a penlight) to inspect skin surfaces or body cavities.
6. Do not hurry inspection. Pay attention to detail.

After inspection of a body part, findings may indicate the need for further examination. Use palpation with or after visual inspection.

Palpation

Palpation involves the use of the hands to touch body parts and make sensitive assessments. It typically occurs right after inspection. However, when examining the abdomen, palpation is performed after auscultation.

Key points to be taken care of:

- Use palpation to examine all accessible parts of the body. For example, palpate the skin for temperature, moisture, texture, turgor, tenderness, and thickness. Palpate the abdomen for tenderness, distention, or masses. Use standard precautions (see Chapter 9) if any body fluids are present.
- Make the patient comfortable and relax because muscle tension during palpation impairs your ability to interpret physical findings. Asking the patient to take slow, deep breaths enhances muscle relaxation.
- *Palpate tender areas last.*
- Do not palpate without considering a patient's overall condition. For example, if a patient has a fractured rib, use extra care to locate the painful area. Do not palpate a vital artery with pressure that obstructs blood flow. Patient safety and doing no harm are top priorities.
- After washing hands, perform palpation slowly, gently, and deliberately. Light palpation of structures such as the abdomen determines areas of irregularity or tenderness (Fig. 7.2A). Place your hand on the area you are examining and depress about 1 cm (1/2 inch).
- Light intermittent pressure is best when palpating; heavy prolonged pressure causes loss of sensitivity in the hand. If a patient reports pain, do not proceed to deep palpation in the area of concern.
- After light palpation, use deeper palpation to examine the condition of organs (Fig. 7.2B) if appropriate. Depress the area that you are examining deeply and evenly

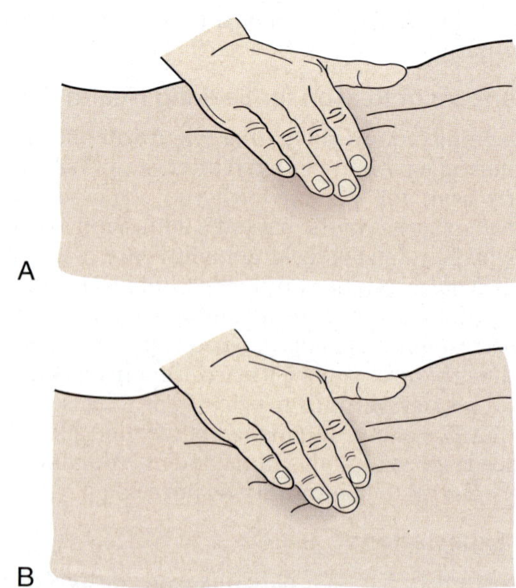

Fig. 7.2 A, During light palpation, gentle pressure against underlying skin and tissues can detect areas of irregularity and tenderness. **B,** During deep palpation, depress tissue to assess condition of underlying organs.

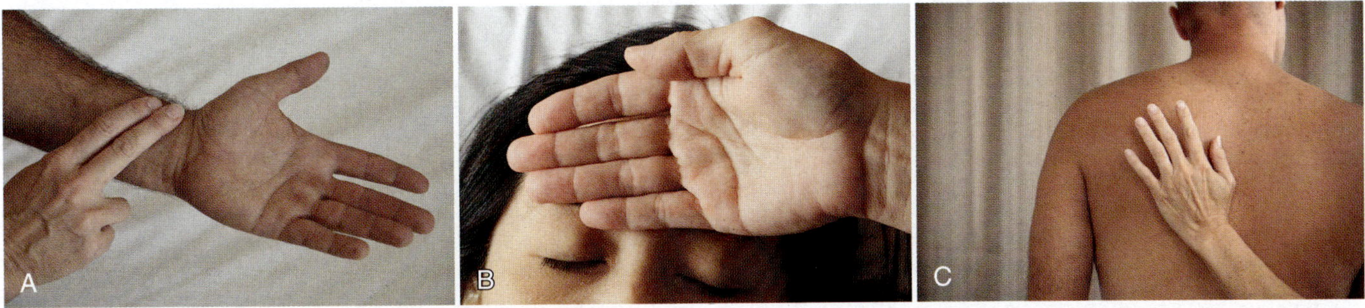

Fig. 7.3 **A,** Radial pulse is detected with pads of fingertips, the most sensitive part of the hand. **B,** Dorsum of hand detects temperature variations in skin. **C,** Bony part of the palm at base of fingers detects vibrations.

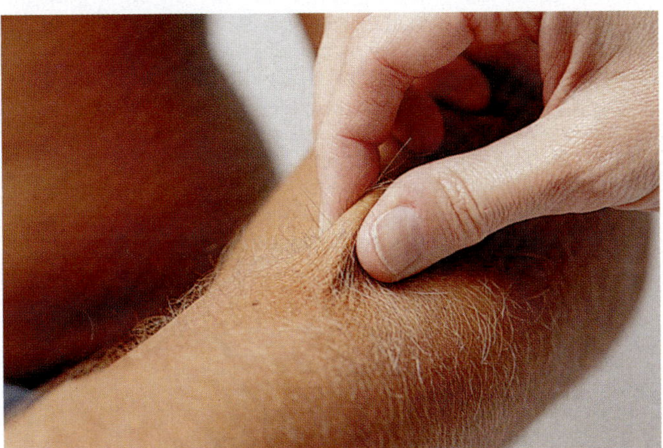

Fig. 7.4 Assessment of skin turgor.

(Ball et al., 2015). Apply deep palpation with one or both hands (bimanually). Bimanual palpation involves one hand placed over the other while applying pressure. The upper hand exerts downward pressure as the other hand feels the subtle characteristics of underlying organs and masses.

- Use the palmar surface of the fingers and finger pads to determine position, texture, size, consistency, masses, fluid, and pulsation (Fig. 7.3A). Assess temperature with the dorsal surface, or back, of the hand (Fig. 7.3B). The palm of the hand is more sensitive to vibration (Fig. 7.3C). Measure position, consistency, and turgor by lightly grasping the body part with the fingertips (see Fig. 7.4).

Percussion

Percussion involves tapping the body with the fingertips to produce a vibration that travels through body tissues. This vibration is transmitted through the body tissues, and the character of the sound heard depends on the density of the underlying tissue. The resulting sounds determine the location, size, and density of underlying structures and help verify abnormalities assessed by palpation and auscultation. The skill of percussion is used more often by advanced practice nurses than by nurses in daily practice at the bedside.

Auscultation

Auscultation is listening for sounds produced by the body. Some sounds such as voice sounds are audible to the human ear. Other sounds such as those made by the cardiovascular, respiratory, and gastrointestinal (GI) systems require use of a stethoscope.

To auscultate, you need good hearing acuity, a good stethoscope, and knowledge of how to use the stethoscope properly. Individuals with a hearing impairment can use a stethoscope with additional sound amplification. Chapter 6 describes the parts of the stethoscope and its general use. The bell is best for low-pitched sounds such as vascular and certain heart sounds, and the diaphragm is best for high-pitched sounds such as bowel and lung sounds. Practice using the stethoscope (Box 7.3). Placing the bell or diaphragm under the gown or clothing, directly on the skin, aids in accurate assessment. By deliberately producing these sounds, you learn to recognize and disregard them during the actual examination. Learn to recognize the following characteristics of sounds such as frequency (number of sound waves generated per second), intensity (amplitude of sound waves to describe as loud or soft), quality (sound characteristics such as blowing or gurling), and duration (short, medium, or long in a minute).

Auscultation requires concentration and practice. The sounds heard over the abdomen are caused by intestinal peristalsis and are heard over all four abdominal quadrants as intermittent "tinkling" sounds. After understanding the cause and character of normal auscultated sounds, it becomes easier to recognize abnormal sounds and their origins.

Olfaction

While assessing a patient, become familiar with the nature and source of body odors (Table 7.1). **Olfaction,** or smelling, helps to detect abnormalities not recognized by other means. Unusual smells lead to detection of serious abnormalities.

PREPARATION FOR EXAMINATION

Preparation of the environment, equipment, and patient ensures a smooth examination. A disorganized approach when preparing for a physical examination causes errors and incomplete findings. Use standard precautions during an examination (see Chapter 9). It is necessary to wear gloves during palpation and percussion when there is a possibility of coming in contact with body fluids to reduce contact with microorganisms. Perform hand hygiene before and after an examination.

BOX 7.3 Using a Stethoscope

1. Ensure that earpiece follows the contour of the ear canals. Learn which fit is best for you by comparing the amplification of sounds with the earpieces in both directions.
2. Place earpieces in both ears with tips of earpieces turned toward the face. *Lightly* blow into the diaphragm. Again, place earpieces in your ears, this time with ends turned toward the back of the head. *Lightly* blow into the stethoscope diaphragm. You find that you hear clearer sounds with the earpiece turned toward the face. After you have learned the right fit for the loudest sound, wear the stethoscope the same way each time.
3. Put the stethoscope on and *lightly* blow into the diaphragm. If sound is barely audible, *lightly* blow into the bell. Sound is carried through only one part of the chest piece at a time. If the sound is greatly amplified through the diaphragm, the diaphragm is in position for use. If sound is barely audible through the diaphragm, the bell is in position for use.
4. Place the diaphragm over the anterior part of your chest. Ask a friend to speak in a normal conversational tone. Environmental noise seriously detracts from hearing the noise created by body organs. When using a stethoscope, the patient and the examiner need to remain quiet.
5. Put the stethoscope on and gently tap the tubing. It is often difficult to avoid stretching or moving the stethoscope tubing. Position yourself so that the tubing hangs free. Moving or touching the tubing creates extraneous sounds.
6. *Care of the stethoscope:* Remove earpieces regularly and clean or remove cerumen (earwax). Keep the bell and diaphragm free of dust, lint, and body oils. Keep the tubing away from your body oils. Avoid draping the stethoscope around the neck next to the skin. To clean, wipe the entire stethoscope (e.g., diaphragm, tubing) with alcohol or soapy water. Be sure to dry all parts thoroughly. Follow manufacturer recommendations.
7. *Infection control:* Harmful bacteria, even antibiotic-resistant microorganisms, transfer from patient to patient when using portable equipment such as stethoscopes. Follow institution infection control guidelines, especially contact precautions, to decrease this risk. Clean the stethoscope (diaphragm/bell) with a disinfectant before reuse on another patient. Using a disinfectant such as isopropyl alcohol (with or without chlorhexidine), benzalkonium, or sodium hypochlorite is effective in reducing the number of bacterial colonies. Earpieces of stethoscopes are sources of transferable bacteria as well when you inadvertently touch your ears and then care for the patient. Potential pathogens could contaminate earpieces. Using hand hygiene before and after patient contact decreases the risk for transmitting microorganisms from your ear to your patient. Do not use cloth stethoscope covers because these have been shown to easily become contaminated.

Table 7.1 Assessment of Characteristic Odors

Odor	Site or Source	Potential Causes
Alcohol	Oral cavity	Ingestion of alcohol, diabetes
Ammonia	Urine	Urinary tract infection, renal failure
Body odor	Skin, particularly in areas where body parts rub together (e.g., under arms and breasts)	Poor hygiene, excess perspiration (hyperhidrosis), foul-smelling perspiration (bromhidrosis)
	Wound site	Wound abscess
	Vomitus	Abdominal irritation, contaminated food
Feces	Vomitus/oral cavity (fecal odor)	Bowel obstruction
	Rectal area	Fecal incontinence
Foul-smelling stools in infant	Stool	Malabsorption syndrome
Halitosis	Oral cavity	Poor dental and oral hygiene, gum disease
Sweet, fruity ketones	Oral cavity	Diabetic ketoacidosis
Stale urine	Skin	Uremic acidosis
Sweet, heavy, thick odor	Draining wound	*Pseudomonas* (bacterial) infection
Musty odor	Casted body part	Infection inside cast
Fetid, sweet odor	Tracheostomy or mucus secretions	Infection of bronchial tree (*Pseudomonas* bacteria)

Environment

A physical examination requires privacy. An examination room is preferable, but often the examination occurs in the patient's room. In a patient's home, the examination could possibly be performed in the patient's bedroom. Adequate lighting is necessary to perform inspection. Ideally an examination room is soundproof so that patients feel comfortable discussing their conditions. Be sure to eliminate other sources of noise, take precautions to prevent interruptions, and ensure that the room is warm enough to maintain comfort.

Patients with mobility impairments require safe transfer to an examination table; assist the patient as needed on and off the table. Consider patient comfort while on the examination table. When a patient lies supine, raise the head of the table about 30°, using a small pillow if needed. Do not leave a confused, combative, or uncooperative patient unsupervised on an examination table.

Equipment

Perform hand hygiene before equipment preparation and the examination. Have equipment readily available and arranged in order for easy use (Box 7.4). Prepare equipment as needed (e.g., warm diaphragm of stethoscope between the hands; be sure to have a proper size earpiece for an

BOX 7.4 **Equipment and Supplies for Physical Assessment**

- Cervical brush or broom (if needed)
- Cotton applicators
- Disposable pad/paper towels
- Drapes
- Eye chart (e.g., Snellen chart)
- Flashlight and spotlight
- Forms (e.g., physical, laboratory)
- Gloves (sterile or clean)
- Gown for patient
- Ophthalmoscope
- Otoscope
- Papanicolaou (Pap) liquid preparation (if needed)
- Percussion (reflex) hammer
- Pulse oximeter
- Ruler
- Scale with height measurement rod
- Specimen containers, slides, wooden or plastic spatula, and cytological fixative (if needed)
- Sphygmomanometer and cuff
- Sterile swabs
- Stethoscope
- Tape measure
- Thermometer
- Tissues
- Tongue depressors
- Tuning fork
- Vaginal speculum (if needed)
- Water-soluble lubricant
- Wristwatch with second hand or digital display

otoscope). Check all equipment to ensure that they function properly. The ophthalmoscope and otoscope require batteries and light bulbs.

Physical Preparation of a Patient

A patient's physical comfort is vital for a successful examination. Before starting, ask whether the patient needs to use the restroom. An empty bladder and bowel make examination of the abdomen, genitalia, and rectum easier.

Physical preparation involves ensuring that a patient is dressed or covered properly. A patient at an office visit or screening event might have to undress and wear a light cover, depending on the body part involved. Provide a patient privacy and plenty of time during undressing, avoiding unnecessary embarrassment. Make sure that the patient stays warm by eliminating drafts, controlling room temperature, and providing warm blankets. Routinely ask whether the patient is comfortable.

Positioning

During the examination, ask the patient to assume proper positions so that body parts are accessible and the patient stays comfortable. Table 7.2 lists and shows the preferred positions for each part of the examination. A patient's ability to assume positions depends on the patient's physical strength, mobility, ease of breathing, age, and degree of wellness. Explain the positions and help patients assume them. Adjust the sheets or drapes so that the area examined is accessible, making sure not to unnecessarily expose a body part. Use extra care when positioning older adults or patients with weak muscles because they are more prone to having limitations.

Psychological Preparation of a Patient

Many patients find an examination tiring or stressful, or they experience anxiety about possible findings. A thorough, simple, and clear explanation of the purpose and steps of each assessment lets patients know what to expect and helps them cooperate with each step. Give a detailed explanation as you examine each body system. Convey an open, professional, and relaxed approach (Ball et al., 2015).

Use a medical interpreter for patients who do not speak or understand English. If a patient has a hearing or speech impairment, identify the communication system that will be used (sign language interpreter, word board, or talk box). If necessary, use Braille, audiotaped information, or three-dimensional anatomical models to help a patient with visual impairments understand information (Ball et al., 2015).

When a patient and nurse are of opposite gender, it helps to have a third person of the patient's gender in the room. The presence of a third person assures the patient that you will behave ethically. During the examination, watch the patient's emotional responses. Watch whether body movements appear stiff from anxiety. Remain calm and explain each step clearly. It is sometimes necessary to stop the examination and ask how the patient feels. Findings are more accurate if you postpone until the patient can cooperate and relax.

ASSESSMENT OF DIFFERENT AGE GROUPS

Different interview styles and approaches are needed to perform a health history and examine patients of different age groups. Routine pediatric examinations focus on health promotion and illness prevention, particularly for the care of well children who receive competent parenting and have no serious health problems (Hockenberry et al., 2017). The examination focuses on growth and development, sensory screening, dental examination, and behavioral assessment. When examining children, the following tips help in data collection:

1. Gain a child's trust before performing any type of examination. Talk and play with the child first. It also helps to perform parts of the examination that you can do visually before actually touching the child.
2. Children feel safer during an examination if it is initiated from the periphery and then moves to the center. For example, examine the extremities before moving to the chest.
3. When obtaining histories of infants and children gather all or part of the information from parents or guardians.

Table 7.2 Positions for Examination

Position	Areas Assessed	Rationale	Limitations
Sitting	Head and neck, back, posterior thorax and lungs, anterior thorax and lungs, breasts, axillae, heart, vital signs, upper extremities	Sitting upright provides full expansion of lungs and better visualization of symmetry of upper body parts.	Physically weakened patient is sometimes unable to sit. Use supine position with head of bed elevated instead.
Supine	Head and neck, anterior thorax and lungs, breasts, axillae, heart, abdomen, extremities, pulses	This is most normally relaxed position. It provides easy access to pulse sites.	If patient becomes short of breath easily, raise head of bed.
Dorsal recumbent	Head and neck, anterior thorax and lungs, breasts, axillae, heart, abdomen	This position is for abdominal assessment because it promotes relaxation of abdominal muscles.	Patients with painful disorders are more comfortable with knees flexed.
Lithotomy[a]	Female genitalia and genital tract	This position provides maximal exposure of genitalia and facilitates insertion of vaginal speculum.	Lithotomy position is embarrassing and uncomfortable; examiner minimizes time that patient spends in it. Keep the patient well draped.
Sims[a]	Rectum and vagina	Flexion of hip and knee improves exposure of rectal area.	Joint deformities hinder patient's ability to bend hip and knee.
Prone	Musculoskeletal system	This position is only for assessing extension of hip joint, skin, and buttocks.	Patients with respiratory difficulties do not tolerate this position well.
Lateral recumbent	Heart	This position helps to detect murmurs.	Patients with respiratory difficulties do not tolerate this position well.
Knee-chest[a]	Rectum	This position provides maximal exposure of rectal area.	This position is embarrassing and uncomfortable.

[a]Patients with arthritis or other joint deformities may be unable to assume this position.

4. Because parents sometimes think they are being tested or judged by the examiner, offer support during examination and do not pass judgment.
5. Call children by their preferred name and address parents formally (e.g., as "Mr and Mrs Brown") rather than by first names.
6. Open-ended questions often allow parents to share more information and describe more of the child's problems.
7. Older children and adolescents tend to respond best when treated as adults and individuals and often can provide details about their health history and severity of symptoms.
8. Remember an adolescent has a right to confidentiality. After talking with parents about historical information, arrange to speak privately with the adolescent.

For Older Adults

During the examination, recognize that with advancing age the body does not respond vigorously to injury or disease. Therefore, older people do not always exhibit the expected signs and symptoms. Characteristically, older adults have blunted or atypical signs and symptoms. Follow these principles described by Touhy and Jett (2018) during examination of an older adult:

1. Do not assume that aging is always accompanied by illness or disability. Older adults are able to adapt to change and maintain functional independence.
2. Allow extra time; be patient, relaxed, and unhurried with older adults and provide adequate space for an examination, particularly if a patient uses a mobility aid.
3. Measure performance under the most favorable conditions. Take advantage of natural opportunities for assessment (e.g., during bathing, grooming, mealtime).
4. Sequence an examination to keep position changes to a minimum. Be efficient throughout the examination to limit patient movement.
5. Be sure that an examination of an older adult includes review of mental status.

ORGANIZATION OF THE EXAMINATION

A physical examination follows the completion of the health history. Health assessment documentation needs to include each body system, including subjective data collected. Electronic or paper physical examination documentation forms allow you to record objective and subjective data in the same sequence that it was gathered. Use common and accepted medical abbreviations to keep documentation accurate and concise. Information from the health history focuses your attention on specific parts of the examination. New objective data from the examination supplement information from the history to confirm or refute the data.

Be systematic and well organized about the examination so that you do not miss important assessments. A complete head-to-toe approach includes all body systems and helps you anticipate each step. In an adult, begin by assessing the head and neck, progressing methodically down the body to include all body systems. Compare both sides of the body for symmetry. If a patient is seriously ill, examine the body system most at risk for being abnormal. Provide rest periods if a patient becomes fatigued. Perform any painful procedures near the end of the examination.

GENERAL ASSESSMENT

When a patient first enters an examination room, observe his or her walk and general appearance and be attentive to his or her behavior and dress. A general survey, or appraisal, of the patient's presentation and behavior provides information about characteristics of an illness, the patient's ability to function independently, body image, emotional state, recent changes in weight, and developmental status. If there are abnormalities or problems, assess the affected body system more closely during the full examination.

General Appearance and Behavior

Assess appearance and behavior while preparing the patient for the examination. For this review include:

- *Gender and race:* A person's gender affects the type of examination performed and the order of the assessments. Different physical features are related to gender and race. Certain illnesses are more likely to affect a specific gender or race (e.g., the incidence of skin cancer is more common in white people than in black people, prostate cancer is higher in black men than in white men, and cancer of the bladder is higher in men than women) (ACS, 2015).
- *Age:* Age influences normal physical characteristics and a person's ability to participate in some parts of the examination.
- *Signs of distress:* Sometimes obvious signs or symptoms indicate pain (grimacing, splinting painful area), difficulty breathing (shortness of breath, sternal retractions), or anxiety. Set priorities and examine the related physical areas first.
- *Body type:* Observe whether the patient appears trim and muscular, obese, or excessively thin. Body type reflects the level of health, age, and lifestyle.
- *Posture:* Normal standing posture shows an upright stance with parallel alignment of the hips and shoulders. Normal sitting posture involves some degree of rounding of the shoulders. Observe whether the patient has a slumped, erect, or bent posture, which reflects mood or pain. Changes in older adult physiology often result in a stooped, forward-bent posture, with the hips and knees somewhat flexed and the arms bent at the elbows.
- *Gait:* Observe as the patient walks into the room or stands at the bedside (if the patient is ambulatory). Note whether movements are coordinated or uncoordinated. A person normally walks smoothly, with the arms swinging freely at the sides and the head and face leading the body.
- *Body movements:* Observe whether movements are purposeful, noting any tremors involving the extremities. Determine whether any body parts are immobile.
- *Hygiene and grooming:* Note the patient's level of cleanliness by observing the appearance of the hair, skin, and fingernails. Determine whether his or her clothes are clean. Grooming depends on the patient's cognitive and emotional function, daily or social activities, and occupation. Observe for excessive use of cosmetics or colognes that could indicate a change in self-perception.
- *Dress:* Culture, lifestyle, socioeconomic level, and personal preference affect the selection and wearing of clothing. However, you should assess whether the clothing is appropriate for the temperature, weather conditions, or setting. Depressed or mentally ill people may not be able to select proper clothing, and an older adult might tend to wear extra clothing because of sensitivity to cold.
- *Body odor:* An unpleasant body odor can result from physical exercise, poor hygiene, or certain disease states. Validate any odors that might indicate a health problem.
- *Affect and mood:* Affect is how a person appears to others. Patients express mood or emotional state verbally and nonverbally. Determine whether verbal expressions match nonverbal behavior and if the mood is appropriate for the situation. By maintaining eye contact, you can observe facial expressions while asking questions.
- *Speech:* Normal speech is understandable and moderately paced and shows an association with the person's thoughts. However, emotions or neurological impairment sometimes causes rapid or slowed speech. Observe whether the patient speaks in a normal tone with clear inflection of words.
- *Signs of patient abuse:* During the examination, observe whether the patient fears his or her spouse or partner, a caregiver, a parent, or an adult child. Abuse of children, women, and older adults is a growing health problem. Consider any obvious physical injury or neglect as signs of possible abuse (e.g., evidence of malnutrition or presence of bruising on the extremities or trunk) (WHO, 2015).
- *Substance abuse:* Unusual or inconsistent behavior may be an indicator of substance abuse, which can affect all socioeconomic groups. Always approach the patient in a caring and nonjudgmental way; substance abuse

involves both emotional and lifestyle issues. Box 7.5 lists characteristics of patients who should be further assessed for potential substance abuse. If you suspect abuse or addiction in people 18 years of age or older, a tool such as the NIDA Quick Screen V1.0 helps to identify the level or risks associated with substance abuse (NIDA, 2012). If you suspect that alcohol abuse is a major problem, the CAGE questionnaire provides a useful set of questions to guide assessment. CAGE is an acronym for the following:

- Have you ever felt the need to **Cut down** on your drinking or drug use?
- Have people **Annoyed** you by criticizing your drinking or drug use?
- Have you ever felt bad or **Guilty** about your drinking or drug use?
- Have you ever used or had a drink first thing in the morning as an **Eye-opener** to steady your nerves or feel normal?

Among older adults, risk factors for development of alcohol-related problems include chronic medical disorders, sleep disorders, social isolation, loneliness, bereavement, and acute or chronic pain. When assessing adolescents, use the T-ACE modification to assess a patient's degree of tolerance (e.g., how many drinks does it take to make you feel high?) (Burns et al., 2010).

Vital Signs

Assessment of vital signs (see Chapter 6) is the first part of the physical examination. Positioning or moving a patient excessively can result in inaccurate values. Be sure to recheck and report any vital signs outside of normal ranges.

BOX 7.5 Red Flags for Suspicion of Substance Abuse

- Patients who frequently miss appointments
- Patients who frequently request written excuses for absence from work
- Patients who have chief complaints of insomnia, "bad nerves," or pain that does not fit a particular pattern
- Patients who often report lost prescriptions (e.g., tranquilizers, pain medications) or ask for frequent refills
- Patients who make frequent emergency department visits
- Patients who have a history of changing health care providers or bring in medication bottles prescribed by several different providers
- Patients with histories of gastrointestinal bleeding, peptic ulcers, pancreatitis, cellulitis, or frequent pulmonary infections
- Patients with frequent sexually transmitted diseases, complicated pregnancies, multiple abortions, or sexual dysfunction
- Patients who complain of chest pains or palpitations or who have a history of admissions to rule out myocardial infarctions
- Patients who give histories of activities that place them at risk for human immunodeficiency virus (HIV) infections (e.g., multiple partners, multiple rapes)
- Patients with family history of addiction; history of childhood sexual, physical, or emotional abuse or social and financial or marital problems

Data from American Psychiatric Association: *Diagnostic and statistical manual of mental disorders,* ed 5, Washington, DC, 2013, The Association; Ries R, Wilford B: *Principles of addiction medicine,* ed 5, Chevy Chase, MD, 2014, Lippincott Williams & Wilkins.

Height and Weight

Height and weight reflect a patient's general level of health. This information may also be important for diagnostic testing and dosing of medications. Weight is routinely measured during health screenings and visits to health care providers' offices or clinics and when patients are admitted to a health care setting. Measuring an infant's or child's height and weight provides data about his or her growth and development. In older adults, height and weight coupled with a nutritional assessment help to identify dietary problems or dental or other functional deficits. Be sure to recognize overall trends in height and weight changes. Frequently adults become shorter with vertebral changes related to aging.

Daily variation in a patient's weight normally occurs as a result of fluid loss or retention. Health assessments screen for abnormal weight changes, using the nursing history data to focus on possible causes for weight changes. Determine the patient's current height and weight, noting weight gains or losses. Assess changes in diet habits, appetite, use of prescription or over-the-counter drugs, or physical symptoms. Standardized tables provide normal expected weights for a patient at a given height.

Several types of scales are available including built-in hospital bed scales, wheelchair scales, and digital or mechanical standing scales. Mechanical scales need to be calibrated regularly. To accurately weigh a patient, use the same scale and weigh the patient at about the same time each day (Ball et al., 2015). Patients capable of bearing their own weight use a standing scale. The scale measures in weight increments to the nearest 0.1 kg or 0.1 lb depending on how the scale is set (Ball et al., 2015). The patient stands on the scale platform and remains still. Electronic scales automatically display weight within seconds. Electronic scales are automatically calibrated each time they are used.

Weigh infants in baskets or on platform scales. Remove the infant's clothing, keeping the room warm to reduce heat loss. A light cloth or paper placed on the scale prevents surface contamination from urine or feces. Hold a hand lightly above the infant to prevent falls. Measure the weight of an infant in ounces, grams, and kilograms.

To measure the height of a weight-bearing patient, have the patient remove his or her shoes. When needed place a paper towel on the scale platform so that the patient's feet remain clean. The platform scale has a metal rod attached to the back of the scale; this swings out and over the crown of the patient's head. Have the patient stand erect. Measure his or her height in centimeters or inches.

Place an infant in the supine position on a firm surface with shoes removed (Fig. 7.5). Portable devices are available that provide a reliable means to measure height. While the caregiver holds the infant's head against the headboard, straighten the legs at the knees and place the footboard against the bottom of the infant's feet. Record the infant's length to the nearest 0.5 cm or 1/8 inch (Hockenberry et al., 2017).

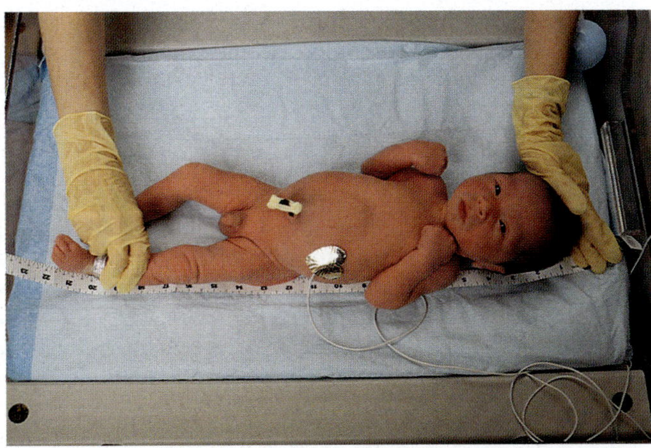

Fig. 7.5 Measuring infant length. (From Murray SS, McKinney ES: *Foundations of maternal-newborn and women's health nursing*, ed 5, St Louis, 2014, Saunders.)

ASSESSMENT OF EACH SYSTEM

Skin, Hair, and Nails

The **integument** consists of the skin, hair, scalp, and nails. First inspect all skin surfaces or assess the skin gradually while examining other body systems. Use the skills of inspection, palpation, and olfaction to assess the function and integrity of the integument.

Skin

Skin assessment reveals changes in oxygenation, circulation, nutrition, local tissue damage, and hydration. In a hospital setting, many patients are older adults, debilitated patients, or young but seriously ill patients. Such patients may be at risk for skin lesions resulting from trauma to the skin during administration of care, prolonged pressure during immobilization, or reactions to medications. Patients at high risk include neurologically impaired, chronically ill, and orthopedic patients. Others at risk include patients with diminished mental status, poor tissue oxygenation, low cardiac output, or inadequate nutrition. In nursing homes and extended care facilities, some patients are at risk for many of the same problems, depending on their level of mobility and the presence of chronic illness. Routinely assess the skin to look for primary or initial lesions that develop. Without proper care, primary lesions often deteriorate to become secondary lesions that require more extensive nursing care.

Be alert for any lesions that show evidence of cancer. Melanoma, an aggressive form of skin cancer, is the cause of most skin cancer deaths (American Cancer Society [ACS], 2016a). Cutaneous malignancies are the most common neoplasms seen in patients. Although it is important to perform a thorough skin assessment for all patients, research demonstrates the effectiveness of patient education and self-examination for prevention and early detection of skin cancers (Box 7.6).

The condition of the patient's skin reveals the need for nursing intervention. Use assessment findings to determine the type of hygiene measures required to maintain integrity of the integument (see Chapter 16). Adequate nutrition

BOX 7.6 Evidence-Based Practice

PICO Question: In individuals who practice high-risk behaviors or have a familial tendency for skin cancers, does monthly systematic skin inspection result in earlier diagnosis of skin cancers than annual examinations with the health provider?

Summary of Evidence

The American Cancer Society (ACS) estimated that 83,510 new cases and 13,650 deaths would result from skin cancers in 2016 (ACS, 2016a). These numbers are not including the most common types of cancer—basal cell and squamous cell skin cancer (also referred to as nonmelanoma). A melanoma is a cancerous (malignant) tumor that begins in the cells that produce the skin coloring (melanocytes). There are several risk factors for melanoma. Major risk factors are positive family history of melanoma, a prior melanoma, and multiple or unusual moles (nevi). Other risk factors include fair skin, freckling, and light hair; immune suppression; age younger than 30 years; and excessive exposure to the sun and ultraviolet light (especially before 18 years of age) (ACS, 2016b).

Research has indicated that when detected early and treated properly, skin cancer is highly curable. Overall survival rates for melanoma at 5 and 10 years are 92% and 89% (ACS, 2016a). Therefore, early intervention is of utmost importance. In July 2014, a call to action to prevent skin cancer by the surgeon general increased awareness and encouraged all Americans to initiate a reduction in skin cancer (USPHS, 2014).

The Skin Cancer Foundation (2015) emphasizes the importance of skin self-examination from the crown of your head to the soles of your feet. Familiarize yourself with all moles on your body; have a loved one help if needed. The deadliest melanomas do not appear in preexisting moles; 70%−80% develop in previously normal skin. Any new or changing lesion needs to be reported to a health care provider.

The current evidence does not demonstrate a benefit for health care providers to complete a visual skin examination to screen for skin cancer (U.S. Preventive Services Task Force [USPSTF], 2016). This does not mean that health care providers should not complete a visual assessment at this time because it is a screening tool; there is not sufficient evidence to support the benefit. A new publication by the US Preventive Services Task Force, *Skin Cancer Prevention: Behavioral Counseling,* is currently in progress and is due for release in 2018 (USPSTF, 2017).

Application to Nursing Practice

- Use a well-lit room and mirrors to examine all skin surfaces. If necessary, have the patient ask a family member and/or significant other to aid in the examination.
- Use visual images to teach patients how to routinely assess their skin and the importance of contacting their health care provider if a skin lesion or mole starts to change, bleed, or ooze or feels different (swollen, hard, lumpy, itchy, or tender to the touch) (McWhirter and Hoffman-Gomez, 2013; Skin Cancer Foundation, 2015). Especially instruct older adults, who tend to have delayed wound healing.
- For adolescents and young adult patients, online programs to teach how to identify and reduce risks for skin cancers are effective (Heckman et al, 2016).
- Inform patients of ways to prevent skin cancer by avoiding overexposure to the sun:
  - Wear sunglasses, wide-brimmed hats, and long sleeves and long pants.
  - Apply broad-spectrum sunscreens with sun protection factor (SPF) 15 or greater to protect against ultraviolet B (UVB) and ultraviolet A (UVA) rays approximately 15 min before going into the sun and after swimming, perspiring, or bathing.

Continued

BOX 7.6 Evidence-Based Practice—cont'd

- Avoid tanning under the direct sun at midday (10 a.m. to 4 p.m.).
- Do not use indoor sunlamps, tanning parlors, or tanning pills.
- Inform patients who are on medications that make the skin more sensitive to the sun (e.g., oral contraceptives, statins, anti-inflammatories, antihypertensives, immunosuppressives) to take extra precautions when spending time in the sun.
- Inform patients to protect their children from the sun. Severe sunburns in childhood greatly increase melanoma risk later in life (ACS, 2016b).

and hydration become goals of therapy if an alteration in the status of the integument is identified.

Provide adequate lighting and comfortable temperatures when assessing the skin. The recommended light is natural sunlight; halogen lighting is another option. A room that is too warm causes superficial vasodilation, resulting in increased skin redness. Patients who are sensitive to cold develop **cyanosis** (bluish color) around the lips and nail beds.

You inspect all skin surfaces during an examination; begin with a brief overall visual review of the entire body. The examination includes inspecting skin color, moisture, temperature, texture, and turgor; vascular changes; **edema;** phlebitis; and lesions. Wear clean gloves when any moisture is present. Carefully palpate any abnormalities. Skin odors are usually noted in skinfolds such as the axillae or under the breasts in female patients.

Nursing History

Ask the patient about history of skin changes including dryness, pruritus, sores, rashes, lumps, color, odor, and nonhealing lesions. Localized changes in skin color are sometimes the first indicators of skin cancer. Inquire about the patient's history of sun exposure, use of sunscreen, and predisposition to develop skin cancer (fair, freckled, light-colored hair or eyes, family history). Assess for use of topical medications, sun lamps, or tanning beds and exposure to creosote, coal, tar, or radium. Ask whether the patient has noticed any changes in skin coloring; then proceed with inspection.

Color

Skin color varies by body part and person. Despite individual variations, skin color is usually uniform over the body. Table 7.3 lists common variations in skin color. Normal skin pigmentation ranges from ivory or light pink to ruddy pink in light skin and from light to deep brown or olive in dark skin. In older adults, the pigmentation increases unevenly, causing discolored skin. While inspecting the skin, be aware that cosmetics or tanning agents sometimes mask color.

Assessment of skin color first involves areas of the skin not exposed to the sun. Usually you see color hues best on the palms of the hands, soles of the feet, lips, tongue, and nail beds. Note whether the skin is unusually pale or dark. Areas of increased color (hyperpigmentation) and decreased color (hypopigmentation) are common. Skin creases and folds are darker than the rest of the body.

Inspect sites where you can more easily identify abnormalities. For example, you can see **pallor** (unusual paleness) more easily in the face, buccal mucosa (mouth), conjunctivae, and nail beds. Observe for cyanosis (bluish discoloration) in the lips, nail beds, palpebral conjunctivae, and palms. To recognize pallor in a dark-skinned patient, observe that normal brown skin appears to be yellow-brown, and normal black skin appears to be ashen gray. Also assess the lips, nail beds, and mucous membranes for generalized pallor that causes them to appear ashen gray. Assessment of cyanosis in dark-skinned patients requires that you observe areas where pigmentation occurs the least (conjunctivae, sclera, buccal mucosa, tongue, lips, nail beds, and palms and soles). A bluish tint of the lips and gums may be a normal finding in dark-skinned patients (Ball et al., 2015).

The best site to inspect for **jaundice** (yellow-orange discoloration) is the patient's sclera. You can see normal reactive hyperemia, or redness, most often in regions exposed to pressure such as the sacrum, heels, and greater trochanter (see Chapter 17). Inspect for any patches or areas of skin

Table 7.3 Skin Color Variations

Color	Condition	Causes	Assessment Locations
Bluish (cyanosis)	Increased amount of deoxygenated hemoglobin (associated with hypoxia)	Heart or lung disease, cold environment	Nail beds, lips, base of tongue, skin (severe cases)
Pallor (decrease in color)	Reduced amount of oxyhemoglobin	Anemia	Face, conjunctivae, nail beds, palms of hands
	Reduced visibility of oxyhemoglobin resulting from decreased blood flow	Shock	Skin, nail beds, conjunctivae, lips
Loss of pigmentation	Vitiligo	Congenital or autoimmune condition causing lack of pigment	Patchy areas on skin over face, hands, arms
Yellow-orange (jaundice)	Increased deposit of bilirubin in tissues	Liver disease, destruction of red blood cells	Sclerae, mucous membranes, skin
Red (erythema)	Increased visibility of oxyhemoglobin caused by dilation or increased blood flow	Fever, direct trauma, blushing, alcohol intake	Face, area of trauma, sacrum, shoulders, other common sites for pressure injuries
Tan-brown	Increased amount of melanin	Suntan, pregnancy	Areas exposed to sun (face, arms), areolae, nipples

Table 7.4 Physical Findings of the Skin Indicative of Substance Abuse

Physical Finding	Commonly Associated Drug
Diaphoresis	Sedative-hypnotic (including alcohol)
Spider angiomas	Alcohol, stimulants
Burns (especially fingers)	Alcohol
Needle marks	Opioids
Contusions, abrasions, cuts, scars	Alcohol, other sedative-hypnotics
"Homemade" tattoos	Cocaine, i.v. opioids (prevents detection of injection sites)
Increased vascularity of face	Alcohol
Red, dry skin	Phencyclidine (PCP)

Modified from Burchum JR, Rosenthal LD: *Lehne's pharmacology for nursing care,* ed 9, St Louis, 2016, Elsevier; Ries R, Wilford B: *Principles of addiction medicine,* ed 5, Chevy Chase, MD, 2014, Lippincott Williams & Wilkins.

color variation. Localized skin changes such as pallor or **erythema** (red discoloration) often indicate circulatory changes or are caused by localized vasodilation resulting from sunburn or fever. To help identify erythema in a dark-skinned patient, palpate the area for heat and warmth to note the presence of skin inflammation. An area of an extremity that appears unusually pale results from an arterial occlusion or edema.

There is a pattern of findings associated with patients who are chemically dependent and i.v. drug abusers (Table 7.4). It is sometimes difficult to recognize signs and symptoms with just one examination. Edematous, reddened, and warm areas along the arms and legs suggest a pattern of recent repeated i.v. injections. Evidence of old injection sites appears as hyperpigmented and shiny or scarred areas.

The hydration of skin and mucous membranes helps to reveal body fluid imbalances, changes in skin environment, and regulation of body temperature. Moisture refers to wetness and oiliness. The skin is normally smooth and dry, whereas areas such as the axillae are normally moist; minimal perspiration or oiliness is present (Ball et al., 2015). Increased perspiration is associated with activity, warm environments, obesity, anxiety, or excitement. Diaphoresis could also occur in patients with certain conditions such as diabetes, fever, menopause, and hyperthyroidism. Use ungloved fingertips to palpate skin surfaces and observe for dullness, dryness, crusting, and flaking. Flaking is the appearance of dandruff when the skin surface is rubbed lightly. Scaling involves fishlike scales that are easily rubbed off the surface of the skin. Both flaking and scaling indicate abnormally dry skin. Other factors causing dry skin include lack of humidity, exposure to sun, smoking, stress, excessive perspiration, and dehydration. Excessive dryness worsens existing skin conditions. In bariatric patients, pay close attention to the areas with minimal airflow such as folds of large breasts, abdomen, and inguinal areas (Ball et al., 2015).

Temperature

The temperature of the skin depends on the amount of blood circulating through the dermis. Increased or decreased skin temperature reflects an increase or decrease in blood flow. An increase in skin temperature often accompanies localized erythema or redness of the skin. A reduction in skin temperature reflects a decrease in blood flow. Remember that a cold examination room affects the patient's skin temperature and color.

Accurately assess temperature by palpating the skin with the **dorsum** or back of the hand. Compare symmetrical body parts. Normally, the skin temperature is warm and consistent throughout the body. Always assess skin temperature for patients at risk for impaired circulation, such as when skin temperature varies in one area or after a cast application or vascular surgery. A stage 1 pressure injury can be identified early by noting warmth and erythema on an area of the skin (see Chapter 17).

Texture

The character of the surface of the skin and the feel of deeper portions are its texture. Determine whether the patient's skin is smooth or rough, thin or thick, tight or supple, or **indurated** (hardened) or soft by stroking it lightly with the fingertips. The texture of the skin is normally smooth, soft, and flexible in children and adults. However, it is usually not uniform. The palms of the hands and soles of the feet tend to be thicker. In older adults, the skin becomes wrinkled and leathery because of a decrease in collagen, subcutaneous fat, and sweat glands.

Localized changes result from trauma, surgical wounds, or lesions. If you find irregularities in texture such as scars or induration, ask the patient whether there has been recent skin injury. Deeper palpation sometimes reveals irregularities such as tenderness or localized areas of induration commonly caused by repeated injections.

Turgor

Turgor is the elasticity of the skin. Normally, the skin loses its elasticity with age. Edema or dehydration diminishes turgor. To assess skin turgor, grasp a fold of skin on the back of the forearm or sternal area with the fingertips and release (Fig. 7.4). Normally, the skin lifts easily and snaps back immediately to its resting position. It stays pinched or tented when turgor is poor. A decrease in turgor predisposes a patient to skin breakdown. When assessing an older adult, skin may hang loosely because of loss of elasticity and loss of adipose tissue. In this case, tenting may be a normal finding when evaluating for skin turgor (Ball et al., 2015).

Vascularity

Skin circulation affects color in localized areas and the appearance of superficial blood vessels. Capillaries become fragile with aging. Localized pressure areas, found after a patient has remained in one position, appear reddened, pink, or pale (see Chapter 17). **Petechiae** are pinpoint-size red or purple spots on the skin caused by small hemorrhages in the skin layers. They do not blanch and may indicate serious blood-clotting disorders, drug reactions, or liver disease.

Edema

Areas of the skin become swollen or edematous from fluid buildup in the tissues. Direct trauma and impairment of venous return are two common causes of edema. Inspect edematous areas for location, color, and shape. The formation of edema separates the surface of the skin from the pigmented and vascular layers, masking skin color. Edematous skin also appears stretched and shiny. Palpate edematous areas to determine mobility, consistency, and tenderness. When pressure from your finger leaves an indentation in the edematous area, it is called *pitting edema.* To assess pitting edema, press the edematous area firmly with the thumb for several seconds and release. The depth of pitting, recorded in millimeters, determines the degree of edema (Ball et al., 2015). For example, +1 edema equals 2 mm depth, and +2 edema equals 4 mm (see Fig. 7.6).

Lesions

The skin is normally free of lesions except for common freckles or age-related changes such as skin tags or senile keratosis (thickening of skin), cherry angiomas (ruby red papules), and atrophic warts. Primary lesions occur as initial spontaneous manifestations of a pathological process such as an insect bite or are secondary and result from later formation of trauma to a primary lesion such as a pressure injury. When you detect a lesion, inspect it for color, location, texture, size, shape, type (Table 7.5), grouping (e.g., clustered or linear), and distribution (localized or generalized). Observe any exudate for color, odor, amount, and consistency. Measure the size of the lesion by using a small, clear, flexible ruler divided in centimeters. Measure lesions in height, width, and depth.

Palpation determines the mobility, contour (flat, raised, or depressed), and consistency (soft or indurated) of the lesion. Palpate gently, covering the entire area of the lesion. If the lesion is moist or has draining fluid, wear

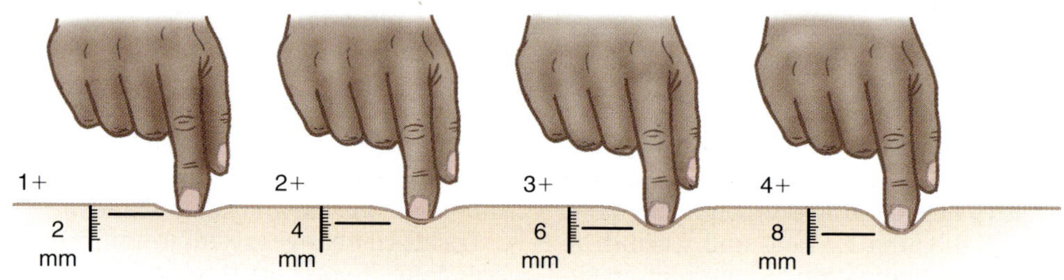

Fig. 7.6 Assessing for pitting edema. (From Ball JW, et al: *Seidel's guide to physical examination,* ed 8, St Louis, 2015, Elsevier.)

Table 7.5 Types of Primary Skin Lesions

Macule: Flat, nonpalpable change in skin color, smaller than 1 cm (e.g., freckle, petechia)

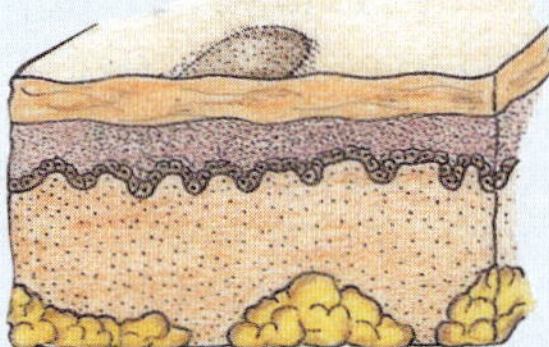

Papule: Palpable, circumscribed, solid elevation in skin, smaller than 0.5 cm (e.g., elevated nevus)

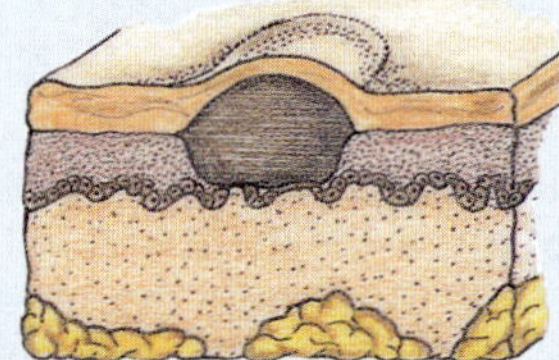

Nodule: Elevated solid mass, deeper and firmer than papule, 0.5–2 cm (e.g., wart)

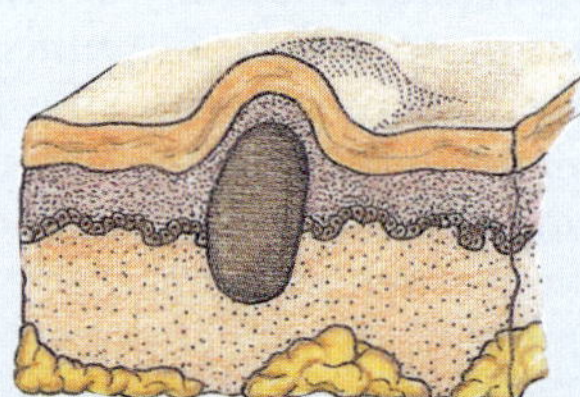

Tumor: Solid mass that extends deep through subcutaneous tissue, larger than 1–2 cm (e.g., epithelioma)

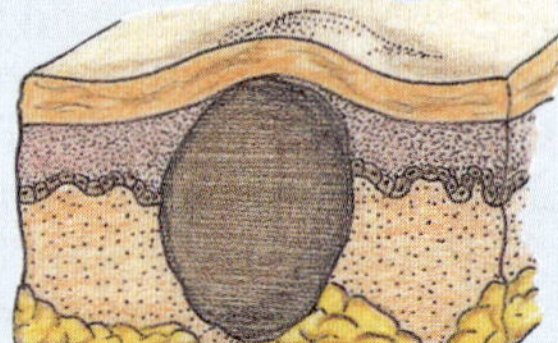

Wheal: Irregularly shaped, elevated area or superficial localized edema, varies in size (e.g., hive, mosquito bite)

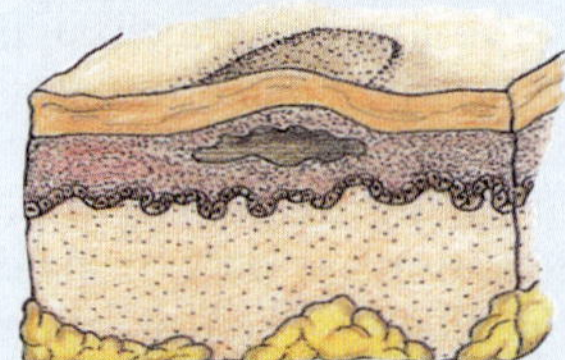

Vesicle: Circumscribed elevation of skin filled with serous fluid, smaller than 1 cm (e.g., herpes simplex, chickenpox)

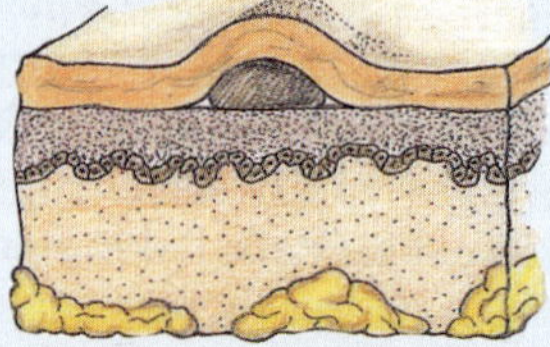

Pustule: Circumscribed elevation of skin similar to vesicle but filled with pus; varies in size (e.g., acne, staphylococcal infection)

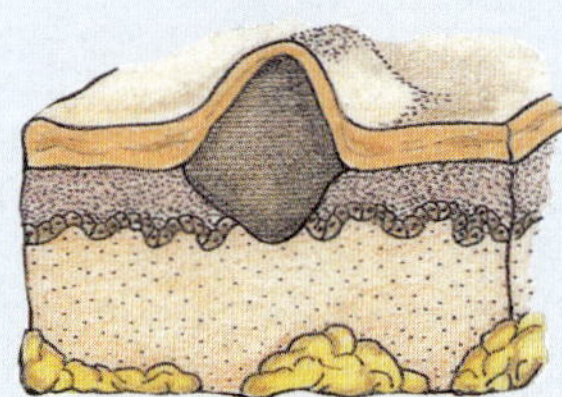

Ulcer: Deep loss of skin surface that sometimes extends to dermis and frequently bleeds and scars; varies in size (e.g., venous stasis ulcer)

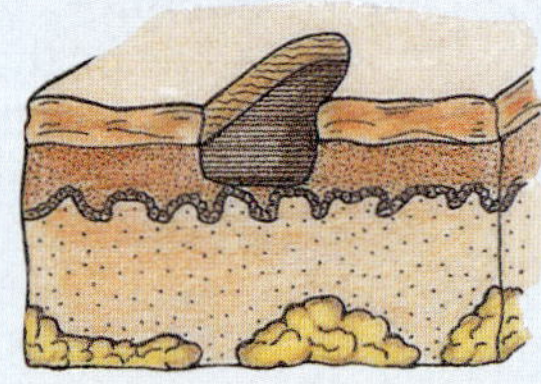

Atrophy: Thinning of skin with loss of normal skin furrow with skin appearing shiny and translucent; varies in size (e.g., arterial insufficiency)

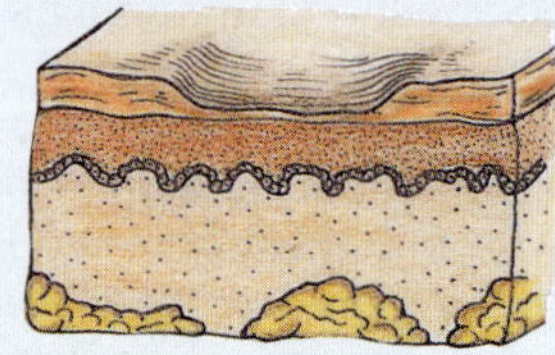

clean gloves during palpation. Note if the patient complains of tenderness during palpation. Cancerous lesions frequently undergo changes in color and size. Report abnormal lesions that have changed in character (e.g., color or size) to a health care provider for further examination.

Hair and Scalp

Inspecting the condition and distribution of body hair and integrity of the scalp requires good lighting. Hair assessment occurs during all portions of the examination. Assess its distribution, thickness, texture, lubrication, and grooming.

Nursing History

Assess whether the patient has noticed a change in growth or loss of hair or change in texture. Determine whether the patient wears a wig or hairpiece, and ask whether he or she is comfortable with it being removed briefly to examine the skin underneath. Determine whether the patient is on a medication or has any medical conditions that possibly alter hair texture or growth (e.g., chemotherapy or vasodilator).

During inspection, explain that it is necessary to separate parts of the hair to detect abnormalities. Wear clean gloves to avoid possible infection from lesions or lice. First inspect the color, distribution, quantity, thickness, texture, and lubrication of body hair. Hair is normally distributed evenly, is neither excessively dry nor oily, and is pliant or flexible. While separating sections of scalp hair, observe for characteristics of color and coarseness. Normal terminal hair (long, coarse, thick hair on the scalp, axillae, and pubic areas) varies in color from light blond to black to gray. In older adults, the hair becomes dull gray, white, or yellow. It also thins over the scalp, axillae, and pubic areas. Older men lose facial hair, whereas older women sometimes develop hair on the chin and upper lip.

Changes occur in the thickness, texture, and lubrication of scalp hair. Disturbances such as a febrile illness or scalp disease sometimes result in hair loss. Conditions such as thyroid disease alter the condition of the hair, making it fine and brittle. Hair loss (alopecia) or thinning of the hair is usually related to genetic tendencies and endocrine disorders such as diabetes and menopause. Poor nutrition causes stringy, dull, dry, and thin hair. The hair is lubricated from the oil of sebaceous glands. Excessively oily hair is associated with androgen hormone stimulation. Dry, brittle hair occurs with aging and excessive use of chemical agents.

The amount of hair covering the extremities is sometimes reduced as a result of aging or a disease process such as arterial insufficiency most commonly over the lower extremities. In women, do not confuse a loss of hair with shaved legs.

Inspect the scalp for lesions, which are not easily noticed in thick hair. The scalp is normally smooth and inelastic with even coloration. Thoroughly examine the scalp for lesions by carefully separating strands of hair. Note the characteristics of any scalp lesions. If you find lumps or bruises, ask whether the patient has experienced recent head trauma. Moles on the scalp are common. Warn the patient that combing or brushing sometimes causes a mole to bleed. Dandruff or psoriasis frequently causes scaliness or dryness.

Careful inspection of hair follicles on the scalp and pubic areas may reveal lice or other parasites. There are head lice, body lice, and crab lice. Head and crab lice attach their eggs to hair. Lice eggs look like oval particles of dandruff. The lice themselves are difficult to see. Observe for bites or pustular eruptions in the follicles and areas where skin surfaces meet such as behind the ears and in the groin. The discovery of lice requires immediate treatment and family education (Box 7.7).

Nails

The condition of the nails reflects general health, state of nutrition, a person's occupation, and level of self-care. The most visible portion of the nails is the nail plate, the transparent layer of epithelial cells covering the nail bed. The vascularity of the nail bed creates the underlying color of the nail. The semilunar, whitish area at the base of the nail bed is called the *lunula,* from which the nail plate develops.

Nursing History

Ask the patient whether there have been any recent changes in the nails (e.g., splitting, breaking, or thickening) or recent

BOX 7.7 Patient Teaching

Hair and Scalp Assessment

Outcome

Patient performs proper hygiene practices for care of the hair and scalp.

Teaching Strategies

- Instruct in basic hygiene practices for care of the hair and scalp (see Chapter 16).
- Instruct patients who have head lice to shampoo thoroughly with pediculicide (shampoo available at drug stores) in cold water, comb thoroughly with fine-tooth comb (following product directions), and discard comb. Caution against the use of products containing lindane, a toxic ingredient known to cause adverse reactions. Repeat shampoo treatment 12–24 h later.
- After combing, remove any detachable nits or nit cases with tweezers or between the fingernails. A dilute solution of vinegar and water helps loosen nits.
- Instruct patients and parents about ways to reduce transmission of lice:
  - Do not share personal-care items with others.
  - Vacuum all rugs, car seats, pillows, furniture, and flooring thoroughly and discard vacuum bag.
  - Seal nonwashable items in plastic bags for 14 days if unable to dry-clean or vacuum.
  - Use thorough hand-hygiene practices.
  - Launder all clothing, linen, and bedding in hot soap and water and dry in a hot dryer for at least 20 min. Dry-clean nonwashable items.
  - Do not use insecticide.
  - Instruct the patient to notify partner if lice were sexually transmitted.
  - Avoid physical contact with individuals who are infested and their belongings, especially clothing and bedding.
  - Soak combs, brushes, and hair accessories in lice-killing products for 1 h or in boiling water for 10 min.

Evaluation

- Use the principles of teach back to evaluate patient/family caregiver learning:
  - "Describe for me the methods you use to care for your hair and scalp."
  - "Tell me the steps we discussed to reduce lice transmission."

trauma. Determine the patient's nail care practices such as use of acrylic nails or risk for exposure to fungi at nail salons. Determine any physiological risk factors for nail problems (e.g., diabetes mellitus, peripheral vascular disease, older age).

Inspect the nail bed color, cleanliness, and length; the thickness and shape of the nail; the texture of the nail; the angle between the nail and the nail bed; and the condition of tissue around the nail. The nails are normally transparent, smooth, well rounded, and convex, with surrounding cuticles smooth, intact, and without inflammation. In light-skinned patients, nail beds are pink with translucent white nail tips. In dark-skinned patients, nail beds are darkly pigmented, have a blue or reddish hue, and have yellow-tinged nail tips. A brown or black pigmentation is normal with longitudinal streaks. Trauma, cirrhosis, diabetes mellitus, and hypertension cause splinter hemorrhages. Vitamin, protein, and electrolyte changes cause various lines or bands to form on nail beds.

Nails normally grow at a constant rate, but direct injury or generalized disease impairs growth. With aging the nails of the fingers and toes become harder and thicker. Longitudinal striations develop, and the rate of nail growth slows. Nails become more brittle, dull, and opaque and turn yellow in older adults because of insufficient calcium. Also with age, the cuticle becomes less thick and wide.

Inspection of the angle between the nail and nail bed normally reveals an angle of 160° (Table 7.6). A larger angle and softening of the nail bed indicate clubbing resulting from chronic oxygenation problems.

Palpate the nail base to determine firmness and condition of circulation. It is normally firm. To palpate, gently grasp the patient's finger and observe its color. An ongoing bluish or purplish cast to the nail bed occurs with cyanosis. A white cast or pallor can result from anemia and/or liver disease. Observe for jaundice (yellow/orange), which can also indicate liver disease.

Calluses and corns often occur on the toes or fingers. A callus is flat and painless, resulting from thickening of the epidermis such as on the finger that supports a pencil or pen or on the bottom of the feet. Friction and pressure from shoes cause corns, usually over bony prominences. During the examination, instruct the patient in proper nail care (Box 7.8).

Table 7.6 Abnormalities of the Nail Bed

Illustration	Description
160°	**Normal nail:** Approximately 160° angle between nail plate and nail
180°; >180°	**Clubbing:** Change in angle between nail and nail base (eventually greater than 180°); nail bed softening with nail flattening; often enlargement of fingertips *Causes:* Chronic lack of oxygen: heart or pulmonary disease
	Beau lines: Transverse depressions in nails indicating temporary disturbance of nail growth (nail grows out over several months) *Causes:* Systemic illness such as severe infection; nail injury
	Koilonychia (spoon nail): Concave curves *Causes:* Iron-deficiency anemia, syphilis, use of strong detergents
	Splinter hemorrhages: Red or brown linear streaks in nail bed *Causes:* Minor trauma, subacute bacterial endocarditis, trichinosis
	Paronychia: Inflammation of skin at base of nail *Causes:* Local infection, trauma

Head and Neck

An examination of the head and neck includes assessment of the head, eyes, ears, nose, mouth, pharynx, and neck

BOX 7.8 Patient Teaching

Nail Assessment

Outcome

Patient properly cares for fingernails, feet, and toenails.

Teaching Strategies

- Instruct the patient to cut nails only after soaking them about 10 min in warm water. (Exception: Patients with diabetes are warned against soaking nails because this dries the hands and feet; dry skin leads to infection.)
- Caution the patient to avoid using over-the-counter preparations to treat corns, calluses, or ingrown toenails.
- Tell the patient to cut nails straight across and even with tops of fingers or toes. If the patient has diabetes, tell him or her to file rather than cut nails (see Chapter 16).
- Instruct the patient to shape nails with file or emery board.
- If the patient has diabetes (ADA, 2014):
  - Set a time to inspect feet each day in good lighting, looking for dry places and cracks in skin.
  - Wash feet daily in warm water and carefully dry them, especially between toes.
  - Soften dry feet. Rub a thin coat of skin lotion over the tops and bottoms of feet.
  - Do not put lotion between toes; moisture between toes promotes growth of microorganisms, leading to infection.
  - Caution patient against using sharp objects to poke or dig under toenail or around cuticle.
  - Wear shoes and socks and do not go barefoot.
  - Protect feet from extreme heat and cold.
  - Keep blood flowing to feet. Elevate feet when sitting, and wiggle toes and move ankles periodically. Do not cross legs for long periods of time.
  - Have the patient see a podiatrist for treatment of ingrown toenails and nails that are thick or tend to split.

Evaluation

- Use the principles of teach back to evaluate patient/family caregiver learning:
  - "Describe to me how you regularly check your nails for problems."
  - "List for me the steps you take to avoid injury to your fingernails, feet, and toenails."

(lymph nodes, carotid arteries, thyroid gland, and trachea). During assessment of peripheral arteries also assess the carotid arteries. Assessment of the head and neck uses inspection, palpation, and auscultation, with inspection and palpation often used simultaneously.

Head

Nursing History

Determine whether your patient has a recent history of head trauma or neurological symptoms such as headache, dizziness, seizures, poor vision, or loss of consciousness. Review the patient's occupation, participation in contact sports, and use of protective head gear.

Inspect the patient's head, noting the position, size, shape, and contour. The head is normally held upright and midline to the trunk. Holding the head tilted to one side is an indication of unilateral hearing or visual loss. A horizontal jerking or bobbing indicates a tremor.

Note facial features looking at the eyelids, eyebrows, nasolabial folds, and mouth for shape and symmetry. It is normal for slight asymmetry to exist. If there is facial asymmetry, note whether all features on one side of the face are affected or whether only part of the face is involved. Various neurological disorders such as a facial nerve paralysis affect different nerves that innervate muscles of the face.

Examine the size, shape, and contour of the skull. Generally, it is round with prominences in the frontal area anteriorly and the occipital area posteriorly. Trauma typically causes local skull deformities. Palpate the skull for nodules or masses. Gently rotate the fingertips down the midline of the scalp and then along the sides of the head to identify abnormalities.

In infants, a large head results from congenital anomalies or the accumulation of cerebrospinal fluid in the ventricles (hydrocephalus). Acromegaly causes an enlarged jaw and facial bones in affected adults.

Eyes

Examination of the eye includes assessment of visual acuity, visual fields, and external and internal eye structures. Fig. 7.7 shows a cross-section of the eye. The assessment detects visual alterations and determines the level of assistance that patients require when ambulating or performing self-care activities. Patients with visual problems need special aids for reading educational materials or instructions.

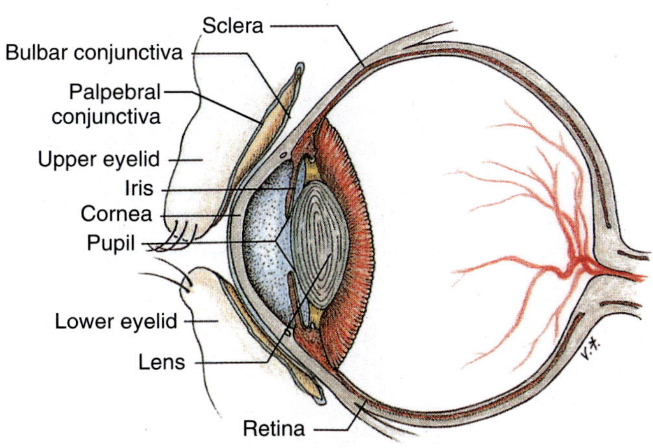

Fig. 7.7 Cross-section of eye.

Nursing History

Review with the patient any history of partial or complete vision loss from eye disease (e.g., glaucoma, cataracts), eye trauma, diabetes, hypertension, or eye surgery. Assess for common symptoms of eye disease such as eye pain, photophobia (sensitivity to light), burning, itching, excessive tearing, diplopia (double vision), blurred vision, or visual disturbances (e.g., flashing lights, halos, "film" over vision field). Review the patient's occupational history, use of glasses or contact lenses, use of safety glasses, and visits to an optometrist (Box 7.9). Determine the patient's current medication use including any eye medication.

Visual Acuity

The assessment of visual acuity (i.e., the ability to see small details) tests central vision. The easiest way to assess visual acuity is to ask the patient to read printed material or a Snellen chart under adequate lighting. Patients need to wear prescription glasses or contact lenses during the assessment. Identify the language the patient speaks and reading ability. Asking the patient to read aloud helps determine literacy. Position the patient 6 m (20 feet) away from the chart. Test each eye separately by covering one eye with a card or gauze square, avoiding pressure on the eye. A patient who has difficulty reading related to vision needs to consult an ophthalmologist or optometrist for further evaluation.

BOX 7.9 Patient Teaching

Eye Assessment

Outcome

Patient follows recommendations for preventive eye care, including regular eye care examinations and protection from injury.

Teaching Strategies

- Tell the patient that people younger than 40 years need to have a complete eye examination every 3–5 years (or more often if family histories reveal risks such as diabetes or hypertension).
- Teach the patients that people older than 40 years need to have a complete eye examination every 2 years to screen for conditions that may develop without patient awareness (e.g., glaucoma); this increases to annual examinations after 65 years of age.
- Describe the typical symptoms of eye disease (see Chapter 27).
- Instruct older adults to take the following precautions because of normal vision changes: avoid or use caution while driving at night, increase lighting in the home to reduce risk for falls, and paint the first and last steps of a staircase and the edge of each step in between a bright color to aid in depth perception.

Evaluation

- Use the principles of teach back to evaluate patient/family caregiver learning:
  - "Please describe to me when your most recent ophthalmologist visit was and what plans you have for future visits."
  - "Describe to me the common symptoms of eye disease that we discussed."
  - "Describe for me the safety measures for eye protection you take when working at home or with tools and equipment."

Visual Fields

Objects in the periphery can normally be seen when a person looks straight ahead. To assess visual fields, remove the patient's eyeglasses. Have the patient stand or sit 60 cm (2 feet) away facing you at eye level. He or she gently closes or covers one eye (e.g., the left) and looks at your eye directly opposite. Close the opposite eye as the field of vision is superimposed on that of the patient. Move a finger equidistant at arm's length from you and the patient outside the field of vision and then slowly bring it back into the visual field. Ask the patient to tell you when the finger is visible. If you see the finger before the patient does, this reveals that a portion of the patient's visual field is reduced.

External Eye Structures

To inspect external eye structures, stand directly in front of the patient at eye level and ask him or her to look at your face. Ask patients to remove glasses or contacts for the remainder of the examination.

Position and Alignment

Assess the position of the eyes in relation to one another. Normally, they are parallel to one another. Bulging eyes (exophthalmos) usually indicate hyperthyroidism. Crossed eyes (strabismus) result from neuromuscular injury or inherited abnormalities. A tumor or inflammation of the orbit may cause abnormal eye protrusion.

Eyebrows

Inspect the eyebrows for size, extension, texture of hair, alignment, and movement. Coarseness of hair and failure to extend beyond the temporal canthus may reveal hypothyroidism. If the brows are thinned, identify whether the patient plucks or waxes the hair. Aging causes loss of the lateral third of the eyebrows. Have the patient raise and lower the eyebrows. They normally raise and lower symmetrically. An inability to move them indicates a facial nerve (cranial nerve VII) paralysis.

Eyelids

Inspect the eyelids for position, color, condition, and direction of lashes; assess the patient's ability to open, close, and blink. When the eyes are open in a normal position, the lids do not cover the pupil, and you cannot see the sclera above the iris. The lids are also close to the eyeball. An abnormal drooping of the lid over the pupil is called *ptosis*, which is caused by edema or impairment of the cranial nerve III. In older adults, ptosis results from a loss of elasticity that accompanies aging. An older adult frequently has lid margins that turn out (ectropion) or in (entropion). An entropion sometimes leads to the lashes of the lid irritating the conjunctiva and cornea, increasing risk for infection. Normally, the eyelashes are distributed evenly and curved outward away from the eye.

The lids close symmetrically. Ask the patient to open the eyes, and observe the blink reflex, during which the cornea is lubricated. Normally, a patient blinks involuntarily and bilaterally up to 20 times a minute. Report absent, infrequent, rapid, or monocular (one-eyed) blinking. Failure of lids to close exposes the cornea to drying. This condition happens in unconscious patients or patients with facial nerve paralysis.

Lacrimal Apparatus

The lacrimal gland (Fig. 7.8), located in the upper, outer wall of the anterior part of the orbit, is responsible for tear production. Tears flow from the gland across the surface of the eye to the lacrimal duct, which is in the nasal corner or inner canthus of the eye. Inspect the lacrimal gland for edema and redness. Palpate the gland area gently to detect tenderness. Normally, the gland cannot be felt. The nasolacrimal duct may become obstructed, blocking the flow of tears. Observe for evidence of excess tearing or edema in the inner canthus. Gentle palpation of the duct at the lower eyelid just inside the orbital rim causes a regurgitation of tears.

Conjunctivae and Sclerae

The bulbar conjunctiva covers the exposed surface of the eyeball up to the outer edge of the cornea. Observe the sclera under the bulbar conjunctiva; it normally has the color of white porcelain in Caucasians and light yellow in dark-skinned patients. To view both structures, gently retract both lids simultaneously with thumb and index finger pressed against the lower and upper bony orbits. For adequate exposure, retract the eyelids without placing pressure directly on the eyeball. Ask the patient to look up, down, and side to side. Inspect for color, texture, and the presence of edema or lesions.

Normally, the conjunctivae are free of erythema. The presence of redness indicates traumatic, allergic, or infectious conjunctivitis. Conjunctivitis is a highly contagious infection, and the crusty drainage that collects on eyelid margins easily spreads from one eye to the other. Perform proper hand hygiene (see Chapter 9) before and after the examination. Wear clean gloves during the examination.

Corneas

The cornea is the transparent, colorless portion of the eye covering the pupil and iris. From a side view, it looks like the crystal of a wristwatch. While the patient looks straight ahead, inspect the cornea for clarity and texture while shining a penlight obliquely across its surface. Normally, the cornea is shiny, transparent, and smooth. In older adults, it loses its luster. Any irregularity in the surface indicates an abrasion or tear that requires further examination by a health care provider. Both conditions are very painful. To test for the corneal blink reflex, see the cranial nerve function section of this chapter.

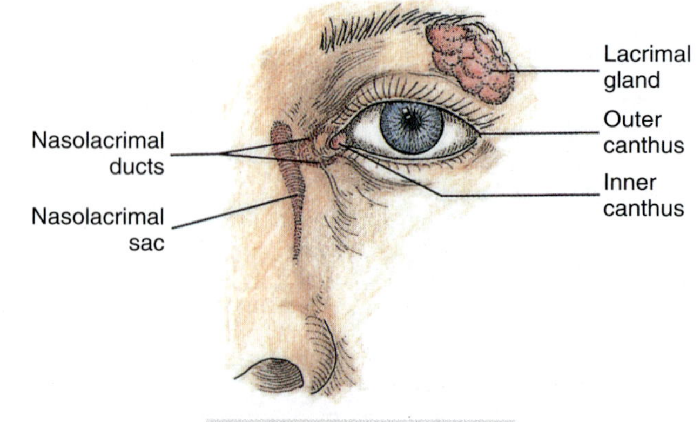

Fig. 7.8 Lacrimal apparatus.

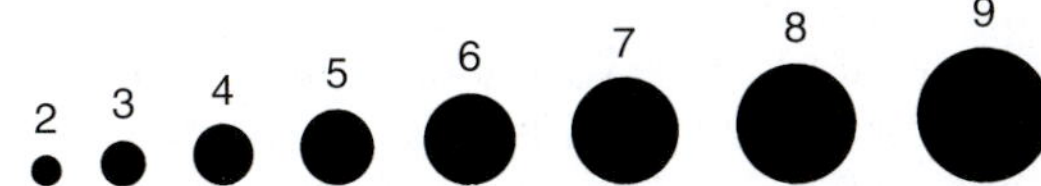

Fig. 7.9 Chart depicting pupillary size in millimeters.

Pupils and Irises

Observe the pupils for size, shape, equality, accommodation, and reaction to light. They are normally black, round, regular, and equal in size (2–6 mm in diameter) (Fig. 7.9). The iris should be clearly visible. Note the color and details of the iris. In an older adult, it becomes faded. A thin white ring along the margin of the iris, called an **arcus senilis,** is common with aging but abnormal in anyone younger than 40 years.

Cloudy pupils indicate cataracts. Continuous dilation of pupils results from neurological disorders, glaucoma, trauma, eye medication, or withdrawal from opioids. Pinpoint pupils are a common sign of opioid intoxication. When shining a beam of light through the pupil and onto the retina, the third cranial nerve is stimulated, causing the muscles of the iris to constrict. Any abnormality along the nerve pathways from the retina to the iris alters the ability of the pupils to react to light. Changes in intracranial pressure, lesions along the nerve pathways, locally applied ophthalmic medications, and direct trauma to the eye alter pupillary reaction.

Test pupillary reflexes (to light and accommodation) in a dimly lit room. Instruct the patient to look straight ahead, bring a penlight from the side of the patient's face, and direct the light onto the pupil (Fig. 7.10A and B). A directly illuminated pupil constricts, and the opposite pupil constricts consensually. Observe the quickness and equality of the reflex. Repeat the examination for the opposite eye.

To test accommodation, ask the patient to gaze at a distant object (the far wall) and then at a test object (finger or pencil) held approximately 10 cm (4 inches) from the bridge of the patient's nose. The pupils normally converge and accommodate by constricting when looking at close objects. The responses of the pupils are equal. If assessment of pupillary reaction is normal in all tests, record the abbreviation PERRLA (pupils equal, round, reactive to light, and accommodation).

Internal Eye Structures

An advanced nurse practitioner or other health care provider usually performs examination of the internal eye structures through the use of an ophthalmoscope.

Ears

The ear assessment determines the integrity of ear structures and hearing acuity. Inspect and palpate external ear structures, inspect middle ear structures with the otoscope, and test the inner ear by measuring the patient's hearing acuity. Assessment of patients with hearing impairment provides useful data in planning effective communication techniques.

Nursing History

Review risk factors for hearing problems with the patient (e.g., intake of aspirin or noise exposure) and assess for history of ear trauma or surgery. Determine whether the patient has ear pain, itching, discharge, tinnitus (ringing in ears), vertigo (loss of balance), or change in hearing. Note behavior that indicates hearing loss such as leaning forward to hear, inattentiveness to speech, and requests to repeat comments. Determine the onset and contributing factors to any hearing problem. Assess whether the patient wears a hearing aid and how he or she normally cleans it and the ears.

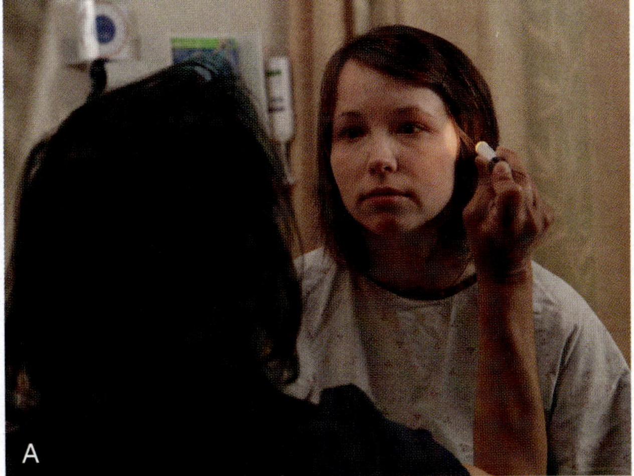

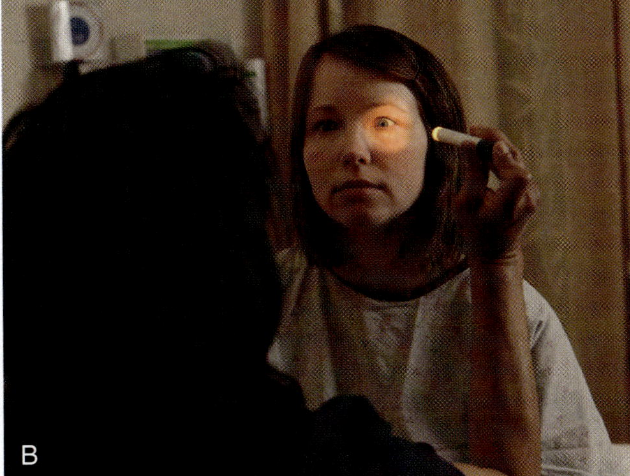

Fig. 7.10 A, To check pupillary reflexes, the nurse first holds the penlight to the side of the patient's face. **B,** Illumination of pupil causes pupillary constriction.

Auricles

With the patient sitting, inspect the size, shape, symmetry, flexibility, landmarks, position, and color of the auricle. The auricles are normally of equal size and level with one another. The upper point of attachment to the head is normally in a straight line with the outer canthus, or corner of the eye. Ears that are low set or at an unusual angle may indicate a chromosome abnormality or renal disorders. Ear color is the same as the face without moles, cysts, deformities, or nodules. Redness is a sign of inflammation or fever.

Palpate the auricles for texture, tenderness, swelling, and skin lesions. Auricles are normally smooth, firm, mobile, and without lesions. If the patient complains of pain, gently pull the auricle, press on the tragus, and palpate behind the ear over the mastoid process. If palpating the tragus increases the pain, an external ear canal infection is likely. If palpating the auricle and tragus does not influence the pain, the patient may have a middle ear infection. Tenderness in the mastoid area indicates mastoiditis.

Inspect the opening of the ear canal for size and presence of discharge. If discharge is present, wear clean gloves during the examination. A swollen or occluded meatus is not normal. A yellow, waxy substance called **cerumen** is common. Yellow or green foul-smelling discharge indicates infection or a foreign body in the canal. The color of cerumen is darker in dark-skinned patients.

Ear Canals and Eardrums

Observe the deeper structures of the external and middle ear with the use of an otoscope. A special ear speculum attaches to the handle of the ophthalmoscope. For best visualization, select the largest speculum that fits comfortably in the patient's ear. Before inserting it, check for foreign bodies in the opening of the auditory canal.

Make sure that the patient avoids moving the head during the examination to avoid damage to the canal and tympanic membrane. Hold the head of moving infants and young children. Lie infants supine with their heads turned to one side and their arms held securely at their sides or wrap them snugly in a blanket. Have young children sit on their parents' laps with their legs held between the parents' knees.

Turn on the otoscope by rotating the dial at the top of the handle. To insert the speculum properly, ask the patient to tip the head slightly to the opposite shoulder. Hold the handle of the otoscope in the space between the thumb and index finger, supported on the middle finger. This leaves the ulnar side of your hand to rest against the patient's head, stabilizing the otoscope as it is inserted into the canal (Ball et al., 2015). Insert the scope while pulling the auricle upward and backward in adults and older children (Fig. 7.11). This maneuver straightens the ear canal. In children younger than 3 years, pull the auricle down and back.

Insert the speculum slightly down and forward, 1–1.5 cm (1/4–3/4 inch) into the ear canal. Take care not to scrape the sensitive lining of the ear canal, which is painful. The ear canal normally has little cerumen and is uniformly colored with tiny hairs in the outer third of the canal. Observe for color, discharge, scaling, lesions, foreign bodies, and cerumen. Normally, cerumen is dry (light brown to gray and flaky) or moist (dark yellow or brown) and sticky. Dry cerumen occurs more often in Asians and Native Americans (Ball et al., 2015). A reddened canal with discharge is a sign of inflammation or infection. In older adults, accumulated cerumen is a common cause of mild hearing loss. During the examination, ask the patient how he or she normally cleans the ear canal (Box 7.10). Caution the patient on the danger of inserting pointed objects into the canal. Avoid the use of cotton-tipped applicators to clean the ears because this causes impaction of cerumen deep in the ear canal.

The light from the otoscope allows visualization of the eardrum (tympanic membrane). Know the common anatomical landmarks and their appearance (Fig. 7.12). Move the auricle to see the entire drum and its periphery. Because the eardrum is angled away from the ear canal, the light from the otoscope appears as a cone shape rather than a circle. The umbo is near the center of the drum, behind

BOX 7.10 Patient Teaching

Ear Assessment

Outcome

Patient follows preventive guidelines for screening hearing loss of voice and environmental sounds.

Teaching Strategies

- Encourage the patients older than 65 years or with noticeable change in hearing to have regular hearing checks. Explain that a reduction in hearing is a normal part of aging (see Chapter 27).
- Instruct family members of patients with hearing losses to avoid shouting, speaking instead with low tones while directly facing the patient.

Evaluation

- Use the principles of teach back to evaluate patient/family caregiver learning:
- "Tell me how often you have your hearing checked."
- "Explain how you adjust with your hearing loss when you interact with family members."

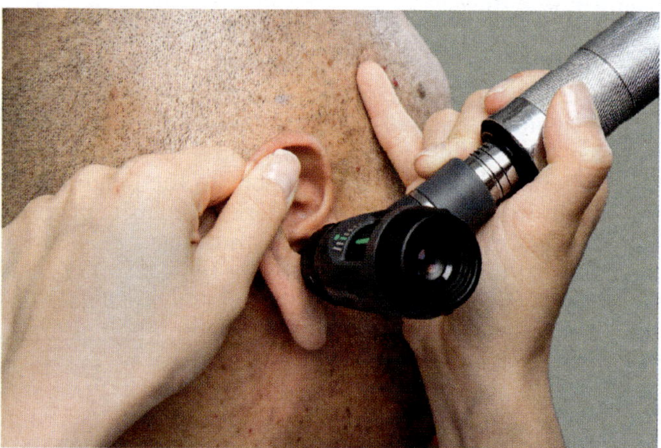

Fig. 7.11 Otoscopic examination. (From Wilson S, Gidden J: *Health assessment for nursing practice*, ed 6, St Louis, 2016, Elsevier.)

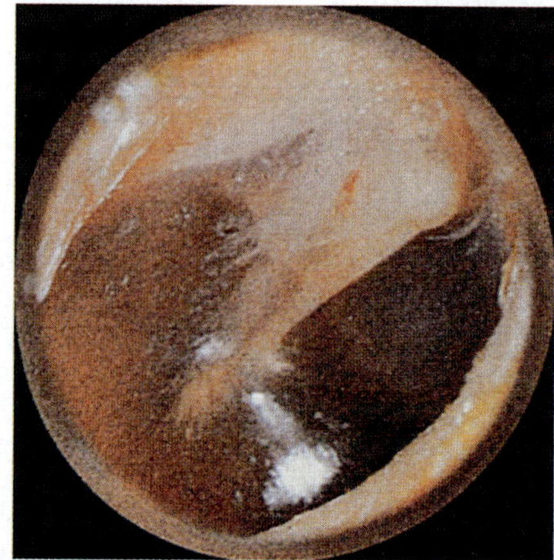

Fig. 7.12 Normal tympanic membrane. (Courtesy Dr. Richard A. Buckingham, Abraham Lincoln School of Medicine, University of Illinois, Chicago.)

which is the attachment of the malleus. The underlying short process of the malleus creates a knoblike structure at the top of the drum. Check carefully to be sure that there are no tears or breaks in the membrane of the eardrum. The normal eardrum is taut, translucent, shiny, and pearly gray. It is free from tears or breaks. A pink or red bulging membrane indicates inflammation. A white color reveals pus behind it. If cerumen is blocking the tympanic membrane, warm water irrigation safely removes the wax.

Hearing Acuity

A patient with hearing loss often fails to respond to conversation. The three types of hearing loss are conduction, sensorineural, and mixed. A conduction loss interrupts sound waves as they travel from the outer ear to the cochlea of the inner ear because they are not transmitted through the outer and middle ear structures. A sensorineural loss involves the inner ear, auditory nerve, or hearing center of the brain. In this instance, sound is conducted through the outer and middle ear structures, but the continued transmission of sound becomes interrupted at some point beyond the bony ossicles. A mixed loss involves a combination of conduction and sensorineural loss.

Patients working or living around loud noises are at risk for hearing loss. Adolescents are at risk for premature hearing loss from continued exposure to loud music through earbuds connected to electronic music devices or loud concerts. Deterioration of the cochlea and thickening of the tympanic membrane cause older adults to gradually lose hearing acuity. Older adults experience an inability to hear high-frequency sounds and consonants (e.g., *s, z, t, g*). Hearing loss can be caused by ototoxicity resulting from high maintenance doses of antibiotics (e.g., aminoglycosides).

To conduct a hearing assessment, have the patient remove any hearing aid, if worn. Note the patient's response to questions. Normally, the patient responds without excess requests to have the questions repeated. If you suspect a hearing loss, check the patient's response to the whispered voice. Test one ear at a time while the patient occludes the other ear with a finger. Ask the patient to gently move the finger up and down during the test. While standing 30–60 cm (1–2 feet) from the testing ear, cover your mouth so the patient is unable to read lips. After exhaling fully, whisper softly toward the nonoccluded ear, reciting random numbers with equally accented syllables such as *nine-four-ten*. Ask the patient to repeat what was heard. If necessary, gradually increase voice intensity until the patient repeats the numbers correctly. Then test the other ear for comparison. If a hearing loss is present, further testing should be recommended with experienced practitioners using a tuning fork or audiometry.

Nose and Sinuses

Assess the integrity of the nose and sinuses by inspection and palpation. The patient sits during the examination. A penlight allows for gross examination of each naris. A more detailed examination requires using a nasal speculum to inspect deeper nasal turbinates. Do not use a speculum unless a qualified practitioner is present.

Nursing History

Determine whether the patient has a history of exposure to dust or pollutants, allergies, nasal obstruction, recent nasal trauma or discharge, frequent infections, headaches, or postnasal drip. Assess for a history of nosebleed (epistaxis) or use of nasal sprays, including frequency and duration (Box 7.11). Ask about breathing difficulties or snoring.

Nose

When inspecting the external nose, observe the shape, size, skin color, and presence of deformity or inflammation. The nose is normally smooth and symmetrical and is the same color as the face (Fig. 7.13). Recent trauma causes edema and discoloration. If swelling or deformities exist, gently palpate the ridge and soft tissue of the nose by placing one finger on each side of the nasal arch and gently moving

BOX 7.11 Patient Teaching

Nose and Sinus Assessment

Outcome

Patient follows good preventive practices to ensure against injury to olfactory organs, or maintenance of safety when there is decreased olfaction.

Teaching Strategies

- Caution patients against overuse of over-the-counter nasal sprays, which can injure nasal olfactory organs.
- Instruct older adults to install smoke detectors on each floor of their home.
- Instruct older adults to always check dated labels on food to ensure against spoilage.

Evaluation

- Use the principles of teach back to evaluate patient/family caregiver learning:
  - "I want you to show me how to use your over-the-counter nasal spray."
  - "Describe the safety practices you use in your home."
  - "Show me how you check whether the foods in your refrigerator are safe to eat."

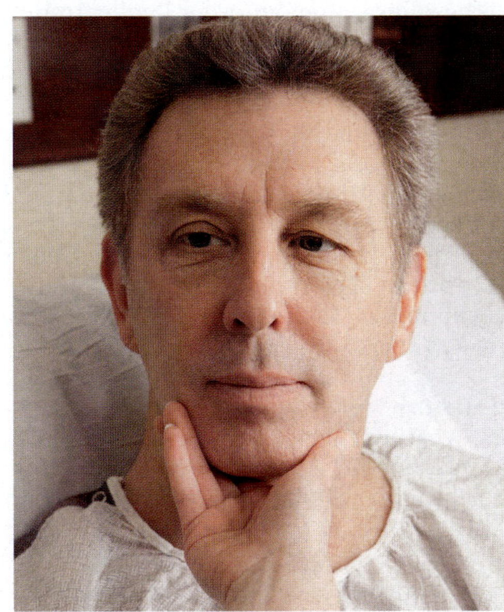

Fig. 7.13 Inspection of nose and facial features for symmetry.

fingers from the nasal bridge to the tip. Note any tenderness, masses, and underlying deviations. Nasal structures are usually firm and stable.

When a person breathes, air normally passes freely and noiselessly through the nose. To assess patency of the nares, place a finger on the side of the patient's nose and occlude one naris. Ask the patient to breathe with the mouth closed. Repeat the procedure for the other naris.

While illuminating the anterior nares, inspect the mucosa for color, lesions, discharge, swelling, and evidence of bleeding. If discharge is present, apply clean gloves. Normal mucosa is pink and moist without lesions. Pale mucosa with clear discharge indicates allergy. A mucoid discharge indicates rhinitis. A sinus infection results in yellowish or greenish discharge. Habitual use of intranasal cocaine and opioids causes puffiness and increased vascularity of the nasal mucosa. For a patient with a nasogastric tube, check for local skin breakdown (excoriation) of the naris, characterized by redness and skin sloughing.

To view the septum and turbinates, have the patient tip the head back slightly to provide a clear view. Illuminate the septum and look for alignment, perforation, or bleeding. Normally, it is close to the midline and thicker anteriorly than posteriorly. Normal mucosa is pink and moist without lesions. A deviated septum obstructs breathing and interferes with passage of an enteral nasal tube. Perforation of the septum often occurs after repeated use of intranasal cocaine. Note any polyps (tumorlike growths) or purulent drainage.

Sinuses

Examination of the sinuses involves palpation. In cases of allergies or infection, the interior of the sinuses becomes inflamed and swollen. The most effective way to assess for tenderness is by externally palpating the frontal and maxillary facial areas. Palpate the frontal sinus by exerting pressure with the thumb up and under the patient's eyebrow. Gentle, upward pressure easily elicits tenderness if sinus irritation is present. Do not apply pressure to the eyes. If tenderness of sinuses is present, ask a nurse or health care provider with advanced experience to transilluminate the sinuses to monitor for fluid within the sinus cavity.

Mouth and Pharynx

Assess the mouth and pharynx to detect signs of overall health; determine oral hygiene needs; and develop therapies for patients with dehydration, restricted intake, oral trauma, or oral airway obstruction. To assess the oral cavity, use a penlight and tongue depressor or single gauze square. Wear clean gloves and have the patient sit or lie during the examination. Assess the oral cavity while administering oral hygiene.

Nursing History

Determine whether the patient wears dentures or retainers and how they fit. Assess for any recent changes in appetite or weight, which indicate problems with chewing and swallowing. Assess the patient's dental hygiene practices. To identify cancer risks, determine whether the patient smokes, chews tobacco, or consumes alcohol. Identify whether he or she still has his or her tonsils and adenoids.

Lips

Inspect the lips for color, texture, hydration, contour, and lesions. With the patient's mouth closed, view the lips from end to end. Normally, they are pink, moist, symmetrical, smooth, and without lesions. Lip color in dark-skinned patients varies from pink to plum. Have female patients remove their lipstick before the examination. Anemia causes pallor of the lips, with cyanosis caused by respiratory or cardiovascular problems. Any lesions such as nodules or ulcerations can be related to infection, irritation, or skin cancer.

Buccal Mucosa, Gums, and Teeth

Ask the patient to clench the teeth and smile to observe teeth occlusion. The upper molars normally rest directly on the lower molars, and the upper incisors slightly override the lower incisors. Assess for symmetry.

Inspect the teeth to determine the quality of a patient's dental hygiene (Box 7.12). Note the position and alignment of the teeth. To examine the posterior surface of the teeth, have the patient open the mouth with lips relaxed. Use a tongue depressor to retract the lips and cheeks, especially when viewing the molars. Note the color of teeth and the presence of dental caries, tartar, and extraction sites. Normal healthy teeth are smooth, white, and shiny. A chalky white discoloration of the enamel is an early sign of caries formation. Brown or black discolorations indicate the formation of caries. An older adult's teeth often feel rough when tooth enamel calcifies, and there may be loose or missing teeth because of increased bone resorption. Yellow and darkened teeth are also common in older adults because of general wear and tear that exposes the darker, underlying dentin.

BOX 7.12 Patient Teaching

Mouth and Pharyngeal Assessment

Outcome

Patient follows good preventive practices to ensure oral and dental health.

Teaching Strategies

- Discuss proper techniques for oral hygiene, including brushing and flossing (see Chapter 16).
- Explain the early warning signs of oral cavity and pharynx cancer, including a sore that bleeds easily and does not heel, a lump or thickening in the throat, red or white patch on the mucosa that persists, ear pain, a neck mass, and coughing up blood. Difficulty chewing, swallowing, and moving the tongue or jaw are late symptoms (ACS, 2016a).
- Encourage regular dental examinations every 6 months for children, adults, and older adults.
- Identify older patients who have difficulty chewing and changes in the teeth. Teach patients to eat soft foods; cut food into small pieces; and eat more frequent, smaller meals.

Evaluation

- Use the principles of teach back to evaluate patient/family caregiver learning:
  - "Show me the proper way to brush your teeth."
  - "Explain to me how often you should visit your dentist each year."
  - "Describe to me the warning signs of oral and throat cancer."

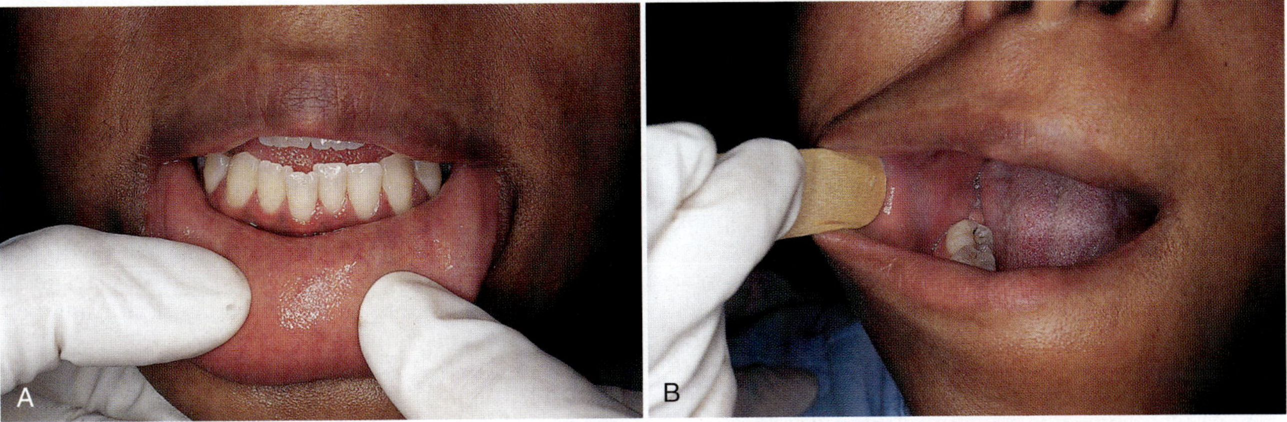

Fig. 7.14 **A,** Inspection of inner oral mucosa of lower lip. **B,** Retraction of buccal mucosa allows for clear visualization.

To view the inner oral mucosa, ask the patient to remove any dental appliance. View the inner oral mucosa by having the patient open the mouth slightly and gently pull the lower lip away from the teeth (Fig. 7.14A). Repeat this process for the upper lip. Inspect the mucosa for color; hydration; texture; and lesions such as ulcers, abrasions, or cysts. Normally, the mucosa is glistening pink, smooth, and moist. Palpate any lesions with a gloved hand for tenderness, size, and consistency.

To inspect the buccal mucosa, ask the patient to open the mouth, and gently retract the cheeks with a tongue depressor or gloved finger covered with gauze (Fig. 7.14B). View the surface of the mucosa from right to left and top to bottom. A penlight illuminates the most posterior portion of the mucosa. For patients with normal pigmentation, the buccal mucosa is a good site to inspect for jaundice and pallor. In older adults, it is normally dry because of reduced salivation. Thick white patches (leukoplakia) are often precancerous lesions seen in heavy smokers and alcoholics. Palpate for any buccal lesions by placing the gloved index finger within the buccal cavity and the thumb on the outer surface of the cheek.

Examine the gums (gingivae) for color, edema, retraction, bleeding, and lesions while retracting the cheeks. Healthy gums are pink, moist, and smooth and fit tightly around each tooth. Dark-skinned patients often have patchy pigmentation. In older adults, the gums are usually pale. With clean gloves, palpate the gums to assess for lesions, thickening, or masses. Normally, there is no tenderness. Spongy gums that bleed easily indicate periodontal disease or vitamin C deficiency.

Tongue and Floor of Mouth

Carefully inspect the tongue on all sides and the floor of the mouth. Have the patient relax the mouth and stick the tongue out halfway. The gag reflex is elicited if the patient protrudes the tongue too far. Using the penlight, examine the tongue for color, size, position, texture, movement, and coating or lesions. A normal tongue appears medium or dull red in color, moist, slightly rough on the top surface, and smooth along the lateral margins. When the tongue protrudes, it remains at midline. To test the tongue for mobility, ask the patient to raise it and move it from side to side. It should move freely.

The undersurface of the tongue and floor of the mouth are highly vascular. Take extra care to inspect this area, a common site of origin for oral cancer lesions. The patient lifts the tongue by placing its tip on the palate behind the upper incisors. Inspect for color, swelling, and lesions such as cysts. The ventral surface of the tongue is pink and smooth, with large veins between the frenulum folds.

Palate

Have the patient extend the head backward, holding the mouth open to allow you to inspect the hard and soft palates. The hard palate, or roof of the mouth, is located anteriorly. The whitish hard palate is dome shaped. The soft palate extends posteriorly toward the pharynx. It is normally light pink and smooth. Observe the palates for color, shape, texture, and extra bony prominences or defects.

Pharynx

Perform an examination of the pharyngeal structures to rule out infection, inflammation, or lesions. Have the patient tip the head back slightly, open the mouth wide, and say "Ah" while the tip of a tongue depressor is placed on the middle third of the tongue. Take care not to press the lower lip against the teeth (Fig. 7.15). By placing the tongue depressor too far anteriorly, the posterior part of

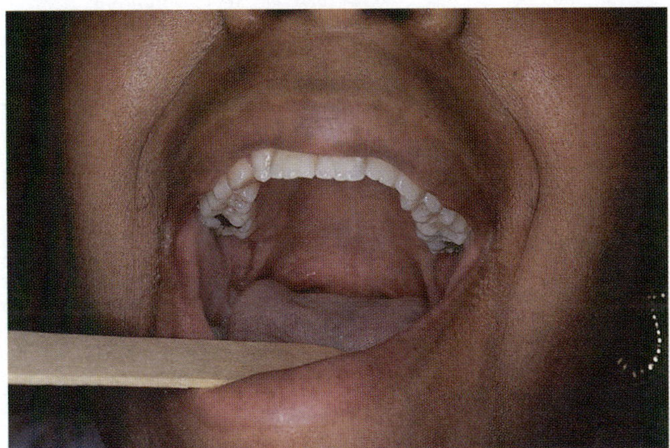

Fig. 7.15 Penlight and tongue depressor allow visualization of uvula and posterior soft palate.

the tongue mounds up, obstructing the view. Placing the tongue depressor on the posterior tongue elicits the gag reflex.

With a penlight, first inspect the uvula and soft palate. Both structures, which are innervated by the cranial nerve X (vagus), rise centrally as the patient says "Ah." Examine the anterior and posterior tonsillar pillars and note the presence or absence of tonsillar tissue. The posterior pharynx is behind the pillars. Normally, pharyngeal structures are smooth, pink, and well hydrated. Small irregular spots of lymphatic tissue and small blood vessels are normal. Note edema, petechiae, lesions, or exudate. Patients with chronic sinus problems frequently exhibit a clear exudate that drains along the wall of the posterior pharynx. Yellow or green exudate indicates infection. A patient with a typical sore throat has a reddened and edematous uvula and tonsillar pillars with possible presence of yellow exudate.

Neck

Assessment of the neck includes assessing the neck muscles, lymph nodes of the head and neck, carotid arteries, jugular veins, thyroid gland, and trachea (Fig. 7.16). Examination of the carotid arteries and jugular veins is addressed as part of the vascular system assessment. Inspect and palpate the neck to determine the integrity of neck structures, and examine the lymphatic system. An abnormality of superficial lymph nodes sometimes reveals the presence of infection or malignancy. Examination of the thyroid gland and trachea also helps to rule out malignancies. Perform this examination with the patient sitting.

Nursing History

Determine whether the patient has a history of a recent cold or infection, enlarged lymph nodes, or exposure to radiation or toxic chemicals. If there is a history of enlarged lymph nodes, inquire about any past history of i.v. drug use, hemophilia, and risk factors for human immunodeficiency virus (HIV) infection. Learn whether the patient takes thyroid medication for a history of hypothyroidism or hyperthyroidism; ask about a family history of thyroid disease. Ask the patient to describe any head or neck injury or pain of head and neck structures.

Neck Muscles

First inspect the gross neck structures with the neck in the usual anatomical position. Observe for symmetry of neck muscles. Ask the patient to flex the neck with the chin to the chest, hyperextend the neck backward, and move the head laterally to each side and then sideways with the ear moving toward the shoulder. This tests the sternocleidomastoid and trapezius muscles. The neck normally moves freely without discomfort.

Lymph Nodes

An extensive system of lymph nodes collects lymph from the head, ears, nose, cheeks, and lips (Fig. 7.17). With the patient's chin raised and head tilted slightly back, first inspect the area where lymph nodes are distributed and compare both sides. This position stretches the skin slightly over any possible enlarged nodes. Inspect visible nodes for edema, erythema, or red streaks. Nodes are not normally visible.

Use a methodical approach to palpate the lymph nodes to avoid overlooking any single node or chain. The patient relaxes with the neck flexed slightly forward. Inspect and palpate both sides of the neck for comparison. During palpation, either face or stand to the side of the patient for easy access to all nodes. Using the pads of the middle three fingers of each hand, gently palpate in a rotary motion over the nodes. Check each node methodically in the following sequence: occipital nodes at the base of the skull, postauricular nodes over the mastoid, preauricular nodes just in front of the ear, retropharyngeal nodes at the angle of the mandible, submandibular nodes, and submental nodes in the midline behind the mandibular tip. Try to detect enlargement and note the location, size, shape, surface characteristics, consistency, mobility, tenderness, and warmth of the nodes. If the skin is mobile, move it over the area of the nodes (Fig. 7.18). It is important to press underlying tissue in each area and not simply move the fingers over the skin.

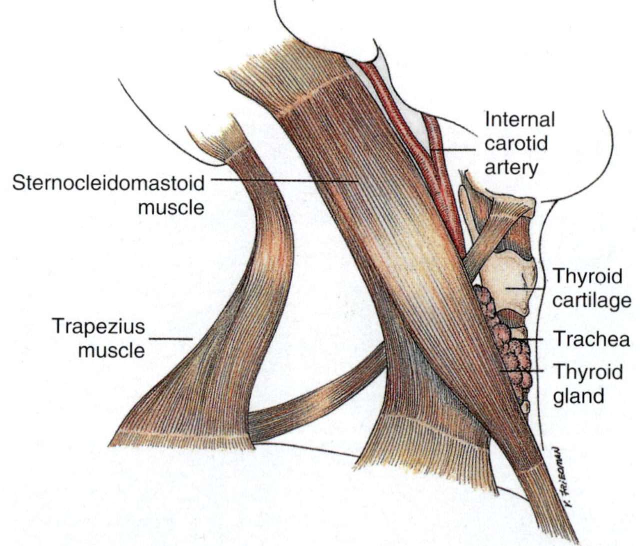

Fig. 7.16 Anatomical position of major neck structures. Note triangles formed by muscles.

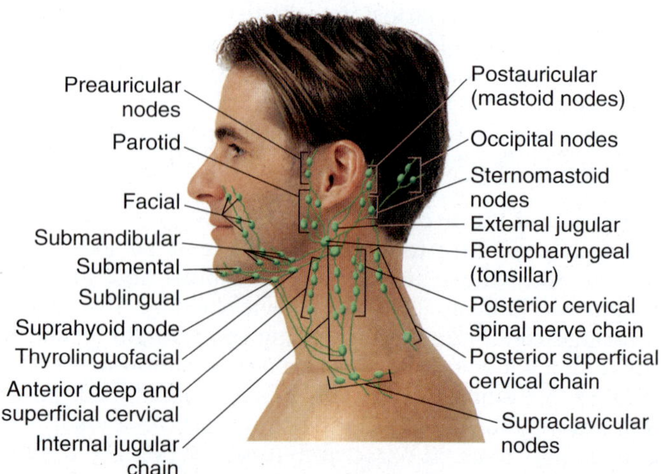

Fig. 7.17 Palpable lymph nodes in head and neck. (From Ball JW, et al: *Seidel's guide to physical examination*, ed 8, St Louis, 2015, Elsevier.)

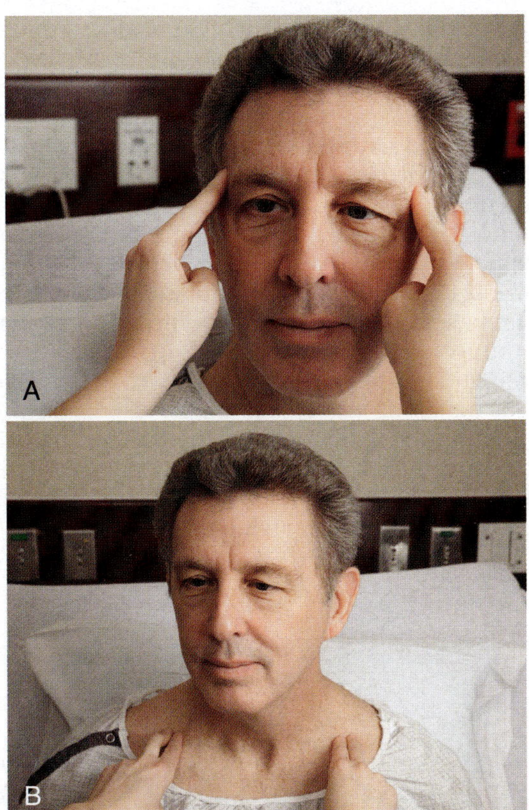

Fig. 7.18 A, Palpation of preauricular lymph nodes. **B,** Palpation for supraclavicular lymph nodes.

To palpate supraclavicular nodes, ask the patient to bend the head forward and relax the shoulders. Palpate these nodes by hooking the index and third finger over the clavicle, lateral to the sternocleidomastoid muscle. Palpate the deep cervical nodes only with the fingers hooked around the sternocleidomastoid muscle.

Normally, lymph nodes are not easily palpable. Lymph nodes that are large, fixed, inflamed, or tender indicate a problem such as local infection, systemic disease, or neoplasm (Ball et al., 2015). Tenderness almost always indicates inflammation (Box 7.13). A problem involving a lymph node of the head and neck means an abnormality in the mouth, throat, abdomen, breasts, thorax, or arms. These are the areas drained by the head and neck nodes.

Thyroid Gland

The thyroid gland lies in the anterior lower neck, in front of and to both sides of the trachea. The gland is fixed to the trachea with the isthmus overlying the trachea and connecting the two irregular, cone-shaped lobes (Fig. 7.19). Inspect the lower neck overlying the thyroid gland for obvious masses, symmetry, and any subtle fullness at the base of the neck. Give the patient a glass of water and observe the neck as the patient swallows. This maneuver helps to visualize an abnormally enlarged thyroid gland. More experienced nurses examine the thyroid by palpating for more subtle masses.

Carotid Artery and Jugular Vein

Examination of these vessels is discussed under examination of the vascular system.

BOX 7.13 Patient Teaching

Neck Assessment

Outcome

Patient takes proper preventive action if a mass is noticed in the neck.

Teaching Strategies

- Stress the importance of regular compliance with medication schedule to patients with thyroid disease.
- Instruct patients about the lymph nodes and how infection commonly causes node tenderness.
- Instruct patients to call a health care provider when they notice a lump or mass in the neck.

Evaluation

- Use the principles of teach back to evaluate patient/family caregiver learning:
  - "Explain to me when you would notify your health care provider about a neck mass."

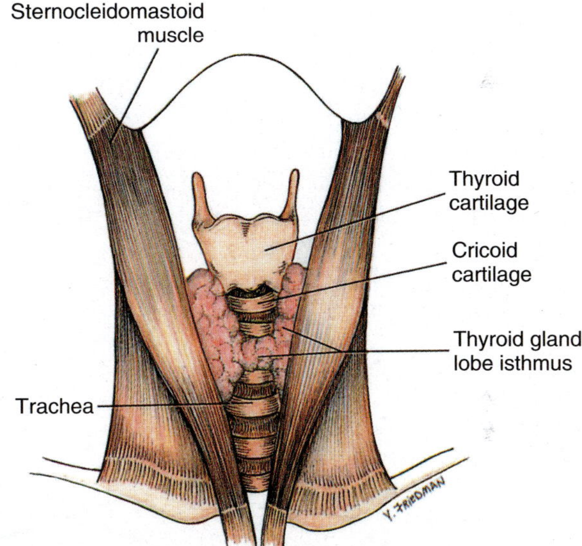

Fig. 7.19 Anatomical position of the thyroid gland.

Trachea

The trachea is a part of the upper respiratory system that requires direct palpation. It is normally located in the midline above the suprasternal notch. Masses in the neck or mediastinum and pulmonary abnormalities cause lateral displacement. Have the patient sit or lie down during palpation. Determine the position of the trachea by palpating at the suprasternal notch, slipping the thumb and index fingers to each side. Note whether your finger and thumb shift laterally. Do not apply forceful pressure to the trachea because this elicits coughing.

Thorax and Lungs

Physical assessment of the thorax and lungs requires an in-depth review of the ventilatory and respiratory functions of the lungs. If disease is affecting the lungs, it affects other body systems as well. For example, reduced oxygenation causes changes in mental alertness because of the sensitivity of the brain to lowered oxygen levels. Use data from all body systems to determine the nature of pulmonary alterations.

Before assessing the thorax and lungs, be familiar with the landmarks of the chest (Fig. 7.20). These landmarks help you locate findings and use assessment skills correctly. The patient's suprasternal notch, manubrium, costal angle, clavicles, angle of Louis, and vertebrae are key landmarks that provide a series of imaginary lines for identification of signs and symptoms. Keep a mental image of the location of the lobes of the lung and the position of each rib (Fig. 7.21A). The proper orientation to anatomical structures ensures a thorough assessment of the anterior, lateral, and posterior thorax.

Locating the position of each rib is critical to visualizing the lobe of the lung being assessed. To begin, locate the angle of Louis at the junction between the manubrium and the body of the sternum. Knowing that the second rib extends from the angle makes it easy to locate and palpate the **intercostal spaces** (between the ribs) in succession. The spinous process of the third thoracic vertebra and the fourth, fifth, and sixth ribs serves to locate the lobes of the lung laterally (Fig. 7.21B). The lower lobes project laterally and anteriorly.

Posteriorly the tip or inferior margin of the scapula lies approximately at the level of the seventh rib. Identify the seventh rib, count upward to locate the third thoracic vertebra, and align it with the inner borders of the scapula to locate the posterior lobes (Fig. 7.21C).

Examination of the lungs and thorax is most effective when the patient is undressed to the waist. Begin with the patient sitting for assessment of the posterior and lateral chest and sitting or lying down for examination of the anterior chest. Have a female patient keep a gown draped loosely over her chest while you examine the posterior chest.

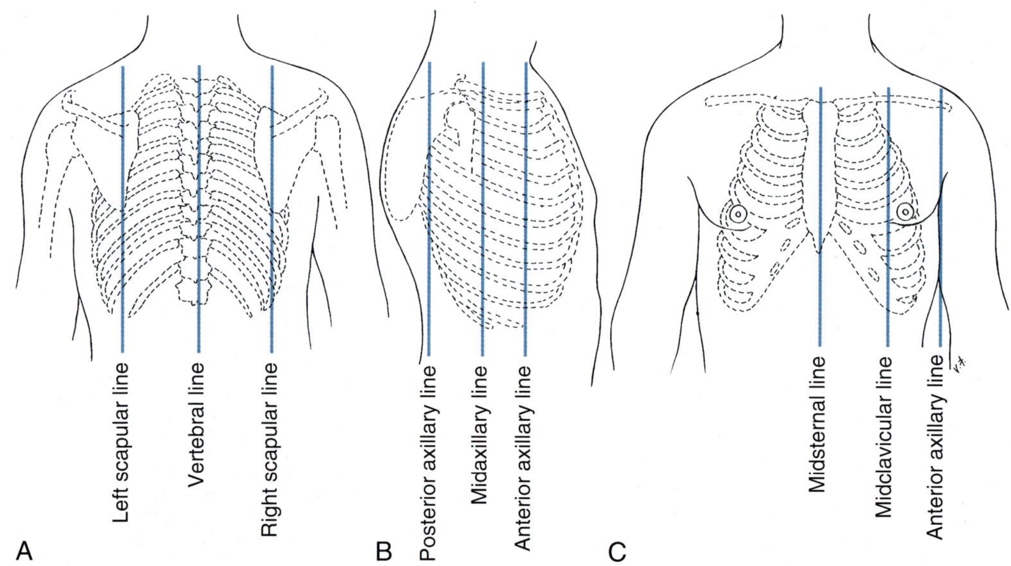

Fig. 7.20 Anatomical chest wall landmarks. **A,** Posterior chest. **B,** Lateral chest. **C,** Anterior chest.

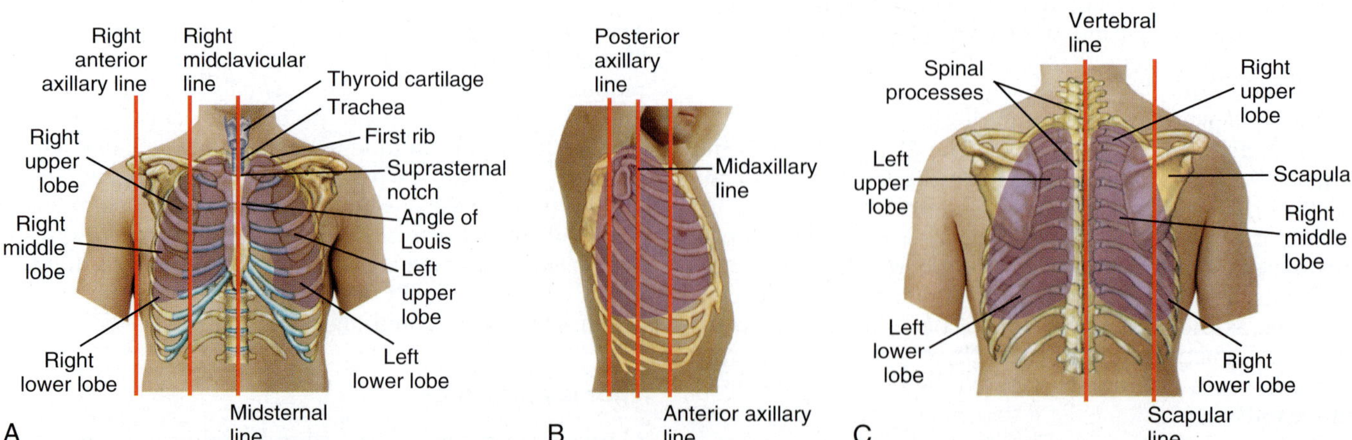

Fig 7.21 A, Anterior position of lung lobes in relation to anatomical landmarks. **B,** Lateral position of lung lobes in relation to anatomical landmarks. **C,** Posterior position of lung lobes in relation to anatomical landmarks. (From Ball JW, et al: *Seidel's guide to physical examination,* ed 8, St Louis, 2015, Elsevier.)

Nursing History

First interview the patient for any recent problems of increased work of breathing. Ask the patient about *persistent cough* (productive or nonproductive), *blood-streaked sputum, voice change, chest pain,* shortness of breath, **orthopnea** (must be in upright position to breathe), **dyspnea** (breathlessness) during exertion or at rest, poor activity tolerance, or *recurrent pneumonia* or *bronchitis*. These reveal cardiopulmonary problems or warning signs for lung cancer (symptoms in italics). Assess for a history of tobacco or marijuana use, including type of tobacco, duration and amount (pack-years = number of years smoking × number of packs per day), age started, efforts to quit, and length of time since smoking stopped. Determine whether your patient works in an environment containing pollutants (e.g., asbestos, coal dust), is exposed to radiation, or resides in an area with high levels of particulate air contaminants. Teach the patient about warning signs of lung disease (Box 7.14).

Review risk factors for tuberculosis (TB) and/or HIV infection, and assess for symptoms including persistent cough, hemoptysis, unexplained weight loss, fatigue, anorexia, night sweats, and fever. Assess history of allergies to airborne irritants, foods, drugs, or chemical substances. Ask whether the patient has had pneumonia or influenza vaccine and a TB test. Review the patient's family history for cancer, TB, allergies, or chronic obstructive pulmonary disease.

Posterior Thorax

Begin examination of the posterior thorax by observing for any signs or symptoms in other body systems that indicate pulmonary problems. Reduced mental alertness, nasal flaring, somnolence (sleepiness), and cyanosis are examples of symptoms or findings that indicate oxygenation problems. Inspect the posterior thorax by observing the shape and symmetry of the chest from the patient's back and sides. Pay close attention to the position of the scapula bilaterally. Note the anteroposterior (AP) diameter. Body shape or posture significantly affects ventilatory movement. Normally the chest contour is symmetrical, with the AP diameter 1/3 to 1/2 the size of the transverse or side-to-side diameter. Infants have an almost round shape with a 1:1 ratio between the AP and transverse diameters. In adults, a barrel-shaped chest (AP diameter = transverse) characterizes chronic lung disease. A more rounded chest is also associated with older age. Congenital and postural alterations cause abnormal contours. Patients with breathing problems may lean over a table or splint the side of the chest. Splinting or holding the chest wall because of pain causes a patient to bend toward the affected side, which impairs ventilatory movement.

With the patient sitting or standing, position yourself at a midline position behind the patient, and look for deformities, position of the spine, slope of the ribs, retraction of the intercostal spaces during inspiration, and bulging of the intercostal spaces during expiration. The scapulae are normally symmetrical and closely attached to the thoracic wall. The normal spine is straight without lateral deviation. Posteriorly, the ribs tend to slope across and down. The ribs and intercostal spaces are easier to see in a thin person. Normally, no bulging or active movement occurs within the intercostal spaces during breathing. Bulging or retraction indicates that the patient is using great effort to breathe.

Also assess the rate and rhythm of breathing at this time (see Chapter 6). Observe the thorax as a whole. It normally expands and relaxes with equality (symmetry) of movement bilaterally. In healthy adults, the normal respiratory rate varies from 12 to 20 respirations/min.

Palpate the posterior thorax beginning with the thoracic muscles and skeleton for lumps, masses, pulsations, and unusual movement. Use caution if you note pain or tenderness. Fractured rib fragments could be displaced against vital organs. If you find a suspicious mass or swollen area, lightly palpate it for size, shape, and typical qualities of a lesion.

BOX 7.14 Patient Teaching

Lung Assessment

Outcome

Patient follows recommendations that improve and protect pulmonary health.

Teaching Strategies

- Explain risk factors for chronic lung disease and lung cancer, including cigarette smoking (most important factor); history of smoking for more than 20 years; exposure to environmental pollution; and radiation exposure from occupational, medical, and environmental sources. Exposure to residential radon and asbestos also increases risk, especially for cigarette smokers. Other risk factors include certain metals (arsenic, cadmium), some organic chemicals, and personal history of tuberculosis. Genetics plays a role as well, especially in patients who develop disease at a young age (ACS, 2016a).
- Share brochures on lung cancer from the American Cancer Society with patient and family caregiver before discharge from the hospital.
- Discuss with patient the warning signs of lung cancer such as a persistent cough, blood-streaked sputum, chest pains, and recurrent attacks of pneumonia or bronchitis.
- Counsel patients on the benefits of receiving appropriate vaccines. Pneumonia vaccines are recommended for all adults 65 years of age or older, and for adults 19–64 years of age who smoke (CDC, 2016). Annual influenza vaccinations are recommended for all individuals 6 months of age and older (Grohskopf et al., 2016).
- Instruct patients with chronic obstructive pulmonary disease (COPD) or other respiratory illnesses in coughing and pursed-lip breathing exercises (see Chapter 24).
- Refer people at risk for tuberculosis for skin testing.

Evaluation

- Use the principles of teach back to evaluate patient/family caregiver learning:
  - "Describe for me the risk factors for lung disease and lung cancer and tell me which risk factors that you have."
  - "List for me the warning signs for lung cancer."
  - "Tell me how often you should have a vaccination for the flu and for pneumonia. Tell me when you were last tested for tuberculosis."
  - "Show me how to do the breathing and coughing exercises that we reviewed."

To measure chest excursion or depth of breathing, stand behind the patient and place the thumbs along the spinal processes at the 10th rib, with the palms lightly contacting the posterior lateral surfaces. Place thumbs about 5 cm (2 inches) apart pointing toward the spine and fingers pointing laterally (Fig. 7.22). Press the hands toward the spine so that a small skinfold appears between the thumbs. Do not slide the hands over the skin. Instruct the patient to take a deep breath after exhaling. Note movement of the thumbs. Expect chest excursion to be symmetrical, separating the thumbs 3−5 cm (1¼ −2 inches). Reduced chest excursion is caused by pain, postural deformity, or fatigue. In older adults, chest excursion normally declines because of costal cartilage calcification and respiratory muscle atrophy.

Auscultation assesses the movement of air through the tracheobronchial tree and detects mucus or obstructed airways. Normally, air flows through the airways in an unobstructed pattern. Recognizing the sounds created by normal airflow allows for detection of sounds caused by airway obstruction. The patient sits during auscultation of the lungs.

Place the diaphragm of the stethoscope firmly on the skin, over the posterior chest wall between the ribs. Ask the patient to take slow, deep breaths with the mouth slightly open. Listen to an entire inspiration and expiration at each position of the stethoscope (Fig. 7.23A). If sounds are faint or distant, as in an obese patient, ask the patient to temporarily breathe harder and faster. Breath sounds are much louder in children because of their thin chest walls. In small children, listen through the bell of a pediatric stethoscope because of their small chest. Use a systematic pattern comparing the sounds in one region on one side of the body with sounds in the same region on the opposite side.

Auscultate for normal breath sounds and abnormal or **adventitious sounds.** Normal breath sounds differ in character depending on the area you auscultate. Bronchovesicular and vesicular sounds normally are heard over the posterior thorax. Bronchovesicular sounds are medium-pitched blowing sounds normally heard between the scapulae. The sounds have equal inspiratory and expiratory phases. The character of bronchovesicular sounds is created by air moving through large airways. Vesicular sounds are normally heard over the periphery of the lungs. Air moving through the smaller airways creates these sounds. Vesicular sounds are soft, breezy, and low pitched; the inspiratory phase is about three times longer than the expiratory phase.

Abnormal sounds result from air passing through moisture, mucus, or narrowed airways. They also result from alveoli suddenly reinflating or from an inflammation between

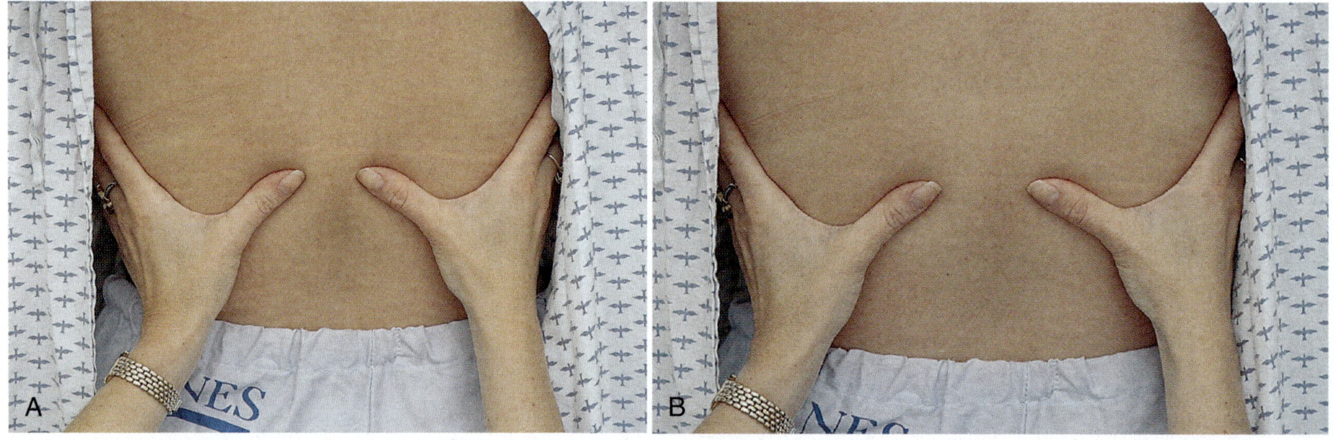

Fig. 7.22 A, Palpating thoracic expansion by placing thumbs at the level of the 10th rib. **B,** As patient inhales, movement of chest excursion separates thumbs.

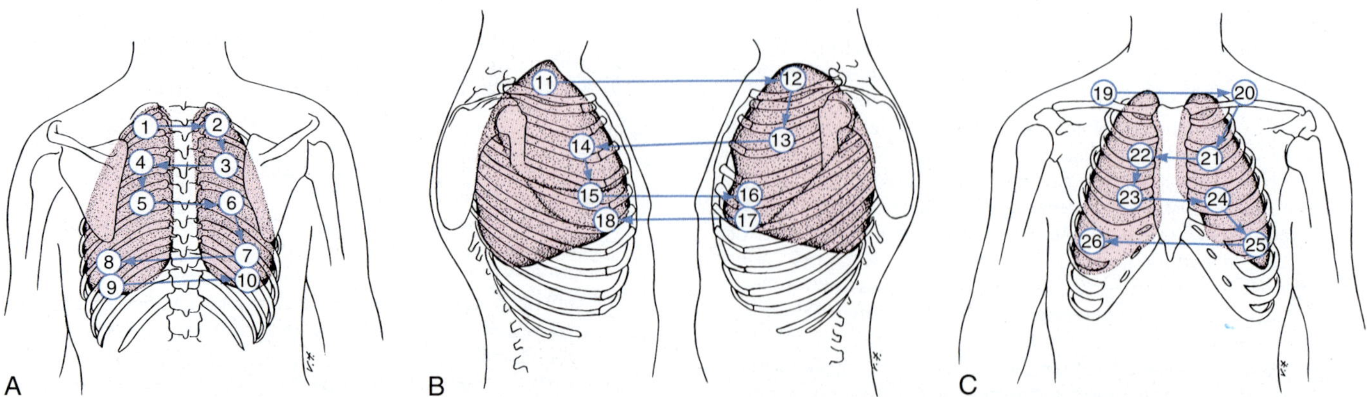

Fig. 7.23 A−C, A systematic pattern (posterior-lateral-anterior) is followed for palpating and auscultating the thorax.

the pleural linings of the lung. Adventitious sounds often occur superimposed over normal sounds. The four types of adventitious sounds are **crackles,** rhonchi, wheezes, and pleural friction rub. Each sound has its own cause and is characterized by typical auditory features (Table 7.7 and Fig. 7.24). During auscultation, note whether the sound is on inspiration, expiration, or both and the location and characteristics of the sounds. Listen for the absence of breath sounds (found in patients with collapsed or surgically removed lobes).

Lateral Thorax

Extend the assessment of the posterior thorax to the lateral sides of the chest (see Fig. 7.23B). Have the patient raise the arms to improve access to lateral thoracic structures. Use inspection, palpation, and auscultation skills to examine the lateral thorax. Normally, the breath sounds you hear are vesicular.

Anterior Thorax

Inspect the anterior thorax for the same features as the posterior thorax. Have the patient sit upright if possible to maximize chest expansion. Observe the accessory muscles of breathing: sternocleidomastoid, trapezius, and abdominal muscles. The accessory muscles move minimally with normal passive breathing. The accessory and abdominal muscles contract when a patient requires effort to breathe as a result of strenuous exercise or disease.

Observe the width of the costal angle. It is usually larger than 90° between the two costal margins. Observe the breathing pattern. Assess respiratory rate and rhythm anteriorly (see Chapter 6). The respirations in male patients are usually diaphragmatic, whereas the respirations in female patients are more costal.

Auscultation of the anterior thorax follows a systematic pattern (see Fig. 7.23C). Pay special attention to the lower lobes, where mucus secretions commonly gather. Listen for

Table 7.7 Adventitious Breath Sounds

Sound	Site Auscultated	Cause	Character
Crackles	Most common in dependent lobes: right and left lung bases	Random, sudden reinflation of groups of alveoli; disruptive passage of air through small airways	Fine crackles: High-pitched fine, short, interrupted crackling sounds heard during end of inspiration; usually not cleared with coughing Moist crackles: Lower, more moist sounds heard during middle of inspiration; not cleared with coughing Coarse crackles: Loud, bubbly sounds heard during inspiration; not cleared with coughing
Rhonchi (sonorous wheeze)	Primarily heard over trachea and bronchi; if loud enough, can be heard over most lung fields	Muscular spasm, fluid, or mucus in larger airways, new growth or external pressure causing turbulence	Loud, low-pitched, rumbling coarse sounds heard during either inspiration or expiration; may be cleared by coughing
Wheezes (sibilant wheeze)	Heard over all lung fields	High-velocity airflow through severely narrowed or obstructed airway	High-pitched, continuous musical sounds such as a squeak heard continuously during inspiration or expiration; usually louder on expiration
Pleural friction rub	Heard over anterior lateral lung field (if the patient is sitting upright)	Inflamed pleura, parietal pleura rubbing against visceral pleura	Has dry, grating quality heard during inspiration; does not clear with coughing; heard loudest over lower lateral anterior surface

Data from Ball JW, et al: *Seidel's guide to physical examination,* ed 8, St Louis, 2015, Elsevier.

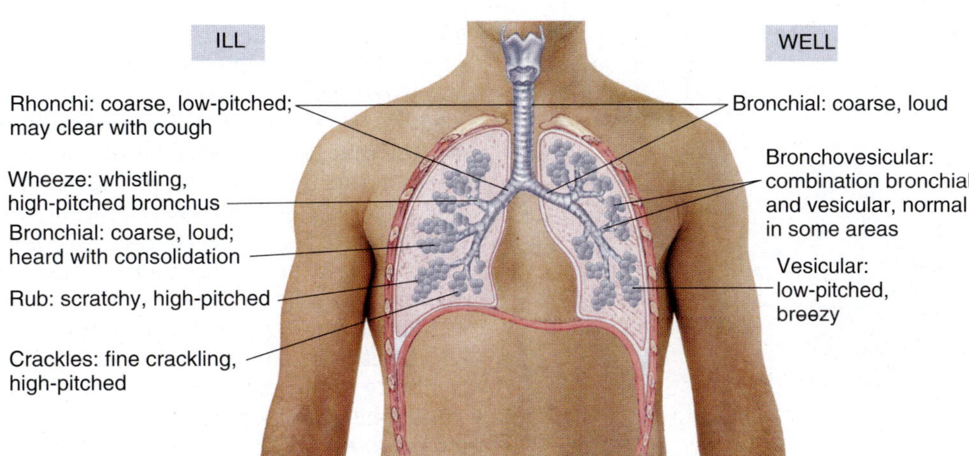

Fig. 7.24 Schema of breath sounds in the ill and well patient. (From Ball JW, et al: *Seidel's guide to physical examination,* ed 8, St Louis, 2015, Elsevier.)

bronchovesicular and vesicular sounds above and below the clavicles and along the lung periphery. Auscultate for bronchial sounds, which are loud, high pitched, and hollow sounding with expiration lasting longer than inspiration (3:2 ratio). You normally hear this sound over the trachea.

Heart

Compare your assessment of heart function with findings from the vascular assessment. Alterations in either system sometimes manifest as changes in the other. Some patients with signs and symptoms of heart (cardiac) problems have a life-threatening condition requiring immediate attention. In this case, act quickly and conduct only the parts of the examination that are absolutely necessary. When a patient is more stable, conduct a more thorough assessment.

Assess cardiac function through the anterior thorax. Form a mental image of the exact location of the heart (Fig. 7.25). In adults, the heart is located in the center of the chest (precordium) behind and to the left of the sternum, with a small section of the right atrium extending to the right of the sternum. The base of the heart is the upper portion, and the apex is the bottom tip. The surface of the right ventricle constitutes most of the anterior surface of the heart. A section of the left ventricle shapes the left anterior side of the apex. The point of maximal impulse (PMI) is palpable at the fifth intercostal space at the left midclavicular line in adults and children older than 7 years. In children younger than 7 years, the PMI is at the fourth intercostal space at the left midclavicular line (Hockenberry et al., 2017).

To assess heart function, you need to understand the cardiac cycle and associated physiological events (Fig. 7.26). The heart normally pumps blood through its four chambers in a methodical, even sequence. Events on the left side occur just before events on the right. As the blood flows through each chamber, valves open and close, pressures within chambers rise and fall, and chambers contract. Each event creates a physiological sign. Both sides of the heart function in a coordinated fashion.

There are two phases to the cardiac cycle: systole and diastole. During systole, the ventricles contract and eject blood from the left ventricle into the aorta and from the right ventricle into the pulmonary artery. During diastole, the ventricles relax, and the atria contract to move blood into the ventricles and fill the coronary arteries.

Heart sounds occur in relation to physiological events in the cardiac cycle. As systole begins, ventricular pressure

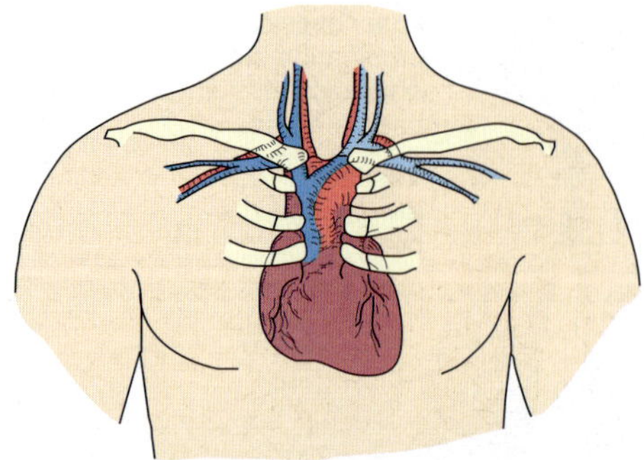

Fig. 7.25 Anatomical position of the heart.

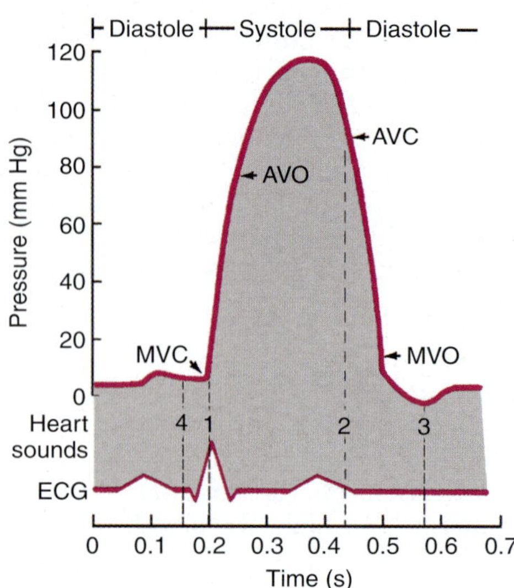

Fig. 7.26 Cardiac cycle. *MVC,* mitral valve closes; *AVO,* aortic valve opens; *AVC,* aortic valve closes; *ECG,* electrocardiogram; *MVO,* mitral valve opens.

rises and closes the mitral and tricuspid valves. Valve closure causes the first heart sound (S_1), often described as "lub." The ventricles then contract, and blood flows through the aorta and pulmonary circulation. After the ventricles empty, ventricular pressure falls below the pressure in the aorta and pulmonary artery. This allows the aortic and pulmonic valves to close, causing the second heart sound (S_2), described as "dub." As ventricular pressure continues to fall, it drops below that of the atria. The mitral and tricuspid valves reopen to allow ventricular filling. Rapid ventricular filling may create a third heart sound (S_3), which is heard more often in children and young adults. S_3 is an abnormal finding in adults older than 30 years and is heard after S_2. A fourth heart sound (S_4) occurs when the atria contract to enhance ventricular filling and is heard before S_1. S_4 may be heard in healthy older adults, children, and athletes; but it is not normal in adults. S_4 needs to be reported to a health care provider.

Nursing History

The nursing history focuses on risk factors for cardiovascular disease (Box 7.15). Determine the patient's history of smoking, alcohol intake, caffeine intake, use of prescription and recreational drugs, exercise habits, and dietary patterns including fat and sodium intake. Ask whether the patient is taking medications for cardiovascular function (e.g., antidysrhythmics or antihypertensives) and whether he or she knows their purpose, dosage, and side effects. Assess for chest pain or discomfort, palpitations, excess fatigue, cough, dyspnea, edema of the feet, cyanosis, fainting, or orthopnea. These are key symptoms of heart disease. If the patient reports chest pain, determine whether it is cardiac in nature; anginal pain is usually a deep pressure or ache that is substernal and diffuse radiating to one or both arms, the neck, or the jaw. Determine whether the patient has a stressful lifestyle. Assess for personal or family history of heart disease, diabetes, high cholesterol, hypertension, stroke, or rheumatic heart disease.

BOX 7.15 Patient Teaching

Heart Assessment

Outcome

Patient chooses healthy heart practices, noting personal risk factors for heart disease.

Teaching Strategies

- Explain risk factors for heart disease including high dietary intake of saturated fat or cholesterol, lack of regular aerobic exercise, smoking, excess weight, stressful lifestyle, hypertension, and family history of heart disease.
- Refer patient to appropriate available resources for controlling or reducing risks (e.g., nutritional counseling, smoking cessation, exercise class, stress-reduction programs).
- Explain that research shows clinical benefit from reducing dietary intake of cholesterol and saturated fats. Teach patient that approximately 70%–75% of saturated fatty acids come from meats, poultry, fish, and dairy products. The American Heart Association (AHA, 2015) recommends a diet that includes a variety of fruits and vegetables, whole grains, low-fat dairy products, skinless poultry and fish, nuts and legumes, and nontropical vegetable oils.
- Encourage regular measurement of total blood cholesterol levels and triglycerides. Desirable levels of total cholesterol are less than 170 mg/dL. More than one cholesterol measurement is needed to assess the blood cholesterol level accurately. Because low-density lipoprotein (LDL) cholesterol is the major component of atherosclerotic plaques, tests should include separate measurement of LDL cholesterol. An LDL cholesterol level of 130 mg/dL or higher indicates high risk for heart disease (Ball et al., 2015).
- Advise patients to minimize alcohol, quit smoking, and avoid secondhand cigarette smoke (AHA, 2015).
- Have patient consult with health care provider regarding the benefit of taking a daily low dose of aspirin.

Evaluation

- Use the principles of teach back to evaluate patient/family caregiver learning:
  - "Tell me the risk factors for heart disease that we discussed."
  - "Show me the meal plan low in saturated fat and cholesterol that you developed for yourself."
  - "Review with me your most recent cholesterol level from your follow-up appointment."

Inspection and Palpation

Ensure that the patient is comfortable and not anxious. Anxiety and discomfort may cause tachycardia, which produces inaccurate findings. Use the skills of inspection and palpation simultaneously. The examination begins with the patient supine and the upper body elevated 45° because patients with heart disease frequently experience shortness of breath while lying flat. Stand at the patient's right side. Discourage the patient from talking, especially when auscultating heart sounds. Good lighting in the room is essential.

Direct your attention to the anatomical sites best suited for assessment of cardiac function. Inspect the angle of Louis; feel the ridge in the sternum approximately 5 cm (2 inches) below the sternal notch. Slip the fingers along the angle on each side of the sternum to feel the adjacent ribs. The intercostal spaces are just below each rib. The second intercostal space allows for identification of each of the six anatomical landmarks (Fig. 7.27). The second intercostal space on the right is the aortic area, and the second intercostal space on the left is the pulmonic area. You need deeper palpation to feel the spaces in obese or heavily muscled patients. After locating the pulmonic area, move the fingers down the patient's left sternal border to the third intercostal space, called the *second pulmonic area*. The tricuspid area is located at the fourth or fifth intercostal space along the sternum. To find the apical or mitral area, locate the fifth intercostal space just to the left of the sternum and move the fingers laterally to the left midclavicular line. Locate the apical area with the palm of the hand or the fingertips. Normally, you feel the apical impulse as a light tap in an area 1–2 cm (1/4–3/4 inch) in diameter at the apex. Another landmark is the epigastric area at the tip of the sternum where you palpate for aortic abnormalities.

Locate the six anatomical landmarks of the heart; inspect and palpate each area. Look for the appearance of pulsations, viewing each area over the chest at an angle to the side. Normally, you do not see pulsations except perhaps at the PMI in thin patients or the epigastric area as a result of abdominal aortic pulsation. Use the proximal halves of the four fingers together and alternate with the ball of the hand to palpate for pulsations. Touch the areas gently to allow movements to lift the hand. Normally, you do not feel any pulsations or vibrations in the second, third, or fourth intercostal spaces. Loud murmurs cause a vibration. Time palpated pulsations or vibrations and their occurrence in relation to systole or diastole by auscultating heart sounds simultaneously.

The apical impulse or PMI should be felt easily. If not, have the patient turn onto the left side, moving the heart closer to the chest wall. Estimate the size of the heart by noting the diameter of the PMI and its position relative to the midclavicular line. In cases of serious heart disease, the cardiac muscle enlarges, with the PMI found to the left of the midclavicular line. The PMI is sometimes difficult to find in older adults because the chest deepens in its AP diameter. It is also difficult to find in muscular or overweight patients. You usually find an infant's PMI at the third or fourth intercostal space more easily because of the infant's thin chest wall.

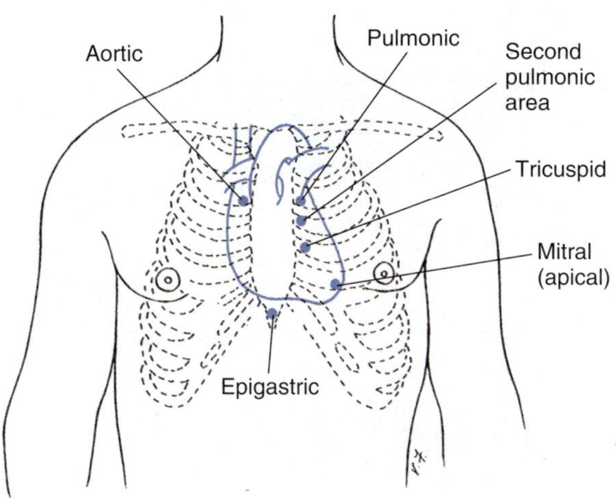

Fig. 7.27 Anatomical sites for assessment of cardiac function.

Auscultation

Auscultation of the heart detects normal heart sounds, extra heart sounds, and murmurs. Concentrate on detecting low-intensity sounds caused by valve closure. To begin auscultation, eliminate all sources of room noise and explain the procedure to reduce the patient's anxiety. Follow a systematic pattern beginning at the aortic area and inching the stethoscope across each of the anatomical sites. Listen for the complete cycle ("lub-dub") of heart sounds clearly at each location. If you suspect a problem, repeat the sequence using the bell of the stethoscope. Sometimes, the patient assumes three different positions during the examination (Fig. 7.28):

- Sitting up and leaning forward—good for all areas and to hear high-pitched murmurs
- Supine—good for all areas
- Left lateral recumbent—good for all areas and best position to hear low-pitched sounds in diastole

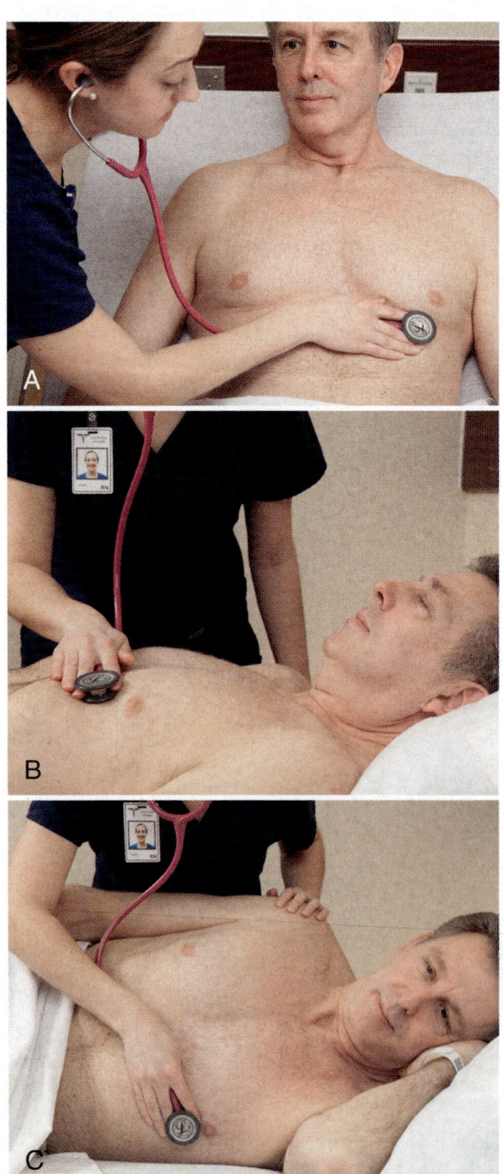

Fig. 7.28 Sequence of patient positions for heart auscultation. **A,** Sitting. **B,** Supine. **C,** Left lateral recumbent.

Learn to identify S_1 and S_2 heart sounds. At normal rates, S_1 occurs after the long diastolic pause and before the short systolic pause. S_1 is high pitched, dull in quality, and heard best at the apex. If it is difficult to hear S_1, time it in relation to the carotid pulse. S_2 follows the short systolic pause and precedes the long diastolic pause; you hear it best at the aortic area.

Auscultate for rate and rhythm after hearing both sounds clearly. Each combination of S_1 and S_2 or "lub-dub" counts as one heartbeat. Count the rate for 1 minute and listen for the interval between S_1 and S_2 and then the time between S_2 and the next S_1. A regular rhythm involves regular intervals of time between each sequence of beats. There is a distinct silent pause between S_1 and S_2. Failure of the heart to beat at regular successive intervals is a **dysrhythmia**. Some dysrhythmias are life-threatening.

When assessing an irregular heart rhythm, compare apical and radial pulse rates simultaneously to determine whether a pulse deficit exists. Auscultate the apical pulse first and then immediately assess the radial pulse (one-examiner technique). Assess the apical and radial rates at the same time when two examiners are present. When a patient has a pulse deficit, the radial pulse is slower than the apical pulse because ineffective contractions fail to send pulse waves to the periphery. Report a difference in pulse rates to the health care provider immediately.

Assess extra heart sounds and murmurs at each auscultatory site. Use the bell of the stethoscope and listen for low-pitched extra sounds such as S_3 and S_4 gallops, clicks, murmurs, and rubs. Clicks can occur when a device such as a prosthetic valve is present. A pericardial friction rub resembles a scratching or raspy sound. If a swooshing sound is heard, this is a murmur that usually represents turbulent blood flow. The presence of extra heart sounds sometimes indicates a pathological condition; therefore, such sounds should be reported to the health care provider immediately. Typically, advanced practice nurses perform this part of the examination.

Vascular System

Examination of the vascular system includes measuring the blood pressure (see Chapter 6) and assessing the integrity of the peripheral vascular system. Use the skills of inspection, palpation, and auscultation. You may perform portions of the vascular examination during other body system assessments. For example, check the carotid pulse after palpating the cervical lymph nodes.

Health History

Determine whether the patient has leg cramps; numbness or tingling in the extremities; sensation of cold hands or feet; pain in the legs; or swelling or cyanosis of the feet, ankles, or hands. These signs and symptoms may indicate vascular disease. If the patient has leg pain or cramping in the lower extremities, ask whether walking or standing for long periods or sleep aggravates or relieves the symptoms. This question helps to clarify whether the problem is musculoskeletal or vascular. Ask patients whether they wear tight-fitting garters or hosiery and whether they sit or lie in bed with legs crossed. These activities impair venous return. Consider previous cardiac risk factors that may predispose to vascular disease (e.g., smoking, nutritional problems). Assess the patient's medical history for heart disease, hypertension, phlebitis, diabetes, or varicose veins.

Carotid Arteries

When the left ventricle pumps blood into the aorta, the arterial system transmits pressure waves. The carotid artery reflects heart function better than peripheral arteries because their pressure correlates with the pressure of the aorta. The carotid artery supplies oxygenated blood to the head and neck (Fig. 7.29). The overlying sternocleidomastoid muscle protects it.

To examine the carotid arteries, have the patient sit or lie supine with the head of the bed elevated 30°. Examine one carotid artery at a time. If both arteries are simultaneously occluded during palpation, the patient loses consciousness as a result of inadequate circulation to the brain. Do not palpate or massage the carotid arteries vigorously because the carotid sinus is in the upper third of the neck. The sinus sends impulses along the vagus nerve. Stimulating the vagus nerve causes a reflex drop in the heart rate and blood pressure, which causes syncope (light-headedness) or circulatory arrest. This is a particular problem for older adults.

Begin inspection of the neck for obvious pulsation of the artery. Have the patient turn the head slightly away from the artery being examined. Sometimes, the wave of the pulse is visible. Absence of a pulse wave may indicate arterial occlusion (blockage) or stenosis (narrowing).

To palpate the pulse, ask the patient to look straight ahead or turn the head slightly toward the side being examined. Turning relaxes the sternocleidomastoid muscle. Slide the tips of your index and middle fingers around the medial edge of the sternocleidomastoid muscle. Gently palpate to avoid occlusion of circulation (Fig. 7.30).

The normal carotid pulse is localized rather than diffuse. As a strong pulse, the carotid has a thrusting quality. As the patient breathes, no change occurs. Rotation of the neck or a shift from a sitting to a supine position does not change the quality of the carotid artery. Both carotid arteries normally are equal in pulse rate, rhythm, and strength and are equally elastic. Diminished or unequal carotid pulsations indicate atherosclerosis (plaque buildup in arteries) or other forms of arterial disease.

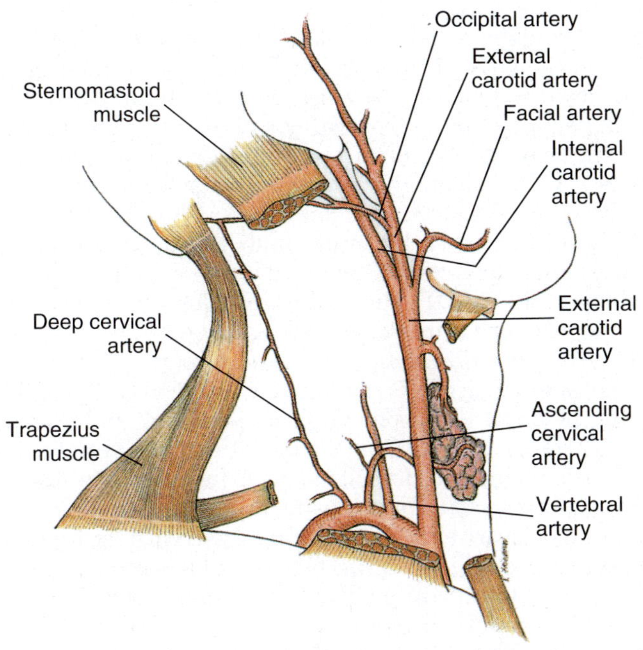

Fig. 7.29 Anatomical position of carotid artery.

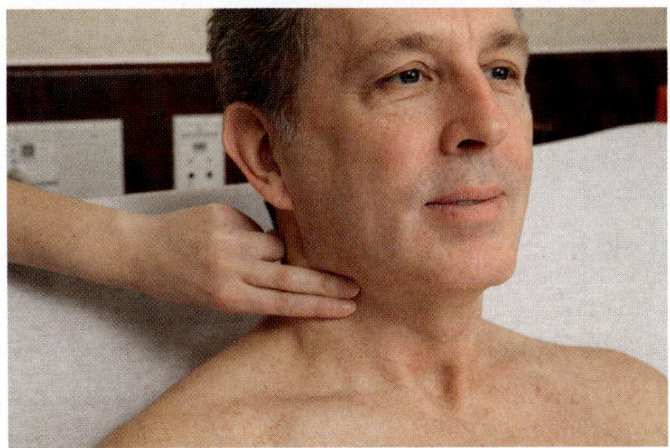

Fig. 7.30 Palpation of internal carotid artery along margin of sternocleidomastoid muscle.

The carotid is the most commonly auscultated pulse. Auscultation is especially important for middle-aged or older adults or patients suspected to have cerebrovascular disease. When the lumen of a blood vessel is narrowed, blood flow is disturbed. As blood passes through the narrowed section, this creates turbulence, causing a blowing or swishing sound. The blowing sound is called a **bruit** (pronounced "brew-ee"). Place the bell of the stethoscope over the carotid artery at the base of the neck and move it gradually toward the jaw. Ask the patient to hold his or her breath for a few heartbeats so that respiratory sounds do not interfere with auscultation. Normally, you do not hear any sound during carotid auscultation. Palpate the artery lightly for a **thrill** (palpable bruit) if you hear a bruit.

Jugular Veins

The most accessible veins for examination are the internal and external jugular veins in the neck. Both veins drain bilaterally from the head and neck into the superior vena cava. The external jugular lies superficially and is just above the clavicle. The internal jugular lies deeper, along the carotid artery (Fig. 7.31). Normally, when a patient lies in the supine position, the external jugular distends and becomes easily visible. In contrast, the jugular veins normally flatten when the patient is in a sitting or standing position. However, some patients with heart disease have distended jugular veins when sitting.

To measure venous pressure, inspect the jugular veins with the patient in the supine position (normally veins protrude), when standing (normally veins are flat), and when sitting at a 45° angle (jugular veins are distended only if the patient has right-sided heart failure). An advanced practice nurse completes the specific measurement of jugular venous pressure.

Peripheral Arteries and Veins

To examine the peripheral vascular system, begin by assessing the adequacy of blood flow to the extremities by

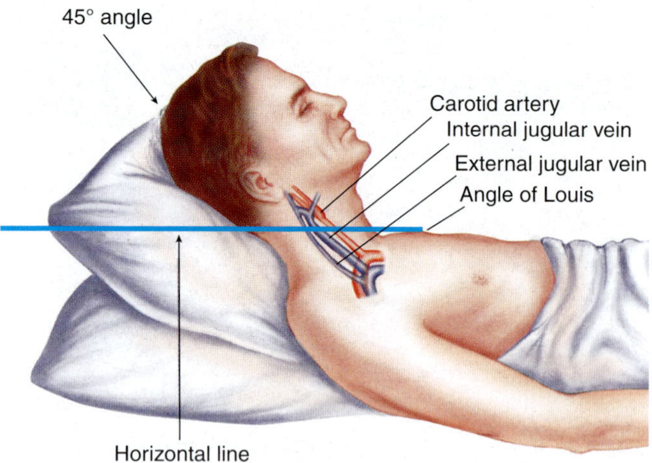

Fig. 7.31 Position of patient to assess jugular vein distention. (From Thompson JM, et al: *Mosby's clinical nursing*, ed 4, St Louis, 1997, Mosby.)

BOX 7.16 Patient Teaching

Vascular Assessment

Outcome

Patient chooses activities that maintain or improve peripheral vascular status.

Teaching Strategies

- Explain the effects of high-fat diet choices, discussing how cholesterol and *trans* fats contribute to the development of atherosclerosis and lead to hypertension.
- Explain high risks for peripheral artery disease including smoking, hypertension, diabetes, stroke, kidney disease with hemodialysis, and heart disease.
- Explain the benefit of regular monitoring of blood pressure (daily, weekly, or monthly) with available home blood pressure monitors.
- Instruct patients with risk or evidence of vascular insufficiency in the lower extremities to avoid tight clothing over the lower body or legs, avoid sitting or standing for long periods, walk regularly, and elevate the feet when sitting.

Evaluation

- Use the principles of teach back to evaluate patient/family caregiver learning:
  - "Explain to me what is the normal blood pressure for your age."
  - "Show me how you take your blood pressure with your home equipment."
  - "Describe to me how you have progressed with smoking cessation practices, worked at controlling your diabetes, and followed treatment for your other health problems."

measuring arterial pulses and inspecting the skin and nails. Then assess the integrity of the venous system. Assess the arterial pulses in the extremities to determine sufficiency of the entire arterial circulation. Factors such as coagulation disorders, local trauma or surgery, constricting casts or bandages, and systemic diseases impair circulation to the extremities. Discuss risk factors for circulatory problems with the patient (Box 7.16).

Peripheral Arteries

Examine each peripheral artery using the distal pads of the second and third fingers. The thumb helps anchor the brachial and femoral arteries. Apply firm pressure, but avoid occluding a pulse. When a pulse is difficult to find, it helps to vary pressure and feel all around the pulse site.

Routine vital signs usually include assessment of the rate and rhythm of the radial artery because it is easily accessible (see Chapter 6). Count the pulse for either 30 or 60 seconds depending on the character of the pulse. Always count an irregular pulse for 60 seconds. With palpation, you normally feel the pulse wave at regular intervals. When an interval is interrupted by an early, late, or missed beat, the pulse rhythm is irregular. In emergencies, health care providers usually assess the carotid artery because it is accessible and most useful in evaluating heart activity. To check local circulatory status of tissues, palpate the peripheral arteries long enough to note that a pulse is present.

Assess each peripheral artery for elasticity of the vessel wall, strength, and equality. Normally, the arterial wall is elastic, making it easily palpable. Depress the artery; it springs back to shape when pressure is released. An abnormal artery is described as hard, inelastic, or calcified.

The strength of a pulse is a measurement of the force with which blood is ejected against the arterial wall. Some examiners use a rating from 0 (absent, not palpable) to 4 (bounding) (Ball et al., 2015).

Measure all peripheral pulses for equality and symmetry. Compare pulses on each side of the body. Lack of symmetry indicates impaired circulation such as a localized obstruction or an abnormally positioned artery.

In the upper extremities, the brachial artery channels blood to the radial and ulnar arteries of the forearm and hand. If circulation in this artery becomes blocked, the hands do not receive adequate blood flow. If circulation in the radial or ulnar artery becomes impaired, the hand still receives adequate perfusion. An interconnection between the radial and ulnar arteries guards against arterial occlusion (Fig. 7.32A).

To locate pulses in the arm, have the patient sit or lie down. Find the radial pulse along the radial side of the forearm at the wrist. Thin individuals have a groove lateral to the flexor tendon of the wrist. Feel the radial pulse with light palpation in the groove (Fig. 7.32B). The ulnar pulse is on the opposite side of the wrist and feels less prominent (Fig. 7.32C). Palpate the ulnar pulse only when evaluating arterial insufficiency to the hand.

To palpate the brachial pulse, find the groove between the biceps and triceps muscle above the elbow at the antecubital fossa (Fig. 7.32D). The artery runs along the medial side of the extended arm. Palpate the artery with the fingertips of the first three fingers in the muscle groove.

The femoral artery is the primary artery in the leg, delivering blood to the popliteal, posterior tibial, and dorsalis pedis arteries (Fig. 7.33A). An interconnection between the posterior tibial and dorsalis pedis arteries guards against local arterial occlusion. Wearing disposable gloves, find the femoral pulse with the patient lying down with the inguinal area exposed (Fig. 7.33B). The femoral artery runs below the inguinal ligament, midway between the symphysis pubis and the anterior superior iliac spine. Sometimes, you use deep palpation to feel the pulse. Bimanual palpation is effective in obese patients. Place the fingertips of both hands on the opposite sides of the pulse site. Feel a pulsatile sensation when the arterial pulsation pushes the fingertips apart.

The popliteal pulse runs behind the knee (Fig. 7.33C). Have the patient slightly flex the knee with the foot resting on the examination table or assume a prone position with the knee slightly flexed. Instruct the patient to keep leg muscles relaxed. Palpate with the fingers of both hands deeply into the popliteal fossa, just lateral to the midline. The popliteal pulse is difficult to locate.

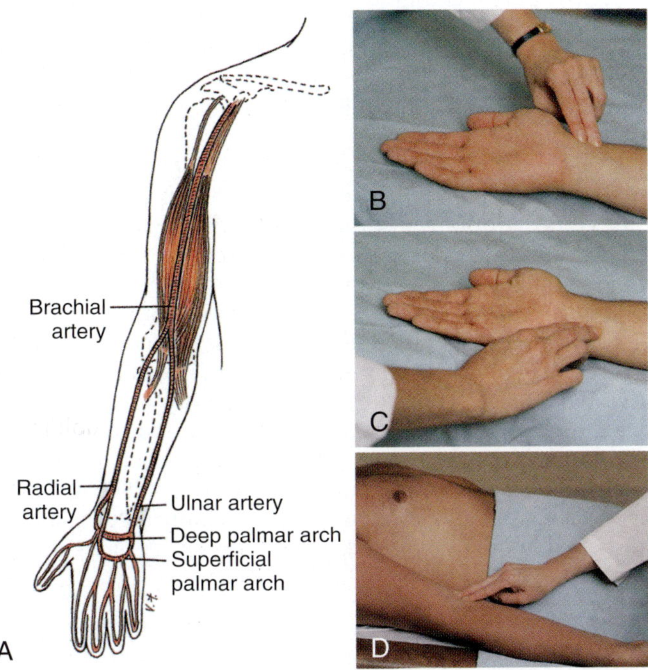

Fig. 7.32 **A,** Anatomical positions of brachial, radial, and ulnar arteries. **B,** Palpation of radial pulse. **C,** Palpation of ulnar pulse. **D,** Palpation of brachial pulse.

With the patient's foot relaxed, locate the dorsalis pedis pulse. The artery runs along the top of the foot in a line with the groove between the extensor tendons of the great and first toes (Fig. 7.33D). To find the pulse, place the fingertips between the great and first toe and slowly move up the dorsum of the foot. This pulse is sometimes congenitally absent.

Find the posterior tibial pulse on the inner side of each ankle (Fig. 7.33E). Place the fingers behind and below the patient's medial malleolus (ankle bone). With the patient's foot relaxed and slightly extended, palpate the artery.

Ultrasound Stethoscopes

If a pulse is difficult to palpate, an ultrasound (Doppler) stethoscope is a useful tool that amplifies sounds of a pulse wave. Apply a thin layer of transmission gel to the patient's skin at the pulse site or directly onto the transducer tip of the probe. Turn on the volume control and place the tip of the probe at a 45–90° angle on the skin. Move the transducer until you hear a pulsating "whooshing" sound, which indicates that arterial blood flow is present. Document in the patient's record that the recorded pulse was obtained by Doppler and at what location.

Tissue Perfusion

The condition of the skin, mucosa, and nail beds offers useful data about the status of circulatory blood flow. Examine the face and upper extremities, looking at the color of skin, mucosa, and nail beds. The presence of cyanosis requires special attention. Heart disease sometimes causes central cyanosis (bluish discoloration of the lips, mouth, and conjunctivae), indicating poor arterial oxygenation. Blue lips, earlobes, and nail beds are signs of peripheral cyanosis, which indicates peripheral vasoconstriction. When cyanosis is present, consult with a health care provider to have laboratory testing of oxygen saturation to determine the severity of the problem. Examination

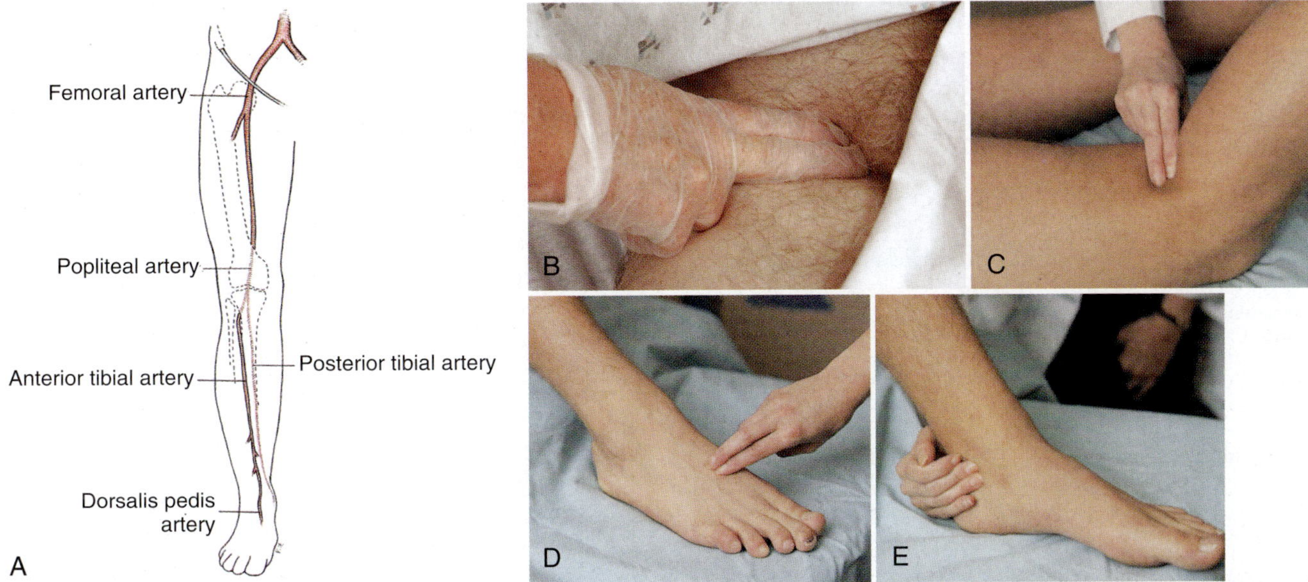

Fig. 7.33 **A,** Anatomical position of femoral, popliteal, dorsalis pedis, anterior tibial, and posterior tibial arteries. **B,** Palpation of femoral pulse. **C,** Palpation of popliteal pulse. **D,** Palpation of dorsalis pedis pulse. **E,** Palpation of posterior tibial pulse.

of the nails involves inspection for clubbing (a bulging of the tissues at the nail base), resulting from insufficient oxygenation at the periphery.

Inspect the lower extremities for changes in color, temperature, and condition of the skin indicating either arterial or venous alterations (Table 7.8). This is a good time to ask the patient about history of pain in the legs. If an arterial occlusion is present, the patient has signs resulting from absence of blood flow. Pain is distal to the occlusion. The 5 *Ps* characterize an occlusion: *p*ain, *p*allor, *p*ulselessness, *p*aresthesias, and *p*aralysis. Venous congestion causes tissue changes indicating inadequate circulatory flow back to the heart.

During examination of the lower extremities, also inspect skin and nail texture; hair distribution on the lower legs, feet, and toes; venous pattern; and scars, pigmentation, or ulcers. Palpate the legs for color and temperature. Assess for capillary refill.

The absence of hair growth over the legs indicates circulatory insufficiency. Do not confuse an absence of hair on the legs with shaved legs. Many men have less hair around the calves because of tight-fitting dress socks or jeans. Chronic recurring ulcers of the feet or lower legs are a serious sign of circulatory insufficiency and require a health care provider's intervention.

Peripheral Veins

Assess the status of the peripheral veins by asking the patient to assume sitting and standing positions. Assessment includes inspection and palpation for varicosities, peripheral edema, and phlebitis. Varicosities are superficial veins that become dilated, especially when legs are in a dependent position. They are common in older adults because the veins normally fibrose, dilate, and stretch. They are also common in people who stand for prolonged periods. Varicosities in the anterior or medial part of the thigh and the posterolateral part of the calf are abnormal.

Dependent edema around the feet and ankles is a sign of venous insufficiency or right-sided heart failure. It is common in older adults and people who spend a lot of time standing (e.g., nurses, waitresses, security guards). To assess for pitting edema, use your thumb to press firmly for several seconds over the medial malleolus or the shins and then release. A depression left in the skin indicates edema. Grading +1 through +4 characterizes the severity of the edema (Fig. 7.6).

Phlebitis (inflammation of a vein) occurs commonly after trauma to the vessel wall, infection, immobilization, or prolonged insertion of i.v. catheters (see Chapter 25). To assess for phlebitis, inspect the calves for localized redness, tenderness, and swelling over vein sites. Gentle palpation of calf muscles reveals warmth, tenderness, and firmness of the muscle. Unilateral edema of the affected leg is one of the most reliable findings of phlebitis. A Doppler study is a noninvasive test that examines venous blood flow and is commonly performed if deep vein thrombosis (DVT) is suspected. The Homan's sign is no longer a reliable indicator of phlebitis or DVT, and it can be present in other conditions (Ball et al., 2015). The Homan's sign test is contraindicated in patients with DVT. If a clot is in the leg, it may dislodge from its original site during a Homan's sign test, resulting in a pulmonary embolus.

Lymphatic System

Assess the lymphatic drainage of the lower extremities during examination of the vascular system or during the female or male genital examination. Superficial and deep lymph nodes drain the legs, but only two groups of superficial nodes are palpable. With the patient supine, palpate the area of the superior superficial inguinal nodes in the groin area (Fig. 7.34). Then move your fingertips toward the inner thigh, feeling for any palpable inferior nodes. Use a firm but gentle pressure when palpating over each lymphatic chain. Multiple nodes are not normally palpable, although a few soft, nontender nodes are not unusual. Enlarged, hardened, tender nodes reveal potential sites of infection or metastatic disease.

Breasts

It is important to examine the breasts of female and male patients. Men have a small amount of glandular tissue, a potential site for the growth of cancer cells, in the breast. In contrast, most of the female breast is glandular tissue.

Female Breasts

An estimated 246,660 new cases of invasive breast cancer in women and 2600 new cases in men in the United States were predicted by the American Cancer Society in 2016

Table 7.8 Signs of Venous and Arterial Insufficiency

Assessment Criterion	Venous	Arterial
Color	Normal or cyanotic	Pale; worsened by elevation of extremity; dusky red when extremity lowered
Temperature	Normal	Cool (blood flow blocked to extremity)
Pulse	Normal	Decreased or absent
Edema	Often marked	Absent or mild
Skin changes	Brown pigmentation around ankles	Thin, shiny skin; decreased hair growth; thickened nails

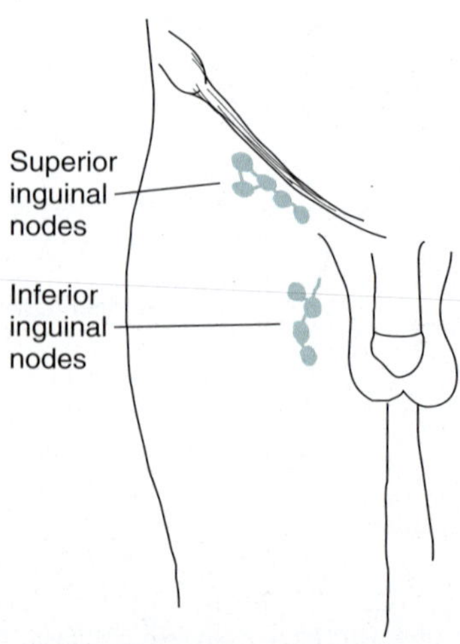

Fig. 7.34 Inguinal lymph nodes.

(ACS, 2016a). Because of this, it is important to know the recommended breast cancer screening guidelines. According to the ACS (2015, 2016c), screening tests and examinations are used to find cancer in people who do not have any symptoms. Although research does not support the clear benefit of regular breast self-examination (BSE), it is important for all women to be familiar with how their breasts look and feel. Experts have concluded that knowing how one's own breasts look and feel is as effective for detecting breast cancer as a structured BSE (ACS, 2015). A BSE is optional for women starting in their 20s (ACS, 2016c). Women should be told about the benefits and limitations of BSE and to report any breast changes to the health care provider right away (Box 7.17).

BSE plays a small role in finding breast cancer compared with finding a breast lump by chance or simply being aware of what is normal for each woman. Some women feel very comfortable doing BSE regularly (usually monthly after their period), using a systematic step-by-step approach to examine the look and feel of their breasts. Other women are more comfortable simply looking at and feeling their breasts in a less systematic approach (e.g., while showering or getting dressed) (ACS, 2016c). Familiarity makes it easier to notice any changes in the breast from one month to another. Early discovery of a change from "normal" is the idea behind regular BSE.

For women who menstruate, the best time to perform BSE is 2 or 3 days after the period ends when breasts are

BOX 7.17 Patient Teaching

Female Breast Assessment

Outcome

Patient performs activities to ensure breast health or provide early identification of breast disease.

Teaching Strategies

- Women who are 20 years of age and older should be told about the benefits of knowing one's own breasts and to evaluate for any changes (Siu, 2016). The more familiar women are with the usual appearance and feel of their breasts, the more likely they are to notice changes that would require a visit to a health care provider. Prompt reporting of any new breast symptoms to a health care professional is important. Provide the following information about breast self-examination (BSE) (ACS, 2015):
  1. BSE should be performed once a month so that the woman becomes familiar with the usual appearance and feel of her breasts.
  2. For women who menstruate, the best time to perform BSE is between the fourth and the seventh day of the menstrual cycle or right after the menstrual cycle ends, when the breasts are least likely to be tender or swollen. Women who no longer menstruate should pick a day such as the first day of the month to remind them to perform BSE.
  3. Men should also examine their breasts, areolas, nipples, and axillae for any swelling, nodules, or ulcerations.
  4. When implants are present, help the patient determine the edges of each implant and demonstrate how to evaluate each breast. At the time of implant, the surgeon usually shows the patient how to identify the edges of the implant. However, it is important to verify that the patient is able to palpate the edges of the implant.
- Teach the steps for performing BSE (ACS, 2015):
  1. Lie down on your back and place your right arm behind your head. This position is recommended because when you lie down the breast tissue spreads evenly over the chest wall and is as thin as possible, making it much easier to feel all the breast tissue.
  2. Use the finger pads of the three middle fingers on your left hand to feel for lumps in the right breast. Use overlapping, dime-sized, circular motions of the finger pads to feel the breast tissue. Use three different levels of pressure to feel all of the breast tissue. Light pressure is needed to feel the tissue closest to the skin, medium pressure is needed to feel a little deeper, and firm pressure is needed to feel the tissue closest to the chest and ribs. It is normal to feel a firm ridge in the lower curve of each breast, but you should tell your health care provider if you feel anything else out of the ordinary. If you are not sure how hard to press, discuss this with your health care provider. Use each pressure level to feel the breast tissue before moving on to the next spot.
  3. Move around the breast in an up-and-down pattern starting at an imaginary line drawn straight down your side from the underarm and moving across the breast to the middle of the chest (sternum, or breastbone). Be sure to check the entire breast area going down until you feel only ribs and up to the neck or collarbone (clavicle).
  4. Repeat the self-examination in the left breast, putting your left arm behind your head and examining the breast as noted in Steps 1–3.
  5. While standing in front of a mirror with your hands pressing firmly down on your hips, look at your breasts, observing for any changes in size, shape, contour, dimpling, or redness or scaliness of the nipple or breast tissue. Pressing down on your hips contracts the chest wall muscles and enhances any breast changes.
  6. Examine each underarm while sitting or standing and with your arm only slightly raised so that you can easily feel in this area for any lumps or changes. Raising your arm straight tightens the tissue in this area, making it harder to examine.
  7. Call your health care provider if you find a lump or other abnormality.
- If the patient is obese, has a family history of breast cancer, or has a history of chest radiation at a young age, she is at higher risk for the disease (Siu, 2016). Diet recommendations are to follow a low-fat diet including limiting meat consumption to well-trimmed, lean beef, pork, or lamb; removing skin from cooked chicken before eating it; selecting tuna and salmon packed in water and not oil; and using low-fat dairy products. In addition, encourage the patient to reduce intake of caffeine. Although this is controversial, many believe that decreasing caffeine intake reduces symptoms of benign (fibrocystic) breast disease.

Evaluation

- Use the principles of teach back to evaluate patient/family caregiver learning:
  - "Tell me when you had your last screening mammogram and how often you should have one."
  - "Describe for me the signs and symptoms of breast cancer compared with benign (fibrocystic) breast disease."
  - "Show me how you would perform BSE."
  - "Describe for me changes that you could make in your diet to reduce the risk of breast disease and cancer."

least likely to be tender or swollen. A pregnant woman should also check her breasts on a monthly basis. Women who no longer menstruate should pick a day such as the first of the month to remind themselves to perform BSE. A clinical breast examination should be part of a regular health examination by a health care provider.

Older women require special attention when reviewing the need for BSE. Fixed incomes limit many older women; thus, they often do not have regular clinical breast examination and mammography. Older women often ignore changes in their breasts, assuming that they are part of aging. Review the patient's history for normal developmental changes and signs of breast disease. Because of the glandular structure, the breast undergoes changes during a woman's life. Knowledge of these changes (Box 7.18) allows you to complete an accurate assessment.

The American Cancer Society (ACS, 2015) and US Preventive Services Task Force (Siu, 2016) recommend the following guidelines for the detection of breast cancer in women who are at average risk (i.e., no personal or strong family history of breast cancer, no genetic mutation such as the *BRCA* gene, or no chest irradiation before the age of 30 years):

1. Monthly BSE is an option for women starting in their 20s.
2. Women 20 years of age and older need to report any breast changes to a health care provider immediately.
3. Health care providers may perform a clinical breast examination every 3 years in women 20–40 years of age and annually in women older than 40 years.
4. Women 40–49 years of age may begin screening mammograms. Women should discuss options with their health care provider.
5. Screening mammograms should take place every 2 years for women 50–74 years of age.
6. For women of any age with an increased risk, the ACS recommends discussion of screening options and additional testing with a health care provider.
   For women with a high risk for breast cancer, the ACS (2016c) recommends an MRI and mammogram every year. This includes women who:
   - Have a lifetime risk of breast cancer of about 20%–25% or greater, according to risk assessment tools that are based mainly on family history
   - Have a known *BRCA1* or *BRCA2* gene mutation
   - Have a first-degree relative (parent, brother, sister, or child) with a *BRCA1* or *BRCA2* gene mutation and have not had genetic testing themselves
   - Had radiation therapy to the chest when they were between the ages of 10 and 30 years

The patient's history may reveal an increased risk for breast cancer, normal developmental changes, or signs of breast disease, and these should be addressed on an individual basis. Knowledge of these risk factors and changes (see Boxes 7.17 and 7.18) are an important aspect of breast health.

Nursing History

The nursing history should explore risk factors for breast cancer such as being a woman older than 40 years or a personal or family history of breast cancer, especially with the *BRCA1* and *BRCA2* inherited gene mutations (ACS, 2015). Early-onset menarche (before 12 years of age) and late-age menopause (after 55 years of age) also affect risk. Other risk factors include never having children, giving birth to the first child after the age of 30 years, recent use of oral contraceptives, previous chest radiation, alcohol use, and being overweight. Ask whether the patient (both male and female) has noticed a lump, thickening, pain, or

BOX 7.18 Normal Changes in the Breast During a Woman's Life Span

Puberty (8–20 Years)

Breasts mature in five stages. One breast may grow more rapidly than the other. The ages at which changes occur and rate of developmental progression vary.

Stage 1 (Preadolescent)

This stage involves elevation of the nipple only.

Stage 2

The breast and nipple elevate as a small mound, and the areolar diameters enlarge.

Stage 3

There is further enlargement and elevation of the breast and areola, with no separation of contour.

Stage 4

The areola and nipple project into the secondary mound above the level of the breast (does not occur in all girls).

Stage 5 (Mature Breast)

Only the nipple projects, and the areola recedes (varies in some women).

Young Adulthood (20–31 Years)

Breasts reach full (nonpregnant) size. Shape is generally symmetrical. Breasts are sometimes unequal in size.

Pregnancy

Breast size gradually enlarges to two to three times the previous size. Nipples enlarge and become erect. Areolae darken, and diameters increase. Superficial veins become prominent. The nipples expel a yellowish fluid (colostrum).

Menopause

Breasts shrink. Tissue becomes softer, sometimes flabby.

Older Adulthood

Breasts become elongated, pendulous, and flaccid as a result of glandular tissue atrophy. The skin of the breasts tends to wrinkle, appearing loose and flabby.
Nipples become smaller and flatter and lose erectile ability.
Nipples invert because of shrinkage and fibrotic changes.

Data from Hockenberry MJ et al. *Essentials of pediatric nursing,* ed 10, St Louis, 2017, Mosby; Ball JW, et al: *Seidel's guide to physical examination,* ed 8, St Louis, 2015, Elsevier; and Touhy TA, Jett KF: *Ebersole and Hess' gerontological nursing and healthy aging,* ed 5, St Louis, 2018, Mosby.

tenderness of the breast; discharge, distortion, retraction, or scaling of the nipple; or change in breast size. Determine the patient's use of medications that increase risk (oral contraceptives, steroids).

Inspection

Research does not show benefit of physical breast examinations performed by a patient or a health care provider in relation to breast cancer screening (ACS, 2015). A full examination needs to be conducted when a patient identifies a change. At that time, it is appropriate to inspect the breasts for size and symmetry. It is common for one breast to be smaller. However, inflammation or a mass can cause a difference in size. With age, the ligaments supporting the breast tissue weaken, causing the breasts to sag and the nipples to lower. To be able to recognize abnormalities, the patient needs to be familiar with the normal appearance of her breasts (Fig. 7.35).

Observe the contour or shape of the breasts and note masses, flattening, retraction, or dimpling. Breasts vary in shape from convex to pendulous or conical. Retraction or dimpling results from invasion of underlying ligaments by tumors. Edema also changes the contour of the breasts. To detect the presence of retraction or changes in the shape of the breasts, ask the patient to assume three positions: raise arms above the head, press hands against the hips, and extend arms straight ahead while sitting and leaning forward. Each maneuver causes a contraction of the pectoral muscles, which accentuates the presence of any retraction.

Carefully inspect the skin for color; venous pattern; and presence of edema, lesions, or inflammation. Lift each breast when necessary to observe lower and lateral aspects for color and texture changes. The breasts are the color of neighboring skin, and venous patterns are the same bilaterally. Venous patterns are easily visible in thin or pregnant women. Women with large breasts often have redness and excoriation of the undersurface caused by rubbing of skin surfaces.

Inspect the nipple and areola for size, color, shape, discharge, and the direction the nipples point. The normal areolae are round or oval and nearly equal bilaterally. Color ranges from pink to brown. In light-skinned women, the areola turns brown during pregnancy and remains dark. In dark-skinned women, the areola is brown before pregnancy (Ball et al., 2015). Normally, the nipples point in symmetrical directions, are everted, and have no drainage. If the nipples are inverted, ask whether this has been present since birth. A recent inversion or inward turning of the nipple indicates an underlying growth. Rashes or ulcerations are not normal on the breast or nipples. Note any bleeding or discharge from the nipple. Clear yellow discharge 2 days after childbirth is common. While inspecting the breasts, explain the characteristics you see. Teach the patient the significance of abnormal signs or symptoms.

Palpation

Once again, palpation is not part of the general assessment process, but further assessment is required if abnormalities are identified by the patient. Palpation assesses the condition of underlying breast tissue and lymph nodes. Breast tissue consists of glandular tissue, fibrous supportive ligaments, and fat. Glandular tissue is organized into lobes that end in ducts opening onto the surface of the nipple. The largest portion of glandular tissue is in the upper outer quadrant and tail of each breast. Suspensory ligaments connect to skin and fascia underlying the breast to support the breast and maintain its upright position. Fatty tissue is located superficially and to the sides of the breast.

A large proportion of lymph from the breasts drains into axillary lymph nodes. Learn the location of supraclavicular, infraclavicular, and axillary nodes (Fig. 7.36). The axillary nodes drain lymph from the chest wall, breasts, arms, and hands. A tumor of one breast sometimes involves nodes on both sides of the body.

To palpate lymph nodes, have the patient sit with arms at her sides and muscles relaxed. While facing the patient and standing on the side you are examining, support her arm in a flexed position and abduct the arm from the chest wall. Place the free hand against her chest wall and high in the

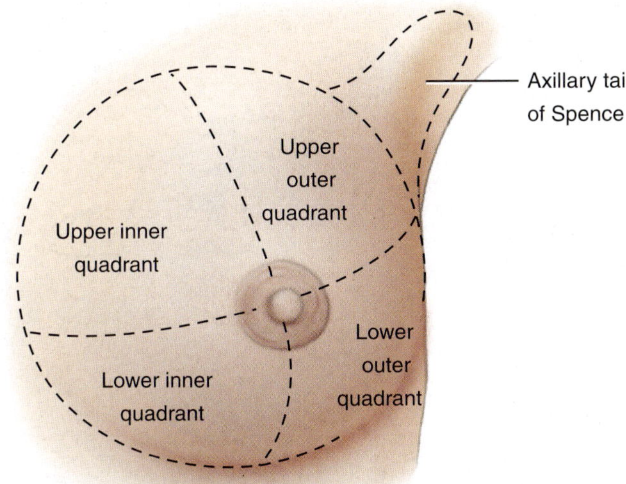

Fig. 7.35 Quadrants of the left breast and axillary tail of Spence. (From Shiland BJ: *Medical terminology and anatomy for coding,* ed 3, St Louis, 2017, Mosby.)

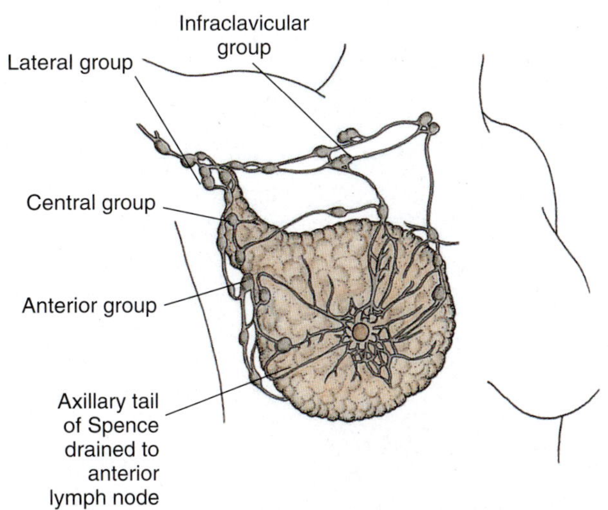

Fig 7.36 Anatomical position of axillary and clavicular lymph nodes.

axillary hollow (Fig. 7.37). With your fingertips, press gently down over the surface of the ribs and muscles. Palpate the axillary nodes with the fingertips gently rolling soft tissue. Palpate four areas of the axilla: the edge of the pectoralis major muscle along the anterior axillary line, the chest wall in the midaxillary area, the upper part of the humerus, and the anterior edge of the latissimus dorsi muscle along the posterior axillary line. Normally, lymph nodes are not palpable. Note the number, consistency, mobility, and size of palpable nodes. A palpable node feels like a small mass that is hard, tender, and immobile. Also palpate along the upper and lower clavicular ridges. Repeat the procedure for the patient's other side.

Perform palpation of breast tissue with the patient lying supine. This position allows the breast tissue to flatten evenly against the chest wall. The patient raises her hand and places it behind the neck to further stretch and position breast tissue evenly. Place a small pillow or towel under her shoulder blade to further position breast tissue (Fig. 7.38).

If the patient complains of a mass, examine the opposite breast first to ensure an objective comparison of normal and abnormal tissue. Use the pads of the first three fingers to compress breast tissue gently against the chest wall, noting tissue consistency. During a clinical breast examination, perform palpation systematically in one of three ways: (1) using a vertical technique with the fingers moving up and down each quadrant; (2) clockwise or counterclockwise, forming small circles with the fingers along each quadrant and the tail; or (3) palpating from center of the breast in a radial fashion, returning to the areola to begin each spoke (Fig. 7.39). Whatever approach you use, be sure to cover the entire breast and tail, directing attention to any areas of tenderness. When palpating large, pendulous breasts, use a bimanual technique. Support the inferior portion of the breast in one hand while using the other hand to palpate breast tissue against the supporting hand.

During palpation, note the consistency of breast tissue. The breasts of a young patient are firm and elastic. In an older patient, the tissue may feel stringy and nodular. The

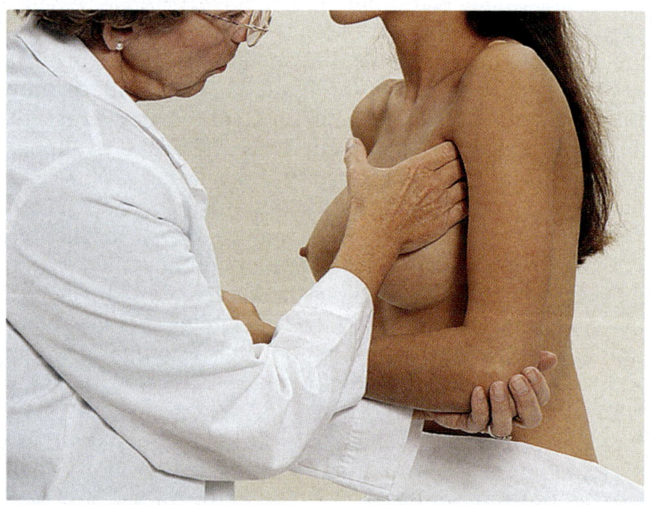

Fig 7.37 Support patient's arm and palpate axillary lymph nodes. (From Wilson S, Gidden J: *Health assessment for nursing practice,* ed 6, St Louis, 2016, Elsevier.)

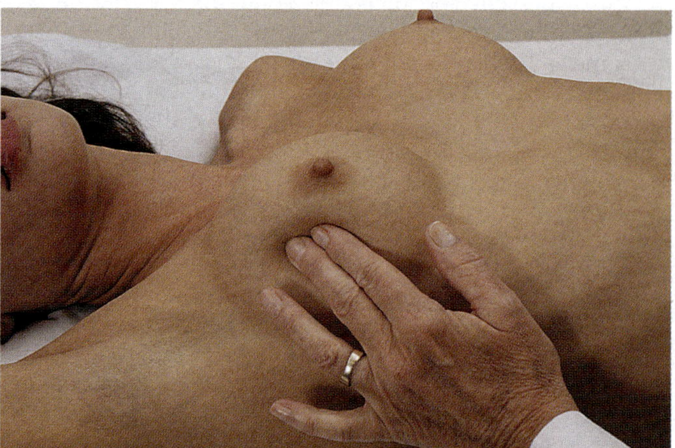

Fig. 7.38 Patient lies flat with arm abducted and hand under head to help flatten breast tissue evenly over the chest wall. (From Wilson S, Gidden J: *Health assessment for nursing practice,* ed 6, St Louis, 2016, Elsevier.)

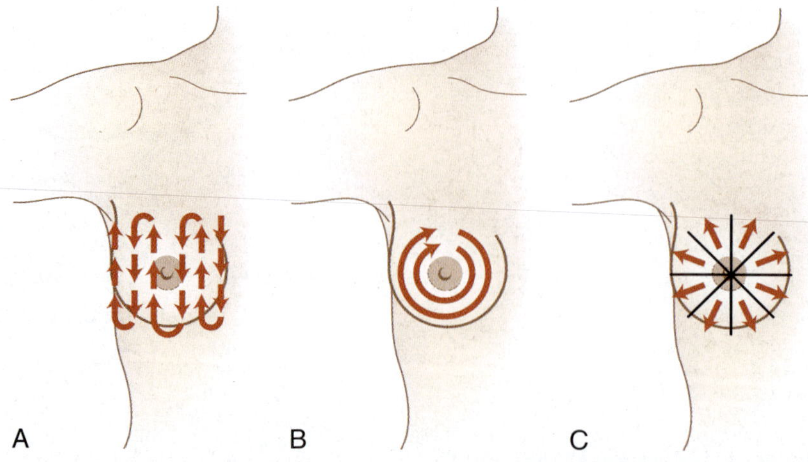

Fig. 7.39 Various methods for breast palpation. **A,** Palpate from top to bottom in vertical strips. **B,** Palpate in concentric circles. **C,** Palpate out from the center in wedge sections.

patient's familiarity with the texture of her own breasts is most important. The lobular feel of glandular tissue is normal. The lower edge of each breast feels firm and hard and indicates the normal inframammary ridge, not a tumor. It helps to move the patient's hand so that she feels normal tissue variations. Palpate abnormal masses to determine location in relation to quadrants, diameter in centimeters, shape (e.g., round or discoid), consistency (soft, firm, or hard), tenderness, mobility, and discreteness (clear or unclear borders). Cancerous lesions are hard, fixed, nontender, irregular in shape, and usually unilateral.

Pay special attention when palpating the nipple and areola. Palpate the entire surface gently. Use the thumb and index finger to compress the nipple and note any discharge. During the examination of the nipple and areola, the nipple may become erect with wrinkling of the areola. These changes are normal.

Male Breasts

Inspect the nipple and areola for nodules, edema, and ulceration. An enlarged male breast results from obesity or glandular enlargement. Steroid use contributes to breast enlargement in young men. Male breast cancer is associated with obesity, Klinefelter syndrome, and gynecomastia (NCI, 2014). Fatty tissue feels soft. Glandular tissue is firm. Use the same techniques to palpate for masses used in examination of the female breast. Because male breast cancer is relatively rare, routine self-examinations are unnecessary. However, men with a first-degree relative (e.g., mother) with breast cancer are at increased risk and should perform regular breast self-examinations.

Abdomen

The abdominal examination is complex because of the number of organs located within and near the abdominal cavity. It includes an assessment of structures of the lower GI tract in addition to the liver, stomach, uterus, ovaries, kidneys, and bladder. Abdominal pain is a common complaint of patients seeking health care. An accurate assessment requires matching patient history data with an assessment of the location of physical symptoms.

Assess the organs anteriorly and posteriorly. A system of landmarks helps to map out the abdominal region. The xiphoid process (tip of the sternum) is the upper boundary of the anterior abdominal region. The symphysis pubis is the lower boundary. Divide the abdomen into four imaginary quadrants to refer to assessment findings (Fig. 7.40A) and record them in relation to each quadrant. Posteriorly the lower ribs and heavy back muscles protect the kidneys, which are located from the T12 to L3 vertebrae (Fig. 7.40B). The **costovertebral angle** formed by the last rib and vertebral column is a landmark used during palpation of the kidney.

During the abdominal examination, use interventions that help the patient to relax. Tight abdominal muscles make palpation difficult. Ask the patient to void before beginning. Be sure that the room is warm and cover the patient's upper chest and legs. The patient lies supine or in a dorsal recumbent position with the arms at the sides and knees slightly bent. Place small pillows beneath the knees. If the patient places the arms under the head, the abdominal muscles tighten. Proceed calmly and slowly, being sure

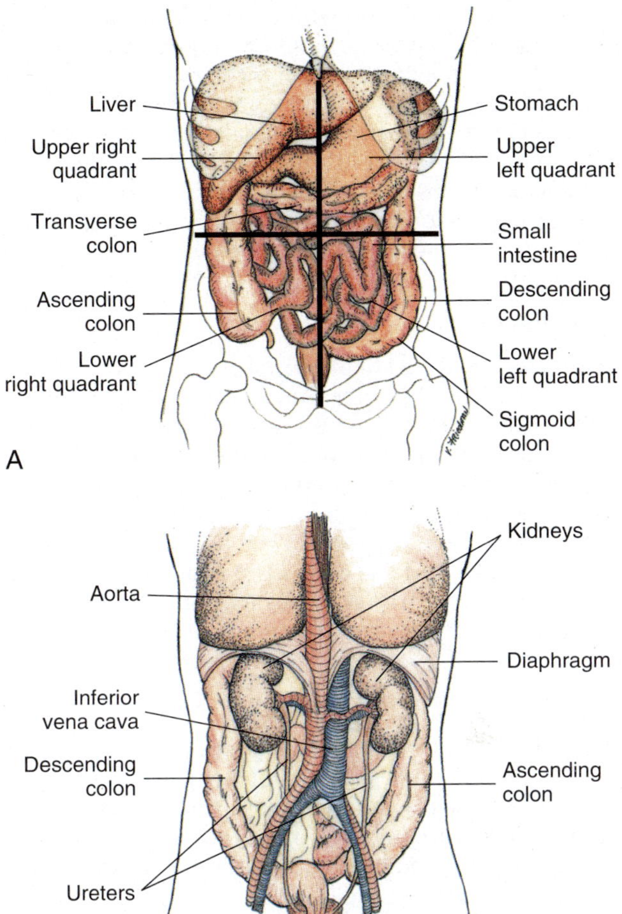

Fig. 7.40 A, Anterior view of abdomen divided by quadrants. **B,** Posterior view of abdominal sections.

that there is adequate lighting. Expose the abdomen from just above the xiphoid process down to the symphysis pubis. Warm hands and stethoscope promote relaxation. Ask the patient to report pain and point out areas of tenderness. Assess tender areas last.

The order for an abdominal examination differs slightly from that for previous assessments. Begin with inspection and then auscultation. By using auscultation before palpation, there is less chance of altering the frequency and character of bowel sounds. Palpation could falsely increase peristalsis. Have a tape measure and marking pen available during the examination.

Nursing History

Ask whether the patient has abdominal or low back pain, and assess the character of the pain in detail (see Chapter 11). Also review the patient's normal bowel habits and stool character, including use of laxatives. Determine whether the patient has had abdominal surgery, trauma, or diagnostic tests of the GI tract. Assess for difficulty swallowing, belching, flatulence (gas), bloody emesis (hematemesis), black or tarry stools (melena), heartburn, diarrhea, or constipation. Assess whether the patient has had a recent weight change or intolerance to diet (e.g., nausea, vomiting, or cramping). If the patient takes anti-inflammatory drugs (e.g., aspirin, ibuprofen, or steroids) and antibiotics, there is risk for GI upset or bleeding. Inquire about a family history of cancer, kidney disease, alcoholism, hypertension, or heart disease. Assess the patient's usual intake of alcohol. Also determine whether a female patient is pregnant and note the date of her last menstrual period. Review the patient's history for risk factors for hepatitis B virus (HBV) exposure (e.g., hemodialysis or i.v. drug use). Finally, ask the patient to locate any tender areas before beginning the examination.

Inspection

Always observe the patient during routine care activities. Note the patient's posture and look for evidence of abdominal splinting, lying with the knees drawn up, or moving restlessly in bed. A patient free from abdominal pain does not guard or splint the abdomen. To inspect the abdomen for abnormal movement or shadows, stand on the patient's right side and inspect the abdomen from above. By sitting down to look across the abdomen, you assess abdominal contour. Direct the examination light over the abdomen. Inspect it for continuity, any retractions, bulging, and symmetry.

Skin

Inspect the skin over the abdomen for color, scars, venous patterns, lesions, and striae (stretch marks). The skin is subject to the same color variations as the rest of the body. Venous patterns are normally faint except in thin patients. Artificial openings indicate drainage sites resulting from surgery or an ostomy (see Chapters 21 and 22). Scars reveal evidence of past trauma or surgery that created permanent changes in underlying organ anatomy. Bruising indicates accidental injury, physical abuse, or a type of bleeding disorder. Ask whether the patient self-administers injections (e.g., insulin or anticoagulants). Unexpected findings include generalized skin color changes such as jaundice or cyanosis. A glistening taut (tight) appearance indicates ascites.

Umbilicus

Note the position; shape; color; and presence of inflammation, discharge, or protruding masses. A normal umbilicus is flat or concave with the color the same as surrounding skin. Underlying masses (e.g., hernias) cause displacement of the umbilicus.

Contour and Symmetry

Inspect for contour, symmetry, and surface motion of the abdomen, noting any masses, bulging, or distention. A flat abdomen forms a horizontal plane from the xiphoid process to the symphysis pubis. A round abdomen protrudes in a convex sphere from a horizontal plane. A concave abdomen appears to sink into the muscular wall. Each of these findings is normal if the shape of the abdomen is symmetrical. In older adults, there is often an overall increased distribution of adipose tissue. The presence of masses on only one side, or asymmetry, indicates an underlying pathological condition.

Intestinal gas, tumor, or fluid in the abdominal cavity causes distention (swelling). When distention is generalized, the entire abdomen protrudes. The skin often appears taut, as if it were stretched over the abdomen. When gas causes distention, the flanks do not bulge. However, if fluid is the source of the problem such as in ascites, the flanks bulge. Ask the patient to roll onto one side. A protuberance forms on the dependent side if fluid is the cause of the distention. Ask the patient if the abdomen feels unusually tight. Be careful not to confuse distention with obesity. In obesity the abdomen is large, rolls of adipose tissue are often present along the flanks, and the patient does not complain of tightness in the abdomen. If abdominal distention is expected, measure the abdomen by placing a tape measure around it at the level of the umbilicus. Consecutive measurements show any increase or decrease in distention. Use a marking pen to indicate where you applied the tape measure.

Enlarged Organs or Masses

Observe the contour of the abdomen while asking the patient to take a deep breath and hold it. Normally, the contour remains smooth and symmetrical. To evaluate abdominal musculature, have the patient raise his or her head. This position causes superficial abdominal wall masses, hernias, and muscle separations to become more apparent.

Movement or Pulsations

Inspect for movement. A patient with severe pain has diminished respiratory movement and tightens abdominal muscles to guard against the pain. Observe for peristaltic movement and aortic pulsation by looking across the abdomen from side to side. These movements are visible in thin patients; otherwise, no movement is present.

Auscultation

In an abdominal examination, always auscultate before you palpate to reduce the risk of altering the frequency and intensity of bowel sounds. Ask the patient not to speak when you auscultate. Patients with GI tubes connected to suction need them temporarily turned off before beginning the examination.

Bowel Motility

Bowel sounds are the audible passage of air and fluid that normal intestinal contractions (peristalsis) create. Place the warmed diaphragm of the stethoscope lightly over each of the four quadrants (Fig. 7.41). Normally, air and fluid move through the intestines, creating soft gurgling or clicking

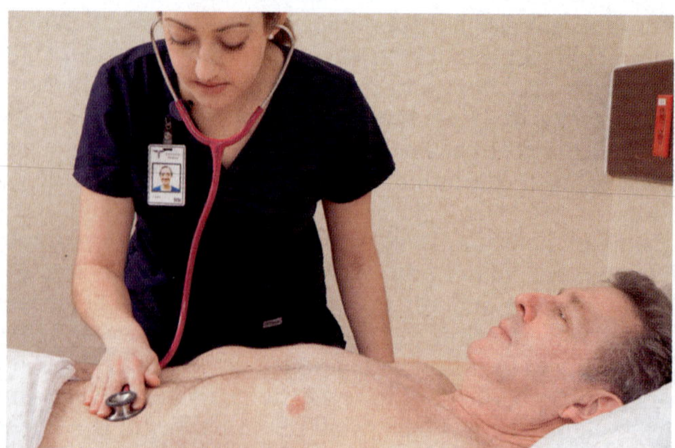

Fig. 7.41 Auscultation of abdomen using diaphragm of stethoscope.

sounds that occur irregularly 5–35 times per minute (Ball et al., 2015). Sounds may last 1/2 second to several seconds. It normally takes 5–20 seconds to hear a bowel sound. However, it takes 5 minutes of continuous listening before determining that bowel sounds are absent. Auscultate all four quadrants, starting in the right lower quadrant, to be sure that you do not miss any sounds. The best time to auscultate is between meals. Sounds are generally described as normal, audible, absent, hyperactive, or hypoactive.

Absent sounds indicate a lack of peristalsis, possibly caused by bowel obstruction, paralytic ileus (decreased or absent peristalsis), or peritonitis (inflammation of the peritoneum). Hyperactive sounds are loud, "growling" sounds (borborygmi) that indicate increased GI motility. Inflammation of the bowel, anxiety, bleeding, excess ingestion of laxatives, and reaction of the intestines to certain foods cause increased motility (Box 7.19).

Vascular Sounds

Bruits auscultated in affected blood vessels indicate narrowing of the blood vessels and turbulent disrupted blood flow. The presence of bruits in the abdominal area reveals aneurysms or stenotic vessels. Use the bell of the stethoscope to auscultate in the epigastric region and each of the four quadrants. Normally, there are no vascular sounds over the aorta (midline through the abdomen) or femoral arteries (lower quadrants). Report a bruit immediately to a health care provider.

Palpation

Palpation primarily detects areas of abdominal tenderness, distention, or masses. As assessment skills improve, learn to palpate for specific organs such as the liver using light and deep palpation.

Use light palpation over each abdominal quadrant. Initially, avoid areas previously identified as problem spots. Lay the palm of the hand with fingers extended and approximated lightly on the abdomen. Explain the maneuver to the patient; with the palmar surface of the fingers, depress 1.3 cm (1/2 inch) in a gentle dipping motion (Fig. 7.42A). Avoid quick jabs and use smooth, coordinated movements. For ticklish patients, first place the patient's hand on the abdomen with your hand on the patient's hand; continue until the patient tolerates palpation. Assess for muscular resistance, tenderness, distention, and superficial organs or masses. Observe for signs of discomfort. The abdomen is

BOX 7.19 Patient Teaching

Abdominal Assessment

Outcome

Patient experiences improved digestion and elimination health.

Teaching Strategies

- Explain factors that promote normal bowel elimination such as diet, regular exercise, limited use of over-the-counter drugs causing constipation, establishment of a regular elimination schedule, and adequate fluid intake (see Chapter 22).
- Caution the patient about dangers of excessive use of laxatives or enemas.
- Instruct the patient with new onset of abdominal pain or discomfort to be evaluated by a health care provider.
- If the patient has chronic pain, explain measures used for pain relief (e.g., relaxation exercises, positioning) (see Chapter 11).
- Instruct the patient about warning signs of colon cancer including rectal bleeding, cramping pain in lower abdomen, black or tarry stools, blood in the stool, and a change in bowel habits (constipation or diarrhea).
- Instruct the patient to report any noticeable yellowing of eyes, mucous membranes, or skin.
- If the patient is a health care worker or has contact with blood or body fluids of affected people, encourage the patient to receive series of three hepatitis B virus (HBV) vaccine doses.

Evaluation

- Use the principles of teach back to evaluate patient/family caregiver learning:
  - "Describe for me a meal plan that includes foods that will improve your bowel habits."
  - "Show me how to perform the relaxation exercise we reviewed to help reduce your abdominal pain."
  - "Explain to me the signs and symptoms of bowel problems that you should report to your doctor."
  - "Tell me the dates that you have had your HBV vaccine."
  - "Describe to me the signs and symptoms of colon cancer."

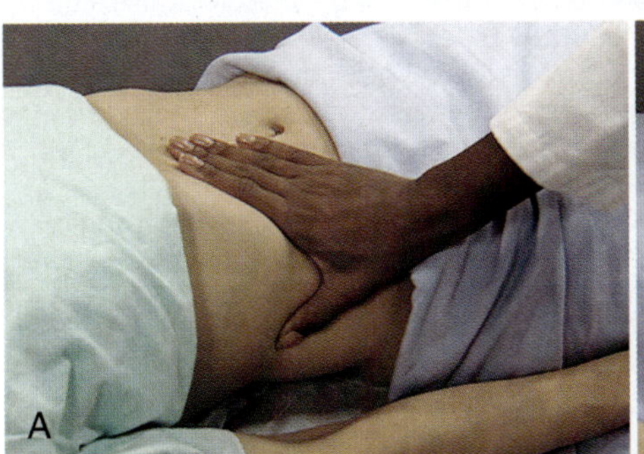

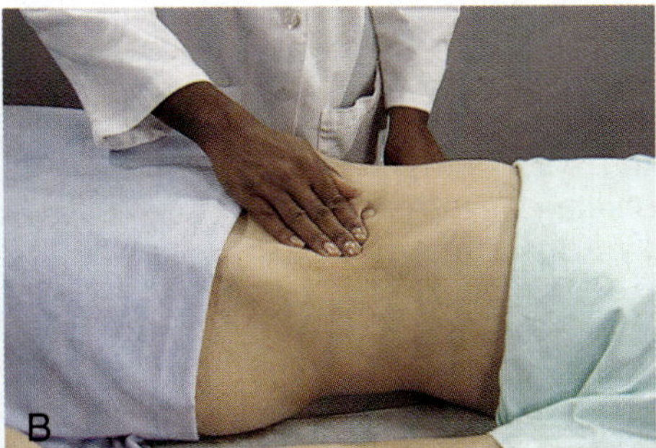

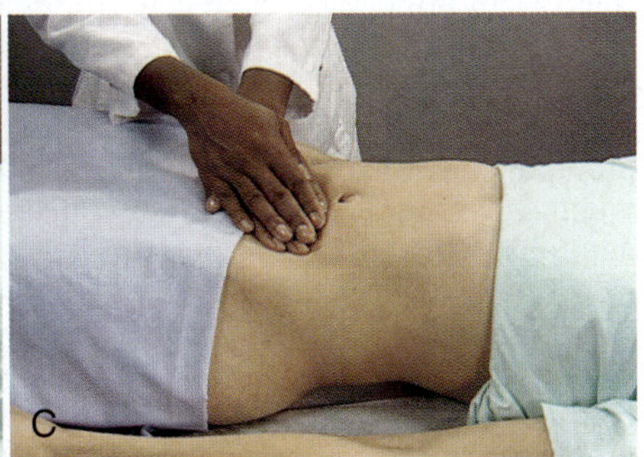

Fig. 7.42 A, Light palpation of abdomen. **B,** Deep palpation of abdomen. **C,** Deep bimanual palpation. (From Ball JW, et al: *Seidel's guide to physical examination*, ed 8, St Louis, 2015, Elsevier.)

normally smooth with consistent softness and nontender without masses. Older adults often lack abdominal tone.

With experience, perform deep palpation (Fig. 7.42B and C) to assess abdominal organs and detect less obvious masses. You need short fingernails. It is important for the patient to be relaxed while the hands depress approximately 2.5–7.5 cm (1–3 inches) into the abdomen. Never use deep palpation over a surgical incision or over extremely tender organs. It is also unwise to use deep palpation on abnormal masses. Deep pressure causes tenderness in the healthy patient over the cecum, sigmoid colon, and aorta and in the midline near the xiphoid process (Ball et al., 2015).

Assess each quadrant systematically. Palpate masses for size, location, shape, consistency, tenderness, pulsation, and mobility. Test for rebound tenderness by pressing a hand slowly and deeply into the involved area and then letting go quickly. The test is positive if the patient feels pain when the hand is released. Rebound tenderness occurs in patients with peritoneal irritation such as in appendicitis; pancreatitis; or any peritoneal injury causing bile, blood, or enzymes to enter the peritoneal cavity.

Aortic Pulsation

To assess aortic pulsation, palpate with the thumb and forefinger of one hand deeply into the upper abdomen just left of the midline. Normally, a pulsation is transmitted forward. If the aorta is enlarged from an aneurysm (localized dilation of a vessel wall), the pulsation expands laterally. Do not palpate a pulsating abdominal mass. In obese patients, it is often necessary to palpate with both hands, one on each side of the aorta.

Female Genitalia and Reproductive Tract

Examination of the female genitalia requires a calm, relaxed approach. The gynecological examination is one of the most difficult experiences for adolescents. Cultural background further adds to apprehension. For example, in some cultural groups, women allow only a female health care provider to perform a physical assessment. Other cultures have a strong social value for modesty. Provide a thorough explanation of the reason for the procedures used in the examination, and ask the patient whether there is a need for a chaperone during the examination. The lithotomy position assumed during the examination is often a source of embarrassment. Make the patient feel comfortable by correctly positioning and draping her. Be sure to explain each portion of the examination in advance so that the patient anticipates each action. Adolescents sometimes choose to have a female parent present in the examination room.

Sometimes, a patient requires a complete examination, including assessing external genitalia and performing a vaginal examination. As a nurse, you can examine external genitalia while performing routine hygiene measures or inserting a urinary catheter. An examination is a part of each woman's preventive health care because ovarian cancer was estimated to cause 14,240 deaths in 2016 and accounts for 5% of cancer deaths among women, more than any other gynecological cancer (ACS, 2016a).

Adolescents and young adults are examined because of the growing incidence of sexually transmitted infections (STIs). The average age of menarche among girls has declined, and most male and female teenagers are sexually active by the age of 19 years (Hockenberry et al., 2017). Because the patient assumes a lithotomy or dorsal recumbent position, rectal and anal assessments are combined with this examination.

Nursing History

Begin by asking what the patient hopes to learn or do as a result of the examination. Establish rapport with her to increase her comfort level, focusing on her feelings about exposing herself to a health care provider. Next, the nursing history reviews the patient's previous illnesses or surgeries involving reproductive organs, including STIs. A review of the menstrual history includes age at menarche, frequency and duration of menstrual cycle, character of flow, presence of dysmenorrhea (painful menstruation), pelvic pain, dates of last two menstrual periods, and premenstrual symptoms. Ask whether the patient has had signs of bleeding, vaginal discharge, or pain outside the normal menstrual period or after menopause. Ask whether she has symptoms or history of genitourinary problems such as burning during urination, frequency, urgency, nocturia, hematuria, incontinence, or stress incontinence.

It is important to remember that this nursing history usually contains sensitive information. The adolescent may be uncomfortable sharing symptoms and other valuable information if a parent or guardian is in the room. Whenever possible, obtain the history with just the patient present.

Ask the patient to describe her obstetrical history, including each pregnancy and history of abortions or miscarriages. Also question her about current and past contraceptive practices and problems encountered. It is important to determine whether the patient uses safe sex practices. Discuss risks of STIs and HIV infection. Also, review a patient's risk for developing cervical, endometrial, or ovarian cancer (Box 7.20).

BOX 7.20 Patient Teaching

Female Genital and Reproductive Tract Assessment

Outcome

Patient follows routine preventive and safety measures for gynecological health.

Teaching Strategies

- Instruct the patient in the purpose and recommended frequency of Papanicolaou (Pap) tests and gynecological examinations. Explain that the Pap test is needed annually for women who are sexually active or older than 21 years. Patients are screened more often if certain risk factors exist such as a weak immune system, multiple sex partners, smoking, and a history of infections (e.g., human papillomavirus [HPV]).
- Counsel women and men about genital HPV infection and the need to receive the HPV vaccine. The vaccine is ideally recommended at the age of 11 or 12 years (ACS, 2016a).
- Counsel patients with sexually transmitted infections (STIs) about diagnosis and treatment.
- Instruct in genital self-examination: Using a mirror, position self to examine the area covered by the pubic hair. Spread the hair apart, looking for bumps, sores, or blisters. Also, look for any warts, which appear as small, bumpy spots and enlarge to

BOX 7.20 Patient Teaching—cont'd

fleshy, cauliflower-like lesions. Next, spread the outer vaginal lips apart and look at the clitoris for bumps, blisters, sores, or warts. Also, look at both sides of the inner vaginal lips. Inspect the area around the urinary and vaginal openings for bumps, blisters, sores, or warts.

- Explain warning signs of STIs: pain or burning on urination, pain during sex, pain in the pelvic area, bleeding between menstrual periods, itchy rash around the vagina, and vaginal discharge.
- Teach measures to prevent STIs: male partner's use of condoms, restricting number of sexual partners, avoiding sex with people who have several other partners, and perineal hygiene measures.
- Tell patients with STIs to inform their sexual partner or partners of the need for an examination.
- Reinforce the importance of perineal hygiene (as appropriate).

Evaluation

- Use the principles of teach back to evaluate patient/family caregiver learning:
  - "Explain to me why routine gynecological examination and Pap test are important."
  - "Describe to me ways to prevent transmission of STIs."
  - "Tell me how you will use safe sex practices."

Preparation of the Patient

It is your responsibility to assist the patient's primary health care provider with the examination. For a complete examination, you need the following special equipment: examination table with stirrups, vaginal speculum of correct size, adjustable light source, sink, clean gloves, plastic or wooden spatula, cervical brush or broom device, glass slides and cytological fixative, culture plates or media, and deoxyribonucleic acid (DNA) probe kits for chlamydia and gonorrhea (Ball et al., 2015).

Make sure that equipment is ready before the examination begins. Ask the patient to empty her bladder; often it is necessary to collect a urine specimen. For an external genitalia assessment, help the patient to the lithotomy position in bed or on an examination table. On the table, place and stabilize her feet into stirrups for a speculum examination and have her slide the buttocks down to the edge of the table. Place a hand at the edge of the table and instruct the patient to move until touching the hand. Her arms should be at her sides or folded across the chest to prevent tightening of abdominal muscles.

Provide a drape or sheet for the patient. A good method is to cover the knees and symphysis, depressing the drape between her knees (Ball et al., 2015). After the examination begins, lift the drape over the perineum. A male examiner always needs to have a female attendant during the examination. A female examiner may prefer to work alone but should have a female attendant if the patient is particularly anxious, is emotionally unsteady, or has requested one.

External Genitalia

Make sure that the perineal area is well illuminated. Apply clean gloves on both hands. The perineum is extremely sensitive and tender; do not touch the area suddenly without warning the patient. It is best to touch the neighboring thigh first before advancing to the perineum.

While sitting at the end of the examination table or bed, inspect the quantity and distribution of hair growth. Preadolescents have no pubic hair. During adolescence, hair grows along the labia, becoming darker, coarser, and curlier. In an adult, hair grows in a triangle over the female perineum and along the medial surface of the thighs. Normally, it is free of nits and lice.

Inspect surface characteristics of the labia majora. The skin of the perineum is smooth, clean, and slightly darker than other skin. The mucous membranes appear dark pink and moist. The labia majora are gaping or closed and appear dry or moist. They are usually symmetrical. After childbirth, the labia majora separate, causing the labia minora to become more prominent. When a woman reaches menopause, the labia majora become thinned. With advancing age, they become atrophied (decrease in size). The labia majora are normally without inflammation, edema, lesions, or lacerations.

To inspect the remaining external structures, use your nondominant hand and gently place the thumb and index finger inside the labia minora and retract the tissues outward (Fig. 7.43). Be sure to have a firm hold to avoid repeated retraction against the sensitive tissues. Use the other hand to palpate the labia minora between the thumb and second finger. On inspection, the labia minora are normally thinner than the labia majora, and one side is sometimes larger. The tissue feels soft on palpation and without tenderness. The size of the clitoris varies, but it normally does not exceed 2 cm (3/4 inch) in length and 0.5 cm (1/4 inch) in diameter. Look for **atrophy,** inflammation, or adhesions. If inflamed, the clitoris is a bright cherry red. In young women, the clitoris is a common site for syphilitic lesions or chancres, which appear as small open ulcers that drain serous material. Some older women have malignant changes that result in dry, scaly, nodular lesions.

Inspect the urethral orifice carefully for color and position. Normally, it is intact and without inflammation. The urethral meatus is anterior to the vaginal orifice and pink.

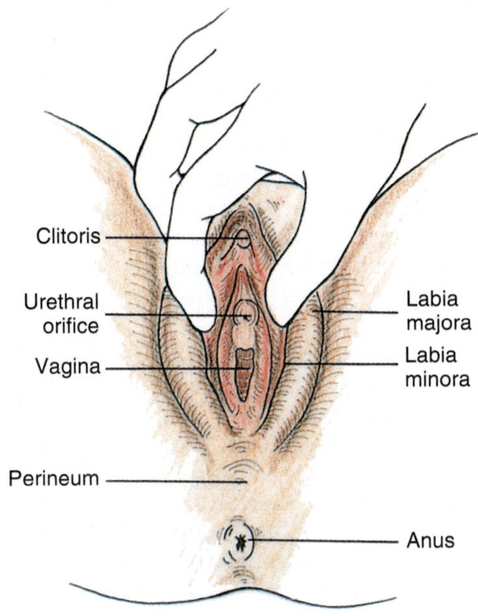

Fig. 7.43 Female external genitalia.

It appears as a small slit or pinhole opening just above the vaginal canal. Note any discharge, polyps, or fistulas.

Inspect the vaginal orifice (introitus) for inflammation, edema, discoloration, discharge, and lesions. Normally, the introitus is a thin vertical slit or large orifice. The tissue is moist. While inspecting the vaginal orifice or introitus, note the condition of the hymen, which is just inside the introitus. In the virgin female, the hymen restricts the opening of the vagina. Only remnants of the hymen remain after sexual intercourse.

Inspect the anus looking for lesions and hemorrhoids (see rectal examination). After completion of the external examination, dispose of examination gloves, offer the patient perineal hygiene, and perform hand hygiene.

Patients who are at risk for contracting STIs need to learn to perform a genital self-examination (see Box 7.20). The purpose of the examination is to detect signs or symptoms of STIs. Many people do not know that they have an STI (e.g., chlamydial infection), and some STIs (e.g., syphilis) can remain undetected for years. Therefore, it is essential to stress the importance of regular screening for STIs in sexually active individuals.

Speculum Examination of Internal Genitalia

An examination of internal genitalia requires much skill and practice. Advanced practice nurses and primary care providers perform this examination. Beginning students more than likely only observe the procedure or assist the examiner by helping the patient with positioning, handing off specimen supplies, and comforting the patient.

The examination involves use of a plastic or metal speculum consisting of two blades and an adjustable thumbscrew. The examiner inserts the speculum into the vagina to assess the vaginal walls and cervix for cancerous lesions and other abnormalities. During the examination, the examiner collects a sample for a Papanicolaou (Pap) test for cervical and vaginal cancer.

Male Genitalia

An examination of the male genitalia assesses the integrity of the external genitalia, inguinal ring, and canal. Because the incidence of STIs in adolescents and young adults is high, an assessment of the genitalia needs to be a routine part of any health maintenance examination for this age group. Use a calm, gentle approach to lessen the patient's anxiety. Offer the patient the option of having a companion or parent available during the examination. Have him void and then lie supine with the chest, abdomen, and lower legs draped or stand during the examination. Apply clean gloves.

Nursing History

Begin by explaining the purpose of the genital examination. Especially for adolescents, discuss the components of the male examination. Review the patient's normal urinary elimination pattern, including frequency of voiding; history of nocturia; character and volume of urine; daily fluid intake; and symptoms of burning, urgency and frequency, difficulty starting stream, and hematuria. The history also includes a review of previous surgery or illness involving urinary or reproductive organs including STIs. The patient's sexual history and use of safe sex habits identify any risks for HIV infection or other STIs. Patients at risk require extensive education. Ask whether the patient has difficulty achieving erection or ejaculation, and review medications that influence sexual performance including diuretics, sedatives, antihypertensives, and tranquilizers. Ask whether the patient has noted penile pain or swelling, genital lesions, or urethral discharge, which indicate signs and symptoms of STIs. The patient's knowledge of testicular self-examination provides a guide for health teaching (Box 7.21). Determine whether the patient has noticed heaviness or painless enlargement of a testis or irregular lumps (warning signs of testicular cancer). If he reports an enlargement in the inguinal area, assess whether it is intermittent or constant; whether it is associated with straining or lifting;

BOX 7.21 Patient Teaching

Male Genitalia Assessment

Outcome

Patient follows routine preventive and safety measures for genital and testicular health.

Teaching Strategies

- Provide the following information about genital self-examination to all male patients 15 years and older:
  - Perform examination monthly after a warm bath or shower when the scrotal sac is relaxed and less thick.
  - Stand naked in front of a mirror, hold the penis in your hand, and examine the head. Pull back the foreskin if uncircumcised to expose the glans (see illustration A).
  - Inspect and palpate the entire head of the penis in a clockwise motion, looking carefully for any bumps, sores, blisters, or unusual discharge. Blisters and bumps may be light colored or red and resemble pimples.
  - Look for genital warts.
  - Look at the opening (urethral meatus) at the end of the penis for discharge.
  - Look along the entire shaft of the penis for the same signs.
  - Be sure to separate pubic hair at the base of the penis and carefully examine the skin underneath.
- Provide the following information about testicular self-examination (TSE) to all men 15 years and older:
  - Look for swelling or lumps in the skin of the scrotum while looking in the mirror.
  - Use both hands, placing the index and middle fingers under the testicles and the thumb on top (see illustration B).
  - Gently roll the testicle, feeling for lumps, swelling, soreness, or change in consistency (hardening).
  - Find the epididymis (a cordlike structure on the top and back of the testicle; it is not a lump).
  - Feel for small, pea-size lumps on the front and side of the testicle. The lumps are usually painless and are abnormal.
  - Call your health care provider about abnormal findings.
  - Counsel patients with sexually transmitted infections (STIs) about diagnosis and treatment.
  - Explain warning signs of STIs: pain on urination and during sex, abnormal penile discharge (different from usual), swollen lymph nodes, or rash or ulcer on skin or genitalia.
  - Teach measures to prevent STIs: use of condoms, avoiding sex with infected partners, restricting number of sexual partners, avoiding sex with people who have multiple partners, using regular perineal hygiene.
  - Tell patients with an STI to inform sexual partner or partners of the need to have an examination.
  - Instruct patient to seek treatment as soon as possible if partner becomes infected with an STI.

BOX 7.21 **Patient Teaching—cont'd**

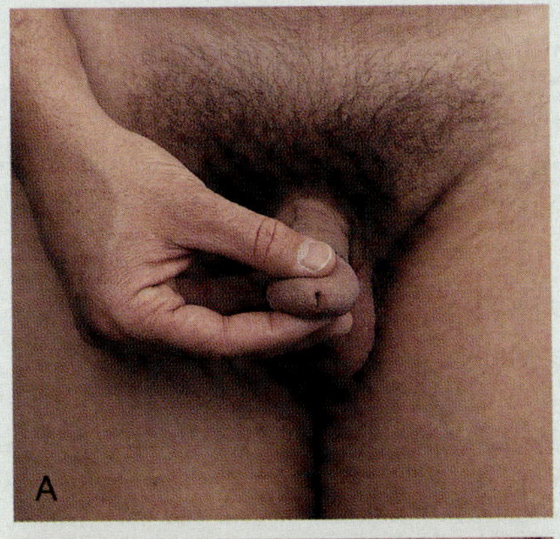

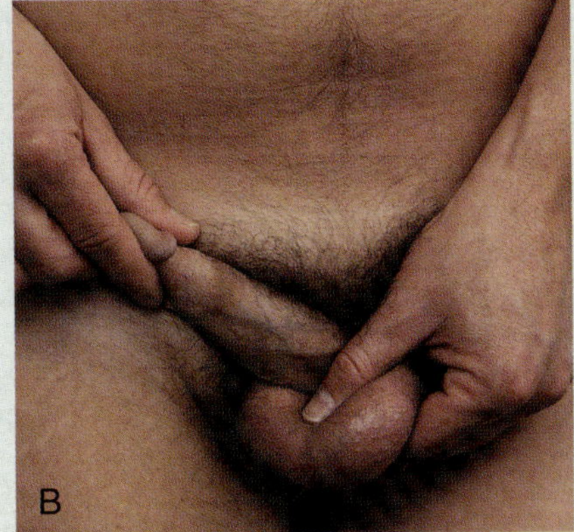

Evaluation

- Use the principles of teach back to evaluate patient/family caregiver learning:
  - "Demonstrate to me how you perform genital self-examination and testicular self-examination."
  - "Describe for me ways you can prevent getting a sexually transmitted disease."

Illustrations from Ball JW, et al: *Seidel's guide to physical examination,* ed 8, St Louis, 2015, Elsevier.

whether it is painful; and whether coughing, lifting, or straining at stool increases the pain. These are all signs and symptoms that indicate an inguinal hernia.

Sexual Maturity

First note the sexual maturity of the patient by observing the size and shape of the penis and testes; the size, color, and texture of scrotal skin; and the character and distribution of pubic hair. The testes first increase in size in preadolescence. By the end of puberty, the testes and penis enlarge to adult size and shape, and scrotal skin darkens and becomes wrinkled. Hair growth occurs with puberty, and hair is coarse and abundant in the pubic area. The penis has no hair, and the scrotum has very little hair. Also inspect the skin covering the genitalia for lice, rashes, excoriations, or lesions. Normally, the skin is clear, without lesions.

Penis

To inspect penile surfaces thoroughly, manipulate the genitalia or have the patient help. Inspect the corona, prepuce (foreskin), glans, urethral meatus, and shaft (Fig. 7.44). In uncircumcised patients, retract the foreskin to reveal the glans and urethral meatus. The foreskin usually retracts easily. A small amount of white, thick smegma sometimes collects under this foreskin. In the circumcised male patient, the glans is exposed. It should look smooth and pink along all surfaces. The urethral meatus is slitlike and normally positioned at the tip of the glans. In some congenital conditions, the meatus is displaced along the penile shaft. The area between the foreskin and glans is a common site for venereal lesions.

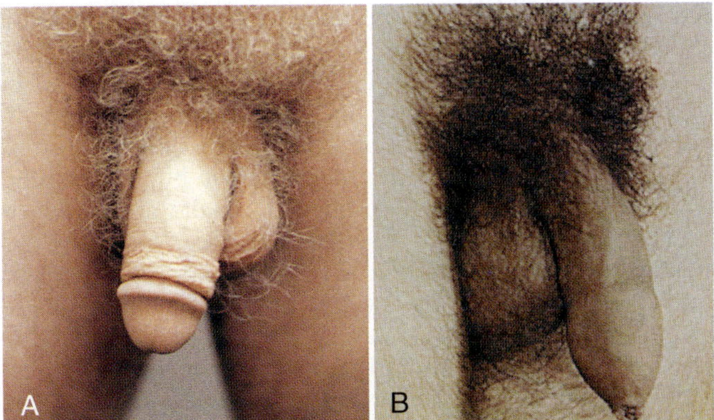

Fig. 7.44 Normal male genitalia. **A,** Circumcised. **B,** Uncircumcised. (From Ball JW, et al: *Seidel's guide to physical examination,* ed 8, St Louis, 2015, Elsevier.)

Gently compress the glans between your thumb and index finger; this opens the urethral meatus for inspection of discharge, lesions, and edema. Normally, the opening is glistening and pink without discharge. Palpate any lesion gently to note tenderness, size, consistency, and shape. When inspection and palpation of the glans are complete, pull the foreskin down to its original position. Continue by inspecting the entire shaft of the penis including the undersurface looking for any lesions, scars, or edema. Palpate the shaft between the thumb and first two fingers to detect localized areas of hardness or tenderness. A patient who has lain in bed for a prolonged time may develop dependent edema in the penile shaft.

It is important for all male patients to learn to perform a genital self-examination to detect signs and symptoms of STIs. Many people who have an STI do not know it. Self-examination is a routine part of self-care (see Box 7.21).

Scrotum

Be especially cautious while inspecting and palpating the scrotum because the structures that lie within the scrotal sac are very sensitive. The scrotum is divided internally into two halves. Each half contains a testicle, epididymis, and the vas deferens, which travels upward into the inguinal ring. Normally, the left testicle is lower than the right. Inspect the size, color, shape, and symmetry of the scrotum while observing for lesions or edema.

Gently lift the scrotum to view the posterior surface. The scrotal skin is usually loose, and the surface is coarse. The skin color is often more deeply pigmented than body skin. Tightening or loss of wrinkling reveals edema. The size of the scrotum normally changes with temperature variations, contracting in cold and relaxing in warm temperature. Lumps in the scrotal skin are commonly sebaceous cysts.

Testicular cancer is a solid tumor commonly found in young men 18–34 years of age. Early detection is critical. Explain testicular self-examination while examining the patient. The testes are normally sensitive but not tender. The underlying testicles are normally ovoid and approximately 2 × 4 cm (3/4 × 1⅝ inches) in size. While the patient retracts the penis upward, gently palpate the testes and epididymis between the thumb and first two fingers (Fig. 7.45). Note the size, shape, and consistency of tissue and ask whether the patient feels any tenderness. The testes feel smooth and rubbery and are free from nodules. The epididymis is resilient. In older adults, the testicles decrease in size and are less firm during palpation. The most common symptoms of testicular cancer are a painless enlargement of one testis and appearance of a palpable small, hard lump about the size of a pea on the front or side of the testicle. Continue to palpate the vas deferens separately as it forms the spermatic cord toward the inguinal ring, noting nodules or swelling. It normally feels smooth and discrete.

Inguinal Ring and Canal

The external inguinal ring provides the opening for the spermatic cord to pass into the inguinal canal. The canal forms a passage through the abdominal wall, a potential site for hernia formation. A hernia is a protrusion of a portion of intestine through the inguinal wall or canal. Sometimes, an intestinal loop enters the scrotum. The patient stands during this portion of the examination.

During inspection, ask the patient to strain or bear down. The maneuver helps to make a hernia more visible. Look for obvious bulging in the inguinal area. Complete the examination by palpating for inguinal lymph nodes. Normally, small, nontender, mobile horizontal nodes are palpable. Any abnormality indicates local or systemic infection or malignant disease.

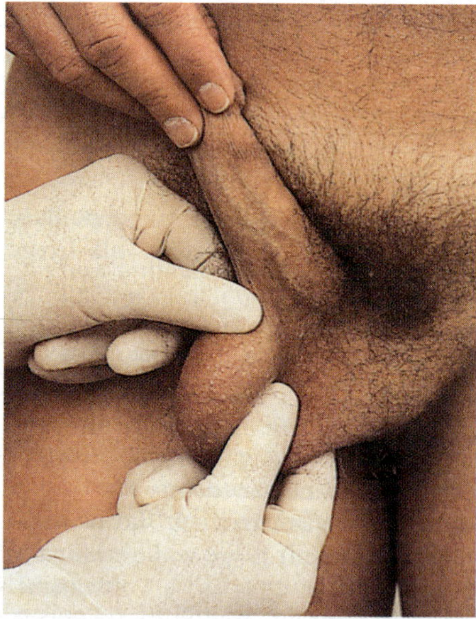

Fig. 7.45 Palpating contents of scrotal sac. (From Ball JW, et al: *Seidel's guide to physical examination*, ed 8, St Louis, 2015, Elsevier.)

Rectum and Anus

A good time to perform the rectal examination is after the genital examination. This examination is not performed in the examination in children or adolescents. The examination can detect colorectal cancer in its early stages. In men, the rectal examination also detects prostatic enlargement and tumors. The rectal examination is uncomfortable; thus, explaining all steps helps the patient relax.

Nursing History

The nursing history reviews a patient's risk factors for colorectal cancer including personal and family history of colorectal cancer, polyps, obesity, physical inactivity, long-term smoking, moderate to heavy alcohol consumption, and diet (ACS, 2016a). Determine whether the patient has experienced bleeding from the rectum, black or tarry stools (melena), rectal pain, or change in bowel habits, all of which are warning signs of colorectal cancer (ACS, 2017). Assess dietary habits including intake of high-fat foods, diet high in processed or red meats, or deficient fiber content, which are linked to colon cancer. Determine whether the patient has undergone screening for colorectal cancer (digital examination, fecal occult blood test, flexible sigmoidoscopy, and colonoscopy). Ask male patients whether they have experienced weak or interrupted urine flow, an inability to urinate, or difficulty starting or stopping the urine flow. In addition, ask whether they have had polyuria; nocturia; hematuria; dysuria; or continuing pain in the lower back, pelvis, or upper thighs. These all are warning signs of prostate cancer. Finally, review the patient's use of laxatives, cathartics, codeine, or iron preparations, which can cause elimination problems (Box 7.22).

BOX 7.22 Patient Teaching

Rectal and Anal Assessment

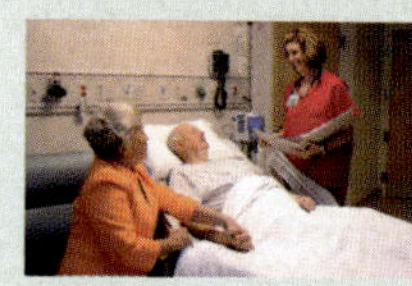

Outcome

Mr Neal follows recommended guidelines for early detection of colorectal cancer and prostate screenings.

Teaching Strategies

- Discuss the ACS guidelines (ACS, 2017; 2016a) for early detection of colorectal cancer. Beginning at 50 years of age both men and women at average risk should use one of these screening tests (ACS, 2017):
  - Fecal occult blood test (FOBT) or fecal immunochemical test (FIT) annually *or*
  - Flexible sigmoidoscopy (FSIG): visual inspection of the rectum and lower colon with a hollow, lighted tube performed by a health care provider every 5 years *or*
  - Double-contrast barium enema every 5 years *or*
  - Colonoscopy every 10 years *or*
  - Computed tomography (CT) colonoscopy every 5 years
- Individuals at increased risk need to discuss options with their health care provider.
- Discuss warning signs of colorectal cancer.
- Discuss dietary planning and healthy lifestyle choices to maintain or improve colon health.
- Warn patients about problems caused by overuse of laxatives, cathartic medications, codeine, or enemas.

BOX 7.22 Patient Teaching—cont'd

- Discuss with male patients the ACS guidelines (ACS, 2016a) for early detection of prostatic cancer:
  - Discuss with male patients the warning signs of prostate cancer.
  - Beginning at 50 years of age, patients should have a conversation with their health care provider discussing risks and screen opportunities.
  - This discussion should start at 45 years of age for men at high risk including African American men and men who have a first-degree relative diagnosed with prostate cancer at an early age (before 65 years of age).
  - The discussion starts at 40 years of age for patients at even higher risk (history of several relatives positive for prostate cancer).

Evaluation

- Use the principles of teach back to evaluate patient/family caregiver learning:
  - "Tell me when you should have your next rectal examination."
  - "Explain to me the warning signs of colorectal and prostate cancer."
  - "Describe to me a meal that would contain the right types of food choices to maintain your colon health."

Inspection

Female patients remain in the dorsal recumbent position after the genitalia examination, or they assume a side-lying (Sims) position. The best way to examine male patients is to have the patients stand and bend over forward with the hips flexed and upper body resting across the examination table. Examine a nonambulatory patient in Sims position.

Using the nondominant hand, gently retract the buttocks to view the perianal and sacrococcygeal areas. Perianal skin is smooth and more pigmented and coarser than skin overlying the buttocks. Inspect anal tissue for skin characteristics, lesions, external hemorrhoids (dilated veins that appear as reddened skin protrusions), ulcers, inflammation, rashes, or excoriation. Anal tissues are moist and hairless, and the anus is held closed by the voluntary external sphincter. Next, ask the patient to bear down as though having a bowel movement. Any internal hemorrhoids or fissures appear at this time. Use clock referents (e.g., 12 o'clock or 5 o'clock) to describe the location of findings. There normally is no protrusion of tissue.

Digital Palpation

Examine the anal canal and sphincters with digital palpation. In male patients, palpate the prostate gland to rule out enlargement. Usually advanced practitioners perform this part of the examination.

Musculoskeletal System

The assessment of the musculoskeletal system focuses on determining ROM, muscle strength and tone, and joint and muscle condition. The examination is conducted as a separate examination as for a sports physical or integrated into other parts of the total physical examination. Assess this system while performing other nursing care measures such as bathing or positioning. Muscular disorders often result from neurological disease. For this reason, health care providers often conduct a neurological assessment simultaneously.

While examining the patient's musculoskeletal function, visualize the anatomy of bone and muscle placement and joint structure (see Chapter 14). Joints vary in their degree of mobility. Some joints such as in the knee are freely movable. The spinal vertebrae are examples of slightly movable joints. For a complete examination, you uncover the limb or area being examined so that the muscles and joints are free to move. Have the patient sit, lie supine or prone, or stand while assessing muscle groups.

Nursing History

Determine the patient's history of musculoskeletal injury or trauma resulting from sports, employment, exercise, or chronic illnesses. Assess for osteoporosis risk factors including use of alcohol and/or caffeine; cigarette smoking; constant dieting; poor calcium or vitamin D intake; thin and light body frame; nulliparous status; menopause before 45 years of age; estrogen deficiency; postmenopause status; family history of osteoporosis; Caucasian, Asian, native American, or Northern European ancestry; advanced age; history of fractures and/or falls; sedentary lifestyle; chronic diseases (e.g., Cushing disease, hyperthyroidism and hypothyroidism, malabsorption and/or malnutrition disorders, neoplasms); long-term use of corticosteroids, methotrexate, phenytoin, and aluminum-containing antacids; and lack of exposure to sunlight.

The nursing history includes a patient's description of problems with bone, muscle, or joint function including history of recent falls, trauma, lifting heavy objects, fractures, and bone or joint disease. It is useful to assess a patient's normal activity pattern including the type of exercise routinely performed (Box 7.23). Also assess the nature and extent of pain or stiffness and determine whether alterations affect the patient's ability to perform ADLs, sleep, and participate in social activities.

General Inspection

Observe the patient's gait and posture when entering the examination room. The gait is more natural when a patient is unaware of being observed. Later, a more formal test has the patient walk in a straight line away, turn, and return to the origin point. Note how the patient walks, sits, and rises from a sitting position. Normally, patients walk with arms swinging freely at the sides and the head leading the body. Older adults walk with smaller steps and a wider base of support. Note foot dragging, limping, shuffling, and the position of the trunk in relation to the legs. Compare extremities bilaterally. Patients in wheelchairs or who use walking assistance are assessed for smooth movements and stability.

Observe the patient from the side in a standing position. The normal standing posture is an upright stance with parallel alignment of the hips and shoulders (Fig. 7.46). There should be an even contour of the shoulders, level scapulae and iliac crests, alignment of the head over the gluteal folds, and symmetry of extremities. With the patient standing sideways, note the normal cervical, thoracic, and lumbar curves. Holding the head erect is normal. As the patient sits, some degree of rounding of the shoulders is normal. Older adults tend to assume a stooped, forward-bent posture, with

BOX 7.23 Patient Teaching

Musculoskeletal Assessment

Outcome

Patient follows measures to prevent or minimize osteoporosis.

Teaching Strategies

- Instruct the patient in correct postural alignment. Consult with a physical therapist to provide the patient with exercises for improving posture.
- Explain that the risk for osteoporosis increases after 50 years of age; women and men should have screening completed by health care providers (NIH, 2015).
- Instruct patients to reduce the risk of fractures by increasing bone density and reducing the risk of falls (NIH, 2015):
  - Building and maintaining bone density: Perform weight-bearing exercises (e.g., walking, climbing stairs, dancing). Perform resistance exercises, such as weight training with free weights or weight machines.
  - Reducing risk of falls: Perform activities to improve balance (yoga, tai chi), flexibility (yoga, tai chi, swimming, stretching exercises), and strength (resistance exercises).
- Encourage intake of calcium and vitamin D to meet the recommended daily allowance. Increased vitamin D aids calcium absorption.
  - Recommendation for calcium supplements is 1000 mg/day for men and women up to the age of 50 and 1200 mg/day for women older than 50 years and men older than 70 years (NIH, 2015).
  - Recommendation for vitamin D supplement is 600 mg/day for men and women up to 70 years of age and increased to 800 mg/day after the age of 70 years (NIH, 2015).
- Explain to patients with low back pain that they will benefit from modification of worker risk factors (e.g., lifting heavy weights, use of protective equipment), regular aerobic exercise, exercises that strengthen the back and increase trunk flexibility, and learning how to lift properly.
- Instruct older adults and adults with osteoporosis in proper body mechanics and ROM and moderate weight-bearing exercises (e.g., swimming, walking) to minimize trauma and subsequent bone fractures.
- Instruct older patients to pace activities to compensate for loss in muscle strength (Touhy and Jett, 2018).

Evaluation

- Use the principles of teach back to evaluate patient/family caregiver learning:
  - "Describe for me the types of exercises you can begin to do that will lessen the risks related to osteoporosis."
  - "Show me how you perform range-of-motion exercises."
  - "Let's review what we discussed about calcium and vitamin D. What are the doses to take each day?"

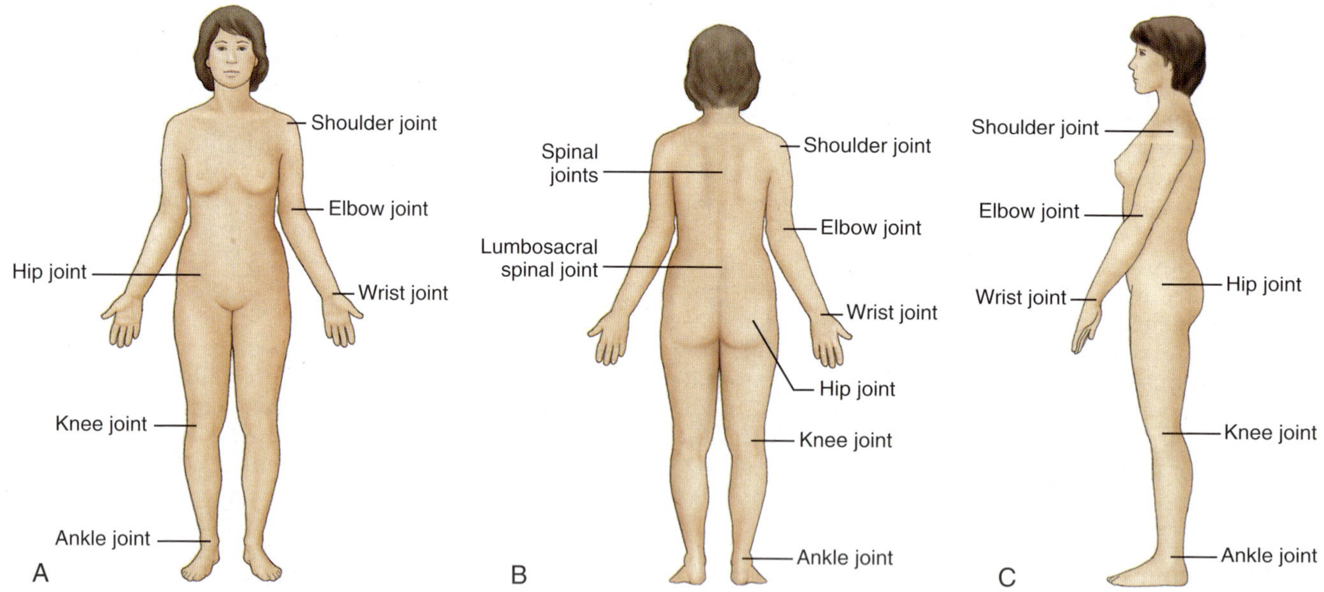

Fig. 7.46 Inspection of overall body posture. **A,** Anterior view. **B,** Posterior view. **C,** Lateral view. (From Muscolino JE: *Kinesiology: the skeletal system and muscle function,* ed 2, St Louis, 2011, Elsevier.)

hips and knees somewhat flexed and arms bent at the elbows, raising the level of the arms.

Common postural abnormalities include lordosis, kyphosis, and scoliosis (Fig. 7.47). Lordosis, or swayback, is an increased lumbar curvature. Kyphosis, or hunchback, is an exaggeration of the posterior curvature of the thoracic spine. This postural abnormality is common in older adults. Scoliosis is a lateral spinal curvature. Loss of height is frequently the first clinical sign of osteoporosis, in which height loss occurs in the trunk as a result of vertebral fracture and collapse. Osteoporosis is a metabolic bone disease that causes a decrease in quality and quantity of bone. The National Institutes of Health (NIH) reports that 53 million Americans already have or are at risk for developing osteoporosis secondary to low bone mass (NIH, 2015). Although a small amount of height loss is expected with aging, if the amount of loss is great, osteoporosis is likely. As men and women age, they are more likely to have osteoporotic fractures of the forearm and/or wrists, hips, and vertebrae.

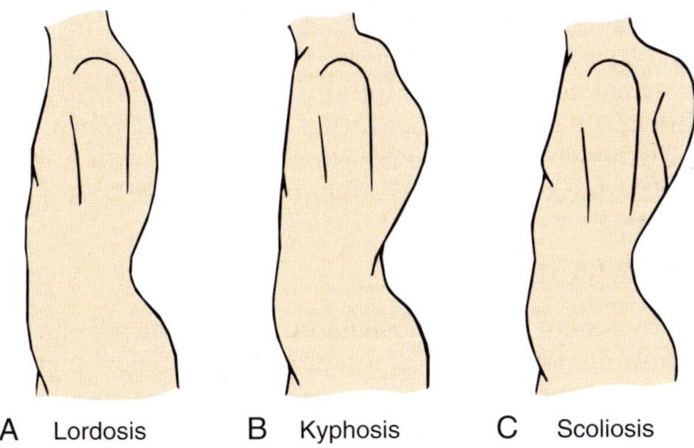

Fig. 7.47 Common postural abnormalities. **A,** Lordosis. **B,** Kyphosis. **C,** Scoliosis.

During general inspection, look at the extremities for overall size, gross deformity, bony enlargement, alignment, and symmetry. Normally, there is bilateral symmetry in length, circumference, alignment, and position and number of skinfolds (Ball et al., 2015). A general review pinpoints the areas requiring specialized assessment.

Palpation

During a complete examination, apply gentle palpation to all bones, joints, and surrounding muscles. In the case of a focused assessment, examine only the involved area. Note any warmth, tenderness, edema, or resistance to pressure. The patient should feel no discomfort when you apply palpation. Muscles should be firm. When assessing the vertebrae, ask the patient to bend at the waist, arms hanging down. Bimanually palpate either side of the spinal column to note any deviations or curvatures.

Range of Joint Motion

The examination includes comparison of both active and passive full ROM. Ask the patient to put each major joint and its muscle groups through full ROM. Learn the terminology for each joint movement (Table 7.9), and teach the patient how to move each joint through ROM. To assess passive ROM, ask the patient to relax, and you then passively move the joints through their ROM. Compare the same body parts for equality in movement. Do not force a joint into a painful position. Know the normal range of each joint and the extent to which you can move the patient's joints. Ideally, assess the patient's normal range to determine a baseline for assessing later change. Joints are typically free from stiffness, instability, swelling, or inflammation. There normally is no discomfort when applying pressure to bones and joints. In older adults, joints often become swollen and stiff, with reduced ROM resulting from cartilage erosion and fibrosis of synovial membranes. If a joint appears swollen and inflamed, palpate it for warmth.

Muscle Tone and Strength

Assess muscle strength and tone during ROM measurement. Note muscle tone (i.e., the slight muscular resistance felt as you move the relaxed extremity passively through its ROM). Ask the patient to allow an extremity to relax or hang limp, which is sometimes difficult if the patient feels pain in the extremity. Support the extremity and grasp each limb, moving it through the normal ROM. Normal tone causes a mild, even resistance to passive movement through the entire range.

If a muscle has increased tone, or hypertonicity, you meet considerable resistance with sudden passive movement of a joint. Continued movement eventually causes the muscle to relax. A muscle that has little tone (hypotonicity) feels flabby. The involved extremity hangs loosely in a position determined by gravity.

For assessment of muscle strength, the patient assumes a stable position. The patient performs maneuvers demonstrating strength of major muscle groups (Table 7.10). Compare symmetrical muscle pairs for strength based on a grading scale of 0−5 (Table 7.11). The arm on the dominant side is normally stronger than the arm on the nondominant side. In older adults, a loss of muscle mass causes bilateral weakness, but muscle strength remains greater in the dominant arm or leg.

Examine each muscle group. Ask the patient first to flex the muscle to be examined and then to resist when you apply opposing force against that flexion (Fig. 7.48). It is important to not allow the patient to move the joint. Gradually increase pressure to a muscle group (e.g., elbow extension). Have the patient resist the pressure applied by attempting to move against resistance (e.g., elbow flexion).

Table 7.9 Terminology for Normal Range-of-Motion Positions

Term	Range of Motion	Examples of Joints
Flexion	Movement decreasing angle between two adjoining bones; bending of limb	Elbow, fingers, knee
Extension	Movement increasing angle between two adjoining bones	Elbow, fingers, knee
Hyperextension	Movement of body part beyond normal resting extended position	Head
Pronation	Movement of body part so that front or ventral surface faces downward	Hand, forearm
Supination	Movement of body part so that front or ventral surface faces upward	Hand, forearm
Abduction	Movement of extremity away from midline of body	Leg, arm, fingers
Adduction	Movement of extremity toward midline of body	Leg, arm, fingers
Internal rotation	Rotation of joint inward	Knee, hip
External rotation	Rotation of joint outward	Knee, hip
Eversion	Turning of body part away from midline	Foot
Inversion	Turning of body part toward midline	Foot
Dorsiflexion	Flexion of toes and foot upward	Foot
Plantar flexion	Bending of toes and foot downward	Foot

Table 7.10 Maneuvers to Assess Muscle Strength

Muscle Group	Maneuver
Neck (sternocleidomastoid)	Place hand firmly against the patient's upper jaw. Ask the patient to turn head laterally against resistance.
Shoulder (trapezius)	Place hand over midline of the patient's shoulder, exerting firm pressure. Have the patient raise shoulder against resistance.
Elbow	
▪ Biceps	Pull down on forearm as the patient attempts to flex arm.
▪ Triceps	Apply pressure against forearm as you flex the patient's arm. Ask the patient to straighten the arm.
Hip	
▪ Quadriceps	When the patient is sitting, apply downward pressure to thigh. Ask the patient to raise the leg up from table.
▪ Gastrocnemius	The patient sits while examiner holds shin of flexed leg. Ask the patient to straighten the leg against resistance.

Table 7.11 Muscle Strength

Muscle Function Level	Grade
No evidence of contractility	0
Trace of movement	1
Full ROM, not against gravity[a]	2
Full ROM against gravity but not against resistance	3
Full ROM against gravity; some resistance but weak	4
Full ROM against gravity; full resistance	5

ROM, range of motion.
[a]Passive movement.
From Ball JW, et al: *Seidel's guide to physical examination,* ed 8, St Louis, 2015, Elsevier.

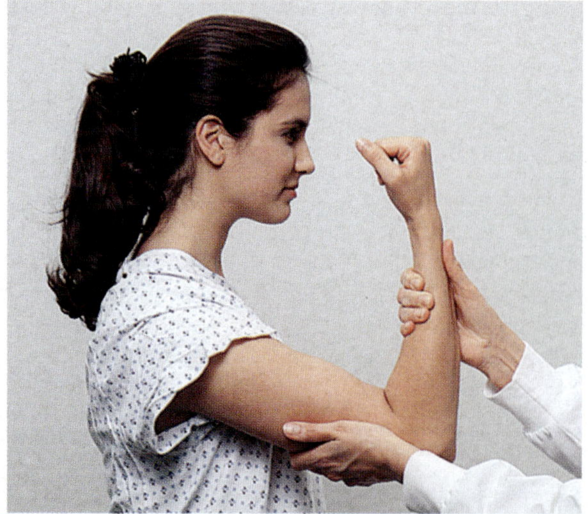

Fig. 7.48 Assess muscle strength: flexion of elbow against opposing force. (From Wilson S, Gidden J: *Health assessment for nursing practice,* ed 6, St Louis, 2016, Elsevier.)

The patient resists until instructed to stop. Vary the amount of pressure applied and observe the joint move. If you identify a weakness, compare the size of the muscle with its opposite counterpart by measuring the circumference of the muscle body with a tape measure. A muscle that has atrophied (reduced in size) feels soft and baggy when palpated.

Neurological System

An assessment of neurological function alone is quite time-consuming. For efficiency, integrate neurological measurements with other parts of the physical examination. For example, test cranial nerve function while assessing the head and neck. Observe mental and emotional status during the initial interview.

Consider many variables when deciding the extent of the examination. A patient's level of consciousness influences the ability to follow directions. General physical status influences tolerance to assessment. A patient's description of signs and symptoms helps to determine the need for a thorough neurological assessment. If a patient complains of headache or a recent loss of function in an extremity, he or she needs a complete neurological assessment. For a complete examination, you need the following special equipment:

- Reading material
- Vials of aromatic substances (e.g., orange, peppermint extract, coffee)
- Opposite tip of cotton swab broken in half or paper clip for testing ability to distinguish sharp from dull
- Snellen eye chart
- Penlight
- Vials containing sugar, salt, and lemon with applicators
- Tongue blade
- Two test tubes containing hot and cold water for temperature sensation testing
- Cotton balls or cotton-tipped applicators
- Tuning fork
- Reflex hammer
- Familiar objects such as coins, keys, or paperclips

Nursing History

Review the patient's use of analgesics, alcohol, sedative-hypnotics, antipsychotics, antidepressants, nervous system stimulants, or recreational drugs. In addition, review the patient's use of over-the-counter sleeping aids. Determine whether the patient has a recent history of seizures and/or convulsions and screen for symptoms of headache, tremors, dizziness, vertigo, numbness or tingling of body parts, visual changes, weakness, pain, or changes in speech. The presence of any symptom requires a more detailed review (e.g., onset, severity, precipitating factors, sequence of events). Discuss with the patient's family any recent changes in the patient's behavior (e.g., increased irritability, mood swings, memory loss, change in energy level). Ask the patient for a history of changes in vision, hearing, smell, taste, and touch. A history of head or spinal cord trauma, meningitis, congenital anomalies, neurological disease, or psychiatric counseling focuses your assessment of select findings. If an older adult patient displays sudden acute confusion (delirium), review history for drug toxicity, serious infections, metabolic disturbances, heart failure, and severe anemia.

Mental and Emotional Status

You learn about mental capacities and emotional state by interacting with a patient. Ask questions during an examination to gather data and observe the appropriateness of emotions and thoughts. Special assessment tools designed to assess a patient's mental status are available. For example, the Mini-Mental State Examination (MMSE) measures a patient's orientation and cognitive function. It asks questions such as "What is the date?" and "Tell me where you are now."

To ensure an objective assessment, consider a patient's cultural and educational background, values, beliefs, and previous experiences. An alteration in mental or emotional status reflects a disturbance in cerebral functioning. The cerebral cortex controls and integrates intellectual and emotional functioning. Primary brain disorders, medications, and metabolic changes are examples of factors that change cerebral function.

Level of Consciousness

A person's level of consciousness exists along a continuum from being fully awake, alert, and cooperative to unresponsiveness to any form of external stimuli. Talk with the patient, asking questions about events involving him or her or concerns about health problems. A fully conscious patient responds to questions quickly and expresses ideas logically. As a patient's consciousness lowers, use the Glasgow Coma Scale (GCS) for an objective measurement of consciousness on a numerical scale (Table 7.12). The patient needs to be as alert as possible before testing. Use caution when using the GCS if a patient has sensory losses (e.g., vision or hearing) or is intubated with mechanical ventilation. The GCS allows evaluation of a patient's neurological status over time. The higher the score, the better the patient's neurological function. Ask short, simple questions such as "What is your name?" or "Where are you?" Also, ask the patient to follow simple commands such as "Move your toes."

If a patient is not conscious enough to follow commands, try to elicit a pain response. Apply firm pressure with the thumb over the root of the patient's fingernail. The normal response to painful stimuli is withdrawal of the body part from the stimulus.

Table 7.12 Glasgow Coma Scale

Action	Response	Score
Eyes open	Spontaneous opening	4
	To verbal stimuli	3
	To pain	2
	No response	1
Verbal response	Oriented to appropriate stimulation	5
	Confused	4
	Inappropriate words	3
	Incoherent	2
	No response	1
Motor response	Obeys commands	6
	Localizes pain	5
	Withdraws from pain	4
	Flexion to pain (decorticate)	3
	Extension to pain (decerebrate)	2
	None	1

Patient's total score ranges from 3 to 15.
The patient's best response is matched to the criteria for scoring.

Behavior and Appearance

Behaviors, moods, hygiene, grooming, and choice of dress reveal pertinent information about mental status. Assess the patient's mannerisms and actions during the entire physical assessment. Note both nonverbal and verbal behaviors. Does the patient respond appropriately to directions? Does his or her mood vary with no apparent cause? Does he or she show concern about appearance? Is the patient's hair clean and neatly groomed, and are the nails trimmed and clean? The patient should behave in a manner expressing concern and interest in the examination. He or she should make eye contact and express appropriate feelings that correspond to the situation. Normally, a patient's appearance shows some degree of personal hygiene.

Choice and fit of clothing reflect socioeconomic background or personal taste rather than deficiency in self-concept or self-care. Avoid being judgmental and focus assessments on the appropriateness of clothing for the weather. Older adults sometimes neglect their appearance because of a lack of energy, finances, or reduced vision.

Language

Normal cerebral function allows a person to understand spoken or written words and express himself or herself through written words or gestures. Assess the patient's voice inflection, tone, and manner of speech. Normally, a patient's voice has inflections, is clear and strong, and increases in volume appropriately. Speech is fluent. When communication is clearly ineffective (e.g., omission or addition of letters and words, misuse of words, hesitations), assess the patient for aphasia.

Injury to the cerebral cortex results in aphasia. The two types of aphasia are sensory (or receptive) and motor (or expressive). With receptive aphasia, a person cannot understand written or verbal speech. With expressive aphasia, a person understands written and verbal speech but cannot write or speak appropriately when attempting to communicate. A patient sometimes suffers from a combination of receptive and expressive aphasia. When communication is ineffective, assess language capabilities with simple assessment techniques. Ask the patient to name familiar objects when pointing at them. Ask him or her to respond to simple verbal commands such as "Stand up." Finally ask the patient to read a simple sentence out loud. Normally, a patient names objects correctly, follows commands, and reads sentences correctly.

Intellectual Function

Intellectual function includes memory, knowledge, abstract thinking, and judgment. Testing each aspect of function involves a specific technique. However, because cultural and educational background influences the ability to respond to test questions, do not ask questions related to concepts or ideas with which the patient is unfamiliar. Validate information with a family member if appropriate.

Memory

Assess immediate recall and recent and remote memory. Patients demonstrate immediate recall by repeating a series of numbers in the order they are presented or reverse order. Patients normally recall five to eight digits forward or four to six digits backward.

First explain that you will test the patient's memory. Then state clearly and slowly the names of three unrelated objects. After stating all three, ask the patient to repeat each. Continue until the patient is successful. Later in the assessment, ask the patient to repeat the three words again. The patient should be able to identify the three words. Another test for recent memory involves asking the patient to recall events occurring during the same day (e.g., what was eaten for breakfast).

To assess past memory, ask the patient to recall the maiden name of the patient's mother, a birthday, or a special date in history. Compare the response with recorded data from the health record. It is best to ask open-ended questions rather than simple yes/no questions. A patient usually has immediate recall of such information. With older adults, do not interpret a hearing loss as confusion.

Knowledge

Assess knowledge by asking how much the patient knows about his or her illness or the reason for seeking health care. You can also ask questions about basic facts (e.g., who is the president?). By assessing a patient's knowledge, you can determine his or her ability to learn or understand. If there is an opportunity to teach, test the patient's mental status by asking for feedback during a follow-up visit.

Abstract Thinking

Interpreting abstract ideas or concepts reflects the capacity for abstract thinking. For an individual to explain common sayings such as "A stitch in time saves nine" or "Don't count your chickens before they're hatched" requires a higher level of intellectual functioning. Note whether the patient's explanations are relevant and concrete. A patient with altered mental state would probably interpret the phrase literally or merely rephrase the words.

Judgment

Judgment requires a comparison and evaluation of facts and ideas to understand their relationships and form appropriate conclusions. Attempt to measure the patient's ability to make logical decisions with questions such as "Why did you decide to seek health care?" or "What would you do if you suddenly became ill at home?" Normally, a patient makes logical decisions.

Cranial Nerve Function

Although cranial nerve function is not commonly completed as part of the bedside assessment, you may test all 12 cranial nerves or a single nerve or related group of nerves to determine function. A dysfunction in one nerve reflects an alteration at some point along the distribution of the cranial nerve. Measurements used to assess the integrity of organs within the head and neck also assess cranial nerve function. A complete assessment involves testing the 12 cranial nerves in order of their numbers. To remember the order of the nerves, using a simple phrase is helpful. One example is: "On old Olympus' towering tops a Finn and German viewed some hops." The first letter of each word in the phrase is the same as the first letter of the names of the cranial nerves listed in order (Table 7.13).

Table 7.13 Cranial Nerve Function and Assessment

Cranial Nerve	Name	Type	Function	Assessment Method
I	Olfactory	Sensory	Sense of smell	Ask the patient to identify different aromas in each nostril such as coffee and vanilla.
II	Optic	Sensory	Visual acuity and visual fields	Use Snellen chart or ask the patient to read printed material while wearing glasses.
III	Oculomotor	Motor	Pupil constriction and dilation	Measure pupil reaction to light reflex and accommodation.
			Extraocular eye movement	Assess directions of gaze.
IV	Trochlear	Motor	Upward and inward eye movement	Assess directions of gaze.
V	Trigeminal	Sensory	Sensory nerve to cornea, eyelids, forehead, skin of face	Lightly touch cornea with wisp of cotton. Assess corneal reflex. Measure sensation of light pain and touch across skin of face.
		Motor	Motor nerve to muscles of jaw	Palpate temples as the patient clenches teeth; observe chewing.
VI	Abducens	Motor	Lateral eye movement	Assess directions of gaze.
VII	Facial	Sensory	Taste	Have the patient identify salty or sweet taste on front of tongue.
		Motor	Facial expression	Look for asymmetry as the patient smiles, frowns, puffs out cheeks, and raises and lowers eyebrows.
VIII	Auditory	Sensory	Hearing and equilibrium	Assess ability to hear spoken word.
IX	Glossopharyngeal	Sensory	Taste	Ask the patient to identify sour or sweet taste on back of tongue.
		Motor	Ability to swallow and speak	Use tongue blade to elicit gag reflex; have the person swallow.
X	Vagus	Sensory	Sensation of pharynx and behind ear	Ask the patient to say "Ah." Observe movement of palate and pharynx.
		Motor	Movement of vocal cords	Assess speech for hoarseness.
XI	Spinal accessory	Motor	Movement of shoulders and head	Ask the patient to shrug shoulders and turn head against passive resistance.
XII	Hypoglossal	Motor	Position of tongue	Ask the patient to stick out tongue to midline and move it from side to side.

Sensory Function

The sensory pathways of the central nervous system conduct the sensations of pain, temperature, position, vibration, and crude and finely localized touch. Different nerve pathways relay the sensations. Most patients require only a quick screening of sensory function unless there are symptoms of reduced sensation, motor impairment, or paralysis.

Normally, a patient has sensory responses to all stimuli tested. The patient feels sensations equally on both sides of the body in all areas. Perform all sensory testing with the patient's eyes closed so that the patient is unable to see when or where a stimulus strikes the skin (Table 7.14). Then apply stimuli in a random, unpredictable order to maintain the patient's attention and prevent detection of a predictable pattern. Ask the patient to describe when, what, and where each stimulus is felt. Compare symmetrical areas of the body while applying stimuli to the arms, trunk, and legs.

Motor Function

An assessment of motor function includes measurements made during the musculoskeletal examination. In addition, you assess cerebellar function. The cerebellum coordinates muscular activity, maintains balance and equilibrium, and helps to control posture. Patients with any degree of motor dysfunction are at risk for injury (Box 7.24).

Coordination

To avoid confusion, demonstrate each maneuver and have the patient repeat it while you observe for smoothness and balance in the patient's movement. In older adults, normally slow reaction time causes movements to be less rhythmical.

BOX 7.24 Patient Teaching

Neurological Assessment

Outcome

Patient and family caregiver learn the warning signs of stroke and follow safety measures needed for reduced neurologic function.

Teaching Strategies

- Teach the patient and family caregiver to seek emergency care to rule out stroke with any of these symptoms: any sudden visual changes; sudden confusion; change in speech; weakness, sudden numbness, tingling, or loss of movement, especially on one side of the body.
- Teach the patient and family caregiver to immediately seek emergency treatment for a sudden, severe headache that is different from past headaches.
- Explain to family or friends the implications of any behavioral or mental impairment shown by the patient.
- If the patient has sensory or motor impairments, explain measures to ensure safety (e.g., use of ambulation aids, use of safety bars in bathrooms or on stairways).
- Teach older adults to plan enough time to complete tasks because their reaction time is slow.

Evaluation

- Use the principles of teach back to evaluate patient/family caregiver learning:
  - "As a family member, describe the patient's behaviors that you would observe if he were to have a stroke."
  - "Explain safety measures that you are using at home to prevent injury from the weakness you have in your left leg."

Table 7.14 Assessment of Sensory Nerve Function

Function	Equipment	Method	Precautions
Pain	End of paper clip or wooden end of cotton applicator	Ask the patient to say when he or she feels dull or sharp sensation. Alternately apply sharp and blunt ends of paper clip or broken cotton swab to surface of skin. Note areas of numbness or increased sensitivity.	Remember that areas where skin is thickened such as heel or sole of foot are less sensitive to pain.
Temperature	Two test tubes, one filled with hot water, one filled with cold water	Touch skin with tube. Ask the patient to identify hot or cold sensation.	Omit test if pain sensation is normal.
Light touch	Cotton ball or cotton-tipped applicator	Apply light wisp of cotton to different points along surface of skin. Ask the patient to say when he or she feels sensation.	Apply at areas where skin is thin or more sensitive (e.g., face, neck, inner aspect of arms, top of feet and hands).
Vibration	Tuning fork	Apply stem of vibrating fork to distal interphalangeal joint of fingers and interphalangeal joint of great toe, elbow, and wrist. Have the patient say when and where he or she feels vibration.	Be sure that the patient feels vibration and not merely pressure.
Position		Grasp finger or toe, holding it by its sides with thumb and index finger. Alternate moving finger or toe up and down. Ask the patient to say when finger is up or down. Repeat with toes.	Avoid rubbing adjacent appendages as you move finger or toe. Do not move joint laterally; return to neutral position before moving again.
Two-point discrimination	Two ends of paper clip	Lightly apply one or both ends of paper clip simultaneously to surface of skin. Ask the patient whether he or she feels one or two pricks. Find the distance at which the patient can no longer distinguish two points.	Apply paper clip tips to same anatomical site (e.g., fingertips, palm of hand, upper arms). Minimum distance at which the patient discriminates two points varies (2–8 mm on fingertips).

To assess fine-motor function, have the patient extend the arms out to the sides and touch each forefinger alternately to the nose, first with eyes open, then with eyes closed (Fig. 7.49). Performing rapid, rhythmical, alternating movements demonstrates coordination in the upper extremities. While sitting, the patient begins by patting the knees with both hands. Then he or she alternately turns up the palm and back of the hands while continuously patting the knees (Fig. 7.50). Test lower extremity coordination with the patient lying supine, legs extended. Place your hand at the ball of the patient's foot. The patient taps the hand with the foot as quickly as possible, alternating feet. The feet do not normally move as rapidly or evenly as the hands.

Balance

Assess balance and gross motor function by asking the patient to stand with feet together, arms at the sides, both with eyes open and with eyes closed. Protect the patient's safety by standing at the side and observe for swaying. Expect slight swaying of the body in the Romberg test. A loss of balance (positive Romberg) causes a patient to fall to the side.

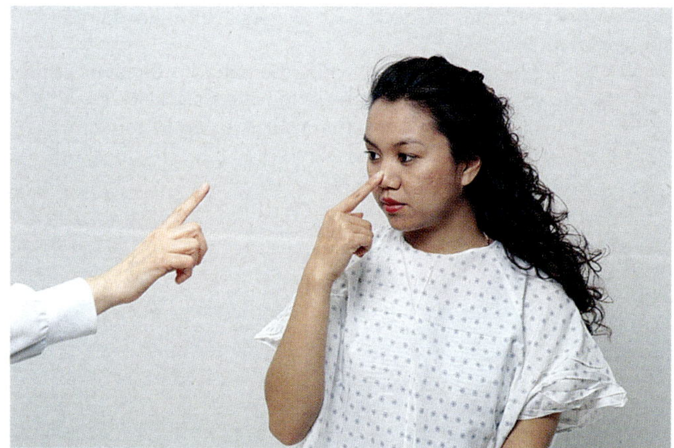

Fig. 7.49 Examination of fine motor function. (From Wilson S, Gidden J: *Health assessment for nursing practice*, ed 6, St Louis, 2016, Elsevier.)

Reflexes

Eliciting reflexes, usually performed by an advanced practice nurse, assesses integrity of sensory and motor pathways. Deep tendon reflexes are elicited by mildly stretching a muscle and tapping a tendon with a reflex hammer. Cutaneous reflexes are tested by stimulating the skin superficially.

After the Examination

Record the physical assessment findings during the examination or at the end. Specific forms are available to record data. Review all findings before helping the patient dress in case of a need to recheck any information or gather additional data. Integrate physical assessment findings into the plan of care.

Give the patient time to dress after completing the assessment. A hospitalized patient often needs help with hygiene and returning to bed. When the patient is comfortable, share a summary of the assessment findings. If the findings show serious abnormalities such as an irregular heart rate, consult the patient's health care provider before revealing any findings. It is the health care provider's responsibility to make definitive medical diagnoses. Explain the type of abnormality found and the need for the health care provider to conduct an additional examination.

The examination space needs to be cleaned when you are finished. Use infection control practices to remove materials or instruments soiled with potentially infectious wastes. If the patient's bedside was the site for the examination, clear away soiled items from the bedside table and make sure the bed linen is dry and clean. The patient will appreciate a clean gown and the opportunity to wash the face and hands. Afterward be sure to perform hand hygiene.

Arrange for ordered ancillary examinations after a physical examination if needed such as X-ray film examinations, laboratory tests, or ultrasonography. These tests provide additional screening information to rule out and help diagnose specific abnormalities found during the examination. Explain the purpose of these tests and the sensations that the patient will experience.

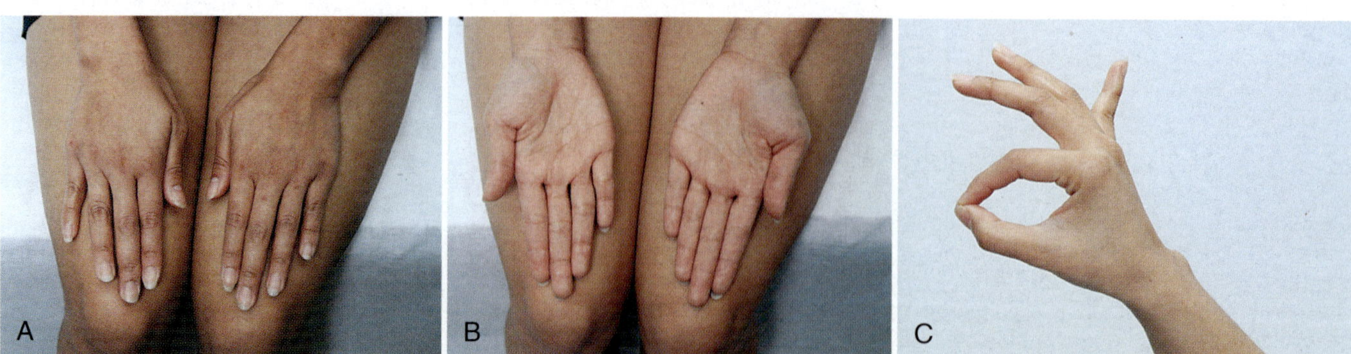

Fig. 7.50 Examination of coordination with rapid alternating movements. **A** and **B,** Alternatively pat knees with back and then palm of both hands. **C,** Touch thumb to each finger in sequence, increasing in speed. (From Wilson S, Gidden J: *Health assessment for nursing practice*, ed 6, St Louis, 2016, Elsevier.)

KEY POINTS

- Baseline assessment findings reflect a patient's functional abilities and serve as the basis for comparison with subsequent assessment findings.
- Physical assessment of a child or infant requires application of the principles of growth and development.
- The normal process of aging affects physical findings collected from an older adult.
- If you suspect substance abuse, conduct a NIDA Quick Screen to determine the patient's need for further intervention.
- Integrate patient teaching throughout the examination to help patients learn about health promotion and disease prevention.
- Inspection requires good lighting, full exposure of the body part, and a careful comparison of the part with its counterpart on the opposite side of the body.
- Palpation involves the use of parts of the hand to detect different types of physical characteristics.
- Use auscultation to assess the character of sounds created in various body organs.
- Perform a physical examination only after properly preparing the environment and equipment and preparing the patient physically and psychologically.
- Keep the patient warm, comfortable, and informed of each step of an examination. Ensure confidentiality.
- Be systematic while combining assessments of different body systems simultaneously.
- Information from the history helps to focus on body systems likely to be affected.
- Creating a mental image of internal organs in relation to external anatomical landmarks enhances accuracy in assessing the thorax, heart, and abdomen.
- When assessing heart sounds, imagine events occurring during the cardiac cycle.
- Never palpate the carotid arteries simultaneously.
- When examining a woman's breasts, explain the techniques for BSE.
- The abdominal assessment differs from other parts of the examination in that auscultation follows inspection.
- During assessment of the genitalia, explain the technique for genital self-examination.
- Assess musculoskeletal function when observing a patient ambulate or participate in other active movements.
- Assess mental and emotional status by interacting with the patient throughout the examination.
- At the end of the examination, provide for the patient's comfort and document a detailed summary of physical assessment findings.

REFERENCES

American Cancer Society (ACS). Breast cancer early detection and diagnosis. 2015. Available from: http://www.cancer.org/cancer/breastcancer/moreinformation/breastcancerearlydetection/breast-cancer-early-detection-acs-recs.

American Cancer Society (ACS). Cancer facts and figures 2016. 2016a. Available from: https://www.cancer.org/research/cancer-facts-statistics/all-cancer-facts-figures/cancer-facts-figures-2016.html.

American Cancer Society (ACS). Risk factors for melanoma skin cancer. 2016b. Available from: http://www.cancer.org/cancer/skincancer-melanoma/detailedguide/melanoma-skin-cancer-risk-factors.

American Cancer Society (ACS). American Cancer Society recommendations for the early detection of breast cancer. 2016c. Available from: https://www.cancer.org/cancer/breast-cancer/screening-tests-and-early-detection/american-cancer-society-recommendations-for-the-early-detection-of-breast-cancer.html.

American Cancer Society (ACS). Recommendations for colorectal early detection: people at average risk. 2017. Available from: https://www.cancer.org/cancer/colon-rectal-cancer/detection-diagnosis-staging/acs-recommendations.html.

American Diabetes Association. Foot care. 2014. Available from: http://www.diabetes.org/living-with-diabetes/complications/foot-complications/foot-care.html.

American Heart Association (AHA). The American Heart Association's diet and lifestyle recommendations. 2015. Available from: http://www.heart.org/HEARTORG/HealthyLiving/HealthyEating/Nutrition/The-American-Heart-Associations-Diet-and-Lifestyle-Recommendations_UCM_305855_Article.jsp#.WU0yoGjyuUk.

Ball JW, Dains J, Flynn J, Solomon B, Stewart R. Seidel's guide to physical examination. 8th ed. St. Louis: Elsevier; 2015.

Burns E, et al: Brief screening questionnaires to identify problem drinking during pregnancy: a systematic review, Addiction 2010;105:601.

Centers for Disease Control and Prevention. Pneumococcal vaccines. 2016. Available from: https://www.cdc.gov/vaccines/vpd/pneumo/index.html.

Grohskopf LA, Sokolow LZ, Broder KR, Olsen SJ, Karron RA, Jernigan DB, et al. Prevention and control of seasonal influenza with vaccines: recommendations of the advisory committee on immunization practices—United States, 2016-2017 influenza season. MMWR Morb Mortal Wkly Rep 2016;65(5):1. Available from: https://www.cdc.gov/mmwr/volumes/65/rr/rr6505a1.htm.

Heckman CJ, Handorf EA, Darlow SD, Ritterband LM, Manne SL. An online skin cancer risk-reduction intervention for young adults: mechanisms of effects. Health Psychol 2016;36(3):215.

Hockenberry MJ, Rodgers C, Wilson D. Essentials of pediatric nursing. 10th ed. St. Louis: Mosby; 2017.

McWhirter JE, Hoffman-Gomez L. Visual images for patient skin self-examination and melanoma detection: a systematic review of published studies. J Am Acad Dermatol 2013;69(1):47.

National Cancer Institute (NCI). NIH study confirms risk factors for male breast cancer. 2014. Available from: https://www.cancer.gov/news-events/press-releases/2014/BreastCancerMalePoolingStudy.

National Institutes of Health (NIH). Once is enough: a guide to preventing future fractures. 2015. Available from: http://www.niams.nih.gov/Health_Info/bone/Osteoporosis/Fracture/default.asp.

National Institute on Drug Abuse (NIDA): Screening for drug use in general medical settings, resource guide, 2012. http://www.drugabuse.gov/publications/resource-guide. Accessed November 21, 2014.

Siu A, U.S. Preventive Services Task Force. Screening for breast cancer: U.S. Preventive Services Task Force Recommendation Statement. Ann Intern Med 2016;164(4):279.

Skin Cancer Foundation. Know your skin, save your life. 2015, Available from: http://www.skincancer.org/publications/sun-and-skin-news/fall-2015-32-4/know.

Touhy T, Jett K. Ebersole and Hess' gerontological nursing & healthy aging. 5th ed. St. Louis: Mosby; 2018.

U.S. Preventive Services Task Force (USPSTF). Screening for skin cancer. U.S. Preventive Services Task Force Recommendation statement. JAMA 2016;316(4):429.

U.S. Preventive Services Task Force (USPSTF). Skin cancer prevention: behavioral counseling. 2017. Available from: https://www.uspreventiveservicestaskforce.org/Page/Document/UpdateSummaryDraft/skin-cancer-counseling2?ds=1&s=counseling%20to%20prevent%20skin%20cancer.

U.S. Public Health Service (USPHS). The surgeon general's call to action to prevent skin cancer. 2014. Available from: http://www.surgeongeneral.gov/library/calls/prevent-skin-cancer/call-to-action-prevent-skin-cancer.pdf.

World Health Organization (WHO): Intimate partner violence, 2015. http://www.who.int/gho/women_and_health/violence/intimate_partner/en/. Accessed April 20, 2015.

8 Equipment and Linen

OBJECTIVES

- To define maintenance of equipment.
- To enumerate purpose of indent and maintenance of equipment.
- To describe methods of indent.
- To describe strategies of maintenance of equipment.
- To enlist techniques of inventory control.
- To discuss general instructions to be kept in mind to maintain good hospital housekeeping.
- To describe care of rubber goods, linen, enamelware, steel articles, sharp instruments, glassware, and furniture.

KEY TERMS

enamelware, p. 175
glassware, p. 175
hospital furniture, p. 176
housekeeping, p. 178
indent, p. 177
inventory, p. 178
linen, p. 175
maintenance, p. 177
rubber goods, p. 175
sharp instruments, p. 176
stainless steel instruments, p. 176

INTRODUCTION

Health care services are the result of a number of materials used in the process. A nurse working in type of health care facility must have awareness about the basic care and handling of equipment, machinery, and housekeeping, so that a nursing care can be provided swiftly and an optimum patient satisfaction can be achieved. The medical materials, such as perfusion materials, surgical disposables, instruments, electrical, civil and engineering items for maintenance, housekeeping materials, linen, biomedical equipment, drugs, food items, play an important role in the quality of health care services. The term equipment is used for more permanent type of article and may be classified as fixed and movables. Fixed equipment is not a structure of the building, but it is attached to the walls or floors. Movable equipment includes furniture, instruments, and so on.

With increased modernization and upgradation of technology, highly sophisticated equipment is in use in modern-day nursing care. Hence, the nurses should be able to use and care for the equipment properly. The training of nurses is essential for maintenance and upkeeping of critical hospital equipment because this helps in prolonging the life of the equipment and smooth implementation of care. Let us understand some of the essential terminologies related to hospital machinery and equipment.

Health Technology

The application of organized knowledge and skills in the form of devices, medicines, vaccines, procedures, and systems developed to solve a health problem and improve quality of life. It is used interchangeably with health care technology.

Medical Devices

An article, instrument, apparatus, or machine that is used in the prevention, diagnosis, or treatment of illness or disease, or for detecting, measuring, restoring, correcting, or modifying the structure or function of the body for some health purpose. Typically, the purpose of a medical device is not achieved by pharmacological, immunological, or metabolic means.

Medical Equipment

Medical devices requiring calibration, maintenance, repair, user training, and decommissioning—activities usually managed by clinical engineers. Medical equipment is used for the specific purposes of diagnosis and treatment of disease or rehabilitation following disease or injury; it can be used either alone or in combination with any accessory, consumable, or other piece of medical equipment. Medical equipment excludes implantable, disposable, or single-use medical devices.

CARE OF LINEN

Hospital management in modern milieu has become patient oriented. It is an established fact that the patient outcome is a result of efficient and appropriate medical, nursing, and allied care along with provision of good hygienic food, clean linen, safe environment, congenial atmosphere, and good interpersonal relationship.

The support services for patient care are indispensable for a hospital to perform in true perspective and facilitate the patient care process. **Linen** and laundry service is a recognized support service that not only ensures prevention and containment of hospital infection but also contributes to widen the image of the hospital in the eyes of public. The dictionary meaning of linen is a flex or an article of cotton. However, in hospital, the term is used for clothing of the patient, medical, nursing, and paramedical staff and also the clothing material used for the patients' care services in operation theatres, beds, trolleys, including the mattresses, pillows, blankets, sheets, and towels, and so on.

Clean linen installs psychological confidence in the patients and the public and enhances their faith in the services rendered by the hospital. Simultaneously, an efficient linen and laundry service is of advantage for hospital marketing and speaks of ability of the medical care service. Hospital housekeepers gather, wash, and iron dirty bed linen, scrubs, and gowns on a daily basis. Housekeepers are also responsible for inspecting linen for wear and tear, mending them when possible and discarding them when they cannot be mended. Following points must be considered for care of linen in hospitals:

- Care of linen should be taken to prevent staining.
- The nature of the fabric itself, as well as the character of the staining agent, must be determined before the material is submitted to any procedure for stain removal.
- Almost all of the materials used for stain removal may be classified as solvents, bleaches, and absorbents.
- The solvents are used to remove stains made by tar, oil, grease, wax, gum, paints, lipstick, chocolate, and so on (e.g., gasoline with benzene, toluene, and xylene). These are very expensive and highly inflammable and therefore dangerous to use.
- Water is also a solvent and can be used to remove stains on a large number of fabrics. It is the safest solvent for unknown dirt or stains.
- Bleaches are oxidizing agents and must be used carefully because they remove color and may weaken the fibers of the material.
- The absorbents such as chalk, magnesium carbonate, corn meal when spread on the stained fabric will often absorb the stain.

CARE OF RUBBER GOODS

Common **rubber goods** used in hospitals are air cushions, mackintoshes, hot water bags, rubber tubes, catheter, gloves, rubber beds, and so on. Following points must be considered for care of rubber goods in hospitals:

- Rubber goods should be washed with a mild soap, rinsed thoroughly, because soap deteriorates rubber, and dried before putting away.
- Rubber should be stored in a cool place, protected from the air by an airtight covering of paper or by storing in a tightly covered metal container to prevent rapid oxidation.
- Repeated folding is likely to cause cracks.
- Sheets and cases of rubber should be rolled or hung over a bar in a cool, dark place.
- Serrated hemostats should never be used on tubing because it cracks.
- For cleaning tubing, plenty of cold water should be forced through the tube.
- Hot water bags, ice caps, and air rings should be partially inflated before being put away.

CARE OF GLASSWARE

The commonly used **glassware** in hospitals are ounce glasses, drainage bottles, suction bottles, and so on. Following points must be considered for effective handling of glassware:

- When buying glassware, select hard glass, which is resistant to heat and mechanical shocks.
- Avoid cleaning the glassware with abrasive material.
- Exposing the glass to sudden variation of temperature may cause cracks.
- When sending the glassware for boiling or autoclaving, they should be adequately padded to prevent breaking by rubbing with hard surface.

CARE OF ENAMELWARE

The material used in the manufacture of nursing care articles must be sturdy, rust resistant, and inexpensive. Pewter, ceramic, and porcelain were the most common materials for much of the 19th century, but nurses found these articles troublesome because of their considerable weight. This problem was minimized by a shift to **enamelware** nursing care2providing articles. The popularity of enamelware increased dramatically in the late 19th century as new industrial machinery made its large-scale application economical. Enamel bonded with a steel base produced a very smooth, pleasant, and durable surface. The longevity, rust resistance, light weight, and wipe-clean ease of use made enamelware the most popular material for nursing care2providing articles until it was superseded by disposable plastics in the 1960s. The common enamelware used in the hospital are kidney tray, bedpan, urinals, sputum mugs, feeding cups and trays, and so on. Following points must be considered for effective handling of enamelware:

- Avoid mishandling or dropping of enamelware because it can chip off and become unsafe for use.
- Do not boil for longer period or cool them rapidly because the enamel may erode.
- Wash enamelware immediately after use, especially when antiseptic reagents are used because the enamelware get stained or damaged with strong acid, alkalis, and dyes.

CARE OF PLASTIC MATERIALS

Use of plastic in health care institutes has exponentially increased in last few decades, especially with emergence of HIV/AIDS. Use of plastic material ranges from plastic furniture, food trays, nursing care trays, kidney trays, jugs, mugs, dressing pack tray, plastic parts in medical machines to single-use plastic in form of syringes, intravenous fluid bags, intravenous tubing, surgical packing, drapes, waterproof surgical gowns, sheets, cap, mask, goggles, and so on. Health care facilities prefer single-use plastic because of cost, durability, convenience, surety of sterility, and so on. It is estimated that 25% of the waste generated by a hospital is plastic. A study documented that a single hysterectomy procedure can produce up to 9 kg of waste, most of which is plastic. However, it is also believed that single-use plastics are the cleanest, most efficient way, to facilitate health and hygiene in hospitals. The specific guidelines for the care of plastic material are as follows:

- Reusable plastic food serving trays can be washed with soap and water to reuse for serving the food to the patients.
- Plastic nursing care trays, kidney tray, jugs, mugs, and other reusable plastic material used for clean nursing procedures can be washed with soap and water and further these should be disinfected with 70% alcohol. In addition, these items must be disinfected with 1% hypochlorite solution, if they are soiled with blood or body fluid of a patient diagnosed with infectious disease such as HIV/AIDS and hepatitis.
- The reusable plastic material used of the sterile health care procedure such as surgical dressing plastic stray, Ambu bags, and plastic specula must be sterilized in ethylene oxide (ETO) or plasma sterilizer.
- Single-use plastic material should be discarded in the appropriate biomedical waste management bin—Red Bin per the Bio-Medical Waste Management (Amendment) Rules, 2019, Government of India. Furthermore, per green hospital initiatives, use of single-use plastic in hospitals must be minimized, and there are some of the plastic items used in patient care that are not soiled and do not have biohazards such as packaging and storage containers, which could be recycled.

CARE OF METAL INSTRUMENTS

The commonly used **stainless steel instruments** in hospitals are forceps, surgical instruments, spatulas, tongue depressor, mouth gag, dilator, sharp surgical instruments, and so on. Instruments represent a significant material asset within the overall investment of a hospital. The care and maintenance these instruments receive are critical to their performance during surgery and to the cost containment efforts of each hospital authority. Having made the investment in a quality product, the authority can expect several years of trouble-free use if the operator uses proper techniques during use, care, and handling of its surgical instruments. Following essential interventions can keep the stainless steel instruments functional for significant longer period without any undue problems:

- All stainless steel items are heat resistant, anticorrosive, and long-lasting but expensive; hence, they should be handled well.
- They can be easily sterilized using chemicals and by autoclaving.
- Immediately after the use, clean the instrument under running water of temperature not more than 45°C because higher temperature may lead to coagulation of tissue protein. A proper cleaning is as essential as the disinfection.
- Disinfect or sterilize the instrument per the manufacture's guidelines or hospital policy. Always use a fresh disinfecting solution and use optimum concentration of disinfectant because higher concentration may lead to corrosion and lower concentration may lead to ineffective disinfection.
- Powdered disinfecting products must be completely dissolved prior to immersing any instrument because undissolved particles may lead to clogging of narrow lumens of instruments.
- Do not boil stainless steel items repeatedly because this can cause corrosion and dullness of the instrument.
- Sharp edges are dulled by rough use and exposure to high temperature and moisture.
- Immerse the **sharp instruments** in chemical disinfectants for prescribed duration because lower contact period could lead to ineffective disinfection and increased length of contact period may lead to corrosion of the instrument.

CARE OF HOSPITAL FURNITURE

A variety of furniture is used in hospitals for the comfortable stay of patients, family, and smooth functioning of health care activities. The commonly used **hospital furniture** includes beds, tables, chairs, cardiac table, bedside storage lockers, wheelchairs, stretchers, operation theatre tables, labor room tables, nursing station, cupboards, and so on. Following points must be considered for effective handling of hospital furniture:

- Metal furniture may be adequately cared for by frequent washing with warm water and soap. Scouring powder may scratch the surface of the furniture and thus should not be used.
- Most wood furniture used in hospitals have a waterproof finish and are made to withstand an excessive amount of wear.
- Report damage or breakage of furniture immediately so it can be repaired before it is damaged further.
- When using the overbed table, raise it high enough to clear the foot of the bed so it will not be damaged when moved.
- Use a mild soap solution to wash the furniture and dry it carefully after it has been washed.
- If anything is spilled on the furniture, be sure that it is immediately mopped up.

MAINTENANCE OF EQUIPMENT

Medical devices are assets that directly affect human lives. They are considerable investments, and in many cases have high maintenance costs. It is important, therefore, to have a well-planned and managed **maintenance** program that is able to keep the medical equipment in a health care institution reliable, safe, and available for use when it is needed for diagnostic procedures, therapy, treatments, and monitoring of patients. In addition, such a program prolongs the useful life of the equipment and minimizes the cost of equipment ownership.

A maintenance strategy includes procedures for inspection, as well as preventive maintenance (PM)and corrective maintenance (CM). Performance inspections ensure that equipment is operating correctly, safety inspections ensure that the equipment is safe for both patients and operators, and PM aims to extend the life of the equipment and reduce failure rates. In addition, some hidden problems may be discovered during a scheduled inspection. However, performing inspections of equipment only ensures that the device is in good operating condition at the time of inspection and cannot eliminate the possibility of failure during future use; the nature of most electrical and mechanical components is that they can potentially fail at any time. CM restores the function of a failed device and allows it to be put back into service.

Equipment maintenance is a set of activities performed to keep equipment in their optimum working condition and consists of routine inspection and maintenance practices. Equipment maintenance policy provides a broad framework of decision to be taken for guiding certain actions that are useful in prolonging the life of equipment. The policies are developed in such a way that these ensure safe usage of the equipment and also the results out of its usage are accurate and reliable.

An effective medical equipment maintenance program consists of adequate planning, management, and implementation. Planning considers the financial, physical, and human resources required to adequately implement the maintenance activities. Once the program has been defined, financial, personnel, and operational aspects are continually examined and managed to ensure the program continues uninterrupted and improves as necessary. Ultimately, proper implementation of the program is the key to ensuring optimal equipment functionality.

Purposes of Equipment Maintenance

The well-planned equipment maintenance may have following main purposes:

- Maximum availability and reliability of the equipment.
- Maximum return on investment done on the equipment.
- Prevention of wastage of consumables and spares.
- Extended useful life of the equipment.
- Readiness of the equipment for emergency use whenever required.

Equipment Maintenance Process

In modern-day nursing care, diagnostic hospital equipment is extremely important in understanding the cause of illness, assessing the severity of injuries, or ruling out possible problems. Patient's condition is established with the help of diagnostic equipment. Hospital diagnostic equipment includes stethoscope, sphygmomanometer, thermometers, proctoscope, bronchoscope, laryngoscope, surgical equipment, and scanning devices such as X-ray machines, computed axial tomography or CAT scanners, and magnetic resonance imaging (MRI).

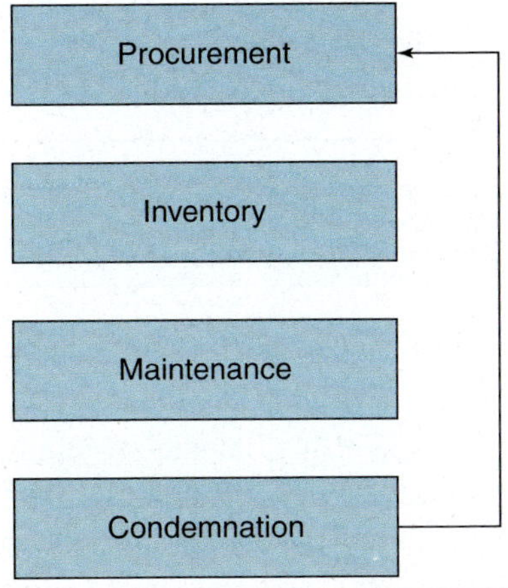

Fig. 8.1 Equipment maintenance process.

All equipment required in the hospital are procured, stocked and annual inventory maintained. Increased dependency on the medical equipment in the hospital for diagnosis and treatment demands their availability in their best working conditions at all time. This is possible only when a comprehensive maintenance of the equipment is carried out (Fig. 8.1).

1. ***Indent/procurement of the equipment:*** For the purpose of procurement or **indent**, equipment is categorized into high-value instruments or low-value instruments. Another classification is sophisticated equipment, electronics and nonelectronic equipment. Indent for routine or low-value equipment can be done weekly, monthly, or annually. Equipment is procured by submitting a statement of case (SOC) or an indent form depending on the hospital policy. The SOC or indent form should be approved by the competent authority. An annual acquisition plan can be prepared, which indicates the outlay for the procurement of specific kind of equipment.
2. ***Equipment maintenance:*** The basic objective of the maintenance is to have increased availability of equipment, with increased safety. Maintenance management involves managing the functions of maintenance. Maintaining equipment has been a challenging task because the hospital equipment are highly sophisticated and expensive; therefore, effective maintenance management is very important in terms of cost optimization. It is essential for any health care facility, regardless of its size, to implement a maintenance program for medical equipment. The complexity of the program depends on the size and type of facility, its location, and the resources required. However, the principles of a

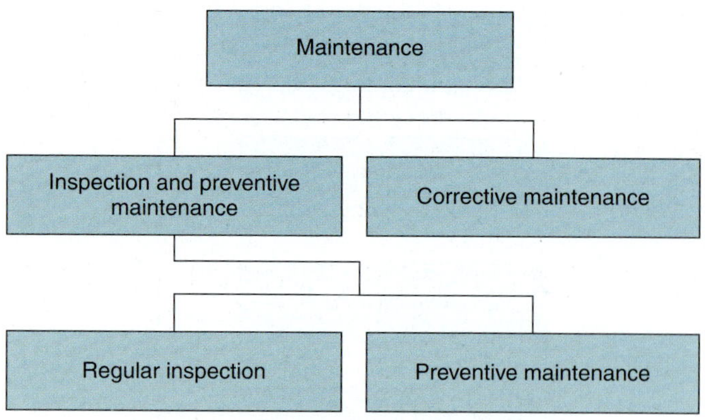

Fig. 8.2 Components of maintenance strategy.

good maintenance program will be the same if it is in an urban area in a high-income country or a rural setting in a low- to middle-income country.

Medical equipment maintenance can be divided into two major categories: inspection and preventive maintenance (IPM) and CM (Fig. 8.2). IPM includes all scheduled activities that ensure equipment functionality and prevents breakdowns or failures. Performance and safety inspections are straightforward procedures that verify proper functionality and safe use of a device. PM refers to scheduled activities performed to extend the life of a device and prevent failure (i.e., by calibration, part replacement, lubrication, and cleaning). Inspection can be conducted as a stand-alone activity and in conjunction with PM to ensure functionality; this is important because PM can be fairly invasive in that components are removed, cleaned, or replaced. Another school of thought categorizes the maintenance strategies as follows:

- Breakdown maintenance or unplanned maintenance
- PM or scheduled maintenance
- Condition-based maintenance

The equipment under breakdown maintenance is allowed to run until it breaks down and then repairing and putting it back to operation. This strategy is suitable for equipment that are not critical and have spare capacity or redundancy available. In PM or scheduled maintenance, maintenance actions such as inspection, lubrication, cleaning, adjustment, and replacement are undertaken at fixed intervals. Condition monitoring detects and diagnoses faults and it helps in planned maintenance based on equipment condition. This condition-based maintenance strategy or predictive maintenance is preferred for critical systems, and for such systems breakdown maintenance should be avoided.

3. ***Inventory:*** **Inventory** management is the assessment of supply and storage of items to ensure adequate supply and prevention of oversupply. It is a system designed for internal control and accounting purpose because this is direct cost to the hospital. There should be a proper procedure for the inventory flow and management to optimize the cost and also to ensure availability of supplies on time. Some of the identified techniques in inventory control are as follows:
   - *First in, first out (FIFO):* It is mostly used for perishable or limited self-life items such as drugs. For example, in a pharmacy, if new stock coming in would get taken immediately, then older stock would expire, causing great loss. Hence, older stock should be arranged in front or stock must be arranged by date received.
   - *Inspection of stock levels:* Minimum stock level should be maintained, which will fill up the gap while the supplies are reordered. Proper consideration should be given to emergencies besides the time that vendors take to replenish the stock. This will help in arriving at just in time (JIT) ordering, where stock is held for a minimum amount of time.
   - *Security of stock:* Security is necessary to control cost. Many times, the tampering of stock is done by employees rather than outsiders. Hence, high-value items should be properly secured and kept and proper periodic inventory should be performed. Security guards, cameras, bar codes, and security devices can be used.

HOSPITAL HOUSEKEEPING

Housekeeping services in a hospital are entrusted with maintaining a hygienic and clean hospital environment conducive to patient care. It is a service function and an all-pervasive activity, which is performed in every department of the hospital. Housekeeping services has a direct effect on the health, comfort, and morale of the patient, staff, and visitors, hence is also an important public relations variable.

Good housekeeping is one of the basic essentials of nursing and is a primary factor in the economic administration of any household. The purpose of housekeeping is to create an environment for the patient that is comfortable, pleasant, and hygienic. Well-managed housekeeping reduces the cost of hospital operation.

The privatization of medical care and emergence of Consumer Protection Act in history of health care organizations have impressed upon legal, economic, and moral obligation to react positively to the demands of the consumers. The endeavor should be to achieve optimal quality in health care both in terms of professional competence and expectation of the consumers. Failure to accomplish this may affect the image and viability of the hospital. A good housekeeping service is an asset that no hospital can afford to neglect. In a free market economy, attractivity of a hospital depends to a great extent on the services provided in terms of good physical environment and facilities of personal comfort. Hospital housekeeping is an activity on which all health-providing services of the hospital depend. An appropriate housekeeping service can reduce man-hours and costs and raise sanitation levels.

General instructions to be kept in mind in good hospital housekeeping:

- Damp dusting is better than dry dusting because dust easily flies out into atmosphere. Dusting should be performed firmly. Use brush when cleaning grooved surface.
- Avoid collection of water in any surface because it may be a favorable place for the growth of microorganisms.

- Wherever possible, provide maximum exposure to sunlight that destroys growth of bacteria.
- Articles should be stored and arranged in proper and clean place, so that these can be conveniently located.
- Friction aids in cleaning. Soap and water are used for cleaning. Do not use rough or abrasive material over painted and polished surface.
- Disinfection depends on correct concentration and duration of exposure.

KEY POINTS

- Equipment maintenance is a set of activities performed to keep equipment in their optimum working condition.
- Inventory management is the assessment of supply and storage of items to ensure adequate supply and prevention of oversupply.
- The purpose of housekeeping is to create an environment for the patient that is comfortable, pleasant, and hygienic.

9 Infection Prevention and Control

OBJECTIVES

- To explain the relationship between the infection chain and transmission of infection.
- To give an example of preventing infection for each element of the infection chain.
- To identify the normal defenses of the body against infection.
- To describe the signs/symptoms of a localized infection and those of a systemic infection.
- To explain conditions that promote the transmission of health care–associated infection.
- To explain the difference between medical and surgical asepsis.
- To explain the rationale for standard precautions.
- To perform proper procedures for hand hygiene.
- To explain how infection control measures differ in the home versus the hospital.
- To properly apply a surgical mask, sterile gown, and sterile gloves.
- To explain procedures for each isolation category.
- To understand the definition of occupational exposure and explain the postexposure process.
- To describe the importance biomedical waste management and ways to segregate hospital waste.

KEY TERMS

airborne precautions, p. 190
antibody, p. 182
antigen, p. 186
asepsis, p. 187
aseptic technique, p. 187
asymptomatic, p. 181
biomedical waste, p. 203
carriers, p. 182
colonization, p. 180
communicable disease, p. 180
contact precautions, p. 190
disinfection, p. 187
droplet precautions, p. 190
endogenous infection, p. 185
exogenous infection, p. 185
flora, p. 185
immunity, p. 182
infection, p. 180
inflammation, p. 185
medical asepsis, p. 187
microorganisms, p. 180
necrotic, p. 185
pathogens, p. 180
reservoir, p. 182
standard precautions, p. 204
sterilization, p. 187
suprainfection, p. 185
surgical asepsis, p. 187
symptomatic, p. 181
virulence, p. 181

INTRODUCTION

Current trends of newer viral infections, public awareness, and rising costs of health care have increased the importance of infection prevention and control (IPC). Increases in drug-resistant microorganisms and health care–acquired infections (HAIs) and concern about occupational exposure to human immunodeficiency virus (HIV) and hepatitis have increased concern about transmission of infections within health care settings. As a nurse, you will participate in cost-effective, quality health care by using strategies that prevent or reduce the risk for infections. This chapter emphasizes techniques for prevention and control of infections and the critical thinking skills necessary to achieve these goals.

NATURE OF INFECTION

An **infection** is the invasion of a susceptible host (e.g., a patient) by potentially harmful **microorganisms** (pathogens), resulting in disease. The principal infecting agents are bacteria, viruses, fungi, and protozoa (Table 9.1). It is important to know the difference between an infection and colonization. **Colonization** is the presence and growth of microorganisms within a host but without tissue invasion or damage (Tweeten, 2015). All people have microorganisms on their skin, but usually no disease or infection develops. Disease or infection results only if the **pathogens** grow or multiply and alter normal tissue function. An infectious disease transmitted directly from one person to another is considered as contagious or **communicable**

Table 9.1 Common Pathogens and Some Infections or Diseases They Produce

Organism	Major Reservoirs	Major Diseases/Infections
BACTERIA		
Escherichia coli	Colon	Gastroenteritis, urinary tract infection
Staphylococcus aureus	Skin, hair, upper respiratory tract	Wound infection, abscess, cellulitis, osteomyelitis, bacteremia, pneumonia, food poisoning, toxic shock syndrome
Streptococcus (beta-hemolytic group A) organisms	Oropharynx, skin, perianal area	"Strep throat," rheumatic fever, scarlet fever, impetigo, wound infection
Streptococcus (beta-hemolytic group B) organisms	Adult genitalia	Urinary tract infection, wound infection, postpartum sepsis, neonatal sepsis
Mycobacterium tuberculosis	Droplet nuclei from lungs	Tuberculosis
Neisseria gonorrhoeae	Genitourinary tract, rectum, mouth	Sexually transmitted infection, pelvic inflammatory disease, septic arthritis, newborn ophthalmitis
Rickettsia rickettsii	Wood tick	Rocky Mountain spotted fever
Staphylococcus epidermidis	Skin	Wound infection, bacteremia
VIRUSES		
Hepatitis A virus	Feces	Hepatitis A
Hepatitis B virus	Blood, certain body fluids, tissues involved in sexual contact	Hepatitis B
Hepatitis C virus	Blood, certain body fluids, tissues involved in sexual contact	Hepatitis C
Herpes simplex virus (type I)	Lesions of mouth, skin, genitals	Cold sores, herpetic whitlow, sexually transmitted disease
Human immunodeficiency virus (HIV)	Blood, semen, vaginal secretions via sexual contact	Acquired immunodeficiency syndrome (AIDS)
FUNGI		
Aspergillus organisms	Soil, dust, mouth, skin, colon, genital tract	Aspergillosis, pneumonia, sepsis
Candida albicans	Skin, mouth, genital tract	Candidiasis, pneumonia, sepsis
PROTOZOA		
Plasmodium falciparum	Blood	Malaria

Data from Brown M: Microbiology basics. In Grota P, editor: *APIC text of infection control and epidemiology,* ed 4, Washington, DC, 2015, Association for Professionals in Infection Control and Epidemiology (APIC).

disease (Tweeten, 2015) such as recent novel coronavirus disease (COVID-19) pandemic. If the pathogens multiply and cause clinical signs and symptoms, the patient is **symptomatic.** If the clinical signs and symptoms of the illness are not present, the patient is **asymptomatic.** For example, hepatitis C is most efficiently transmitted through the direct entry of blood into the skin through a percutaneous exposure, even if the source (patient) is asymptomatic (Centers for Disease Control and Prevention [CDC], 2016a).

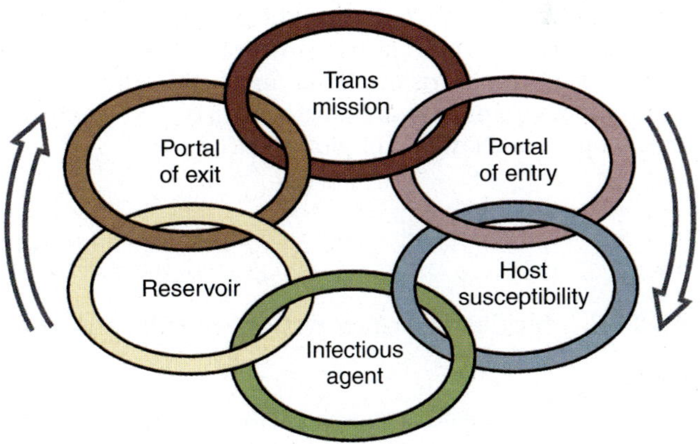

Fig. 9.1 Chain of infection.

CHAIN OF INFECTION

The presence of a pathogen does not mean that an infection develops. The process resulting in an infection is referred to as the *chain of infection*. Components of the chain of infection include the infectious agent or pathogen, reservoir or place for pathogen growth, portal of exit from the reservoir, mode of transmission or vehicle, portal of entry into the reservoir, and a susceptible host (Fig. 9.1). Infection develops if the links in this chain remain intact. Preventing infections involves breaking the chain of infection.

Infectious Agent

The development of an infection depends on the number of microorganisms present; their **virulence,** or the ability to produce disease; their ability to enter and survive in a host; and the susceptibility of the host. Resident skin microorganisms are not virulent. However, they can cause serious infection when surgery or an invasive procedure allows them to enter deep inside tissues or when a patient is severely immunocompromised. Patients become immunocompromised when their immune system is impaired. Some factors that increase a patient's risk for being immunocompromised include chemotherapy and organ transplant antirejection medications, or acquired immunodeficiency syndrome (AIDS).

Reservoir

A place where microorganisms survive, multiply, and wait to transfer to a susceptible host is called a **reservoir.** Common reservoirs are humans and animals (hosts), insects, food, water, and organic matter on inanimate surfaces (fomites). Frequent reservoirs for HAIs include health care workers (HCWs) (especially their hands), body excretions and secretions of patients, equipment, and the health care environment. There are two types of human reservoirs: humans with acute or symptomatic disease and humans who show no signs of disease but are **carriers** of it. Transmission of microorganisms can occur in either case.

Portal of Exit

After microorganisms find a site in which to grow and multiply, they must find a portal of exit if they are to enter another host and cause disease. They exit through a variety of sites such as the skin and mucous membranes, respiratory tract, gastrointestinal (GI) tract, urinary tract, reproductive tract, and blood.

Modes of Transmission

By practicing IPC techniques such as hand hygiene, you can interrupt the mode of transmission (Box 9.1). The same microorganism is sometimes transmitted by more than one route. For example, the virus that causes chickenpox spreads by airborne route in droplet nuclei and by direct contact with vesicle fluid. When the hands of an HCW contact infectious material directly, the microorganisms will spread to the HCW. This mode of transmission is called *direct transmission*. Indirect transmission occurs when microorganisms are transferred to an HCW's hands from contaminated items that are part of patient care such as a stethoscope or a dirty pair of gloves (CDC, 2012).

Portal of Entry

Organisms are able to enter the body through the same routes that they use for exiting. Common portals of entry include broken skin, mucous membranes, genitourinary tract, GI tract, and respiratory tract. For example, obstruction to the flow of urine caused by the presence of a blocked urinary catheter allows organisms to go up into the urethra.

Susceptible Host

Susceptibility to an infection depends on an individual's degree of resistance to pathogens. Although everyone is constantly in contact with large numbers of microorganisms, an infection does not develop until an individual becomes susceptible to the strength and numbers of these microorganisms. The amount of pathogen required to cause an infection in the host is defined as the dose. The more virulent an organism, the greater the dose, and the more likely it is that a person will develop an infection. Some factors that influence a person's susceptibility (degree of resistance) to infection include age, nutritional status, presence of chronic disease, trauma, and smoking. Organisms with resistance to key antibiotics are common in all health care settings, but especially acute care. This is associated with the frequent and sometimes inappropriate use of antibiotics over the years in all settings (i.e., acute care, ambulatory care, clinics, and long-term care). A person's natural defenses against infection and certain risk factors affect susceptibility (Box 9.2).

A host is not considered susceptible if it has acquired **immunity** through either a natural or an artificially induced event. Natural active immunity results from having a certain disease such as measles and mounting an immune response that usually lasts a lifetime. Active immunity also results from the administration of a vaccine. Natural passive immunity is the acquisition of an **antibody** by one person from another such as an infant born with the mother's antibodies. The infant acquires this short-term immunity from antibodies through the placenta during the last months of pregnancy (Dalal and Roifman, 2015).

BOX 9.1 Modes of Transmission: Routes and Means

Contact

- *Direct:* Person-to-person or physical contact between source and susceptible host (e.g., touching patient feces and then touching own face or mouth or consuming contaminated food)
- *Indirect:* Personal contact of susceptible host with contaminated inanimate object (e.g., needles or sharps, dressings)
- *Droplet:* Large particles that travel up to 3 feet and come in contact with susceptible host (e.g., from coughing, sneezing, talking)
- *Airborne:* Droplet nuclei, residue or evaporated droplets suspended in air (e.g., from coughing, sneezing, talking)

Vehicles

- Contaminated items
- Water
- Drugs, solutions
- Blood
- Food (improperly handled, stored, cooked; fresh or thawed meats)

Vector

- External mechanical transfer (flies)
- Internal transmission such as with parasitic conditions between vector and host, for example:
  - Mosquito
  - Louse
  - Tick
  - Flea

Data from Tweeten S: General principles of epidemiology. In Grota P, editor: *APIC text of infection control and epidemiology,* ed 4, Washington, DC, 2015, Association for Professionals in Infection Control and Epidemiology.

BOX 9.2 Factors Affecting Susceptibility to Infection

Age

- Infants have immature immune systems.
- Children acquire more immunity but are susceptible to infectious diseases such as mumps and measles if unvaccinated.
- Young and middle-aged adults have refined body system defenses and immunity.
- Older adults experience decline in immune responses, and the structure and function of major organs change.

Heredity

- Certain congenital and genetic chromosome disorders affect humoral or cellular immunity.
- Patients with diabetes and patients with a hereditary predisposition to diabetes are at increased risk for infections and delayed wound healing.

Cultural Practices

- Cultural or religious beliefs or practices influence patients' decisions to seek treatment for an infection or the type of methods used to prevent infections.

Nutritional Status

- A reduction in protein, carbohydrates, and fats as a result of illness, inadequate diet, or debility increases a patient's susceptibility to infection and delays wound repair.

Stress

- Increased stress elevates cortisol levels, causing decreased resistance to infection.
- Continuous stress exhausts energy stores.

Rest and Exercise

- Inadequate rest and exercise increase stress and decrease bodily functions such as elimination and circulation.

Inadequate Defenses

- Primary and secondary defenses can be altered by broken skin or mucosa, traumatized tissue, or suppressed immune response.

Personal Habits

- Smoking reduces respiratory ciliary action and decreases resistance to respiratory infections.
- Alcohol ingestion impairs the effect of antibiotics.
- Risky sexual behavior such as multiple sex partners increases the chance for exposure to HIV and agents of other sexually transmitted diseases.

Environmental Factors

- Crowded living conditions and adequacy and safety of water supply influence a patient's susceptibility to infections.
- Inadequate refrigeration and cooking facilities increase a patient's exposure to foodborne illness such as salmonellosis or campylobacteriosis.

Immunization/Disease History

- Patients who have not received recommended immunizations are at risk for vaccine-preventable diseases such as measles, mumps, and rubella.
- Older adults with underlying medical conditions decrease their susceptibility to influenza and pneumococcal pneumonia when they receive immunizations.

Medical Therapies

- Certain drugs such as cortisone and certain invasive therapies such as i.v. catheters or surgeries increase the risk for infection.

Clinical Appearance and Data

- Localized infections usually manifest with redness, swelling, and pain or tenderness. There is sometimes a purulent drainage from wounds or lesions.
- Systemic infections manifest with fever, chills, nausea and vomiting, loss of appetite, or lymph node enlargement.
- Clinical data may show an increase in WBCs, a positive culture, or an abnormal X-ray film examination.

HIV, human immunodeficiency virus; *WBC*, white blood cell.

TYPES OF INFECTION

On the Basis of Body Part Involvement

Localized Infection

If the infection is localized such as in a wound, antibiotic therapy and proper wound care control the spread of the infection and minimize the illness. The patient usually experiences only localized symptoms such as pain, tenderness, and swelling at the wound site.

Systematic Infection

An infection that affects the entire body instead of just a single organ or part is systemic, characterized by a fever and increase in white blood cells (WBCs). Systemic infections can cause further complications including organ damage and are associated with higher mortality rates.

On the Basis of Causative Organism

- Bacterial infection
- Viral infection
- Fungal infection
- Parasitic infection
- Prions

Health Care–Associated Infections

Patients in health care settings, especially hospitals and long-term care facilities (LTCFs), are at a higher risk for infection than patients seen in the home. When a patient develops an infection that was not present or incubating at the time of admission to a health care setting, it is called an **HAI. HAIs** result from the delivery of health services in a health care facility. They occur as the result

BOX 9.3 Examples of Sites for and Causes of Health Care–Acquired Infections

Improperly performing hand hygiene increases patient risk for all types of health care–acquired infections.

Urinary Tract

- Unsterile insertion of urinary catheter
- Improper positioning of catheter drainage tubing
- Open drainage system
- Disconnection of catheter and tube
- Contact between drainage bag port and contaminated surface
- Improper specimen collection technique
- Obstruction or interference with urinary drainage
- Urine in catheter or drainage tube being allowed to reenter bladder (reflux)
- Repeated catheter irrigations

Surgical or Traumatic Wounds

- Improper skin preparation before surgery (i.e., shaving versus clipping hair; not performing a preoperative bath or shower)
- Failure to cleanse skin surface properly
- Failure to use aseptic technique during dressing changes
- Use of contaminated antiseptic solutions

Respiratory Tract

- Contaminated respiratory therapy equipment
- Failure to use aseptic technique while suctioning airway
- Improper disposal of secretions

Bloodstream

- Contamination of i.v. fluids by tubing
- Adding medications to i.v. fluid
- Addition of connecting tube or stopcocks to i.v. system
- Improper care of needle insertion site
- Contaminated needles or catheters
- Failure to change i.v. access site when inflammation first appears
- Improper technique during administration of multiple blood products
- Improper care of peritoneal or hemodialysis shunts
- Improperly accessing an i.v. port

of invasive procedures, antibiotic administration, the presence of **multidrug-resistant organisms** (MDROs), and breaks in IPC activities. The number of health care employees having direct contact with a patient, the type and number of invasive procedures, the therapy received, and the length of hospitalization influence the risk of infection. Major sites for HAIs include surgical or traumatic wounds, urinary and respiratory tracts, and the bloodstream (Box 9.3).

HAIs significantly increase costs of health care. Older adults have increased susceptibility to these infections because of their affinity to chronic disease and the aging process itself. Extended stays in health care institutions, increased disability, increased costs of antibiotics, and prolonged recovery times add to the expenses both of the patient and the health care institution and funding bodies (e.g., Medicare). Costs for HAIs are often not reimbursed; as a result, prevention has a beneficial financial impact and is an important part of managed care. TJC lists several national safety goals focusing on the care of older adults (e.g., ensuring that older adults receive influenza and pneumonia vaccines, preventing infection after surgery).

Patients who develop HAIs often have multiple illnesses, are older adults, or are poorly nourished and may have a compromised immune system; thus, they are more susceptible to infections. In addition, many patients have a lowered resistance to infection because of underlying medical conditions (e.g., diabetes mellitus or cancer) that impair or damage the immune response of the body. Invasive treatment devices such as intravenous (i.v.) catheters or indwelling urinary catheters impair or bypass the natural defenses of the body against microorganisms. Critical illness increases patients' susceptibility to infections, especially multidrug-resistant bacteria. Meticulous hand hygiene practices, the use of chlorhexidine washes for bathing and personal hygiene care, and advances in intensive care unit (ICU) infection prevention (Fig. 9.2) help to prevent these infections.

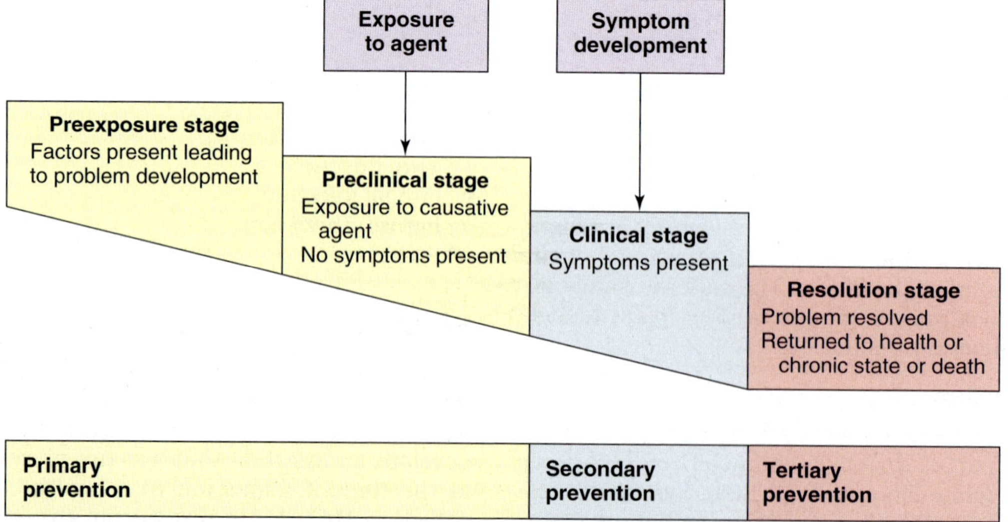

Fig. 9.2 Stages of the natural history of a condition and their relationship to primary, secondary, and tertiary levels of prevention. (From Clark MJ: Community health nursing: caring for populations, ed 4, Upper Saddle River, NJ, 2003, Pearson Education.)

Exogenous and Endogenous Infection

HAIs are exogenous or endogenous. An **exogenous infection** comes from microorganisms found outside the individual such as *Salmonella, Clostridium tetani,* and *Aspergillus.* They do not exist as normal flora. An **endogenous infection** occurs when part of a patient's flora becomes altered and overgrowth results (e.g., staphylococci, enterococci, yeasts, streptococci). This often happens when a patient receives broad-spectrum antibiotics that alter normal flora. When sufficient numbers of microorganisms normally found in one body site move to another site, an endogenous infection develops. The number of microorganisms needed to cause an HAI depends on the virulence of the organism, susceptibility of the host, and body site affected.

Iatrogenic Infections

Iatrogenic infections are a type of HAI caused by an invasive diagnostic or therapeutic procedure. For example, procedures such as a bronchoscopy and treatment with broad-spectrum antibiotics increase the risk for certain infections. Use critical thinking when practicing aseptic techniques during the performance of procedures. Follow basic IPC policies and procedures to reduce the risk of HAIs. Always consider the patient's risks for infection and anticipate how the approach to care increases or decreases the risk.

Community-Acquired Infection

A community-acquired infection is one that was present at the time of admission to a health care setting.

COURSE OF INFECTION BY STAGE

By understanding the chain of infection, you have knowledge that is vital in preventing infections. When the patient acquires an infection, observe for signs and symptoms of infection and take appropriate actions to prevent its spread. Infections follow a progressive course (Box 9.4).

BOX 9.4 Course of Infection by Stage

Incubation Period

Interval between entrance of pathogen into body and appearance of first symptoms (e.g., chickenpox, 14–16 days after exposure; common cold, 1–2 days; influenza, 1–4 days; measles, 10–12 days; mumps, 16–18 days; Ebola, 2–21 days.

Prodromal Stage

Interval from onset of nonspecific signs and symptoms (malaise, low-grade fever, fatigue) to more specific symptoms. (During this time, microorganisms grow and multiply, and patient may be capable of spreading disease to others.) For example, herpes simplex begins with itching and tingling at the site before the lesion appears.

Illness Stage

Interval when the patient manifests signs and symptoms specific to type of infection. For example, strep throat is manifested by sore throat, pain, and swelling; mumps is manifested by high fever, parotid and salivary gland swelling.

Convalescence

Interval when acute symptoms of infection disappear. (Length of recovery depends on severity of infection and patient's host resistance; recovery may take several days to months.)

BODY DEFENSES AGAINST INFECTION

The body has normal defenses against infection, including normal flora, body system defenses, and the immune system. Intact skin protects from pathogens, and linings of the nasal passages act to prevent organisms from entering the lungs. Each organ system has defense mechanisms to prevent exposure to infection. In addition, the **inflammatory response** of the body is a protective reaction that neutralizes pathogens and repairs body cells.

Normal Flora

The normal **flora** of the body is made up of a large number of microorganisms residing on the surface and deep layers of the skin, in the saliva, and on the oral mucosa and intestinal walls. Normal flora usually does not cause disease but instead maintains health. For example, skin flora reduces multiplication of organisms landing on the skin. The number and variety of flora maintain a sensitive balance with other microorganisms to prevent infection. Any factor that disrupts this balance increases the risk for infection. For example, the use of broad-spectrum antibiotics for the treatment of infection eliminates or changes normal bacterial flora, often leading to **suprainfection.** Microorganisms resistant to antibiotics cause serious infection (Arnold, 2015).

Body System Defenses

Microorganisms easily enter the skin, respiratory tract, and GI tract. However, these body systems also have unique defenses against infection that are physiologically suited to their structure and function (Table 9.2). Any condition that impairs the specialized defenses of an organ increases susceptibility to infection.

Inflammation

The cellular responses of the body to injury or infection is **inflammation.** Inflammation is a protective vascular reaction that involves a cascade of physiological responses that neutralize and eliminate pathogens or **necrotic** tissues and establishes a means of repairing body cells and tissues. Acute inflammation is usually a short-lived process, lasting only a few days (e.g., inflammation around a cut or surgical incision). If inflammation lasts longer, it is referred to as chronic inflammation. Chronic inflammation may last weeks, months, or longer. Along with abnormal laboratory values, there are multiple signs and symptoms of inflammation. Many physical agents (e.g., temperature extremes

Table 9.2 Normal Body System Defense Mechanisms Against Infection

Defense Mechanisms	Action	Factors That May Alter Defense
SKIN		
Intact multilayered surface, first line of defense of body against infection	Provides mechanical barrier to microorganisms and antibacterial activity	Cuts, abrasions, puncture wounds, areas of maceration
Shedding of outer layer of skin cells	Removes organisms that adhere to outer layers of skin	Failure to bathe regularly, improper hand-hygiene techniques
Sebum	Contains fatty acid that kills some bacteria	Excessive bathing
MOUTH		
Intact multilayered mucosa	Provides mechanical barrier to microorganisms	Lacerations, trauma, extracted teeth
Saliva	Washes away particles containing microorganisms	
Contains microbial inhibitors (e.g., lysozyme)	Poor oral hygiene, dehydration	
EYE		
Tearing and blinking	Provide mechanisms to reduce entry (blinking) or help wash away (tearing) particles containing pathogens	Injury, exposure—splash, splatter of blood or other potentially infectious material into the eye
RESPIRATORY TRACT		
Cilia lining upper airways, coated by mucus	Trap inhaled microbes and sweep them outward in mucus to be expectorated or swallowed	Smoking, high concentration of oxygen and carbon dioxide, decreased humidity, cold air
Macrophages	Engulf and destroy microorganisms that reach alveoli of lung	Smoking, immunosuppression
URINARY TRACT		
Flushing action of urine flow	Washes away microorganisms on lining of bladder and urethra	Obstruction to normal flow by indwelling urinary catheter placement, obstruction from growth or tumor, or delayed micturition
Intact multilayered epithelium	Provides barrier to microorganisms	Introduction of urinary catheter, continual movement of catheter in urethra
GASTROINTESTINAL TRACT		
Acidity of gastric secretions	Chemically destroys microorganisms incapable of surviving low pH	Administration of antacids, histamine-2 blockers
Rapid peristalsis in small intestine	Prevents retention of bacterial contents	Delayed motility from fecal impaction in large bowel or mechanical obstruction by masses
VAGINA		
At puberty, normal flora causes vaginal secretions to achieve low pH	Inhibits growth of many microorganisms	Antibiotics and birth control pills that disrupt normal flora

and radiation), chemical agents (e.g., gastric acid or poisons), and microorganisms trigger inflammation.

Immune Response

When a foreign material **(antigen)** enters the body, a series of responses changes the biological makeup of the body. The next time that the same antigen enters the body, antibodies bind to the antigens they find and neutralize, destroy, or eliminate them.

Vascular and Cellular Responses

Acute inflammation is an immediate response to cellular injury. Rapid vasodilation occurs, allowing more blood near the location of the injury. The increase in local blood flow causes the redness and localized warmth at the site of inflammation.

Injury causes tissue damage and possibly necrosis. As a result, the body releases chemical mediators that increase the permeability of small blood vessels, and fluid, protein, and cells enter interstitial spaces. The accumulation of fluid appears as localized swelling (**edema**). Another sign of inflammation is pain, which is caused by the swelling of inflamed tissues that increases pressure on nerve endings. As a result of the physiological inflammatory response, the involved body part may have a temporary loss of function. For example, a localized infection of the hand causes the fingers to become swollen, painful, and discolored. Joints become stiff as a result of swelling, but function of the fingers returns when inflammation subsides.

The cellular response of inflammation involves WBCs arriving at the site. WBCs pass through blood vessels and into the tissues. Phagocytosis is a process that involves the destruction and absorption of bacteria. Through the process of phagocytosis, specialized WBCs, called neutrophils and monocytes, ingest and destroy microorganisms or other small particles. If inflammation becomes systemic, other signs and symptoms develop. Leukocytosis, or an increase in the number of circulating WBCs, is the response of the body to WBCs leaving blood vessels. In an adult, a serum WBC count is normally $5000-10{,}000/mm^3$ but typically rises to $15{,}000-20{,}000/mm^3$ and higher during inflammation. Fever is caused by phagocytic release of pyrogens from bacterial cells, which causes a rise in the hypothalamic set point.

Inflammatory Exudate

Accumulation of fluid, dead tissue cells, and WBCs forms an exudate at the site of inflammation. Exudate may be **serous** (clear, like plasma), **sanguineous** (containing red blood cells), or **purulent** (containing WBCs and bacteria). Usually the exudate is cleared away through lymphatic drainage. Platelets and plasma proteins such as fibrinogen form a meshlike matrix at the site of inflammation to prevent its spread.

Tissue Repair

When there is injury to tissue cells, healing involves the defensive, reconstructive, and maturative stages. Damaged cells eventually are replaced with healthy new cells. The new cells undergo a gradual maturation until they take on the same structural characteristics and appearance as the previous cells. If inflammation is chronic, tissue defects sometimes fill with fragile **granulation tissue** that eventually takes the form of a scar at the completion of the healing process. The scar and surrounding tissues are not as strong as normal tissue and may be more susceptible to injury from pressure, shear, or friction, which increase the risk for pressure ulcer development.

CONCEPT OF ASEPSIS

Efforts to minimize the onset and spread of infection to patients are based on the principles of **aseptic technique.** The term **asepsis** means the absence of disease-producing microorganisms. The two types of aseptic technique are medical asepsis and surgical asepsis.

Medical asepsis, or clean techniques, includes procedures used to reduce the number and prevent the spread of microorganisms. Hand hygiene, use of barrier techniques such as gloving and gowning, and routine environmental cleaning are examples of medical asepsis.

Surgical asepsis, or sterile technique, includes procedures to eliminate all microorganisms from an area. **Sterilization** destroys all microorganisms and their spores (CDC, 2008). Nurses in the operating room, in labor and delivery, and at the bedside practice sterile technique when using sterile instruments and supplies for patient care. Surgical asepsis demands the highest level of aseptic technique and requires that all areas be kept free of infectious microorganisms (Association of periOperative Nurses, 2016).

MEDICAL ASEPSIS

Basic medical aseptic techniques break the infection chain. Use these techniques for all patients, even when no infection is diagnosed. Aggressive preventive measures are highly effective in reducing HAIs.

Control or Elimination of Infectious Agents

With the common use of disposable equipment, nurses are sometimes less aware of disinfection and sterilization procedures. The proper cleaning, disinfection, and sterilization of contaminated objects (e.g., surgical instruments or blood pressure cuffs) significantly reduce and/or eliminate microorganisms (CDC, 2008; Rutala and Weber, 2015).

Cleaning

Cleaning involves removing organic material such as blood or inorganic material such as soil from objects. For example, nurses will often clean the surfaces of bed mattresses when there has been excess soiling. Generally, this involves the use of soap and water and proper mechanical scrubbing action. Cleaning occurs before disinfection and sterilization procedures (CDC, 2008; Rutala and Weber, 2015). Best practice recommends that surfaces should be physically clean before disinfection for any disinfectant to be effective (Royal College of Nursing, 2011). Check the policy of the health care agency before cleaning. In most institutions, technicians clean equipment. When cleaning objects soiled with blood or body fluids, use personal protective equipment (PPE) such as gloves, goggles, and mask to protect yourself from splashing fluids.

Disinfection and Sterilization

Disinfection and sterilization use both physical and chemical processes. Both processes disrupt the internal functioning of microorganisms by destroying cell proteins. **Disinfection** eliminates almost all pathogenic organisms, with the exception of bacterial spores. Nurses commonly use disposable disinfectant cloths (e.g., alcohols and bleach) to wipe off soiled surfaces such as bedside tables and the outer surfaces of equipment. The solutions in these cloths have exposure or dwell times needed for a disinfectant to achieve full efficacy. How well a disinfectant is applied over a surface also affects efficacy (Royal College of Nursing, 2011). There are cloths with solutions specific for destroying certain microorganisms. For example, *Clostridium difficile* is one of the most difficult microorganisms to kill and is becoming a common HAI. The only disinfectants that work against *C. difficile* are accelerated hydrogen peroxide and bleach-based products.

Sterilization eliminates or destroys all forms of microbial life including spores (Rutala and Weber, 2015). Sterilization methods include processing items using steam, dry heat, hydrogen peroxide plasma, or ethylene oxide (ETO). The level of disinfection and sterilization required depends on the type and use of the contaminated item (Box 9.5). Always check package integrity and/or expiration dates before using an object designated as sterile. Dispose of items not meeting the criteria for being sterile or return them to the sterilization-processing department (CDC, 2008).

Control or Elimination of Reservoirs

To control or eliminate infection in reservoir sites, eliminate sources of body fluids, drainage, or solutions that possibly harbor microorganisms. For example, carefully discard disposable articles that become contaminated with infectious material in the proper receptacles (Box 9.6).

Control of Portals of Exit

To control organisms exiting through the respiratory tract, it is important to avoid talking, sneezing, or coughing directly over a surgical wound or sterile dressing field. Also, teach patients to protect others when they sneeze or cough and

BOX 9.5 Categories of Items Requiring Sterilization, Disinfection, and Cleaning

Critical Items

Items that enter sterile tissue or the vascular system present a high risk for infection if they are contaminated with microorganisms, especially bacterial spores. *Critical* items must be *sterile.* Some of these items include:

- Surgical instruments
- Cardiac or intravascular catheters
- Surgical implants

Semicritical Items

Items that come in contact with mucous membranes or nonintact skin also present a risk. These objects must be free of all microorganisms (except bacterial spores). *Semicritical items* must be *high-level disinfected (HLD)* or *sterilized.* Some of these items include:

- Respiratory and anesthesia equipment
- Endoscopes
- Endotracheal tubes
- Gastrointestinal endoscopes
- Diaphragm fitting rings

After rinsing, items must be dried and stored in a manner to protect from damage and contamination.

Noncritical Items

Items that come in contact with intact skin but not mucous membranes must be clean. *Noncritical items* must be *disinfected.* Some of these items include:

- Bedpans
- Blood pressure cuffs
- Bed rails
- Linens
- Stethoscopes
- Bedside trays and patient furniture
- Food utensils

BOX 9.6 Infection Prevention and Control to Reduce Reservoirs of Infection

Bathing

- Use soap and water to remove drainage, dried secretions, or excess perspiration.

Dressing Changes

- Change dressings that become wet and/or soiled.

Contaminated Articles

- Place tissues, soiled dressings, or soiled linen in fluid-resistant bags for proper disposal.

Contaminated Sharps

- Place all needles—safety needles and needleless systems—into puncture-proof containers located at the site of use.
  Federal law requires use of needle safety technology. Blood tube holders are single-use only (OSHA, 2015).

Bedside Unit

- Keep table surfaces clean and dry.

Bottled Solutions

- Do not leave bottled solutions open.
- Keep solutions tightly capped.
- Date bottles when opened and discard in 24 h.

Surgical Wounds

- Keep drainage tubes and collection bags patent to prevent accumulation of serous fluid under skin surface.

Drainage Bottles and Bags

- Wear gloves and protective eyewear if splashing or spraying with contaminated blood or body fluids is anticipated.
- Empty and dispose of drainage suction bottles according to agency policy.
- Empty all drainage systems on each shift unless otherwise ordered by health care provider.
- Never raise drainage system (e.g., urinary drainage bag) above level of site being drained unless it is clamped off.

give patients disposable wipes or tissues to control spread of microorganisms. Try not to work with patients who are highly susceptible to infection if you have a cold or other communicable infection.

Another way of controlling the exit of microorganisms is by using standard precautions when handling body fluids such as urine, feces, and wound drainage. Wear clean gloves if there is a chance of contact with any blood or body fluids and perform hand hygiene after providing care. Be sure to bag contaminated items appropriately.

Control of Transmission

Effective IPC requires knowledge of the modes of transmission of microorganisms and the methods of control. In any health care setting, a patient usually has a personal set of care items. Sharing graduated containers for measuring urine, bath basins, and eating utensils among patients creates routes for transmission of infection. Research supports that the contamination level of a stethoscope is substantial. When using a stethoscope, always wipe off the bell, diaphragm, and ear tips with a disinfectant such as an alcohol wipe before proceeding to the next patient (Longtin et al., 2014).

Because certain microorganisms travel easily through the air, do not shake linens or bedclothes. Dust surfaces within a patient's room with a treated or dampened cloth to prevent dust particles from entering the air.

To prevent transmission of microorganisms through indirect contact, do not allow soiled items and equipment to touch your clothing. A common error is to carry dirty linen in the arms against the uniform. Use special linen bags or carry soiled linen with the hands held out from the body. Never put clean or soiled linens on the floor.

Hand Hygiene

The most effective basic technique in preventing and controlling transmission of infection is hand hygiene (Box 9.7).

BOX 9.7 Procedural Guidelines

Hand Hygiene

Steps

1. Inspect surface of hands for breaks or cuts in skin or cuticles. Cover any skin lesions with a dressing before providing care. If lesions are too large to cover, you may be restricted from direct patient care.
2. Inspect hands for visible soiling.
3. Inspect condition of nails. Natural tips should be no longer than 0.625 cm (1/4 inch). Be sure that fingernails are short, filed, and smooth. If nails are polished, there should be no chips, and artificial nails or applications are contraindicated.
4. Push wristwatch and long uniform sleeves above wrists. Avoid wearing rings. If worn, remove during hand hygiene.
5. **Antiseptic hand rub**
    a. According to manufacturer directions, dispense ample amount of alcohol-based waterless antiseptic product into palm of one hand (usually an amount the size of a dime) (see illustration).
    b. Rub hands together, covering all surfaces of hands and fingers with antiseptic (see illustration).
    c. Rub hands together for 30 s to allow your hands to completely absorb the product and the hand sanitizer to completely dry. Allow hands to completely dry before applying gloves. If it takes less than 30 s for hands to dry, you likely have not used enough antiseptic.
6. **Handwashing using antimicrobial soap**
    a. Stand in front of sink, keeping hands and uniform away from sink surface. (If hands touch sink during handwashing, repeat sequence.)
    b. Turn on water. Turn faucet on (see illustration) or push knee pedals laterally or press pedals with foot to regulate flow and temperature.
    c. Avoid splashing water against uniform.
    d. Regulate flow of water so that temperature is warm.
    e. Wet hands and wrists thoroughly under running water. Keep hands and forearms lower than elbows during washing.
    f. Apply 3–5 mL of antiseptic soap and rub hands together (see illustration).

Clinical decision point: The most effective basic technique in preventing and controlling transmission of infection is hand hygiene (CDC, 2002).

    g. Perform hand hygiene using plenty of lather and friction for at least 15–20 s, making sure you clean all areas of the hands (CDC, 2016b). A tip is to sing the "Happy Birthday" song twice. Interlace fingers and rub palms and back of hands with circular motion at least five times each using friction. Keep fingertips down to facilitate removal of microorganisms.
    h. Areas underlying fingernails are often soiled. Clean them with fingernails of other hand and additional soap or with disposable nail cleaner.
    i. Rinse hands and wrists thoroughly, keeping hands down and elbows up (see illustration).
    j. Dry hands thoroughly from fingers to wrists with paper towel, single-use cloth, or warm air dryer.
    k. If used, discard paper towel in proper receptacle.
    l. To turn off hand faucet, use clean, dry paper towel; avoid touching handles with hands (see illustration). Turn off water with foot or knee pedals (if applicable).
    m. If hands are dry or chapped, use a small amount of lotion or barrier cream dispensed from an individual-use container.
7. Inspect surface of hands for obvious signs of dirt or other contaminants.
8. Inspect hands for dermatitis or cracked skin.
9. **Use teach back:** "I want to be sure you remember what we discussed earlier. Explain to me when you and your family should wash your hands at home." Revise your instruction now or develop a plan for revised patient,Äâ/family caregiver teaching if patient,Äâ/family caregiver is not able to teach back correctly.

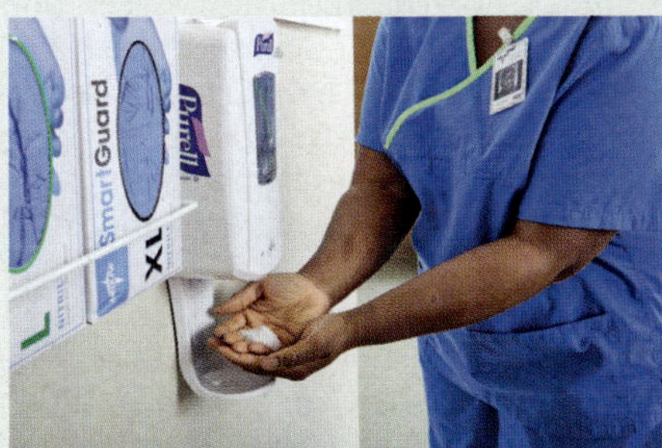

Step 5a Apply waterless antiseptic to hands.

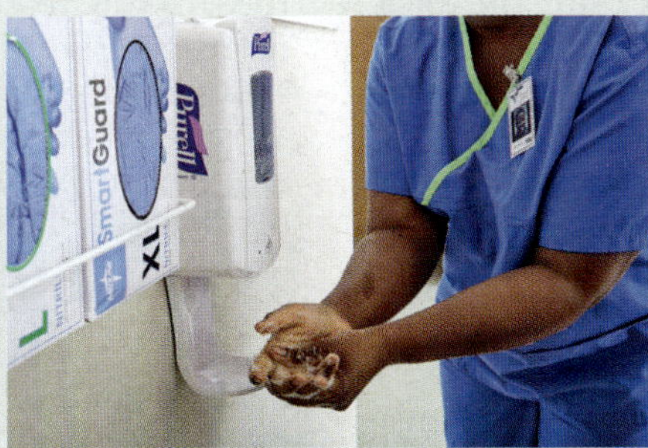

Step 5b Rub hands thoroughly, making sure to cover all surfaces of the fingers and hands.

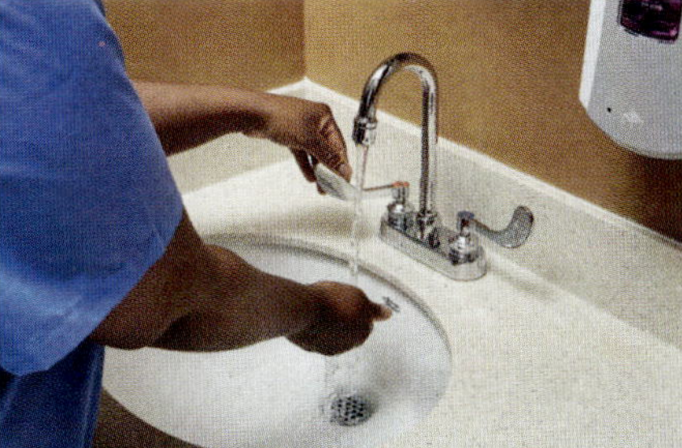
Step 6b Regulate flow of water.

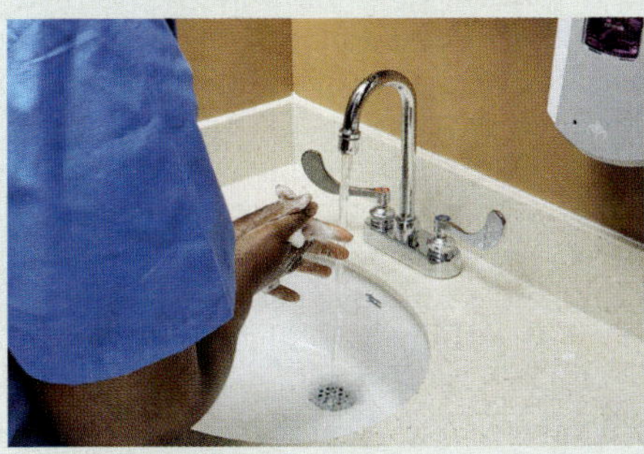
Step 6f Wet hands; apply soap and lather hands thoroughly.

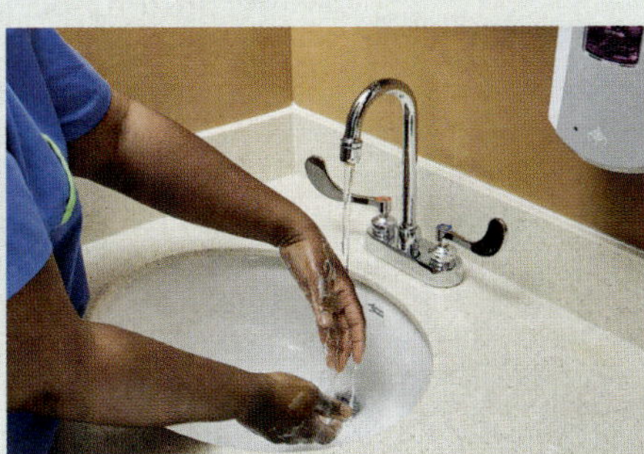
Step 6i Rinse hands.

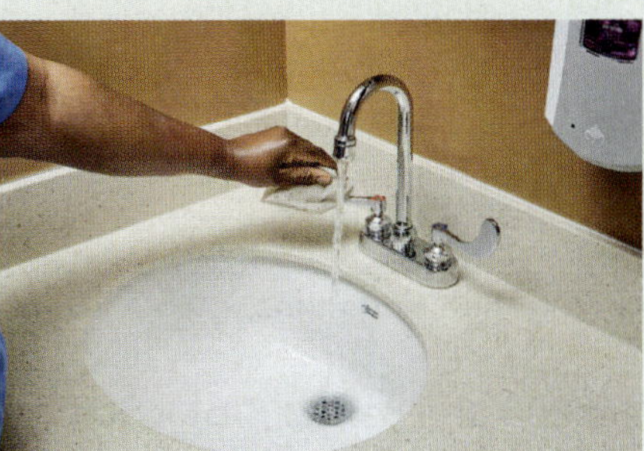
Step 6l Turn off faucet with clean, dry paper towel.

Hand hygiene is a general term that applies to four techniques: handwashing, antiseptic hand wash, antiseptic hand rub, and surgical hand antisepsis. Handwashing is defined by the CDC (2009) as the vigorous, brief rubbing together of all surfaces of lathered hands, followed by rinsing under a stream of warm water. The fundamental principle behind handwashing is removal of microorganisms mechanically from the hands and rinsing with water. Handwashing with soap and water does not kill microorganisms but does remove visible soiling of the hands.

An antiseptic hand wash involves handwashing with warm water and an antiseptic agent. Some antiseptics kill bacteria and some viruses. An antiseptic hand rub involves applying an antiseptic hand-rub product to all surfaces of the hands to reduce the number of microorganisms present. An alcohol-based hand sanitizer is the preferred method for cleaning the hands when working in a health care agency when the hands are not visibly dirty (CDC, 2016b). Ethanol-based hand antiseptics containing 60%−90% alcohol appear to be the most effective against common pathogens found on the hands (CDC, 2009). Alcohol-based products are more effective for standard handwashing or hand antisepsis (nonsoiled hands) by HCWs than regular soap or antimicrobial soaps (CDC, 2002). Surgical hand antisepsis is an antiseptic hand-wash or hand-rub technique that surgical personnel perform before surgery to eliminate transient hand flora and reduce resident flora. Antiseptic detergent preparations have persistent antimicrobial activity (CDC, 2002; World Health Organization [WHO], 2009).

Alcohol-based hand antiseptics are not effective on hands that are visibly dirty or are contaminated with organic materials (Haas, 2015). Thus, when hands are visibly dirty or contaminated with proteinaceous material or visibly soiled with blood or other body fluids, wash them with either a plain soap or an antimicrobial soap and water. Handwashing is also indicated before eating and after using the toilet. Wash hands with soap and water if they are exposed to spore-forming organisms such as *C. difficile or Bacillus anthracis* (CDC, 2008).

If hands are not visibly soiled, you may use an alcohol-based hand rub to decontaminate the hands during the Five Moments for Hand Hygiene (World Health Organization [WHO], 2017):

1. Before touching a patient.
2. Before clean/aseptic procedures (e.g., insertion of invasive devices, hygiene care).
3. After body fluid exposure/risk (e.g., contact during bathing, dressing changes, specimen collection).
4. After touching a patient.
5. After touching patient surroundings (e.g., overbed table, bed linen, i.v. pump).

This evidence-based, field-tested, user-centered approach is designed to be easy to learn, logical, and applicable to a wide range of health care settings (WHO, 2017) (Fig. 9.3). You may also wash hands with an antimicrobial soap and water in these situations.

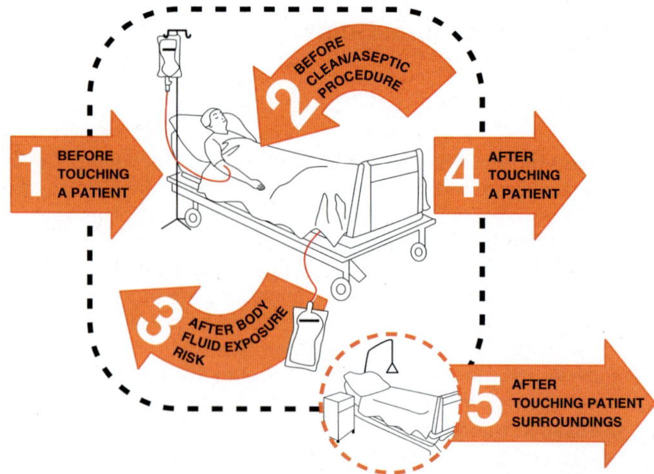

Fig. 9.3 Five Moments for Hand Hygiene. (From World Health Organization: About SAVE Lives: Clean Your Hands: 5 moments for hand hygiene, 2017, http://www.who.int/gpsc/5may/background/5moments/en/.)

Isolation and Barrier Protection

HICPAC published revised guidelines for isolation precautions in 2007 (CDC, 2007). HICPAC recommends that agencies modify these guidelines according to need and as dictated by federal, state, or local regulations. The guidelines contain recommendations for respiratory hygiene/cough etiquette as part of standard precautions. The CDC recommendations contain two tiers of precautions (Table 9.3). The first and most important tier is called standard precautions; the CDC designed it to be used for care of all patients, in all settings, regardless of risk or presumed infection status. Standard precautions are the primary strategies for prevention of infection transmission and apply to contact with blood, body fluids, nonintact skin, mucous membranes, and equipment or surfaces contaminated with these potentially infectious materials. The strategy of respiratory hygiene/cough etiquette applies to any person with signs of respiratory infection including cough, congestion, rhinorrhea, or increased production of respiratory secretions when entering a health care site. Educating health care staff, patients, and visitors to cover the mouth and nose with a tissue when coughing, dispose of used tissues properly, and perform hand hygiene is among the elements of respiratory hygiene. These precautions protect patients and HCWs (Box 9.8).

Assess the need for standard precautions based on the potential for transmission of infection, regardless of a patient's diagnosis. For example, when suctioning a patient with a tracheostomy, wearing gloves, eyewear, and a mask is appropriate protection regardless of the presence of known respiratory infection.

The second tier of precautions (see Table 9.3) includes precautions designed for the care of patients who are known or suspected to be infected or colonized with microorganisms transmitted by the droplet, airborne, or contact route (Berends and Walesa, 2015; CDC, 2007). There are three types of transmission-based precautions: **airborne precautions, droplet precautions,** and **contact precautions.** They are used singly or in combination for diseases that have multiple routes of transmission (e.g., chickenpox). Use them in addition to standard precautions.

One important aspect of care for patients on isolation is compliance with hand hygiene and changing gloves between exposure to body sites and patient equipment. Inadequate glove changes and hand hygiene often lead to

Table 9.3 Centers for Disease Control and Prevention Isolation Guidelines

STANDARD PRECAUTIONS (TIER 1) FOR USE WITH ALL PATIENTS

- Standard precautions apply to blood, blood products, all body fluids, secretions, excretions (except sweat), nonintact skin, and mucous membranes.
- Perform hand hygiene before, after, and between direct contact with patients. (Examples of between contact: cleaning hands after a patient care activity, moving to a non–patient care activity, then cleaning hands again before returning to perform patient contact.)
- Perform hand hygiene after contact with blood, body fluids, secretions, and excretions; after contact with surfaces or articles in a patient's room; and immediately after gloves are removed.
- When hands are visibly soiled or contaminated with blood or body fluids, wash them with either a nonantimicrobial soap or an antimicrobial soap and water.
- When hands are not visibly soiled or contaminated with blood or body fluids, use an alcohol-based hand rub to perform hand hygiene.
- Wash hands with antimicrobial soap and water if contact with spores (e.g., *Clostridium difficile*) is likely to have occurred.
- Do not wear artificial fingernails or extenders if duties include direct contact with patients at high risk for infection and associated adverse outcomes.
- Wear gloves when touching blood, body fluids, secretions, excretions, nonintact skin, mucous membranes, or contaminated items or surfaces. Remove gloves and perform hand hygiene between patient care encounters and when going from a contaminated to a clean body site.
- Wear PPE when the anticipated patient interaction indicates that contact with blood or body fluids may occur.
- A private room is unnecessary unless the patient's hygiene is unacceptable (e.g., uncontained secretions, excretions, or wound drainage).
- Discard all contaminated sharp instruments and needles in a puncture-resistant container. Health care agencies must make needleless devices available. Any needles should be disposed of uncapped, or a mechanical safety device is activated for recapping.
- Respiratory hygiene/cough etiquette: Have patients cover the nose/mouth when coughing or sneezing; use tissues to contain respiratory secretions, and dispose of in nearest waste container; perform hand hygiene after contacting respiratory secretions and contaminated object/materials; contain respiratory secretions with procedure or surgical masks; sit at least 3 feet away from others if coughing.

TRANSMISSION-BASED PRECAUTIONS (TIER 2) FOR USE WITH SPECIFIC TYPES OF PATIENTS

Category	Disease	Barrier Protection
Airborne precautions (droplet nuclei smaller than 5 microns)	Measles, chickenpox (varicella), disseminated varicella zoster, pulmonary or laryngeal tuberculosis	Private room, negative-pressure airflow of at least 6–12 exchanges per hour via HEPA filtration Mask or respiratory protection device, N95 respirator (depending on condition)
Droplet precautions (droplets larger than 5 microns; being within 3 feet of the patient)	Examples include *Bordetella pertussis,* influenza virus, adenovirus, rhinovirus, *Neisseria meningitidis,* group A *Streptococcus* (until first 24 h of antimicrobial therapy); refer to agency policy	Private room or cohort patients Mask or respirator required depending on condition (refer to agency policy)
Contact precautions (direct patient or environmental contact)	Colonization or infection with multidrug-resistant organisms such as VRE and MRSA, *Clostridium difficile, Shigella,* and other enteric pathogens; major wound infections; herpes simplex; scabies; varicella zoster (disseminated); respiratory syncytial virus in infants, young children, or immunocompromised adults	Private room or cohort patients (see agency policy), gloves, gowns (patients may leave their room for procedures or therapy if infectious material contained or covered, placed in a clean gown, and if hands are cleaned)
Protective environment	Allogeneic hematopoietic stem cell transplants	Private room; positive-pressure airflow with 12 or more air exchanges per hour; HEPA filtration for incoming air Mask to be worn by the patient when out of room during times of construction in area

HEPA, high-efficiency particulate air; *MRSA,* methicillin-resistant *Staphylococcus aureus; PPE,* personal protective equipment; *VRE,* vancomycin-resistant enterococci.
Modified from Centers for Disease Control and Prevention, Hospital Infection Control Practice Advisory Committee: 2007 Guideline for isolation precautions in hospitals, *MMWR Morb Mortal Wkly Rep* 57(RR-16):39, 2007.

BOX 9.8 Procedural Guidelines

Caring for a Patient on Isolation Precautions

Equipment

Personal protective equipment (PPE) determined by type of isolation required; clean gloves, mask, eyewear or goggles, face shield, and gown (gowns may be disposable or reusable, depending on agency policy); other patient care equipment (as appropriate; e.g., hygiene items, medications, dressing supplies, sharps container, disposable blood pressure cuff); soiled linen bag and trash receptacle, sign for door indicating type of isolation and/or for visitors to come to the nurses' station before entering room. Tuberculosis (TB) isolation: room with negative airflow, N95 or P100 respirator.

Steps

1. Assess patient's medical history for possible indications for isolation (e.g., risk factors for TB, major draining wound, or purulent productive cough). Review precautions for the specific isolation system, including appropriate barriers to apply (see Table 9.3).
2. Review laboratory test results (e.g., wound culture, acid-fast bacillus [AFB] smears, changes in white blood cell [WBC] count).
3. Review agency policies and isolation precautions necessary for type of isolation ordered, and consider types of care measures that you will perform while in patient's room (e.g., medication administration or dressing change).
4. Review nursing care plan notes or confer with colleagues regarding patient's emotional state and reaction/adjustment to isolation. Also, assess the patient's understanding of purpose of isolation.
5. Assess whether the patient has a known latex allergy. If an allergy is present, refer to agency policy and resources available to provide full latex-free care.

Continued

BOX 9.8 Procedural Guidelines—cont'd

6. Perform hand hygiene (see Box 9.7).
7. Prepare all equipment to be taken into the patient's room. In many cases, dedicated equipment such as stethoscopes, blood pressure equipment, and thermometers should remain in the room until the patient is discharged. If the patient is infected or colonized with a resistant organism (e.g., vancomycin-resistant enterococcus [VRE], methicillin-resistant *Staphylococcus aureus* [MRSA]), equipment remains in room and is thoroughly disinfected before removal from room (see agency policy).
8. Prepare for entrance into isolation room. Ideally, before applying PPE, step into the patient's room and stay by door. Introduce yourself and explain the care that you are providing. If this is not possible, apply PPE outside of the room.
   a. Apply cover gown, being sure that it covers all outer garments. Pull sleeves down to wrist. Tie securely at neck and waist (see illustration).
   b. Apply either surgical mask or a fitted respirator around mouth and nose (type and fit-testing depend on type of isolation and agency policy). You must have a medical evaluation and be fit-tested before using a respirator mask. You are allowed to pick the most acceptable respirator from a sufficient number of respirator models and sizes so that the respirator is acceptable to you and fits correctly (OSHA, n.d.). Comfort of a respiratory mask includes position of the mask on the nose, room for eye protection, room to talk, and position of mask on the face and cheeks.
   c. If needed, apply protective eyewear or goggles snugly around face and eyes. If you wear prescription glasses, side shields may be used.
   d. Apply clean gloves. (Note: Wear unpowdered, latex-free gloves if you, the patient, or another health care worker has a latex allergy.) As of January 19, 2017, the FDA has banned powdered medical gloves (FDA, 2016). If gloves are worn with gown, bring glove cuffs over edge of gown sleeves (see illustration).
9. Enter the patient's room and identify the patient using at least two personal identifiers, for example, full name and date of birth (TJC, 2018). Then confirm this information with the patient's identification bracelet. Arrange supplies and equipment. (Note: If equipment will be reused, place on a clean paper towel.)
10. Explain purpose of isolation and the precautions for the patient and family to follow. Offer opportunity to ask questions and assess for evidence of emotional problems. If the patient is on TB precautions, instruct the patient to cover mouth with tissue when coughing and to wear disposable surgical mask when leaving room.
11. Assess vital signs.
    a. If the patient is infected or colonized with a resistant organism (e.g., VRE, MRSA), equipment remains in the room including the stethoscope and blood pressure cuff.
    b. If stethoscope is to be reused, clean earpieces and diaphragm or bell with 70% alcohol or agency-approved germicide. Set aside on clean surface.
    c. Use individual or disposable thermometers and blood pressure cuffs when available.

Clinical decision point: If disposable thermometer indicates a fever, assess for other signs and/or symptoms. Confirm fever using an alternative thermometer. Do not use electronic thermometer if the patient is suspected or confirmed to have *Clostridium difficile* infection (Surawicz et al., 2013).

12. Administer medications (see Chapter 26).
    a. Give oral medication in unit dose wrapper or cup.
    b. Dispose of wrapper or cup in plastic-lined receptacle.
    c. Wear gloves when administering an injection.
    d. Discard needleless syringe or safety sheathed needle into designated sharps container.
    e. Place reusable syringe (e.g., carpuject) on a clean towel for eventual removal and disinfection.

Clinical decision point: If gloves are torn and hands come in contact with contaminated article or body fluids, perform hand hygiene as soon as possible and reapply gloves.

13. Administer personal hygiene care, encouraging the patient to ask any questions or express concerns about isolation. Provide informal teaching at this time.
    a. Avoid allowing isolation gown to become wet; carry washbasin outward away from gown; avoid leaning against wet tabletop.

Clinical decision point: When there is a risk for excess soiling, wear a gown impervious to moisture.

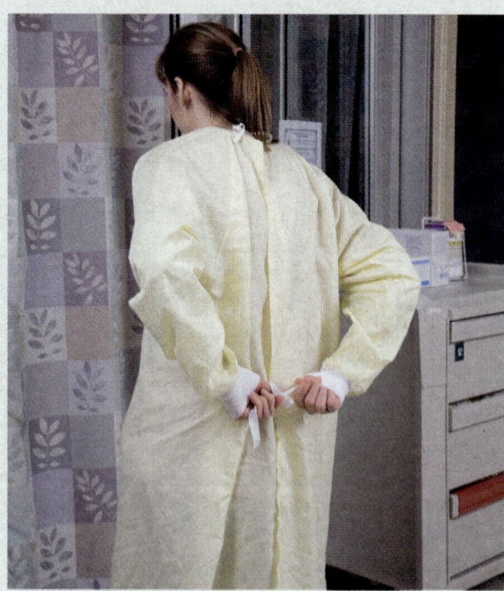

Step 8a Tie gown at waist and neck.

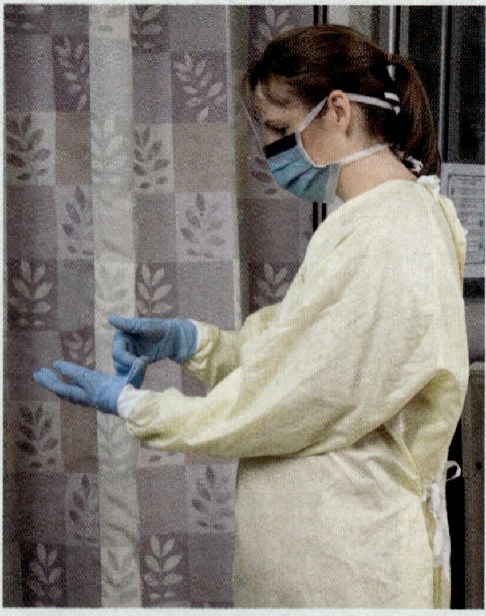

Step 8d Apply gloves over gown sleeves.

BOX 9.8 Procedural Guidelines—cont'd

b. Help the patient remove own gown; discard in leak-proof linen bag.
c. Remove linen from bed; avoid contact with isolation gown. Place in leak-proof linen bag.
d. Provide clean bed linen.
e. Change gloves. Perform hand hygiene if gloves become excessively soiled and further care is necessary. Reapply gloves.

14. Collect specimens.
    a. Place specimen container on clean paper towel in the patient's bathroom and follow procedure for collecting specimen of body fluids.
    b. Follow agency procedure for collecting specimen of body fluids.
    c. Transfer specimen to container without soiling outside of container. Place container in plastic bag, and place label on outside of bag or per agency policy. Label specimen in front of the patient (TJC, 2018). Place containers of blood or body fluids in a biohazard bag (see illustration). Perform hand hygiene. Reapply gloves if additional procedures are needed.
    d. Check label on specimen for accuracy. Send to laboratory. (**Note:** Additional warning labels are often used, depending on agency policy.)
15. Dispose of linen, trash, and disposable items.
    a. Use sturdy moisture-impervious bags to contain soiled articles. Use double bag, if necessary, for heavily soiled linen or heavy wet trash.
    b. Tie bags securely at top in knot (see illustration).
16. Remove all reusable pieces of equipment. Clean any contaminated surfaces with hospital-approved disinfectant (CDC, 2009) (see agency policy).
17. Resupply room as needed. Have staff colleague hand new supplies to you.
18. Leave isolation room. Order of removal of PPE depends on what you wear in room. The following sequence describes steps to take if all barriers were worn. PPE worn in the isolation room must be removed before leaving the room.
    a. Remove gloves. Remove one glove by grasping cuff and pulling glove inside out over hand. Place used glove in gloved hand. With ungloved hand, tuck thumb inside cuff of remaining glove and pull it off, inside out (see illustration).
    b. Remove eyewear, face shield, or goggles. Handle by headband or earpieces. Discard in proper container.
    c. Untie neck strings and then untie back strings of gown. Allow gown to fall from shoulders (see illustration); touch inside of gown only. Remove hands from sleeves without touching outside of gown. Hold gown inside at shoulder seams and fold inside out into a bundle; discard in laundry bag.
    d. Remove mask. If mask loops over ears, remove elastic from ears and pull mask away from face. For a tie-on mask, untie *top* mask strings, hold strings, untie *bottom* strings, pull mask away from face (see illustration), and drop into trash receptacle. (Do not touch outer surface of mask.)

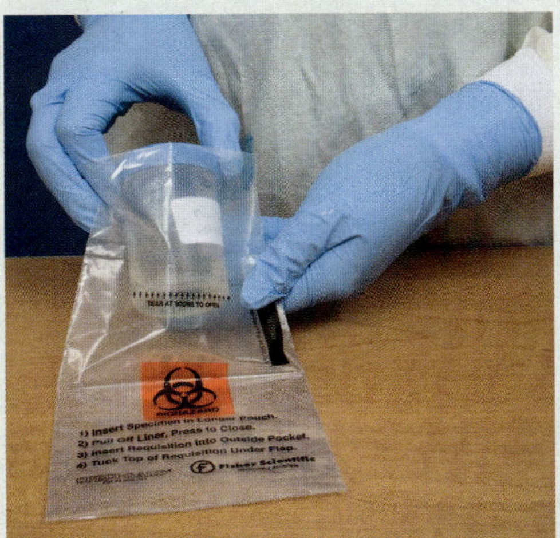

Step 14c Specimen container placed in biohazard bag and sealed.

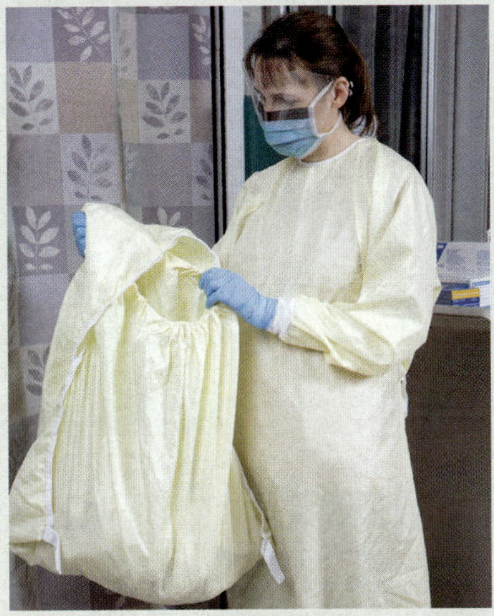

Step 15b Tie trash bag securely.

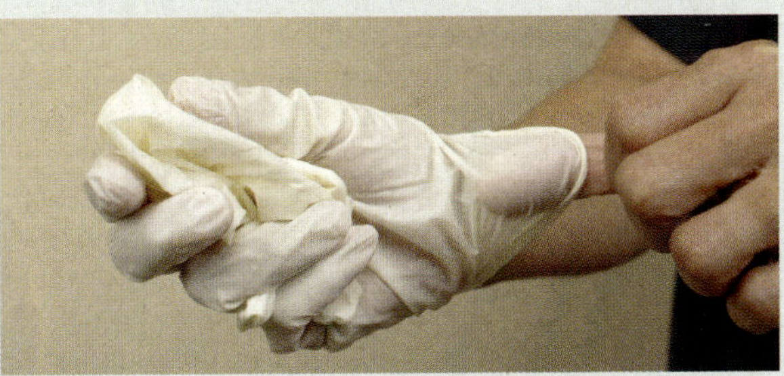

Step 18a Remove gloves.

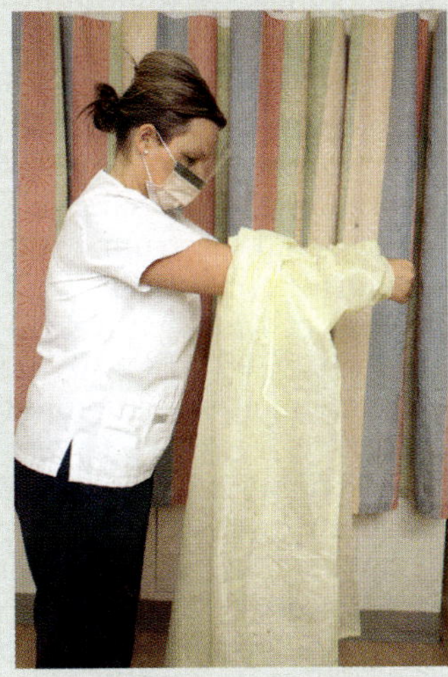

Step 18c Remove gown by allowing it to fall from shoulders and remove so that outside of gown is now inside.

Continued

BOX 9.8 Procedural Guidelines—cont'd

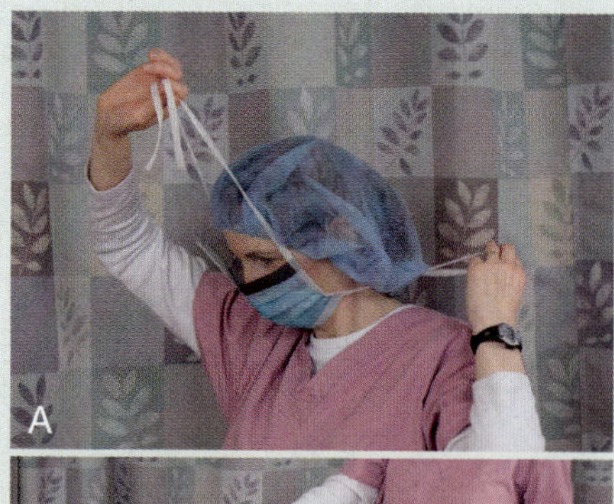

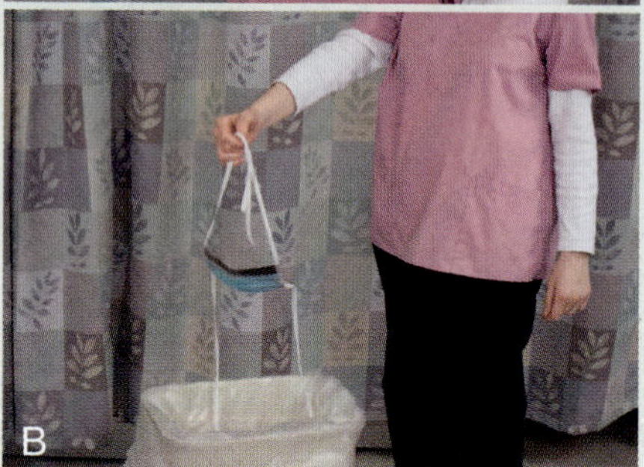

Step 18d Remove mask.

Clinical decision point: If the patient is on TB precautions, place reusable mask in labeled paper bag for storage, being careful not to crush mask (check agency policy for number of times reusable masks can be used).

e. Perform hand hygiene.
f. Explain to the patient when you plan to return to room. Ask whether the patient requires any personal care items. Offer books, magazines, or audiotapes.
g. Leave room and close door if necessary. Close door if the patient is on airborne precautions or in negative airflow room.
h. Dispose of all contaminated supplies and equipment in proper manner (see agency policy). Perform hand hygiene.

19. Observe the patient and family members' use of isolation precautions when visiting.
20. While in room, ask whether the patient has had a sufficient opportunity to discuss health problems, course of treatment, or other topics important to him or her.
21. **Use teach back:** "I want to be sure I explained why you need to wear the protective clothing. Tell me why you think you need to wear the gown, gloves, and mask." Revise your instruction now or develop a plan for revised patient/family caregiver teaching if patient/family caregiver is not able to teach back correctly.

contamination of previously colonized sites (Haas, 2015). Noncompliance with these practices increases the risk of HAIs.

Because of the resurgence of tuberculosis (TB), the CDC (2005) developed guidelines to prevent its transmission to HCWs and stresses the importance of isolation for patients with known or suspected TB in a special negative-pressure room. Close the doors to the patient's room to control direction of airflow. Wear a special high-filtration particulate respirator on entering a respiratory isolation room. Health care organizations must provide fit-testing to be sure a respirator fits each HCW with different facial sizes and characteristics (OSHA, n.d.). When worn correctly, particulate respirators and masks (Figs 9.4 and 9.5) have a tighter face seal and filter at a higher level than routine surgical masks (OSHA, 2009).

MDROs such as methicillin-resistant *Staphylococcus aureus* (MRSA) and vancomycin-resistant *Enterococcus* (VRE) have become more common as a cause of colonization and HAIs. MDROs are organisms that have developed a resistance to one or more broad-spectrum antibiotics, making the organism hard to treat effectively. MRSA is a highly virulent organism that can frequently lead to sepsis and death (Becker and Kock, 2015; CDC, 2016c). VRE poses a risk to patients who are immune-compromised and debilitated (Archibald, 2015; CDC, 2011). *C. difficile* infection is one of the most common and costly HAIs. Patient susceptibility to *C. difficile* usually results from prior treatment with antibiotics (particularly clindamycin). In contrast to MRSA and VRE, *C. difficile* is harder to eliminate from the environment because it is a spore-forming organism, meaning it can remain on surfaces in a dormant state for long periods and is resistant to the contents in commercial hand sanitizers (CDC, 2011). For this reason, when caring for patients with *C. difficile*, it is recommended that vigorous handwashing using soap and water be used to clean hands. To reduce the risk of cross-contamination among patients, use contact precautions in addition to standard precautions when caring for patients with MDROs.

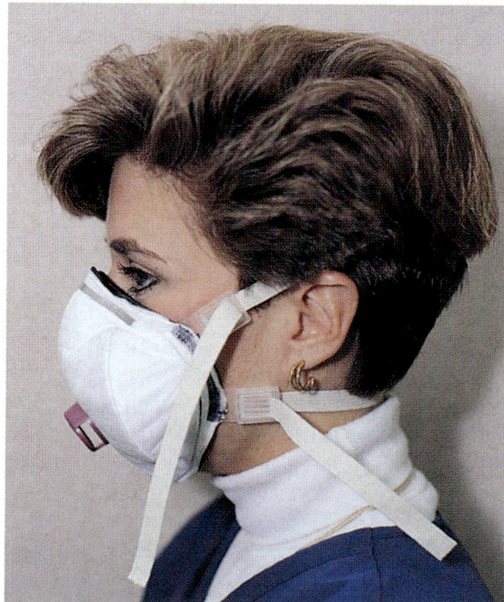

Fig. 9.4 Disposable high-efficiency particulate air (HEPA)–purifying respirator.

Regardless of the type of isolation or barrier protection used, follow certain basic principles when delivering care in a patient's room. Understand how certain diseases are transmitted and which barriers you need to prevent transmission. For example, you do not routinely need to wear a gown or gloves when giving oral medications, but you do need these barriers when changing a dressing from a draining wound.

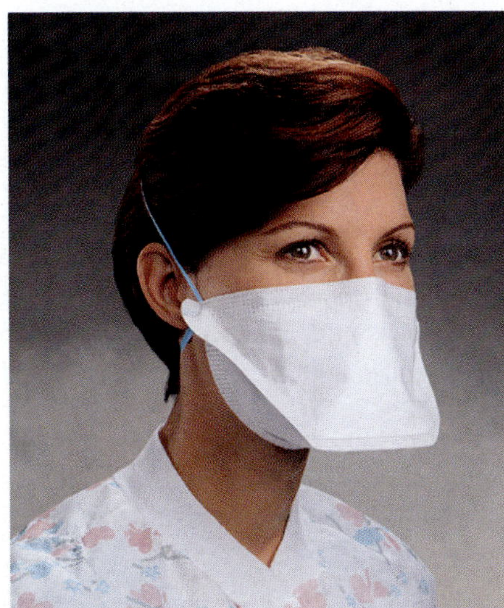

Fig. 9.5 N95 respirator mask with protective eyewear. (Courtesy Halyard Health, Inc., Alpharetta, GA.)

Gloves are appropriate when helping a patient with an oral medication if the patient needs assistance putting the medication in the mouth.

Take care to avoid exposing an article brought into a patient's room to any infectious material. Bag or decontaminate any contaminated article (e.g., glucose meter, blood pressure cuff) according to agency policy. Decontaminate equipment that is shared among patients.

Before you institute isolation measures, explain to a patient and family members the nature of the patient's condition, the purpose of the isolation barriers, and ways to carry out specific precautions. Teach them the proper way to perform hand hygiene and apply gloves, masks, or gowns. Demonstrate each procedure, and give the patient and family an opportunity to practice. Always reinforce the specific reasons why these steps are important in the care of the patient. Explain methods of transmission of infectious organisms so they understand the difference between contaminated and clean objects.

Provide for a patient's sensory stimulation during isolation. Encourage the family to bring the patient reading materials, puzzle books, music, and similar items. Take the opportunity to listen to the patient's concerns or interests. If you rush care or show a lack of interest in the patient's needs, he or she will feel rejected and even more isolated. Explain the patient's potential risk for depression or loneliness to family members. Encourage visitors to avoid negative expressions or actions concerning isolation. Advise family members on ways to provide meaningful stimulation.

Protective Environment

In some situations, special isolation rooms are used for highly susceptible patients such as organ transplant recipients and patients with neutropenia (low WBC count). Post a card on the patient's room door with a list of the precautions in use when a private room is recommended (check agency policy). The card is a handy reference for HCWs and visitors and alerts all who enter the room of any special precautions in use. Make sure that you follow agency policies on isolation practice (CDC, 2007).

The isolation room or an adjoining anteroom, if present, needs to contain hand-hygiene supplies, bathing facilities, and toilet facilities. Personnel and visitors need to perform hand hygiene before entering and on exiting a patient's room. Store PPE in an anteroom between the room and hallway or in a location convenient to where the PPE is needed.

Each patient care room, including rooms used for isolation, contains a trash container with plastic liners. Rooms used for isolation also contain a soiled linen hamper. These containers prevent transmission of microorganisms by preventing leakage and waste from contaminating the outside surface. Have a disposable, rigid container available in the room to discard used needles, sharps, and syringes.

Depending on the microorganisms identified and the mode of transmission, critically evaluate which articles or equipment to take into an isolation room. For example, HICPAC recommends taking only dedicated articles into an isolation room when VRE is present (CDC, 2007).

PERSONAL PROTECTIVE EQUIPMENT

Gowns or cover-ups protect HCWs from contacting infected blood and body fluids or materials during procedures or when patients have uncontained secretions. Gowns used for barrier protection are made of a fluid-resistant material. Change a gown immediately if it is damaged or heavily contaminated. Isolation gowns usually open at the back and have ties or snaps at the neck and waist to keep the gown closed and secure. A gown is long enough to cover all outer garments. Long sleeves with tight-fitting cuffs provide added protection.

Wear a mask or respirator if you anticipate splashing or spraying of blood or body fluids. The mask also protects you from inhaling microorganisms from a patient's respiratory tract and prevents the transmission of pathogens from your respiratory tract. Occasionally, a patient who is susceptible to infection wears a mask to avoid inhaling pathogens. Patients requiring respiratory precautions wear surgical masks when ambulating or being transported outside of their room to protect other patients and personnel.

Masks prevent the transmission of infections caused by direct contact with mucous membranes. A mask discourages the wearer from touching the nose or mouth. A properly applied mask fits snugly over the mouth and nose so that the pathogens and body fluids cannot enter or escape through the sides (Box 9.9). If a person wears glasses, the top edge of the mask fits below the glasses so that they do not cloud over as the person exhales. Keep talking to a minimum while wearing a mask. Discard a mask that has become moist because it is ineffective. Discard the mask when leaving a patient's room. Warn patients and family members that a mask sometimes causes a sensation of smothering. If family members become uncomfortable, have them leave the room and discard their masks.

Apply disposable gloves when there is a risk for exposing the hands to blood, body fluids, mucous membranes, nonintact skin, or potentially infectious material on objects or surfaces. In addition, use gloves when you have scratches or breaks in your skin and when performing venipuncture, fingersticks, or heelsticks. You wear gloves alone or

BOX 9.9 Procedural Guidelines

Applying an Isolation Mask

Equipment

Disposable mask

Steps

1. Find top edge of mask, which usually has thin metal strip along edge.
2. Hold mask by top two strings or loops, keeping top edge above bridge of nose. Tie two top strings at top of back of head, over cap (if worn), with strings above ears (see illustration). Alternatively place loops over ears.
3. Tie two lower ties snugly around neck with mask well under chin (see illustration).
4. Gently pinch upper metal band around bridge of nose.

Clinical decision point: Change mask if wet, moist, or contaminated.

5. Remove mask by untying bottom mask strings and then top strings; pull mask away from face and drop into trash receptacle (see illustrations in Box 9.9, Step 18d). (Do not touch outer surface of the mask.)

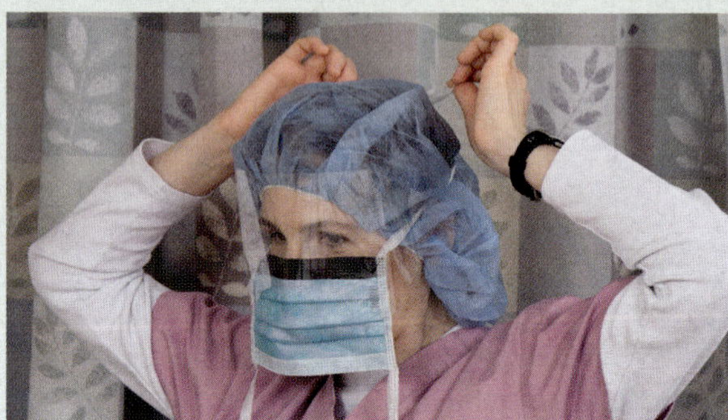

Step 2 Attaching top two ties of a tie-on mask.

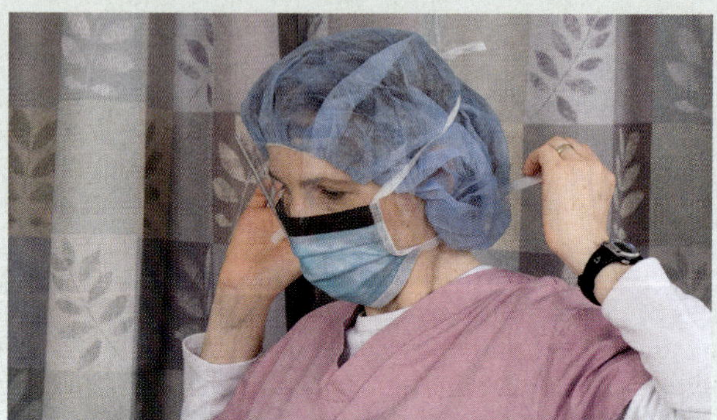

Step 3 Securing bottom two ties of a tie-on mask.

in combination with other PPE. When other PPE is necessary, first put on a mask and eyewear (if required), apply a gown (if required), and then apply gloves. Pull the glove cuffs up over the wrists or cuffs of a gown.

After contacting infectious material, change gloves and perform hand hygiene even if you have not finished caring for the patient. If your actions do not involve more patient contact, it is not necessary to reapply gloves. Teach patients and their families the reasons for wearing gloves and the correct method for applying them.

Most gloves used for barrier protection or surgical asepsis are latex-free. However, when you wear gloves made of latex follow these precautions. Before applying latex gloves, assess a patient's potential for having a latex allergy. Individuals most at risk include individuals with a history of spina bifida, congenital or urogenital defects, indwelling urinary catheterization, use of condom catheters, multiple childhood surgeries, and food allergies. A history of occupational exposure to latex is another risk for a patient. The symptoms of a reaction to latex range from mild dermatitis to severe anaphylactic shock. The Food and Drug Administration (FDA, 2016) has banned the use of powdered gloves. The powder had been a factor in causing latex sensitivity because of repeated contact or by inhaling aerosolized latex allergens. The Association of PeriOperative Registered Nurses (AORN, 2016) provides the following suggestions for nurses to avoid becoming allergic to latex:

1. Wear gloves only when indicated.
2. Wash with a pH-balanced soap immediately after removing gloves.
3. Apply only non–oil-based hand care products (oil-based products break down latex allergens).
4. If a reaction or dermatitis occurs, report to employee health service and/or seek medical treatment immediately.

Wear protective eyewear and face shields properly fitted during procedures in which it is possible to splatter the eyes or face with blood or other infectious material. In many instances, caregivers purchase their own eyewear with prescription lenses. Regular glasses are insufficient. Protective eyewear needs to have side shields to prevent material from entering the eye between the glasses and face.

Role of PPE has significant importance during recent COVID-19 pandemic.

Specimen Collection

A patient with a suspected or actual infectious disease sometimes has many laboratory studies. Body fluids and materials suspected to contain infectious organisms are collected for culture and sensitivity tests. In the laboratory, the specimen is placed in a special medium that promotes the growth of organisms. A laboratory technologist then identifies the type of microorganisms growing in the culture and the broad-spectrum antibiotics that may kill those organisms. Additional sensitivity test results indicate the antibiotics to which the organisms are resistant or sensitive. Thus, proper medications are ordered.

Obtain all culture specimens with sterile equipment. Collecting fresh material (e.g., wound drainage) from the site of an infection ensures that resident flora does not contaminate the specimen. Seal all specimen containers tightly to prevent spillage and contamination of the outside of the containers (Box 9.10). After you transfer specimens to containers, label each specimen properly with the patient's

BOX 9.10 Specimen Collection Techniques

Ensure that each specimen container or the bag in which it is placed has a biohazard symbol on the outside. Before collecting specimen, identify the patient using at least two identifiers, for example, full name and date of birth (TJC, 2018). Confirm this information on the patient's identification bracelet.

Wound Specimen

Perform hand hygiene and apply clean gloves. Clean area around wound edges with antiseptic swab. Wipe from edges outward to remove old exudate (see Chapter 17). Remove gloves, perform hand hygiene, and reapply gloves. Use a cotton-tipped swab or syringe to collect as much drainage as possible. Have clean test tube or culture tube ready on clean paper towel. After swabbing center of wound site, grasp collection tube with paper towel. Carefully insert swab without touching outside of tube and secure top of tube. For some specimens, you need to crush end of tube and push swab into fluid. Transfer tube into biohazard bag for transport and perform hand hygiene.

Blood Specimen Culture[a]

Wearing gloves, clean venipuncture site with antiseptic swabs, with first swab moving back and forth on horizontal plane, another swab on vertical plane, and last swab in a circular motion from site outward for 5 cm (2 inches) lasting a total of 30 s. Allow to dry. Clean tops of culture bottles for 15 s with agency-approved cleansing solution. Use 20-mL needle-safe syringe and collect 10–15 mL of blood per culture bottle (check health care agency policy). Perform venipuncture at two different sites to decrease likelihood of both specimens being contaminated with skin flora. Place blood culture bottles on clean paper towel on bedside table or other surface; swab off bottle tops with alcohol. Inject appropriate amount of blood into each bottle. Transfer specimen into clean, labeled biohazard bag for transport. Remove gloves and perform hand hygiene.

Stool Specimen

Wearing gloves, use clean cup with seal top (need not be sterile) and tongue blade to collect small amount of stool, approximately 2–3 cm (approximately 1 inch). Place cup on clean paper towel in the patient's bathroom. Using tongue blade, collect needed amount of feces from the patient's bedpan. Transfer feces to cup without touching outside surface of cup. Dispose of tongue blade and place seal on cup. Transfer specimen into clean biohazard bag for transport. Remove gloves and perform hand hygiene.

Urine Specimen

Apply gloves; cleanse needleless port on urinary catheter and use needleless syringe to collect 1–5 mL of urine. Fill sterile specimen cup or specimen tube, and place on clean towel in the patient's bathroom. If the patient is not catheterized, have the patient follow procedure to obtain clean voided specimen (see Chapter 21). Secure top of transfer container and place in biohazard bag. Remove gloves and perform hand hygiene.

Note: Health care agency policies may differ on type of containers and amount of specimen material required. For all specimens, label containers for specimens in the presence of the patient (TJC, 2018).

[a]This procedure is usually performed by a laboratory technician.
From Pagana KD, Pagana TJ: *Mosby's diagnostic and laboratory test reference*, ed 11, St Louis, 2012, Mosby.

name, patient identifier, date and time, and type of specimen. Label specimens in the presence of the patient (TJC, 2018). Place specimen containers in labeled leak-proof biohazard bags before transporting them to the laboratory (see agency policy).

Bagging

In general, bagging articles is the same for all patients regardless of whether they are on isolation (see agency policy). Bagging articles prevents accidental exposure of personnel to contaminated articles and contamination of the surrounding environment.

Place all soiled linen in a designated waterproof bag in a patient's room. Do not overfill the bag. Handle, transport, and process linen soiled with blood or body fluids in a way that prevents exposure of skin or mucous membrane and/or contamination of the HCW's clothing. Some hospitals still require double bagging. A standard-size linen bag, not overfilled, tied securely and intact is adequate to prevent infection transmission. Consult agency policy and any applicable regulations.

Biohazardous waste includes both infectious and medical waste that must be disposed of in special red bags or per agency policy. These disposal procedures are a large expense for health care agencies. Consider the following waste materials to be infectious or medical waste (WHO, 2015):

- Infectious waste such as cultures of infectious organisms or waste from highly infectious patients
- Pathological waste such as discarded human tissue, organs, and body parts
- Blood and blood products
- Sharps, including discarded needles, syringes, scalpels, and blood vials
- Chemicals used for laboratory preparation and disinfectants
- Genotoxic waste from cytotoxic drugs used in cancer treatment
- Radioactive diagnostic material

Removal of Protective Equipment

The method of removing protective clothing, gloves, eyewear, gown, and mask before leaving an isolation room depends on the protective equipment worn at the time. If you wear all four protective items, first remove the gloves because they are most likely to be contaminated. If you untie a gown while wearing gloves, there is a chance of contaminating your hair or a portion of your uniform. See Box 9.8 for steps for removing PPE.

Transporting Patients

Patients infected with highly communicable organisms such as the TB bacillus may leave their rooms only for essential purposes such as diagnostic procedures or surgery. Before transferring a patient to a wheelchair or stretcher, provide the patient with appropriate barrier protection. For example, patients infected by an organism transmitted by the respiratory tract need to wear surgical masks. Personnel transporting patients practice the appropriate precautions while in a patient's room and remove PPE when leaving the room. Notify personnel in diagnostic areas or the operating room that the patient is on isolation precautions. Record the type of isolation on the patient's chart, and explain ways to avoid transmitting infection during transport (CDC, 2007).

Control of Portals of Entry

Many measures that control the exit of microorganisms also control the entrance of pathogens. Provide interventions to control and prevent organisms from gaining a portal of entry (Box 9.11).

Protection of the Susceptible Host

A patient's resistance to infection improves by using measures that protect normal body defense mechanisms, including supporting existing body defense mechanisms or controlling exposure to microorganisms. For example, regular bathing removes transient microorganisms from the skin. Bathing with chlorhexidine gluconate has been shown to significantly decrease acquired infection of MRSA or VRE (Donskey and Deshpande, 2016). Lubrication keeps the skin hydrated and intact. Regular oral hygiene removes proteins in the saliva that attract microorganisms. Flossing removes tartar and plaque that cause infection. Adequate fluid intake promotes normal urine formation and a resultant outflow of urine to flush the bladder and urethra of microorganisms. For patients who are immobilized or dependent, regular coughing and deep-breathing exercises remove mucus from lower airways.

BOX 9.11 Infection Control of Portals of Entry

Intact Skin and Mucosa

- Keep skin clean and well lubricated. Use chlorhexidine gluconate for daily bathing of hospitalized patients (Denny and Munro, 2016).
- Avoid positioning the patients on tubes or objects that might cause breaks in skin.
- Use dry, wrinkle-free linen.
- Offer frequent oral hygiene (see Chapter 16).
- Provide frequent position changes for patients with impaired mobility.
- Clean skin of patients who are incontinent with nonabrasive agent; avoid drying with abrasive towel or tissue.

Urinary Tract

- Teach women to clean perineum and rectum by wiping from area of least contamination (urinary meatus) toward area of most contamination (rectum).
- Do not allow urine in drainage bags and tubes to flow back into bladder. Never raise drainage system above level of bladder.
- Keep points of connection between catheter or drain and tubing closed.

Invasive Tubes and Lines

- When obtaining specimens from drainage tubes or inserting safety needles into i.v. lines, disinfect tube ports by wiping them liberally with disinfectant solution before entering system. **Scrub the hub** before accessing site. Before inserting an i.v. line, cleanse the skin with antiseptic. Cleansing the skin and tubing removes and, in some cases, kills microorganisms.

Wound Care

- Keep draining wounds covered to contain drainage.
- Clean outward from wound site using clean swab for each application (see Chapter 38).

SURGICAL ASEPSIS

Surgical asepsis, or aseptic technique, is designed to eliminate all microorganisms including spores and pathogens from an object and to protect an area from these microorganisms. Surgical asepsis requires more precautions than medical asepsis. Breaks in technique result in contamination, increasing a patient's risk for infection (Murphy, 2015).

Surgical asepsis is commonly practiced in the operating room, labor and delivery area, and major diagnostic or procedural areas, but nurses also use surgical aseptic techniques at a patient's bedside (e.g., when inserting i.v. or urethral catheters). Use surgical asepsis during procedures that require intentional perforation of a patient's skin (e.g., i.v. insertion), when the integrity of the skin is broken from trauma or burns, and during procedures that involve insertion of a catheter or surgical instruments into sterile body cavities (AORN, 2016).

Multiple steps involving application of PPE for use of sterile technique are used in the operating room in this order: applying a mask, protective eyewear, and a cap; performing a surgical scrub; and applying a sterile gown and gloves. In contrast, performing a sterile dressing change at a patient's bedside requires only hand hygiene, applying a clean gown if splashing of fluid is likely, and applying sterile gloves (Box 9.12). It is important for you to refer to agency policy and procedure whenever there is a question about a procedure requiring sterile technique. Regardless of the procedures followed in different settings, the use of surgical asepsis depends on developing an aseptic conscience. Always recognize the importance of strict adherence to aseptic principles. In addition, be an excellent role model and patient advocate, reinforcing proper practice for other caregivers (AORN, 2016).

Preparation for Sterile Procedures

In treatment rooms and at the bedside, it is important to have a patient's full cooperation in maintaining aseptic technique. Therefore, assess the patient's understanding of sterile procedure and the reasons for not moving or interfering with the procedure. Special precautions such as masking the patient or changing his or her position are sometimes necessary to prevent contamination during procedures. Determine whether a patient has undergone a sterile procedure in the past. Explain how you will perform the procedure and what the patient can do to avoid contaminating sterile objects:

1. Avoid sudden movements of body parts covered by sterile drapes.
2. Do not touch sterile supplies, drapes, or your sterile gloves and gown.
3. Avoid coughing, sneezing, or talking over a sterile area.

BOX 9.12 Procedural Guidelines

Putting on Sterile Gloves

Equipment

Pair of proper-sized sterile gloves (latex or synthetic neolatex)

Steps

1. Consider the type of procedure to be performed, and consult agency policy on use of sterile gloves.
2. Consider the patient's risk for infection (e.g., a preexisting condition and size or extent of area being treated).
3. Select correct size and type of gloves and then examine glove package to determine whether it is dry and intact with no water stains.
4. Inspect condition of hands for cuts, hangnails, open lesions, or abrasions. In some settings, you are allowed to cover any open lesion with a sterile, impervious transparent dressing (check agency policy). In some cases, the presence of such lesions may prevent you from participating in a procedure.
5. Assess the patient for the following risk factors before applying latex gloves:
   a. Previous reaction to the following items within hours of exposure: adhesive tape, dental or face mask, golf club grip, ostomy bag, rubber band, balloon, bandage, elastic underwear, i.v. tubing, rubber gloves, condom
   b. Personal history of asthma, contact dermatitis, eczema, urticaria, or rhinitis
   c. History of food allergies, especially avocado, banana, peach, chestnut, raw potato, kiwi, tomato, or papaya
   d. Previous history of adverse reactions during surgery or dental procedure
   e. Previous reaction to latex product

Clinical decision point: Synthetic nonlatex gloves must be used when patients are at risk or if nurse has sensitivity or allergy to latex.

6. Apply sterile gloves.
   a. Perform thorough hand hygiene. Place glove package near work area.
   b. Remove outer glove package wrapper by carefully separating and peeling apart sides (see illustration).
   c. Grasp inner package and lay on clean, dry, flat surface at waist level. Open package, keeping gloves on inside surface of wrapper.
   d. Identify right and left glove. Each glove has a cuff approximately 5 cm (2 inches) wide. Glove dominant hand first.
   e. With thumb and first two fingers of nondominant hand, grasp glove for dominant hand by touching only inside surface of cuff.
   f. Carefully pull glove over dominant hand, leaving a cuff and being sure that cuff does not roll up wrist. Be sure that thumb and fingers are in proper spaces (see illustration).

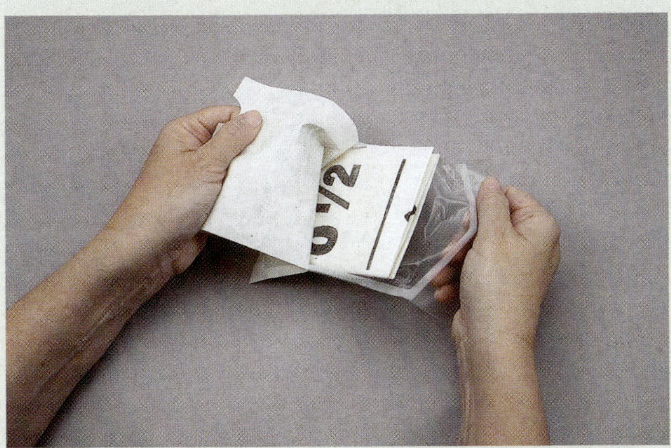

Step 6b Open outer glove package wrapper.

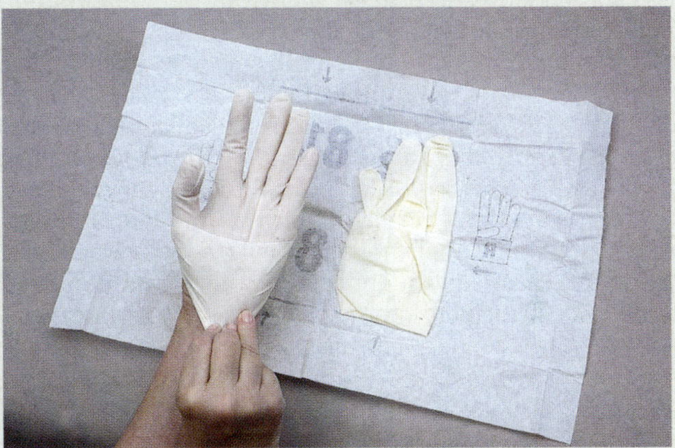

Step 6f Pick up glove at cuff of dominant hand and insert fingers; pull glove completely over dominant hand (example is for a left-handed person).

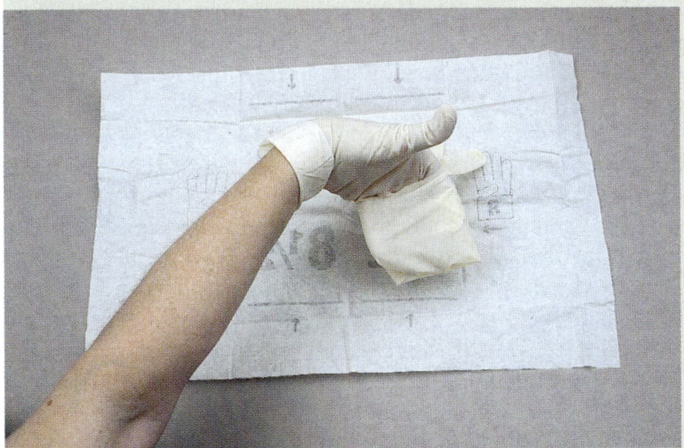

Step 6g Pick up glove for nondominant hand.

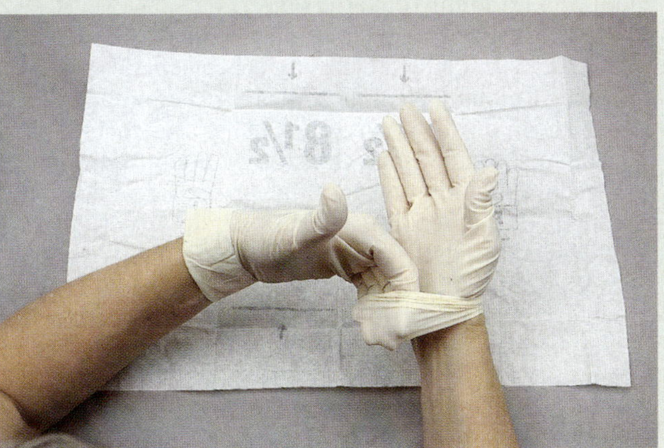

Step 6h Pull second glove over nondominant hand.

Continued

BOX 9.12 Procedural Guidelines—cont'd

g. With gloved dominant hand, slip fingers underneath cuff of second glove (see illustration).

h. Carefully pull second glove over fingers of nondominant hand (see illustration).

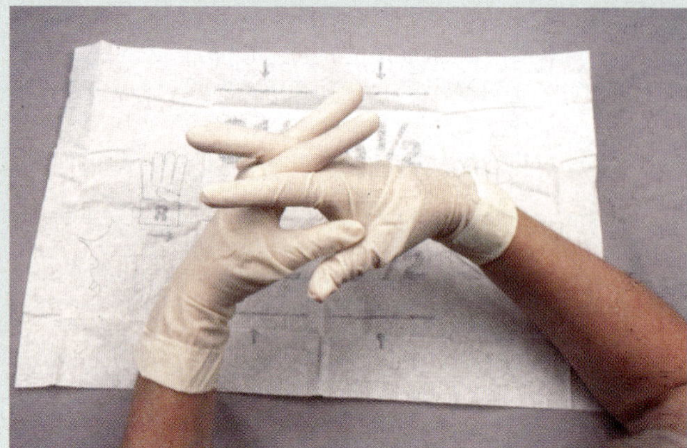

Step 6i Interlock gloved hands.

Clinical decision point: Do not allow fingers and thumb of gloved dominant hand to touch any part of exposed nondominant hand. Keep thumb of dominant hand abducted back.

i. After second glove is on, interlock hands and hold away from body above waist level until beginning the procedure (see illustration).

7. Remove gloves.
   a. Grasp outside of one cuff with other gloved hand; avoid touching wrist.
   b. Pull glove off, turning it inside out, and place it in gloved hand.
   c. Take fingers of bare hand and tuck inside remaining glove cuff. Peel glove off inside out and over previously removed glove. Discard both gloves in receptacle.
   d. Perform thorough hand hygiene.
8. Assess the patient for signs of infection, focusing on area treated.
9. Assess the patient for signs of latex allergy.

Certain sterile procedures last for an extended time. Assess each patient's needs (e.g., pain control or elimination) in advance and anticipate factors that will disrupt a procedure. If a patient is in pain, administer prescribed analgesics no more than 30 minutes before a sterile procedure begins. Patients often are placed in relatively uncomfortable positions during sterile procedures. Help the patient assume the most comfortable position possible. Finally, the patient's condition sometimes results in events that contaminate a sterile field. For example, a patient with a respiratory infection coughs, transmitting organisms that contaminate the sterile field. Anticipate such a problem and offer a mask to the patient before the procedure begins.

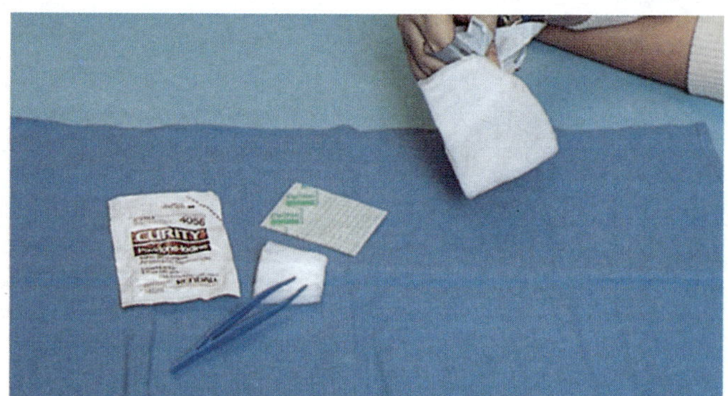

Fig. 9.6 Adding item to a sterile field.

Principles of Surgical Asepsis

Principles of surgical asepsis include the following:

1. *A sterile object remains sterile only when touched by another sterile object.* The following principles guide you in placement and handling of sterile objects:
   - Sterile touching sterile remains sterile (e.g., wear sterile gloves to handle objects on a sterile field).
   - Sterile touching clean becomes contaminated (e.g., if the sterile tip of a syringe touches the surface of a clean disposable glove, the syringe is contaminated).
   - Sterile touching contaminated becomes contaminated (e.g., when you touch a sterile object with an ungloved hand, the object is contaminated).
   - Sterile touching questionable is contaminated (e.g., when you find a tear or break in the covering of a sterile object, discard or reprocess it, regardless of whether the object appears untouched).
2. *Place only sterile objects on a sterile field.* Be sure the item is sterile before use. The package or container holding a sterile object must be intact and dry. A package that is torn, punctured, wet, or open is unsterile. When placing sterile items on a sterile field (e.g., sterile drape), do not reach over the field (Fig. 9.6).
3. *A sterile object or field out of the range of vision or an object held below a person's waist is contaminated.* Never turn your back on a sterile tray or leave it unattended. Any object held below waist level is considered contaminated because you cannot view it at all times. Keep sterile objects either on or out over the sterile field.
4. *A sterile object or field becomes contaminated by prolonged exposure to the air.* Avoid activities that create air currents such as excessive movements or rearranging linen after a sterile object or field becomes exposed. Minimize the number of individuals walking into an area where sterile packages are being opened or are open. Microorganisms also travel by droplet through the air. No one should talk, laugh, sneeze, or cough over a sterile field or when gathering and using sterile equipment. Wear a mask when opening a tray and adding sterile equipment. Microorganisms traveling through the air can fall on sterile items or fields if you reach over the work area (Box 9.13).

BOX 9.13 **Procedural Guidelines**

Opening Wrapped Sterile Items

Equipment

Sterile kit or package, waist-high countertop or table surface

Steps

1. Perform hand hygiene (see Box 9.7).
2. Apply PPE as needed (consult agency policy) (see Boxes 9.8 and 9.9).
3. Open sterile commercial kit or pack containing sterile items. Place sterile kit or pack on clean, dry, flat work surface above waist level.
4. Open outside cover (see illustration) and remove package from dust cover. Place on work surface.
5. Grasp outer surface of tip of top outermost flap.
6. Open outermost flap away from body, keeping arm outstretched and away from sterile field (see illustration).
7. Grasp outside surface of edge of first side flap.
8. Open side flap, pulling to side, allowing it to lie flat on table surface. Keep arm to side and not over sterile surface (see illustration).
9. Repeat Steps 7 and 8 for second side flap (see illustration).
10. Grasp outside border of last and innermost flap.
11. Stand away from sterile package and pull flap back, allowing it to fall flat on table (see illustration).
12. Use inner surface of package (except for 1-inch border around edges) as a sterile field to add items because it is sterile. Grasp the 1-inch border to move field over the work surface.

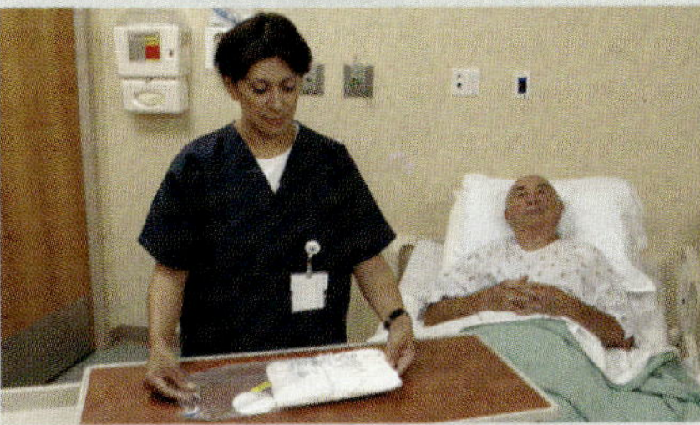

Step 4 Open outside cover of sterile kit.

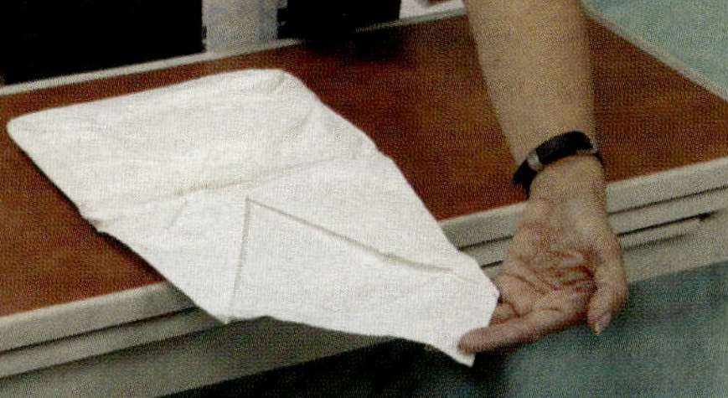

Step 6 Open outermost flap of sterile kit away from body.

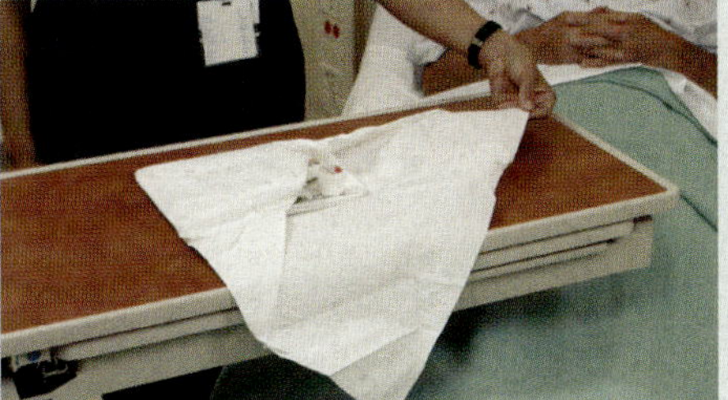

Step 8 Open first side flap, pulling to side.

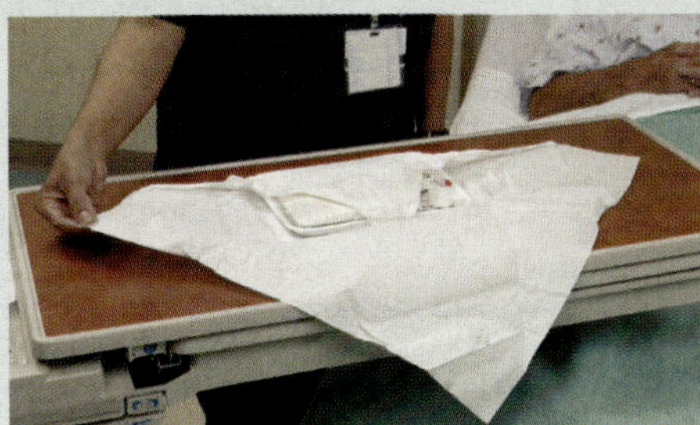

Step 9 Open second side flap, pulling to side.

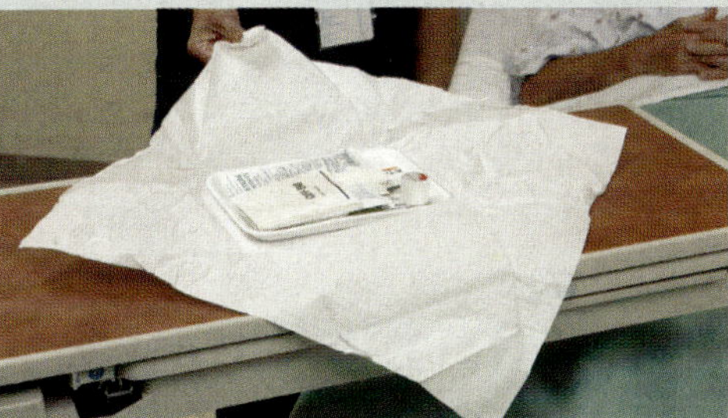

Step 11 Open last and innermost flap.

5. *A sterile object or field becomes contaminated by capillary action when a sterile surface comes in contact with a wet contaminated surface.* Moisture seeps through the protective covering of a sterile package, allowing microorganisms to travel to the sterile object. When stored sterile packages become wet, discard the objects immediately or send the equipment to be sterilized again. Spilling solution over a sterile drape contaminates the field unless the drape cannot be penetrated by moisture.
6. *Because fluid flows in the direction of gravity, a sterile object becomes contaminated if gravity causes a contaminated liquid to flow over the surface of an object.* To avoid contamination during a surgical hand scrub, hold your hands above the elbows. This allows water to flow downward without contaminating your hands and fingers. Because gravity makes water flow downward, this is also the reason for drying from fingers to elbows with the hands held up after the scrub.
7. *The edges of a sterile field or container are contaminated.* A 2.5-cm (1-inch) border around a sterile towel or drape is considered contaminated (Box 9.14). The edges of sterile containers become exposed to air after they are open and are thus contaminated. After you remove a sterile needle from its protective cap or after you remove forceps from a container, the objects must not touch the edge of the container. The lip of an opened bottle of solution also becomes contaminated after it is exposed to air. When pouring a sterile liquid, first pour a small amount of solution and discard it. The solution washes away any microorganisms on the bottle lip. Then pour the liquid a second time to fill a sterile container with the amount of solution you need.

ROLE OF THE INFECTION PREVENTION AND CONTROL DEPARTMENT

Most health care agencies employ health professionals who are specially trained in the area of IPC. Their responsibilities

BOX 9.14 **Procedural Guidelines**

Preparation of a Sterile Field

Equipment

Sterile pack, sterile gloves *(optional)*

Steps

1. Perform hand hygiene.
2. Place pack containing sterile drape on flat, dry surface and open as described in Box 9.13.
3. Apply sterile gloves (*optional*, see agency policy). You may touch outer 2.5-cm (1-inch) border of drape without wearing gloves.
4. Using fingertips of one hand, pick up folded top edge of drape along 1-inch border.
5. Gently lift drape up from its wrapper and let it unfold by itself without touching any object. Discard wrapper with other hand.
6. With other hand, grasp an adjacent corner of drape and hold it straight up and away from body (see illustration).
7. Holding drape, position bottom half over top half of intended work surface (see illustration).
8. Allow top half of drape to be placed over bottom half of work surface (see illustration).
9. Grasp 1-inch border around edge to position drape as needed.

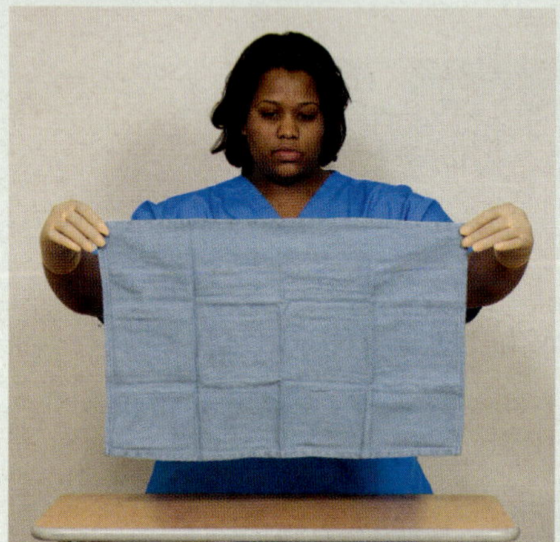

Step 6 Hold corners of sterile drape up and away from body.

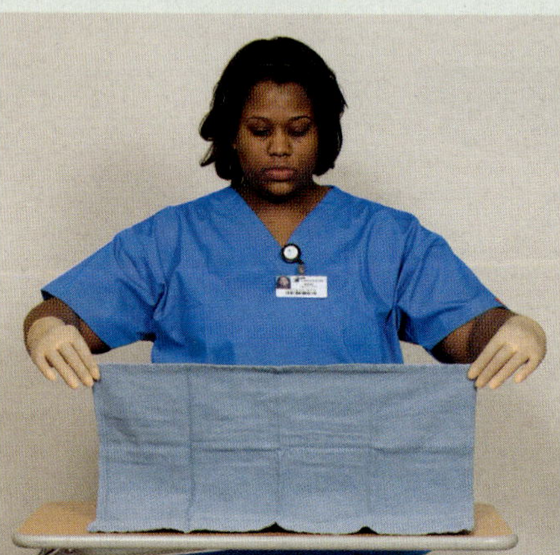

Step 7 Position bottom half of sterile drape over top half of work space.

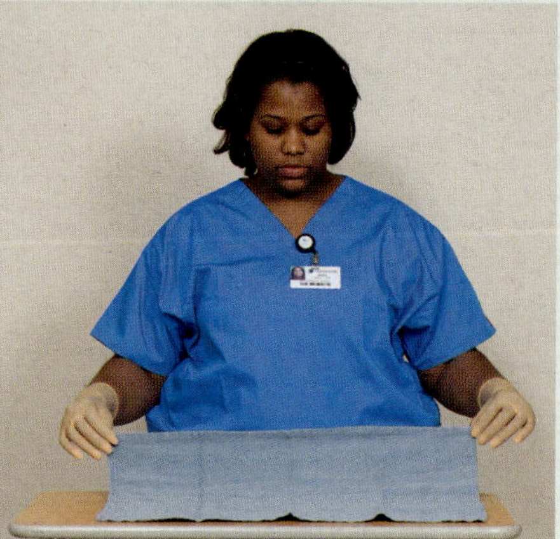

Step 8 Allow top half of drape to be placed over bottom half of work surface.

include collection and analysis of data about HAIs, surveillance of MDROs, implementation of evidence-based protocols for infection prevention, and providing consultation and education to staff and others about IPC.

COVID-19 AND SPECIFIC INFECTION PREVENTION AND CONTROL PRACTICES

Sever acute respiratory syndrome coronavirus-2 (SARS-CoV-2) is highly contagious and found to be transmitted through respiratory droplets and contact routes (Box 9.15). The virus-laden aerosol might travel up to 4-m distance from infected patient (higher positivity in ICUs as compared with wards—66.7% vs. 8.3%), where highest concentration of aerosols was in patient room (44.4%), followed by air outlets (35.7%), doctor's room (12.5%), and outside isolation room (0%). Therefore, HCWs must strictly follow appropriate IPC precautions. The essential IPC precautions recommended to be followed by HCWs while caring patients infected with SARS-CoV-2 are listed as follows (Sharma et al, 2020):

BOX 9.15 **Mode of Transmission and Incubation Period of COVID-19**

Mode of Transmission

- Aerosolized droplets generated through coughing, sneezing, or breathing
- Direct contact with patient and his or her body fluids including feces
- Indirect contact with surfaces and fomites (virus can survive on surfaces for longer period: plastic/stainless steel, 2–3 days; cardboard, 24 h, and copper, 4 h)
- Airborne transmission is suspected but not yet confirmed (virus can survive in droplet particle in air up to 3 h and is found up to 4-m distance from the patient)
- Fecal−oral route of transmission is also suspected (SARS-CoV-2 is detected in feces but no reports of fecal−oral transmission till date)

Incubation Period

2–14 days (most cases occurring within 5 days of exposure)

- Proactive meticulous hand hygiene practices. Wash hands with soap and water or alcohol hand rub when hands are not visibly soiled.
- Provide the patients with a triple-layer surgical masks and ask them to follow coughing and sneezing etiquettes.
- Deploy minimum required HCWs in the isolation room and practice bundling of nursing interventions to reduce the need of PPEs and risk of infections to HCWs.

- Disposal or dedicated equipment (e.g., stethoscopes, blood pressure cuffs, and thermometers) should be used to prevent cross-infection and should be disinfected with 70% alcohol in between use.
- PPE, gloves, gowns, eye protectives (goggles or eye shield), head covers, shoe covers, and face masks preferably 95 respirators when exposed to aerosol-generating procedures (e.g., nebulization, open suctioning, intubation, extubation, and noninvasive mechanical ventilation) should be used rationally.
- Touching surfaces around patients must be minimized and practice meticulous hand hygiene with soap and water or alcohol-based hand rub when hands are not visibility soiled.
- Do not touch nose, eyes, mouth, face and maintain possibility 1- to 2-m distance with others, but new study has found that even virus might travel up to 4 m.
- Floors should be cleaned every 4 hours, by first mopping with 5% phenolic solution followed by 0.5% sodium hypochlorite solution (NaOCl).
- High touch surfaces such as doorknobs, bedrails, overbed table, computer mouse, telephone, nursing trolley, nursing station, light switches, wall areas around the toilet, and so on, should be cleaned every 4 hours with 1% NaOCl solution.
- Metallic surfaces around the patient should be cleaned with 70% alcohol, and furniture, machines, instrument, and surfaces in isolation room should be cleaned and disinfected with 1% NaOCl solution.
- Linen should be soaked in 0.05% NaOCl solution for 30 minutes before sending to laundry in a leak-proof plastic bag.
- Blood or body fluid spillage should be treated with 1% NaOCl solution for 30 minutes before wiping.
- Biomedical waste should be treated with 1%–2% NaOCl solution and discarded in color-coded bins per local or national biomedical waste management policy.

BIOMEDICAL WASTE MANAGEMENT

Biomedical waste is taken into account as any sort of waste that is generated throughout the diagnosing, treatment, or protection of individuals or animals or analysis activities pertaining to it or within the production or testing of biological or in health camps, together with the classes mentioned in Schedule I appended to those rules.

Infectious waste includes all those medical wastes that are potential to transmit infectious agent, bacteria, flora, or parasitic diseases. It includes each human and animal infectious waste that is generated in any of the healthcare setting including veterinary care. Any waste with a possibility to create a threat to human health and life is named unsafe waste. Infectious waste is unsafe in nature, and if the infectious part mixes up with the final noninfectious waste within the black bag, the whole bulk of that black bag waste becomes probably infectious and should be treated as infectious waste. Therefore, the hospital waste poses a significant threat to public health and atmosphere.

Classification of Health Care Waste

The medicinal services offices while producing the waste are liable for isolation, assortment, in-house transportation, pretreatment of waste, and capacity of waste, before such waste is gathered by Common Bio-clinical Waste Treatment Facility (CBWTF) operator.

Thus, for proper management of the waste inside the care facilities, the technical necessities of waste handling area unit required to be understood and practiced by every class of the workers in accordance with the Biomedical Waste Management Rules, 2016. Waste generated is classified as:

- Biomedical waste
- General waste
- Other wastes

Biomedical waste is categorized into four categories—yellow, red, white, and blue on the basis of segregation pathway and color code per Biomedical Waste Management Rules, 2016. Detail description of color code and waste under each category is mentioned in Table 9.4.

General waste

General waste is the type of waste other than biomedical waste and consists of 85%–90% of total hospital

Table 9.4 Categories of Biomedical Waste and Recommended Color-Coded Bins for Segregation

Category	Type of Waste
Yellow Bin	**Item contaminated with blood, body fluids** ▪ Human anatomical waste (organ, body part, fetus, etc.) ▪ Routine mask, cap and gown ▪ Dressings, bandages, gauze, linen ▪ Soiled plaster casts, cotton swabs ▪ Expired and discarded medicines ▪ Bags containing residual or discarded blood, blood component including tubings **Cytotoxic-labelled yellow bin** ▪ All cytotoxic drugs, glass, plastics, ampules, vials
Red Bin	**Contaminated plastic waste** ▪ All plastic tubings ▪ Plastic and i.v. bottles ▪ Catheter ▪ Drains ▪ Urobag ▪ Syringes without needles ▪ I.v. cannula ▪ Gloves and shoe covers (disposable) ▪ Vacutainer without needle
Blue Bin	**Glassware items** ▪ Broken or discarded and contaminated glass including medicine vials and ampules ▪ Glass slides ▪ Metallic body implants ▪ Keep cardboard box inside the bag
White Bin	**Contaminated sharps** ▪ Needles ▪ Syringes with fixed needles ▪ Scalpels, blades, suture needles

Biomedical Waste Management Rules, 2016, as amended.
Guidelines for Management of Healthcare Waste Management Rules, 2016 by health care Facilities.

wastes. In simple terms, it is the type of waste that had not been in contact with any hazardous or infectious, chemical or biological secretions. It is collected under two categories—dry waste and wet waste.

Dry waste: Newspapers, card boxes, plastic water bottles, aluminum cans of soft drinks, packaging materials.

Wet waste: Food containers of empty residual food, organic/biodegradable waste, construction and demolition wastes.

Other wastes

Other wastes include used electronic wastes, used batteries, and radioactive wastes that are not lined underneath medical specialty wastes, however ought to be disposed as and once such wastes are generated per the provisions arranged down underneath E-Waste (Management) Rules, 2016, Batteries (Management & Handling) Rules, 2001, and rules/guidelines underneath Energy Act, 1962.

Biomedical Waste Segregation

Biomedical waste generated from a medical building is needed to be quarantined at the purpose of generation per the color writing stipulated underneath Schedule I of Biomedical Waste Management Rules, 2016. Following activities should be followed to confirm correct waste segregation:

- Waste must be segregated at the point of generation of source and not in later stages. "Point of Generation" means the place where wastes initially generate, accumulate and is under the control of doctor/nursing staff, and so on, who is providing treatment to the patient and within the process generating biomedical waste.
  Posters/placards for biomedical waste segregation should be provided in all the wards and in waste segregation area.
- Adequate number of color-coded bins/containers and bags should be available at the purpose of generation of biomedical waste.
- Color-coded plastic luggage ought to be in line with the Plastic Waste Management Rules, 2016.
- Give personnel protecting instrumentation to the biomedical waste handling employees.

KEY POINTS

- Normal body flora helps the body resist infection by reducing the reproduction of pathogenic microorganisms.
- Immunity to infection depends on the capacity to produce antibodies in response to exposure to an antigen.
- An infection can develop if the six elements of the infection chain are present and uninterrupted.
- The virulence of a microorganism depends on its ability to resist attack by normal bodily defenses.
- Increasing age, poor nutrition, stress, inherited conditions, chronic disease, and treatments or conditions that compromise the immune response increase susceptibility to infection.
- Wear gloves when in contact with blood or potentially infectious material. Wear a gown and mask in combination with an eye protection device such as goggles or glasses with solid side shields whenever you anticipate splashes or spray of blood or potentially infectious material.
- The main cause of HAIs is nonadherence to hand hygiene.
- Invasive procedures, medical therapies, long hospitalization, and contact with health care personnel increase a hospitalized patient's risk for acquiring an HAI.
- Surgical asepsis requires more stringent techniques than medical asepsis.
- The CDC recommends that all patients be considered as potentially infected with HIV and other bloodborne pathogens; therefore, health care workers reduce the risk for exposure to blood and body fluids by following standard precautions.
- Following aseptic principles is the key to your success in preventing patients from acquiring infections.
- A patient on isolation precautions is subject to sensory deprivation because of the restricted environment.
- If the skin is broken or if you perform an invasive procedure into a body cavity normally free of microorganisms, use surgical aseptic practices.
- A sterile object becomes contaminated by direct contact with a clean or contaminated object, exposure to airborne microorganisms, or contact with a wet surface.

REFERENCES

Archibald L. Enterococci. In: Grota P, Allen V, Boston KM., editors: APIC text of infection control and epidemiology. 4th ed. Washington, DC: Association for Professionals in Infection Control and Epidemiology (APIC); 2015.

Arnold F. Antimicrobials and resistance. In: Grota P, Allen V, Boston KM., editors: APIC text of infection control and epidemiology. 4th ed. Washington, DC: Association for Professionals in Infection Control and Epidemiology (APIC); 2015.

Association of periOperative Nurses (AORN): 2016 guidelines for perioperative practice. Denver CO: AORN, Inc; 2016.

Becker K, Kock R. Staphylococci. In: Grota P, Allen V, Boston KM., editors: APIC text of infection control and epidemiology. 4th ed. Washington, DC: Association for Professionals in Infection Control and Epidemiology (APIC); 2015.

Berends C, Walesa B. Isolation precautions (transmission based precautions). In: Grota P, Allen V, Boston KM., editors: APIC text of infection control and epidemiology. 4th ed. Washington, DC: Association for Professionals in Infection Control and Epidemiology (APIC); 2015.

Centers for Disease Control and Prevention (CDC). Guideline for hand hygiene in health-care settings: recommendations of the Healthcare Infection Control Practices Advisory Committee and the HICPAC/SHEA/APIC/IDSA Hand Hygiene Task Force. MMWR Morb Mortal Wkly Rep 2002;51 (RR-16). Available from: http://www.cdc.gov/mmwr/PDF/rr/rr5116.pdf.

Centers for Disease Control and Prevention (CDC). Guidelines for preventing the transmission of *Mycobacterium tuberculosis* in health care facilities. MMWR Recomm Rep 2005;54:RR–17.

Centers for Disease Control and Prevention (CDC), Hospital Infection Control Practice Advisory Committee. 2007 Guideline for isolation precautions: preventing transmission of infectious agents in healthcare settings, Healthcare Infection Control Practices Advisory Committee (HICPAC). 2007. Available from: https://www.cdc.gov/hicpac/2007IP/2007isolation Precautions.html.

Centers for Disease Control and Prevention (CDC): OPRP—general information on hand hygiene. 2009. Available from: http://www.cdc.gov/nceh/vsp/cruiselines/hand_hygiene_general.htm.

Centers for Disease Control and Prevention (CDC). VRE in healthcare settings. 2011. Available from: http://www.cdc.gov/hai/organisms/vre/vre.html.

Centers for Disease Control and Prevention (CDC). Principles of epidemiology in public health practice, third edition: an introduction to applied epidemiology and biostatistics. 2012. Available from: http://www.cdc.gov/ophss/csels/dsepd/SS1978/Lesson1/Section10.html.

Centers for Disease Control and Prevention (CDC). Viral hepatitis. 2016a. Available from: http://www.cdc.gov/hepatitis/hcv/hcvfaq.htm#b1.

Centers for Disease Control and Prevention (CDC). Hand hygiene in healthcare settings: show me the science. 2016b. Available from: https://www.cdc.gov/handhygiene/science/index.html.

Centers for Disease Control and Prevention (CDC). Precautions to prevent the spread of MRSA. 2016c. Available from: https://www.cdc.gov/mrsa/healthcare/clinicians/precautions.html.

Dalal I, Roifman CM. Immunity of the newborn. 2015. Available from: http://www.uptodate.com/contents/immunity-of-the-newborn.

Denny J, Munro CL. Chlorhexidine bathing effects on health-care-associated infections. Biol Res Nurs 2016;19(2):123.

Donskey CJ, Deshpande A. Effect of chlorhexidine bathing in preventing infections and reducing skin burden and environmental contamination: a review of the literature. Am J Infect Control 2016;44:e17–21.

Food and Drug Administration (FDA), Department of Health and Human Services. Banned Devices; powdered surgeon's gloves, powdered patient examination gloves, and absorbable powder for lubricating a surgeon's glove. 2016. Available from: https://s3.amazonaws.com/public-inspection.federalregister.gov/2016-30382.pdf.

Haas J. Hand hygiene. In: Grota P, Allen V, Boston KM., editors: APIC text of infection control and epidemiology. 4th ed. Washington, DC: Association for Professionals in Infection Control and Epidemiology (APIC); 2015.

Longtin Y, Schneider A, Tschopp C, Renzi G, Gayet-Ageron A, Schrenzel J, et al. Contamination of stethoscopes and physicians' hands after a physical examination. Mayo Clin Proc 2014;89:291–9.

Murphy R. Surgical services. In: Grota P, Allen V, Boston KM., editor: APIC text of infection control and epidemiology. 4th ed. Washington, DC: Association for Professionals in Infection Control and Epidemiology (APIC); 2015.

Occupational Safety and Health Administration (OSHA). Respiratory infection control: respirators versus surgical masks, OSHA Fact Sheet. 2009. https://www.osha.gov/Publications/OSHA3219.pdf.

Occupational Safety and Health Administration (OSHA). Disposal of contaminated needles and blood tube holders used for phlebotomy. OSHA Safety and Health Information Bulletin; 2015. Available from: https://www.osha.gov/dts/shib/shib101503.html.

Occupational Safety and Health Administration (OSHA). Fit testing procedures: part I, OSHA-accepted fit test protocols. n.d. Available from: https://www.osha.gov/pls/oshaweb/owadisp.show_document?p_table=standards&p_id=9780.

Royal College of Nursing. Wipe it out: one chance to get it right. London: Royal College of Nursing; 2011. Available from: https://www.rcn.org.uk/professional-development/publications/pub-005940.

Rutala WA, Weber DJ. CDC guidelines for disinfection and sterilization in healthcare facilities, 2008. Available at: https://www.cdc.gov/infectioncontrol/pdf/guidelines/disinfection-guidelines-H.pdf.

Rutala WA, Weber DJ. Cleaning, disinfection, and sterilization. In: Grota P, editor: APIC text of infection control and epidemiology. 4th ed. Washington, DC: Association for Professionals in Infection Control and Epidemiology (APIC); 2015.

Sharma SK, Nuttall C, Kalyani V, Hemlata. Clinical nursing care guidance for management of patient with COVID-19. J Pak Med Assoc 2020;70(5 Suppl. 3):S118–23.

Surawicz CM, Brandt LJ, Binion DG, Ananthakrishnan AN, Curry SR, Gilligan PH, et al. Guidelines for diagnosis, treatment, and prevention of *Clostridium difficile* infections. Am J Gastroenterol 2013;108:478–98.

The Joint Commission (TJC). 2018 National Patient Safety Goals. Oakbrook Terrace, IL: The Commission; 2018. Available from: https://www.jointcommission.org/hap_2017_npsgs/.

Tweeten S. General principles of epidemiology. In Grota P, editor: APIC text of infection control and epidemiology. 4th ed. Washington, DC: Association for Professionals in Infection Control and Epidemiology (APIC); 2015.

World Health Organization (WHO). WHO guidelines on hand hygiene in health care. Geneva: WHO; 2009.

World Health Organization (WHO): Health-care waste: fact sheet no 253. 2015. Available from: http://www.who.int/mediacentre/factsheets/fs253/en/.

World Health Organization (WHO). About SAVE Lives: Clean Your Hands: 5 moments for hand hygiene. 2017. Available from: http://www.who.int/gpsc/5may/background/5moments/en/.

10 Comfort, Rest, and Sleep

OBJECTIVES

After reading this chapter, the student should be able to:

- Define the concept of rest and comfort.
- Explain the factors influencing comfort including physical and psychological conditions.
- Enlist the purpose of comfort devices and different types of comfort devices used for patients' comfort.
- Describe principles and importance of bed making.
- Define common therapeutic positions and its associated purposes.
- Discuss mechanisms that regulate sleep and 24-hour sleep−wake cycle.
- Describe the normal stages of sleep and functions of sleep.
- Compare and contrast the characteristics of sleep for different age groups.
- Identify factors that promote or disrupt sleep.
- Discuss characteristics of common sleep disorders.
- Summarize the elements of a sleep history and assessment.
- Describe interventions appropriate to promoting sleep for patients with various sleep disorders.
- Discuss differences in sleep interventions for patients of different age groups.

KEY TERMS

circadian rhythm, p. 213
hypnotics, p. 222
insomnia, p. 218
narcolepsy, p. 219
nocturia, p. 217
nonrapid eye movement (NREM) sleep, p. 214
rapid eye movement (REM) sleep, p. 214
sedatives, p. 222
sleep, p. 213
sleep apnea, p. 219
sleep deprivation, p. 220

INTRODUCTION

Physical and emotional health depends on adequate rest and sleep. Without proper amounts of rest and sleep, a person's ability to concentrate, make judgments, promote healing, and participate in daily activities decreases. To help patients gain needed rest and sleep, you need to understand the nature of sleep, the factors influencing it, and patients' sleep habits. Nurses care for patients who often have preexisting sleep disturbances and who develop sleep problems as a result of illness or being in the health care environment. Individualize your care based on patients' personal sleep habits and patterns of sleep to provide effective sleep therapies.

COMFORT

Comfort is somewhat related with physical and mental relaxation or it is freedom from pain, tension, and anxiety. Comfort is an integral part of patients' experience in hospital during their treatment. Satisfactory stay of patients during their care is the quality indicator of overall care provided to them. Physical comfort is one of the key components in holistic health care approach. Thus, comfort is more commonly associated with nursing care. Patients' response to treatment is majorly depending on comfortable environment.

Comfort may be defined as any supportive aid that is used to provide comfort and relaxation to the patient during his or her hospital stay and helps in maintaining correct body posture is known as comfort device.

Factors Influencing Comfort

There are large number of factors that may influence the comfort of the patient during their stay in health care facility. Some of the key factors under physical and psychological domains have been listed below.

Physical Conditions

a) Painful procedures
b) Movement restriction
c) Dirty linen
d) Self-unhygienic conditions
e) Extreme temperature, and humidity
f) Inadequate ventilation
g) Bright light
h) Noisy environment

Psychological Conditions

a) Sleep disturbances
b) Frequent bladder and bowel movement
c) Uncomfortable position
d) Disturbed daily routine

Purposes for Use of Comfort Devices

Patients receiving care in health care facility may require different type of comfort devices for several purposes, some of these are listed as follows:

- To make patient comfortable
- To relieve pressure on affected body parts
- To prevent any accidental injury
- To maintain correct body posture
- To prevent mobilization of body parts
- To facilitate easy breathing
- To prevent pressure sore

Types of Comfort Devices

As comfort is the state of physical and mental peace with self and surroundings, some of the commonly used comfort devices in health care facilities are as follows:

1. *Comfortable bed:* Patient's bed should be tidy, firm and bedsheet must be wrinkle-free and clean. Mattress should be according to need of the patient, which could be of cotton, foam, or air.
2. *Back rest:* Patients who are unable to sit themselves need back rest. It is supportive in making the patient sit in bed without other's assistance. It is helpful during procedures such as mouth care, oral care, and steam inhalation and in respiratory difficulties. It can be used separately; however, in modern hospital beds, it is an integral part of bed itself, which could be manually or electronically operable.
3. *Bed cradle:* It is used for patients with burns or open wound area, where top bedsheet should not touch the body. Bed cradle is positioned in such a way over the patient that the affected area must be free from the weight of top bedsheet. The purpose is to avoid friction and irritation due to bedsheet cloth. Bed cradle could be made of wood, or metal, which may be electronically equipped to keep the patient warm.
4. *Bed board:* It is used to make bed firm and hard for those patients who need support to spine and during cardiopulmonary resuscitation (CPR) procedure. Bed board is placed over the mattress to make surface rigid.
5. *Sand bags:* These are rubber or plastic bag with sand inside. They are useful in immobilization of body parts. They are also used for providing pressure over the certain areas to prevent the risk of hemorrhage from post-angiography sites.
6. *Air mattress:* Air mattress are used in obese and thin patients who are long bedridden and having risk of developing pressure ulcers. It is helpful in improving circulation by relieving pressure on bony prominences.
7. *Cardiac table:* It is an overbed table that is kept in front of patient while sitting in Fowler's position. Table has lots of uses including to lean forward to ease breathing during cardiac position, to help in writing, and to eat food, and so on.
8. *Pillows:* Pillows are comfortable devices while sleeping to raise head slightly and to support any body part. It maintains the body in good alignment and supports the specific body part.
9. *Footboard:* It is usually made up of wood, plastic, and hard canvas. It is placed toward the foot of the patient to support the feet and prevent foot drop in patients who are neurologically deficit, unconscious for a significant longer period.
10. *Side rails:* These are used for safety of the patient and to prevent fall and accidental injury. These are positioned alongside of the bed.
11. *Air cushion:* These are made up of rubber material and filled with air. These are used to provide comfort by relieving pressure on various body parts.
12. *Knee rest:* These are used to relieve back pain and improve circulation. It is kept underneath the knees and user can lie on the back.

Maintaining Comfort

Depending on a patient's age and physical condition, maintain the room temperature between 20°C and 23°C (68°F and 73.4°F). Infants, older adults, and acutely ill patients often need a warmer room. However, patients with certain illnesses benefit from cooler room temperatures to help reduce the body's metabolic demands. Protect acutely ill patients, infants, and older adults from drafts by ensuring that they are adequately dressed and covered with a lightweight blanket.

An effective ventilation system prevents stale air and odors from lingering in the room. Good ventilation reduces lingering odors caused by draining wounds, emesis, bowel movements, and used bedpans and urinals. Always empty and cleanse bedpans and urinals promptly. Room deodorizers help remove many unpleasant odors; however, be sure that your patient is not allergic or sensitive to the deodorizer itself.

Make every effort to limit the noise level, especially when patients are trying to sleep. Explain the source of unfamiliar noises such as an i.v. pump or a pulse oximeter alarm.

Proper lighting helps ensure safety and comfort. A brightly lit room usually stimulates the patient, whereas a darkened room promotes rest and sleep. Adjust room lighting by closing or opening drapes, regulating overbed and floor lights, and closing or opening room doors. When entering a patient's room at night, avoid abruptly turning on the overhead light unless necessary.

BEDS

Patients who are seriously ill may remain in bed for a long time. The typical hospital bed has a firm mattress on a metal frame that you can raise and lower horizontally and that can be placed in various positions. You vary the bed positions to promote patient comfort, minimize symptoms, promote lung expansion, and improve access during procedures. You change the position of an electric bed by using electrical controls usually incorporated into the nurse call system or in a panel on the side or foot of the bed. Become familiar with use of the bed controls. Instruct patients in the proper use of controls and caution them against raising the bed to a position that causes harm. Maintain the bed height at the lowest horizontal position when a patient is unattended.

Patients who are at risk for falling often are placed on low beds in the hospital (see Chapter 12). Special beds and mattress options (e.g., low-pressure mattresses, rotation beds) may be used with patients who are at risk for pressure injuries (see Chapter 17).

All beds contain safety features such as locks on the wheels or casters. Lock the wheels when a bed is stationary to prevent accidental movement. Side rails help patients to move more efficiently in bed and prevent accidents. Do not use side rails to restrict a patient from moving in bed. Using side rails as a restraint requires a health care provider's order (see Chapter 12). You can remove the headboard from most beds. This is important when the medical team needs easy access to the head such as during CPR.

BED MAKING

Keep a patient's bed clean and comfortable by regularly checking linen to ensure it is clean, dry, and free of wrinkles. When patients are diaphoretic, have draining wounds, or experience incontinence, check frequently for wet or soiled linen.

You usually make the bed in the morning after the patient's bath or while the patient is bathing, in a shower, sitting in a chair eating, or out of the room for procedures or tests. Throughout the day, straighten linen that becomes loose or wrinkled. In addition, check the bed linen for food particles after meals and for wetness or soiling. Change linen that becomes soiled or wet.

When changing bed linen, follow basic principles of medical asepsis by keeping soiled linen away from your uniform. Place soiled linen in linen bags before placing in the linen hamper. To avoid air currents that spread microorganisms, never shake linen. To avoid transmitting infection, do not place soiled linen or linen bags on the floor. Immediately place any clean linen that touches the floor or any unclean surface into a dirty linen container.

During bed making, use safe patient–handling procedures and proper body mechanics. Always raise the bed to the appropriate height before changing linen so that you do not have to bend or stretch over the mattress.

A patient's privacy, comfort, and safety are important when you make a bed. If the patient is confined to bed, organize bed-making activities to conserve time and energy. Use side rails, keep the nurse call system within a patient's reach, and maintain the proper bed position. After making a bed, return the bed to its lowest horizontal position and verify that the wheels are locked to prevent falls.

When you make an unoccupied bed, follow the same basic principles used for making an occupied bed (Box 10.1). When possible, make the bed while it is unoccupied (Box 10.2). The surgical, recovery, or postoperative

BOX 10.1 Procedural Guidelines

Making an Occupied Bed

Equipment

Linen bags, mattress pad (*optional* depending on agency practice; needs to be changed only when soiled), bottom sheet (flat or fitted), drawsheet *(optional)*, top sheet, blanket (*optional* depending on patient preference), bedspread, waterproof pads and/or bath blankets *(optional)*, pillowcases, bedside chair or table, clean gloves *(optional)*, paper towels or washcloth, disinfectant.

Steps

1. Review medical record and assess restrictions concerning patient mobility and/or positioning.
2. Perform hand hygiene and gather needed supplies, being sure not to let clean linen touch your uniform. Arrange equipment on bedside chair or overbed table. Remove unnecessary equipment such as a dietary tray or items used for hygiene. Pull curtain and close door.
3. Make sure equipment is working properly and that bed is in locked position and appropriate number of side rails are raised.
4. Explain procedure to the patient including that he or she will be asked to turn on side and roll over linen.
5. Perform hand hygiene. Apply clean gloves if the patient was incontinent or if drainage is present on linen.
6. Adjust bed height to comfortable working position with bed flat if the patient can tolerate. Lower raised side rail on side where you will be standing. Loosen all top linen. Remove bedspread and blanket separately, leaving the patient covered with top sheet. Place soiled bedspread and/or blanket in linen bag and discard. If bedspread to be reused, fold and place and/or blanket over back of chair.
7. Cover the patient with bath blanket in the following manner: unfold bath blanket over top sheet. Ask the patient to hold top edge of bath blanket. If the patient cannot help, tuck top of bath blanket under shoulders. Grasp top sheet under bath blanket at the patient's shoulders and bring sheet down to foot of bed. Remove sheet and discard in linen bag.
8. Position the patient on far side of bed, turned onto side and facing away from you. **Note:** This is when another caregiver can help by standing at bedside across from you. Be sure that side rail in front of the patient is up. Encourage the patient to use side rail to turn. Adjust pillow under the patient's head.
9. Loosen bottom linens, moving from head to foot. With seam side down (facing the mattress), fanfold soiled drawsheet and bottom sheet toward the patient. Tuck edges of linen just under buttocks, back, and shoulders. Do not fanfold mattress pad if it is to be reused (see illustration).

BOX 10.1 **Procedural Guidelines—cont'd**

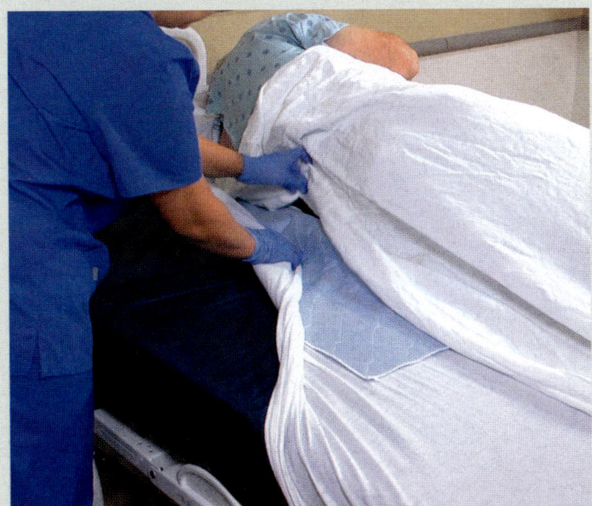

Step 9 Tuck all soiled linen from one side of bed alongside the patient's back.

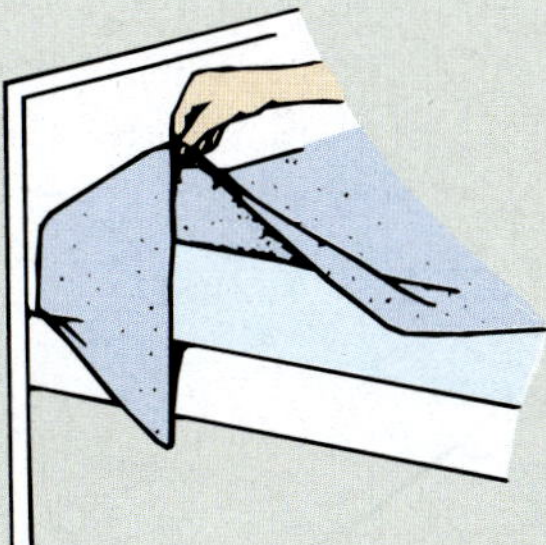

Step 12c Top edge of sheet picked up.

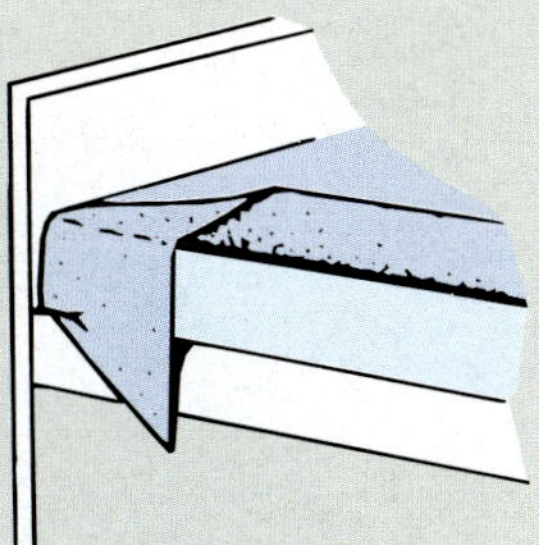

Step 12d Sheet on top of mattress in a triangular fold.

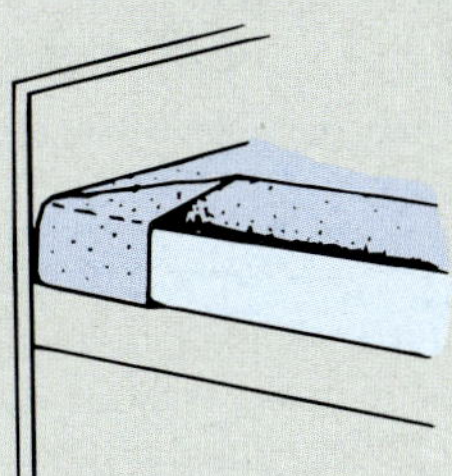

Step 12e Lower edge of sheet tucked under mattress.

10. Wipe off any moisture on exposed mattress with paper towel. Clean and disinfect and dry mattress surface (check agency policy).
11. Apply clean linen to exposed half of bed:
    a. Place clean mattress pad (if used) on bed by folding it lengthwise with center crease in middle of bed. Fanfold top layer over mattress. (If pad is reused, simply smooth out any wrinkles.)
    b. If using flat sheet for bottom sheet, unfold sheet lengthwise so that center crease is situated lengthwise along center of bed. Fanfold top layer of sheet toward center of bed alongside patient. Smooth bottom layer of sheet over mattress and bring edge over closest side of mattress. If using fitted sheet, pull sheet smoothly over mattress ends.
    c. Allow edge of flat unfitted sheet to hang about 25 cm (10 inches) over mattress edge. Make sure that lower hem of bottom flat sheet lies seam down and even with bottom edge of mattress.
12. If flat sheet is used for bottom sheet, miter bottom flat sheet at head of bed:
    a. Face head of bed diagonally. Place hand away from head of bed under top corner of mattress, near mattress edge, and lift.
    b. With other hand, tuck top edge of bottom sheet smoothly under mattress so that side edges of sheet above and below mattress meet when brought together.
    c. Face side of bed and pick up top edge of sheet at approximately 45 cm (18 inches) from top of mattress (see illustration).
    d. Lift sheet and lay it on top of mattress to form a neat triangular fold, with lower base of triangle even with mattress side edge (see illustration[D339]).
    e. Tuck lower edge of sheet, which is hanging free below the mattress, under mattress. Tuck with palms down without pulling triangular fold (see illustration).
    f. Hold part of sheet covering side of mattress in place with one hand. With the other hand, pick up top of triangular linen fold and bring it down over side of mattress. Tuck this part under mattress (see illustrations).
    g. Tuck remaining part of sheet under mattress, moving toward foot of bed. Keep linen smooth.

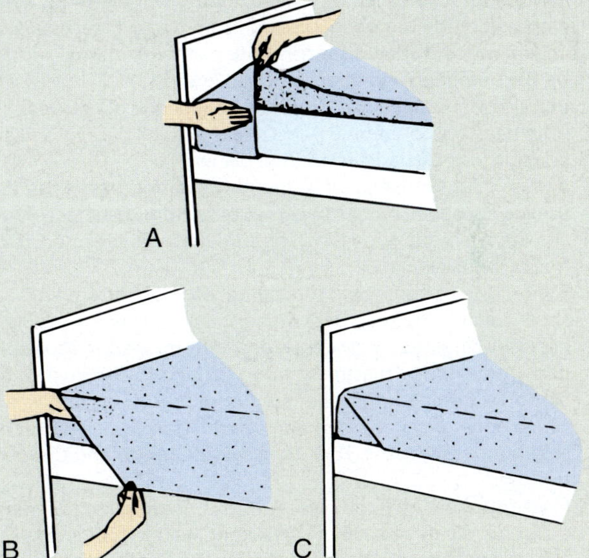

Step 12f Triangular fold placed over side of mattress, sheet tucked under mattress.

13. *Optional:* Open clean drawsheet so that it unfolds in half. Lay centerfold along middle of bed lengthwise and position sheet so that it is under patient's buttocks and torso. Fanfold top layer of drawsheet toward the patient with edge along patient's back. Smooth bottom layer out over mattress and tuck excess edge under mattress (keep palms down).
14. Place single waterproof pad over drawsheet *(optional)* with centerfold against the patient's side. Fanfold top layer toward the patient.

Continued

BOX 10.1 Procedural Guidelines—cont'd

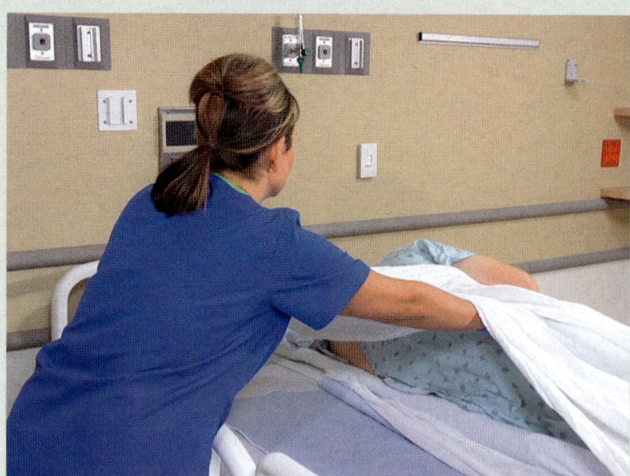

Step 15 Patient begins rolling over layers of linen.

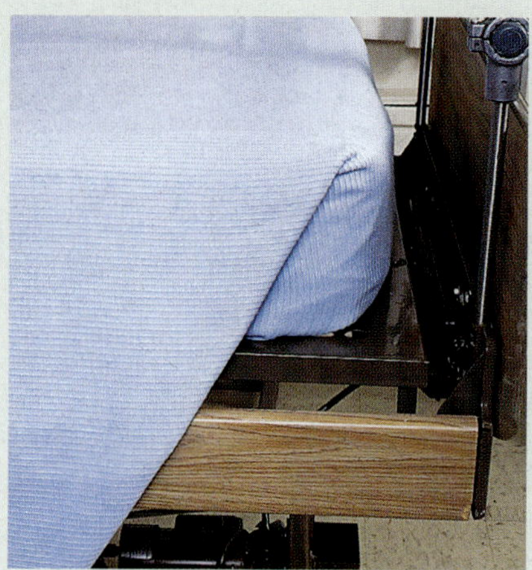

Step 27 Modified mitered corner.

15. Advise the patient that rolling over thick layer of linens is necessary and that he or she will feel a lump. Have the patient roll slowly toward you over the layers of linen, rolling like a log (see illustration). Have the patient lie still and raise side rail on working side before going to other side of bed.
16. Lower side rail. Help the patient to comfortable position on other side as needed. Loosen edges of soiled linen from under mattress.
17. Remove all soiled linen by folding it into a bundle or square with soiled side turned in. Discard in linen bag. If necessary, wipe mattress with antiseptic solution and dry mattress surface before unfolding and applying clean linen.
18. Pull clean, fanfolded linen smoothly over edge of mattress from head to foot of bed. Help the patient roll back into supine position (if preferred). Reposition pillow.
19. If using a fitted sheet, pull it smoothly over mattress ends. If using a flat sheet, miter top corner of bottom sheet (see Step 12a–g). When tucking corner, be sure that sheet is smooth and free of wrinkles.
20. Facing side of bed, grasp remaining edge of bottom flat sheet. Lean back, keep back straight, and pull while tucking excess linen under mattress. Proceed from head to foot of bed. (Avoid lifting mattress during tucking to ensure fit.)
21. Smooth fanfolded drawsheet out over bottom sheet. Grasp edge of sheet with palms down, lean back, and tuck sheet under mattress. Tuck from middle to top and then to bottom.
22. Place top sheet over the patient with centerfold lengthwise down middle of bed. Open sheet from head to foot and unfold over the patient. Ask the patient to hold clean top sheet or tuck sheet around his or her shoulders. Remove bath blanket and discard in linen bag.
23. Place blanket on bed, unfolding it so that crease runs lengthwise along middle of bed. Unfold blanket to cover the patient. Make sure that top edge is parallel with edge of top sheet and 15–20 cm (6–8 inches) from edge of top sheet.
24. Place spread over bed according to Step 22. Be sure that top edge of spread extends about 2.5 cm (1 inch) above edge of blanket. Tuck top edge of spread over and under top edge of blanket.
25. Make cuff by turning edge of top sheet down over top edge of blanket and spread.
26. Standing on one side at foot of bed, lift mattress corner slightly with one hand and tuck sheet and blanket together under mattress. Be sure that lines are loose enough to allow movement of the patient's feet. Making a horizontal toe pleat is an option.
27. Make modified mitered corner with top sheet, blanket, and spread (follow Step 12a–e). After making the triangular fold, do not tuck tip of the triangle under the mattress (see illustration).
28. Raise side rail. Make other side of bed. Spread out sheet, blanket, and bedspread evenly. Fold top edge of spread over blanket and make cuff with top sheet (see Step 25); make modified mitered corner (see Step 27).
29. Change pillowcase:
    a. Have the patient raise head. While supporting neck with one hand, remove pillow. Allow the patient to lower head.
    b. Remove soiled case by grasping pillow open end with one hand and pulling case back over pillow with other hand. Discard case in linen bag.
    c. Grasp clean pillowcase at center of closed end. Gather case, turning it inside out over the hand holding it. With same hand pick up middle of one end of pillow. Pull pillowcase down over pillow with other hand.
    d. Be sure that pillow corners fit evenly into corners of pillowcase. Place pillow under the patient's head.
30. Place nurse call system in an accessible location within the patient's reach. Return bed to comfortable position and height. Open room curtains and rearrange furniture. Place personal items within easy reach on overbed table or bedside stand.
31. Place dirty linen in hamper or chute. Remove gloves (if worn); dispose of the gloves and perform hand hygiene.
32. Ask whether the patient feels comfortable.
33. Use this time to inspect skin for areas of irritation.

BOX 10.2 **Procedural Guidelines**

Making an Unoccupied Bed

Equipment

Linen bag, mattress pad (change only when soiled), bottom sheet (flat or fitted), drawsheet *(optional)*, top sheet, blanket, bedspread, waterproof pads *(optional)*, special linens for support surface mattress *(optional)*, pillowcases, bedside chair or table, clean gloves (if linen is soiled), washcloth or paper towel, antiseptic cleanser.

Steps

1. Perform hand hygiene and arrange supplies at bedside.
2. Assess environment for safety (e.g., check room for spills, make sure equipment is working properly and that bed is in locked position).
3. Assess activity orders or restrictions in mobility to determine whether the patient can get out of bed for procedure. Help the patient to bedside chair or recliner.
4. If the patient has been incontinent or if excess drainage is on linen, gloves are necessary.
5. Lower side rails on both sides of bed and raise bed to comfortable working position.
6. Remove soiled linen and place in laundry bag. Avoid shaking or fanning linen.
7. Reposition mattress and wipe off any moisture with a washcloth or paper towel moistened in antiseptic solution. Dry thoroughly.
8. Apply all bottom linens on one side of bed (before moving to opposite side):
   a. Be sure that fitted sheet is placed smoothly over mattress.
   b. To apply a flat unfitted sheet, allow about 25 cm (10 inches) to hang over sides of mattress edges. Make sure that lower hem of sheet lies seam down, even with bottom edge of mattress. Pull remaining top part of sheet over top edge of mattress.
9. While standing at head of bed, miter top corner of bottom sheet (see Box 10.1, Step 12a–g).
10. Tuck remaining part of unfitted sheet under mattress from head to foot of bed.
11. *Optional:* Apply drawsheet, laying centerfold along middle of bed lengthwise. Smooth drawsheet over mattress and tuck excess edge under mattress, keeping palms down.
12. Move to opposite side of bed and spread bottom sheet smoothly over edge of mattress from head to foot of bed.
13. Apply fitted sheet smoothly over each mattress corner. For an unfitted sheet, miter top corner of bottom sheet (see Step 9), making sure that corner is taut.
14. Grasp remaining edge of unfitted bottom sheet and tuck tightly under mattress while moving from head to foot of bed.
15. Smooth folded drawsheet over bottom sheet and tuck under mattress, first at middle, then at top, and then at bottom.
16. If needed, apply single waterproof pad over bottom sheet or drawsheet.
17. Place top sheet over bed with vertical centerfold lengthwise down middle of bed. Open sheet out from head to foot, being sure that top edge of sheet is even with top edge of mattress.
18. Make horizontal toe pleat: stand at foot of bed and make fanfold in sheet 5–10 cm (2–4 inches) across bed. Pull sheet up from bottom to make fold approximately 15 cm (6 inches) from bottom edge of mattress.
19. Tuck in remaining part of sheet under foot of mattress. Place blanket over bed with top edge parallel to top edge of sheet and 15–20 cm (6–8 inches) down from edge of sheet. (*Optional:* Apply additional spread over bed.)
20. Make cuff by turning edge of top sheet down over top edge of blanket and spread.
21. Standing on one side at foot of bed, lift mattress corner slightly with one hand; with other hand tuck top sheet, blanket, and spread under mattress. Be sure that toe pleats have not been pulled out.
22. Make modified mitered corner with top sheet, blanket, and spread. Standing on one side at foot of bed, lift mattress corner slightly with one hand and tuck sheet and blanket together under mattress. Be sure that lines are loose enough to allow movement of the patient's feet. Making a horizontal toe pleat is an option (see Box 10.1, Step 26).
23. Go to other side of bed. Spread out sheet and blanket evenly. Make cuff with top sheet and blanket. Make modified corner at foot of bed.
24. Apply clean pillowcase (see Box 10.1, Step 29).
25. Be sure nurse call system is in an accessible location within the patient's reach on bedrail or pillow, and return bed to height allowing for the patient transfer. Help the patient to bed.
26. Arrange the patient's room. Remove and discard supplies. Perform hand hygiene.

bed is a modified version of the unoccupied bed. Fold the top covers of the surgical bed to one side or fanfold them to the bottom third of the bed so that you can easily transfer the patient into the bed after a procedure. When a patient is discharged, send all bed linen to the laundry. Housekeeping personnel usually clean and disinfect the mattress and bed and apply new bed linen after discharge. Many agencies have "nurse servers" either within or just outside the patient's room where a daily supply of linen is stored. To help control costs and prevent infection transmission, avoid bringing excess linen into the patient's room. Once you bring linen into a patient's room, even if the linen has not been used, it must be laundered before being used by another patient.

COMMON THERAPEUTIC POSITIONS

Positioning of the patient is important to provide rest, to perform procedures and immobilization of the effected body parts whenever required. Positions are dependent on disease conditions of the patient and it is vital to change patients' position frequently especially among chronic bedridden patients, unconscious patients, and immobilized patients.

Nursing care involves providing positions to the patients either in bed or during any examination. There are several positions described in Table 10.1, which can be provided to patients according to his or her needs. Sometimes, patients

Table 10.1 Common Therapeutic Positions

Position	Description	Uses
Fowler's 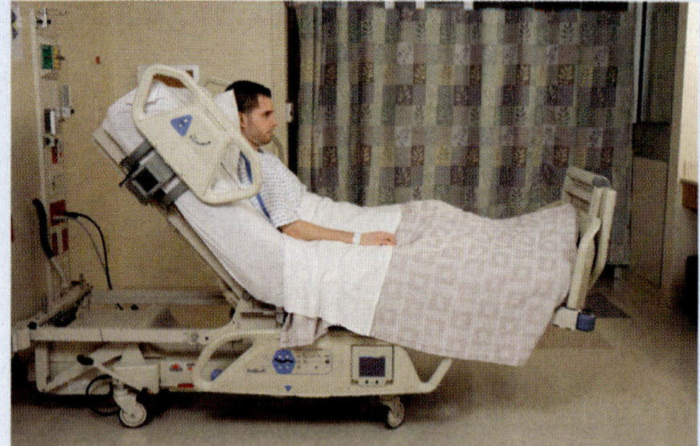	Head of bed raised to angle of 45° or more; semisitting position; foot of bed may also be raised at knee	Used during meals and oral medication administration, nasogastric tube insertion, and nasotracheal suction. Promotes lung expansion.
Semi-Fowler's 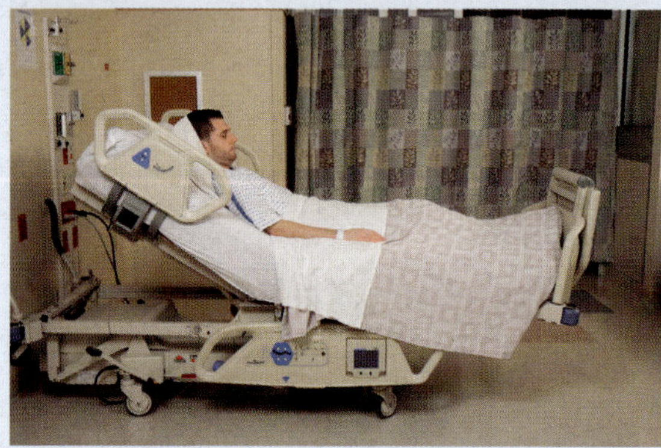	Head of bed raised approximately 30°; incline less than Fowler's position; foot of bed may also be raised at knee	Promotes lung expansion. Used when patients receive gastric feedings to reduce regurgitation and risk for aspiration.
Trendelenburg's 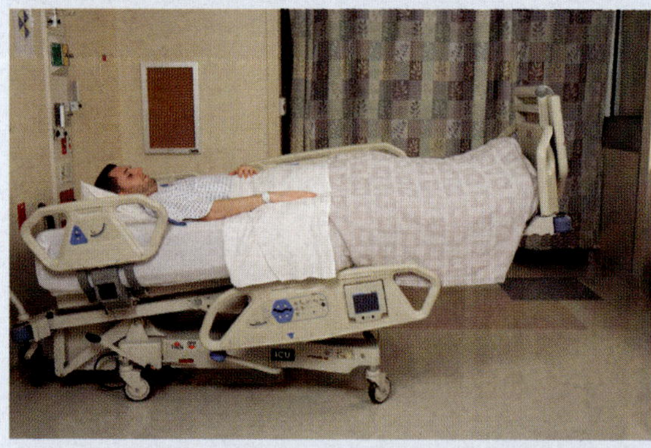	Entire bed tilted with head of bed down	Used for postural drainage. Facilitates venous return in patients with poor peripheral venous perfusion.
Reverse Trendelenburg's 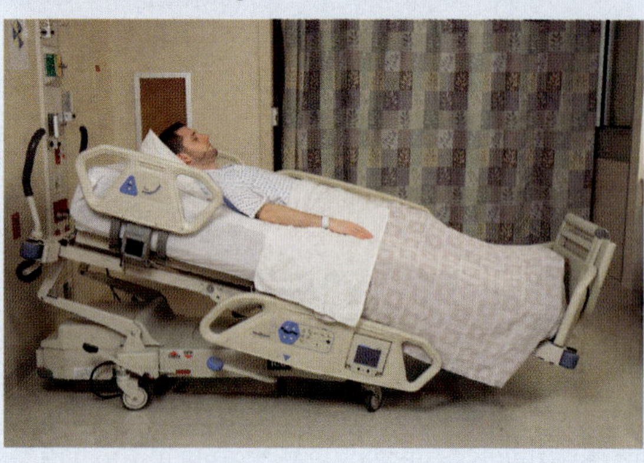	Entire bedframe tilted with foot of bed down	Used infrequently. Promotes gastric emptying. Prevents esophageal reflux.

Table 10.1 Common Therapeutic Positions—cont'd

Position	Description	Uses
Supine also known as dorsal decubitus	Entire bedframe horizontally parallel with floor	Used for patients with vertebral injuries and in cervical traction. Used for patients who are hypotensive. Generally preferred by patients for sleeping.
Prone	Entire bedframe horizontally parallel with floor Patient lies on her or his stomach and face turn to the one side	Used for spinal and neck surgeries, neurosurgeries, and colorectal surgeries
Sim's	Patient will turn to left side with left leg straight and right leg is bent from the knee	Access to anus
Lithotomy	Patient lies on her back with legs placed in stirrups	Used in gynecological examination, baby delivery, copper T insertion, perineal and pelvic procedures

can be hesitant or not cooperative while providing positions but this may lead to poor body alignment and difficulty in performing examinations or procedures. It is important for nurses to consider indications and contraindication of each position to prevent any harm to patient.

PHYSIOLOGY OF SLEEP

Sleep is a cyclical physiological process that alternates with longer periods of wakefulness. The sleep–wake cycle influences and regulates physiological function and behavioral responses.

Circadian Rhythms

People experience cyclical rhythms as part of their everyday life. The most familiar rhythm is the 24-hour, day–night cycle known as the diurnal or **circadian rhythm.**

- The suprachiasmatic nucleus nerve cells in the hypothalamus control the rhythm of the sleep–wake cycle and coordinate it with other circadian rhythms (Huether and McCance, 2017).
- Circadian rhythms influence the 24-hour pattern of major biological and behavioral functions such as predictable changes in body temperature, heart rate, blood pressure, hormone secretion, sensory acuity, and mood (Kryger et al., 2017).

Light and temperature affect all circadian rhythms including the sleep–wake cycle. External factors such as social activities and environmental stressors also affect circadian rhythms. Every person has a **biological clock** that is normally synchronized by exposure to light and activity. This explains why some people fall asleep at 8 p.m., whereas others go to bed at midnight or early in the morning. It also explains why people function best at different times of the day.

Hospitals or extended care facilities usually do not adapt care to an individual's sleep–wake cycle preferences. Typical hospital routines require nurses to interrupt patients' sleep to complete assessments or provide nursing care such as administering medications and changing dressings. Poor quality of sleep results when a person's sleep–wake cycle changes. Reversals in the sleep–wake cycle, such as when a person who is normally awake during the day falls asleep during the day, sometimes indicate a serious illness.

When the sleep–wake cycle becomes disrupted (e.g., by working rotating shifts), other physiological functions change as well. For example, a new nurse who starts working the night shift experiences a decreased appetite and loses weight. Anxiety, restlessness, irritability, and impaired judgment are other common symptoms of sleep cycle disturbances. Failure to maintain a usual sleep–wake cycle negatively influences overall health.

Sleep Regulation

Sleep is a series of physiological states maintained by highly integrated central nervous system (CNS) activity that is associated with changes in the peripheral nervous, endocrine, cardiovascular, respiratory, and muscular systems (Huether and McCance, 2017). Specific sequential physiological responses and patterns of brain activity identify each sleep cycle. Instruments that measure physiological aspects of sleep include the electroencephalogram

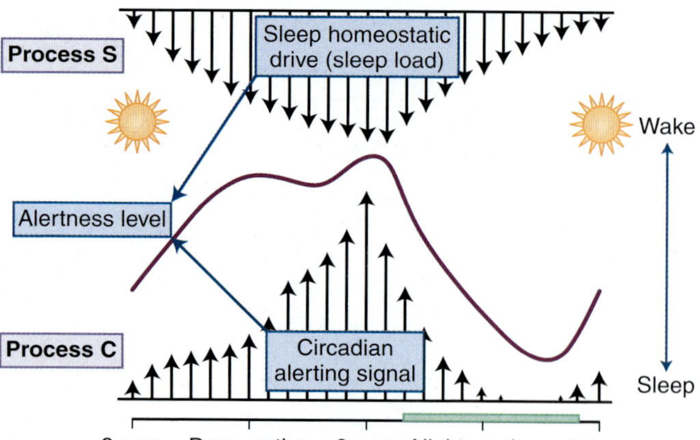

Fig 10.1 Two-process model of sleep regulation shows the time course of the homeostatic process (Process S) and the circadian process (Process C). Process S rises during waking and declines during sleep. The intersection of Process S and Process C defines the time of wake-up. (From Daroff RB, et al: Bradley's neurology in clinical practice, ed 6, Philadelphia, 2012, Saunders.)

(EEG), which measures electrical activity in the cerebral cortex; the electromyogram (EMG), which measures muscle tone; and the electrooculogram (EOG), which measures eye movements.

The major sleep center is in the hypothalamus. Hypocretins (a form of peptide) secreted by the hypothalamus promote wakefulness and rapid eye movement (REM) sleep. Prostaglandin D_2, L-tryptophan, and growth factors also control sleep (Huether and McCance, 2017).

Researchers believe that several neuron groups within and next to the pontine and midbrain reticular formation work together to maintain alertness and wakefulness. Arousal, wakefulness, and maintenance of consciousness result from neurons in these areas releasing serotonin, norepinephrine, histamine, acetylcholine, and orexin (Kryger et al., 2017). Each of the neurotransmitters works on a distinct receptor to control sleep–wake patterns.

The homeostatic process (Process S), which primarily regulates the length and depth of sleep, and the circadian rhythms (Process C—"biological time clocks"), which influence the internal organization of sleep and timing and duration of sleep–wake cycles, operate simultaneously to regulate sleep and wakefulness (Kryger et al., 2017). Time of wake-up is the intersection of Process S and Process C (Fig. 10.1).

STAGES OF SLEEP

There are two sleep phases: **nonrapid eye movement (NREM) sleep** and **rapid eye movement (REM) sleep** (Box 10.3). In the classical definition of NREM sleep, an individual progresses through four stages during a typical 90-minute sleep cycle. The American Academy of Sleep Medicine defines three stages in NREM sleep, combining stages 3 and 4 (Kryger et al., 2017). The quality of sleep from stage 1 through stage 4 becomes increasingly deep. Lighter sleep is characteristic of stages 1 and 2, when a person is more easily arousable. Combined stages 3 and 4 involve a deeper sleep called *slow-wave sleep*, from which a person is more difficult to arouse (Kryger et al., 2017). REM sleep is the phase at the end of each 90-minute sleep cycle. During REM sleep, there is increased brain activity associated with REMs and muscle atonia.

BOX 10.3 Stages of the Sleep Cycle

Stage 1: NREM

- Stage lasts a few minutes.
- It includes lightest level of sleep.
- Decreased physiological activity begins with gradual fall in vital signs and metabolism.
- Sensory stimuli such as noise easily arouse person.
- When awakened, person feels as though daydreaming has occurred.

Stage 2: NREM

- Stage lasts 10–20 min.
- It is a period of sound sleep.
- Relaxation progresses.
- Body functions continue to slow.
- Arousal remains relatively easy.

Stage 3: NREM

- Stage lasts 15–30 min.
- It involves initial stages of deep sleep.
- Muscles are completely relaxed.
- Vital signs decline but remain regular.
- Sleeper is difficult to arouse and rarely moves.

Stage 4: NREM

- Stage lasts approximately 15–30 min.
- It is the deepest stage of sleep.
- If sleep loss has occurred, sleeper spends considerable part of night in this stage.
- Vital signs are significantly lower than during waking hours.
- Sleepwalking and enuresis (bed-wetting) sometimes occur.
- It is very difficult to arouse the sleeper.

REM Sleep

- Stage usually begins about 90 min after the sleep has begun.
- Duration increases with each sleep cycle and averages 20 min.
- Vivid, full-color dreaming occurs; less vivid dreaming occurs in other stages.
- Stage is typified by rapidly moving eyes, fluctuating heart and respiratory rates, increased or fluctuating blood pressure, loss of skeletal muscle tone, and increase of gastric secretions.
- It is very difficult to arouse the sleeper.

NREM, nonrapid eye movement; *REM*, rapid eye movement.

Sleep Cycle

Normally an adult's routine sleep pattern begins with a presleep period, during which the person is aware only of a gradually developing sleepiness. This period normally lasts 10–30 minutes. Individuals experiencing difficulty falling asleep often remain in this stage for an hour or more. Once asleep, a person usually passes through four to six complete sleep cycles, each cycle consisting of four stages of NREM sleep and a period of REM sleep, for a total of 90–110 minutes (Huether and McCance, 2017).

With each successive cycle, stage 3 (combined stages 3 and 4) of NREM sleep shortens, and REM sleep lengthens. REM sleep lasts up to 60 minutes during the last sleep cycle.

Not all people progress consistently through the usual stages of sleep. For example, a sleeper fluctuates back and forth for short intervals between NREM stages 2 and 3 before entering REM sleep. The amount of time spent in each stage varies. The number of sleep cycles depends on the total amount of time that the person spends sleeping.

FUNCTIONS OF SLEEP

- Sleep functions as a time of restoration, memory consolidation, and preparation for the next period of wakefulness (Huether and McCance, 2017).
- During NREM sleep, biological functions slow down. A healthy adult's heart rate decreases from a normal average of 70–80 beats/min to 60 beats/min or less during sleep, thus preserving cardiac function.
- Other biological functions that decrease during sleep are respirations, temperature, blood pressure, and muscle tone (Kryger et al., 2017).
- Sleep restores biological processes. During NREM stage 3 sleep, the body releases human growth hormone for the repair and renewal of epithelial and specialized cells such as brain cells (Huether and McCance, 2017). Protein synthesis and cell division for the renewal of tissues also occur during rest and sleep. The basal metabolic rate lowers during sleep, which conserves the energy supply of the body (Huether and McCance, 2017).
- REM sleep appears to be important for early brain development, cognition, and memory. Researchers associate REM sleep with changes in the brain including cerebral blood flow and increased cortical activity. In addition, there is increased oxygen consumption and epinephrine release. These changes are associated with memory storage and learning.

The benefits of sleep often go unnoticed until a person develops a problem resulting from sleep deprivation. Current estimates show that 50–70 million adults in the United States have some type of sleep–wake problem (Centers for Disease Control and Prevention [CDC], 2015). Sleep deprivation affects immune function, metabolism, nitrogen balance, and protein catabolism. A loss of REM sleep often leads to confusion and suspicion. Prolonged sleep loss alters various body functions (e.g., mood, motor performance, memory, equilibrium) (National Sleep Foundation, 2016b). Individuals with sleep problems are also more likely to have chronic diseases such as hypertension, diabetes, and obesity. They sometimes also experience poorer quality of life and productivity (Kohansieh and Makaryus, 2015). Millions of health care dollars are spent on indirect costs related to sleep deprivation such as motor vehicle and industrial accidents, litigation, property damage, hospitalization, medical errors, and death (Liu et al., 2016).

DREAMS

Dreams during REM sleep are more vivid and elaborate than dreams during NREM sleep. Researchers believe REM dreams are functionally important to learning, memory processing, and adaptation to stress (Kryger et al., 2017). REM dreams progress throughout the night from dreams about current events to emotional dreams of childhood or the past. Personality influences the quality of dreams (e.g., a creative person may have very vivid, unusual dreams, whereas a depressed person may have dreams of helplessness). Dreams help people sort out immediate concerns or erase certain fantasies or nonsensical memories. Because most dreams are forgotten, many people have little dream recall and do not believe they dream at all. People who recall dreams vividly usually awaken just after a period of REM sleep.

NORMAL SLEEP REQUIREMENTS AND PATTERNS

Neonates

Sleep duration and quality vary among people of all age groups. Neonates and infants up to the age of 3 months average about 16–18 hours of sleep a day. Approximately 50% of this sleep is REM sleep, which stimulates higher brain centers (Hockenberry and Wilson, 2015).

Infants

Infants usually develop a nighttime pattern of sleep by the age of 3–4 months. They sometimes take several naps during the day but usually sleep an average of 9–11 hours during the night. Infants spend about 30% of sleep time in the REM cycle. Infants commonly awake early in the morning, although they sometimes also awaken during the night.

Toddlers and Preschoolers

By the age of 2 years, children usually sleep through the night and take daily naps. Total recommended sleep is 11–14 hours a day (Hirshkowitz et al., 2015). Some children stop taking naps altogether at the age of 3 years. Toddlers commonly awaken during the night, and the percentage of REM sleep continues to fall. Toddlers are often unwilling to go to bed at night. A preschooler sleeps an average of 12 hours a night (about 20% is REM). By the age of 5 years, preschoolers rarely take daytime naps (Hockenberry and Wilson, 2015), except in cultures in which a siesta is the custom. Preschoolers usually have difficulty relaxing or quieting down after long, active days and often have problems with bedtime fears, waking during the night, and nightmares.

School-Age Children

A school-age child usually does not require a nap. A 6-year-old child averages 11–12 hours of sleep nightly, whereas an 11-year-old sleeps about 9–10 hours (Hockenberry and Wilson, 2015). Encouraging quiet activities usually persuades a 6- or 7-year-old child to go to bed. An older child often resists sleeping because of an unawareness of fatigue or a need to be independent.

Adolescents

Adolescents need 8–10 hours of sleep each night; however, the typical teenager gets less than 8½ hours of sleep (National Sleep Foundation, 2016d). At a time when sleep needs actually increase, the typical adolescent is subject to a number of changes that often reduce the time spent sleeping (e.g., early start times for school; after-school social events, part-time jobs, worrying before sleep, and personal habits such as caffeine intake and viewing electronic devices) (Wheaton et al., 2016). Adolescents typically stay up much later and may develop a circadian disorder called sleep phase delay. Adolescents with delayed sleep phase want to go to bed later, usually after midnight, and sleep later than what is typical, but this may not be possible with early school start times. The shortened sleep time in adolescents often results in excessive daytime sleepiness (EDS), which can impair waking, reduce performance in school, increase the risk of motor vehicle accidents and sports injuries, increase the use of alcohol, and lead to behavior and mood problems (Bartel et al., 2015).

Young Adults

Most young adults average 6–8½ hours of sleep a night, but this varies. Young adults rarely take regular naps. They spend approximately 20% of sleep time in REM sleep, which remains consistent throughout the remainder of life. Healthy young adults require adequate sleep (7–9 hours per day) to participate in daily busy activities (Hirshkowitz et al., 2015). However, lifestyle demands and family relationships sometimes lead to insomnia. It is important that young adults learn to effectively cope with stressors and avoid unhealthy coping strategies. Pregnancy increases the need for rest and sleep. Common problems during the third trimester of pregnancy include restless legs syndrome (RLS), insomnia, periodic limb movements, and sleep-disordered breathing (Kryger et al., 2017).

Middle-Age Adults

During middle adulthood, the total time spent sleeping at night declines. Health care providers often initially diagnose sleep disturbances among people in this age range even when the symptoms of a disorder have been present for several years. Because of stresses experienced in middle age, insomnia is a common occurrence. It is often experienced by menopausal women who may also develop restless leg syndrome (RLS) or periodic limb movements as a result of iron deficiency from menorrhagia.

Older Adults

Sleeping difficulties increase with age. Approximately 40% of older adults report problems with sleep (Kryger et al., 2017; National Sleep Foundation, 2016a). Older adults spend more time in stage 1 and less time in stages 3 and 4 (NREM sleep); some older adults have almost no NREM stage 4 sleep. Episodes of REM sleep tend to shorten. Older adults experience fewer episodes of deep sleep and more episodes of lighter sleep. They tend to awaken more often during the night, and it takes more time for them to fall asleep. Older adults increase the number of naps taken during the day to compensate. Older adults with insomnia often have comorbid psychiatric illnesses or medical conditions, take medications that disrupt sleep patterns, or use drugs or alcohol (Touhy and Jett, 2018).

FACTORS AFFECTING SLEEP

A number of factors (physical, psychological, and environmental) affect the quantity and quality of sleep. Often more than one factor combines to cause a sleep problem.

Physical Illness

Any illness or condition that causes pain, difficulty breathing, nausea, or mood problems such as anxiety or depression can result in sleep problems (Table 10.2). Individuals with such problems have trouble falling or staying asleep or may wake early. Illnesses or diseases also sometimes force patients to sleep in positions to which they are unaccustomed. For example, it is difficult for a patient with a leg immobilizer to rest comfortably.

Table 10.2 Illnesses and Conditions That Can Alter Sleep

Illness/Condition	Nature of Sleep Alteration
Respiratory disease (e.g., emphysema, asthma, bronchitis, allergic rhinitis, common cold)	Shortness of breath requires the use of two to three pillows to raise head and alters rhythm of breathing. Nasal congestion and sore throat impair breathing and ability to relax.
Coronary heart disease with episodes of chest pain and irregular heart rates	Heart disease causes frequent awakenings, sleep stage changes during sleep, and significant alterations in all stages of sleep.
Hypertension	Reduced length and depth of NREM sleep and a shortened REM latency period cause arousals and early morning awakening, resulting in fatigue.
Hypothyroidism	Decreases in slow-wave and REM sleep and increased movements during sleep contribute to daytime sleepiness.
Hyperthyroidism	Increase in metabolism causes insomnia resulting from increased time needed to fall asleep.
Nocturia (reduced bladder tone, heart failure, diabetes, urethritis, prostate disease)	Waking at night to urinate results in difficulty returning to sleep.
Gastric reflux	Burning pain in lower esophagus or nocturnal coughing increases when lying flat in bed.
Depression	Early morning awakenings with inability to return to sleep are worsened by anxiety or agitation.
Perimenopause	Waking at night is caused by hot flashes and sweating.
Pain	Delay in sleep onset, increased waking from sleep, and decreased slow-wave activity during sleep result in poor sleep quality. Pain is worsened by increased sympathetic activity, resulting in high cardiac heart rate.

NREM, nonrapid eye movement; *REM,* rapid eye movement.

Sleep-related breathing disorders are linked to increased incidence of nocturnal angina (chest pain), increased heart rate, electrocardiogram changes, high blood pressure, and risk of heart diseases and stroke (Huether and McCance, 2017).

Nighttime urination **(nocturia)** disrupts sleep and the sleep cycle. It is difficult to return to sleep after repeated awakenings, and a complete sleep cycle is prevented from occurring. Although this condition is most common in older people, it also affects a significant portion of younger people (Madhu et al., 2015). Nocturia also occurs in people with obstructive sleep apnea (OSA) because of release of atrial natriuretic peptide.

RLS is a neurological sensorimotor disorder that causes an irresistible urge to move the legs while they are at rest, sitting, or lying. Symptoms are most severe in the evening and night and can severely disrupt a patient's sleep (National Sleep Foundation, 2016c).

Drugs and Substances

Numerous drugs cause sleepiness, insomnia, or fatigue as a side effect (Box 10.4). Medications prescribed for sleep often cause more problems than benefits. L-Tryptophan is a natural protein found in foods such as milk, cheese, and meats (e.g., turkey and chicken) and sometimes helps a person sleep. It is a precursor, or forerunner, to the neurotransmitter serotonin, which has a role in the sleep–wake cycle.

Lifestyle

A person's daily routine influences sleep patterns. For example, an individual who alternately works day and night shifts often has difficulty adjusting to an altered sleep schedule. Lifestyle changes that contribute to decreased quantity and quality of sleep include working an increased number of hours per day or week or at multiple jobs and spending more time on the internet. Other alterations in routine that disrupt sleep patterns include performing unaccustomed heavy work or exercise, engaging in late-night social activities, and changing evening mealtime. Travel across time zones is a common factor associated with insomnia.

Usual Sleep Patterns and Excessive Daytime Sleepiness

Only 35% of adults report getting 8 hours of sleep a day regularly (University of Maryland Medical Center, 2016). The average American adult gets 7½ hours of sleep a night, but 35% of those report that their sleep quality is fair or poor (Liu et al., 2016; National Sleep Foundation, 2014). This leads to EDS during the day. A contributor to EDS is the use of technology close to bedtime, such as watching television, talking or texting on a cell phone, or reading information on electronic devices.

Sleepiness becomes pathological when it occurs at times when people need or want to be awake. People who temporarily experience sleep deprivation as a result of an active social evening or lengthened work schedule usually feel sleepy the next day. However, they are usually able to overcome these feelings even though they have difficulty performing tasks and remaining attentive. Chronic lack of sleep is much more serious than temporary sleep deprivation and causes serious alterations in the ability to perform daily activities. EDS is most difficult to overcome during sedentary tasks (e.g., driving).

Emotional Stress

Worry over personal problems or situations interferes with sleep. Emotional stress causes tension and often leads to frustration when sleep does not come. Stress also causes a person to try too hard to fall asleep, to awaken frequently during the sleep cycle, or to oversleep. Continued stress causes poor sleep habits in some cases.

BOX 10.4 Effect of Medications and Other Substances on Sleep

Hypnotics

- Interfere with reaching deeper sleep stages
- Provide only temporary (1 week) increase in quantity of sleep
- Sometimes cause "hangover" feeling during day
- In some cases, worsen sleep apnea in older adults

Diuretics (Administered Late in the Day)

- Cause nocturia, which leads to nighttime awakenings

Antidepressants and Stimulants

- Suppress REM sleep and decrease total sleep time

Alcohol

- Speeds onset of sleep and disrupts REM sleep
- Awakens person during night and causes difficulty returning to sleep

Caffeine

- Stimulant; prevents person from falling asleep
- Causes person to awaken during night

Nicotine

- Causes decrease in sleep time
- Causes nighttime awakenings
- Causes difficulty staying asleep

Beta-Adrenergic Blockers

- Cause nightmares and insomnia
- Cause awakening from sleep

Benzodiazepines

- Increase sleep time
- Increase daytime sleepiness

Opiates

- Suppress REM sleep
- Cause increased daytime drowsiness

Antihistamines

- Cause drowsiness
- Cause insomnia when used in excess

Anticonvulsants

- Decrease REM sleep
- Cause daytime drowsiness

REM, rapid eye movement.

Environment

The physical environment in which a person sleeps influences the ability to fall and remain asleep. Proper ventilation, a comfortable (usually cooler versus warmer) temperature, and a quiet, darkened or softly lit room are essential for restful sleep. A comfortable bed also affects sleep quality. Hospital beds are often harder than beds at home. If a person usually sleeps with another individual, sleeping alone during times of illness causes wakefulness. However, sleeping with a restless or snoring bed partner also disrupts sleep. It is best for older adults to avoid using beds for nonsleep activities such as watching television or reading.

Noise easily disturbs all patients, especially older adults because most of their sleep is in lighter sleep stages. This problem is greatest the first night a patient stays in a hospital or other agency, and often he or she experiences increased total wake time, increased awakening, and decreased REM sleep and total sleep time. Nursing activities are a source of increased sound levels. Noise from confused and ill patients and ringing of alarm systems and telephones are new and strange noises and make the hospital environment noisy and disruptive to sleep (Vincensi et al., 2016).

Exercise and Fatigue

Exercise and fatigue affect the ability to fall asleep and stay asleep. People who have a relatively inactive lifestyle may not feel sleepy at bedtime, especially if they have spent extended periods in bed. A person who is moderately fatigued usually achieves restful sleep, especially if the fatigue results from enjoyable work or exercise. Exercising at least 2 or more hours before bedtime allows time for the body to cool and maintain a state of fatigue that promotes relaxation. However, excessive fatigue can make falling asleep difficult. This is common in adolescents who stay active with long hours involving school, extracurricular activities, and work.

Food and Caloric Intake

Following good eating habits is important for proper health including sleep. Eating a large, heavy, or spicy meal within 3–4 hours of bedtime sometimes results in indigestion. Alcohol consumed in the evening has insomnia-producing and diuretic effects. Coffee, tea, cola, and chocolate contain caffeine and xanthines that cause sleeplessness as a result of CNS stimulation.

Weight loss or weight gain influences sleep patterns. Weight gain contributes to OSA because of the increased size of the soft tissue structures in the upper airway (Kryger et al., 2017). Weight loss caused by semistarvation diets sometimes causes sleep disorders such as reduced sleep and insomnia.

SLEEP DISORDERS

Sleep disorders are conditions that, if left untreated, cause disturbed nighttime sleep as well as potentially serious physiologic alterations. Many adults in the United States have significant sleep problems from inadequacies in either the quantity or the quality of their nighttime sleep and experience hypersomnolence on a daily basis (American Sleep Association [ASA], 2016). The American Academy of Sleep Medicine developed the International Classification of Sleep Disorders version 3 (ICSD-3), which classifies sleep disorders into eight major categories (Box 10.5).

Insomnia

Insomnia is a symptom rather than the name of a disease and is experienced by patients who have chronic difficulty falling asleep, frequent awakenings from sleep, or nonrestorative sleep (Maness and Khan, 2015). It is commonly experienced by patients diagnosed with depression (Trauer et al., 2015). Insomnia leads to insufficient quantity and quality of sleep. It sometimes signals

BOX 10.5 Classification of Select Sleep Disorders

Insomnias

- Adjustment sleep disorder (acute insomnia)
- Inadequate sleep hygiene
- Behavioral insomnia of childhood
- Insomnia caused by medical condition

Sleep-Related Breathing Disorder

Central Sleep Apnea Syndromes

- Primary central sleep apnea
- Central sleep apnea caused by medical condition
- Obstructive sleep apnea syndromes

Hypersomnias Not Caused by a Sleep-Related Breathing Disorder

- Narcolepsy (four specified types)
- Menstrual-related hypersomnia
- Hypersomnia caused by a medical condition

Parasomnias

Disorders of Arousal

- Sleepwalking
- Sleep terrors

Parasomnias Usually Associated With REM Sleep

- Nightmare disorder
- REM sleep behavior disorder

Other Parasomnias

- Sleep-related hallucinations
- Sleep-related eating disorder
- Sleep-related enuresis (bed-wetting)

Circadian Rhythm Sleep Disorders

Primary Circadian Rhythm Sleep Disorders

- Delayed sleep phase type
- Advanced sleep phase type

Behaviorally Induced Circadian Rhythm Sleep Disorders

- Jet lag type
- Shift work type
- Drug or substance use

BOX 10.5 Classification of Select Sleep Disorders—cont'd

Sleep-Related Movement Disorders

- Restless legs syndrome
- Periodic limb movements
- Sleep-related bruxism (teeth grinding)

Isolated Symptoms, Apparently Normal Variants, and Unresolved Issues

- Long sleeper
- Short sleeper
- Sleep talking

Other Sleep Disorders

- Physiological (organic) sleep disorders
- Environmental sleep disorder

REM, rapid eye movement.

Data from American Academy of Sleep Medicine: International classes of diseases and international classification of sleep disorders. In Kryger HM et al: *Principles and practice of sleep medicine,* ed 5, St Louis, 2011, Saunders.

an underlying physical or psychological disorder and is more common in older adults and women.

Often people experience acute transient or temporary insomnia following situational stresses such as work or family problems, illness, or grief. Insomnia sometimes recurs, but between episodes a person is able to sleep well. However, a temporary case of insomnia caused by a stressful event can lead to chronic difficulty in getting enough sleep. Insomnia is often associated with poor sleep hygiene, which negates behaviors that promote sleep (Badin et al., 2016). If the condition continues, the fear of not being able to sleep is enough to cause wakefulness. During the day, a person with chronic insomnia feels sleepy, fatigued, depressed, and anxious.

Sleep Apnea

Sleep apnea is a disorder characterized by a lack of airflow through the nose and mouth for periods ranging from 10 seconds to 1–2 minutes during sleep. The person stops breathing during sleep. There are three types of sleep apnea: obstructive, central, and mixed, which has both an obstructive component and a central component.

The most common form of sleep apnea is OSA, which is a cessation or stopping of airflow despite the effort to breathe. It occurs when muscles or soft structures of the oral cavity or throat relax during sleep. The upper airway becomes partially or completely blocked, and nasal airflow diminishes (hypopnea) or stops (apnea). The person tries to breathe because chest and abdominal movements continue, which often results in loud snoring sounds. When breathing is partially or completely diminished, the person becomes sufficiently hypoxic and must awaken to breathe. Structural abnormalities such as a deviated septum, nasal pharyngeal alterations, a narrow lower jaw, enlarged tonsils, or obesity predispose a patient to OSA. Smoking, increasing age (older than 65 years), heart failure, alcohol use, large neck circumference, and menopause are increased risk factors (Schub, 2016; Qaseem et al., 2014). Serious OSA can lead to heart failure, hypertension, and coronary artery disease. About 10%–17% of adults in the United States are affected by OSA (Qaseem et al., 2014). However, a large majority of people are undiagnosed and untreated (Kryger et al., 2017). Research shows that the risk for OSA is similar among African Americans, Asians, and Caucasians (Kryger et al., 2017).

Central sleep apnea (CSA) involves dysfunction in the respiratory control center of the brain. Pauses in breathing happen in the respiratory and pulmonary systems at the same time. The brain stops sending signals to muscles that control breathing. Conditions that are associated with CSA include stroke, degeneration of the cervical spine, obesity, and encephalitis. People with CSA tend to awaken during sleep and therefore complain of insomnia.

EDS is a common complaint in people experiencing OSA and CSA. Other common symptoms of OSA include fatigue, morning headaches, irritability, depression, difficulty concentrating, and decreased sex drive (Kryger et al., 2017). Lifestyle changes (including a weight-reduction program in people who are obese and improved sleep hygiene), bilevel positive airway pressure (BPAP or BiPAP), continuous positive airway pressure (CPAP), surgery, and oral repositioning devices for the jaw and tongue are treatment options (Rotenberg et al., 2016; Schub, 2016).

Narcolepsy

Narcolepsy is a rare CNS dysfunction of mechanisms that regulate sleep and wake states. EDS is the most common symptom. During the day, a person suddenly feels an overwhelming wave of sleepiness and falls asleep, often at inappropriate times. This is commonly referred to as a sleep attack. Involuntary sleep episodes may be brief, lasting only a few seconds to minutes. It is possible for REM sleep to occur within 15 minutes of falling asleep. Unless recognized, others often mistake a person who suddenly and inappropriately falls asleep as being lazy, disinterested, or possibly drunk. Typically, symptoms first occur in adolescence and are sometimes confused with EDS. Narcolepsy can occur with or without cataplexy. **Cataplexy** is a sudden muscle weakness during intense emotions such as anger or laughter that can occur at any time during the day. In a severe cataplectic attack, a patient loses voluntary muscle control and falls to the floor. Narcolepsy commonly includes frightening dreamlike experiences during the transition from a wake to a sleep state.

Narcolepsy is treated with stimulants or wakefulness-promoting drugs (e.g., sodium oxybate, modafinil) that only partially increase wakefulness and reduce sleep attacks. Prescribed antidepressants suppress cataplexy and other REM-related symptoms. Short daytime naps (no longer than 20 minutes) help reduce feelings of sleepiness. Exercising regularly, maintaining a regular nighttime sleep schedule, eating light meals high in protein, deep breathing, chewing gum, and taking vitamins are other management methods (Barateau et al., 2016; Kryger et al., 2017). People with narcolepsy need to avoid situations and activities that increase drowsiness (e.g., alcohol, heavy meals, exhausting activities, long-distance driving).

Sleep Deprivation

Sleep deprivation can be acute or chronic and results from insufficient or disrupted sleep. Causes include illness (e.g., fever, difficulty breathing, pain), emotional stress, medications, environmental disturbances (e.g., frequent interruptions in sleep during nursing care, noisy neighbors or pets), and variability in the timing of sleep as a result of shift work. Sleep disorders such as sleep apnea or insomnia can cause sleep deprivation. With sleep deprivation, there is a decrease in the quantity or quality of sleep and/or an inconsistency in the timing of sleep. Interrupted or fragmented sleep changes the normal sequencing of the sleep cycle. Cumulative sleep deprivation develops over time.

Individuals respond to sleep deprivation differently. Some patients experience a variety of physiological and psychological symptoms such as blurred vision, decreased reflexes, slow response time, headaches, memory problems, confusion, and irritability. The severity of symptoms is often related to the duration of sleep deprivation. The most effective treatment for sleep deprivation is elimination or correction of environmental factors and patient care activities that disrupt the sleep pattern. Nurses play an important role in identifying treatable sleep deprivation problems. Evidence suggests that chronic sleep deprivation is associated with obesity, type 2 diabetes, poor memory, depression, digestive problems, and development of cardiovascular disease (Kohansieh and Makaryus, 2015).

Parasomnias

Parasomnias are sleep disorders that can occur during arousal from REM sleep or partial arousal from NREM sleep. These disorders include

- Sleepwalking
- Sleep eating
- Night terrors
- Nightmares
- Teeth grinding
- Bed-wetting

Most parasomnias are more common in children, possibly because of brain immaturity, but they can also occur in adults. An individual often experiences more than one parasomnia. In all cases, it is important to support patients experiencing a sleep disorder and maintain their safety.

NURSING INTERVENTIONS TO PROMOTE SLEEP AND REST

Your nursing interventions for improving the quality of a person's sleep largely focus on health promotion. In an acute care setting, your focus becomes managing the environment to support a patient's normal sleep habits and keeping the patient safe. In long-term care or nursing home environments, give special considerations for promoting adequate sleep and rest.

SLEEP ASSESSMENT

The focused nursing assessment for the sleep and rest has been illustrated in Table 10.3.

Health Promotion

Helping patients to develop good sleep hygiene practices is important. Educational interventions offer individuals in the community information for improving sleep hygiene practices. Your specific interventions promote a person's normal sleep and rest pattern.

Environmental Controls

All patients require a sleeping environment with a comfortable room temperature and proper ventilation, minimal noise, a comfortable bed, and proper lighting. Infants sleep best when the room temperature is 18–21°C (64–70°F). Place healthy infants on their backs to sleep (Hockenberry and Wilson, 2015). Children and adults vary more in regard to comfortable room temperature but usually sleep best in cooler environments. Some individuals prefer to sleep without covers. Older adults often require extra blankets, covers, or socks (Box 10.6).

Eliminate or reduce distracting noise so that the bedroom is as quiet as possible. In the home, the television or the ringing of the telephone disrupts a patient's sleep. The television is too stimulating to watch before sleep and should not be watched in bed or immediately before going to bed (Brockmann et al., 2016). The cooperation of several people living with the patient is often required to reduce noise. Wearing ear plugs may help to reduce or eliminate distracting noises. Some patients sleep better with inside noises such as the hum of a ceiling fan.

Table 10.3 Focused Patient Assessment

Factors to Assess	Questions	Physical Assessment
Bedtime routines	How do you prepare for bed? Tell me what time you typically go to bed each night.	Observe for dark circles under patient's eyes. Observe the number of times the patient yawns.
Bedtime environment	How much light is in your bedroom at night? What is the temperature of your room during the night? Do you listen to music to go to sleep?	Ask the patient or sleeping partner about multiple patient position changes during sleep or frequent reawakenings.
Current life events	Tell me what hours do you normally work. Have you experienced any recent changes in your job or home responsibilities? Which activities do you do to relax outside of work? What hobbies do you have?	Observe the patient's ability to concentrate on the conversation.

BOX 10.6 Care of the Older Adult

Sleep Disturbances

Sleep–Wake Pattern

- Maintain a regular rising time and bedtime.
- Eliminate early morning and late afternoon naps.
- If the patient takes naps, limit to 20–30 min or less twice a day.
- Go to bed when sleepy.
- Use relaxation techniques and a regular bedtime routine to promote sleep.
- If unable to sleep in 15–30 min, get out of bed and do routine quiet activities.

Environment

- Expose to natural light or bright interior lights for 30 min to 2 h daily, preferably soon after waking.
- Sleep where you sleep best.
- Keep noise to a minimum; use soft music to mask noise if necessary.
- Use night-light and keep path to bathroom free of obstacles.
- Set room temperature to preference.

Medications

- Use sedatives and hypnotics as last resort; then, use only for a short time if needed.
- Adjust medications being taken for other conditions and look for drug interactions that cause insomnia or EDS.

Diet

- Limit alcohol, caffeine, and nicotine in late afternoon and evening.
- Eat a light snack such as cereal and milk or cheese and crackers before bedtime.
- Decrease fluids 2–4 h before sleep.

Physiological/Illness Factors

- Elevate head of bed, and provide extra pillows as preferred.
- Use analgesics 30 min before bed to ease aches and pains.
- Use prescribed medications to control symptoms of chronic conditions.

EDS, excessive daytime sleepiness.

Make sure that the bed and mattress provide support and comfortable firmness. Place a bed board under the mattress to add support. Sometimes, extra pillows help a person position more comfortably in bed. The position of the bed in the room also makes a difference for some patients.

For a patient prone to confusion or falls, safety is critical. In the home, a small night-light helps the patient become oriented to the room environment before arising to go to the bathroom. Beds set lower to the floor reduce the risk for falls when a patient stands. Remove clutter from the path a patient uses to walk from the bed to the bathroom. If a patient needs help in ambulating from the bed to the bathroom, have a small bell at the bedside to call family members or obtain a bedside commode.

Patients vary in regard to the amount of light that they prefer at night. Infants and older adults sleep best in softly lit rooms. Do not have light shining directly on their eyes. Small table lamps or night-lights prevent total darkness. For older adults, this reduces the chance of confusion when arising from bed. If streetlights shine through windows or when patients nap during the day, a sleep mask or heavy shades, drapes, or slatted blinds are helpful.

Promoting Bedtime Routines

Bedtime routines and sleep hygiene measures relax patients in preparation for sleep. A person should go to sleep when he or she feels tired or sleepy. Patients and their bed partners need to learn techniques that promote sleep and conditions that interfere with it. Encourage patients in the hospital to follow their at-home bedtime routine as much as possible.

Adults need to avoid excessive mental stimulation just before bedtime. Reading a light novel, watching a relaxing television program, or listening to music helps a person relax. Progressive muscle relaxation exercises and praying induce calm in patients.

Promoting Comfort

People fall asleep only after feeling comfortable and relaxed. You offer strategies that can reduce the minor irritants that keep people awake. Have family members change diapers before placing infants in bed. An extra blanket prevents chilling when trying to fall asleep. Encourage a patient to wear loose-fitting nightwear and to void before bedtime. Have family members give a relaxing back rub.

Patients with painful illnesses may benefit from the application of dry or moist heat, use of supportive dressings or splints, and proper positioning with the use of extra pillows for support. Patients with temporary acute pain (e.g., following surgery) may sleep better if the bed partner lets the patient sleep alone until the pain subsides. Also, encourage the patient to take pain medications 30–60 minutes before going to bed.

Promoting Activity

Increasing daytime activity lessens problems with falling asleep. Always plan rigorous exercise at least 2–3 hours before bedtime. Research indicates that exercise is beneficial, particularly for older adults, to improve nighttime sleep. However, older adults with chronic diseases that influence their functional abilities are likely to have limited activity (Touhy and Jett, 2018). Recommend activities that are safe for older patients to perform, such as walking, swimming, wheelchair propulsion, and cycling on a stationary bike. Weight lifting using light weights (e.g., ≈0.90–2.3 Kg) builds upper body strength and endurance. Activity and exercise often prove to be beneficial by improving activity endurance, mobility, and sense of well-being.

Stress Reduction

When patients feel emotionally upset, urge them to try not to force sleep. Otherwise insomnia often develops, and soon they will associate bedtime with the inability to relax. Encourage a patient who has difficulty falling asleep to get up and pursue a relaxing activity rather than staying in bed and thinking about sleep. When the emotional problem is ongoing and the patient finds little relief, encourage referral to an appropriate counselor.

Children often have problems going to bed and falling asleep. Have parents enter their children's rooms immediately after nightmares and talk to them briefly about their fears to provide a cooling-down period. Comforting children while they lie in their own bed is reassuring. Keeping a light on in the room also helps. Usually experts do not recommend that a child be allowed to sleep with parents; however, families approach sleep practices differently based on cultural traditions.

Bedtime Snacks

Some people enjoy bedtime snacks, whereas others cannot sleep after eating. A bedtime snack containing protein and carbohydrates such as cereal and milk or cheese and crackers, which contain l-tryptophan, may help to promote sleep. A full meal before bedtime often causes gastrointestinal upset and interferes with the ability to fall asleep.

Make sure that patients avoid drinking excess fluids or ingesting caffeine before bedtime. Coffee, tea, cola, and chocolate cause a person to stay awake or wake up throughout the night. Alcohol interrupts sleep cycles and reduces the amount of deep sleep. Caffeinated drinks and alcohol act as diuretics, which cause nocturia.

Pharmacological Approaches to Promoting Sleep

Melatonin is a neurohormone produced in the brain that helps control circadian rhythms. It is a popular nutritional supplement in the United States used to aid sleep. The recommended dose is 0.3 – 3 mg taken 2 hours before bedtime to improve sleep onset. Older adults with decreased levels of melatonin find it aids sleep (Emet et al., 2016). The short-term use of melatonin is considered safe with infrequent mild side effects of nausea, headache, and dizziness. Melatonin is a dietary supplement, not a drug, and is not regulated by the US Food and Drug Administration (FDA).

Sedatives and **hypnotics** are groups of drugs that induce and/or maintain sleep. However, long-term use of these drugs disrupts sleep and leads to more serious problems. Benzodiazepines are a common classification of drug used to treat sleep problems when a change in sleep hygiene is not effective. Examples of benzodiazepines include temazepam, flurazepam, and triazolam. Benzodiazepines may cause psychological and physical dependence, and physical withdrawal symptoms may occur if the drug is not carefully tapered following long-term use (Burchum and Rosenthal, 2016). The use of benzodiazepines in older adults is potentially dangerous. Long-term use and high doses in older adults are associated with sedation and cognitive impairment leading to falls (Burchum and Rosenthal, 2016).

Trazodone is a serotonin antagonist and reuptake inhibitor (SARI) antidepressant often used in patients with depression or anxiety and insomnia. The most common side effects are daytime grogginess and orthostatic hypotension. Low-dose trazodone is often used as an alternative to benzodiazepines, especially in older patients.

Nonbenzodiazepine receptor agonists appear to have better safety profiles and fewer adverse effects than benzodiazepines. They are also associated with a lower risk of abuse and dependence than benzodiazepines, although abuse and dependence do occur. Examples of medications in this class include zolpidem, zaleplon, and eszopiclone (Burchum and Rosenthal, 2016). A low dose of a short-acting medication such as zolpidem can be effective for short-term use (no longer than 2 – 3 weeks). Patients should avoid drinking alcohol while taking these drugs.

The use of nonprescription over-the-counter sleeping medications is not advisable. Over the long-term, these drugs lead to further sleep disruption even when they initially seem effective. Help patients with optional sleep interventions that do not require the use of drugs.

Regular use of any sleep medication leads to tolerance, and withdrawal causes rebound insomnia. Make sure that all patients understand the possible side effects of sleep medications. In 2007, the FDA released a warning related to complex sleep-related behaviors such as sleep driving or sleep eating that have occurred with prescription sleep medications (FDA, 2016). Routine monitoring of patient response to sleeping medications is important.

NURSING INTERVENTIONS TO PROMOTE SLEEP AND REST IN ACUTE CARE

The nursing interventions described for health promotion are applicable to a patient requiring acute care. The nature of the acute care setting requires you to be creative in finding ways to maintain the patient's normal sleep pattern.

Managing Environmental Stimuli

A challenge in the hospital is controlling noise. Implement ways to reduce noise such as conducting conversations and reports in a private area away from patient rooms and keeping necessary conversations to a minimum, especially at night (Flynn Makic et al., 2014). Provide patients with ear plugs or eye masks to decrease noise and light stimulation (Caple and March, 2016; Litton et al., 2016). Because many patients spend only a short time in hospitals, it is easy to forget the importance of establishing good sleep conditions. In a hospital setting, plan nursing care activities to avoid waking patients. Try to schedule assessments, treatments, procedures, and routines for times when patients are awake. Perform nursing activities before the patient receives sleeping medication or begins to fall asleep. For example, you have a patient who had surgery. Before the patient gets ready for bed, change the surgical dressing, reposition the patient, administer pain medication, and check vital signs. Give medications and draw blood during waking hours when possible (Caple and March, 2016). Plan with other departments and services to schedule therapies at intervals that give patients time to rest. Whenever it becomes necessary to wake a patient, perform the activity as quickly as possible so the patient can fall back to sleep as soon as possible.

Safety

Safety precautions are important for patients who wake up during the night to use the bathroom and for patients with EDS. Set beds lower to the floor to lessen the chance of the patient falling when first standing. Remove clutter and move equipment from the path that a patient uses to walk from the bed to the bathroom. If a patient needs assistance in ambulating from the bed to the bathroom, make sure that the nurse call system is accessible within the patient's reach. Be sure that the patient knows how to turn the light on correctly.

If patients normally use a CPAP machine at home because of sleep apnea, it is important that they bring their home equipment with them to the hospital and use it every night. Check to make sure the mask is snug fitting and put on correctly so that the positive pressure is maintained (Schub, 2016) (see Chapter 24). In patients with sleep apnea who have surgery and receive general anesthesia, the anesthesia in combination with opioid medications used after surgery reduces the patient's defenses against airway obstruction. After surgery, the patient achieves very deep levels of REM sleep that lead to muscle relaxation and airway obstruction. Use pain medication carefully in these patients. These patients need ventilator support in the postoperative period because OSA is linked to increased postoperative respiratory complications. Monitor the patient's breathing and oxygen saturation levels regularly (see Chapter 6). Notify the health care provider right away if the patient is difficult to arouse or is having trouble breathing.

Patients who experience EDS can fall asleep while sitting up in a chair or wheelchair. Position patients so that they do not fall out of the chair when sleeping. Elevating their feet on an ottoman or small bench may help to position them safely. A pillow placed in the patient's lap provides some support. If a patient enjoys leaning over an overbed table while sitting in a chair, be sure that the table is locked and secure. Avoid using safety belts because they are considered restraints (see Chapter 12).

Comfort Measures

You make the patient more comfortable in an acute care setting by providing personal hygiene before bedtime. A warm bath or shower is very relaxing. Offer patients restricted to bed the opportunity to wash their face and hands. Toothbrushing and care of dentures also help to prepare the patient for sleep. Have patients void before going to bed so they are not kept awake by a full bladder. While a patient prepares for bed, help to position him or her off any potential pressure sites.

Removal of irritating stimuli also improves a patient's comfort for a restful sleep. Changing or removing moist dressings, repositioning drainage tubing, reapplying wrinkled compression hose, and changing tape on nasogastric tubes eliminate constant irritants to the patient's skin. When an i.v. site becomes irritated and painful, reinsertion of the i.v. line is usually recommended. Cleanse the perineal or anal area thoroughly for patients who are incontinent. Diaphoretic patients benefit from a cool bath and dry clothes or linens.

KEY POINTS

- The 24-hour sleep–wake cycle is a circadian rhythm that affects physiological function and behavior.
- During a typical night's sleep, a person fluctuates between NREM stages 2, 3, and 4 before entering REM sleep. The amount of time in each stage varies.
- The number of hours of sleep needed by each person to feel rested varies.
- Long-term use of sleeping medications leads to difficulty in initiating and maintaining sleep.
- The hectic pace of a person's lifestyle, emotional and psychological stress, and drug and alcohol ingestion disrupt the sleep pattern.
- An environment with a darkened room, reduced noise, comfortable bed, appropriate temperature, and good ventilation promotes sleep.
- The most common type of sleep disorder is insomnia. Characteristics of insomnia include the inability to fall asleep, to remain asleep during the night, or to go back to sleep after waking up earlier than desired.
- Use your patient's self-report to determine whether the sleep is restful.
- When using environmental controls to promote sleep, consider the usual characteristics of the patient's home environment and normal lifestyle.
- Noise can disrupt sleep and enhance pain perception.
- The HCAHPS survey measures patients' perspectives on hospital care after discharge including quietness of the hospital environment.
- A bedtime routine of relaxing activities prepares a person physically and mentally for sleep.
- Important nursing interventions for promoting sleep in a hospital are establishing periods for uninterrupted sleep and decreasing noise.

REFERENCES

American Sleep Association (ASA). What is insomnia? 2016. Available from: https://www.sleepassociation.org/patients-general-public/insomnia/insomnia.

Badin E, Haddad C, Shatkin JP. Insomnia: the sleeping giant of pediatric public health. Curr Psychiatry Rep 2016;18:47.

Barateau L, Lopez R, Dauvilliers Y. Treatment options for narcolepsy. CNS Drugs 2016;30:369.

Bartel KA, Gradisar M, Williamson P. Protective and risk factors for adolescent sleep: a meta-analytic review. Sleep Med Rev 2015;21:72.

Brockmann PE, Diaz B, Damiani F, Villarroel L, Núñez F, Bruni O. Impact of television on the quality of sleep in preschool children. Sleep Med 2016;20:140.

Burchum JR, Rosenthal LD. Lehne's pharmacology for nursing care. 9th ed. St. Louis: Elsevier; 2016.

Caple C, March P. Evidence-based care sheet: sleep and hospitalization. Glendale: Cinahl Information Systems; 2016.

Centers for Disease Control and Prevention (CDC). Insufficient sleep is a public health problem. 2015. Available from: https://www.cdc.gov/sleep/index.html.

Emet M, Ozcan H, Ozel L, Yayla M, Halici Z, Hacimuftuoglu A. A review of melatonin, its receptors and drugs. Eurasian J Med 2016;48(2):135.

Flynn Makic MB, Rauen C, Watson R, Poteet AW. Examining the evidence to guide practice: challenging practice habits. Crit Care Nurse 2014;34(2):28.

Hirshkowitz M, Whiton K, Albert SM, Alessi C, Bruni O, DonCarlos L, et al. National Sleep Foundation's sleep time duration recommendations: methodology and results summary. Sleep Health 2015;1:40.

Hockenberry MJ, Wilson D. Wong's nursing care of infants and children. 10th ed. St. Louis: Mosby; 2015.

Huether SE, McCance K, editors. Understanding pathophysiology. 6th ed. St. Louis: Elsevier; 2017.

Kohansieh M, Makaryus AN. Sleep deficiency and deprivation leading to cardiovascular disease. Int J Hypertens 2015;2015:615681.

Kryger MH, Roth T, Dement W. Principles and practice of sleep medicine. 6th ed. St. Louis: Elsevier; 2017.

Litton E, Carnegie V, Elliott R, Webb SA. The efficacy of earplugs as a sleep hygiene strategy for reducing delirium in the ICU: a systematic review and meta-analysis. Crit Care Med 2016;44(5):992.

Liu Y, Wheaton AG, Chapman DP, Cunningham TJ, Lu H, Croft JB. Prevalence of healthy sleep duration among adults: United States, 2014. MMWR Morb Mortal Wkly Rep 2016;65(6):1.

Madhu C, Coyne K, Hashim H, Chapple C, Milsom I, Kopp Z. Nocturia: risk factors and associated comorbidities findings from the EpiLUTS study. Int J Clin Pract 2015;69(12):1508.

Maness DL, Khan M. Nonpharmacologic management of chronic insomnia. Am Fam Physician 2015;92(12):1058.

National Sleep Foundation. Lack of sleep is affecting Americans, finds the National Sleep Foundation. 2014. Available from: https://sleepfoundation.org/media-center/press-release/lack-sleep-affecting-americans-finds-the-national-sleep-foundation.

National Sleep Foundation. Aging and sleep. 2016a. Available from: https://sleepfoundation.org/sleep-topics/aging-and-sleep.

National Sleep Foundation. Depression and sleep. 2016b, http://sleepfoundation.org/article/sleep-topics/depression-and-sleep.

National Sleep Foundation. Restless legs syndrome (RLS) and sleep. 2016c. Available from: https://www.sleepfoundation.org/restless-legs-syndrome. Accessed October 4, 2017.

National Sleep Foundation. Teens and sleep. 2016d. Available from: https://sleepfoundation.org/sleep-topics/teens-and-sleep.

Qaseem A, Dallas P, Owens DK, Starkey M, Holty JE, Shekelle P, et al. Diagnosis of obstructive sleep apnea in adults: a clinical practice guideline from the American College of Physicians. Ann Intern Med 2014;161(3):210.

Rotenberg BW, Vicini C, Pang EB, Pang KP. Reconsidering first-line treatment for obstructive sleep apnea: a systematic review of the literature. J Otolaryngol Head Neck Surg 2016;45:23.

Schub T, Buckley L. Obstructive sleep apnea in adults. Available at: http://dx.doi.org/. Accessed Jan 12, 2021.

Touhy T, Jett K. Ebersole & Hess'gerontological nursing and healthy aging. 5th ed. St. Louis: Elsevier; 2018.

Trauer JM, Qian MY, Doyle JS, Rajaratnam SM, Cunnington D. Cognitive behavioral therapy for chronic insomnia. Ann Intern Med 2015; 163(3):191.

University of Maryland Medical Center. Insomnia. 2016. Available from: https://www.medschool.umaryland.edu/news/2016/UM-SOM-Sleep-Experts-Explore-the-Massive-Financial-Toll-of-Insomnia.html.

U.S. Food and Drug Administration (FDA). Sleep problems. 2016. Available from: https://www.fda.gov/forconsumers/byaudience/forwomen/ucm118563.htm.

Vincensi B, Pearce K, Redding J, Brandonisio S, Tzou S, Meiusi E. Sleep in the hospitalized patient: nurse and patient perceptions. Medsurg Nurs 2016;25(5):351.

Wheaton AG, Olsen OE, Miller G, Crofft JB. Sleep duration and injury-related risk behaviors among high school students—United States, 2007-2013. MMWR Morb Mortal Wkly Rep 2016;65(13):1.

11 Pain Management

OBJECTIVES

After reading this chapter, the student should be able to:

- Define pain and describe the nature and physiology of pain including transduction, transmission, perception, modulation, and neurotransmitters.
- Identify components of the pain experience and understand gate control theory of pain.
- Describe different types of pain such as acute pain, chronic pain, chronic and persistent noncancer pain, cancer pain, and idiopathic pain.
- Identify physiological, social, psychological, spiritual, and cultural factors influencing pain.
- Explore meaning of pain, anxiety, depression, and coping styles.
- Perform assessment of pain and develop appropriate nursing diagnoses for a patient experiencing pain.
- Discuss older adult consideration for pain and its management.
- Describe guidelines for selecting and individualizing pain therapies.
- Enumerate nonpharmacological nursing interventions to manage pain.
- Discuss nursing implications for administering analgesics.
- Describe the sequence of interventions recommended in pain management.

KEY TERMS

acupuncture, p. 238
analgesics, p. 232
biofeedback, p. 238
cutaneous stimulation, p. 237
endorphins, p. 227
epidural infusion, p. 236
guided imagery, p. 238
local anesthesia, p. 235
opioid, p. 233
pain management, p. 232
pain, p. 225
patient-controlled analgesia (PCA), p. 233
prostaglandins, p. 226
palliative care, p. 239
relaxation, p. 237
transcutaneous electrical nerve stimulation (TENS), p. 237

INTRODUCTION

You will encounter patients experiencing pain in all health care settings. Physiological, sociocultural, spiritual, psychological, and environmental factors influence the way patients interpret and experience pain. According to McCaffery's classic definition, "Pain is whatever the experiencing person says it is, existing whenever he says it does" (Pasero and McCaffery, 2011). Pain relief is not always achievable; however, nurses implement interventions to decrease pain, which can increase quality of life. Pain management involves more than administering analgesics. You need to understand how the pain experience affects a patient's ability to function and then use interventions that meet the unique needs of the patient (Pasero and McCaffery, 2011).

Pain is a leading public health problem in the United States. Many organizations have declared that pain management is a basic right of patients who are seriously ill. As a nurse, you are legally and ethically responsible for managing patients' pain. Effective pain management improves quality of life, promotes return to the previous level of activity, and decreases health care costs.

DEFINITION

The International Association for the Study of Pain (IASP) defines **pain** as "an unpleasant, subjective sensory *and* emotional experience associated with actual or potential tissue damage, or described in terms of such damage" (IASP, 2014b).

NATURE OF PAIN

Pain is more than a single physiological sensation caused by a specific stimulus. It is subjective and highly individualized. The person experiencing pain is the only person who can confirm the existence of the pain and describe it. Pain is a physiological mechanism that protects an individual from a harmful stimulus. Pain warns of tissue damage and alerts the body to protect itself. Inability to express pain because of aphasia, airway intubation, or mental status changes does not mean that a patient is not experiencing pain. Carefully assess a patient's pain to identify the severity and effects of pain. Some patients such as patients with spinal cord injuries are unable to sense painful stimuli. You must take special precautions to protect these patients from additional injury (Pasero and McCaffery, 2011).

PHYSIOLOGY OF PAIN

There are four physiological processes of normal pain: transduction, transmission, perception, and modulation (Huether and McCance, 2017). Understanding each process helps you recognize factors that cause pain, symptoms that result, and the rationale for interventions for pain management.

Transduction

A thermal, mechanical, or chemical stimulus usually activates a pain event. Transduction converts energy produced by these noxious stimuli into electrical impulses. The process begins in the periphery when the pain-producing stimulus sends an impulse across a sensory peripheral pain nerve fiber, known as a nociceptor. Once transduction is complete, transmission of a pain impulse begins (Huether and McCance, 2017).

Transmission

Cellular damage from thermal, mechanical, or chemical injuries results in the release of excitatory neurotransmitters such as **prostaglandins,** histamine, bradykinin, and substance P (Fig. 11.1). These pain-sensitizing substances surround the pain fibers in the extracellular fluid, spreading the pain message and causing an inflammatory response. The pain stimulus enters the spinal cord via the dorsal horn and travels one of several routes until ending within the gray matter of the spinal cord. At the dorsal horn, substance P is released, causing a synaptic transmission from the afferent (sensory) nerve to spinothalamic tract nerves, which cross to the opposite side (Fig. 11.2) (Pasero and McCaffery, 2011).

Nerve impulses travel along afferent peripheral nerve fibers. Two types of peripheral nerve fibers conduct painful stimuli: the large, fast, myelinated A-delta fibers and the small, slow unmyelinated C fibers. The A fibers send sharp, localized, and distinct sensations that specify the source of the pain and detect its intensity. The C fibers relay slower impulses that are poorly localized, visceral, and persistent. For example, after stepping on a sharp object without shoes, a person initially feels a sharp localized pain, which is the result of A-fiber transmission, or first pain. Within a few minutes, the entire foot aches from C-fiber stimulation, or second pain.

Pain impulses travel up the spinal cord (see Fig. 11.2). When the impulse reaches the thalamus, the primary relay station of sensory impulses, it transmits information to higher centers in the brain where pain perception occurs.

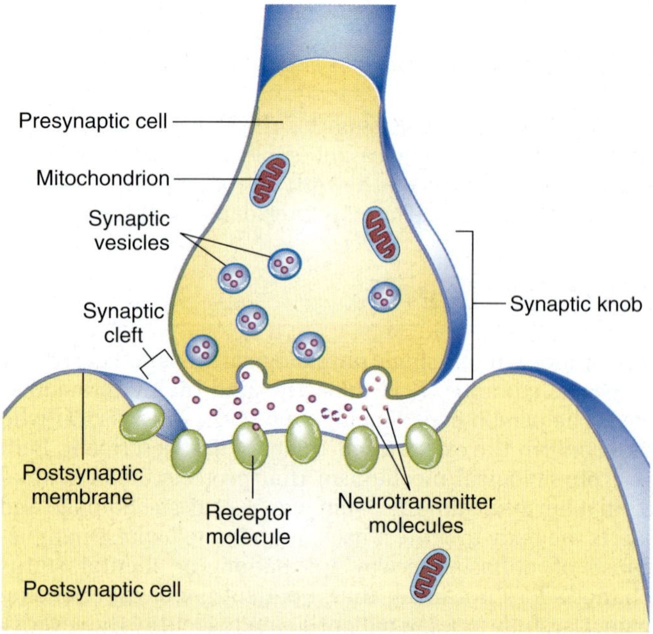

Presynaptic cell
Mitochondrion
Synaptic vesicles
Synaptic cleft
Synaptic knob
Postsynaptic membrane
Receptor molecule
Neurotransmitter molecules
Postsynaptic cell

Fig. 11.1 Chemical synapses involve transmitter chemicals (neurotransmitters) that signal postsynaptic cells. (From Patton KT, Thibodeau GA: *Anatomy & Physiology,* ed 7, St Louis, 2010, Mosby.)

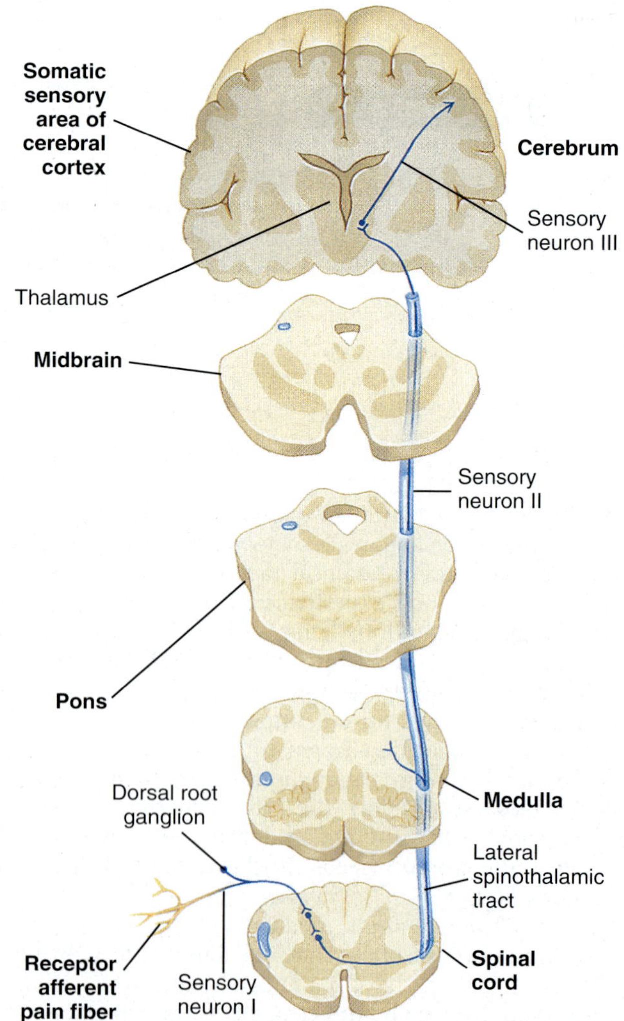

Fig. 11.2 Spinothalamic pathway that conducts pain stimuli to the brain.

Perception

As a pain impulse moves up the spinal cord toward the brain, the central nervous system extracts information such as location, duration, and quality of the pain impulse. Psychological and cognitive factors interact with neurophysiological factors. The thalamus is the first structure in the brain to process the impulse. It sends the impulse to many areas in the brain including the cerebral cortex, hypothalamus, and limbic system. Perception is that point in time when a patient becomes aware of the pain and attaches meaning to it. There is no one pain center in the brain that supports the complex nature of pain. Any factor that interrupts or influences normal pain perception, such as fatigue, depression, or an analgesic, affects a person's awareness and response to pain.

Modulation

The fourth and final phase of the pain process is modulation. When a person perceives a harmful impulse, the brain releases inhibitory neurotransmitters such as endogenous opioids, serotonin, norepinephrine, and gamma-aminobutyric acid (GABA). The neurotransmitters hinder the transmission of pain to help produce an analgesic effect (Huether and McCance, 2017).

A protective reflex response also occurs with pain (Fig. 11.3). When a person is injured, a noxious stimulus from the skin travels along sensory neurons to the dorsal horn of the spinal cord where it synapses with spinal motor neurons. The impulse continues to travel along the spinal nerve to the skeletal muscle, creating a reflex arc and causing the person to withdraw from the source of the pain. For example, when you accidentally touch a hot iron, your hand reflexively withdraws from the hot surface. Pain processes require an intact peripheral nervous system and spinal cord.

Neurotransmitters

Neurotransmitters are substances that affect the sending of nerve stimuli (Box 11.1). They either excite or inhibit nerve transmission. Excitatory neurotransmitters such as substance P enhance transmission of the painful impulse. Inhibitory neurotransmitters such as **endorphins** decrease neuron activity through a synapse. Pain perception is influenced by balancing neurotransmitters and by the descending pain-control fibers originating from the cerebral cortex (Huether and McCance, 2017).

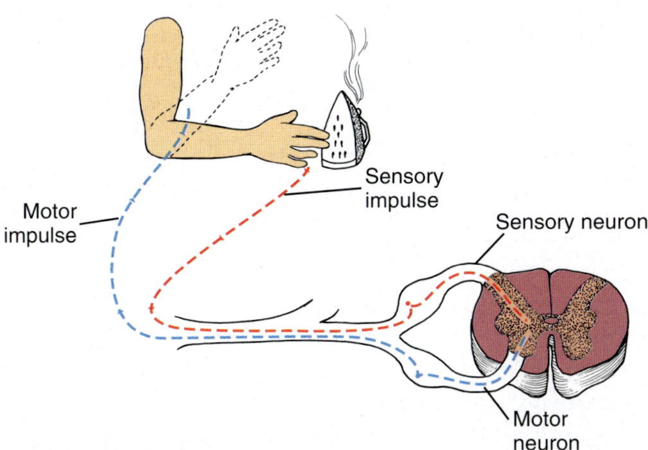

Fig. 11.3 Protective pain reflex. Sensory impulse directly stimulates motor nerves, bypassing brain and causing withdrawal from pain stimulus.

BOX 11.1 Neurophysiology of Pain: Neurotransmitters

Neurotransmitters (Excitatory)

Bradykinin

- Released from plasma that leaks from surrounding blood vessels at site of tissue injury
- Binds to receptors on peripheral nerves, increasing pain stimuli
- Binds to cells that cause chain reaction producing prostaglandins

Substance P

- Found in pain neurons of the dorsal horn (excitatory peptide)
- Needed to transmit pain impulses from periphery to higher brain centers
- Causes vasodilation and edema

Serotonin

- Released from brain stem and dorsal horn to inhibit pain transmission

Prostaglandins

- Generated through breakdown of phospholipids in cell membranes
- Increase sensitivity to pain

Neurotransmitters (Inhibitory)

Endorphins, Enkephalins, and Dynorphins

- Natural supply of morphine-like substances in the body
- Activated by stress and pain
- Located within brain, spinal cord, and gastrointestinal tract
- Cause analgesia when they attach to opiate receptors in the brain
- Present in high levels in people who have less pain than others with a similar injury

Gate Control Theory of Pain

The gate control theory suggests that gating mechanisms along the central nervous system can regulate and possibly block pain impulses (Mendell, 2014). The gating mechanism occurs within the spinal cord, thalamus, reticular formation, and limbic system. The brain determines whether the gate will be open or closed, either increasing or decreasing the intensity of the ascending pain impulse. The theory suggests that pain impulses pass through when the gate is open and not while it is closed. Closing the gate is the basis for nonpharmacological pain-relief interventions. The gate control theory suggests the importance of psychological variables (thoughts and feelings) and physiological sensations in the perception of pain. Using psychological, physiological, and pharmacological interventions to close the gate lowers pain intensity. For example, therapies such as exercise, heat, cold, massage, and transcutaneous electrical nerve stimulation (TENS) are thought to release endorphins, which close the gate and reduce perception of pain (Mendell, 2014).

Physiological Responses

When acute pain impulses travel up the spinal cord toward the brain stem and thalamus, the autonomic nervous system is stimulated as part of the stress response. Acute pain of low-to-moderate intensity and superficial pain cause the fight-or-flight response from the sympathetic branch of the autonomic nervous system and results in transient physiological responses (Table 11.1). If pain is unrelenting, severe, or deep, typically involving visceral organs, the parasympathetic nervous system is activated. Most patients adapt quickly, with physical signs such as vital signs returning to normal. As a result, your patient in pain does not always present with physical signs (Huether and McCance, 2017).

It is important to understand that patients with chronic pain do not have the same physiological responses as patients with acute pain. They may not demonstrate autonomic or sympathetic nervous system reactions. In addition, if you do not treat acute pain adequately, it can progress to chronic pain. It appears that unrelieved pain sensitizes and changes nerves (neuroplasticity), resulting in enhanced intensity, duration, and distribution of pain. These permanent neuroplastic changes contribute to the development of chronic pain syndromes. Chronic pain is not simply acute pain that lasts a long time (Huether and McCance, 2017).

Behavioral Responses

The response to pain is complex and variable, influenced by such factors as a person's culture, experiences with pain, meaning of pain, and ability to cope with stress. Be familiar with behavioral responses to pain. Clenching the teeth, facial grimacing, holding or guarding the painful part, and bent posture are common indications of acute pain. Chronic pain affects a patient's activity (eating, sleeping, hygiene, social interactions), thinking (confusion, forgetfulness, helplessness), or emotions (anger, depression, irritability, frustration) and quality of life (Huether and McCance, 2017). Recognizing a patient's unique response to pain is important in assessing the success of the pain management plan. Some patients choose not to report pain if they believe that it inconveniences others or if it signals loss of self-control. Encourage your patients to accept pain-relieving measures so that they remain active and involved in daily activities. In contrast, other patients seek relief before pain occurs, having learned that prevention is easier than treatment. Help patients communicate their pain response effectively and do not question their report of pain (Pasero and McCaffery, 2011).

TYPES OF PAIN

The two types of pain that you most frequently observe in patients are acute (transient) and chronic (persistent). Millions of people experience pain every year. Pain results in increased health care costs and loss of income from being unable to work.

Acute/Transient Pain

Acute pain is protective, usually has an identifiable cause, is of short duration, and has limited tissue damage and emotional response. It is common after acute injury, disease, or surgery. Acute pain warns people of injury or disease; thus, it is protective. It eventually resolves after the damaged tissue heals. Patients in acute pain are frightened, are anxious, and expect relief quickly. Acute pain is self-limiting; therefore, the patient knows that an end is in sight. Because it usually has an identifiable cause and is usually of short duration, health care providers are willing to treat acute pain aggressively.

Acute pain often slows recovery because it interferes with a patient's ability to become active and involved in self-care.

Table 11.1 Physiological Reactions to Acute Pain

Response	Cause or Effect
SYMPATHETIC STIMULATION[a]	
Dilation of bronchial tubes and increased respiratory rate	Provides increased oxygen intake
Increased heart rate	Provides increased oxygen transport
Peripheral vasoconstriction (pallor, elevation in blood pressure)	Elevates blood pressure with shift of blood supply from periphery and viscera to skeletal muscles and brain
Increased blood glucose level	Provides additional energy
Diaphoresis	Controls body temperature during stress
Increased muscle tension	Prepares muscles for action
Dilation of pupils	Affords better vision
Decreased gastrointestinal motility	Frees energy for more immediate activity
PARASYMPATHETIC STIMULATION[B]	
Pallor	Causes blood supply to shift away from periphery
Muscle tension	Results from fatigue
Decreased heart rate and blood pressure	Results from vagal stimulation
Rapid, irregular breathing	Causes body defenses to fail under prolonged stress of pain
Nausea and vomiting	Causes return of gastrointestinal function
Weakness or exhaustion	Results from expenditure of physical energy

[a]Pain of low-to-moderate intensity and superficial pain.
[b]Severe or deep pain.

This decrease in self-care ability results in prolonged hospitalization and recovery from complications such as immobility, sleep deprivation, delayed wound healing, and pulmonary issues. Patients often focus all their energy on pain relief when acute pain persists. Efforts aimed at teaching and motivating a patient toward self-care are often hampered until pain is managed successfully. If not adequately controlled, acute pain can progress to chronic pain. When you relieve acute pain, a patient can direct full attention toward recovery.

Chronic/Persistent Pain

In contrast to acute pain, chronic pain is not protective. Chronic pain is prolonged, varies in intensity, and usually lasts longer than 3–6 months and beyond the expected or predicted healing time (Huether and McCance, 2017). It does not always have an identifiable cause and can greatly affect a person. Examples of chronic pain include arthritis, low back pain, myofascial pain, headache, and peripheral neuropathy. Chronic pain such as low back pain often results from nonprogressive or healed tissue injury. The pain is ongoing and often does not respond to treatment. Chronic pain is a major cause of psychological and physical disability, leading to problems such as job loss, sexual dysfunction, and social isolation. A person with chronic pain often does not show obvious symptoms and does not adapt to the pain. Associated symptoms include fatigue, insomnia, anorexia, weight loss, apathy, hopelessness, and anger. Sometimes, patients with chronic pain consult with many health care providers to seek adequate pain relief. When this occurs, patients may inaccurately be judged as drug seekers. Nurses need to discourage patients from having multiple health care providers for treating pain and refer them to specialists. Pain centers use nonpharmacological and pharmacological strategies for a holistic approach to pain management (Pasero and McCaffery, 2011).

Chronic Episodic Pain

Pain that occurs sporadically over an extended period of time is episodic pain. Pain episodes last for hours, days, or weeks. Examples are migraine headaches and pain related to sickle cell crisis.

Cancer Pain

Not all patients with cancer have pain. For patients who do experience pain, 90% are able to have their pain managed with simple interventions (Burchum and Rosenthal, 2016). Some patients with cancer have acute and chronic pain. The pain is nociceptive or neuropathic. Nociceptive pain is more common and is the result of tissue injury. Neuropathic pain is related to peripheral nerve injury. Cancer pain is usually caused by tumor progression and related pathological processes, invasive procedures, treatment toxicities, infection, and physical limitations. A patient senses pain at the actual tumor site or distant to the site (called referred pain). Always assess reports of new pain by a patient with existing pain. Although the treatment of cancer pain has improved, undertreatment continues. Inadequate education of health care providers and fear of addiction lead to undertreatment of cancer pain (Burchum and Rosenthal, 2016).

Idiopathic Pain

Idiopathic pain is chronic pain in the absence of an identifiable physical or psychological cause or pain perceived as excessive for the extent of an organic pathological condition. An example of idiopathic pain is complex regional pain syndrome (CRPS). Research is needed to better identify the cause of idiopathic pain, thus leading to more effective treatment (Pasero and McCaffery, 2011).

FACTORS INFLUENCING PAIN

To accurately assess and then treat a patient's pain, be aware of the various factors that influence the pain experience.

Physiological Factors

Age

Developmental differences influence how patients of all ages react to pain. Infants demonstrate pain through crying, changes in vital signs, facial expression, and movement of extremities. Children have trouble understanding pain and any treatments or procedures that cause pain. Children without full vocabularies have difficulty verbally describing and expressing pain to parents or caregivers. Toddlers and preschoolers are unable to recall explanations about pain, or they associate it with experiences that occur in various situations. A child's personality affects coping with pain.

Pain management for children is challenging and frequently results in undertreatment (Krauss et al., 2016). Children often describe treatments and procedures as the most difficult part of being sick or in a hospital. Analgesic doses are often ineffective because they are too small or given too infrequently. It is necessary for you to understand a child's response to pain. Self-reporting pain is the most accurate assessment, but if a child is too young or unable to speak, observe behavioral changes such as crying, whining, grimacing, muscle tension, unusual inactivity, and inconsolability as signs of pain (Burchum and Rosenthal, 2016). If a behavior such as crying changes after a child receives an analgesic, pain probably caused the behavior.

Pain in adolescents is usually related to an acute condition. Consider an adolescent's cognitive development, language skills, and growth and development needs when assessing pain and providing patient education.

Adults experience pain from acute and chronic conditions. Some health care providers are less accepting of reports of severe pain from younger adults than older adults. There may be an expectation of higher tolerance of pain in adults. Concern about drug-seeking behaviors and prescription drug abuse is also common among health care providers (Pasero and McCaffery, 2011).

Pain is not a natural part of aging. Likewise, pain perception does not decrease with age. However, older adults have a greater likelihood of developing pathological conditions, which are accompanied by pain. The older adult in pain, his or her family, and health care providers frequently take these conditions for granted or underestimate the pain. Serious impairment in functional status often accompanies pain in older adults. It reduces mobility, activities of daily living (ADLs), social activities, and activity tolerance in some older adults (Pasero and McCaffery, 2011).

Fatigue

Fatigue heightens pain perception. If it occurs along with sleeplessness, the perception of pain is even greater. Restful sleep often reduces pain perception.

Neurological Function

A patient's neurological function influences his or her pain experience. Any factor that interrupts or influences normal pain reception or perception (e.g., spinal cord injury, peripheral neuropathy) affects a patient's awareness of and response to pain.

Gender

Research on pain in men and women demonstrates differences in occurrence and response to pain related to gender. Chronic pain conditions occur more often in women than men. This is because some chronic pain conditions such as endometriosis occur only in women, and some such as chronic fatigue syndrome and fibromyalgia occur predominately in women. Reports of headache and joint pain are more common in women than men (Institute of Medicine [IOM], 2011).

Social Factors

Attention

The degree to which a patient focuses attention on pain influences pain perception. Increased attention frequently increases a person's pain, whereas distraction often decreases pain. By focusing a patient's attention and concentration on other stimuli such as having a patient listen to music or breathe rhythmically, you help turn his or her focus away from the pain. Usually increased tolerance for pain lasts only during the time of distraction.

Previous Experience

People learn from painful experiences. Previous experience includes pain that a patient has experienced personally and pain that a patient has heard about from someone else. Prior experience does not mean that a person accepts pain more easily in the future. Frequent episodes of pain without relief or bouts of severe pain produce anxiety or fear. In contrast, if a person repeatedly experiences the same type of pain that was successfully relieved in the past, it is easier for him or her to interpret the sensation. As a result, the person is better prepared to take steps to relieve the pain. A patient who has had no experience with a particular type of pain sometimes has an impaired ability to cope with it. You need to prepare your patient with a clear explanation of the type of pain to expect and methods to reduce it.

Family and Social Support

Patients often depend on the support and assistance of family members or friends when coping with pain. Family caregivers sometimes have misconceptions about pain and pain management. Some caregivers think patients should wait as long as possible before receiving pain medication and fear the possibility of addiction. It is your responsibility to educate the patient and family caregivers about the importance of early assessment and treatment of pain. The presence of a loved one usually minimizes anxiety and fear when a patient is experiencing pain. Absence of social support often makes the pain experience more stressful. The presence of parents is especially important for children in pain.

Spiritual Factors

Spirituality is an active searching for meaning to situations in which one finds oneself. Spiritual questions include, "Why has this happened to me?" and "Why am I suffering?" Often spiritual concerns include the loss of independence and becoming a burden to one's family. Be sensitive to a patient's spiritual needs and consider referral to a pastoral care professional (see Chapter 10).

Cultural Factors

Culture influences how people perceive the causes and meaning of pain as well as their reactions to and expressions of pain. Understanding cultural background and personal characteristics helps you more accurately assess pain and its meaning for patients. People from some cultures appear to have a higher pain tolerance and avoid vocalizing to express their pain, whereas people from other cultures are more expressive with moaning and crying. The words used to describe pain may vary in different cultures. When patients do not speak the same language as you, you may find that their language does not have a word equivalent to "pain."

Psychological Factors

Meaning of Pain

The meaning that a patient attributes to pain affects the pain experience. Patients perceive pain differently if it suggests a threat, loss, punishment, or challenge. The degree and quality of pain perceived by a patient are related to its meaning.

Anxiety

High anxiety levels often increase pain perception, and pain usually causes anxiety. Autonomic arousal patterns are similar in pain and anxiety. Patients who worry about symptoms that are minor or nonexistent have health anxiety. The presence of health anxiety in patients who have pain negatively influences their response to pain and its associated treatments. Lowering a patient's health anxiety helps lower the patient's pain perception.

Depression

Patients with chronic pain are at a high risk of experiencing depression because they often experience many losses such as their ability to enjoy life, be in control, work, socialize, and be independent. Suicidal thoughts are relatively common; therefore, you need to routinely assess for suicidal tendencies and reports of sleep disruption and deteriorating ability to function. As a nurse, be aware of the possibility of depression in patients with persistent pain and suggest a referral if symptoms of major depression emerge (Cheatle, 2014).

Coping Style

Pain sometimes causes feelings of loneliness. Frequently patients in pain feel a loss of control over their environment or the outcome of events, especially when their pain is difficult to manage. A patient's coping style influences the ability to cope with pain. Patients with internal loci of control perceive themselves as having personal control over their environments and the outcome of events. They ask questions, desire information, and like choices of treatment. In contrast, patients with external loci of control perceive other factors in their environments (e.g., nurses) as being responsible for the outcome of events. These patients tend to be less demanding, follow directions, and are more passive in managing their pain. They want specific instructions. Frequently patients with internal loci of control report less severe pain than patients with external loci.

PAIN ASSESSMENT

A comprehensive assessment of pain gathers information about the cause of a person's pain and determines its effect on the person's ability to function. Accurate and factual pain assessment is necessary for determining a patient's responses, arriving at proper nursing diagnoses, and selecting appropriate therapies (Table 11.2). Pain assessment is one of the most frequent and difficult activities you perform. It is important to carefully interpret pain cues, and remember that psychological and physical components of pain influence a patient's reaction to it.

When assessing pain, be sensitive to a patient's level of discomfort and determine which level will allow your patient to function. For example, ask a patient in pain, "Which level of pain on a scale of 0–10 (with 0 being no pain and 10 being the worst pain you can imagine) (see Fig. 11.7) allows you to walk down the hall?" If the patient answers that walking is possible when pain is at a level of 2, you then focus efforts on decreasing pain to that level. If pain is acutely severe, it is unlikely that the patient will provide detailed information. During an episode of acute pain, you primarily assess its location, severity, and quality. Collect a more detailed assessment when the patient is more comfortable, using the PQRSTU characteristics of pain (Table 11.3). A more comprehensive pain assessment takes time; you do this when the patient becomes more alert and attentive.

Pain always changes; it does not stay the same. Thus, monitor pain on a regular basis along with vital signs. Many institutions now treat pain as the fifth vital sign. Pain assessment is *not* simply a number. Although pain assessment is a nursing function, nursing assistive personnel (NAP) also screen for pain and are responsible for informing a nurse immediately when a patient is having pain. This allows the nurse to confirm the assessment and provide appropriate therapy.

For patients with chronic pain, focus your assessment on the emotional impact and meaning of the experience and on its history and context. In addition, include level of function in your assessment because it is sometimes impossible to achieve complete pain relief. Teach family caregivers of

Table 11.2 Focused Patient Assessment

Factors to Assess	Questions	Physical Assessment
Location of pain	Where is your pain located? Use your finger and point to where the pain is.	Depending on area of pain, use inspection to determine whether body part is swollen, discolored, or warm to touch. Have the patient use hand to locate area where pain originates and then spreads. Use light palpation over area identified by the patient.
Aggravating factors	Describe your pain when you move. Do you do other things that make your pain worse? Tell me what makes the pain better.	When positioning body part aggravates pain, determine whether range of motion is altered. Observe the patient's facial expression and movement when the patient attempts activity that typically aggravates pain.

Table 11.3 Implications of Pain Assessment for Nursing Interventions

Assessment Criteria (PQRSTU)	Nursing Interventions
Palliative or **P**rovocative factors—What makes your pain worse or better?	Avoid activities that cause or aggravate pain. Teach the patient or family to avoid these activities.
Quality—How do you describe your pain?	Suggest changing pharmacological interventions if the quality of pain (neuropathic versus nociceptive) changes.
Relief measures—What do you do at home to gain pain relief?	Use measures that patient uses to relieve pain if they are safe and appropriate.
Region (location)—Show me where you hurt.	Position the patient off affected area. Apply local treatments (e.g., elastic bandage, cold, heat, splinting) directly over painful site.
Severity—On a scale of 0–10, with 0 being no pain and 10 being the worst, how bad is your pain now?	Change or revise interventions, depending on success of one intervention in reducing severity.
Timing (onset, duration, and pattern)—Is your pain constant, intermittent, or both?	Administer analgesics so that peak action occurs when pain is most acute (e.g., during dressing change or exercise therapy).
U (effect of pain on patient)—What are you unable to do because of your pain?	Schedule activities that are important to the patient during time of day when he or she feels least pain.

BOX 11.2 Routine Clinical Approach to Pain Assessment and Management (ABCDE)

A ***Ask*** about pain regularly.
B ***Believe*** patients and family caregivers in their report of pain and what relieves it.
C ***Choose*** pain control options appropriate for patient, family, and setting.
D ***Deliver*** interventions in timely, logical, and coordinated fashion.
E ***Empower*** patients and their families.

From Maryniak K: Pain assessment and management, *RN.com*, 2013, https://lms.rn.com/courses/1773/presentation_html5.html.

patients with cancer how to assess pain so that they promote continuity of effective pain management (Box 11.2). In the home setting, involving family caregivers in pain assessment offers patients and families control over their experience. Be aware of possible errors in pain assessment. Bias (overestimating or underestimating level of pain), vague or unclear assessment questions, and use of unreliable or invalid pain assessment tools do not provide accurate data. Family caregivers' estimates of a patient's pain are not always accurate and should be used only when the patient is unable to verbalize or indicate pain intensity.

Older Adult Considerations

The ability of older adults to interpret pain is complicated. Older adults tend to use words such as *hurting* or *aching* instead of the word *pain* to describe their pain. In addition, older adults sometimes have more than one painful site. They often hesitate to discuss their pain because of concerns about bothering their health care providers. Frequently older adults believe they cannot change their pain and they simply must endure it. These barriers contribute to inadequate pain assessment and management (Lewis et al., 2014). Patients with a cognitive impairment or who are nonverbal (e.g., patients with aphasia or mental status changes) have trouble communicating pain and providing a detailed description. Thus, you need to observe physical and behavioral cues when assessing pain (Huether and McCance, 2017).

Multiple diseases and vague symptoms affecting similar parts of the body further complicate the ability of older adults to interpret pain. When older patients have more than one source of pain, be sure to gather detailed assessments. Different diseases cause similar symptoms. For example, a patient who has a below-knee amputation continues to perceive pain from the foot that has been amputated (phantom pain) and has suture-line pain from the surgery. A patient who has a stroke sometimes has pain in the paralyzed arm and in areas of the body unaffected by the stroke.

PAIN MANAGEMENT

When providing pain-relief measures, choose therapies suited to a patient's unique pain experience. Box 11.3 includes guidelines that are applicable for individualizing pain therapy (Pasero and McCaffery, 2011).

BOX 11.3 Guidelines for Individualized Pain Therapy

- *Use different types of pain-relief measures.* This produces an additive effect in reducing pain and allows for changes in the character of pain.
- *Provide pain-relief measures before pain becomes severe.* It is easier to prevent severe pain than to try to relieve it after it occurs.
- *Use measures that a patient believes are effective.* A patient's beliefs make pain therapy successful; therefore, include these remedies unless they are harmful.
- *Some patients have ideas about pain-relief measures they are willing to use and times to use them.* Consider a patient's ability or willingness to participate in pain-relief measures.
- *Do not force participation.* Suggest measures that require little physical effort for patients unable to actively assist with pain therapy because of fatigue or altered levels of consciousness.
- *Choose pain-relief measures based on patient behavior that reflects the severity of pain.* Never administer a potent analgesic for mild pain. Only a patient can determine the potency of an effective therapy.
- *Depending on the therapy, ensure that you attempt a sufficient trial before abandoning it.* Pharmacological interventions particularly often need ATC administration for several days to attain and maintain therapeutic level and provide pain relief.
- *Keep an open mind about ways to relieve pain.* Rejecting nonconventional therapy leads to mistrust. Be sure that all therapies are safe.
- *Keep trying.* When efforts at pain relief fail, do not abandon the patient, but reassess the situation and consider alternative therapies.
- *Protect the patient.* Pain therapy does not cause more distress than the pain itself; you want to relieve pain without disabling the patient mentally, emotionally, or physically.
- *Educate the patient about pain.* Explain the cause of pain, times when you will give analgesics, and alternative therapies.

ATC, around-the-clock.

Pharmacological Pain Therapy

All pharmacological agents require a health care provider's order. Your judgment in the use and management of analgesics with or without other pain therapies ensures the best pain relief possible. A systematic approach to pain assessment and appropriate treatment choices ensures a quick response for managing patient discomfort.

Analgesics

The most common treatment for pain relief is **analgesics.** However, health care providers still tend to undertreat patients because of incorrect drug information, concerns about addiction, anxiety over errors in using opioid analgesics, and administration of less medication than was ordered. Make sure that you understand the drugs available for pain relief and their pharmacological effects. Reassure patients that treatment of pain is necessary to aid recovery and that addiction is highly unlikely when analgesics are taken correctly.

There are three types of analgesics: (1) nonopioids including acetaminophen and nonsteroidal anti-inflammatory drugs (NSAIDs); (2) opioids (traditionally called *narcotics*); and (3) adjuvants or coanalgesics, medications that enhance analgesics or analgesic properties (Burchum and Rosenthal, 2016).

Acetaminophen (Tylenol) is considered one of the most tolerated and safest analgesics available. It has no anti-inflammatory effects, and its action is unknown. Its major adverse effect is toxicity to the liver. Acetaminophen is in a variety of over-the-counter (OTC) cold, flu, and allergy remedies. The maximum 24-hour dose is 4 g (the same limitation as aspirin). It is often combined with opioids (e.g., oxycodone [Percocet], hydrocodone [Vicodin], tramadol [Ultracet]) because it reduces the dose of opioid needed.

Nonselective NSAIDs such as aspirin and ibuprofen provide relief for mild-to-moderate acute intermittent pain such as pain from headache or muscle strain. Treatment for mild-to-moderate postoperative pain begins with an NSAID unless contraindicated (Burchum and Rosenthal, 2016). In contrast to opioids, NSAIDs do not depress the central nervous system, and they do not interfere with bowel and bladder function. However, chronic NSAID use is not recommended because it is associated with gastrointestinal bleeding, renal insufficiency, and bleeding tendencies. NSAIDs have anti-inflammatory properties and work with opioids to relieve pain better than when given alone (Burchum and Rosenthal, 2016).

Opioid or opioid-like analgesics such as codeine, morphine, fentanyl, and hydromorphone are prescribed for moderate-to-severe pain. These analgesics act on higher centers of the brain and spinal cord by binding with opiate receptors to modify pain perception. Opioid-naïve patients have used opioids around-the-clock (ATC) less than approximately 1 week. A rare adverse effect of opioids in opioid-naïve patients is respiratory depression. Respiratory depression is clinically significant only if there is a decrease in the rate *and* depth of respirations from a patient's baseline assessment (Pasero and McCaffery, 2011). Patients who breathe deeply rarely have clinical respiratory depression. Sedation always occurs before respiratory depression. Closely monitor for sedation in opioid-naïve patients. If a patient develops respiratory depression, administer naloxone (Narcan) 0.4 mg diluted with 9 mL saline i.v. push at a rate of 0.5 mL every 2 minutes until the respiratory rate is greater than 8 breaths/min with good depth. Evaluate patients who receive naloxone every 15 minutes for 2 hours because its duration is less than that of the opioid and respiratory depression can return. Additional adverse effects of opioids include nausea, vomiting, constipation, itching, urinary retention, and altered mental processes.

One way to maximize pain relief while potentially decreasing drug use is to administer analgesics on an ATC rather than as-needed (prn) basis (Burchum and Rosenthal, 2016). There are also a variety of extended-release or controlled-release oral opioid formulations with dosing intervals of 8, 10, 12, or 24 hours and transdermal patches with a dosing interval of 72 hours. These formulations maintain constant serum opioid concentration, minimizing toxic and subtherapeutic concentrations. They also lessen the severity of end-of-dose pain, allowing a patient to sleep through the night.

The current pharmacological approach to pain management is to provide multimodal analgesia. This approach combines drugs with at least two different mechanisms of action to optimize pain control. Medications are combined to target different sites in the peripheral or central pain pathways. Multimodal analgesia allows for lower-than-usual doses of each medication, thereby lowering the risk of side effects while providing good or better pain relief than giving each medication alone.

When a patient is converted from an i.v. to an oral form of opioid, know that the dose of the oral opioid is usually much higher than the i.v. dose because of the first-pass effect (Pasero and McCaffery, 2011). When a patient takes oral opioids, the opioids go to the liver first, where most of the medication is inactivated. Thus, the body needs larger doses of oral opioids to achieve the same level of pain relief as the same opioid given intravenously. Know the comparative potencies of analgesics in oral and i.v. form. Also, know the route of administration that is most effective for a patient to achieve controlled, sustained pain relief. Equianalgesic charts show the conversion of one opioid to another and of parenteral forms of opioids to oral forms. These charts are available on nursing units, in the pharmacy, and in printed and online drug resources. Nurses on succeeding shifts need to know the route of administration that is most effective for a patient so that the patient has controlled, sustained pain relief.

Adjuvants or coanalgesics are drugs (e.g., steroids, anticonvulsants, antidepressants, muscle relaxants) originally developed to treat conditions other than pain that also have analgesic properties. For example, tricyclic antidepressants (e.g., nortriptyline), anticonvulsants (e.g., gabapentin), and infusional lidocaine successfully treat neuropathic pain. Corticosteroids relieve pain associated with inflammation and bone metastasis. Adjuvants have analgesic properties, enhance pain control, or relieve other symptoms associated with neuropathic pain such as anxiety, depression, and nausea. You give these alone or with analgesics (Burchum and Rosenthal, 2016). Sedatives, antianxiety agents, and muscle relaxants have no analgesic effect; however, they often cause drowsiness and impaired coordination, judgment, and mental alertness. Be aware of the risk for falls when a patient is taking these medications.

The proper use of analgesics requires careful assessment, application of pharmacological principles, and critical thinking (Box 11.4). Not all patients react the same way to analgesics. An orally administered analgesic usually brings the same relief as an injectable form.

Children require careful calculation of drug doses (see Chapter 26). Equianalgesia charts that convert recommended adult doses to children's doses are available. These charts consider age and body size. In addition, older adults require special dosing considerations (Box 11.5).

Patient-Controlled Analgesia

Patients benefit from having control over their pain therapy. **Patient-controlled analgesia (PCA)** is a safe method for a variety of painful conditions including but not limited to postoperative, traumatic, sickle cell crisis, cancer, and burn pain (Pasero and McCaffery, 2011). PCA is a drug-delivery system that allows patients to self-administer opioids with minimal risk of overdose, when they need medication, and without repeated parenteral injections (see Skill 11.1). The goal is to maintain a constant plasma level of analgesic to avoid the problems of intermittent dosing. Systemic PCA traditionally involves i.v. or subcutaneous administration.

BOX 11.4 Nursing Principles for Administering Analgesics

Know the Patient's Previous Response to Analgesics

- Determine whether the patient obtained pain relief.
- Ask whether a nonopioid was as effective as an opioid.
- Identify previous doses and routes of administration to avoid undertreatment.
- Determine whether the patient has allergies.
- Know whether the patient is at risk for using NSAIDs (e.g., history of gastrointestinal bleeding or renal insufficiency) or opioids (e.g., history of obstructive sleep apnea).

Select Proper Medications When More Than One Is Ordered

- Use nonopioid analgesics or opioid combination drugs (e.g., oxycodone with acetaminophen) for mild-to-moderate pain.
- Give opioids with nonopioids.
- In older adults, avoid combinations of opioids.
- Fentanyl patches, morphine, or hydromorphone are opioids of choice for long-term severe pain.
- I.v. medications act more quickly and usually relieve severe, acute pain within 1 h, whereas oral medications take up to 2 h to relieve pain.
- Avoid intramuscular analgesics, especially in older adults.
- For chronic pain, give oral extended-release formulations for longer, more sustained relief.

Know Accurate Dosage

- Remember that patients with severe pain generally need higher doses of analgesics.
- Adjust doses as appropriate for children and older patients.
- Large doses of opioids are acceptable in patients who are opioid tolerant but not in patients who are opioid naïve.
- When titrating opioids, it is important to titrate to effect or to uncontrollable side effects.
- Dosage typically requires adjustment over time.

Assess Right Time and Interval for Administration

- Administer analgesics as soon as pain occurs and before it increases in severity.
- An ATC administration schedule is best.
- Give analgesics *before* pain-producing procedures or activities.
- Know average peak and duration of action for drug so that you time drug administration to peak when pain is most intense.
- Give extended-release opioid formulations on an ATC basis and not prn.
- Avoid abruptly stopping opioids in patients who are opioid tolerant.

Choose Right Route

- Oral route is generally preferred; i.v. route is preferred if the patient is unable to swallow or has gastrointestinal problems.
- Avoid intramuscular and subcutaneous administration because these routes are painful and absorption is not reliable.

ATC, around-the-clock; *NSAIDs*, nonsteroidal anti-inflammatory drugs.
Modified from Pasero C, McCaffery M: *Pain assessment and pharmacological management*, St Louis, 2011, Mosby.

BOX 11.5 Care of an Older Adult

Principles of Pain Management in an Older Adult

- The presence of pain requires aggressive assessment and management.
- Older adults are at high risk for pain-inducing situations.
- Sometimes, several pain-producing conditions coexist.
- Older adults are often fearful that pain will result in loss of independence, making them a burden to their family.
- Age-related changes in pain perception are most likely not clinically significant.
- Older patients experience faster onset, longer duration of action, and adverse effects from analgesics because of lower serum protein levels and reduced liver, renal, and cardiac function.
- Older adults may be more sensitive to analgesic and adverse effects of opioids. Thus, start with low doses of opioids and increase dose slowly as needed (Pasero and McCaffery, 2011).
- There is an increased risk for gastric and renal toxicity from NSAIDs among older adults.

NSAIDs, nonsteroidal anti-inflammatory drugs.

PCA infusion pumps are portable and contain a cassette or chamber for a syringe. The PCA delivers a small preset dose of opioid. To receive a demand dose, a patient pushes a button attached to the PCA device. Systems are programmed to deliver a specified number of doses every 1−4 hours (depending on the pump settings) given every 5−15 minutes to avoid overdoses. On-demand doses typically add 1 mg of morphine every 10 minutes, with a limit set for every hour or every 4 hours. Most pumps have locked safety systems that prevent tampering by patients or family caregivers and are generally safe to be managed in the home. The typical PCA prescription relies on a series of "loading" doses (e.g., 3−5 mg of morphine repeated every 5−10 minutes until initial pain diminishes). A low-dose basal infusion (0.5−1 mg/h) at night allows uninterrupted sleep; this option is commonly used for cancer pain. Use continuous basal infusions with caution in patients who are opioid naïve during the first 24−48 hours after surgery because of the possibility of respiratory depression from the combination of anesthetics with opioids (Pasero and McCaffery, 2011).

Benefits of PCA include better pain control, a need for less medication, and pain relief that does not depend on nurses' availability. Small PCA doses delivered at short intervals stabilize serum drug concentrations for sustained pain relief.

Patient preparation and teaching are critical to the safe and effective use of PCA. If PCA is ordered, patients having surgery receive teaching and demonstration of the PCA pump before surgery. Patients need to understand PCA and be able to physically locate and press the button to deliver the dose (Pasero and McCaffery, 2011). PCA therapy is not appropriate for patients who are confused, have altered levels of consciousness, or are unable to understand how to use the equipment. Be sure to instruct family members not to "push the button" for patients. Use American Society for Pain Management Nursing (ASPMN) and Authorized Agent Controlled Analgesia (AACA) guidelines to authorize a family member or nurse to administer the analgesic when appropriate (Cooney et al., 2013). In these cases, you select one family member or significant other to be the patient's primary pain manager. Check the patient's i.v. line or subcutaneous needle placement and PCA device regularly to ensure proper functioning. Most PCA devices track cumulative dosages and show the information when needed. Document drug doses carefully and record any wasted or unused opioid. Monitor the patient for adverse drug effects and pain management effectiveness. Use of PCA gives nurses and patients more flexibility in pain management.

Perineural Local Anesthetic Infusion

Perineural infusion pumps are an option for managing pain for a variety of adult and pediatric surgical procedures. An unsutured catheter from a surgical wound placed near a nerve or groups of nerves connects to a pump containing a local anesthetic. You set the pump on demand or continuous mode, and it is usually left in place for 48 hours. Patients learn how to discontinue the pump at home by pulling out the catheter and bringing it to their next health care provider visit.

Local Anesthetics

The loss of sensation to a localized body part is termed **local anesthesia.** Health care providers use local anesthetics including lidocaine, bupivacaine, and ropivacaine during brief surgical procedures such as suturing a wound. Local anesthetics are applied topically on skin and mucous membranes or are injected subcutaneously, perineurally, or intradermally to anesthetize a body part. The drugs produce temporary loss of sensation by inhibiting nerve conduction. Local anesthetics may also block motor and autonomic functions, depending on the amount used and the location and depth of an injection. Smaller sensory nerve fibers are more sensitive than large motor fibers. Thus, a patient loses sensation before losing motor function; conversely, motor function returns before sensation.

Local anesthetics cause side effects depending on their absorption into the circulation. Itching or burning of the skin or a localized rash is common after topical applications. Application to vascular membranes increases the chance of systemic effects such as a change in heart rate. Protect patients from injury until full sensory and motor function return because they can easily injure themselves without knowing it. You need to educate patients receiving local anesthesia by explaining insertion sites and warning them that they will temporarily lose sensory function. Injection is painful unless the health care provider first numbs the injection site. Prepare patients for such discomfort. Before a patient receives an anesthetic, assess for any medication allergies. Assess vital signs to monitor for systemic effects.

Epidural Analgesia

Epidural analgesia is a form of regional anesthesia and an effective therapy for the treatment of postoperative, labor and delivery, and chronic cancer pain. Epidural medications block transmission of pain stimuli in the spinal cord. Analgesia is short or long term, depending on a patient's condition and pain management needs. Short-term epidural analgesia is especially effective for pain after intrathoracic, abdominal, and orthopedic surgery. Long-term epidural therapy is effective for pain unresponsive to oral or parenteral medications. The advantages of epidural analgesia include the following:

- Production of excellent analgesia
- Occurrence of minimal sedation
- Long-lasting pain relief with fewer opioid doses
- Facilitation of early ambulation
- Avoidance of repeated injections
- No significant effect on sensation
- Little effect on blood pressure or heart rate
- Fewer pulmonary complications

Epidural analgesia is administered into the epidural space to block a group of sensory nerve fibers. It is administered through a catheter, which is usually placed in the operating room, postanesthesia care unit, or intensive care unit. The patient lies in the fetal position (lateral decubitus) to open the space between the vertebrae. The health care provider administers a local anesthetic into the skin at the needle insertion site and then inserts a blunt-tip needle into the level of the vertebral interspace nearest to the area requiring analgesia (usually L4–L5). The health care provider advances a plastic catheter into the epidural space and then removes the needle (Fig. 11.4). The remainder of the catheter is secured with an occlusive dressing and

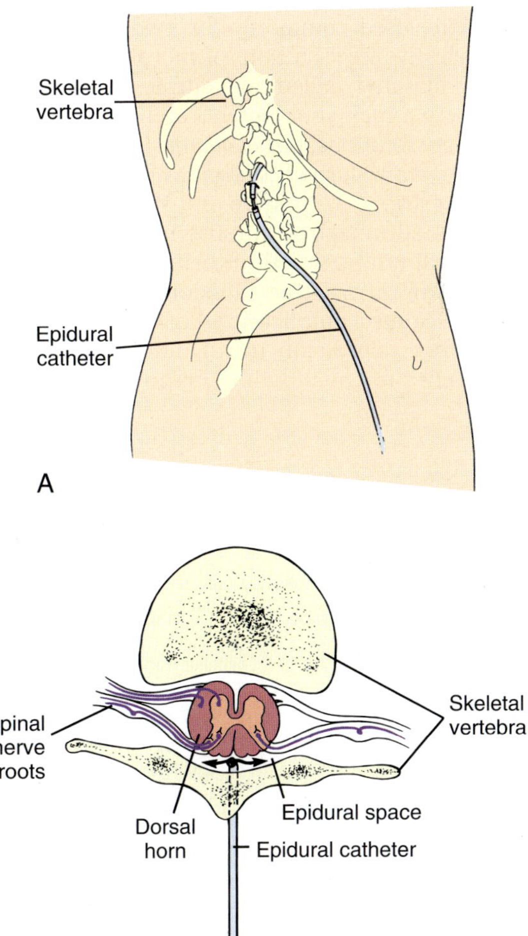

Fig. 11.4 A, Epidural catheter inserted into L4–L5 space. **B,** Anatomical drawing of epidural space.

taped up the back of the patient. A temporary catheter is sometimes connected to tubing positioned along the spine and over the patient's shoulder. You can place the end of the catheter on the patient's chest for easier access. Permanent catheters are tunneled through the skin and exit at the patient's side. Assessment of the insertion site and patency of the tubing are important nursing responsibilities (Pasero and McCaffery, 2011).

The epidural catheter is connected to a continuous **epidural infusion** pump, a port, or a reservoir, or it is capped for bolus injections. In many hospitals, only anesthesiologists or nurse anesthetists administer epidural anesthesia. Some institutions allow patients to deliver epidural analgesic doses (patient-controlled epidural analgesia [PCEA]) via a pump. To reduce the risk for accidental epidural injection of drugs intended for i.v. use, always place a brightly colored intermittent injection cap on the catheter tubing. You should label the catheter "epidural catheter" or use color-coded catheters and tubing to prevent accidental connections of i.v. tubing to the epidural catheter. Hospitals use tubing that has no access ports to minimize accidental introduction of i.v. medications. Administer continuous infusions through electronic infusion devices for proper control. Because of the catheter location, follow strict surgical aseptic technique when handling tubing to prevent a potentially fatal infection. Notify a health care provider immediately if any signs or symptoms of infection or pain at the insertion site develop (Pasero and McCaffery, 2011).

Medications used commonly for epidural analgesia include preservative-free solutions of morphine sulfate, hydromorphone, fentanyl, sufentanil citrate, bupivacaine, and clonidine. Sometimes, your patient receives the combination of two of these solutions. *Do not administer supplemental doses of opioids or sedative/hypnotics because of possible additive central nervous system effects* (Pasero and McCaffery, 2011).

Table 11.4 summarizes nursing implications for managing epidural analgesia. Monitoring for drug effects differs, depending on whether infusions are intermittent or continuous. Some complications of epidural opioid use are respiratory depression (rare), nausea and vomiting, urinary retention, constipation, orthostatic hypotension, and pruritus (Pasero and McCaffery, 2011). When you start patients on epidural analgesia, monitor respiratory rate, respiratory effort, and skin color as often as every 15 minutes. Pulse oximetry is also a standard measurement. If a patient remains stable, monitoring takes place every hour (see agency policy). Inform patients about the potential for respiratory depression, and instruct them to notify you if breathing difficulty develops. If respiratory depression develops, turn off the infusion immediately and notify the health care provider.

Nonpharmacological Pain-Relief Measures

There are many nonpharmacological or complementary therapies for pain relief that nurses use to promote health as well as manage acute and restorative care needs. Examples include massage, guided imagery, music, prayer, journaling, exercise, and relaxation techniques. Complementary therapies such as biofeedback and acupuncture require special training to perform. Use other therapies such as massage and relaxation to lessen the perception of pain, perhaps in combination with pharmacological measures (Burchum and Rosenthal, 2016). Combine pharmacological therapy with nonpharmacological therapies. Guidelines for chronic pain management from the CDC recommend using nonpharmacological therapy before opioids (Dowell et al., 2016). If opioids are needed, health care providers can add opioids, but only in combination with nonpharmacological approaches and nonopioid analgesics.

Reducing Pain Reception and Perception

One simple way to promote comfort is to remove or prevent painful stimuli. This is especially important for patients who are immobilized or have difficulty expressing themselves. For example, tighten and smooth wrinkled bed linen and be sure to position patients so that they are not lying on tubing and other equipment. Change wet dressings or bed linen immediately. Do not allow tubing from a Foley catheter to become kinked because bladder distention is uncomfortable. Remember to use safe patient-handling techniques when repositioning and lifting patients. Do not pull when

Table 11.4 Nursing Care of Patients With Epidural Infusions

Goal	Actions
Prevent catheter displacement	Secure catheter (if not connected to implanted reservoir) carefully to skin.
Maintain catheter function	Check external dressing around catheter site for dampness or discharge. (Leak of cerebrospinal fluid may develop.) Use transparent, adhesive dressing to aid inspection. Inspect catheter for breaks.
Prevent infection	Use aseptic technique when caring for catheter. Do *not* routinely change dressing over site. Change tubing every 24 h or per agency policy.
Monitor for respiratory depression	Monitor vital signs, especially respirations, per policy. Use pulse oximetry and apnea monitoring when necessary. Maintain head of bed at 30–45°.
Prevent undesirable complications	Assess for pruritus (itching) and nausea and vomiting. Administer antihistamines and antiemetics as ordered. Verify that tubing is connected to epidural catheter; label appropriately.
Maintain urinary and bowel function	Monitor intake and output. Assess bladder and bowel for distention. Assess for discomfort, frequency, and urgency.

positioning patients in correct anatomical alignment. Minimize exposure to skin irritants such as diarrhea stool or wound drainage. Many of these measures are easy for family caregivers to learn. Removing noxious stimuli is especially important for patients who are immobile. You can prevent pain by anticipating painful activities (e.g., ambulation or turning). Before performing a procedure, consider the patient's condition, aspects of the procedure that are painful, and ways to avoid causing pain. Consideration of the patient's comfort and a little extra time are needed to avoid pain-producing situations.

Anticipatory Guidance

Modifying anxiety directly associated with pain relieves the pain and adds to the beneficial effects of other pain-relief measures. Giving patients detailed descriptions of all medical procedures and expected postprocedural discomfort and giving instruction for decreasing treatment-related and mobility-related pain decrease pain and analgesic use. Provide patients with sufficient procedural and sensory information (e.g., prick of the needle during blood draw or burning during urinary catheter insertion) to satisfy their curiosity and enable them to prepare for and communicate pain.

Distraction

The reticular activating system inhibits painful stimuli if a person receives sufficient or excessive sensory input. With meaningful sensory stimuli, a patient can ignore or become unaware of pain. Pleasurable sensory stimuli reduce pain perception by the release of endorphins. Distraction directs a patient's attention to something else, thus reducing the awareness of pain. Distraction works best for short, intense pain lasting a few minutes such as during an invasive procedure or while waiting for an analgesic to become effective. Useful forms of distraction include singing, praying, describing photos out loud, telling jokes, and playing games. Music is helpful for managing acute and chronic discomfort, stress, anxiety, and depression by diverting a patient's attention and creating a relaxation response. Always let patients select the type of music they prefer. Patients may use earphones to enhance their concentration on the music. Evidence shows that music decreases the use of analgesics in some postoperative patients (Cole and LoBiondo-Wood, 2014).

Cutaneous Stimulation

Stimulation of the skin helps to relieve pain. A massage, warm bath, ice pack, and **TENS** are simple ways to reduce pain perception (Chou et al., 2016). How **cutaneous stimulation** works is unclear, but it may cause release of endorphins, thus blocking transmission of painful stimuli. The gate control theory suggests that cutaneous stimulation activates larger, faster A-beta sensory nerve fibers that are sensitive to touch, pressure, and warmth. This decreases pain transmission through small-diameter A-delta and C fibers. Synaptic gates thus close to pain transmission.

Cutaneous stimulation gives patients and families some control over pain symptoms and treatment in the home. Using it properly helps to reduce muscle tension, resulting in less pain. When using cutaneous stimulation, eliminate environmental noise, help patients to assume comfortable positions, and explain the purpose of therapies. Do not use cutaneous stimulation directly on sensitive skin areas (e.g., burns, bruises, skin rashes, inflammation, underlying bone fractures).

Massage

It is effective for producing physical and mental relaxation, reducing pain, and enhancing the effectiveness of pain medication. Massaging the back, shoulders, hands, and/or feet relaxes muscles and promotes sleep. Massage conveys caring, and family caregivers can learn how to do this easily.

Cold and Heat Applications

Cold and heat applications relieve pain and promote healing (see Chapter 17). The choice to use heat or cold is based on the origin of the pain and a patient's preferences and past experiences with pain relief using these methods. For example, moist heat often relieves the pain from a tension headache, and a cold pack reduces acute pain from inflammation. The use of heat or cold applications in the acute care setting requires a health care provider's order. When using any form of heat or cold application, instruct a patient to avoid injury to the skin by checking the temperature and not applying it directly to the skin. Older adults, confused patients, and patients with spinal cord or other neurological injuries and decreased sensation are at risk for burns from heating devices.

Transcutaneous Electrical Nerve Stimulation

It stimulates the skin by passing mild electrical currents through external electrodes, blocking pain stimuli from reaching the brain. A patient places the electrodes directly over or near the site of pain and turns on a battery-powered transmitter to create a tingling electrical current when feeling pain. TENS is useful in reducing postoperative procedural pain (e.g., removing drains). The research evidence on the use of TENS for pain relief is often conflicting; however, TENS is safe, noninvasive, nonaddictive, inexpensive, and easy to use. It requires a health care provider's order (Chou et al., 2016).

Relaxation and Guided Imagery

Relaxation and guided imagery allow patients to alter affective motivational and cognitive pain perception. **Relaxation** is mental and physical freedom from tension or stress that provides individuals a sense of self-control. Potential physiological and behavioral changes associated with relaxation include decreased pulse, blood pressure, and respirations; heightened awareness; decreased oxygen consumption; a sense of peace; and decreased muscle tension and metabolic rate. Relaxation strategies include meditation, yoga, Zen, guided imagery, and progressive relaxation. Sometimes, a combination is needed to achieve pain relief. The techniques require periodic reinforcement through encouragement and coaching.

For effective relaxation, a patient needs to be able to concentrate, participate, and cooperate. Teach relaxation techniques only when a patient is not anxious, in acute discomfort, or in severe pain. Explain the technique in detail. It sometimes takes several teaching sessions before patients effectively feel less pain. Patients can practice relaxation training indefinitely and usually with no side effects. Remove any noises or other irritating stimuli such as bright lights from the environment. Have a patient sit in a comfortable chair in proper alignment or lie in bed. A light sheet or blanket keeps the patient warm and comfortable. Describe common sensations that the patient will experience (e.g., decrease in temperature, feeling of heaviness, numbness of a body part). The patient uses these sensations as feedback. Acting as the coach, guide the patient slowly through the steps of the exercise.

In **guided imagery,** a patient creates an image in the mind, concentrates on that image, and gradually becomes less aware of pain. Initially, ask the patient to think of a pleasant scene or experience that promotes using all senses. The patient describes the image, and you record it for later use. Use only specific information given by the patient and make no changes in the image. The following is an example of a portion of a guided imagery exercise:

Imagine yourself lying on a cool bed of grass with the sounds of water trickling over stones in a nearby stream. It's a warm day. You turn to see a patch of blue wildflowers in bloom, and you smell their fragrance.

Sit close enough so the patient can hear you but not so close that you are intrusive. A calm, soft voice helps the patient focus more completely on the suggested image. You speak continuously while the patient relaxes and focuses on the image. If the patient shows signs of agitation, restlessness, or discomfort, stop the exercise and begin again later when the patient is more at ease.

Progressive relaxation exercises involve the combination of controlled breathing exercises and a series of contractions and relaxation of muscle groups. A patient begins by breathing slowly from the diaphragm, allowing the abdomen to rise slowly. The chest remains still while fully expanding. Often a patient closes the eyes to focus on the exercise. When the patient establishes a regular breathing pattern, coach him or her to locate any area of muscular tension, think about how it feels, gently tense the muscles, and then completely relax them. This creates the sensation of removing all discomfort and stress. Gradually the patient relaxes the muscles without first tensing them. After achieving full relaxation, pain perception is lowered, and anxiety toward the pain experience lessens. If the patient becomes agitated or uncomfortable, stop the exercise. If the patient reports difficulty relaxing part of the body, slow the progression of the exercise and concentrate on the tensed body part. If the patient reports increased pain, focus on relaxing areas of muscle tension instead of consciously tensing the muscle. The patient may stop the exercise at any time. With practice the patient learns to perform relaxation exercises independently. Relaxation techniques are particularly effective for chronic pain, labor pains, and relief of procedure-related pain. The techniques are less effective for episodes of acute or severe pain.

Biofeedback

Biofeedback is a mind–body technique that uses instruments to teach self-regulation and voluntary self-control over specific physiological responses. Electronic or electromechanical instruments measure, process, and provide information to patients about their muscle tension, cardiac activity, respiratory rates, brain-wave patterns, and autonomic nervous system activity. This feedback is given in physical, physiological, auditory, or visual feedback signals that increase a person's awareness of internal processes that are linked to illness and distress. Several biofeedback therapies can change thinking, emotions, and behaviors, which support beneficial physiological changes, resulting in improved health and well-being. For example, patients connected to a biofeedback device sometimes hear a sound if their pulse rate or blood pressure increases out of their therapeutic zone. Practitioners then help patients interpret these sounds and use a variety of breathing, relaxation, and imaging exercises to gain voluntary control over their racing heart or their increasing systolic blood pressure.

Biofeedback is an effective addition to more traditional relaxation programs because it immediately demonstrates to patients their ability to control some physiological responses and the relationship among thoughts, feelings, and physiological responses. It helps individuals focus on and monitor specific body parts by providing immediate feedback about which stress-relaxation behaviors work most effectively. Eventually patients notice positive physiological changes without the need for instrument feedback. One of the most critical components of any behavioral program is adherence to a treatment regimen. Patients who follow their treatment plans have more positive results.

Biofeedback is a noninvasive intervention used in numerous situations (Fig. 11.5). Although biofeedback produces effective outcomes in many patients, there are several precautions to consider. During biofeedback sessions, repressed emotions or feelings sometimes surface. For this reason, practitioners who offer biofeedback need to be trained in more traditional psychological methods or have qualified professionals available for referral. In addition, long-term use of biofeedback sometimes lowers blood pressure, heart rates, and other physiological parameters. As with other biobehavioral interventions, monitor patients closely to determine the need for medication adjustments.

Acupuncture

As a key component of (TCM) Traditional Chinese Medicine, **acupuncture** is one of the oldest practices in the world. When used outside of TCM, it is viewed as a mind–body therapy and is called *medical acupuncture*. In the United States, medical acupuncture is often provided by specially trained health care providers.

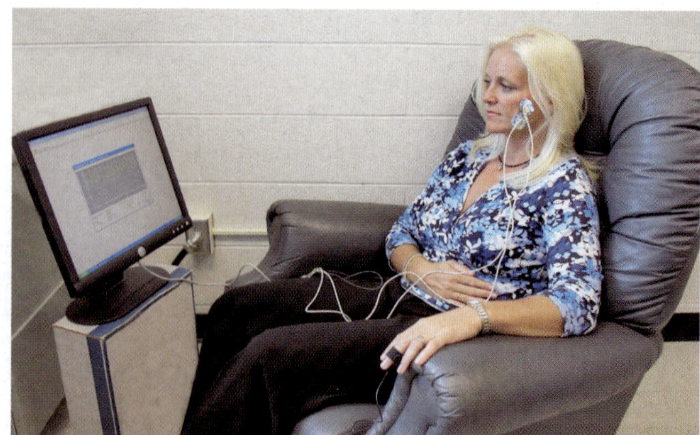

Fig. 11.5 A patient using biofeedback can visually see how relaxation affects physiological functions. (From Okeson JP: ***Management of temporomandibular disorders and occlusion,*** ed 7, St Louis, 2013, Elsevier.)

Acupuncture regulates or realigns the **vital energy (qi)**, which flows like a river through the body in channels that form a system of 20 pathways called meridians. An obstruction in these channels blocks energy flow in other parts of the body. Acupuncturists insert needles into the skin in specific areas along the channels called **acupoints**, through which the qi can be influenced and flow reestablished.

Current evidence shows that acupuncture modifies the response of the body to pain and how pain is processed by central neural pathways and cerebral function. Acupuncture has helped control symptoms related to PTSD and to manage tinnitus symptoms in war veterans.

Acupuncture is a safe therapy when the practitioner has the appropriate education and training. Therapists should use sterilized needles. Although needle complications occur (e.g., infection, fainting), they are rare if the practitioner takes appropriate precautions. In addition, caution pregnant patients and patients with a history of seizures or immunosuppression about the use of acupuncture. Treatment is contraindicated in people who have bleeding disorders and skin infections.

Palliative Care

Palliative care offers treatments to help patients live perhaps years with a variety of incurable conditions including persistent pain. The goals of palliative care are to relieve suffering and support the best possible quality of life for patients with chronic and life-threatening conditions and their family members (ONS, 2016). Palliative care is not the same as end-of-life or hospice pain management.

Patients with chronic pain require a different approach to pain management than patients with acute pain. Health care providers cannot eliminate all pain, and learning to live with daily pain is difficult. It is important for patients with chronic pain to gain control of their pain versus allowing the pain to control them. Consider making a referral to the palliative care team when you care for patients diagnosed with incurable conditions that have persistent pain. These teams are composed of a variety of health care professionals who help patients achieve the level of pain control that allows them to function and enjoy life (ONS, 2016). The patient is an active participant in pain management. Without patient involvement, adequate pain control is not possible.

Hospice

Hospice programs care for patients who are terminally ill by helping them continue to live at home in comfort and privacy with the help of a health care team. The emphasis is on quality of life over quantity, and pain control is a priority. Under the guidance of hospice nurses, family caregivers learn to monitor a patient's symptoms and become the primary caregivers. Chapter 28 discusses hospice in detail.

Hospice programs help nurses overcome their fears of contributing to a patient's death when administering large doses of opioids. The American Nurses Association (ANA, 2015) and the ASPMN (Reynolds et al., 2013) support aggressive treatment of pain and suffering at the end of life. Current evidence suggests that moderate opioid dose increases in patients who are terminally ill do not hasten death (Reynolds et al., 2013). The disease, not the opioid, is ending the life of the patient.

Patients With Cancer Pain

Some cancer pain is intractable and difficult to treat. It becomes so debilitating that patients will try anything to gain relief. National Comprehensive Cancer Network (NCCN) guidelines promote treating cancer pain in a more comprehensive and aggressive manner, providing patients and family caregivers more options for pain relief. The best choice of treatment often changes when a patient's condition and the characteristics of pain change. Both nonpharmacological and pharmacological therapies are beneficial (NCCN, 2017).

Various medications and routes of administration provide relief for patients with cancer pain. Long-acting or controlled-release medications are very successful. These controlled-release medications (e.g., morphine [MS Contin, Roxanol SR], oxycodone [OxyContin]) relieve pain for 8–12 hours. A 72-hour fentanyl transdermal patch is also available. You can manage most cancer pain with oral or transdermal medications.

Administering analgesics to treat cancer-related pain requires applying principles different from the principles used to treat acute pain. The World Health Organization (WHO) recommends a three-step approach to managing cancer pain (Fig. 11.6) (Burchum and Rosenthal, 2016). Therapy begins with NSAIDs and/or adjuvants and progresses to strong opioids if pain persists. Side effects of opioids such as nausea and constipation are treated aggressively so that patients are able to continue using the opioids. Patients usually become tolerant to the side effects except for constipation. Health care providers should routinely order stimulant laxatives, not simple stool softeners, to prevent and treat constipation.

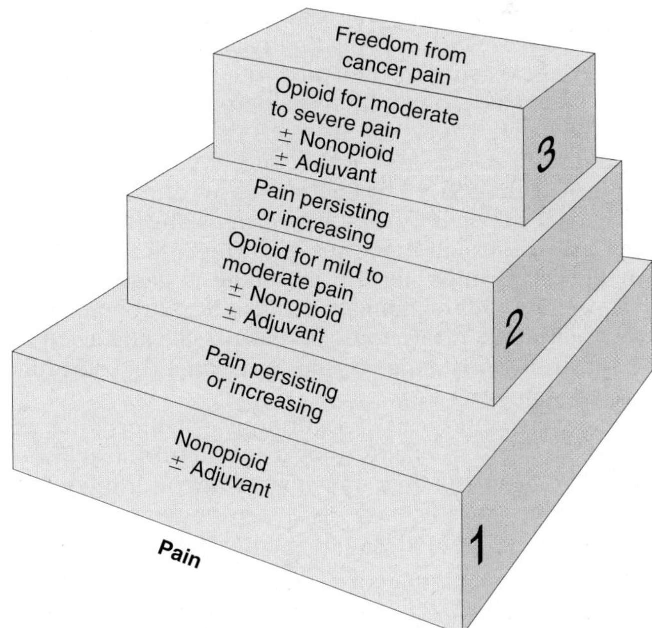

Fig. 11.6 World Health Organization analgesic ladder is a three-step approach to treating cancer pain. (From http://www.who.int/cancer/palliative/painladder/en/.)

When a patient with cancer first has pain, it is best to begin with a higher dosage than what will be routinely needed. This provides a patient with immediate pain relief. The health care provider then slowly decreases the dosage to the amount that successfully controls pain. Patients receiving long-term opioids often develop a drug tolerance. Therefore, they require higher dosages to attain pain relief. Higher dosages are not dangerous because most patients also develop tolerance to life-threatening side effects (Burchum and Rosenthal, 2016).

For patients with cancer, the aim of drug therapy is to anticipate and prevent or minimize pain. Therefore, you give required analgesic dosages regularly, even when pain subsides. Regular administration maintains blood levels for ongoing pain control. However, patients still have flares of pain or "breakthrough pain" that require additional bolus doses of medication (rescue doses). Breakthrough pain is a transient flare of moderate-to-severe pain superimposed on continuous or persistent pain. A decrease in the duration of pain relief or an increase in the intensity of pain relief provided by the regular analgesia therapy and the need for an increased number of rescue doses are indications that a patient needs a higher opioid dose (Burchum and Rosenthal, 2016). A transmucosal fentanyl "unit" given buccally is available to treat breakthrough pain in opioid-tolerant patients.

Transdermal drug systems administer drugs via a patch placed on the skin. Patches are useful when patients are unable to take drugs orally. Self-adhesive patches deposit the opioid into the subcutaneous tissue. The subcutaneous tissue releases the drug slowly at predetermined rates for 72 hours. This results in effective analgesia throughout the day and night. Inform patients that it sometimes takes 12−24 hours for analgesia to take effect when they first begin to use an analgesic patch (Burchum and Rosenthal, 2016). Therefore, it is important for you to obtain an order for an immediate-release opioid for any breakthrough pain. Because heat causes more rapid drug absorption, warn patients to avoid external heat sources such as heating pads, hot showers, and prolonged exposure to the sun while using patches. Patients who have chronic stable pain are candidates for the fentanyl patch.

Another measure for treating severe persistent cancer pain is morphine given by continuous i.v. drip or intermittently by a PCA pump. Continuous infusions provide uniform pain control at lower dosages. Thus, there are fewer side effects. Continuous-drip morphine is given in acute care settings and the home. An infusion control pump delivers morphine intravenously to ensure safe and accurate administration. Each agency has guidelines for morphine dose and infusion rates.

When a patient receives continuous-drip morphine, assess the i.v. site to ensure that it is patent and without complications (e.g., no redness, swelling, or drainage). A central line catheter such as a Groshong or Hickman catheter, an implanted venous access port, or a peripherally inserted central catheter (PICC) is usually best for long-term i.v. infusion. When a patient starts on continuous i.v. morphine, you need to monitor for and prevent overdose and central nervous system depression. Record baseline blood pressure and respiratory rates before the infusion begins. Monitor the patient frequently and closely per agency policy. If the patient's blood pressure or respirations decrease, reduce the infusion rate per the health care provider's order or agency policy. Small i.v. doses of naloxone can be ordered for severe respiratory depression and to increase respiratory rate and depth but not to reverse the pain relief. Patients who are placed on continuous analgesic infusions become opioid tolerant; thus, respiratory depression is rare.

CHARACTERISTICS OF PAIN

Only the patient can describe pain characteristics. Each characteristic presents implications for how you help to manage a patient's pain. The PQRSTU model is an effective tool for assessing pain in adults and determining interventions to relieve the pain (see Table 11.3).

Timing (Onset, Duration, and Pattern)

Ask questions to determine the start, duration, and time sequence of pain. When did it begin? How long has it lasted? Does it occur at the same time each day? How often does it recur? It is sometimes easier to diagnose the nature of pain by identifying time factors. The onset of sudden and severe pain is easier to assess than gradual, mild discomfort. Knowing the time cycle of a patient's pain helps you intervene before the pain occurs or worsens.

Precipitating Factors

Determine the specific events or conditions that precipitate or aggravate pain. Ask a patient to describe activities that cause pain such as sitting, bending over, drinking coffee or alcohol, urination, swallowing, or stress. Ask the patient to demonstrate actions that cause painful responses such as coughing or turning in a certain manner. After identifying specific factors, it is easier to plan interventions to avoid worsening the pain.

Quality

There is no common pain vocabulary in general use. Patients describe pain in their own way. Patients often use *hurt* and *ache* to describe their pain, reserving the word *pain* for severe discomfort. Knowing the quality of pain helps to select appropriate therapies to treat it. When assessing the quality of pain, do not provide descriptive words for a patient. Assessment is more accurate if a patient describes the sensation in his or her own words in response to open-ended questions. For example, say, "Tell me what your pain feels like." When a patient's description fits the pattern forming in your assessment, you are able to make a clearer analysis of the nature and type of pain. This leads to more appropriate pain management because you treat different types of pain differently.

Relief Measures

Learn whether a patient has an effective way of relieving pain such as changing position, pacing, rocking, eating, praying, or applying heat or cold to a painful site. A patient's methods are often ones that you can use for treatment.

Determine whether patients use relief measures safely in their home. Patients gain trust when they know you are willing to try their relief measures. They also gain a sense of control over the pain instead of the pain controlling them. Identify all health care providers. Patients with chronic pain are likely to try alternative health care methods.

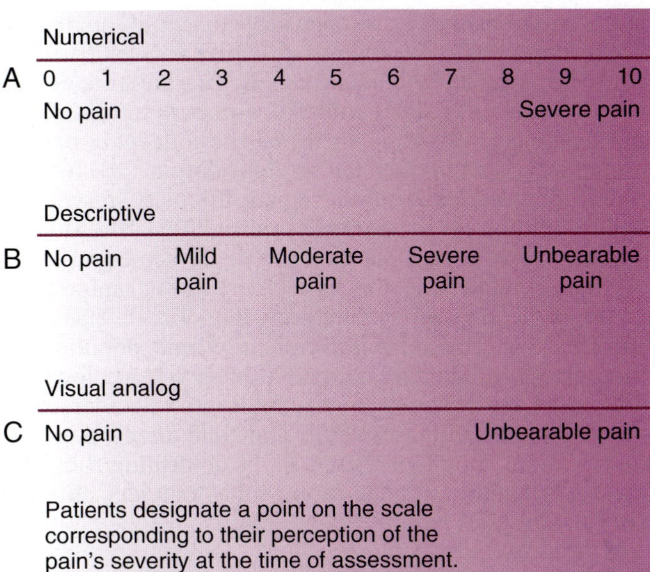

Fig. 11.7 Sample pain scales. **A,** Numerical. **B,** Descriptive. **C,** Visual analog.

Region/Location

To assess pain location, ask a patient to point to all areas of discomfort. To localize the pain more specifically, have the patient trace the area from the most severe point outward. This is difficult to do if the pain is diffuse, involves several sites, or involves large parts of the body. Use a drawing showing the location of pain as the baseline if the pain changes. Use anatomical landmarks and descriptive terminology to record the pain location (e.g., "Pain is in the right upper quadrant of the abdomen"). Pain classified by location is also superficial or cutaneous, deep or visceral, localized or diffuse, referred or radiating.

Severity

One of the most subjective and therefore most useful characteristics for reporting pain is its severity or intensity. Nurses use a variety of pain scales to help patients communicate pain intensity. Many are available in foreign languages. Examples of pain intensity scales include the verbal descriptor scale (VDS), the numerical rating scale (NRS), and the visual analog scale (VAS) (Fig. 11.7). Use a scale to measure the current severity of a patient's pain. In addition, ask patients to rate their average pain and the worst pain they have had over the past 24 hours. This helps to determine an average pain intensity, allowing you to see trends. An NRS requires patients to rate pain on a line scale of 0–10, with 0 representing no pain and 10 representing the worst pain the patient can imagine. These scales work best when assessing pain intensity before and after a therapy (e.g., ambulation or an analgesic). A VDS consists of a line with three- to six-word descriptors equally spaced along the line. Show the patient the scale and ask him or her to choose the descriptor that best represents the severity of pain. A VAS consists of a straight line without labeled subdivisions. The straight line shows a continuum of intensity and has labeled end points (no pain to pain as bad as it could possibly be). The patient indicates pain by marking the appropriate point on the line (Pasero and McCaffery, 2011). An effective pain scale is easy to use, understandable, and not time-consuming. If a patient can read and understand a scale easily, the description of pain is more accurate. If patients use a hearing aid or glasses, be sure that they are using them when answering pain assessment questions or marking the pain scale. Descriptive scales are useful in assessing pain severity and evaluating changes in a patient's condition. Once you select a scale that works for a patient, be sure to use it consistently. Do not use pain scale ratings to compare one patient with another but only to compare one patient's current pain level with what it was previously. Several pain scales are available to assess pain in children. Wong and Baker (Wong-Baker FACES Foundation, 2016) developed the FACES pain rating scale to assess pain in children (Fig. 11.8). The scale shows drawings of six faces ranging from a very happy, smiling face for "no

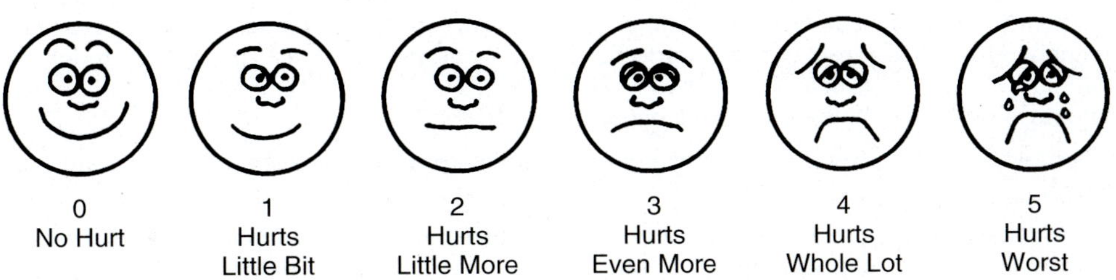

Fig. 11.8 Wong–Baker FACES pain rating scale. (Retrieved May 3, 2017, with permission from http://www.WongBakerFACES.org. Originally published in *Whaley & Wong's Nursing Care of Infants and Children*. © Elsevier Inc.)

pain" to increasingly less happy faces to a final sad, tearful face for "worst pain." Children as young as 3 years of age can use the scale. The advantage is that patients do not have to interpret the meaning of numbers or adjectives. The faces clearly and quickly depict the concept of pain or discomfort (Wong-Baker FACES Foundation, 2016). Another tool designed to measure pain intensity in children is the Oucher pain scale (Beyer et al., 1992). The Oucher consists of two separate scales: the 0–10 scale on the left for older children and the six-picture photographic scale on the right for younger children (Fig. 11.9). There are Oucher scales for several common ethnic populations. Photographs of the face of a child in increasing levels of discomfort are designed to cue children into understanding what pain is and its severity. The child merely points to the selection, simplifying the task of describing the pain. There are additional pain rating tools for older children with verbal skills, neonates, and infants.

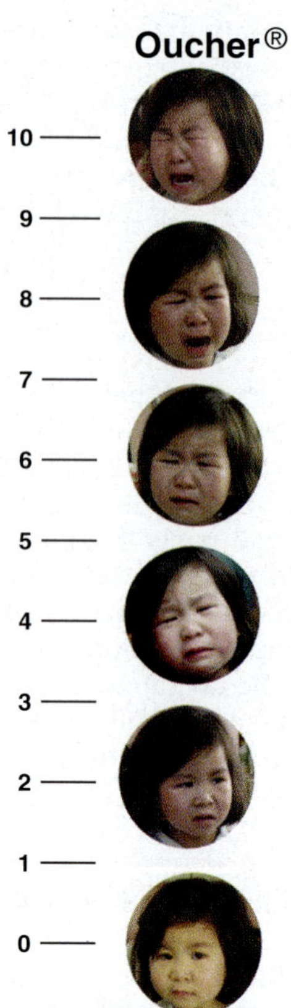

Fig. 11.9 Asian girl version of Oucher pain scale. (The Asian versions of the Oucher scale [male and female] were developed and copyrighted in 2003 by CH Yeh [University of Pittsburgh] and CH Wang, Taiwan.)

Effect of Pain on a Patient

Pain alters a person's lifestyle and psychological well-being. For example, chronic/persistent pain often causes loss of control, loneliness, and an impaired quality of life. To understand a patient's pain experience, ask the patient what the pain prevents him or her from doing. Patients who live with daily pain or who have prolonged pain during a hospitalized illness are less able to participate in routine activities, which often leads to physical deconditioning. This deconditioning slows recovery of a patient who is hospitalized.

SKILL 11.1 Patient-Controlled Analgesia

Equipment

- PCA system and tubing
- Identification label and time tape (may come attached and completed by pharmacy)
- Needleless connector
- Alcohol swab
- Adhesive tape
- Clean gloves (when applicable)
- Equipment for vital signs and pulse oximeter, capnography (carbon dioxide) monitoring equipment

STEP	RATIONALE
Assessment	
1. Check accuracy and completeness of memory address register (MAR) or computer printout with health care provider's order for the patient's name, name of medication, dose, frequency of medication (continuous or demand or both), and lockout period.	Health care provider order required for administration of opioid medication. Ensures patient receives right medications.
2. Check medical record for the patient's history for drug allergies and typical reactions.	Avoids placing the patient at risk for allergic reaction.
3. Review medication information in drug reference manual or consult with pharmacist if uncertain about any medications to be administered.	Understanding medications before administering them prevents medication errors (Adhikari et al., 2014).
4. Perform hand hygiene. Assess severity and character of the patient's pain. Use a standard pain scale. If the patient is unable to provide a self-report, select an appropriate scale for assessing pain in patients who are nonverbal or not cognitively alert.	Reveals source and nature of pain and factors that may increase pain.

STEP	RATIONALE
5. Assess environment for factors that could contribute to pain (e.g., noise, room temperature).	Elimination of irritating stimuli may help to reduce pain perception.
6. Assess for conditions that predispose patients to unwanted effects from opioids. Known, untreated, or unknown obstructive sleep apnea (OSA) poses a significant risk for respiratory depression. Use the STOP-BANG questionnaire to assess for OSA (Lockhart et al., 2013) (see Chapter 33 and agency policy).	Assessment should be completed preoperatively by anesthesia. Identification allows treatment teams (surgeon, respiratory therapy, anesthesia) to take appropriate precautions such as making continuous positive airway pressure or bilevel positive airway pressure ventilation devices available.
7. Perform hand hygiene. Apply clean gloves. Assess patency of i.v. access and surrounding tissue for inflammation or swelling.	Reduces transmission of infection. I.v. line needs to be patent for safe administration of pain medication. Confirmation of placement of i.v. catheter and integrity of surrounding tissues ensures that medication is administered safely.
8. If the patient had surgery, inspect incision while still wearing clean gloves. Gently palpate around area for tenderness. Use sterile gloves if necessary to place hand directly on incision. Remove gloves and perform hand hygiene.	Reveals evidence of tissue trauma or damage, which stimulates peripheral pain receptors to transmit impulses to cortex to create conscious awareness of pain.
Clinical decision point: Be aware that nausea is not an allergic reaction and it can be treated; pruritus alone is not an allergic reaction and is common to opioid use. Pruritus is treatable and does not rule out the use of PCA.	
9. Assess the patient's knowledge and perceived effectiveness of previous pain management strategies, especially previous PCA use.	Response to pain control strategies helps identify learning needs and affects the patient's willingness to try therapy.
Planning	
1. Collect appropriate equipment. Draw curtains around the patient's bed or close door to room.	Aids in organization. Maintains patient privacy.
2. Prepare and organize equipment.	
3. Explain procedure to the patient and family.	Reduces anxiety and fear.
Implementation	
1. Perform hand hygiene.	Reduces transmission of infection.
2. Obtain PCA analgesic in cartridge prepared by pharmacy. Check label of medication against the MAR two times: when removing from storage and when preparing for assembly.	Follows the six rights of medication administration to be sure of correct medication. *This is the first and second check for accuracy.*
3. At the bedside, identify the patient using at least two identifiers (e.g., name and birthday or name and medical record number) according to agency policy. Compare identifiers with information on the patient's MAR or medical record.	Minimizes risk for medication error and harm to the patient. Ensures correct patient. Complies with The Joint Commission standards and improves patient safety (TJC, 2018).
4. At the bedside, compare the MAR or computer printout with the name of medication on the drug cartridge. Have a second RN confirm health care provider's order and correct setup of the PCA. The second RN checks the order and the device independently and does not just look at existing setup.	Ensures the correct patient receives the right medication. *This is the third check for accuracy.*
5. Before initiating analgesia, explain purpose and demonstrate function of PCA to the patient and family as follows:	Allows patient participation in care and independence in pain control. Preoperative education about PCA therapy improves postoperative pain relief (Pasero and McCaffery, 2011).
a. Explain type of medication in device.	
b. Explain that device safely administers self-initiated small but frequent amounts of medication when needed to provide comfort and minimizes side effects from analgesia.	
c. Explain that self-dosing will aid in repositioning, walking, or coughing and deep breathing.	
d. Explain that device is programmed to deliver ordered type and dose of pain medication, lockout interval, and 1- to 4-h dosage limits. Explain how lockout time prevents overdose.	
e. Demonstrate to the patient how to push medication demand button (see illustration).	
f. Instruct the patient to notify a nurse for possible side effects, problems in gaining pain relief, changes in severity or location of pain, alarm sounding, or questions.	
6. Apply clean gloves. Check infuser and patient-controlled module for accurate labeling or evidence of leaking.	Avoids medication error and injury to the patient.

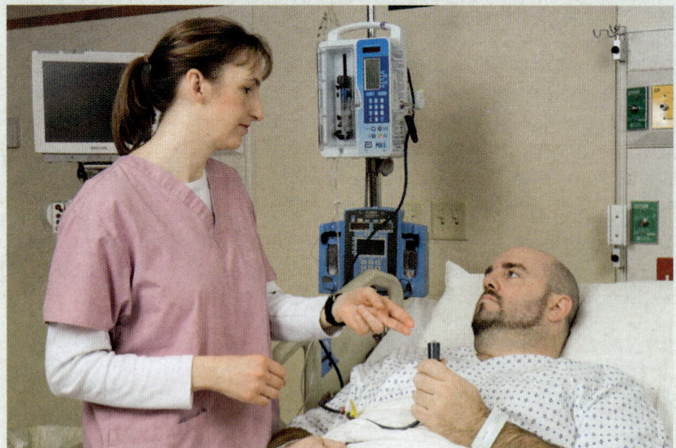

Step 5e Patient learns how to press PCA device button.

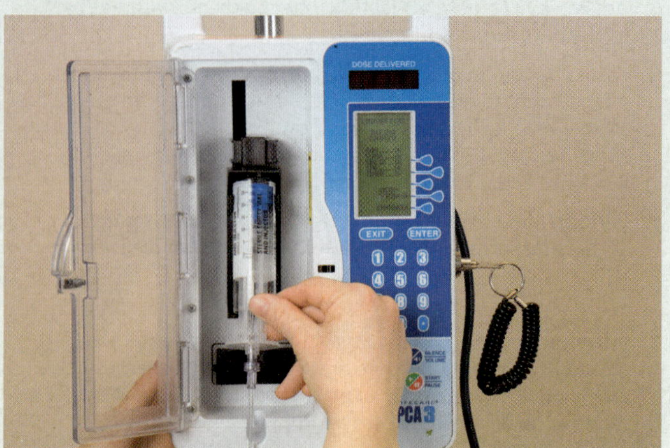

Step 8 Nurse inserting drug cartridge into PCA device.

STEP	RATIONALE
7. Position the patient comfortably to be sure that venipuncture or central line site is accessible.	Ensures unimpeded flow of infusion.
8. Insert drug cartridge into infusion device (see illustration) and prime tubing.	Locks system and prevents air from infusing into i.v. tubing.
9. Attach needleless adapter to tubing adapter of patient-controlled module.	Needed to connect with i.v. line.
10. Wipe injection port of maintenance i.v. line vigorously with alcohol or antiseptic for 15 s and allow to dry.	Minimizes entry of surface microorganisms during needle insertion, reducing risk of catheter-related bloodstream infection.
11. Insert needleless adapter into injection port nearest patient (at Y-site of peripheral i.v. or central line, or connect to its own i.v. site). There should not be a chance to use the PCA tubing for administering an i.v. push with another drug.	Establishes route for medication to enter main i.v. line. Needleless systems prevent needlestick injuries. Prevents medication interaction and incompatibility.
12. Secure connection and anchor PCA tubing with tape. Label PCA tubing.	Prevents dislodging of needleless adapter from port. Facilitates the patient's ability to ambulate. Label prevents error from connecting tubing from different device to PCA.
13. Program computerized PCA pump as ordered to deliver prescribed medication dose and lockout interval. Have second RN check setting. (**Note:** Recheck with oncoming RN during shift hand-off to ensure line reconciliation.)	Ensures safe, therapeutic drug administration. With appropriate dose intervals (e.g., 10 min), usually an appreciable analgesic effect and/or mild sedation is achieved before the patient can access the next dose, and thus there is a lower chance for oversedation and respiratory depression (Burchum and Rosenthal, 2016).
14. Administer loading dose of analgesia as prescribed. Manually give a one-time dose or turn on pump and program dose into pump.	Establishes initial level of analgesia.
15. Remove and discard gloves and supplies in appropriate containers. Dispose of empty cassette or syringe in compliance with institutional policy. Perform hand hygiene.	Reduces transmission of microorganisms. The Federal Controlled Substances Act regulates control and dispensation of opioids for all institutions.
16. If experiencing pain, have the patient demonstrate use of PCA system; if not, have the patient repeat instructions given earlier.	Repeating instructions reinforces learning. Checking the patient's understanding through return demonstration helps you determine the patient's level of understanding and ability to manipulate device.
17. Be sure venipuncture or central line site is protected, and recheck before leaving the patient. Perform hand hygiene.	Ensures patency of i.v. line. Reduces transmission of infection.
18. **To discontinue PCA:**	
a. Check health care provider order for discontinuation. Obtain necessary PCA information from pump for documentation; note date, time, amount infused, and amount of drug wasted, and reason for wastage.	Ensures correct documentation of a Schedule II drug. Two RNs must witness waste of opioids (narcotics) and document to meet requirements of the Controlled Substances Act for scheduled drugs. **Note:** Some agencies have a specific controlled substance disposal program (CsRx), which facilitates disposal of controlled substances in a safe, efficient manner and prevent diversion (check agency policy).

STEP	RATIONALE
b. Perform hand hygiene and apply clean gloves. Turn pump off. Disconnect PCA tubing from primary i.v. line, but maintain i.v. access.	Reduces transmission of infection. Ensures continuation of i.v..
c. Dispose of empty cartridge, tubing, and gloves according to agency policy. Perform hand hygiene.	
Evaluation	
1. Use pain rating scale to evaluate the patient's pain intensity after treatments and procedures according to agency policy.	Determines response to PCA dosing. Documenting "PCA in use" or "PCA effective" is not an adequate record of patient's pain level.
2. Observe the patient for nausea or pruritus.	Common side effects of opioid.
3. Monitor the patient's level of sedation, vital signs, and pulse oximetry or capnography every 1 – 2 h for the first 12 h. Monitor more often at the start, during first 24 h, and at night when hypoventilation and hypoxia tend to occur (Burchum and Rosenthal, 2016). Follow agency policy.	The patient is at highest risk the first 24 h of use. Excess sedation (difficult to arouse) precedes respiratory depression.
4. Have the patient demonstrate dose delivery.	Evaluates skill in use of PCA.
5. According to agency policy, evaluate number of attempts (number of times the patient pushed the button), delivery of demand doses (number of times drug actually given and total amount of medication delivered in a particular time frame), and basal dose if ordered.	Assists in evaluating effectiveness of PCA dose and frequency in relieving pain. Maintains compliance with Controlled Substances Act.
6. Observe the patient initiate self-care.	Demonstrates pain relief.
7. **Use teach back:** "I want to be sure I explained how PCA will help with your pain and how you should use the device. Explain to me how you should use the PCA device. What will you do if you find PCA is not relieving your pain?" Revise your instruction now or develop a plan for revised patient/family caregiver teaching if patient/family caregiver is not able to teach back correctly.	Determines the patient's/family caregiver's level of understanding of instructional topic.

Recording and Reporting

- Record drug, concentration, dose (basal and/or demand), time started, lockout time, and amount of i.v. solution infused and remaining solution in nurses' notes in electronic health record (EHR) or chart. Many agencies have special PCA documentation forms.
- Document your evaluation of patient/family caregiver learning.
- Record regular assessment of the patient response to analgesia on PCA medication form, in nurses' notes in EHR, on pain assessment flow sheet, or on other documentation according to agency policy. Assessment includes vital signs, oximetry or capnography, sedation status, pain rating, and status of vascular access site.

Unexpected Outcomes and Related Interventions

- The patient verbalizes continued or worsening discomfort or displays nonverbal behaviors indicative of pain.
  - Perform complete pain reassessment.
  - Assess for possible complications other than pain.
  - Inspect i.v. site for possible catheter occlusion or infiltration.
  - Evaluate number of attempts and deliveries initiated by the patient.
  - Check that maintenance i.v. fluid is running continuously.
  - Evaluate pump for operational problems.
  - Consult with health care provider.
- The patient is sedated and not easily aroused.
  - Stop PCA and notify health care provider.
  - Elevate head of bed 30° unless contraindicated.
  - Instruct the patient to take deep breaths.
  - Apply oxygen at 2 L/min per nasal cannula (if ordered).
  - Assess vital signs.
  - Evaluate amount of opioid delivered within past 4 – 8 hours.
  - Ask the family members whether they pressed the button without patient's knowledge.
  - Review MAR for other possible sedating drugs.
  - Prepare to administer opioid-reversing agent.
  - Observe the patient frequently (Burchum and Rosenthal, 2016).
- The patient is unable to manipulate PCA device to maintain pain control.
  - Consult with health care provider regarding alternative medication route or possibly a basal (continuous) dose.
  - If agency allows, determine whether reliable family caregiver can responsibly manipulate PCA device (Pasero and McCaffery, 2011).

KEY POINTS

- Acute pain, a protective mechanism that warns a person of tissue injury, is completely subjective.
- Misconceptions about pain lead to undertreatment.
- A patient's age, gender, anxiety, culture, previous experience, and meaning of pain influence the pain experience.

- The difference between acute and chronic pain involves the duration of discomfort, physical signs and symptoms, and the patient's perceptions regarding relief.
- A comprehensive assessment of a patient's pain must be performed to understand the extent to which pain affects the patient's ability to function.
- The patient's family and friends are a key resource in pain assessment.
- Eliminating sources of painful stimuli is a basic nursing measure for promoting comfort.
- Nonpharmacological therapies are effective in altering a patient's perception of pain, promoting muscle relaxation, and giving the patient control over pain.
- When administering opioids, know that respiratory depression is clinically significant only if there is a decrease in the rate and depth of respirations from a patient's baseline assessment. Give i.v. naloxone (Narcan) to reverse respiratory depression.
- For patients unable to self-report pain, be alert for subtle behaviors that indicate pain.
- Using a regular around-the-clock (ATC) schedule for analgesic administration is more effective than an as-needed schedule.
- A patient-controlled analgesia (PCA) device gives patients pain control with a low risk for overdose.
- Your primary role in caring for a patient who receives local anesthesia is to protect the patient from injury.
- The goal of therapy for patients with chronic pain is to anticipate and prevent pain.
- When a patient is receiving epidural analgesia, do not administer supplemental doses of opioids or sedatives because of possible additive central nervous system effects.

REFERENCES

Adhikari R, Tocher J, Smith P, Corcoran J, MacArthur J. A multi-disciplinary approach to medication safety and the implication for nursing education and practice. Nurse Educ Today 2014;34(2):185.

American Nurses Association (ANA). Code of ethics for nurses with interpretive statements. 2015. Available from: http://www.nursingworld.org/MainMenuCategories/EthicsStandards/CodeofEthicsforNurses/Code-of-Ethics-For-Nurses.html.

Beyer JE, Denyes MJ, Villarruel AM. The creation, validation, and continuing development of the Oucher: a measure of pain intensity in children. J Pediatr Nurs 1992;7(5):335.

Burchum JR, Rosenthal LD. Lehne's pharmacology for nursing care. St. Louis: Elsevier; 2016.

Cheatle MD. Assessing suicide risk in patients with chronic pain and depression. J Fam Pract 2014;63(6):S6.

Chou R, Gordon DB, de Leon-Casasola OA, Rosenberg JM, Bickler S, Brennan T, et al. Guidelines on the management of postoperative pain. J Pain 2016;17(2):131.

Cole LC, LoBiondo-Wood G. Music as an adjuvant therapy in control of pain and symptoms in hospitalized adults: a systematic review. Pain Manag Nurs 2014;15(1):406.

Cooney MF, Czarnecki M, Dunwoody C, Eksterowicz N, Merkel S, Oakes L, et al. American Society for Pain Management Nursing Position Statement with Clinical Practice Guidelines: authorized agent controlled analgesia. Pain Manag Nurs 2013;14(3):176.

Dowell D, Haegerich TM, Chou R. CDC Guideline for prescribing opioids for chronic pain—United States, 2016. MMWR Recomm Rep 2016;65(RR-1):1.

Huether SE, McCance KL. Understanding pathophysiology. St. Louis: Elsevier; 2017.

Institute of Medicine (IOM). Relieving pain in America: a blueprint for transforming prevention, care, education, and research. Washington, DC: National Academies Press; 2011.

International Association for the Study of Pain (IASP): Pain taxonomy, 2014b, https://www.iasp-pain.org/Education/Content.aspx?ItemNumber=1698. Accessed July 10, 2019.

Krauss BS, Calligaris L, Green SM, Barbi E. Current concepts in management of pain in children in the emergency department. Lancet 2016;387:83.

Lewis SL, Dirksen SR, Heitkemper MM, Bucher L, Harding M. Medical-surgical nursing: assessment and management of clinical problems. 9th ed. St. Louis: Elsevier; 2014.

Lockhart EM, Willingham MD, Abdallah AB, Helsten DL, Bedair BA, Thomas J, et al. Obstructive sleep apnea screening and postoperative mortality in a large surgical cohort. Sleep Med. 2013;14(5):407.

Mendell LM. Constructing and deconstructing the gate theory of pain. Pain 2014;155(2):210.

National Comprehensive Cancer Network (NCCN). Adult cancer pain. 2017. Available from: https://www.nccn.org/professionals/physician_gls/pdf/pain.pdf.

Oncology Nursing Society (ONS). Palliative care for people with cancer. 2016. Available from: https://www.ons.org/make-difference/ons-center-advocacy-and-health-policy/position-statements/palliative-care-people.

Pasero C, McCaffery M. Pain assessment and pharmacologic management. St. Louis: Mosby; 2011.

Reynolds J, Drew D, Dunwoody C. American Society for Pain Management Nursing Position Statement: pain management at the end of life. Pain Manag Nurs 2013;14(3):172.

The Joint Commission (TJC). 2018 National Patient Safety Goals. Oakbrook Terrace, IL: TJC; 2018. Available from: https://www.jointcommission.org/standards_information/npsgs.aspx.

Wong-Baker FACES Foundation. Wong-Baker FACES Pain Rating Scale. 2016. Available from: http://www.WongBakerFACES.org.

12 Promoting Safety in Health Care Environment

OBJECTIVES

After reading this chapter, the student should be able to:

- Define concept of patient safety.
- Describe common physical hazards that pose risks to patient safety such as motor vehicle accident, poison, fire, falls, disaster, pathogen transmission, immunization, and pollution.
- Explain the factors influencing patient safety among all age group.
- Discuss the importance of national patient safety resources and standards for promoting patient safety.
- Describe the nurse's role in prevention of hazards and ensuring patient safety in care.
- Assess risks to patients' safety within health care settings and the home including acute and restorative care.
- Explain different types of restraints used for patient safety and approaches for establishing a restraint-free environment.
- Describe developmentally appropriate nursing interventions for reducing risks for falls, fires, poisonings, and electrical hazards.
- Describe methods or safety devices to evaluate interventions designed to maintain or promote patient safety.

KEY TERMS

basic human needs, p. 249
carbon monoxide, p. 249
chemical restraints, p. 260
grab bars, p. 261
heat exhaustion, p. 249
hypothermia, p. 249
immunization, p. 251
pathogen, p. 251
physical hazards, p. 249
restraint, p. 260
safety, p. 247
serious reportable events (SREs), p. 247
workplace violence, p. 253

INTRODUCTION

Safety, often defined as freedom from psychological and physical injury, is a basic human need. Health care provided in a safe manner and a safe community environment is essential for a patient's survival and well-being. A safe environment reduces the risk for illness and injury and helps to contain the cost of health care by preventing extended lengths of treatment and/or hospitalization, improving or maintaining a patient's functional status, and increasing a patient's sense of well-being. The Institute of Medicine's report *To Err Is Human: Building a Safer Health System* (IOM, 2000) was a pivotal publication that brought patient safety to the forefront of health care. This report indicated that 44,000–98,000 people die each year as a result of preventable medical errors. In an effort to improve patient safety, many organizations became devoted to developing and monitoring key health care safety initiatives and providing information to health care organizations and the public. Health care organizations foster a patient-centered safety culture by continually focusing on performance improvement endeavors, risk management findings, and safety reports; providing current reliable technology; integrating evidence-based practice into procedures; designing a safe work environment and atmosphere; and providing continuing education and access to appropriate resources for staff.

Much of the force behind the changes for improving safety in health care settings comes from regulatory and accreditation agencies. The National Accreditation Board for Hospitals and Healthcare Providers (NABH) and The Joint Commission (TJC) stress the importance of error prevention and patient safety. The Speak Up Campaign encourages patients to take a role in preventing health care errors by becoming active, involved, and informed participants in their health care (TJC, 2017b). For example, patients are encouraged to ask health care workers whether they have washed their hands before providing care. The 2017 TJC National Patient Safety Goals are specifically directed at reducing the risk of medical errors.

The National Quality Forum (NQF, 2017a) has the mission of improving the quality of health care. The NQF focuses on building consensus on national priorities and goals for performance improvement in health care. The NQF also endorses an updated list of 29 **serious reportable events (SREs)** (Box 12.1) that are a major focus for patient safety

Box 12.1 National Quality Forum List of Serious Reportable Events

Surgical or Invasive Procedure Events

- Surgery or other invasive procedure performed on a wrong site
- Surgery or other invasive procedure performed on a wrong patient
- Wrong surgical or other invasive procedure performed on a patient
- Unintended retention of foreign object in a patient after surgery or other invasive procedure
- Intraoperative or immediately postoperative/postprocedure death in ASA class 1 patient

Product or Device Events

- Patient death or serious injury associated with use of contaminated drugs, devices, or biologicals provided by health care setting
- Patient death or serious injury associated with use or function of a device in patient care in which device is used for functions other than intended
- Patient death or serious injury associated with intravascular air embolism that occurs while being cared for in health care setting

Patient Protection Events

- Discharge or release of patient/resident of any age who is unable to make decisions to other than authorized person
- Patient death or serious injury associated with patient elopement (disappearance)
- Patient suicide, attempted suicide, or self-harm that results in serious injury while being cared for in health care setting

Care Management Events

- Patient death or serious injury associated with medication error (e.g., errors involving wrong drug, wrong dose, wrong patient, wrong time, wrong rate, wrong preparation, or wrong route of administration)
- Patient death or serious injury associated with unsafe administration of blood products
- Maternal death or serious injury associated with labor or delivery in low-risk pregnancy while being cared for in health care setting
- Death or serious injury of neonate associated with labor or delivery in low-risk pregnancy
- Patient death or serious injury associated with a fall while being cared for in health care setting
- Any stage 3, stage 4, and unstageable pressure injuries acquired after admission/presentation to health care setting
- Artificial insemination with wrong donor sperm or wrong egg
- Patient death or serious injury resulting from irretrievable loss of irreplaceable biological specimen
- Patient death or serious injury resulting from failure to follow up or communicate laboratory, pathology, or radiology test results

Environmental Events

- Patient or staff death or serious injury associated with electric shock in the course of patient care process in health care setting
- Any incident in which system that is designated for oxygen or other gas to be delivered to patient contains no gas or wrong gas or is contaminated by toxic substances
- Patient or staff death or serious injury associated with a burn incurred from any source in the course of patient care process in health care setting
- Patient death or serious injury associated with use of physical restraints or bedrails while being cared for in health care setting

Radiologic Events

- Death or serious injury of patient or staff associated with introduction of metallic object into magnetic resonance imaging (MRI) area

Potential Criminal Events

- Any instance of care ordered or provided by someone impersonating physician, nurse, pharmacist, or other licensed health care provider
- Abduction of patient/resident of any age
- Sexual abuse/assault on patient or staff member within or on grounds of health care setting
- Death or serious injury of patient or staff member resulting from physical assault (i.e., battery) that occurs within or on grounds of health care setting

initiatives (NQF, 2017b). The insurance agencies now deny payment to hospitals for any hospital-acquired conditions resulting from or complicated by the occurrence of certain SREs that were not present on admission (Box 12.2). Some hospital-acquired conditions are nurse-sensitive indicators, meaning that nursing interventions directly affect their development.

As part of the health care team, you have the professional responsibility to engage in activities that support a patient-centered safety culture. Quality and Safety Education for Nurses (QSEN) was developed to meet the challenge of preparing future nurses to have the knowledge, skills, and attitudes needed to continuously improve the quality and safety of the health care systems where they work (QSEN Institute, 2017). The QSEN safety competency requires you to "minimize risk of harm to patients and providers through both system effectiveness and individual performance." Use of critical thinking skills (see Chapter 18) coupled with application of the nursing process (see Chapter 19) enables you to become a provider of safe patient care and an active participant in health promotion.

PHYSICAL ENVIRONMENT

Health care provided in a safe manner and within a safe community environment is essential for well-being of patients. Vulnerable groups that require help in achieving a safe environment include infants, children, older adults, ill or injured people, people with physical and mental disabilities, people who are illiterate, and people who live in poverty. To be effective, you need to understand factors that contribute to a safe environment in the home or health care agency and be able to thoroughly assess the environment for threats to safety. Understanding how alterations in mobility, sensory function, and cognition affect patients' safety is also important (see Chapters 14 and 27). A safe environment includes meeting basic human

Box 12.2 2016 Centers for Medicare and Medicaid Services Hospital-Acquired Conditions and Present-on-Admission Indicators

- Foreign object retained after surgery
- Air embolism
- Blood incompatibility
- Stage 3 and stage 4 pressure ulcers
- Falls and trauma: fracture, dislocation, intracranial injury, crushing injury, burn, other injuries
- Manifestations of poor glycemic control: diabetic ketoacidosis, nonketotic hyperosmolar coma, hypoglycemic coma, secondary diabetes with ketoacidosis, and secondary diabetes with hyperosmolarity
- Catheter-associated urinary tract infections
- Vascular catheter-associated infections
- Surgical site infection, mediastinitis, following coronary artery bypass graft (CABG)
- Surgical site infection following bariatric surgery for obesity: laparoscopic gastric bypass, gastroenterostomy, laparoscopic gastric restrictive surgery
- Surgical site infection following certain orthopedic procedures: spine, neck, shoulder, elbow
- Surgical site infection following cardiac implantable electronic device (CIED)
- Deep vein thrombosis and pulmonary embolism following certain orthopedic procedures: total knee replacement or hip replacement
- Iatrogenic pneumothorax with venous catheterization

From Centers for Medicare and Medicaid Services (CMS): *Hospital-acquired conditions,* 2012, http://www.cms.gov/Medicare/Medicare-Fee-for-Service-Payment/HospitalAcqCond/Hospital-Acquired_Conditions.html.

needs, reducing physical hazards, and reducing transmission of pathogens.

Basic Human Needs

The physiological needs of adequate oxygen, nutrition, and favorable temperature and humidity are basic human needs often at risk from various environmental hazards. People need to meet these basic needs before physical and psychological safety and security can be addressed.

Oxygen

Patients who require supplemental oxygen in health care settings can be at risk because oxygen is highly flammable. Fire can occur when oxygen therapy is combined with smoking or exposure to a heat source, which can cause severe burns or death. Strict codes regulate the use and storage of medical oxygen in health care agencies. This is not the case in the home environment. In the home, smoking combined with home oxygen use is by far the leading cause of burns, reported fires, deaths, and injuries. Be sure to administer oxygen safely and provide patients and family caregivers the information needed to manage oxygen in the home (see Chapter 24).

Know factors in a patient's environment that decrease the amount of available oxygen. For example, an improperly functioning heating system is a hazard in the home. A furnace, stove, or fireplace that is not properly vented introduces carbon monoxide into the environment. **Carbon monoxide** affects a person's oxygenation by binding strongly with hemoglobin, preventing the formation of oxyhemoglobin, and reducing the supply of oxygen delivered to the tissues (see Chapter 24). Low concentrations of oxygen cause nausea, dizziness, headache, and fatigue. Higher concentrations are often fatal. Unintentional, non–fire-related (UNFR) carbon monoxide poisoning is one of the most common causes of poisoning in the United States and results in approximately 15,000 emergency department visits annually (Centers for Disease Control and Prevention [CDC], 2011).

Nutrition

Meeting nutritional needs requires knowledge about healthy food and food safety. Chapter 20 details the principles of balanced nutrition and therapeutic diets. Health care agencies are required to meet State Board of Health regulations for storage, preparation, and provision of food. In the home, some patients do not know how to properly refrigerate, store, and prepare food. A patient needs a refrigerator with a freezer compartment to keep perishable foods fresh. An adequate, clean water supply is necessary for drinking and to wash fresh produce and dishes. Regular garbage collection is necessary to maintain sanitary conditions. Foods need to be adequately cooked to kill any residing organisms. If a patient does not prepare or store foods properly, it increases the risk for infections and food poisoning from bacteria such as *Escherichia coli, Salmonella,* or *Listeria.* Groups at highest risk for food poisoning are children, pregnant women, older adults, and people with compromised immune systems.

Temperature

A person's comfort zone is usually between 18.3°C and 23.8°C (65°F and 75°F). Temperature extremes, which often occur during the winter and summer, affect comfort, productivity, and safety. Exposure to severe cold for prolonged periods may cause frostbite and accidental **hypothermia** (see Chapter 6). Older adults, infants, young children, patients with cardiovascular conditions, patients who have ingested drugs or excess alcohol, and people who are homeless are at high risk for hypothermia. Prolonged exposure to extreme heat changes body electrolyte balance and raises the core body temperature, resulting in heatstroke or **heat exhaustion.** People of any age can be at risk for heat exhaustion when the weather is extremely hot, regardless of humidity.

Physical Hazards

More than 31.7 million nonfatal injuries take place each year, with most occurring inside or outside of the home (CDC, 2017c). Physical hazards in the environment threaten a person's safety and often result in physical or psychological injury or death. Unintentional injuries are the fourth leading cause of death of all ages (Kochanek et al., 2016). Motor vehicle accidents are the leading cause, followed by poisonings and falls. Additional environmental hazards include fire and disasters. Your role as a nurse is to educate patients about common safety hazards and how to prevent injury, while placing emphasis on hazards to which patients are more vulnerable.

Motor Vehicle Accidents

Vehicle design and equipment such as seat belts, air bags, and laminated windshields that remain in one piece when impacted have improved vehicular safety. State laws relating to licensing of young drivers, safety belt use, child restraint use, and motorcycle helmets exist for protection of drivers. It is important that children ride in child safety seats and booster seats appropriate for their age and weight and the type of car. The American Academy of Pediatrics (AAP, 2017) recommends the following:

1. All infants and toddlers should ride in a rear-facing car safety seat (CSS) until they are 2 years of age or until they reach the highest weight or height allowed by the manufacturer of their CSS.
2. Children who have outgrown the rear-facing weight or height limit for their CSS should use a forward-facing CSS with a harness for as long as possible, up to the highest weight or height allowed by the manufacturer of their CSS.
3. All children whose weight or height exceeds the forward-facing limit for their CSS should use a belt-positioning booster seat until the vehicle seat belt fits properly, typically when they have reached 4 feet 9 inches in height and are between 8 and 12 years of age. All children younger than 13 years of age should ride in the back seat.
4. When children are old enough and large enough for the vehicle seat belt to fit them correctly, they should always use lap-and-shoulder seat belts for the best protection.

Nearly all cars and trucks made after September 2002 are equipped with a LATCH (lower anchors and tethers for children) system for installing child safety seats (Fig. 12.1). There are lower anchors in the back seat where the seat cushions meet and tether anchors located behind the seat either on the panel behind the seat or seat back, ceiling or floor. All lower anchors are rated for a maximum weight of 65 lb (total weight includes car seat and child) (AAP, 2017).

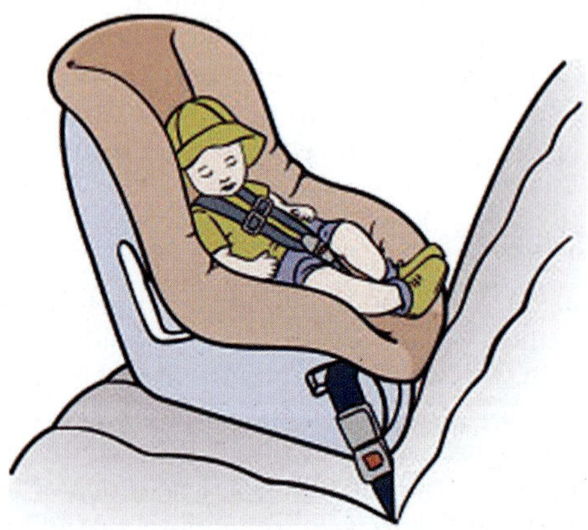

Fig 12.1 Rear-facing infant car seat. (Courtesy Brian and Mayannyn Sallee, Las Vegas, NV.)

According to CDC, the risk of motor vehicle accidents is higher among 16- to 19-year-old drivers than any other age group (CDC, 2017b). Teens tend to underestimate dangerous situations or are unable to recognize hazardous situations (e.g., texting while driving). In addition, they tend to speed and allow shorter headways, ride with intoxicated drivers, and drive after using alcohol and drugs. Teens have the lowest rate of seat belt use. Elderly drivers are keeping their licenses longer and driving more miles than in the past. Age-related decline in vision and cognitive functioning (ability to reason and remember) and physical changes affect driving abilities of some older adults (CDC, 2017d). On the positive side, older adults have a higher incidence of seat belt usage, they tend to drive when road conditions are the safest, and they are less likely to drive under the influence of alcohol.

Poison

A poison is any substance that impairs health or destroys life when ingested, inhaled, or absorbed by the body. Almost any substance is potentially poisonous if too much is taken. Poisons impair the function of every major organ system. Health care providers are at risk from chemicals such as chemotherapy drugs and toxic cleaning agents. Sources of poison in people's homes include medicines, other solid and liquid substances, gases, and vapors. Toddlers, preschoolers, and young school-age children have a greater risk for accidental poisoning in the home because they often ingest household cleaning solutions, medications, or personal hygiene products. Emergency treatment is needed when a person ingests a poisonous substance or comes in contact with a chemical that is absorbed through the skin. A poison control center is the best resource for patients and parents needing information about the treatment of an accidental poisoning. Poison centers offer free, confidential medical advice 24 hours a day, 7 days a week through the Poison Helpline.

Fire

Home fires are a major cause of death and injury. In 2014, US fire departments responded to 367,500 home structure fires, which caused 11,825 civilian injuries and 2745 civilian deaths (Ahrens, 2015). Smoking materials such as cigarettes, cigars, and pipes are a primary source of home fires. Many fatal fires result from individuals falling asleep while smoking in bed or a failure to keep fresh batteries in home smoke detectors. The improper use of cooking equipment and appliances, particularly stoves, is another source for in-home fires. Smoke detectors and carbon monoxide detectors need to be placed strategically throughout a home. Multipurpose fire extinguishers need to be near the kitchen and any workshop areas.

Falls

Among adults 65 years of age and older, falls in the home are the leading cause of unintentional death (CDC, 2017a). Common physical hazards that lead to falls in the home include inadequate lighting, barriers along normal walking paths and stairs, and a lack of safety devices (e.g., walkers or handrails). Falls often involve accidental contact with objects on stairs or floors and low-standing furniture. Falls can result in serious injury such as fractures or internal bleeding depending on the height of the fall, body position on impact, and impact surface.

Disasters

Serious injury or death may result when a natural disaster such as a flood, hurricane, tornado, or wildfire strikes. These types of disasters can also leave many people homeless. Bombings, another type of disaster, are a likely form of a terrorist attack to occur (Terrorism Research, n.d.). National preparedness for all disasters has progressed during the last decade. Hospitals have plans and drills for internal and external disasters (Veenema et al., 2016). Medical and public health professionals have joined the disaster preparedness community, the US federal government has increased investment in preparedness, and community partners and participants are involved in disaster preparedness (Inglesby, 2011).

Pathogen Transmission

Pathogens and parasites pose a threat to patient safety. A **pathogen** is any microorganism capable of producing an illness. The most common means of transmission of pathogens is by the hands. The most effective way to limit the transmission of pathogens is the medical aseptic practice of hand hygiene. Pathogens are also transmitted through human blood and body fluids and by insects (e.g., mosquitoes carrying malaria) and rodents (see Chapter 9).

Health care agencies need to properly process biohazardous wastes (e.g., needles, surgical dressings, sharps, and syringes) to prevent the risk for pathogen exposure to the general population and employees. You also need to clean or dispose of bed linens and patient gowns contaminated by body fluids in proper containers to reduce potential exposure to pathogens.

Immunization

Immunization is the process by which resistance to an infectious disease is produced or increased. The body acquires active immunity after a small amount of weakened or dead organisms and modified toxins from the organism (toxoids) are injected into the body. Passive immunity occurs when antibodies produced by other people or animals are introduced into a person's bloodstream for protection against a pathogen. Nurses must know immunization guidelines and inform members of the public about the importance of immunization in maintaining the health of their children and themselves.

Pollution

A healthy environment is free of pollutants (i.e., harmful chemical or waste materials discharged into the water, soil, or air). Air pollution is the contamination of the atmosphere with a harmful chemical. Prolonged exposure to air pollution increases the risk of pulmonary disease. In urban areas, industrial waste and vehicle exhaust commonly contribute to air pollution. Cigarette smoke is another primary air pollutant. Improper disposal of radioactive and bioactive waste products can cause land pollution. Water pollution is the contamination of lakes, rivers, and streams, usually by industrial pollutants. If the public water supply becomes contaminated, the public must use bottled or boiled water for drinking and cooking. Flooding often damages water treatment stations and thus requires use of bottled or boiled water. Excessive noise is another form of pollution that presents significant health risks.

FACTORS INFLUENCING PATIENT SAFETY

A person's developmental level, lifestyle habits, mobility status, sensory and cognitive function, and safety awareness all influence threats to safety (Table 12.1). As a nurse, be familiar with each patient's risks and the risks that are present within a health care setting.

Developmental Level

Infant, Toddler, and Preschooler

Injuries are a major cause of death during infancy, especially for children 6–12 months old (Hockenberry and Wilson, 2015). The leading causes of injury to infants are falls, ingestion injuries (poison, foreign body ingestion, and medication), and burns. Aspiration often occurs from the ingestion of foreign material such as small toys and food items. The nature of an injury is closely related to an infant's normal growth and development. Children at these early stages are curious; they explore their environment and because of an increase in oral activity put objects in their mouths. Accidents involving young children are largely preventable. Accident prevention requires targeted health education for parents and the removal of dangers whenever possible.

School-Age Child

When children enter school, their environment expands to include the school itself, transportation to and from school, and after-school activities. Although school-age children

Table 12.1 Focused Patient Assessment

Factors to Assess	Questions	Physical Assessment
Environment	Describe times you have fallen in the past. Where do the falls commonly happen? Have you ever burned yourself?	Inspect the home environment both inside and outside for potential hazards; focus on the kitchen and bathroom.
Sensory	When do you wear your glasses? When was the last time you had your eyes checked? Can you easily hear during phone conversations?	Observe patient's ability to read printed material accurately and ability to move about within the home. Assess ability to hear normal spoken word.
Physical mobility	How does your arthritis/surgery/impaired gait affect the way you walk and move around? Do you exercise? Describe how you exercise each day. Are you able to move around safely at home?	Observe patient's posture, gait, and balance during activities of daily living.

learn how to perform more complicated motor activities, they are often uncoordinated. Instruct parents and teachers about safe practices to follow at school and during play. Teach school-age children who are involved in team and contact sports how to use protective safety equipment. Head injuries resulting from falls, motor vehicle injuries, and bicycle injuries are a major cause of pediatric deaths (Hockenberry and Wilson, 2015). Playground safety is especially important during the summer months.

Adolescent

As children enter adolescence, they develop greater independence and a sense of identity. The adolescent begins to separate emotionally from the family, and the peer group begins to have a stronger influence. Adolescents typically have wide variations that swing from childlike to mature behavior (Hockenberry and Wilson, 2015). Adolescents often engage in risk-taking behaviors such as smoking, drinking alcohol, and using drugs. Environmental clues of substance abuse include the presence of drug-oriented magazines, beer and liquor bottles, drug paraphernalia, blood spots on clothing, and wearing long-sleeved shirts in hot weather and dark glasses indoors. Psychosocial clues include failing grades, change in dress, increased absenteeism from school, isolation, increased aggressiveness, and changes in interpersonal relationships. Substance abuse increases the risk for accidents such as drowning and motor vehicle accidents. According to the Insurance Institute for Highway Safety (IIHS, 2016), the fatal crash rate per mile driven for 16- to 19-year-olds in the United States is nearly three times the rate for drivers 20 years of age and older. Teens are at higher risk for fatal crashes because of their immaturity and driving inexperience.

Adult

Threats to an adult's safety are often related to lifestyle habits. For example, a patient who uses alcohol or drugs excessively is at greater risk for motor vehicle accidents. Adults experiencing high levels of stress are at a greater risk for accidents and stress-related illnesses such as headaches, depression, gastrointestinal disorders, and infections.

Older Adult

The physiological changes associated with aging, effects of multiple medications, psychological factors, and acute or chronic disease increase an older adult's risk for falls and other types of accidents. More than one-fourth of adults 65 years of age and older falls each year, but less than half tell their health care providers (CDC, 2017a). Falls are the major cause of injury leading to death among adults 65 years of age and older. They are also the most common cause of nonfatal injuries and hospital admissions for trauma.

Most falls occur within or around the home, specifically in the bedroom, bathroom, and kitchen. Environmental factors such as broken stairs, icy sidewalks, inadequate lighting, throw rugs, and exposed electrical cords cause many accidents. Older adults typically fall while transferring from beds, chairs, and toilets; getting into or out of bathtubs; tripping over carpet edges or doorway thresholds; slipping on wet surfaces; or descending stairs. Fear of falling is common among older adults both with and without a history of falling (Chang et al., 2016). As a result of their fear, many older adults avoid activities or change the way in which they walk and position themselves, making them more at risk for falling. It is important to ask what specific conditions increase an individual's fear of falling so hazards in the home can be removed.

Other Risk Factors

Lifestyle

Lifestyle choices increase safety risks. People who drive or operate machinery while under the influence of chemical substances or work at jobs that are dangerous are at greater risk for injury. People who are preoccupied by stress or anxiety are more accident-prone because they fail to recognize the source of potential accidents such as a cluttered stair or stop sign.

Impaired Mobility

A patient with impaired mobility has many kinds of safety risks. Immobilization predisposes a patient to physiological and emotional hazards, which further restrict mobility and independence (see Chapter 14). Patients with disabilities are at greater risk for injury when entering motor vehicles and buildings that are not accessible.

Sensory Impairments

Patients with visual, hearing, tactile, or communication impairments such as aphasia or language barrier are at greater risk for injury. Such patients are not always able to perceive a potential danger or express need for assistance (see Chapter 27).

Cognitive Impairments

Cognitive impairments associated with delirium, dementia, and depression place patients at greater risk for injury. These conditions contribute to altered concentration and attention span, impaired memory, and orientation changes. Patients with these alterations become easily confused about their surroundings and are more likely to experience falls and burns.

Lack of Safety Awareness

Some patients are unaware of safety precautions such as keeping medicine, poisonous plants, or other poisons away from children or reading the expiration date on food products. This may be the result of their educational background, low health literacy, health beliefs, or access to informational resources.

RISKS IN THE HEALTH CARE ENVIRONMENT

Environmental safety pertains not only to a patient's home and community but also to a health care agency. There are risks in health care agencies that you need to address.

Chemical Exposure

Various forms of chemicals used in patient care can be an environmental risk. Chemicals found in some medications such as chemotherapy agents, anesthetic gases, cleaning solutions, and disinfectants are potentially toxic if ingested or inhaled. Safety data sheets (SDSs) are resources available in any health care agency. These sheets provide information about the chemical composition of a material, first aid measures for exposure, proper disposal methods, and technical information such as the physical and chemical properties of the material (Occupational Safety and Health Administration [OSHA], n.d.-a).

Falls

Falls often occur in health care settings. Up to 50% of patients are at risk for falls while hospitalized, and 30%–35% of patients who fall sustain an injury (The Joint Commission Center for Transforming Healthcare [TJCCTH], 2017). Falls contribute to a patient's functional decline and increased health care use. A fall can cause lasting pain and suffering and may limit physical, psychological, and social function, placing additional burdens on families and society. According to TJC (2014), approximately 11,000 fatal falls occur in the hospital annually. Inpatient falls add about 6.3 days to a patient's stay and cost about 10 lakh rupees (TJCCTH, 2017). Every health care institution has initiatives in place to reduce falls including use of special fall risk assessment tools, fall-prevention protocols, fall alert signs, and identification bands. Causes of falls are multifactorial. Common risk factors for falls in hospital settings are broken down into two categories: intrinsic and extrinsic.

- *Intrinsic factors* are patient related and include physiological conditions such as vision disturbances, urinary/stool frequency or incontinence, mental impairment, gait and balance disorders, polypharmacy, and older age.
- *Extrinsic factors* are environmentally related and include room clutter, loose electrical cords, and liquid spills.

Effectively preventing falls requires an interdisciplinary, evidence-based approach (ECRI Institute, 2016).

Patient-Inherent Accidents

Patient-inherent accidents are accidents (other than falls) in which a patient is the primary reason for the event. Examples are self-inflicted cuts, injuries, and burns; ingestion or injection of foreign substances; self-mutilation or setting fires; and pinching fingers in drawers or doors. Diagnosis of a seizure disorder places a patient at risk for a patient-inherent accident. Place patients with seizure disorders on seizure precautions, which include protecting a patient from harm during a seizure, assisting with airway management if indicated, and administering antiseizure medications as ordered.

Procedure-Related Accidents

Health care providers cause procedure-related accidents. These accidents include medication and fluid administration errors, incorrect placement of external devices, and improper performance of procedures such as dressing changes. Always follow the policies and procedures of an organization and standards of nursing practice to prevent procedure-related accidents. For example, correct use of body mechanics and transfer techniques reduces the risk for injuries when moving and lifting patients (see Chapter 14). All staff need to be aware that distractions and interruptions contribute to procedure-related accidents and need to be limited.

Equipment-Related Accidents

Equipment-related accidents result from an electrical hazard or malfunction, disrepair, or misuse of equipment. To avoid rapid infusion of i.v. fluids, all general-use and patient-controlled analgesic pumps need to have free-flow protection devices. To avoid accidents, do not operate medical equipment without adequate instruction. If you discover a faulty piece of equipment, replace it with the proper working equipment, place a tag on the faulty one, take it out of service, and promptly report any malfunctions. Assess potential electrical hazards to reduce the risk of electrical fires, electrocution, or injury from faulty equipment. In health care settings, the clinical engineering staff make regular safety checks of equipment. Facilities must report all suspected medical device–related deaths to both the Food and Drug Administration (FDA, 2016) and the product manufacturer.

Workplace Violence

Violence is becoming a familiar occurrence in hospitals, nursing homes, and other health care settings. The sources of violence include patients, visitors, intruders, and coworkers. The National Institute for Occupational Safety and Health (NIOSH, 2017) defines **workplace violence** as the act or threat of violence, ranging from verbal abuse to physical assault, directed toward persons at work or on duty. The impact of workplace violence ranges from psychological issues (e.g., posttraumatic stress disorder [PTSD], compassion fatigue) to physical injury or death. In a study involving 6300 RNs and nursing staff, workplace violence–induced anger, frustration, fear, stress, and irritability are most often reported, with 13% of staff reporting long-term difficulty with these symptoms following an event (Gerberich et al., 2004).

From 2002 to 2013, incidents of serious workplace violence (incidents requiring victims to take days off to recuperate) were four times more common in health care than in private industry (OSHA, n.d.-c). However, workplace violence occurs on a continuum. Bullying, verbal threats, and name calling are common. Patients are most commonly the source of violence in health care settings resulting from hitting, kicking, beating, and shoving (OSHA, n.d.-c). Risk factors for workplace violence caused by patients include overcrowded waiting areas in health care agencies, working in isolation from coworkers, working in high-crime areas, having a mobile workplace, transporting patients, poor environmental design, access to firearms, and working with volatile patients (McPhaul et al., 2008). Many incidents of violence are not reported (OSHA, n.d.-c). Patients who exhibit violent behavior are often repeat offenders. Although situations can escalate quickly, they can often be minimized or prevented before they can get out of control (Crisis Prevention Institute [CPI], 2016).

RISK OF FALL ASSESSMENT

Assessment of patients' risk factors for falling is a priority in health care settings. Many different fall assessment instruments are available such as the Morse Fall Scale (Morse, 2009); use the one chosen by your health care agency. Assess both intrinsic and extrinsic factors that increase a patient's risk. Intrinsic factors include a previous history of falling, age 65 years or older, reduced vision, orthostatic hypotension, gait instability, lower limb weakness, balance problems, urinary incontinence, frequency or need for assisted toileting, use of walking aids, agitation or confusion, and effects of medications (e.g., sedatives, hypnotics, anticonvulsants, certain analgesics) (Plaksin, 2014). Extrinsic factors include factors within the hospital environment. Does the placement of equipment pose barriers when a patient attempts to ambulate? Does positioning of a patient's bed allow the patient to safely reach items on a bedside table? Does a patient need assistance with ambulation? Are self-care items at the bedside, and is the nurse call system arranged for accessibility? Another area of risk includes wheelchair-related falls involving older adults and people with disabilities. Patients are at risk for falls during transfer tasks and reaching while seated in a wheelchair. Finally, be sure that equipment is safe to use. Collaborate with the hospital clinical engineering staff if you have any questions about equipment functions.

Your nursing history includes data about a patient's level of wellness to determine whether any underlying conditions pose a further threat to safety. Patients with conditions such as osteoporosis and bleeding disorders are more at risk for injury from falls. When you believe that a patient is a fall risk, assess for a fear of falling. Signs that a person is fearful of falling include concern or worry during walking, sweating or shaking while walking, clutching people or objects while walking, and reluctance to change position or walk. Other fall risk factors to assess include a patient's activity tolerance, level of cognition, presence of painful conditions, muscle strength in extremities, balance, and vision (see Chapter 16). Consider a patient's developmental level when you analyze your data. Review the type and number of medications that a patient is taking and whether the patient is undergoing any procedures that pose risks.

Fall Prevention

TJC recommends that hospitals have formal fall-reduction programs (TJC, 2015). A fall-reduction program includes a fall risk assessment of every patient conducted on admission and routinely (see hospital policy) until a patient's discharge. Many health care organizations are implementing hourly rounding to reduce falls. In addition, most organizations apply yellow color–coded wristbands to patients' wrists to communicate to all health care providers that a patient is a fall risk. In 2008, the American Hospital Association issued an advisory recommending that hospitals standardize wristband colors: red for patient allergies, yellow for fall risk, and purple for do-not-resuscitate preferences (American Hospital Association, 2008). This recommendation came after a near-miss incident in which a nurse working in two different hospitals placed a wrong-colored band on a patient. Many state hospital associations and communities are now standardizing colors to reduce confusion both within and across the health care organizations.

Patient-centered care is important, with nurses making patients and families their partners in recognizing fall risks and taking preventive action. Most hospitals and long-term care facilities have fall-prevention protocols for those patients at risk for falling. A patient assessed as being at fall risk receives a fall risk identification bracelet (yellow in color), is given information about personal fall risks, and receives additional individualized nursing interventions (**see Skill 12.1 on pp. 261**). For example, if a patient has postural hypotension, a nurse chooses a low bed and the practice of dangling the patient for 5 minutes on the side of the bed before ambulating; or a patient with a history of urinary urgency or incontinence benefits from a bedside commode instead of being expected to walk to the bathroom unassisted. Other interventions include established elimination schedules, placement of a fall pad on the floor along the bed, and use of bed safety alarms or motion detectors. A gait belt provides a secure way to steady or guide patients who need assistance with ambulation when transferring or walking. Use additional safety equipment as needed when moving patients.

When patients use assistive aids such as canes, crutches, or walkers, it is important to routinely check the condition of rubber tips and the integrity of the aid. Also, be sure that patients use their devices correctly. Remove excess furniture and equipment and make sure that patients wear rubber-soled shoes or slippers for walking or transferring. Safety bars near toilets (Fig. 12.2), locks on beds and wheelchairs (Fig. 12.3), and call lights are additional safety features found in health care settings.

Another area of fall risk includes wheelchair-related falls involving older adults or patients with disabilities. Patients are at risk for falls during transfer tasks and reaching while seated in a wheelchair. An example of a

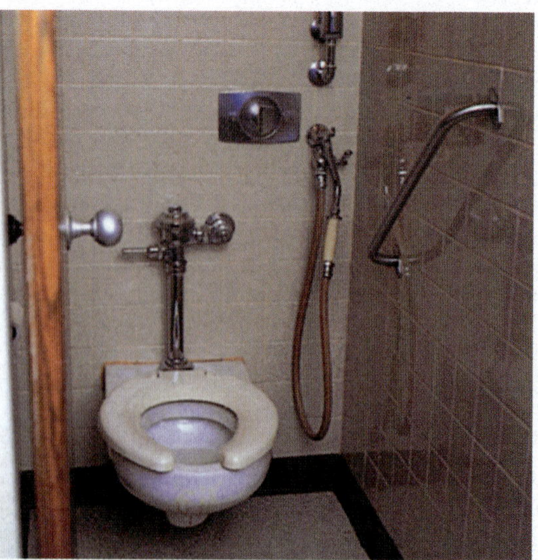

Fig. 12.2 Safety bars around toilets and showers.

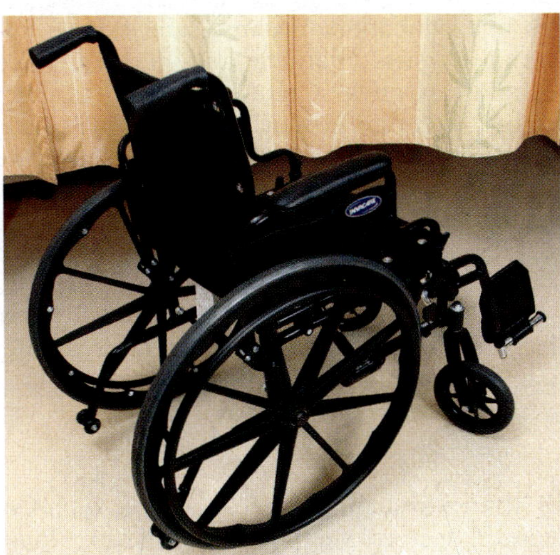

Fig. 12.3 Wheelchair with safety locks and anti-tip bars.

wheelchair characteristic that increases risk for falls is having smaller and harder front wheels that cause a chair to tip when striking uneven terrain (e.g., uneven floor surface moving into an elevator). Tripping over the front foot or leg rest and leaning over the back of a wheelchair to engage or disengage the wheel lock are common causes of injury.

Box 12.3 Care of an Older Adult

Physical Assessment Findings in Older Adults That Increase the Risk for Accidents

Musculoskeletal Changes

- Muscle strength decreased
- Joints becoming less mobile
- Brittle bones caused by osteoporosis
- Posture changes; some kyphosis common
- Limited range of motion (ROM)
- Change in walking/gait

Nervous System Changes

- Slower voluntary or autonomic reflexes
- Decreased ability to respond to multiple stimuli
- Decreased sensitivity of touch

Sensory Changes

- Decreased peripheral vision and lens accommodation
- Decreased night vision and ability to adjust to changes in light
- Development of opacity (cataracts) in lens
- Increased stimuli threshold for light touch and pain
- Impaired hearing because high-frequency tones are less perceptible

Genitourinary Changes

- Increased nocturia
- Increased occurrence of incontinence

Modified from Touhy TA, Jett K: *Ebersole and Hess' toward healthy aging*, ed 9, St Louis, 2016, Mosby.

Older Adult Considerations

When you assess older adults, recognize the types of physical changes that increase their risk for injury (Box 12.3). Research shows that even slight changes in walking speed and stride length can be a strong predictor for a patient fall (Mignardot et al., 2014). An assessment approach used within health care agencies is the timed "get up and go" test (Mathias et al., 1986). Have the older adult wear regular footwear, sit back in a comfortable chair with an armrest, and use his or her normal assist device (if needed). Have a watch with a second hand or a digital second display ready. On the word "go," time the person as he or she performs the following:

1. Stands up from the arm chair
2. Stands still momentarily
3. Walks 10 feet (3 m) (in a line)
4. Turns around
5. Walks back to chair
6. Turns around
7. Sits down

Time the effort and observe the patient for postural stability, steppage, stride length, and sway.

Normally, a person completes the task in less than 10 seconds; an abnormal response is more than 20 seconds.

ROLE OF NURSE IN PROVIDING SAFE ENVIRONMENT

QSEN (2017) outlines recommended skills to ensure nurse competency in patient safety. These include skills involving safe nursing practice during direct care, as follows:

- Demonstrate effective use of technology and standardized practices that support safety and quality.
- Demonstrate effective use of strategies to reduce risk of harm to self or others.
- Use appropriate strategies to reduce reliance on memory (e.g., forcing functions, checklists).

Direct nursing interventions toward maintaining a patient's safety in all settings. Always be safety conscious when you intervene to promote health, implement illness prevention measures, and prevent patient harm and injury.

Health Promotion

Health promotion requires a person to be in a safe environment and practice a lifestyle that minimizes risk of injury. There are both passive and active strategies aimed at health promotion. Passive strategies include public health measures and government legislative interventions (e.g., sanitation and clean water laws). Active strategies require an individual to be actively involved through changes in lifestyle (e.g., wearing seat belts or installing outdoor lighting along walking paths) and participation in wellness programs. As a nurse, you can participate in health promotion activities by supporting legislation; acting as a positive role model; and recommending safety measures in the home, school, neighborhood, and workplace.

Developmental Interventions

Infant, Toddler, and Preschooler

Growing, curious children need adults to protect them from injury. Educate parents or guardians about reducing risks of injuries to children, and teach ways to promote safety in the home. Some examples are preventing access to poisonous substances; creating a safe sleeping environment; using car seats correctly; using safe, age-appropriate toys; and teaching young children safety rules (e.g., proper use of scissors, how to walk in parking lots with parents). Children typically trust their environment and never perceive that they are in danger. Health promotion begins with well-informed parents or guardians. Educate parents about the importance of immunizations and how they protect a child from life-threatening diseases.

School-Age Child

School-age children increasingly explore their environment. They have friends outside their immediate neighborhood, and they become more active in school, church, and the community. Educate parents about the importance of children wearing seat belts whenever riding in a car; wearing helmets when riding a bicycle, skateboard, or scooter; and keeping adults informed of where they are. A child needs to know how to cross a street safely and to refrain from talking to or accepting rides or gifts from strangers. Teach children what to do if a stranger approaches and how to get help as well as how to avoid unsafe and isolated areas.

Adolescent

Risks to an adolescent's safety involve many factors outside the home because adolescents spend much of their time away from home and with their peer group. Adults serve as role models for adolescents, and they can help teens minimize safety risks by setting expectations and providing examples and education. Because adolescence is a time when sexual physical characteristics develop, adolescents often begin to have physical relationships with others. They need prompt, accurate instructions about abstinence and safe sexual practices. It is also important to educate them and their families about signs of school violence including bullying, fighting, weapon use, gang violence, and electronic aggression (CDC, 2017e). Adolescents may benefit from developing better social skills and social problem-solving with peers. Although most schools have drivers' education programs, when teens learn to drive, they need education about complying with rules and regulations regarding safe driving and the use of a car.

Adult

Risks to young and middle-age adults frequently result from lifestyle factors such as childrearing, high-stress states, inadequate nutrition, use of firearms, and abuse of drugs or alcohol. In this fast-paced society, there also appears to be more expression of anger. This anger can quickly precipitate motor vehicle collisions resulting from "road rage." Help adults understand their safety risks and guide them in making lifestyle modifications by referring them to resources such as classes to help quit smoking and for stress management or employee assistance programs. Encourage them to exercise regularly, maintain a healthy diet, practice relaxation techniques, and get adequate sleep (see Chapters 10, 11, and 14).

Older Adult

Elimination of threats to the safety of the older adult focuses primarily on accident prevention. Advancing age and concurrent physiological changes predispose older adults to falls. Table 12.2 lists nursing interventions designed to prevent falls and compensate for the physiological changes of aging. Certain disease states common to older adults such as arthritis or strokes increase the chance of

Table 12.2 Measures to Prevent Falls in Older Adults

Measure	Rationale
HOME OR HEALTH CARE AGENCY	
Stairs	
Install treads with uniform depth of 25.4–28 cm (10–11 inches) and 19–19.7 cm (7½–7¾ inches) risers (vertical face of steps).	When stairs are of uniform size, older adults do not have to continually look at the stairs and adjust their gait.
Install uniform-textured or plain-colored surfaces on each tread, and mark edge of tread with contrasting color.	Uniform textures or color help to decrease vertigo. Marking edge of tread provides obvious visual clue to end of stair.
Ensure proper lighting of each tread. Block sun or light bulb glare with translucent shades or screen or use lower wattage bulbs.	Older adults' vision is unable to adjust quickly to changes in lighting.
Ensure adequate head room so that user does not have to duck to avoid hitting his or her head while going up or down the stairs.	Sudden changes in head position often result in dizziness, which increases risk for falling.
Remove protruding objects from staircase walls.	Decreased peripheral vision prevents older adults from seeing objects at their sides. Moving to avoid protruding objects disrupts balance.
Maintain outdoor walkways and stairs in good condition and free of holes, cracks, and splinters.	Decreased visual acuity prevents the patient from seeing any structural defect. If older adults shuffle their feet when walking, it is easy to trip on uneven surfaces.
Handrails	
The space between the handrail and wall should be 40–50 mm for smooth walls and 60 mm for rough texture walls and 0.85–0.95 m (33½–37½ inches) from the floor (United Nations Enable [UNE], 2004).	Ample distance needed to allow older adults to grasp handrail firmly for support.

Table 12.2 Measures to Prevent Falls in Older Adults—Cont'd

Measure	Rationale
Secure handrail firmly to support user's weight, especially at bottom and top of stairway.	Older adults have greatest risk for falling at top and bottom of stairs because they shift their center of gravity, making balance unstable.
Install grab bars in bathroom near toilet and tub (ADABathroom.com, 2017).	Enables the patient to have support while rising from sitting to standing position.
Floors	
Ensure that patients wear properly fitting shoes or slippers with nonskid surface.	Reduces chances of slipping.
Secure all carpeting, mats, and tile; place nonskid backing under small rugs.	Sudden slip causes dizziness and inability to regain balance.
Place bath mats or nonskid strips on bathtub or shower stall floors.	Wet surfaces increase the risk for falling.
Secure electrical cords against baseboards.	Prevents tripping.
HEALTH CARE AGENCY	
Orientation	
Admit disoriented patients to a room near nurses' station.	Provides for more frequent observation by nursing staff.
Maintain close supervision of confused patients.	Confused patients often attempt to wander out of bed or room.
Show the patient how to use nurse call system at bedside and in bathroom and place in an accessible location within patient's reach. Instruct the patient to call for assistance with movement as needed.	Convenient location and use of the nurse call system are essential to patient safety.
Place bedside tables and overbed tables close to the patient. Place articles within easy reach.	Prevents patients from searching or overreaching for items.
Keep bed in low position. Have the patient rise from bed or chair slowly.	Prevents dizziness resulting from postural hypotension.
Leave one side rail up and one down on side where oriented and ambulatory patient gets out of bed.	Patients are able to use side rail for support when getting in and out of bed and to position self once in bed.
Transport	
Lock bed and wheelchair when transferring the patient from bed to wheelchair or back to bed.	Provides stability and support during transfer.
Place side rails in up position and secure safety straps around the patient on stretcher.	Prevents patients from rolling off stretchers.

injury. The effects of many medications such as sedatives, diuretics, and anticoagulants also increase the chance of injury.

Provide information about neighborhood resources to help an older adult maintain an independent lifestyle. Older adults frequently relocate to new neighborhoods and must get acquainted with new resources such as modes of transportation, church schedules, and food resources (e.g., Meals on Wheels). Information about assistance resources such as daily "hello" programs, emergency services, and elder-abuse hotlines is also helpful.

Environmental Interventions

Nursing interventions directed at eliminating environmental threats include interventions associated with a person's basic needs as well as general preventive measures.

Basic Needs

Nurses contribute to a safer environment by helping patients meet their basic needs. When administering oxygen, follow the principles of medication administration and use precautions to prevent accidental fires. Contact with heat or a spark is needed to trigger combustion. When oxygen is in use, post "No Smoking" and "Oxygen in Use" signs in patients' hospital rooms and in their homes. Do not use oxygen around electrical equipment or flammable products. Store oxygen tanks upright in carts or stands to prevent tipping or falling over. Chapter 24 outlines guidelines for proper oxygen administration. A home medical provider and home health nurse educate patients who require oxygen in the home about safe oxygen use.

Food safety requires a patient and family to understand the following principles of food preparation:

- Proper refrigeration, storage, and preparation of food decrease risk of foodborne illnesses. Store perishable foods in refrigerators to maintain freshness.
- Thaw frozen foods in the refrigerator.
- Wash hands for at least 15 seconds before preparing food.
- Rinse fruits and vegetables thoroughly.
- Avoid cross-contamination of one food with another during preparation, especially with poultry.
- Use separate cutting boards for vegetables, meat, and poultry.
- Cook foods adequately to kill any residual organisms.
- Refrigerate foods at 4°C (40°F) within 2 hours of cooking; label leftovers with the date.

General Preventive Measures

Adequate lighting and security measures in and around a home including the use of night-lights, exterior lighting, and locks on doors and windows reduce a person's risk for injury from falls or crime. Local police departments and community organizations often hold safety classes on how not to become a victim of crime.

Help parents reduce the risk of accidental poisoning by teaching them to keep hazardous substances out of children's reach. Older adults are also at risk for poisoning because diminished eyesight may cause an accidental ingestion of toxic substances. When older adults have impaired memory, accidental overdose of prescription medications may occur. Educate patients or family caregivers about keeping medications in original containers that are labeled in large print. Recommend the use of medication organizers that are filled once a week. Have patients keep poisonous substances out of the bathroom and properly discard old and unused medications.

To control pathogen transmission, teach patients how and when to wash hands (e.g., following toileting, before and after food preparation, before eating, before wound care). Nurses use Standard Precautions when caring for all patients to protect themselves from contact with blood and body fluids (see Chapter 9). Patients also need to know how to dispose of infected material such as wound dressings and used needles in the home. The Environmental Protection Agency (EPA) encourages disposal of used needles by way of community drop-off programs, household hazardous waste facilities, or sharps mail-back programs or by using home needle destruction devices (Illinois EPA, 2015). Encourage patients to contact their local community governments for guidelines on waste disposal methods.

Acute and Restorative Care

Within hospital and long-term care settings, nurses take various measures to maintain patient safety, including fall-prevention strategies, prevention of injuries from use of restraints and side rails, and precautions to prevent fires and exposure to poisoning and electrical hazards. Special precautions are also necessary to prevent injury in patients susceptible to having seizures. Radiation injuries are also a specific safety concern in hospitals.

Nurses use standard precautions for all patients to protect themselves from contact with blood and other potentially infectious body fluids. Additional specific safety measures are applicable to patients in the acute care environment. Nurses are responsible for making a patient's bedside safe. Explain and demonstrate to patients how to use the call light or intercom system and always place the call device close to the patient at the conclusion of every nurse–patient interaction. Respond quickly to call lights and bed/chair alarms. Keep the environment free from clutter around the bedside.

Fires Safety

Although smoking is usually not allowed in health care settings, smoking-related fires continue to pose a significant risk because of unauthorized smoking in beds or bathrooms. Institutional fires typically result from an electrical or anesthetic-related fire. The best intervention is to prevent fires. Nursing measures include complying with the smoking policies of an agency and keeping combustible materials away from heat sources. Box 12.4 highlights fire intervention guidelines in health care agencies. Regardless of where a fire occurs, always have an evacuation plan in place. Know where fire extinguishers and gas shut-off valves are located and how to activate a fire alarm.

Box 12.4 **Fire Intervention Guidelines in Health Care Agencies**

- Keep phone number for reporting fires visible on the telephone at all times.
- Know fire drill and evaluation plan of an agency.
- Know location of all fire alarms, exits, extinguishers, and oxygen shut-off.
- Use the mnemonic **RACE** to set priorities in case of fire:
  - **R**—Rescue and remove all patients in immediate danger.
  - **A**—Activate the alarm. Always do this before trying to extinguish even a minor fire.
  - **C**—Confine a fire by closing doors and windows and turning off oxygen and electrical equipment.
  - **E**—Extinguish a fire with an appropriate extinguisher.

Some health care agencies have fire doors that are held open by magnets and close automatically when a fire alarm sounds. It is important to keep equipment from blocking these doors. All personnel evacuate patients when appropriate. Patients who are close to the fire, regardless of its size, are at risk of injury and need to be moved to another area. If a patient requires oxygen but not life support, discontinue the oxygen, which is combustible and will fuel an existing fire. If the patient is on life support, maintain the patient's respiratory status manually with a bag-valve mask (e.g., Ambu bag) (see Chapter 24) until you move the patient away from the fire. Direct patients who can walk by themselves to move to a safe area or have them help move patients in wheelchairs. Move patients who are bedridden from the scene by a stretcher, their bed, or a wheelchair or have one or two rescuers carry them. If you have to carry a patient, do so correctly (e.g., two-man carry). Another two-rescuer technique is the chair carry, in which the patient is seated in a chair and both rescuers carry the chair. If you must carry a patient, be careful not to overextend your physical limits for lifting because an injury to you can result in further injury to the patient. If fire department personnel are on the scene, they help to evacuate patients.

After a fire has been reported and patients are out of danger, you and other personnel need to take measures to contain or put out the fire such as closing doors and windows, turning off oxygen and electrical equipment, and using a fire extinguisher. There are three types of extinguishers based on causes of fires: type A for paper and rubbish, type B for grease and anesthetic gas, and type C for electrical. There is also a multipurpose extinguisher (ABC) to use for all types of fires. To use an extinguisher correctly, remember the word **PASS** and follow these steps:

- **P**ull the pin. Hold the extinguisher with the nozzle pointing away from you and release the locking mechanism.
- **A**im low. Point the extinguisher at the base of the fire.
- **S**queeze the lever slowly and evenly.
- **S**weep the nozzle from side to side.

Prevention of Electrical Accidents

Electrical equipment used in health care settings is regularly inspected and maintained. The clinical engineering departments of hospitals inspect biomedical equipment such as beds, i.v. infusion pumps, and ventilators. You know that a piece of equipment is safe to use when you see a safety inspection sticker with an expiration date. Decrease the risk for electrical injury and fire by using properly grounded and functional equipment. The ground prong in an electrical outlet carries any stray electrical current back to the ground. Remove equipment that is not in proper working order or that sparks when plugged in or is out of service, and notify appropriate hospital staff.

Radiation Safety

Radiation is a health hazard in health care settings where radiation and radioactive materials are used in the diagnosis and treatment of patients. Hospitals have strict guidelines concerning the care of patients who are receiving radiation and radioactive materials. Know your agency-established protocols. To reduce your exposure to radiation, limit the time spent near the source, make the distance from the source as great as possible, and use shielding devices such as lead aprons. Staff who work near radiation must wear devices that track the cumulative exposure to radiation.

Workplace Violence Prevention

Being able to work in a safe environment is central to job satisfaction. As a nurse, it is important to be aware of your risks of being exposed to violence in the setting where you work. Nurses do not always know what acts constitute violence (Stene et al., 2015). A study involving nurses in emergency departments found that nurses often underreport violence, and as a direct result resources are not recognized or provided (Stene et al., 2015). It is important to recognize the patients who are most likely to enact violence. Research has shown that the five most common predictors of patient violence are confusion/cognitive impairment, anxiety, agitation, shouting/demanding, and a history of physical aggression (Kim et al., 2012).

An assessment tool is available for nurses to use to predict patients who are likely to act violently. The Aggressive Behavior Risk Assessment Tool (ABRAT) is a simple, easy-to-use assessment tool with acceptable interrater reliability, sensitivity, and specificity that may identify patients likely to commit an act of violence while on a medical–surgical unit and in long-term care (Kim et al., 2012; Berry et al., 2017). Behaviors in patients who may become violent include staring, eye contact, threatening tone and volume of voice, anxiety, mumbling, and pacing. If you face a violent situation, use the following tips for reducing violence (CPI, 2016):

1. Be nonjudgmental and empathic of patient's feelings.
   - Whatever the patient's problem is, it can be highly important to him or her.
2. Respect personal space.
   - Stand 1.5–3 feet away from a patient who is escalating. Allowing personal space helps reduce a patient's anxiety and can help you prevent acting-out behavior.
     - If you must enter personal space to administer care, first explain what you are doing and why.
3. Use nonthreatening nonverbal communication.
   - As a patient loses control, he or she does not listen to what you have to say. Instead, the patient reacts to your nonverbal communication (see Chapter 4).
   - Keep your voice tone, facial expressions, and movements neutral.
4. Do not overreact.
   - Stay calm, rational, and professional. Use positive thoughts such as, "I can manage this," and "I know what to do."
5. Focus on feelings.
   - Some people have trouble identifying how they really feel in a situation. Watch and listen carefully for the patient's real message.
6. Redirect or refocus any challenging questions, such as "Why does it always take so long for the doctor to see me?" or "Who's going to make me go to that test?"
   - Restate your request or directive; do not ignore the patient.
   - Bring the discussion back to how you can work together.
7. Set limits.
   - If patients become belligerent, defensive, or disruptive, give them *clear, simple, and enforceable limits*.
   - Speak clearly and offer a positive choice first.
8. Choose wisely what you insist on.
   - Be thoughtful in deciding *which rules are negotiable and which are not*. For example, if a patient is unwilling to walk at a given time, can you allow the patient to choose a time best for them?
   - When patients have options and flexibility, you may be able to avoid an altercation.
9. Allow silence for reflection.
   - Silence gives a person a chance to reflect on what is happening and how to proceed.
10. Allow time for the patient to make a decision.
    - Give patients a few moments to *think through what you have said*. A person's stress increases when they feel rushed.

If you find that you work in a setting where violence occurs, be sure to take care of yourself. Dealing with potentially violent patients is very stressful and sometimes dangerous. Find positive ways to care for yourself away from work. Use stress-management strategies.

SAFETY DEVICES

Restraints

Patients who are confused or disoriented or who repeatedly try to remove medical devices (e.g., i.v. lines or dressings) may temporarily need restraints to keep them safe. Restraints are not a solution to a patient problem but rather a temporary means to maintain patient safety. You must exhaust all alternatives before placing patients in restraints. Federal and state laws prohibit Medicare- and Medicaid-certified nursing homes from using restraints unless they are medically needed.

Types of Restraints

Physical Restraint

A physical **restraint** is any manual method, physical or mechanical device, material, or equipment that immobilizes or reduces the ability of a patient to move arms, legs, body, or head freely. A restraint does not include devices such as orthopedically prescribed devices, protective helmets, or methods that involve physically holding a patient to conduct an examination or test, protecting a patient from falling out of bed, or permitting a patient to participate in activities without the risk of physical harm (TJC, 2017a).

Chemical Restraint

Chemical restraints are medications such as anxiolytics and sedatives used to manage a patient's behavior and are not a standard treatment for a patient's condition.

Purposes

The main purposes for the use of restraints are to:

- Reduce the risk of patient injury from falls
- Prevent interruption of therapy such as traction, i.v. infusions, nasogastric (NG) tube feeding, or Foley catheterization
- Prevent patients who are confused or combative from removing life-support equipment
- Reduce the risk of injury to others by the patient

Problems Associated With Restraints

The use of restraints is associated with serious complications resulting from immobilization such as pressure injuries, pneumonia, constipation, and incontinence. Loss of self-esteem, humiliation, and agitation are also serious concerns. Because of these risks, legislation emphasizes reducing the use of restraints. Regulatory agencies such as TJC and CMS enforce standards for the safe use of restraint devices. A restraint-free environment (neither physical nor chemical restraints) is your first goal for all patients. Always try alternatives before using restraints (Box 12.5).

Legal Implications

For legal purposes, know agency-specific policies and procedures for appropriate use and monitoring of restraints. The use of a restraint must be clinically justified and part of a patient's prescribed medical treatment and plan of care. A physician's order based on a face-to-face assessment of a patient is required. The order must be current, stating the type and location of the restraint, and specify the duration and circumstances under which it will be used. The orders need to be renewed within a specific time frame according to agency policy. In hospitals, each original restraint order and renewal is limited to 4 hours for adults (18 years of age and older), 2 hours for children 9 through 17 years of age, and 1 hour for children younger than 9 years of age (CMS, 2015; TJC, 2017a). Orders may be renewed to the time limits for a maximum of 24 consecutive hours. Restraints are not to be ordered prn. Always make ongoing assessments of patients who are restrained. Properly document the behaviors that led to application of restraints, the procedure used in restraining, the condition of the body part restrained (e.g., color and pulse of extremity), and the evaluation of the patient response. Always remove a restraint periodically and assess if it continues to be necessary.

Box 12.5 Alternatives to Restraints

- Orient patients and family members to the environment; explain all procedures and treatments.
- Provide companionship and supervision; use trained sitters; adjust staffing and involve family.
- Offer diversionary activities such as music, puzzles, crocheting, activity aprons, and folding towels. Enlist ideas and support from family.
- Assign confused or disoriented patients to rooms near nurses' stations and observe them frequently.
- Use calm, simple statements, and physical cues as needed.
- Use de-escalation, time-out, and other verbal intervention techniques when managing aggressive behaviors.
- Provide appropriate visual and auditory stimuli (e.g., family pictures, clock, calendar).
- Remove cues that promote leaving the room (e.g., close doors to block view of stairs, do not wear street clothes).
- Promote relaxation techniques and normal sleep patterns.
- Institute exercise and ambulation schedules as allowed by patient's condition; consult physical therapist for mobility and exercise program.
- Attend frequently to needs for toileting, food and liquid, and pain management.
- Camouflage i.v. lines with clothing, stockinette, or Kling dressing.
- Evaluate all medications and ensure timely and effective pain management.
- Eliminate bothersome treatments as soon as possible. For example, discontinue tube feedings and begin oral feedings as quickly as patient's condition allows.
- Use protective devices such as hip pads, helmet, skid-proof slippers, and nonskid strips near bed.

Applications of Restraints

Follow specific guidelines when using physical restraints (see Skill 12.2).

Side Rails

When used correctly, side rails help to increase a patient's mobility and/or stability when in bed or moving from a bed to chair. Although they are the most commonly used physical restraint, side rails increase the occurrence of falls when patients attempt to get out of bed and crawl over a rail. There are a variety of beds with different side rail designs. A patient needs to have a route to exit a bed safely and maneuver freely within the bed; in this case, side rails are not considered a restraint. For example, raising only the two side rails at the top of the bed so that the lower part of the bed is open gives a patient room to exit a bed safely. Side rails used to prevent a patient such as one who is sedated from falling out of bed are not considered a restraint. Always know agency policy about the use of side rails. Be sure that a bed is in the lowest position possible when side rails are raised. Always assess the risk of using side rails compared with not using them. Check their condition; bars between the bedrails need to be spaced close together to prevent entrapment. A potential exists for trapping a person's head and body in gaps and openings between the bedframe and mattress.

The use of side rails alone for a patient who is disoriented often causes more confusion and further injury. Frequently a patient who is confused or determined to get out of bed because of pain, toileting needs, or anxiety tries to climb over a side rail or out at the foot of the bed. Either attempt often results in a fall. To reduce a patient's confusion, focus your interventions first on the cause, such as a response to a new medication, dehydration, or pain. Frequently nurses mistake a patient's attempt to explore his or her environment or to self-toilet as confusion. Use of a low bed reduces the distance between the bed and floor, facilitating a roll rather than a fall from the bed. If all efforts to reduce confusion or restlessness fail and the patient is at risk for serious injury to self or others, a restraint is sometimes necessary. However, remember that the goal is to remove the restraint at the earliest possible time.

OTHER SAFETY DEVICES

Grab Bars

These are also devices used to prevent a patient from fall and maintain their balance, reducing fatigue while standing. Patient can put some of their weight while standing or sitting or use grab bars to hold in case of a climb, slip or fall. Installation of grab bars depends on the requirement of the patient and usually installed vertically and horizontally. Vertical bars provide assistance when standing while horizontal bars help when sitting or rising (Fig. 12.2).

Sensor Mats

In keeping with current safety trends, electronic devices are alternatives to restraints. Weight- and motion-sensor mats placed on patients' beds or chairs emit silent or audible alarms when pressure is released off the mat. An alarm signals at the central nurses' station or sends a text message to a staff member's phone so that the staff is alerted quickly when a patient is moving and getting up and out of bed. Alarms on doors also alert staff or family members when a patient who is confused, disoriented, or prone to wandering opens a door.

Posey Bed

A less restrictive restraint is the Posey bed (Fig. 12.4). It is a soft-sided, self-contained enclosed bed that is much less restrictive than chemical or physical restraints. It allows for freedom of movement and thus reduces the side effects such as pressure ulcers and loss of dignity caused by physical restraints. A vinyl top covers the padded upper frame of the bed, and the nylon net canopy surrounds the mattress and completely encloses the patient in the bed. Zippers on the four sides of the enclosure provide access to the patient. The Posey bed enclosure works well for patients who are restless and unpredictable, cognitively impaired, and at risk for injury if they were to fall or get out of bed such as patients on anticoagulant therapy at risk for intracranial bleeding. The bed is also a safer alternative to side rails.

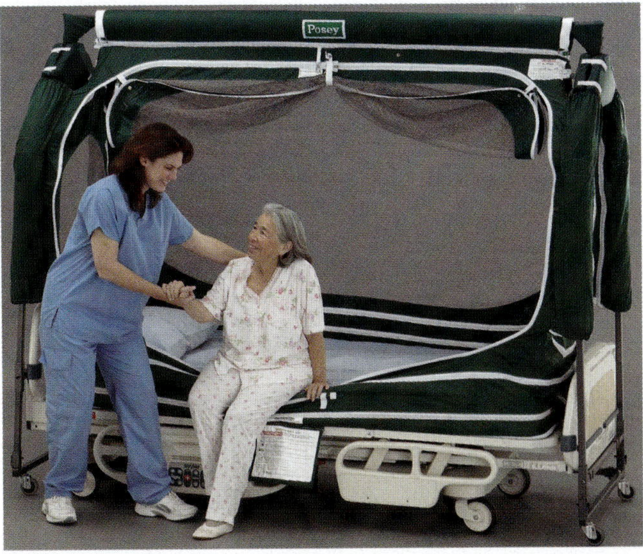

Fig. 12.4 Posey bed all-care model. (Courtesy JT Posey Co, Arcadia, CA.)

Nonskid Slippers

These are slippers that have slip-resistant quality, soft and comfortable insoles. As a nurse, you should advise elderly people to select slippers that are properly fitted, accommodate swelling, and support heel.

SKILL 12.1 Fall Prevention in Health Care Settings

STEP	RATIONALE
Assessment	
1. Identify the patient by using two identifiers (e.g., name and birthday or name and medical record number) according to agency policy.	Ensures correct patient. Complies with The Joint Commission standards and improves patient safety (TJC, 2016).
2. Assess the patient's fall risks using an agency fall risk assessment tool. Assess the patient's age (over 65), number of comorbidities, impaired memory and cognition, incontinence or urinary frequency/urgency, decreased hearing, decreased vision, orthostatic hypotension, impaired gait, weak lower extremities, poor balance, fatigue, need for transfer assistance, decreased peripheral sensation (Spoelstra, 2011; Viera et al., 2011).	A variety of physiological factors predispose patients to fall.

STEP	RATIONALE
3. Determine whether the patient has a history of recent falls or other injuries within the home. Assess previous falls, using the acronym SPLATT (Touhy and Jett, 2014). ■ *S*ymptoms at time of fall ■ *P*revious fall ■ *L*ocation of fall ■ *A*ctivity at time of fall ■ *T*ime of fall ■ *T*rauma after fall	*Key symptoms are helpful in identifying cause for falls. Onset, location, and activity* associated with a fall provide further details on causative factors and how to prevent future falls.
4. Review the patient's medications (including over-the-counter [OTC] medications and herbal products) for use of antidepressants, anticonvulsants, antipsychotics, hypnotics (especially benzodiazepines), anxiolytics, diuretics, antihypertensives, antihistamines, anti-Parkinson drugs, hypoglycemics, muscle relaxants, analgesics, and laxatives. Also assess for polypharmacy (i.e., over six medications, duplicate medications, drugs inappropriate for condition) (Bushardt et al., 2008).	Effects of certain medications and use of multiple medications increase risk for falls and injury (Chang et al., 2011; Gribbin et al., 2010; Kojima et al., 2011).

Clinical decision point: ***If the patient takes multiple medications, confer with health care provider on possibility of reducing or adjusting number of medications.***

STEP	RATIONALE
5. Assess the patient for fear of falling: those higher at risk are patients older than 75 years, female patients, patients with lower income, or single patients and have poor perceived general health or history of falling in last 3 months (Boyd and Stevens, 2009).	Fear of falling is interrelated with incidence of falls.
6. Perform the "Timed Get-up and Go" (TUG) if the patient is able to ambulate. At a minimum, observe the patient walk in room (with or without assistance). Steps for TUG dual assessment: ■ Give the patient verbal instructions to stand up from a chair, walk 10 feet (3 m) as quickly and safely as possible (cross a line marked on the floor), turn around, walk back, and sit down. ■ Have the patient rise from straight back chair without using arms for support. ■ Begin counting. ■ Look for unsteadiness in patient's gait. ■ Have the patient return to chair and sit down without using arms for support. Check time elapsed. For accuracy, a patient should have one practice trial that is not included in the score. The patient must use the same assistive device each time he or she is tested to be able to compare scores.	The Timed Get-up and Go (TUG) is a revision to the original Get-up and Go test (Podsiadlo and Richardson, 1991). It quantifies a patient's functional mobility. Observing a patient walk allows you to determine if gait and posture are normal. The TUG is a measure of physical and cognitive performance. A patient's ability to follow simple instructions measures cognitive function. An older adult who takes 12 s or longer to complete the TUG is at high risk for falling (CDC, 2015). Balance function is scored on a five-point scale: 1 = normal; 2 = very slightly abnormal; 3 = mildly abnormal; 4 = moderately abnormal; 5 = severely abnormal (Mathias et al., 1986). A score of 3 or more on the balance scale indicates a patient is at risk for falling (Mathias et al., 1986). **Note:** The TUG has been found to have limited ability to predict falls in community-dwelling elderly and should not be used in isolation to identify individuals at high risk for falls in this setting (Barry et al., 2014).
7. Assess risk factors for falls in health care facility (e.g., being attached to equipment such as sequential compression hose, intravenous [i.v.] line, or oxygen tubing; improperly lighted room; clutter; obstructed walkway to bathroom; and frequently needed items that are difficult to reach).	Environmental barriers pose risk for falls.
8. Assess condition of equipment (i.e., legs on bedside commode, tips of walker).	Equipment in poor repair increases the risk for fall.
9. Assess the patient's medical history for osteoporosis, being on anticoagulants, history of previous fracture, cancer, and recent chest or abdominal surgery.	Factors increase likelihood of injury from a fall.
10. Use a patient-centered approach. Determine what the patient knows about risks for falling and steps that he or she can take to prevent falls.	Knowledge of fall risks influences one's ability to take needed precautions in reducing falling.
11. If the patient is assessed to be a fall risk, apply color-coded wristband (see illustration). Some agencies institute fall risk signs on doors.	Color-coded yellow bands are easily recognizable.

Planning

STEP	RATIONALE
1. Gather equipment and perform hand hygiene.	Organizes care. Reduces transmission of microorganisms.
2. Explain what you plan to do. Specifically discuss reasons that the patient is at risk for falling. Include family caregivers (as appropriate) in discussion. Provide privacy. Be sure that the patient is comfortable.	Reduces patient anxiety and promotes cooperation. Results in fall-prevention measures that are patient centered and not just routine. Younger patients are very independent and often believe that they are not likely to fall.

STEP	RATIONALE
Implementation	
1. Adjust bed to low position with wheels locked (see illustration). *Option:* Place nonslip padded floor mats at exit side of bed.	Height of the bed allows ambulatory patient to get in and out of bed easily and safely. Pads provide nonslippery surface on which to stand.
2. Encourage the use of properly fitted skid-proof footwear.	Prevents falls from slipping on floor.
3. Orient the patient to surroundings, call light, and routines to expect in plan of care.	Orientation to room and plan of care provides familiarity with environment and activities to anticipate.
a. Provide patient's hearing aid and glasses. Be sure that each is functioning/clean.	Enables the patient to remain alert to conditions in environment.
b. Be sure that call light/bed control system is in an accessible location within patient's reach. Explain and demonstrate how to turn call light/intercom system on and off at bedside and in bathroom (see illustration). Have the patient perform a return demonstration.	Knowledge of location and use of call light is essential for the patient to be able to call for assistance quickly. Reaching for an object when in bed can lead to an accidental fall.
c. Explain to the patient/family caregiver when and why to use call system (e.g., report pain, get out of bed, go to bathroom). Provide clear instructions to the patient/family caregiver regarding mobility restrictions.	Increases likelihood that the patient will call for help and of nurse being able to respond to the patient's needs in a timely way.
4. Safe use of side rails	
a. Explain to the patient and family members the reason for using side rails: moving and turning self in bed.	Promotes cooperation.
b. Check agency policy regarding side rail use.	
▪ Dependent, less mobile patients: In a two-side rail bed, keep both rails up. (**Note:** Rails on newer hospital beds allow for room at foot of bed for the patient to safely exit bed.) In a four-side rail bed, leave two upper rails up.	Side rails are restraint devices if they immobilize or reduce ability of a patient to move his or her arms, legs, body, or head freely.
▪ Patient able to get out of bed independently: In a four-side rail bed, leave two upper side rails up. In a two-side rail, keep only one rail up.	Allows for safe exit from bed.
5. Make the patient's environment safe.	
a. Remove excess equipment, supplies, and furniture from rooms and halls.	Reduces likelihood of falling or tripping over objects.
b. Keep floors clutter- and obstacle-free, particularly the path to the bathroom.	Reduces likelihood of falling or tripping over objects.
c. Coil and secure excess electrical, telephone, and any other cords or tubing.	Reduces the risk of entanglement.
d. Clean all spills promptly. Post a sign indicating a wet floor. Remove the sign when the floor is dry (usually done by housekeeping).	Reduces the risk of falling on slippery, wet surfaces.
e. Ensure adequate glare-free lighting; use a night-light at night.	Glare may be a problem for older adults because of vision changes.
f. Have assistive devices (e.g., cane, walker, bedside commode) on exit side of bed. Have chair back of commode placed against wall of room if possible.	Provides added support when transferring out of bed. Stabilizes commode.
g. Arrange personal items (e.g., water pitcher, telephone, reading materials, dentures) within patient's easy reach and in a logical way.	Facilitates independence and self-care; prevents falls related to reaching for hard-to-reach items.
h. Secure locks on beds, stretchers, and wheelchairs.	Prevents accidental movement of devices during patient transfer.
6. **Additional interventions for patients at moderate-to-high risk for falling** (based on fall risk assessment)	
a. Prioritize call light responses to patients at high risk, using a team approach with all staff knowing responsibility to respond.	Ensures rapid response by a health care provider when patient calls for assistance.
b. Establish elimination schedule, using bedside commode when appropriate.	Proactive toileting keeps patients from being unattended with sudden urge to use toilet.

STEP	RATIONALE
Clinical decision: *Getting out of bed for toileting is a common event leading to a patient's fall (Tzeng, 2010), especially during evening or night hours when a room is darkened.*	
c. Stay with the patient during toileting (standing outside bathroom door).	Patients often try to get up to stand and walk back to their bed from the bathroom without assistance.
d. Place the patient in a Geri chair or wheelchair with wedge cushion. Use wheelchair only for transport, not for sitting an extended time.	Maintains alignment and comfort and makes it difficult to exit chair.
e. Use a low bed that has low height above floor and apply floor mats.	Reduces fall-related injuries.
f. Activate a bed alarm for the patient.	Alarm activates when the patient rises off a sensor. Alarm sends an alert to staff.
g. Confer with physical therapy on feasibility of gait training, weight-bearing activities, balance exercise, and strengthening exercises.	Exercise can reduce falls, fall-related fractures, and several risk factors for falls in individuals with low-bone density and in older adults (deKam et al., 2009; Schubert, 2011).
h. Use sitters or restraints only when alternatives are exhausted.	A sitter is a nonprofessional staff member or volunteer who stays in a patient room to closely observe patients who are at risk for falling. Restraints should be used only as a final option.
7. When ambulating a patient, have the patient wear a gait belt and walk along patient's side (see Chapter 14).	Gait belt gives you a secure hold on the patient during ambulation.
8. **Safe transport using a wheelchair**	
a. Determine level of assistance needed to transfer the patient to wheelchair. Position wheelchair on same side of bed as patient's strong or unaffected side (see Chapter 14).	Patient's condition may require more than a one-person assist. Positioning of chair facilitates the patient's ability to assist in transfer.
b. Place wedge cushion in chair (see illustration.)	Prevents the patient from slipping out of chair.
c. Securely lock brakes on both wheels when transferring the patient into or out of wheelchair.	Keeps chair steady and secure.
d. Raise footplates before transfer to chair; then lower footplates, placing the patient's feet on them after he or she is seated.	Prevents tripping over footplate.
e. Have the patient sit with buttocks well back in seat. *Option:* Apply a quick-release seat belt.	Prevents the patient from sliding out of chair.
f. Back wheelchair into and out of elevator or door, leading with large rear wheels first (see illustration).	Prevents smaller front wheels from catching in crack between elevator and floor, causing chair to tip.
9. Remove unnecessary supplies. Perform hand hygiene.	Reduces transmission of microorganisms.
Evaluation	
1. Conduct hourly rounds.	Hourly rounding programs reduce patient falls, and call light use increases the patients' perception of nursing responsiveness.
2. Evaluate the patient's ability to use assistive devices such as walker or bedside commode.	Adjustments in devices may become necessary.
3. Evaluate for changes in motor, sensory, and cognitive status and review whether any falls or injuries have occurred.	May require different interventions to be added. Fall outcomes determine success of plan.
4. **Use teach back:** State to the patient and family caregiver, "I want to be sure I explained clearly to you why you are more likely to fall than other patients. Can you tell me some of those reasons?" Evaluate whether the patient/caregiver is able to explain fall risks. Revise your instruction now or develop plan for revised patient teaching to be implemented at an appropriate time if the patient/caregiver is not able to teach back correctly.	Evaluates what the patient and family caregiver are able to explain or demonstrate.

Unexpected Outcomes and Related Interventions

1. The patient starts to fall while ambulating with a nurse.
   - Put both arms around the patient's waist or grasp gait belt.
   - Stand with feet apart to provide a broad base of support.
   - Extend one leg and let the patient slide against it to the floor.
   - Bend knees and lower body as the patient slides to floor.

2. The patient falls.
   - Call for assistance. Assess the patient for injury and stay with the patient until assistance arrives to help lift him or her to bed or wheelchair.
   - Reinforce explanation of identified risks with the patient and review safety measures needed to prevent a fall.
   - Monitor the patient closely after the fall since injuries are not always immediately apparent.
3. The patient/family caregiver is unable to explain fall risks.
   - Offer reexplanation, using plain language, and consider use of printed materials if available.

Recording and Reporting

- Record in plan of care specific interventions to prevent falls and promote safety.
- Document your evaluation of patient learning.
- Report the patient's fall risks and measures taken to reduce risks to all health care personnel.
- Report immediately to physician or health care provider if the patient sustains a fall or an injury.
- Complete an agency safety event or incident report noting objective details of fall (time, location, patient's condition, treatment, treatment response). Do not place report in patient medical record.
- Record events related to the fall and treatment in medical record.

Home Care Considerations

- Assess the patient's home environment for hazards and institute safety measures as appropriate, with the patient and family partnering on decisions.
- Keep personal items in their familiar positions and within easy reach in rooms frequently used.
- If the patient has a history of falls and lives alone, recommend that he or she wear an electronic Safe Patient Care device. The device is turned on by the wearer to alert a monitoring site to call emergency services for help.

SKILL 12.2 Applying Physical Restraints

Equipment

- Proper restraint (e.g., belt, wrist, mitten)
- Padding (if needed)

STEP	RATIONALE
Assessment	
1. Identify the patient by using at least two identifiers (e.g., name and birthday or name and medical record number) according to agency policy.	Ensures correct patient. Complies with The Joint Commission standards and improves patient safety (TJC, 2018).
2. Perform hand hygiene.	**Prevents the spread of microorganisms.**
3. Assess for underlying causes of agitation and cognitive impairment leading to patient-initiated medical device removal.	
a. Assess for life-threatening physiological impairments.	Conditions might lead to patient-initiated medical device removal. Identification of life-threatening impairments might lead to more appropriate medical or pharmacological treatment, eliminating need for restraints.
b. Assess for respiratory impairments, neurological impairments, fever and sepsis, hypoglycemia and hyperglycemia, alcohol or substance withdrawal, and fluid and electrolyte imbalance.	
c. Notify physician of change in mental status and compromised physiological status.	
d. Obtain baseline or premorbid cognitive function from family caregivers.	Family caregivers provide excellent source of information about the patient's behavior patterns and past history.
e. Establish whether the patient has history of dementia or depression.	
f. Review medications that cause risk for falling to identify drug–deka interactions, adverse effects.	
g. Review current laboratory values.	
4. Assess the patient's current behavior (e.g., confusion; disorientation; agitation; restlessness; combativeness; inability to follow directions; repeated removal of tubing, dressing, or other therapeutic devices). Does the patient create a risk to other patients?	If the patient's behavior continues despite treatment or restraint alternatives, use of restraint is indicated. You use the least restrictive type of restraint.

STEP	RATIONALE
5. If restraint alternatives failed earlier, confer with health care provider. Review agency policies and state laws regarding restraints. Obtain a current health care provider's order. Order must include purpose, type, location, and time or duration of restraint. Determine whether the signed consent for use of restraint is necessary (long-term care). Orders for nonviolent or non–self-destructive patients are written and renewed according to agency policy. Orders for self-destructive or violent patients are limited to select time limits and renewed only for a maximum of 24 consecutive hours (TJC, 2017a).	A health care provider's order for the least restrictive type of restraint is required.
Clinical decision point: A licensed independent health care provider responsible for the care of the patient evaluates the patient in person within 1 h of initiation of restraint used for management of violent or self-destructive behavior that jeopardizes the physical safety of the patient, staff, or others. An RN or a physician assistant may conduct the in-person evaluation if trained in accordance with the requirements and consults with the aforementioned health care provider after the evaluation as determined by hospital policy (TJC, 2017a). *Always use the least restrictive restraint possible (e.g., mitts, elbow extenders)* (TJC, 2017a).	
6. Review manufacturer's instructions for restraint application before entering the patient's room. Determine most appropriate size restraint.	You need to be familiar with all devices used for the patient care and protection. Incorrect application of restraint device results in patient injury or death.
7. Assess the patient's or family caregiver's knowledge of restraints and the reasons for use.	Encourages cooperation; minimizes risks and anxiety. Identifies teaching needs.
Planning	
1. Provide privacy.	Reduces the patient anxiety and promotes cooperation.
2. Prepare and gather restraint equipment.	Ensures an organized approach for application of restraints.
3. Instruct the patient and family about the use of restraints and associated nursing care.	Promotes the patient and family cooperation and increases understanding of need for restraints.
Implementation	
1. Perform hand hygiene. Adjust the bed to proper height and lower side rail on side of the patient contact. Be sure that the patient is comfortable and in proper body alignment.	Allows you to use proper body mechanics and prevents injury during restraint application. Positioning prevents contractures and neurovascular injury while restraint is in place.
2. Inspect area where restraint is to be placed. Note whether there is any nearby tubing or device. Assess condition of skin, sensation, adequacy of circulation, and range of joint motion.	Restraints sometimes compress and interfere with functioning of devices or tubes. Assessment provides baseline to monitor the patient's response to restraint.
3. Pad skin and bony prominences (as necessary) that will be under restraint.	Reduces friction and pressure from restraint to skin and underlying tissue.
4. Apply proper-size restraint. **Note:** Refer to manufacturer's directions.	
a. *Mitten restraint:* Thumbless mitten device restrains the patient's hands. Place hand in mitten, being sure Velcro strap is around wrist and not forearm (see illustration).	Prevents patient from dislodging or removing medical device, removing dressings, or scratching but allows greater movement than a wrist restraint. It is considered a restraint alternative if untethered and the patient is physically and cognitively able to remove it.
b. *Elbow restraint (freedom splint):* Restraint consists of rigidly padded fabric that wraps around the arm and is closed with Velcro. The upper end has a clamp that hooks to the sleeve of a patient's gown or shirt (see illustration). Insert arm so that elbow joint rests against padded area, keeping joint extended.	Commonly used with infants and children to prevent elbow flexion (e.g., with i.v. line placed in antecubital fossa). Restraint keeps elbow extended, making it difficult to remove or disrupt a medical device.
c. *Belt or body restraint:* Have the patient in sitting position in bed. Apply belt over clothes, gown, or pajamas. Be sure to place restraint at waist, not chest or abdomen. The slot in belt may be positioned in the front for limited movement or rear for increased movement. Remove wrinkles or creases in clothing. Bring ties through slots in belt. Help the patient lie down in bed. Have the patient roll to side and avoid applying belt too tightly. Ensure that straps secured to bedframe are snug so that belt does not slide to sides of bed (see illustrations). *Option:* Apply restraint net if the intent is to limit patient turning.	Restrains center of gravity and prevents the patient from rolling off stretcher or sitting up while on stretcher or from falling out of bed. Tight application interferes with ventilation if belt moves up over abdomen or chest.

STEP	RATIONALE

Step 4a Mitten restraint. (Courtesy Posey Company, Arcadia, CA.)

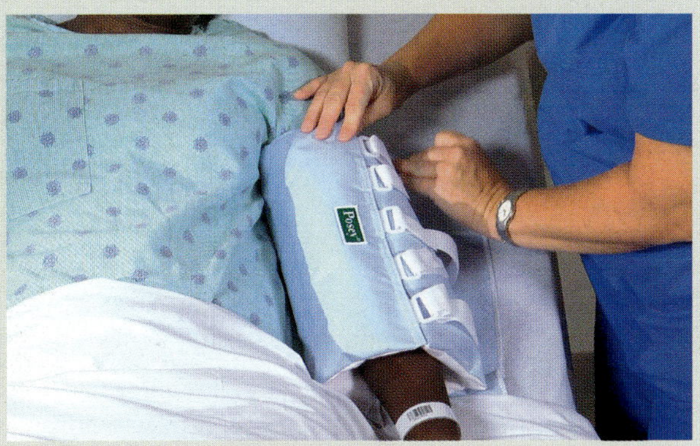

Step 4b Freedom elbow restraint.

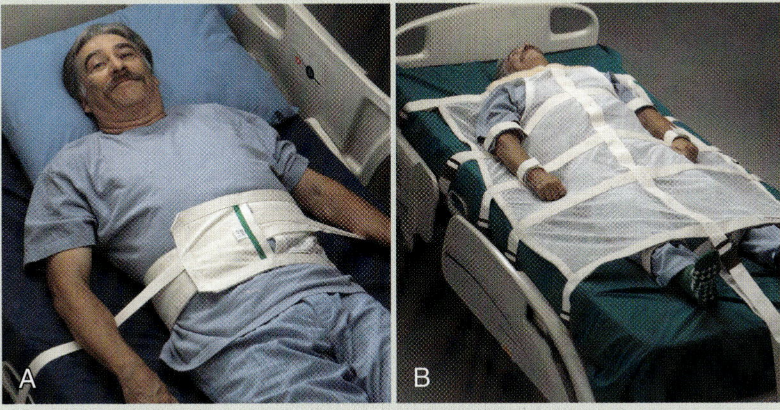

Step 4c **A,** Properly applied belt restraint allows patient to turn in bed. **B,** Option: Restraint with net limits patient's ability to turn.

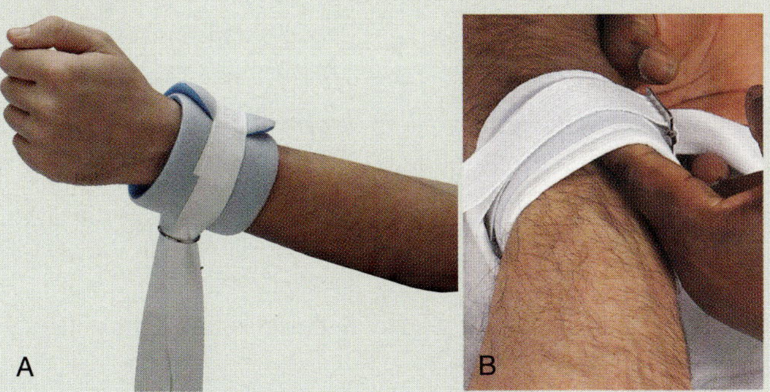

Step 4d **A,** Extremity restraint. **B,** Check restraint for constriction by inserting two fingers under restraint.

STEP	RATIONALE
d. *Extremity (ankle or wrist) restraint:* Restraint made of soft quilted material or sheepskin with foam padding. Wrap limb restraint around wrist or ankle with soft part toward skin and secure snugly (not tightly) in place by Velcro strap (see illustration). Insert two fingers under secured restraint (see illustration).	Restraint designed to immobilize one or all extremities. Maintain immobilization of extremity to protect the patient from fall or accidental removal of therapeutic device (e.g., i.v. tube, Foley catheter). Tight application interferes with circulation and potentially causes neurovascular injury.

Clinical decision point: Patient with wrist and ankle restraints is at risk for aspiration if positioned supine. Place the patient in lateral position or with head of bed elevated rather than supine.

STEP	RATIONALE
5. Attach restraint straps to portion of bedframe that moves when raising or lowering head of bed. Be sure straps are secure. *Do not attach to side rails.* Attach restraint to chair frame for the patient in chair or wheelchair, being sure buckle is out of the patient's reach.	Properly positioned strap does not tighten and restrict circulation when bed is raised or lowered.

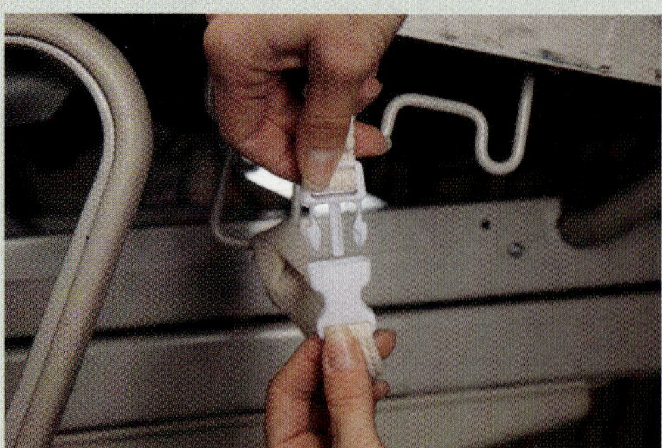

Step 6 Quick-release buckle makes it easier to disconnect and evacuate patients in an emergency.

STEP	RATIONALE
6. Secure restraints on bedframe with quick-release buckle (see illustration). *Do not tie strap in a knot*. Be sure that buckle is out of the patient's reach.	Allows for quick release in an emergency.
7. Double check and insert two fingers under secured restraint one more time. Assess proper placement of restraint including skin integrity, pulses, skin temperature and color, and sensation of restrained body part.	Provides baseline to later evaluate if injury develops from restraint.
8. Reposition the patient, provide comfort and toileting measures, provide nutrition and fluids, and evaluate the patient condition. If the patient is violent or noncompliant, remove one restraint at a time and/or have staff assistance while removing restraints.	Provides an opportunity to attend to the patient's basic needs and determine need for continuation.
Clinical decision point: Do not leave a patient who is violent or aggressive unattended while restraints are off.	
9. Secure nurse call or intercom system within the patient's reach.	Allows the patient, family, or caregiver to obtain assistance quickly.
10. Leave bed or chair with wheels locked. Keep bed in lowest position.	Prevents bed or chair from moving if the patient tries to get out. If the patient falls with bed in lowest position, this reduces chance of injury.
11. Perform hand hygiene.	Reduces transmission of microorganisms.
Evaluation	
1. After application, evaluate the patient for signs of injury every 15 min (e.g., circulation, vital signs, ROM, physical and psychological status, and readiness for discontinuation). Perform visual checks if the patient is too agitated to approach.	Frequent evaluation prevents injury to the patient and ensures removal of restraint at earliest possible time. Frequency of monitoring guides staff in determining appropriate intervals for evaluation based on the patient's needs and condition, type of restraint used, risk associated with use of chosen intervention, and other relevant factors.
2. Evaluate the patient's need for toileting, nutrition and fluids, hygiene, and elimination/release of restraints at least every 2 h.	Prevents injury to the patient and attends to basic needs.
3. Evaluate the patient for any complications of immobility.	Early detection of skin irritation, restricted breathing, or reduction in mobility prevents serious adverse events.
4. Licensed health care provider or RN trained according to CMS requirements needs to evaluate the patient within either 1 h or 4 h after initiation of restraints, depending on Medicare status of hospital (see agency policy).	Determines the patient's immediate situation, reaction to restraints, medical and behavioral condition, and need to continue or terminate restraints (CMS, 2015).
5. After 24 h, before writing a new order, the health care provider who is responsible for the patient's care must see and reassess the patient.	Ensures that restraint application continues to be medically appropriate.
6. Observe i.v. catheters, urinary catheters, and drainage tubes to determine that they are positioned correctly and that therapy remains uninterrupted.	Reinsertion is uncomfortable and increases risk for infection or interrupts therapy.
7. Observe the patient's behavior and reaction to presence of restraint.	Restraints can increase restlessness and agitation, resulting in harm.
8. **Use teach back:** "We have talked about the reason we are using restraints on your father. Can you tell me that reason? I want to be sure you understand." Revise your instruction now or develop a plan for revised patient/family caregiver teaching if the patient/family caregiver is not able to teach back correctly.	Determines the patient's/family caregiver's level of understanding of instructional topic.

Recording and Reporting

- Record nursing interventions and restraint alternatives tried on restraint flow sheet or in nurses' notes in electronic health record (EHR) or chart.
- Record the patient's behavior before restraints were applied, level of orientation, and patient's/family caregiver's understanding of explanation of purpose of restraint and consent (when required).
- Record the purpose for restraint, type and location, time applied, time ending the restraints, and routine observations made every 15 min (e.g., skin color, pulses, sensation, vital signs, behavior) in the flow sheets or nurses' notes.
- Record the patient's level of orientation and behavior after restraint application. Record times the patient was evaluated, attempts to use alternatives, and patient's response when restraint was removed.

Unexpected Outcomes and Related Interventions

- The patient experiences impaired skin integrity.
  - Evaluate need for continued use of restraint and whether alternatives can be used.
  - If restraint still needed, be sure it is applied correctly and provide adequate padding.
  - Check skin under restraint for abrasions and remove restraints more often. Provide appropriate skin care, and change wet or soiled restraints.
- The patient becomes more confused or agitated.
  - Determine cause of the behavior and eliminate if possible; consult with health care provider.
  - Determine need for more or less sensory stimulation and make any stimulation meaningful.
  - Reorient as needed, and try restraint-free options.
- The patient has neurovascular injury (e.g., cyanosis, pallor, and coldness of skin or complains of tingling, pain, or numbness).
  - Remove restraint immediately, stay with the patient, and notify health care provider.
  - Protect extremity from further injury.

KEY POINTS

- A culture of safety requires a commitment that acknowledges the high-risk nature of the activities of an organization, the determination to achieve consistently safe operations, a blame-free environment, and an organizational commitment to resources.
- Vulnerable groups that require help in achieving a safe environment include infants, children, older adults, people who are ill or injured, people with physical and mental disabilities, people with poor literacy skills, and people who live in poverty.
- Your role as a nurse is to educate patients about common safety hazards and how to prevent injury while placing emphasis on hazards to which patients are more vulnerable.
- In the community, a safe environment means that basic needs are achievable, physical hazards are reduced, transmission of pathogens and parasites is reduced, pollution is controlled, and sanitation is maintained.
- Caring for patients requires assessment of safety risks based on their developmental stage.
- Threats to an adult's safety are frequently associated with lifestyle habits.
- In older adults, the physiological changes associated with aging, effects of multiple medications, psychological factors, and acute or chronic disease increase risk for falls and other types of accidents.
- Risks to patient safety within a health care agency include falls and patient-inherent, procedure-related, and equipment-related accidents.
- Common risk factors for falls in hospital settings are broken down into two categories: intrinsic (patient related) and extrinsic (environmentally related).
- Nurses are responsible for making patients' hospital rooms safe.
- Restraints are not a solution to a patient problem. Exhaust all alternatives before placing patients in restraints.
- A medical order for a restraint must be current, stating the type and location of restraint, and specify the duration and circumstances under which it will be used.
- Side rails are the most commonly used physical restraint and increase the occurrence of falls when patients attempt to get out of bed by crawling over a rail.
- Continually evaluate the nursing care plan to promote safety to identify new or continued risks to a patient.

REFERENCES

Ahrens M. Home structure fires. National Fire Protection Association; 2015. Available from: http://www.nfpa.org/news-and-research/fire-statistics-and-reports/fire-statistics/fires-by-property-type/residential/home-structure-fires.

American Academy of Pediatrics (AAP). Car seats: information for families. 2017. Available from: http://www.healthychildren.org/English/safety-prevention/on-the-go/pages/Car-Safety-Seats-Information-for-Families.aspx.

American Hospital Association (AHA). Quality advisory: implementing standardized colors for patient alert wristbands. 2008. Available from: http://www.aha.org/advocacy-issues/tools-resources/advisory/2008/080904-quality-adv.pdf.

ADABathroom.com. Your source for ADA compliance in the bathroom. 2017. Available from: http://www.adabathroom.com.

Barry E, et al: Is the Timed Up and Go test a useful predictor of risk of falls in community dwelling older adults: a systematic review and meta-analysis, *BMC Geriatr* 14: 14, 2014.

Berry B, Young L, Kim SC. Utility of the Aggressive Behavior Risk Assessment Tool in long-term care homes. Geriatr Nurs 2017. Available from: http://www.gnjournal.com/article/S0197-4572(17)30041-1/abstract.

Bushardt RL, et al: Polypharmacy: misleading but manageable, *ClinInterv Aging* 3 (2): 383, 2008.

Boyd R, Stevens JA: Falls and fear of falling: burden, beliefs and behaviors, *Age Ageing* 38 (4): 423, 2009.

Centers for Disease Control and Prevention (CDC). Carbon monoxide exposures—United States, 2000-2009, Atlanta, GA: CDC; 2011. Available from: https://www.cdc.gov/mmwr/preview/mmwrhtml/mm6030a2.htm.

Centers for Disease Control and Prevention (CDC). Check for safety: a home fall prevention checklist for older adults. 2015. Available from: https://www.cdc.gov/steadi/pdf/check_for_safety_brochure-a.pdf.

Centers for Disease Control and Prevention (CDC). Important facts about falls. 2017a. Available from: https://www.cdc.gov/homeandrecreationalsafety/falls/adultfalls.html.

Centers for Disease Control and Prevention (CDC). Teen drivers: get the facts (motor vehicle safety). 2017b. Available from: https://www.cdc.gov/motorvehiclesafety/teen_drivers/teendrivers_factsheet.html.

Centers for Disease Control and Prevention (CDC). Nonfatal injury reports. 2017c. Available from: https://webappa.cdc.gov/sasweb/ncipc/nfirates.html.

Centers for Disease Control and Prevention (CDC). Older adult drivers. 2017d. Available from: http://www.cdc.gov/motorvehiclesafety/older_adult_drivers/.

Centers for Disease Control and Prevention (CDC). About school violence. 2017e. Available from: http://www.cdc.gov/ViolencePrevention/youthviolence/schoolviolence/index.html.

Centers for Medicare and Medicaid Services (CMS). State operations manual. Appendix A: survey protocol, regulations, and interpretive guidelines for hospitals. 2015. Available from: https://www.cms.gov/Regulations-and-Guidance/Guidance/Manuals/Downloads/som107ap_a_hospitals.pdf.

Chang CM, et al: Medical conditions and medications as risk factors of falls in inpatient older people: a case-controlled study, *Int J Geriatr Psychiatry* 26 (6): 602, 2011.

Chang HT, Chen HC, Chou P. Factors associated with fear of falling among community-dwelling older adults in the Shih-Pai study in Taiwan. PLoS One 2016;11(3):e0150612.

Crisis Prevention Institute (CPI). CPI's top 10 de-escalation tips. 2016. Available from: https://www.crisisprevention.com/CPI/media/Media/download/PDF_DT.pdf.

deKam D, et al: Exercise interventions to reduce fall-related fractures and their risk factors in individuals with low bone density: a systematic review of randomized controlled trials, *OsteoporosInt* 20 (12): 2111, 2009.

ECRI Institute. Falls. 2016. Available from: https://www.ecri.org/components/HRC/Pages/SafSec2.aspx?tab=1.

Food and Drug Administration (FDA). Report a problem to the FDA. 2016. Available from: http://www.fda.gov/safety/reportaproblem/.

Gerberich SG, Church TR, McGovern PM, Hansen HE, Nachreiner NM, Geisser MS, et al. An epidemiological study of the magnitude and consequences of work related violence: the Minnesota Nurses' Study. Occup Environ Med 2004;61(6):495.

Gribbin J, et al: Risk of falls associated with antihypertensive medication: population-based case-control study, *Age Ageing* 39 (5): 592, 2010.

Hockenberry M, Wilson D. Wong's nursing care of infants and children. 10th ed. St. Louis: Mosby; 2015.

Illinois Environmental Protection Agency (EPA). Safe options for home needle disposal. 2015. Available from: https://www2.illinois.gov/epa/Documents/iepa/waste-management/medication-disposal/sharps-fact-sheet.pdf.

Inglesby TV. Progress in disaster planning and preparedness since. JAMA 2011;306(12):1372.

Institute of Medicine (IOM) Committee on Quality of Health Care in America. To err is human: building a safer health system. Washington, DC: National Academies Press; 2000.

Insurance Institute for Highway Safety (IIHS). Fatality facts: teenagers 2015. Arlington, VA: The Institute; 2016. Available from: http://www.iihs.org/iihs/topics/t/teenagers/fatalityfacts/teenagers.

Kim SC, Ideker K, Todicheeney-Mannes D. Usefulness of Aggressive Behaviour Risk Assessment Tool for prospectively identifying violent patients in medical and surgical units. J Adv Nurs 2012;68(2):349.

Kochanek KD, Murphy SL, Xu J, Tejada-Vera B. Deaths: final data for 2014. Natl Vital Stat Rep 2016. Available from: https://www.cdc.gov/nchs/data/nvsr/nvsr65/nvsr65_04.pdf.

Kojima T, et al: Association of polypharmacy with fall risk among geriatric outpatients, *GeriatrGerontolInt* 11 (4): 438, 2011.

Mathias S, et al. Balance in elderly patients: the "get-up and go" test. Arch Phys Med Rehabil. 1986 ;67(6):387-9.

McPhaul KM, London M, Murrett K, Flannery K, Rosen J, Lipscomb J. Environmental evaluation for workplace violence in healthcare and social services. J Safety Res 2008;39:237.

Mignardot JB, Deschamps T, Barrey E, Auvinet B, Berrut G, Cornu C, et al. Gait disturbances as specific predictive markers of the first fall onset in elderly people: a two-year prospective observational study. Front Aging Neurosci 2014;6:22.

Morse JM. Preventing patient falls: establishing a fall intervention program. 2nd ed. New York: Springer Publishing; 2009.

National Institute for Occupational Safety and Health (NIOSH). Occupational violence. 2017. Available from: https://www.cdc.gov/niosh/topics/violence/default.html.

National Quality Forum (NQF). Mission and vision. Washington DC: NQF; 2017a. Available from: http://www.qualityforum.org/About_NQF/Mission_and_Vision.aspx.

National Quality Forum (NQF). List of SREs. 2017b. Available from: http://www.qualityforum.org/Topics/SREs/List_of_SREs.aspx#sre1.

Occupational Safety and Health Administration (OSHA). Hazard communication standard: safety data sheets. n.d.-a. Available from: https://www.osha.gov/Publications/HazComm_QuickCard_SafetyData.html.

Occupational Safety and Health Administration (OSHA). Workplace violence in healthcare. n.d.-c. Available from: https://www.osha.gov/Publications/OSHA3826.pdf.

Plaksin J. Falls in older adults—risk factors and strategies for prevention. Clinical Correlations: The NYU Langone Online Journal of Medicine; 2014. Available from: http://www.clinicalcorrelations.org/?p=8114.

Podsiadlo D, Richardson S: The timed "Up & Go": a test of basic functional mobility for frail elderly persons, *J Am GeriatrSoc* 39 (2): 142, 1991.

QSEN Institute. QSEN Institute. 2017. Available from: http://qsen.org/.

Schubert TE: Evidence-based exercise prescription for balance and falls prevention: a current review of the literature, *J GeriatrPhysTher* 34 (3): 100, 2011.

Spoelstra SL, et al: Fall prevention in hospitals: an integrative review, *ClinNurs Res published online*, 2011, http://cnr.sagepub.com/content/21/1/92. Accessed October 14, 2019.

Stene J, Larson E, Levy M, Dohlman M. Workplace violence in the emergency department: giving staff the tools and support to report. Perm J 2015;19(2):e113.

Terrorism Research. Types of terrorist incidents. n.d. Available from: http://www.terrorism-research.com/incidents/.

The Joint Commission (TJC): *2016 National Patient Safety Goals*, Oakbrook Terrace, IL, 2016, The Commission, http://www.jointcommission.org/standards_information/npsgs.aspx. Accessed November 2019.

The Joint Commission (TJC). Center for Transforming Healthcare aims to prevent inpatient falls with injury. Joint Commission Online; 2014. Available from: http://www.jointcommission.org/assets/1/23/jconline_April_30_14.pdf.

The Joint Commission (TJC). Preventing falls and fall-related injuries in health care facilities. 2015. Available from: http://www.jointcommission.org/assets/1/18/SEA_55.pdf.

The Joint Commission (TJC). Comprehensive accreditation manual for hospitals. Chicago: TJC; 2017a.

The Joint Commission (TJC). Speak up initiatives. 2017b. Available from: http://www.jointcommission.org/speakup.aspx.

The Joint Commission (TJC). 2018 National Patient Safety Goals. Oakbrook Terrace, IL: The Joint Commission; 2018. Available from: https://www.jointcommission.org/standards_information/npsgs.aspx.

The Joint Commission Center for Transforming Healthcare (TJCCTH). Targeted solutions tool for preventing falls. 2017. Available from: http://www.centerfortransforminghealthcare.org/tst_pfi.aspx.

Touhy T, Jett K: *Ebersole and Hess' Gerontological nursing & health care*, ed 4, St Louis, 2014, Elsevier.

Tzeng HM: Understanding the prevalence of inpatient falls associated with toileting in adult acute care settings, *J Nurs Care Qual* 25 (1): 22, 2010.

United Nations Enable (UNE). Accessibility for the disabled—a design manual for a barrier free environment. 2004. Available from: http://www.un.org/esa/socdev/enable/designm/AD2-05.htm.

Veenema TG, Griffin A, Gable AR, MacIntyre L, Simons RN, Couig MP, et al. Nurses as leaders in disaster preparedness and response—a call to action. J Nurs Scholarsh 2016;48(2):187.

Viera ER, et al: Risk factors for geriatric patients falls in rehabilitation hospital settings: a systematic review, *ClinRehabil* 25 (9): 788, 2011.

13 Hospital: Admission and Discharge

OBJECTIVES

- To discuss the meaning and indications of admission in hospital.
- To describe the purposes of admission procedure.
- To discuss the types and methods of admission in hospital.
- To understand the basics of preparation of the unit for admission and help the patient to occupy the bed and orient the patient to the ward.
- To explain the steps of admission procedure in the ward.
- To discuss the emotional responses of patient, because of hospitalization, and special considerations nurses must keep in mind while admitting the patient in a ward.
- To understand the medicolegal issues considered during admission of the patient in hospitals.
- To discuss the meaning of discharge from hospital.
- To discuss the types of discharge from hospital.
- To understand the basics of planning for discharge from hospital.
- To explain the steps of discharge procedure from hospital.
- To understand the medicolegal issues considered during discharge of the patient in hospitals.

KEY TERMS

diagnostic admission, p. 272
discharged against medical advice, p. 274
discharge planning, p. 274
emergency admission, p. 272
left against medical advice (LAMA), p. 274
long-term admission, p. 272
routine admission, p. 272
short-term admission, p. 272
therapeutic admission, p. 272

ADMISSION TO THE HOSPITAL

DEFINITION

Admission of a patient means allowing and facilitating a patient to stay in the hospital unit or ward for observation, investigation, and treatment of the diseases he or she is suffering from (Handy, 2016).

INDICATIONS

A person can be admitted to a health care facility with several reasons, including (Baranova, 2019):

- Therapeutic aspect for treatment of any acute or chronic disease
- For observation of the status of client
- For diagnostic need
- For surgical interventions
- On an emergency basis
- For conditions requiring expert care

PURPOSES OF ADMISSION PROCEDURE

- To welcome the patient
- To provide immediate care
- To provide comfort and safety to the patient
- To receive the patient in ward for admission according to his or her condition
- To be ready for any emergency
- To assist the patient in adjusting to the hospital environment
- To obtain information about the client so as to establish therapeutic nurse–patient relationship
- To involve the patient and family in care
- To assist in proper discharge planning

TYPES OF ADMISSION

Admission to the hospital can be divided into different types depending on presence or absence of preplanning, time period, and purposes of admission (www.betterhealth.vic/gov/au, 2019).

A. ***Depending on planning***
   - *Routine admission:* These are planned for clients suffering from clinical disorders and who need to undergo any treatment modality or diagnostic procedure.
   - *Emergency admission:* These are done for clients suffering from acute conditions or life-threatening conditions such as cardiac arrest, stroke, poisoning, and accidents.

B. ***Depending on time spent in hospital***
   - *Long-term admission:* **Long-term admission** is required for clients suffering from pathological conditions having a long-term recovery period.
   - *Short-term admission:* **Short-term admission** is required if clients need less time in health care system.

C. ***Depending on purposes of admission***
   - *Diagnostic admission:* **Diagnostic admission** is usually a short-term admission meant to undergo some investigation.
   - *Therapeutic admission:* In **therapeutic admission**, patients suffering from any medical condition requiring continuous medical care are admitted to hospital for better management.

METHOD OF ADMISSION

Routine Admission

In **routine admission**, client reaches the out-patient department (OPD) first. The clerical staff gathers information to start patient's record and is escorted to doctor's office, where doctor makes the decision for admission (Patel, 1971).

In the admission office, detailed information is gathered regarding identification data, insurance coverage, possible allergies, and so on. The client is issued an identification number. From admission office, the client is taken to nursing unit by an auxiliary person.

OPD → Doctor's office → Admission office → Ward

Emergency Admission

In **emergency admission**, safety and immediate care of the client are essential to save life. From the emergency department, the client is admitted directly to special care units such as intensive care unit, cardiac care unit, burns unit, and emergency operation theatre. In these situations, relatives go to the admitting office to provide necessary information (Patel, 1971).

Emergency department → OT, ICU, CCU, burns unit or a ward

STEPS OF ADMISSION PROCEDURE

- Prepare a clean and neat admission room with all the necessary items per the need of the patient.
- Prepare an appropriate type of bed with adequate adjusted height of the bed.
- Welcome the patient and his or her family with warm approach and check his or her identity to ensure that right patient is admitted in unit.
- Make the patient comfortable in bed and provide him or her with hospital clothes and ensure adequate privacy.
- Assess the vital signs, obtain brief initial nursing assessment and make an observation for significant clinical findings. The laboratory samples also may be sent per physician's prescription and prescribed hospital policy.
- Orient the patient and family with ward, ward routines, supportive hospital facilities, and hospitals policies.
- Record all the basic information in patient's record and report the relevant information to physician or immediate supervisor, if needed. Clearly mention admission date, time, patient's details, complaints of the clients, informed consent, where valuables are given, any allergies, patient's mental status, and progress after being intervened.
- Record in admission register, treatment book, report book, medicolegal case (MLC) register, update ward census and nurse's notes.

SPECIAL CONSIDERATIONS DURING ADMISSION

The following considerations should be paid special attention while admitting a patient to the hospital (Clumbia Asia India, 2019):

- When the patient is admitted in critical condition, collect only the most pertinent information.
- Arrange for trolley, wheel chair, and so on, if a sick patient is expected to be admitted.
- In case of unknown client, keep their clothing and valuables safely and label them. Inform the police department.
- Never leave the patient alone in the casualty. A female client should never be left alone with male attendant.
- All jewelry should be removed at the time of admission. Keep all the valuables (white and yellow metals) with labels and under custody.
- MLCs should have the "MLC" stamp and the notified MLC number in the case's sheet.
- While admitting an infant or a small child, provide emotional support for both the child and the parents.
- Speak slowly and clearly when talking to the elderly clients because of their decreased hearing sense.

MEDICOLEGAL ISSUES RELATED TO ADMISSION

During admission procedure, nurses must keep the following medicolegal issues under consideration, so that they can safeguard themselves and the health care institution (Waghmode, 2020):

- Physician must be informed immediately on the arrival of the patient to OPD, so that undue waiting time for the patient in OPD may be avoided.
- Patient's OPD records such as patient's OPD visit slip, admission cards must be kept under lock and key.
- Ensure the adequate privacy of the patient. During physical examination, a female patient has the right to refuse the physical examination by a male doctor or male nurse; if a female patient is examined by a male health care worker, a female member or a nurse must stay with the patient ensuring adequate privacy.
- Patient's record must be kept confidential; other than the treating physician, no one should have the access to the patient's records.

- Patient's belongings should be kept under custody per the hospital policy. Furthermore, before handing over the belongings to the family or police, permission must be taken from treating physician, and signatures, name, and address of the receiver of the belongings must be taken on a document, which has complete details of all the belongings.
- A complete record about the description of the patient's body fluid must be maintained such as color, amount, and consistency, and these body fluids should not be discarded without confirming with the treating physician.
- It must be ensured that no evidence related to the patient gets destroyed or lost, especially in MLCs.
- A written consent must be taken from the patient (if conscious) or relative before performing any invasive procedure.
- If the patient needs a member from family or friends, they may be allowed to stay with the patient.
- Keep the patient's information confidential; do not convey any information related to the patient to anyone outside the patient's treating health care team.
- It is compulsory for the nurse to provide the information to the police officer, to the press reporter, or any agent of the public. In case of any difficulty, the immediate higher authority may be informed.

ROLES AND RESPONSIBILITIES OF THE NURSE

Preparation of the Unit for Admission

A well-prepared unit makes the patient feel expected and welcomed.

Activities to be completed before patients arrive include the following (https://resources.nure.com, 2020):

- Position the bed at low level if the client is ambulatory, or at the level of the stretcher.
- Open the bed by folding back the linen.
- Assemble the necessary equipment and supplies, including hospital admission pack (basin, water pitcher, tissues, glass, soap, etc.), hospital dress, vital signs tray, weighing machine, specimen bottle, and so on.
- Assemble special equipment and supplies—oxygen cylinder, suction apparatus, and so on.
- Adjust the physical environment—proper lighting, ventilation, and so on.

Helping the Patient to Occupy the Bed

A nurse should observe the following while helping the patient to occupy a bed (see Chapter 10):

- Receive the ambulatory patient in the admission bed and greet him or her with name and introduce yourself.
- Adjust the height of the bed depending on the patient's condition.
- Accompany the patient to his or her bed.
- Arrange for the assistance if the patient arrives in a trolley for shifting.
- Remove extra furniture in the room for smooth transportation.
- Put on hospital clothes per the hospital routine.
- Maintain privacy.
- Check doctor's order for stat medication, tests, or special orders.

Orientation of the Patient to the Ward

The following needs to be taken care of when a nurse orients the patient to the ward:

- Introduce the patient to the hospital staff and other patients.
- Show him or her bathroom facilities.
- Arrange personal belongings.
- Valuables are listed and handed over to the relatives after taking signature (white metal and yellow metals are counted and listed).
- Show the communication system and keep the bed alarm on.
- Explain adjustment of bed, lighting, and ventilation.
- Inform meal timing, visiting time, doctor's rounds, and ward routine.

Emotional Responses to Hospitalization

Irrespective of the cause of hospitalization, all the clients experience apprehension while being admitted to the hospital. Anxiety, fear of unknown, threats to their body image, fear of financial burden, and superstitions add on to the strange environment of hospital. Stress can aggravate the already worsened health status.

Female clients may be worried about their children, lack of care takers, decreased pain threshold, disruption of family routines, and disruption of marital relationship.

Males clients may be worried about the treatment, financial burden, pain, and discomfort due to pathological conditions.

Children develop feeling of mistrust, fear of pain, and strange environment.

Nurse's Response

The nurse's attitude to a newly admitted client should be friendly and unhurried. Make the patient feel at ease and trust you. The patient should be received like a guest in a courteous manner. Thus, much of the client's fear can be alleviated by skilled admission. Confidence and competence from nurses have a positive influence on the patients.

DISCHARGE FROM THE HOSPITAL

DEFINITION

"Discharge of a patient from the hospital is a departure process, which could be because of the attending doctor's advice to leave the hospital on required completion of treatment or patient may leave against medical advice (LAMA) because of personal reasons or patient's body sent after the demise (Alper, 2017)."

TYPES OF DISCHARGE

Discharge can be of several different types, discussed as follows:

- **Planned discharge:** Planned discharge is a process of reliving the patient from the hospital after the due completion of the desired treatment for the patient admitted to hospital.
- **LAMA:** The patient also may leave the hospital on his or her own wish because of his or her personal reasons but against the medical advice, which is known as **left against medical advice (LAMA)**, but now the terminology is redefined as **discharged against medical advice (DAMA)**. During LAMA, when the patient is in critical condition, it is the nurse's responsibility to explain about the critical condition of the patient to family, and signatures must be taken on the patient's medical record (Devit, 2000).
- **Referrals and transfer:** Sometimes, when the patient's diseased condition is not manageable at a particular hospital due to reasons such as infrastructure and expertise, the patient is needed to be referred or transferred to the higher level medical institution. This is known as referrals or transfer.

Special circumstances in which patient leaves the hospital:

- *Parole:* In psychotic hospitals, a patient who has not been discharged from the hospital can be sent home for 2, 3, or more days if requested by the relatives and approved by the psychiatrist in charge. If the patient does not come back after parole, the discharge procedure should be carried out per the hospital policy.
- *Absconding:* If the patient runs away from the ward/hospital, it becomes a major responsibility of the nurse on duty. To avoid this problem, nurses must regularly check the number of patients admitted with the actual number of patients present in the ward, while handing and taking over charges in each shift. If any patient is reported absconding, the chief medical officer is informed immediately in writing. This has also to be signed by the officer. The record of absconding patient must be kept under lock and key.

ROLES AND RESPONSIBILITIES OF THE NURSE

The patient, the family, physician, nurses, social workers, physiotherapist, and all other health team members usually involve and work together to plan and carryout discharge of the patient from the unit. The patient and family members may have great concern about postdischarge care at home. Therefore, nurses have some of the key roles and responsibilities while discharging a patient as detailed in the subsequent text.

Discharge Planning

Discharge planning *begins the moment a patient is admitted to a health care facility.* Nurses play an important role in discharge planning in the hospital, where continuity of care is important. To achieve continuity of care, nurses use critical thinking skills and apply the nursing process. To anticipate and identify the patient's needs, nurses work with all members of the interdisciplinary health care team. They take the lead to develop a plan of care that moves the patient from the hospital to another level of health care such as the patient's home or a nursing home. Discharge planning is a centralized, coordinated, interdisciplinary process that ensures that the patient has a plan for continuing care after leaving a health care agency (Lin, 2012).

Because patients leave hospitals as soon as their physical conditions allow, they often have continuing health care needs when they go home or to another facility. For example, a surgical patient requires wound care at home after surgery. A patient who has had a stroke requires ambulation training. Patients and families worry about how they will care for unmet needs and manage over the long term. Nurses help by anticipating and identifying patients' continuing needs before the actual time of discharge and by coordinating health care team members in achieving an appropriate discharge plan.

Some patients are more in need of discharge planning because of the risks they present (e.g., patients with limited financial resources, limited family support, and long-term disabilities or chronic illness). However, any patient who is being discharged from a health care facility with remaining functional limitations or who has to follow certain restrictions or therapies for recovery needs discharge planning. All caregivers who care for a patient with a specific health problem participate in discharge planning. The process is truly interdisciplinary. For example, patients with diabetes visiting a diabetes management center require the group effort of a diabetes nurse educator, dietician, and physician to ensure that they return home with the right information to manage their condition. A patient who has experienced a stroke will not be discharged from a hospital until the team has established plans with physical and occupational therapists to begin a program of rehabilitation.

Effective discharge planning often requires referrals to various health care disciplines. In many agencies, a health care provider's order is necessary for a referral, especially in planning specific therapies (e.g., physical therapy). It is best to have patients and families participate in referral processes so that they are involved early in any necessary decision-making.

Some tips on making the referral process successful include the following:

- Make a referral as soon as possible.
- Give the care provider receiving the referral as much information about the patient as possible. This avoids duplication of effort and exclusion of important information.
- Involve the patient and family in the referral process, including selecting the necessary referral. Explain the service that the referral will provide, the reason for the referral and what to expect from the services of the referral.
- Determine what the referral discipline recommends for the patient's care and include this in the treatment plan as soon as possible.

Patient and Family Teaching

The nurse provides resources to improve the long-term outcomes of patients with limitations. Discharge planning depends on comprehensive patient and family education. Patients need to know what to do when they get home, how to do it, and for what to observe when problems develop (Shyu, 2008).

A patient requires the following instructions before he or she leaves the health care facility:

- Safe and effective use of medications and medical equipment.
- Instruction in potential food–drug interactions and counseling on nutrition and modified diets.
- Rehabilitation techniques to support adaptation to and/or functional independence in the environment.
- Access to available and appropriate community resources.
- When and how to obtain further treatment.
- The patient's and family's responsibilities in the patient's on-going health care needs and the knowledge and skills needed to carry out those responsibilities.
- When to notify their health care provider for changes in functioning or new symptoms.

Discharge Procedure

- The patient must be duly assessed for the readiness of discharge, and nurse must ensure that there is written order of the discharge or referral from the hospital.
- When the patient is DAMA, then ensure that the patient and family understand the consequence of this and they must duly sign the record for the same.
- Provide adequate discharge teaching to the patient and family so that they may be ensured that the patient and family understand the treatment, medicines, diet, and exercises to be continued at home (Box 13.1).
- Also, ensure that the patient and family understand the follow-up protocol and schedule; make sure that the patient and family get sufficient opportunity to clarify their queries and doubts.
- Ensure arrangement of ambulance or a transporting vehicle is made and also make sure that the patient, along with family, is transferred from hospital ward to the vehicle comfortably on wheelchair or stretcher.
- After the discharge, make sure that the patient's bed, bedside locker, and other utility are appropriately cleaned and disinfected, so that it will be ready to use for next patient.

Discharge Documentation

When discharging a patient, following details must be charted in nurses' notes:

- Date and time of patient discharge.
- How the client left the hospital and if needed arrange the transport.
- Special instructions provided to the client.
- Patient's personal belongings handed over with his or her signature.

BOX 13.1 Before Going Home, the Patient Must Know

- When and whom to follow-up?
- What symptoms to be observed for at home?
- How to take the prescribed medication?
- Which side effects of medication to watch for?

MEDICOLEGAL ISSUES RELATED TO DISCHARGE

During discharge procedure, nurses must keep the following medicolegal issues under consideration, so that they can safeguard themselves and the health care institution (Meera, 2016):

- Transfer of the patient from one ward to another ward or hospital must be carefully entered and signed in the ward records as well as duly recorded in the patient's file.
- Patient's records should not be handed over to police or legal authority without a written permission of the treating physician.
- Name and address of the relative or a person should be entered in hospital record with whom the patient has left the hospital.
- Physician and nurse should inform the chief medical officer about any special condition of discharge of patient such as LAMA or death. Now, LAMA is redefined as DAMA, and the patient must be handed over all the records and discharge notes.
- On discharge, each patient has full right to seek his or her medical records, including investigation reports.
- Discharge note should be kept under lock and key until handed over to the concerned patient and department.

MEDICOLEGAL ISSUES RELATED TO DISCHARGE OF MENTALLY ILL PATIENTS

Per the Indian Mental Health Act, 1987 (which is an amendment of the Indian Lunacy Act, 1912), "Mentally ill patient gets admitted on a voluntary basis (except a minor). After 24 hours, a board should decide regarding continuation of treatment or discharge of the patient." Admission can be made under special conditions where the patient is brought by relatives, friends, or neighbor. Application form for the admission is accompanied by report of two medical officers, of which one should be in government service. But a patient admitted on involuntary basis cannot be discharged with patient's wish but requires a due approval from psychiatrist and order of court.

MEDICOLEGAL ISSUES RELATED TO DISCHARGE OF A DEAD BODY

In case of death of the patient in hospital, the following issues must be kept under consideration:

- In case of death of the patient in hospital, physician should inform the chief medical officer or medical director and ensure that the body is appropriately kept in mortuary for the postmortem examination per the institutional policy.
- A written order should be obtained by the nurse before handing over the body to the mortuary staff/relatives/police officer with complete name, address, indemnification proof, and signature of the person receiving the body.

- Before handing over the articles belonging to the patient to the relatives, it should be ensured that a complete list of items is prepared and duly signed by the person receiving it.
- Ensure an appropriate privacy and dignity of the dead body during last office care.

Unclaimed dead body must be handed over to police after the due permission from the chief medical officer.

CARE OF THE UNIT AFTER DISCHARGE

- The room or unit must be cleaned or decontaminated per the hospital policy.
- Change all the linen and send them to laundry per the protocol. Mattress, pillows, blankets should be cleaned and exposed to sunlight.
- The bed, furniture, doors, and windows should be cleaned and decontaminated using disinfectant per the hospital policy.
- All articles used for patient care should be cleaned, washed, disinfected, or sterilized and send to utility room.
- All disposable items such as used tubing, cotton, dressing must be discarded per the hospital biomedical waste management policy.
- Prepare the room or unit for receiving the next patient, such as ventilate the room properly and prepare admission bed.
- If the patient had any contagious disease, then room or unit must be decontaminated or fumigated per the hospital policy.

KEY POINTS

- Admission facilitates a patient to stay in the hospital for investigation and treatment of the diseases he or she is suffering or for surgical interventions or on emergency basis.
- The purpose of admission procedure is to provide comfort and safety to the patient and to provide immediate care.
- Admission to the hospital can be divided into different types depending on *planning, time spent in hospital, on purposes of admission*.
- During admission, help the patient to occupy the bed and orient him or her to the ward.
- On admission, patients have various emotional responses.
- Discharge of a patient from the hospital is a departure process, which may be *planned discharge or patient may LAMA*.
- Under special conditions, the patients may be referred, transferred, or may be released on parole or absconding.
- Nurses must keep the medicolegal issues under consideration for admission and discharge, so that they can safeguard themselves and the health care institution.

REFERENCES

Alper E, O'Malley TA, Greenwald J, Aronson MD, Park L. Hospital discharge and readmission. UpToDate. Waltham, MA: UpToDate. 2017. Available from https://www.uptodate.com/contents/hospital-discharge-and-readmission.

Baranova K, Torti J, Goldszmidt M. Explicit Dialogue About the Purpose of Hospital Admission Is Essential: How Different Perspectives Affect Teamwork, Trust, and Patient Care. Academic Medicine. 2019 Dec 1;94(12): 1922-30.Avaiable from https://journals.lww.com/academicmedicine/fulltext/2019/12000/explicit_dialogue_about_the_purpose_of_hospital.29.aspx.

Devitt PJ, Devitt AC, Dewan M. Does identifying a discharge as "Against Medical Advice" confer legal protection? J Fam Pract 2000;49:224–227.

Discharge planning starts at admission. Nurse.com. 2021. Available from https://resources.nurse.com/discharge-planning-starts-admission.

Handy K. The admission and discharge nurse role: a quality initiative to optimize unit utilization, patient satisfaction, and nurse perceptions of collaboration, 2016. Available from https://sigma.nursingrepository.org/handle/10755/613233.

Lin C, Cheng S, Shih S, Chu C, Tjung J. Discharge Planning. International Journal of Gerontology. 2012;6(4):237–240.

Meera T. Medicolegal cases: What every doctor should know. J Med Soc 2016;30:133–4.

Preparing for admission. Columbia Asia. India. Available from https://www.columbiaindiahospitals.com/patient-guide/preparing-admission.

Patel AR. Modes of admission to hospital: A survey of emergency admissions to a general medical unit. Br Med J. 1971 Jan 30;1(5743):281–3. Available from https://www.jstor.org/stable/25413271?seq=1.

Shyu YI, Chen MC, Chen ST, Wang HP, Shao JH. A family caregiver-oriented discharge planning program for older stroke patients and their family caregivers. Journal of clinical nursing. 2008 Sep;17(18):2497–508. Available from https://onlinelibrary.wiley.com/doi/full/10.1111/j.1365-2702.2008.02450.x?casa_token=dlE2uLxgTwMAAAAA%3AY_HBIIxPtFwfxWrTbrYDF-oeBvhb8VNOOqgVEXmzCRj9O9NF7JnyFB2bnnoG-pNo9KRjsB3tjEeh90s.

Types of hospital admission. Better Health Channel. 2020. Available from https://www.betterhealth.vic.gov.au/health/servicesandsupport/types-of-hospital-admission.

Waghmode AH, Bodkha P, Chavan RR. Study of medico-legal cases admitted at tertiary care hospital. Bull Horn Injury. 2020 May 15; 4:0–58. Available from https://www.researchgate.net/publication/341252424_Study_of_medico-legal_cases_admitted_at_tertiary_care_hospital.

14 Mobility and Immobility

OBJECTIVES

After reading this chapter, the student should be able to:

- Describe the concepts of mobility and immobility.
- Explain elements of normal movement, body alignment, body balance, posture, and coordinated body movements.
- Enumerate the principles of transfer and positioning techniques.
- Discuss the physiological and psychosocial changes associated with immobility, and identify the impact changes have on nursing interventions.
- Describe how to assess patient body alignment and levels of activity and exercise.
- Formulate nursing diagnoses for patients experiencing alterations with activity and exercise.
- Describe complications associated with the physiological changes of immobility.
- Explain the techniques for assessing body alignment and impaired mobility.
- Discuss the importance of no-lift policies for patients and health care providers.
- Discuss the appropriate decision-making process when choosing equipment needed for safe patient handling and movement.
- Develop an individualized nursing care plan for patients with impaired mobility.
- Compare and contrast active and passive range-of-motion exercises.
- Evaluate patient outcomes of nursing care for improving or maintaining mobility.

KEY TERMS

activity tolerance, p. 295
active range-of-motion (ROM) exercises, p. 287
antagonistic muscles, p. 282
antigravity muscles, p. 282
bed rest, p. 281
body alignment, p. 278
body mechanics, p. 278
cartilage, p. 282
center of gravity, p. 278
crutch gait, p. 285
extension, p. 282
exercise, p. 279
footboards, p. 281
foot boot, p. 288
gait, p. 295
hemiplegia, p. 279
hand-wrist splints, p. 290
hyperextension, p. 289
isometric contraction, p. 280
isotonic contraction, p. 280
joint, p. 282
ligaments, p. 282
mechanical lift, p. 291
muscle tone, p. 278
mobility, p. 277
orthostatic hypotension, p. 292
osteoporosis, p. 279
prone, p. 289
posture, p. 278
proprioception, p. 282
range of motion (ROM), p. 293
synergistic muscles, p. 282
tendons, p. 282
trapeze bar, p. 290
trochanter rolls, p. 288

INTRODUCTION

People are mobile for many purposes (e.g., expression of emotions with nonverbal gestures and meeting basic needs). **Mobility** is also essential for self-defense, activities of daily living (ADLs), and recreational activities. Many functions of the body depend on mobility. Intact musculoskeletal and nervous systems are necessary for optimal physical mobility and functioning. Clinical nursing practices related to mobility and immobility require the incorporation of scientific and nursing knowledge and skills to provide competent care.

NATURE OF MOVEMENT

Movement is a complex process that requires coordination between the musculoskeletal and nervous systems. As a nurse, you will consider how a patient's physical and psychological condition affect body movement. **Body mechanics** is a term that describes the coordinated efforts of the musculoskeletal and nervous systems. Knowing how patients initiate movement and understanding your own movements require a basic understanding of the physics surrounding body mechanics. The body mechanics applied in the lifting techniques historically used in nursing practice often cause debilitating injuries to nurses and other health care staff (Burnfield et al., 2013; Griffis, 2012). Nowadays, nurses use evidence-based information about body alignment, balance, gravity, and friction when implementing nursing interventions such as positioning patients, determining the risk of patient falls, and selecting the safest way to move or transfer patients (Healey and Darowski, 2012).

ELEMENTS OF NORMAL MOVEMENT

The coordinated efforts of the musculoskeletal and nervous systems provide the foundation for body mechanics to maintain balance, **posture,** and body alignment during lifting, bending, moving, and performing **ADLs.** Performing these activities correctly decreases the risk for musculoskeletal system injury, preventing muscle strain and excessive use of muscle energy.

Body Alignment

Body alignment refers to the relationship of one body part to another along a horizontal or vertical line. Correct alignment reduces strain on musculoskeletal structures, maintains adequate **muscle tone,** and contributes to balance.

Body Balance and Posture

You achieve body balance when you balance a relatively low **center of gravity** over a wide, stable base of support. A vertical line falls from the center of gravity through the base of support. The base of support is the foundation. When the vertical line from the center of gravity does not fall through the base of support, the body loses balance.

Posture also enhances body balance. The term *posture* means maintaining optimal body position. It means a position that most favors function; requires the least muscular work to maintain; and places the least strain on muscles, ligaments, and bones (Huether and McCance, 2017).

Maintain proper body alignment and posture. First, widen your base of support by separating your feet to a comfortable distance. Second, bring the center of gravity closer to your base of support to increase balance. Bend your knees and flex the hips until squatting, and maintain proper back alignment by keeping your trunk erect.

Coordinated Body Movement

Weight is the force exerted on a body by gravity. When you lift an object, you must overcome the weight of the object and be aware of its center of gravity. In symmetrical objects, the center of gravity is located at the exact center of the object. The force of weight is always directed downward. An object that is unbalanced has its center of gravity away from the midline and falls without support. Similar to unbalanced objects, patients who fail to maintain balance with their center of gravity are unsteady, placing them at risk for falling. Promptly intervene with patients with an unbalanced center of gravity.

PRINCIPLES OF BODY MECHANICS OR TRANSFER AND POSITIONING TECHNIQUES

Using principles of safe patient transfer and positioning during routine activities decreases work effort and places less strain on musculoskeletal structures (Box 14.1). In addition to following these principles in your own practice, it is important to teach these principles to patients and family caregivers. Teaching family caregivers how to properly transfer or position a family member who is hospitalized increases and reinforces the family's knowledge about proper transfer and position techniques once the patient returns home.

Manual lifting is the last resort. Do *not* use manual lifting when you need to lift most or all of a patient's weight. Before lifting, assess the weight to be lifted, the assistance needed, and the resources available. Use safe patient–handling equipment and refer to algorithms for safe handling and movement in conjunction with agency lift teams to reduce the risk of injury to a patient and health care team members (Table 14.1).

BOX 14.1 Principles of Safe Patient Transfer and Positioning

- Mechanical lifts and lift teams are essential when a patient is unable to assist.
- When a patient is able to assist, remember the following principles:
  - The wider the base of support, the greater the stability of the nurse.
  - The lower the center of gravity, the greater the stability of the nurse.
  - The equilibrium of an object is maintained as long as the line of gravity passes through its base of support.
  - Facing the direction of movement prevents abnormal twisting of the spine.
  - Dividing balanced activity between arms and legs reduces the risk of back injury.
  - Leverage, rolling, turning, or pivoting requires less work than lifting.
  - When friction is reduced between the object to be moved and the surface on which it is moved, less force is required to move it.

Table 14.1 Preventing Lift Injuries in Health Care Workers

Action	Rationale
When planning to move a patient, arrange for adequate help. If your institution has a lift team, use it as a resource.	A lift team is properly trained in techniques to prevent musculoskeletal injuries.
Use patient-handling equipment and devices such as height-adjustable beds, ceiling-mounted lifts, friction-reducing slide sheets, and air-assisted devices (Stevenson, 2014).	These devices reduce caregiver muscular strain during patient handling.
Encourage the patient to help as much as possible during repositioning or transfer.	Promotes the patient's independence and strength while minimizing workload.
Keep back, neck, pelvis, and feet aligned. Avoid twisting.	Reduces risk of injury to lumbar vertebrae and muscle groups. Twisting increases risk of injury.
Flex knees; keep feet wide apart and aligned with shoulders.	A broad base of support increases stability.
Position yourself close to the patient (or object being lifted).	Reduces horizontal reach and stress on caregiver's back.
Use arms and legs (not back).	Leg muscles are stronger, larger muscles capable of greater work without injury.
Slide the patient toward yourself with a slide board or pull sheet. When transferring a patient onto a stretcher or bed, a slide board is more appropriate.	Sliding requires less effort than lifting. Pull sheet minimizes shearing forces, which can damage patient's skin.
Person with the heaviest load coordinates efforts of team involved by counting to three.	Simultaneous lifting minimizes the load for any one lifter.
Perform manual lifting as last resort and only if it does not involve lifting most or all of a patient's weight (Stevenson, 2014).	Lifting is a high-risk activity that causes significant biochemical and postural stressors.

FACTORS AFFECTING BODY ALIGNMENT, MOBILITY, AND ACTIVITY

Many conditions affect body alignment and mobility, including congenital defects; disorders of bones, joints, and muscles; central nervous system damage; and musculoskeletal trauma.

Congenital Defects

Congenital abnormalities can affect the musculoskeletal system by altering alignment, balance, and appearance. Osteogenesis imperfecta is an inherited disorder that affects bone. Some characteristics of this disorder are fractures and bone deformity (Hockenberry and Wilson, 2015). Bones are porous, short, bowed, and deformed; as a result, children experience curvature of the spine and shortness of stature. Scoliosis is a structural curvature of the spine associated with vertebral rotation. Muscles, ligaments, and other soft tissues become shortened. This affects balance and mobility in proportion to the severity of abnormal spinal curvatures (Huether and McCance, 2017).

Disorders of Bones, Joints, and Muscles

Osteoporosis is a common disorder of aging in which bone mass or density is reduced. The bone remains biochemically normal but has difficulty maintaining integrity and support. Many factors cause this, varying from hormonal imbalances to insufficient intake of nutrients (foods that contain calcium and vitamin D) (Huether and McCance, 2017).

Inflammatory and noninflammatory joint diseases and articular disruption all alter joint mobility. Some characteristics of inflammatory joint disease (e.g., arthritis) are inflammation or destruction of the synovial membrane and articular cartilage and systemic signs of inflammation. Noninflammatory diseases such as those resulting from a traumatic injury have none of these characteristics, and the synovial fluid is normal (Huether and McCance, 2017).

Central Nervous System Damage

Damage to any component of the central nervous system that regulates voluntary movement results in impaired body alignment and mobility. For example, you are caring for a patient who experienced head trauma with damage to the motor strip in the cerebrum. As a result, the patient could experience symptoms of limited or complete loss of movement based on where the damage occurred. The amount of voluntary motor impairment is directly related to the amount of destruction of the motor strip. A patient with a right-sided cerebral hemorrhage and damage to the right motor strip usually has left-sided **hemiplegia** or paralysis.

Musculoskeletal Trauma

Trauma to the musculoskeletal system sometimes results in bruises, contusions, sprains, and fractures. A fracture is a disruption of bone tissue continuity. Fractures most commonly result from direct external trauma. They also occur because of some deformity of the bone, as with pathological fractures of osteoporosis.

EXERCISE

Exercise is a physical activity. It can be used for body conditioning, improving health, maintaining fitness, providing therapy for correcting a deformity, or restoring the body to a maximal state of health. During assessment, determine a patient's level and frequency of exercise (Box 14.2). Your assessment of the patient's activity provides baseline information for both exercise and activity tolerance. In addition, baseline information is beneficial when establishing a patient's exercise and rehabilitation plan after an illness or injury. It is crucial to educate patients and family caregivers about the importance of regular physical activity and exercise and how these activities can be incorporated into daily routines (see Box 14.2 and Skill 14.1). Encourage patients to exercise daily; moderate 15- to 30-minute exercise is beneficial to maintain fitness, weight levels, and glycemic (blood sugar) control. CDC (2015) recommends adults need at least 2 hours and 30 minutes (150 minutes) of moderate-intensity aerobic activity each week. If a patient is actively exercising, be sure the patient is setting an adequate target heart rate for vigorous exercise. The AHA (2015) recommends that a person's target heart rate should be between 50% and 85% of his or her maximum heart rate. Maximum heart rate is approximately 220 minus age.

BOX 14.2 General Guidelines for Initiating an Exercise Program

Step 1: Assess Fitness Level

- Seek approval from a health care provider to begin. Are there any limitations to consider before determining the exercises in the fitness program?
- Record baseline fitness scores such as pulse rate, how long it takes to walk 1 mile, waist circumference, and body mass index.

Step 2: Design the Fitness Program

- Consider fitness goals. Make goals attainable.
- Plan a logical progression of activities (e.g., walk 1 mile and gradually increase the pace).
- Build the program into a daily routine.
- Plan the fitness program with creativity and different activities.

Step 3: Assemble Equipment

- Choose athletic shoes designed for the chosen exercise.
- Try equipment at a fitness center before purchasing to make sure that it fits into the fitness program.
- Buy used fitness equipment.
- Try homemade equipment (e.g., half-gallon milk jugs filled with sand for weights).

Step 4: Get Started

- Start slowly, including a warm-up and cool-down period.
- Divide exercise time throughout the day if time or fatigue is a barrier. Ten minutes of exercise three times a day instead of a single 30-min workout may be better for some patients' schedules and medical conditions.

Step 5: Monitor Progress

- Repeat fitness assessment at 6 weeks and then every 3–6 months.
- If losing motivation: set new goals, exercise with a friend, or try new activities.

Modified from the American Academy of Orthopaedic Surgeons: *Rehabilitation exercise and conditioning handouts,* 2012, http://orthoinfo.org/topic.cfm?topic=A00672; and Mayo Clinic Tools for Healthier Lives: *Fitness programs: 5 steps to getting started,* 2014, http://www.mayoclinic.org/healthy-lifestyle/fitness/in-depth/fitness/art-20048269?pg=1.

Always encourage older adults or patients with underlying medical conditions to consult with their health care provider before beginning a vigorous exercise program. Direct patient-centered health promotion activities toward maintaining and/or improving exercise and activity that help return a patient to independence and a maximal state of health after trauma or illness. Although some patients require formal rehabilitation, many of these activities are implemented in a patient's home or neighborhood. Recommend approaches that help older adults increase exercise and activity, use proper body mechanics, and prevent injury (Box 14.3).

Types of Exercise

Three categories of exercise are isotonic, isometric, and resistive isometric.

Isotonic exercises

Isotonic exercises (e.g., walking, swimming, jogging, bicycling) cause muscle contraction and change in muscle length (**isotonic contraction**). Isotonic exercises enhance circulatory and respiratory functioning; increase muscle mass, tone, and strength; and promote osteoblastic activity that combats osteoporosis.

Isometric exercises

Isometric exercises (e.g., quadriceps set exercises, contraction of the gluteal muscles) involve tightening or tensing muscles without moving body parts (**isometric contraction**). This form of exercise is ideal for patients who do not tolerate increased activity. A patient who is immobilized in bed can perform isometric exercises. The benefits are increased muscle mass, tone, and strength, thus decreasing the potential for muscle wasting; increased circulation to the involved body part; and increased osteoblastic activity.

BOX 14.3 Care of an Older Adult

General Guidelines for Initiating an Exercise Program With an Older Adult

- Encourage older adults to avoid prolonged sitting and to get up and stretch. Frequent stretching decreases joint contractures. Supervised resistance and aerobic exercise training in older adults both significantly improved physical function (Parreira et al., 2014; Chmelo et al., 2015).
- Maintain proper body alignment when sitting. Proper alignment minimizes joint and muscle stress.
- Teach older adults how to use stronger joints or larger muscle groups to manipulate items such as spray cans and container lids. Efficient distribution of workload decreases joint stress and pain.
- Provide resources for planned exercise programs. Proper exercise activities slow further bone loss and prevent fractures in older adults with osteoporosis (Wallace et al., 2014).
- It is never too late to begin an exercise program (Edelman et al., 2014). Be sure that older adults consult a health care provider before beginning an exercise program, particularly if they have heart, lung, or other illnesses.

Resistive Isometric

Resistive isometric exercises are exercises in which an individual contracts the muscle while pushing against a stationary object or resisting the movement of an object (Kim et al., 2015). A gradual increase in the amount of resistance and length of time that the muscle contraction is held increases muscle strength and endurance. Examples of resistive isometric exercises are push-ups and hip lifting, in which a patient in a sitting position pushes with the hands against a surface such as a chair seat and raises the hips. In some health care settings, **footboards** are placed on the end of beds; patients push against them to move up in bed. Resistive isometric exercises help promote muscle strength and provide sufficient stress against bone to promote osteoblastic activity.

Benefits of Exercises

Exercise improves muscle tone, size, and strength and cardiopulmonary conditioning. As a result, an individual is able to exercise longer with each strengthening of the muscles. Exercise also enhances joint mobility because the exercise itself requires movement of body parts (Box 14.4).

IMMOBILITY AND EFFECT OF IMMOBILITY

In addition to the effects of trauma and disease, a patient's mobility can be restricted for therapeutic reasons such as when **bed rest** is ordered. Therapeutic reasons for bed rest include decreasing the oxygen needs of the body, reducing cardiac workload and pain, and allowing the debilitated or ill patient to rest. The duration of bed rest depends on the type and nature of an illness or injury and the patient's prior state of health. For example, a patient returning from major surgery might be ordered to remain on bed rest for only a few hours. A patient with a serious systemic infection and cardiac complications might require bed rest for several days. Whatever the cause of a patient's immobility, the extent of the immobilization depends on the length and severity of illness, presence of pain, cognitive and emotional status such as depression, and overall physical condition. It is essential to remember that the hazardous effects of immobility are imposed on each of the systems of a patient's body (Box 14.5) (Huether and McCance, 2017). The greater the extent and longer the duration of immobility, the more pronounced the effects.

BOX 14.4 Benefits of Exercise

Cardiovascular System

- Increased cardiac output
- Improved myocardial contraction, thereby strengthening cardiac muscle
- Decreased resting heart rate
- Improved venous return

Pulmonary System

- Increased respiratory rate and depth followed by a quicker return to resting state
- Improved alveolar ventilation
- Decreased work of breathing
- Improved diaphragmatic excursion

Metabolic System

- Increased basal metabolic rate
- Increased use of glucose and fatty acids
- Increased triglyceride breakdown
- Increased gastric motility
- Increased production of body heat

Musculoskeletal System

- Improved muscle tone
- Increased joint mobility
- Improved muscle tolerance to physical exercise
- Possible increase in muscle mass
- Reduced bone loss

Activity Tolerance

- Improved tolerance
- Decreased fatigue

Psychosocial Factors

- Improved tolerance to stress
- Reports of "feeling better"
- Reports of decrease in illness (e.g., colds, influenza)

Data from Huether SE, McCance KL: *Understanding pathophysiology,* ed 6, St Louis, 2017, Mosby.

BOX 14.5 Effects of Immobility

Physiological Outcomes

- ↓ Basal metabolic rate
- ↓ Gastrointestinal motility
- ↓ Nutrients/fluids
- ↓ Appetite
- Shift in electrolyte balance
- ↓ O_2 availability/ischemia
  - ↓ O_2/CO_2 exchange
  - ↑ Respiratory muscle weakness
  - ↓ Lung expansion
  - ↑ Atelectasis/hypostatic pneumonia
- ↓ Cardiac output
  - ↑ Cardiac workload
  - ↑ Oxygen demand
  - ↑ Dependent edema
  - ↑ Clot formation (deep vein thrombosis)
- ↑ Muscle atrophy
  - ↓ Strength/flexibility/endurance
  - ↑ Joint contractures
- ↑ Disuse osteoporosis
- ↑ Bone resorption

Psychological Outcomes

- ↑ Stressors
- ↑ Depression
  - ↓ Self-identity
  - ↓ Self-esteem
- ↑ Behavioral changes
- ↑ Changes in sleep−wake cycles
- ↓ Coping successes
- ↑ Isolation
- ↑ Passive behaviors
- ↑ Sensory deprivation/overload

Developmental Outcomes

- ↑ Dependence
- ↑ Regression in development

MAINTENANCE OF NORMAL BODY ALIGNMENT AND MOBILITY

Coordinated body movement involves the integrated functioning of the skeletal, muscular, and nervous systems. Because these three systems cooperate so closely in mechanical support of the body, they are often considered as a single functional unit.

Skeletal System

Bones perform five functions in the body: support, protection, movement, mineral storage, and hematopoiesis (blood cell formation). To provide support, bones serve as the framework and contribute to the shape, alignment, and positioning of body parts. Bones provide movement, using their joints as levers for muscle attachment (Huether and McCance, 2017).

Joints

An articulation, or **joint,** is the connection between bones. Each joint is classified according to its structure and degree of mobility. Joints are classified as fibrous, cartilaginous, or synovial connective structures (Huether and McCance, 2017). Fibrous joints have a ligament or membrane that unites two bony surfaces such as the paired bones of the tibia and fibula. They are flexible and permit limited movement. The cartilaginous joint has little movement but is elastic. This type of joint allows for bone growth while providing stability, such as the joint between the sternum and second rib. The synovial, or true, joint is a freely movable joint. Bony surfaces are covered by cartilage and connected by ligaments lined with a synovial membrane. An example is the hip joint.

Ligaments, Tendons, and Cartilage

Ligaments are white, shiny, flexible bands of fibrous tissue that bind joints and connect bones and cartilages. They are elastic and aid joint flexibility and support. In some areas of the body, they also have a protective function. **Tendons** are white, glistening, fibrous bands of tissue that connect muscle to bone. Tendons are strong, flexible, and inelastic and occur in various lengths and thicknesses. **Cartilage** is nonvascular, supporting connective tissue with the flexibility of a firm, plastic material. The gristle-like nature of cartilage permits it to sustain weight and serve as a shock-absorber pad between articulating bones (Huether and McCance, 2017).

Skeletal Muscles

In addition to facilitating movement, muscles determine body form and contour. Skeletal muscles span at least one joint and attach to both articulating bones. When contraction occurs, one bone is fixed, while the other moves. The origin is the point of attachment that remains still; the insertion is the point that moves when the muscle contracts (Huether and McCance, 2017).

Muscles Concerned With Movement

The muscles of movement are near the skeletal region, where a lever system causes movement (Huether and McCance, 2017). The lever system makes the work of moving a weight or load easier. Movement occurs when specific bones such as the humerus, ulna, and radius and the associated joints such as the elbow act as levers. Thus, the force applied to one end of a bone to lift a weight at another point tends to rotate the bone in the opposite direction of the applied force. Muscles that attach to bones of leverage provide the necessary strength to move an object.

Muscles Concerned With Posture

Gravity pulls on parts of the body all the time; muscles exert pull on bones in the opposite direction to keep the body in position. Muscles accomplish this counterforce by maintaining a low level of sustained contraction. Poor posture places more work on muscles to counteract the force of gravity. This leads to fatigue and eventually interferes with bodily functions and causes deformities.

Muscle Groups

The nervous system coordinates the antagonistic, synergistic, and antigravity muscle groups that maintain posture and initiate movement. **Antagonistic muscles** bring about movement at the joint. During movement, the active mover muscle contracts, while its antagonist relaxes. For example, during **extension** of the arm, the active mover, the triceps brachii, contracts, and the antagonist, the biceps brachii, relaxes.

Synergistic muscles contract to accomplish the same movement. For example, when you flex your arm, you increase the strength of the contraction of the biceps brachii by contracting the synergistic muscle, the brachialis.

Antigravity muscles stabilize joints. These muscles continuously oppose the effect of gravity on the body and permit a person to maintain an upright or sitting posture. In an adult, the antigravity muscles are the extensors of the leg, the gluteus maximus, the quadriceps femoris, the soleus muscles, and the muscles of the back.

Skeletal muscles support posture and carry out voluntary movement. The muscles are attached to the skeleton by tendons, which provide strength and permit motion.

Nervous System

The nervous system regulates movement and posture. The motor strip, the major voluntary motor area, is located in the cerebral cortex (precentral gyrus) of the brain. Most motor fibers descend from the motor strip and cross at the level of the medulla. The motor fibers from the right motor strip initiate voluntary movement for the left side of the body, and motor fibers from the left motor strip initiate voluntary movement for the right side of the body. Transmission of the impulse from the nervous system to the musculoskeletal system is an electrochemical event that requires a neurotransmitter (i.e., a chemical that transfers the electrical impulse from the nerve to the muscle).

Proprioception

The nervous system also regulates posture. Posture requires coordination of proprioception and balance. **Proprioception** is the awareness of the position of the body and its parts and depends on impulses from the inner ear and receptors in joints and ligaments (Huether and McCance, 2017). Proprioceptors located on nerve endings in muscles, tendons, and joints monitor proprioception. While a person carries out ADLs, proprioceptors monitor muscle activity and body position. When a person walks, the proprioceptors on the bottom of the feet monitor pressure changes. Thus, when the bottom of the moving foot comes in contact with the walking surface, the individual automatically moves the stationary foot forward.

Balance

The cerebellum and the inner ear control balance through the nervous system. The major function of the cerebellum is to coordinate all voluntary movement. Within the inner ear are the fluid-filled semicircular canals. When you rotate your head suddenly in one direction, the fluid remains stationary for a moment while the canal turns with the head. This allows a person to change position suddenly without losing balance. Conditions affecting the cerebellum or inner ear impair balance and increase patients' risk for falling.

NURSING INTERVENTIONS FOR IMPAIRED BODY ALIGNMENT AND MOBILITY

Assistive Devices for Walking

Walkers

Walkers are extremely light, movable devices, approximately waist high and made of metal tubing (Fig. 14.1). They have four widely placed, sturdy legs. A walker is fitted correctly by having the patient step inside the walker. The person's elbow should bend comfortably, approximately 15–30°, while holding onto the handgrips. When the person relaxes the arms at the side of the body, the top of the walker should line up with the crease on the inside of the wrist (Pierson and Fairchild, 2013; American Academy of Orthopaedic Surgeons, 2015). Box 14.6 describes steps for instructing a patient on use of a walker.

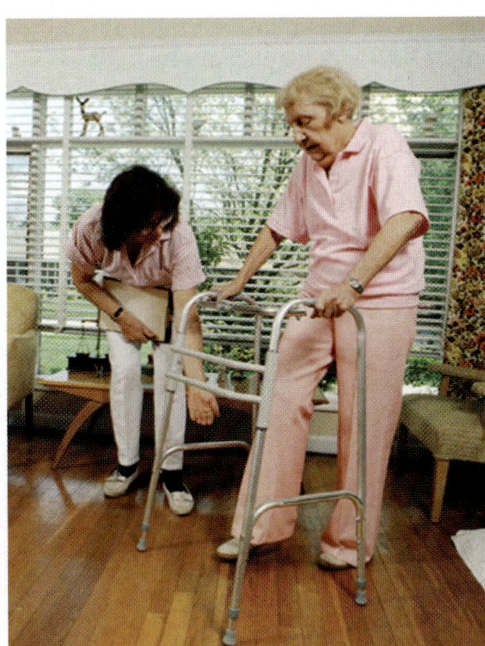

Fig. 14.1 Patient using walker.

Canes

Canes are lightweight, easily movable devices, held approximately waist high, made of wood or metal. Two common types of canes are the single straight-legged cane and the quad cane. The single straight-legged cane is used to support and balance a patient with decreased leg strength. Make sure that a patient keeps the cane on the stronger side of the body (Pierson and Fairchild, 2013). Stand on the patient's weak side to provide support (Pierson and Fairchild, 2013). For maximum support when walking, the patient places the cane forward 15–25 cm (6–10 inches), keeping the body weight on both legs. The patient moves the weaker leg to the cane, which divides body weight between the cane and the stronger leg. The patient then advances the stronger leg past the cane so that the weaker leg and the body weight are supported by the cane and weaker leg. During walking, the patient continually repeats these same three steps. Teach the patient that two points of support such as both feet

BOX 14.6 Patient Teaching

Walker Safety

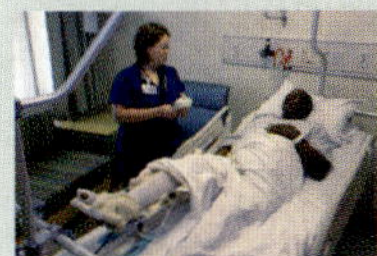

The physical therapist (PT) told Marilyn that Mr Girish Kumar will need a walker for a short time because of limited weight bearing on the affected knee. It is important that Mr Girish Kumar begins to use the walker before discharge. Marilyn and the PT work together to develop the following teaching plan.

Outcome

Patient states the steps needed for safe walker use.

Teaching Strategies

- Ensure patient's elbow bends at approximately 30° while holding onto walker grips.
- Ensure the top of the walker aligns with the crease on the inside of the wrist when patient relaxes the arms at the side of the body (Pierson and Fairchild, 2013).
- Instruct the patient to not lean over the walker or walk behind it so as to not lose balance and fall.
- The patient should walk upright and place one leg, or the injured leg, into the middle area of the walker. Caution the patient to not step close to the front bar. Have the patient keep the walker still as walking into it.
- Have the patient push straight down on the grips of the walker as he or she brings the other leg forward. Have the patient repeat the process by moving the walker forward and stepping into it one leg at a time.
- The patient or family caregiver should inspect walker regularly for worn tips or missing screws in the metal frame.

Evaluation

- Use the principles of teach back to evaluate the patient/family caregiver learning:
  - "Tell me what we discussed about the proper placement of your wrist and arms when using the walker."
  - "Tell me what we discussed about the correct way to walk when using the walker."
  - "Tell me what we discussed about ways to maintain walker safety."

or one foot and the cane need to be touching the ground at all times.

The quad cane provides the most support and is used when there is partial or complete leg paralysis or some hemiplegia (Fig. 14.2). You teach the patient the same three steps used with the straight-legged cane.

Crutches

The use of crutches is usually temporary, such as after ligament damage to the knee or a fracture to the leg. A crutch is a wooden or metal staff. The two types of crutches are the double adjustable Lofstrand or forearm crutch (Fig. 14.3) and the axillary wooden or metal crutch. The forearm crutch has a handgrip and a metal band that fits around a patient's forearm. The metal band and the handgrip are adjustable to fit a patient's height. The axillary crutch has a padded curved surface at the top, which fits under the axilla. The patient holds a handgrip in the form of a crossbar at the level of the palms to support the body. It is important to measure crutches for the appropriate length and teach patients to use their crutches safely. This includes teaching a patient to achieve a stable gait, ascend and descend stairs, and rise from a sitting position. You, or a physical therapist, teach the patient safety measures and guidelines associated with the use of crutches including maintenance of the crutches themselves as follows:

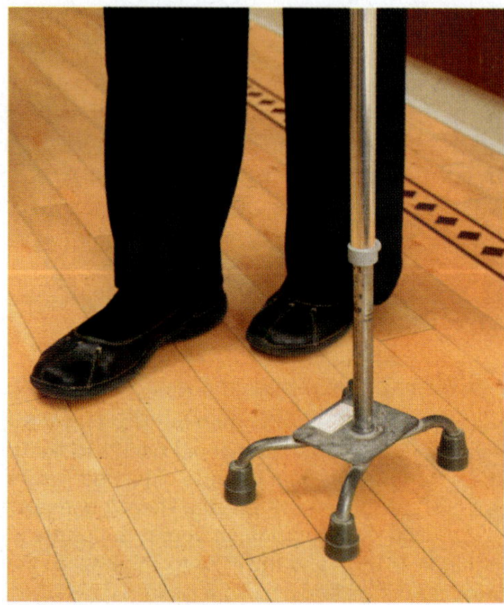

Fig. 14.2 Base of quad cane.

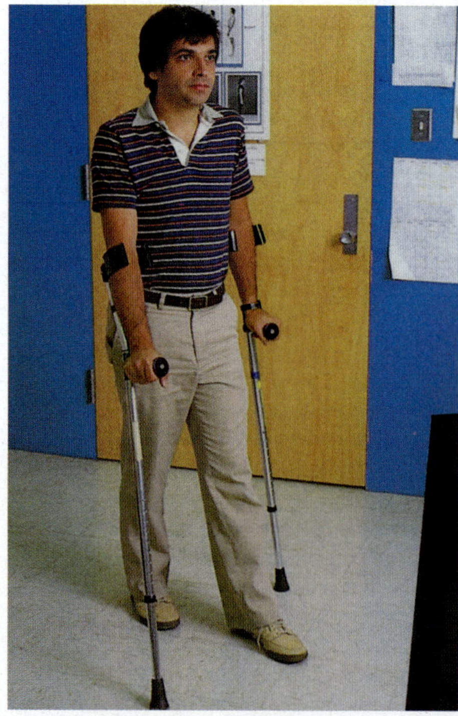

Fig. 14.3 Double adjustable Lofstrand or forearm crutch.

- Make sure that the rubber tips are attached securely to the crutches. Worn tips should be replaced immediately because they increase surface friction and prevent crutches from slipping.
- Inform the patient about the importance of keeping the crutch tips dry. Water decreases surface friction and increases the risk of crutches slipping.
- Show the patient how to inspect the structure of wooden crutches for cracks that decrease the ability of the crutch to support weight. Bends in aluminum crutches alter body alignment, increasing the risk for further damage to the musculoskeletal system.
- Give the patient a list of medical suppliers in the community to obtain repairs, new rubber tips, handgrips, and crutch pads as need arises.
- Suggest that the patient investigate the possibility of having a set of spare crutches and tips.

Measuring for Crutches

The axillary crutch is the more common crutch used. Measurement of a patient for a crutch includes the patient's height, the angle of elbow flexion, and the distance between the crutch pad and the axilla. When fitting a crutch, ensure that the length of the crutch is two to three finger widths from the axilla, and position the tips approximately 2 inches lateral and 4–6 inches anterior to the front of the patient's shoes (Fig. 14.4) (Pierson and Fairchild, 2013).

Position the handgrips so that the axillae are not supporting the patient's body weight. Pressure on the axillae increases risk to underlying nerves, which sometimes results in partial paralysis of the arm. Determine correct position of the handgrips with the patient upright, supporting weight by the handgrips with the elbows slightly flexed at 20–25° (Pierson and Fairchild, 2013). Elbow flexion may be verified with a goniometer by a physical therapist (Fig. 14.5). When you determine the height and placement of the handgrips, verify that the distance between the crutch pad and the patient's axilla is approximately 2 inches (two to three finger widths) (Fig. 14.6).

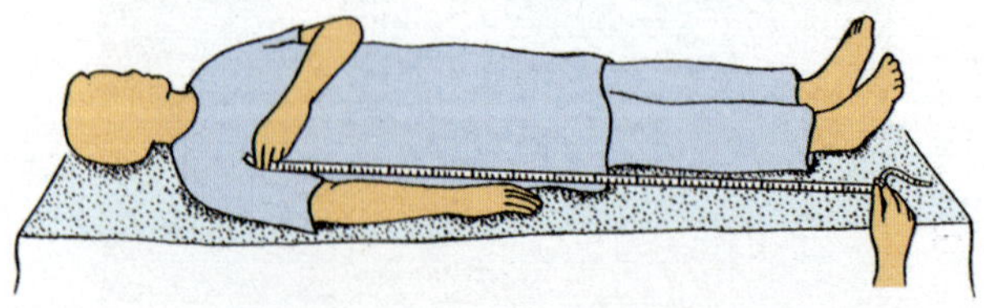

Fig. 14.4 Measuring for crutch length.

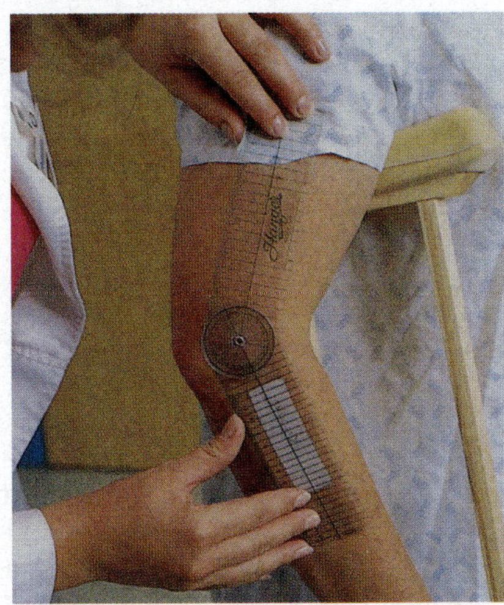

Fig. 14.5 Using goniometer to verify correct degree of elbow flexion for crutch use.

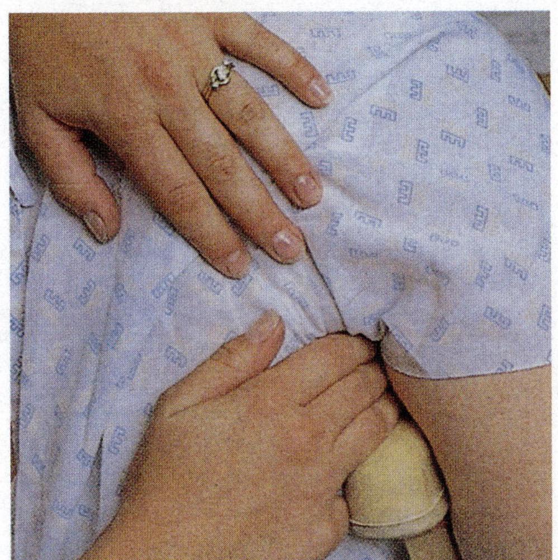

Fig. 14.6 Verifying correct distance between crutch pad and axilla.

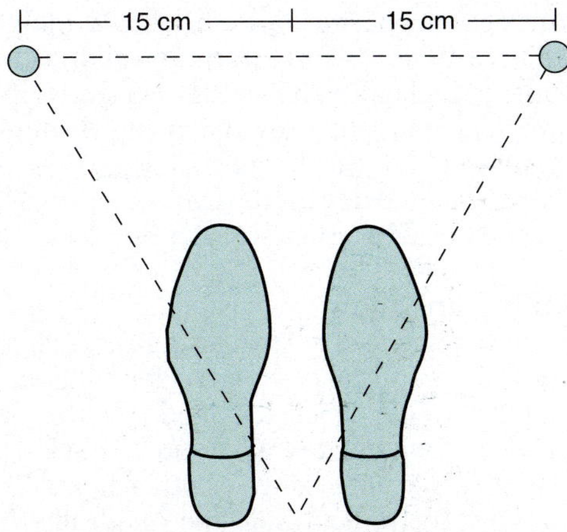

Fig. 14.7 Tripod position, basic crutch stance.

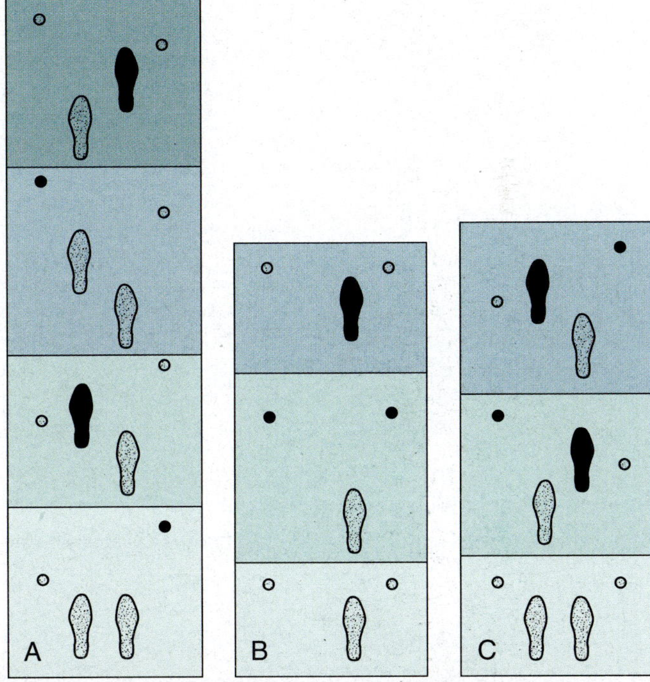

Fig. 14.8 A, Four-point alternating gait. Solid feet and crutch tips show foot and crutch tip moved in each of the four phases. (Read from bottom to top.) **B,** Three-point gait with weight borne on unaffected leg. Solid foot and crutch tips show weight bearing in each phase. **C,** Two-point gait with weight borne partially on each foot and each crutch advancing with opposing leg. Solid areas indicate leg and crutch tips bearing weight.

Crutch Gait

A patient assumes a **crutch gait** by alternately bearing weight on one or both legs and then on the crutches. The physical therapist determines the appropriate gait by assessing a patient's functional abilities, strength and weight-bearing ability, and the disease or injury that resulted in the need for crutches.

This section summarizes the basic crutch stance and the three standard gaits: four-point alternating gait, three-point alternating gait, and two-point gait. The basic crutch stance is the tripod position, formed when the crutches are placed 15 cm (6 inches) in front of and 15 cm to the side of each foot (Fig. 14.7). This position improves the patient's balance by providing a wider base of support. The body alignment of the patient in the tripod position includes erect head and neck, straight vertebrae, and extended hips and knees. No weight should be borne by the axillae. The tripod position is used before crutch walking.

The four-point alternating or four-point gait gives stability to a patient but requires weight bearing on both legs. Each leg is moved alternately with each opposing crutch so that three points of support are on the floor at all times (Fig. 14.8A).

Three-point alternating or three-point gait requires a patient to bear all of the weight on one foot. In a three-point gait, a patient puts weight on both crutches and then on the uninvolved leg and repeats the sequence (Fig. 14.8B). The affected leg does not touch the ground during the early phase of the three-point gait. Gradually, the patient progresses to touchdown and full weight bearing on the affected leg.

The two-point gait requires at least partial weight bearing on each foot (Fig. 14.8C). The patient moves a crutch at the same time as the opposite leg so the crutch movements are similar to arm motion during normal walking.

People with paraplegia who wear weight-supporting braces on their legs frequently use the swing-through gait. With weight placed on the supported legs, the patient places the crutches one stride in front and then swings to or through the crutches while they support his or her weight.

Crutch Walking on Stairs

Walking upstairs or downstairs with a single crutch and using the support of a handrail poses a risk for patients to fall. Perform this skill carefully. Apply a gait belt securely around the patient's waist. Be sure there are no obstacles on the stairs, such as stacks of magazines or other items. To walk up the stairs, have the patient hold the handrail with one hand (strong leg next to railing) (Fig. 14.9). You carry the crutch positioned next to the handrail in your nondominant hand as the patient holds the other crutch. Stay behind the patient holding the gait belt with your dominant hand. Then have the patient support his or her weight evenly between the handrail and crutch. The patient next places some weight on the crutch and then steps up on the first step with the weight-bearing foot. Have the patient get his or her balance. Next, instruct the patient to straighten the uninvolved knee and lift his or her body weight, bringing the crutch and affected leg up the stair. The patient repeats the sequence of steps until patient reaches the top of the stairs. Observe the patient's balance and level of fatigue.

Walking down steps basically involves the same steps with the patient holding the handrail with the involved leg next to the railing. You again carry the other crutch in your hand that is not grasping gait belt. Have the patient bend his or her strong knee while moving the crutch and involved leg down a step (Fig. 14.10, Step 1). The patient then supports his or her

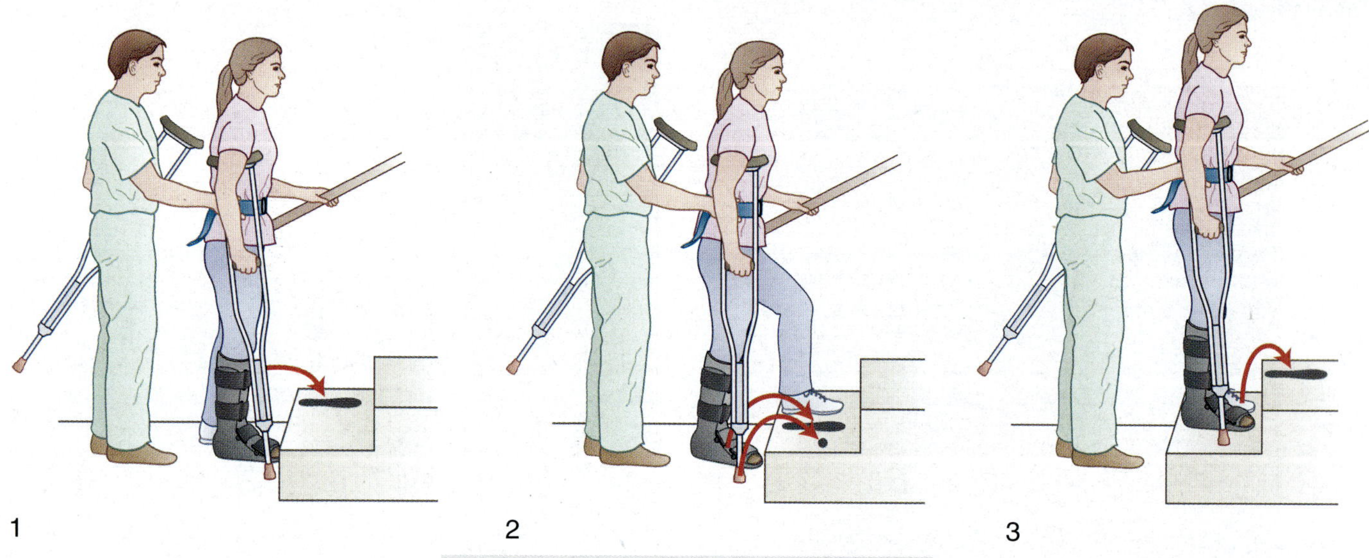

Fig. 14.9 Patient position to begin ascending stairs.

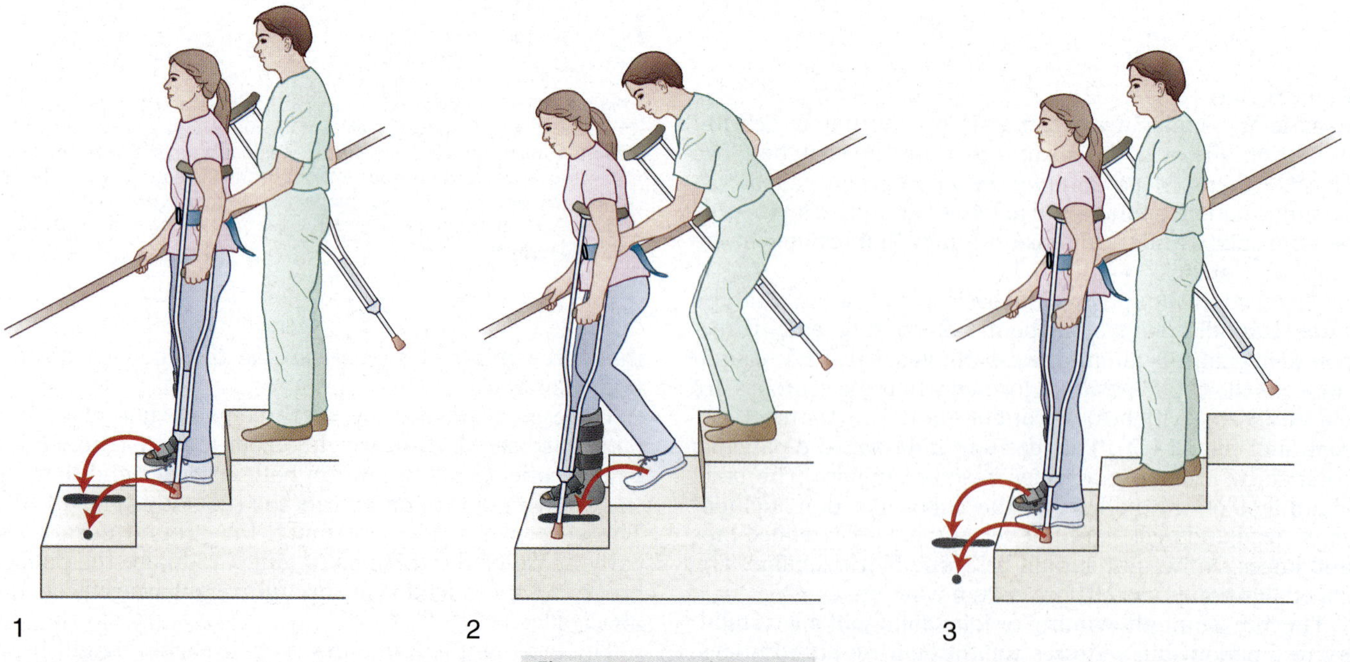

Fig. 14.10 Descending stairs.

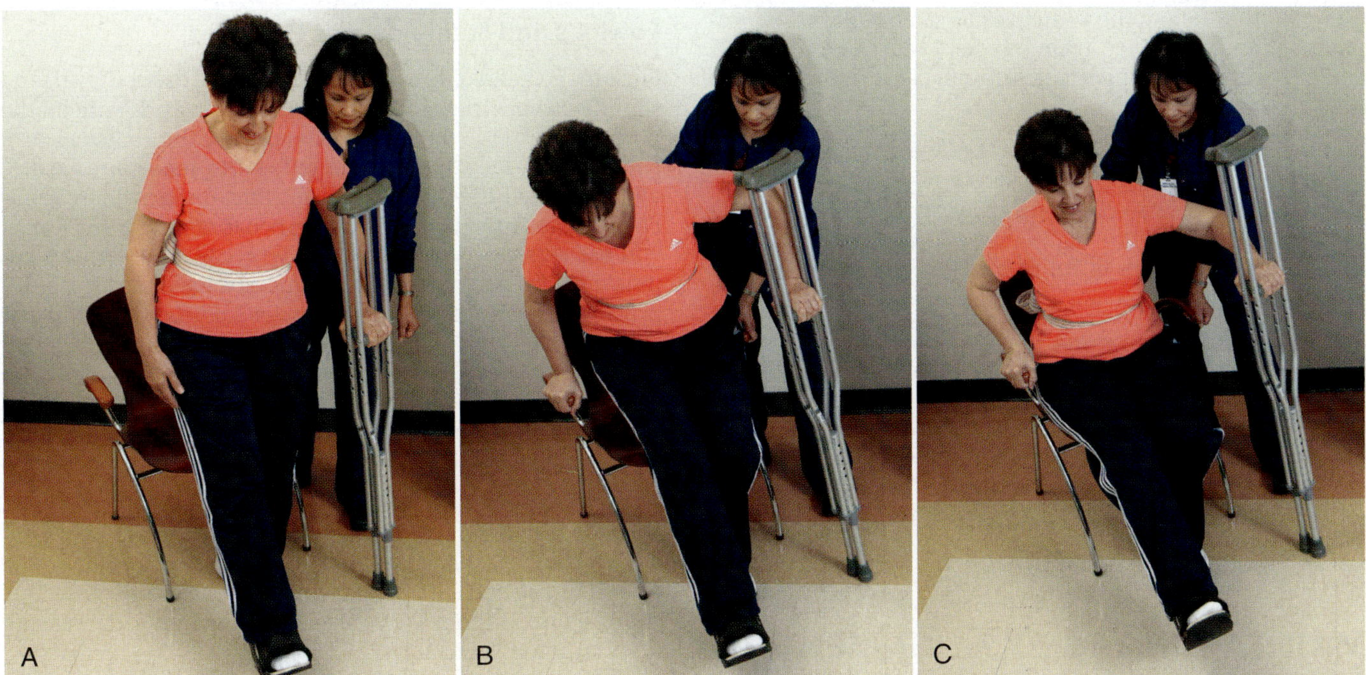

Fig. 14.11 Sitting on chair. **A,** Both crutches are held by one hand. Patient transfers weight to crutches and unaffected leg. **B,** Patient grasps arm of chair with free hand and begins to lower herself into chair. **C,** Patient completely lowers herself into chair.

weight evenly between the handrail and crutch. Hold onto the patient's gait belt at all times. Be sure that the patient has good balance. Have the patient slowly bring the uninvolved or stronger leg down a step and caution the patient not to hop (Fig. 14.10, Step 2). Continue sequence (Fig. 14.10, Step 3).

The American College of Foot and Ankle Surgeons (ACFAS, 2016) recommends a safer method for patients to move up and down steps with crutches. Basically, the patient sits on the stairs and uses both arms and the weight-bearing foot and leg to lift himself or herself up or down, one step at a time. A family caregiver or nurse places the crutches at the top or bottom of the stairs before the patient begins.

Sitting in a Chair With Crutches

Sitting in a chair with crutches also involves phases and requires a patient to transfer weight (Fig. 14.11). First, the patient gets positioned at the center front of the chair with the posterior aspect of the legs touching the chair. Then, the patient holds both crutches in the hand opposite the affected leg. If both legs are affected (e.g., a person who wears weight-supporting braces), the patient holds the crutches in the hand on the stronger side. With both crutches in one hand, the patient supports his or her body weight on the unaffected leg and crutches. While still holding the crutches, the patient grasps the arm of the chair with the remaining hand and lowers the body into the chair. To stand, the patient reverses the procedure and, when fully erect, assumes the tripod position before beginning to walk.

RANGE-OF-MOTION EXERCISES

The easiest intervention to maintain or improve joint mobility for patients—and one that you are able to coordinate with other activities—is the use of ROM exercises. In **active range-of-motion (ROM) exercises,** a patient is able to move his or her joints. In contrast, you move the patient's joints in passive ROM exercises. The use of these exercises enables you to evaluate a patient's response to improve the patient's joint mobility. Unless contraindicated, the nursing care plan includes exercising each joint through as nearly a full ROM as possible. Initiate passive ROM exercises as soon as a patient loses the ability to move the extremity or joint.

Joints that are not moved periodically develop contractures, a permanent shortening of a muscle followed by the eventual shortening of associated ligaments and tendons. Over time, the joint becomes fixed in one position, and a patient loses normal use of it. For a patient who does not have voluntary motor control, passive ROM exercises are the exercises of choice.

Older adults experiencing a decline in physical activity and changes in joints often have limited mobility and joint flexibility. Use a variety of recommended approaches to help older adults maximize movement and prevent injury.

At times, mechanical devices are available to move joints through continuous passive motion (CPM). A physician orders this machine to be set at certain degrees of joint mobility with increasing flexion and extension as the goal. Patients who have historically used the CPM machine have had total joint replacement surgery. However, use of the CPM has decreased in practice over the last 10 years with implementation of fast-track rehabilitation following total knee arthroplasty.

MUSCLE STRENGTH EXERCISES

The main intervention to enhance or maintain the muscle strength, power, activity tolerance, and muscle mass of patient is to practice of muscle strength exercise. These are exercises that follow the principles of strength exercise, resistance, and tolerance training. As a nurse, you should teach three important variables of muscle strengthen exercise. These are as follows:

a. *Intensity:* It refers to the amount of work needed to complete the activity.
b. *Volume:* It refers to counting of exercises sets in a single session.
c. *Frequency:* It refers to number of exercise sessions carried out in a week.

It is important for a nurse to assess baseline fitness level of an older adult and know his or her limitations before initiating an exercise program. An exercise schedule should have an objective to enhance strength. The schedule should be based on patient's ability to perform exercise. The use of these exercises improves the patient's joint mobility, muscle strength, bone density, mass, and activity tolerance.

MAINTAINING BODY ALIGNMENT: POSITIONING TECHNIQUES

Patients with impaired nervous or musculoskeletal system functioning, patients with increased weakness, and patients restricted to bed rest benefit from therapeutic positioning. During patient positioning, determine areas of bony prominences where pressure, **friction,** and shear cause the most wear and tear. Through the use of proper positioning and pressure-relief methods, you are able to protect these areas (see Chapter 17).

In general, you reposition patients as needed and at least every 2 hours if they are in bed and every 15–20 minutes if they are sitting in a chair or wheelchair (AHRQ, 2014; Swafford et al., 2016). Improper positioning increases patients' risk for developing pressure injuries or contractions, especially patients who have underlying conditions such as diabetes mellitus or peripheral vascular diseases.

Reposition patients with contractures or patients who are at greater risk for skin breakdown over bony prominences more often than every 2 hours. New sensor devices are now being used in hospital settings. The devices are applied over bed mattresses and provide a visual image of the interface pressure between a patient's body and support surface or mattress (Wong et al., 2015). The images inform clinicians about areas of the skin under pressure and the need for repositioning strategies. Use of the pressure sensor devices has shown promise in the reduction of hospital-acquired pressure injuries (Behrendt et al., 2014).

Placing patients in positions that compromise peripheral blood flow also damages nerves. Every time you reposition a patient, make certain to check total body alignment, placement of extremities, skin condition, and joint ROM. The following also influence the frequency of position changes: level of comfort, amount of spontaneous movement, presence of edema, loss of sensation, and overall physical and mental status. Several devices are available to maintain a patient's body alignment after positioning. Select the therapeutic position that maximizes your patient's comfort, safety, and ability to still use remaining function (see Skill 14.2).

Fowler's and Semi-Fowler's Positions

Elevate the head of the patient's bed to the desired level, and slightly elevate the patient's knees, avoiding pressure on the popliteal vessels. The head rests against the mattress or a small pillow for support. Use pillows to maintain natural alignment of the hands, wrists, and forearms. In semi-Fowler's position, the head of the bed is at a 30–45° angle; you use this position for patients who cannot tolerate a supine position such as patients with cardiac and respiratory problems. In Fowler's or high-Fowler's position, the head of the bed is 60–90°. Patients with severe respiratory distress breathe more easily in a high-Fowler's position. A patient who remains in place in Fowler's or semi-Fowler's position for more than 2 hours (sometimes less) can develop common problems including the following:

- Increased cervical flexion because the pillow at the head is too thick and head thrusts forward
- Extension of the knees, allowing a patient to slide to the foot of the bed causing shear against the skin
- Pressure on the posterior aspect of the knees, decreasing circulation to the feet
- External rotation of the hips
- Arms hanging unsupported at a patient's sides
- Unsupported feet or pressure on the heels
- Unprotected pressure points at the sacrum and heels
- Increased shearing force on the back and heels when you raise the head of the bed more than 60°

Supine Position

Position a patient supine by placing him or her flat on the back. A small, flat pillow supports the head, neck, and upper shoulders (Perry et al., 2017). When a patient is immobile, use pillows, **trochanter rolls**, heel boots, hand rolls, or arm splints to increase comfort and reduce injury to the skin or musculoskeletal system. The risk for aspiration into the tracheobronchial tree (see Chapter 24) is greater with this position; avoid the supine position when the patient is confused, agitated, experiencing a decreased level of consciousness, or at risk for aspiration. Make sure that the mattress is firm enough to support the cervical, thoracic, and lumbar vertebrae. Avoid pressure on the back of the legs and heels. Use a **foot boot** to prevent footdrop (Fig. 14.12),

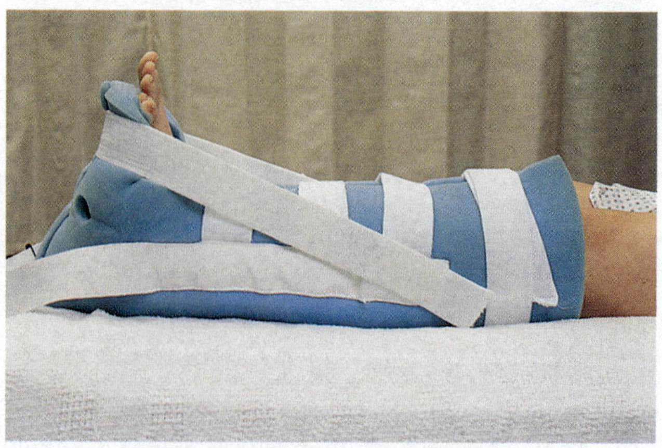

Fig. 14.12 Foot boot with lower leg extension.

maintain proper alignment, and provide freedom of movement for the feet. Patients who remain in the supine position for too long can develop the following problems:

- Cervical flexion from a too thick pillow being placed under the head
- Pressure over the occiput from the head staying flat on the mattress
- Shoulders unsupported and internally rotated
- Elbows extended
- Thumb not in opposition to the fingers
- Hips externally rotated
- Feet unsupported
- Unprotected pressure points at the vertebrae, coccyx, elbows, heels, and occipital region of the head

Prone Position

When **prone,** a patient is in the face-down position. Although it is not a position commonly used for patients, it is used for critically ill patients on mechanical ventilation and who have acute respiratory distress syndrome (ARDS). Use of prone position ventilation has been shown to improve oxygenation in selected patients with ARDS (Henderson et al., 2014). Before placing a patient in the prone position, assess his or her medical record for any possible complications such as increasing intracranial pressure or cardiopulmonary disease. Also assess current vital signs.

Help the patient lie on the abdomen. Have the patient turn the head to the side; this facilitates respiration and drainage of oral secretions. Place a pillow under the head for comfort and relief from pressure. As an alternative, place a wedge under the patient's chest or arms flexed over the head if it is more comfortable. Place a pillow under the lower leg; this promotes relaxation. If a pillow is unavailable, make sure that a patient's ankles are in dorsiflexion over the end of the mattress. Body alignment is poor when the ankles are continuously in plantar flexion and the lumbar spine remains in **hyperextension.** Sometimes, lung expansion is compromised in this position, especially in patients who are obese. Monitor your patient for signs of respiratory distress. You assess for and correct any of the following potential trouble points:

- Neck hyperextension
- Hyperextension of the lumbar spine
- Plantar flexion of the ankles
- Unprotected pressure points at the chin, elbows, hips, knees, and toes

Thirty-Degree Lateral Position

In the 30° lateral position, a patient is supported on the right or left side with the opposite arm, thigh, and knee flexed and resting on the bed. Place a pillow under the patient's head to keep the head, neck, and spine in alignment. Both arms are placed in slightly flexed positions with the upper arm supported with a pillow. The dependent hip is brought forward so that the angle from hip to mattress is approximately 30°. Less pressure is placed directly on the bony prominence compared with just a side-lying position. The upper leg is flexed at the hip and knee and positioned on a small pillow (Perry et al., 2017). The 30° lateral position is recommended as a position to avoid development of pressure injuries (Swafford et al., 2016). A patient placed in the side-lying position instead of 30° lateral position can develop:

- Lateral flexion of the neck
- Spinal curves out of normal alignment
- Shoulder and hip joints internally rotated, adducted, or unsupported
- Lack of support for the feet
- Lack of protection for pressure points at the ear, shoulder, anterior iliac spine, trochanter, and ankles
- Excessive lateral flexion of the spine if the patient has large hips and a pillow is not placed superior to the hips at the waist

Sims' Position

In Sims' position, a patient is semiprone on the right or left side with the opposite arm, thigh, and knee flexed and resting on the bed. Sims' position differs from the side-lying position in the distribution of the patient's weight. In this position, you place the patient's weight on the anterior ilium, humerus, and clavicle. Trouble points common in Sims' position include the following:

- Lateral flexion of the neck
- Internal rotation, adduction, or lack of support to the shoulders and hips
- Lack of support for the feet
- Lack of protection for pressure points at the ilium, humerus, clavicle, knees, and ankles

Several devices are available for maintaining proper patient positioning. Pillows are commonly used to support body alignment. Before using a pillow, determine whether it is the proper size and consistency. A thick pillow under a patient's head causes excessive cervical flexion. A thin pillow under bony prominences is inadequate to protect skin and tissue from damage. When additional pillows are unavailable, use folded sheets, blankets, or towels as positioning aids. Elevate a patient's calves on pillows or use a heel protector to avoid pressure on the heels. A trochanter roll prevents external rotation of the hips when the patient is in a supine position (Fig. 14.13). Hand rolls

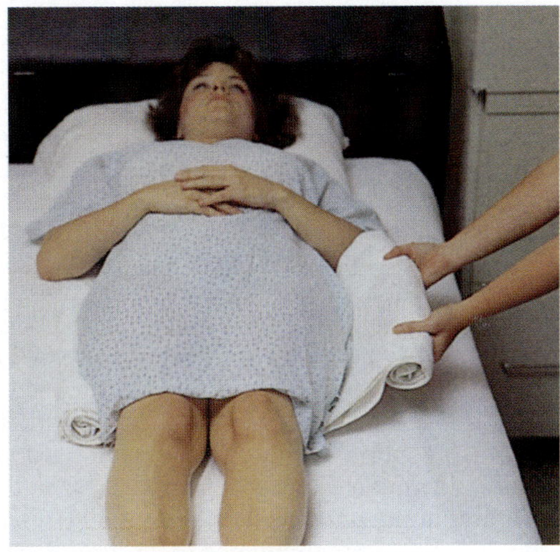

Fig. 14.13 Trochanter roll.

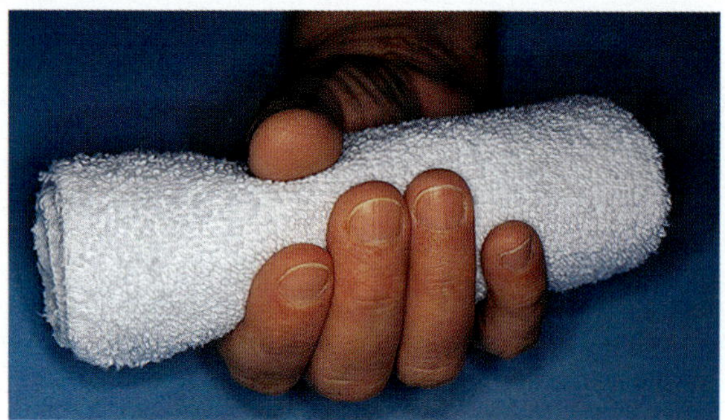

Fig. 14.14 Hand roll.

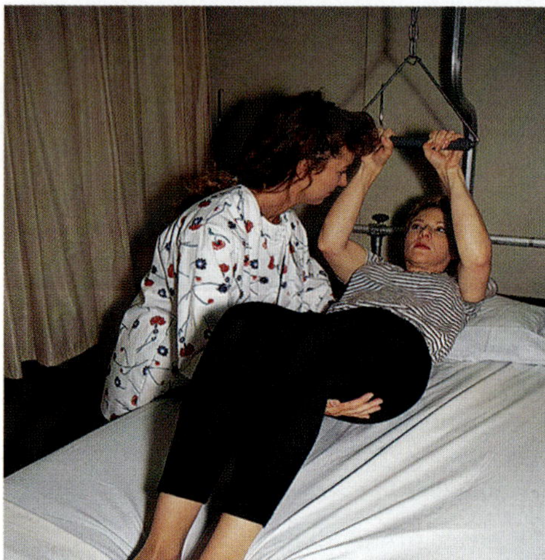

Fig. 14.15 Patient using a trapeze bar.

maintain the hand, thumb, and fingers in a functional position (Fig. 14.14). **Hand-wrist splints** are individually molded for a patient to maintain proper alignment of the thumb. A **trapeze bar** is a triangular device that hangs from a securely fastened overhead bar that is attached to the patient's bedframe (Fig. 14.15). It is a useful device for helping to increase patient independence when moving in bed, maintain upper body strength, and reduce friction from movement in bed.

ASSISTING PATIENT IN AMBULATION

Early Mobility

Recently concerted efforts have been made in hospitals to increase inpatients' activity and mobility levels as soon as possible to prevent deconditioning and other complications of immobilization (see Skill 14.1). The AACN (2013) now recommends an early progressive mobility protocol for critical care patients (refer to agency policy for protocols). When patients are transferred out to general nursing units, early mobility protocols should continue. This is often a challenge because staff nurses on general units often have difficulty routinely ambulating patients because of overall patient care demands, access to equipment, or unfamiliarity with transfer skills (see Skill 14.3). However, early mobilization has been found to be a nursing intervention that provides positive outcomes for critical care, cardiovascular, neurological (stroke), and orthopedic patient populations (Pashikanti and Von Ah, 2012). Early mobility protocols typically involve a progressive series of specific mobility interventions (e.g., ROM, sitting on side of bed, ambulating to chair, ambulating) to help patients attain and/or maintain their baseline mobility status. Some hospitals have designated special mobility teams or mobility assistants to engage patients in early ambulation and activity.

Walking

Walking increases exercise tolerance, circulation, and joint mobility. In the normal walking posture, the head is erect; the cervical, thoracic, and lumbar vertebrae are aligned; the hips and knees have appropriate flexion; and the arms swing freely in alternation with the legs. Illness or trauma reduces activity tolerance, sometimes requiring you to assist the patient with walking or having the patient use assistive devices such as crutches, canes, or walkers.

Helping a patient walk requires preparation. Your initial assessment should have included a patient's activity tolerance, strength, coordination, and balance to determine the type of assistance needed. Also, reassess a patient's orientation and determine whether there are any signs of distress before you assist the patient with ambulation.

Also assess the environment for safety before ambulation. Remove obstacles and be sure that the floor is clean and dry. Establish rest points in case the patient's activity tolerance decreases or the patient becomes dizzy. Also, make sure that the patient wears supportive, nonslip shoes.

When preparing a patient who is in bed for ambulation, dangling is an important technique. You help the patient to a sitting position with the legs dangling off the side of the bed and have him or her rest for 1–2 minutes before standing (see Skill 14.1). The longer the period of immobility, the greater are the physiological changes. This is especially true with changes in circulation. When a patient has been flat for extended periods, blood pressure drops when the patient stands. Dangling helps to prevent this. After standing, have the patient remain stationary for 1–2 minutes before moving. If the patient becomes dizzy, the bed is still nearby, and you are able to quickly ease him or her back to bed.

There are several methods to help a patient with ambulation. Always apply a gait belt to support a patient and maintain a midline center of gravity. Make sure that he or she does not lean to one side while walking because this causes the center of gravity to no longer be at midline, which distorts balance and increases risk for falling.

Return a patient who appears unsteady or complains of dizziness to the closest bed or a chair. If the patient has a syncopal episode or begins to fall, assume a wide base of support with one foot in front of the other, thus supporting the patient's body weight. Gently lower the patient to the floor, protecting his or her head. Although lowering a patient to the floor is not difficult, practice this technique with a friend or classmate before attempting it in a clinical setting (Fig. 14.16). Assess the patient for injuries at this time and notify the patient's health care provider. Even if the patient is stable, obtain the assistance of a lift team to help you get the patient off the floor and back in the bed or a chair.

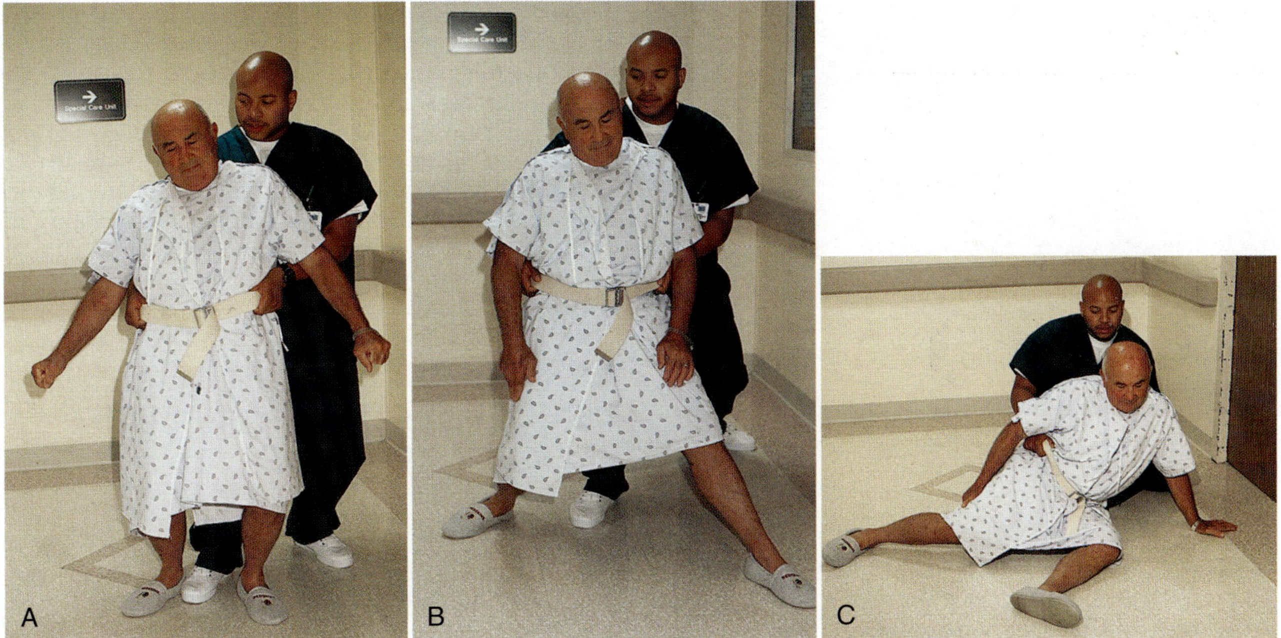

Fig. 14.16 **A,** Stand with feet apart to provide broad base of support. **B,** Extend one leg and let patient slide against it to floor. **C,** Bend knees to lower body as patient slides to floor.

Lifting Techniques

In the clinical setting, patient care activities place health care providers at risk for injury during patient handling. Recently, the rate of injuries in occupational settings has increased dramatically. The most common back injury is strain on the lumbar muscle group, which includes the muscles around the lumbar vertebrae. Injury to these areas affects the ability to bend forward, backward, and side to side and to rotate the hips and lower back.

Lifting activities are necessary in acute care and restorative care settings. For example, you may care for an individual who is wheelchair dependent and healthy but needs assistance moving from bed to chair or chair to commode, or you may care for an individual who is unable to assist with any transfer and needs to be lifted from bed to chair or bed to stretcher. In any setting, you need to know and use proper lifting techniques. Before lifting, assess the weight that you will lift and what assistance, if any, you need. If you need help, assess if a second person is adequate or if you need to use a **mechanical lift**. Once you determine the amount of assistance you need, follow these steps:

1. Keep the weight you are lifting as close to your body as possible; this action places the object in the same plane as the lifter and close to the center of gravity for balance.
2. Bend at the knees; this maintains the center of gravity and uses the stronger leg muscles to do the lifting (Fig. 14.17). Avoid twisting. Twisting overloads the spine and leads to serious injury.
3. Tighten abdominal muscles and tuck the pelvis; this provides balance and helps protect the back.
4. Keep your trunk erect and knees bent so that multiple muscle groups work together in a coordinated manner.

Remember that injuries are not only related to lifting. You spend time in many activities involving bending and twisting that also cause injury (e.g., lifting and carrying supplies and equipment and pushing and pulling equipment) (Anderson et al., 2014).

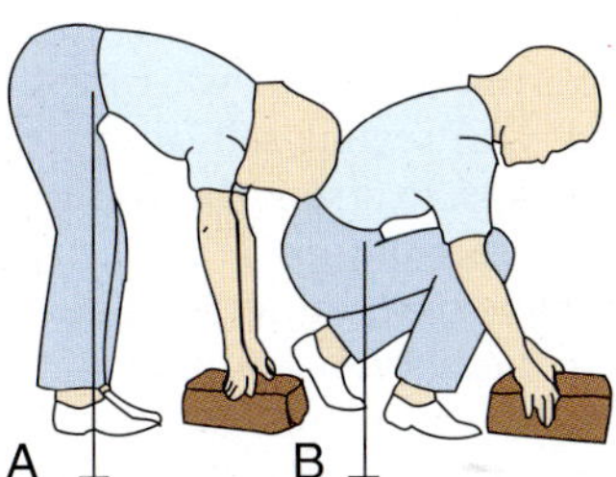

Fig. 14.17 Incorrect **(A)** and correct **(B)** body position for lifting.

Moving and Transferring Patients

Patients require various levels of assistance to move up in bed, move to the side-lying position, or sit up at the side of the bed. For example, a young, healthy woman needs only a little support as she sits at the side of the bed for the first time after childbirth, whereas an older man needs help from two or more nurses to do the same task 1 day after abdominal surgery. When moving or transferring a patient, always ask the patient to help to the fullest extent possible. To determine what the patient is able to do alone and how many people are needed to help move the patient in bed, assess whether the patient's illness contradicts exertion (e.g., cardiovascular disease). As a rule of thumb, *get help* to transfer a patient. If you or any other caregiver needs to lift more than 15.9 kg (35 lb) (Anderson et al., 2014; NIOSH, 2016), use assistive devices for the transfer (Fig. 14.18). Through the use of assessment tools and patient movement algorithms, you determine the safest method by which to move the patient. Explain the assistive device and procedure

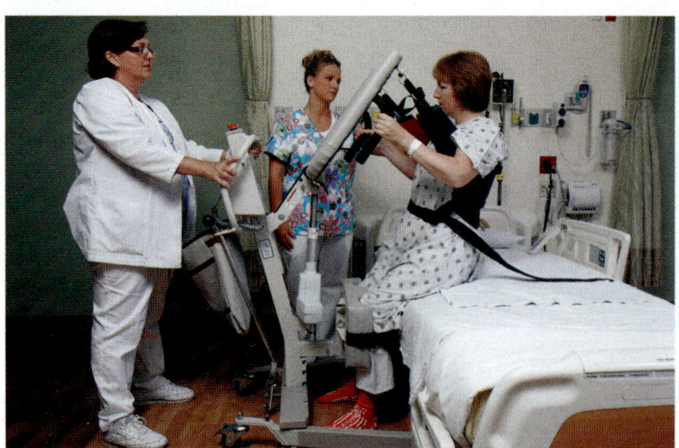

Fig. 14.18 Patient grasps handles as nurse enables motorized lift.

and determine the patient's understanding before the transfer. For example, a patient recently medicated for postoperative pain is too lethargic to understand instruction; thus, to ensure safety, two nurses are necessary to move him or her. Then, determine the patient's level of comfort. It is also important to evaluate your personal strength and knowledge of the procedure.

A safe transfer (e.g., moving from chair to bed, from bed to wheelchair) is the first priority. Proper use of body mechanics enables you to move, lift, or transfer patients safely and protects you from injury to your musculoskeletal system (see Skill 14.3). Prevent self-injury by using correct posture, minimal muscle strength, and effective body mechanics and lifting techniques Transferring is a skill that helps patients regain optimal independence as quickly as possible. Physical activity maintains and improves joint motion, increases strength, promotes circulation, relieves pressure on skin, and improves urinary and respiratory functions. It also benefits the patient psychologically by increasing social activity and mental stimulation and providing a change in environment. Thus, mobilization plays a crucial role in a patient's rehabilitation.

When preparing to transfer patients, consider the type of problems that can develop. A patient who has been immobile for several days or longer is often weak or dizzy or sometimes develops initial **orthostatic hypotension** (a drop in blood pressure of 40 mm Hg or more systolic or 20 mm Hg or more diastolic when rising from a sitting position within 15 seconds of standing) when transferred (Frith et al., 2014; Lewis et al., 2014; Mills and Gray, 2014). A patient with neurological deficits sometimes has paresis (muscle weakness) or paralysis unilaterally or bilaterally, which complicates safe transfer. A flaccid arm sustains injury during transfer if unsupported. As a general rule, use a gait belt and obtain assistance for mobilization of patients with neurological deficits.

CARE OF PATIENT WITH IMMOBILITY USING NURSING PROCESS APPROACH

Assessment

An assessment includes a patient's regular activity level and tolerance and information about preillness functioning. Assess body alignment and posture with a patient standing, sitting, or lying down. Table 14.2 presents examples of factors to assess, related questions, and physical assessment techniques for assessing activity tolerance.

Through assessment, you are able to determine patients' normal physiological changes in growth and development; deviations related to poor posture, trauma, muscle damage, or nerve dysfunction; and any learning needs. In addition, assessment provides opportunities for you to observe patients' posture and obtain important information about other factors that contribute to poor alignment such as fatigue, malnutrition, and psychological problems.

Body Alignment

The first step in assessing body alignment is to help a patient feel at ease so that the patient does not assume unnatural or rigid positions. Begin by having the patient stand if he or she is able, then have the patient sit. Place the patient in the **supine** position by removing pillows and positioning supports from the bed (if not contraindicated) to assess alignment in the recumbent position.

Table 14.2 Focused Patient Assessment

Factors to Assess	Questions	Physical Assessment
ROM	To what extent you have limited movement in your joints? Do you have a history of connective tissue disorders, fractures, or damage to ligaments or tendons?	Observe the patient's gait and ability to carry out ADLs. Inspect joints for deformity. Measure ROM of affected joints.
Pain	Do you experience pain or discomfort on movement? Do you need pain medication before ambulating (with assistance) or other exercise? Please rate your pain on a scale of 0–10 with 10 representing the worst pain.	Inspect joints for redness or swelling indicating potential inflammatory process. Observe for objective signs of pain such as grimacing, moaning, increasing respiratory rate, pulse, and blood pressure. (**Note:** These objective signs are not always present, and it is best to ask the patient whether pain is present.)
Activity tolerance	Do you feel fatigued? Tell me in what way muscle weakness affects your ability to perform daily activities. Do you feel short of breath, palpitations, light-headed, or dizzy?	Observe for signs of fatigue. Observe the patient's performance of ADLs. Observe the patient for paleness, obtain vital signs, and compare with baseline measures.

ADLs, activities of daily living; *ROM*, range of motion.

Standing

Assessment of the patient's alignment normally reveals the following:

- The head is erect and midline.
- Body parts are symmetrical.
- The spine is straight with normal curvatures (cervical concave, thoracic convex, and lumbar concave).
- The abdomen is comfortably tucked in.
- The knees are in a straight line between the hips and ankles and slightly flexed.
- The feet are flat on the floor and pointed directly forward and slightly apart to maintain a wide base of support.
- The arms hang comfortably at the sides (Fig. 14.19).

A patient's center of gravity is in the midline, and the line of gravity is from the middle of the forehead to a midpoint between the feet. Laterally, the line of gravity runs vertically from the middle of the skull to the posterior third of the foot (Ball et al., 2015; Patton and Thibodeau, 2016).

Sitting

Assess your patient for the following: The head is erect, and the neck and vertebral column are in straight alignment; the body weight is distributed on the buttocks and thighs; the thighs are parallel and in a horizontal plane (be careful to avoid pressure on the popliteal nerve and blood supply); the feet are supported on the floor; and the forearms are supported on the armrest, in the lap, or on a table in front of the chair.

Assessment of alignment in the sitting position is particularly important for patients with neuromuscular disorders, muscle weakness, muscle paralysis, or nerve damage. A patient with these alterations has diminished sensation in affected areas and is unable to perceive pressure or decreased circulation. Proper sitting alignment reduces the risk for musculoskeletal system damage.

Recumbent

Position your patient in the lateral side-lying position with all but one pillow and all positioning supports removed from the bed. Make sure that the vertebrae are in straight alignment without observable curves. This assessment provides baseline data concerning a patient's body alignment while in bed. Conditions that create a risk for damage to the musculoskeletal system when lying down include impaired mobility (e.g., spinal curvature), use of immobilization devices (e.g., traction), decreased sensation (e.g., hemiparesis from a stroke), impaired circulation (e.g., diabetes), and lack of voluntary muscle control (e.g., spinal cord injuries).

When a patient is unable to change position voluntarily, assess the position of body parts while the patient is lying down. Make sure that the vertebrae are in straight alignment without any observable curves. Normally, the extremities are in alignment and do not cross over one another. The head and neck are aligned without excessive flexion or extension.

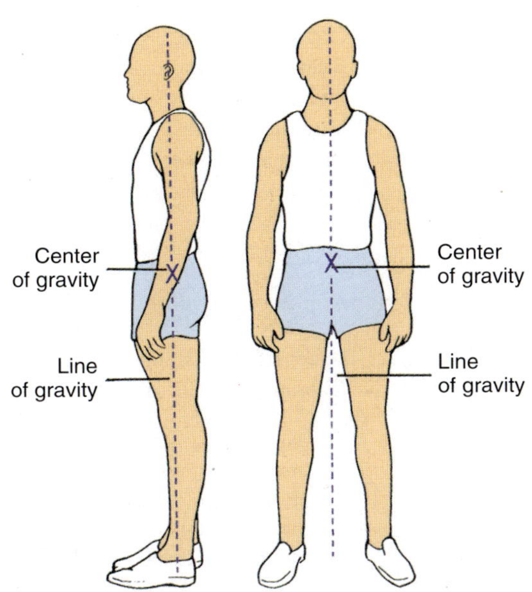

Fig. 14.19 Correct body alignment with standing.

Mobility

The adequacy of a patient's mobility affects his or her coordination and balance while sitting, standing, and walking; the ability to carry out ADLs; and the ability to participate in an exercise program. The assessment of mobility has five components: sitting, standing, range of motion (ROM), gait, and exercise.

Sitting

Your observation includes noting whether a patient can sit on the side of the bed or in a chair upright. A patient's ability to do so affects his or her ability to perform self-care activities such as feeding self and performing hygiene activities. When assessing the ability of patients to sit, allow them to use a side rail (when present). Skill 14.3 describes the Banner Mobility Assessment Tool (BMAT), a validated tool that includes a component for assessment of a patient's mobility while sitting (Boynton et al., 2014). Success with the sitting maneuver indicates good sitting mobility.

Standing

Do not rely on a patient's self-report that he or she is able to stand independently without support. This commonly occurs when nurses rush to admit or transfer patients to their care units. When you assess a patient's ability to stand, it is appropriate to have them use an assistive device for support. The BMAT (Boynton et al., 2014) includes a measure for assessing a patient while standing. A patient should be able to raise the buttocks off the bed and hold for a count of five (Boynton, et al., 2014). The ability to achieve this maneuver indicates good mobility and balance (see Skill 14.3).

Range of Motion

Observing **ROM** is one of the first assessment techniques used to determine the degree of limitation or injury to a joint. Assess ROM to clarify the extent of joint stiffness, swelling, pain, limited movement, and unequal movement. Limited ROM indicates inflammation such as arthritis, fluid in the joint, altered nerve supply, or contractures. Increased mobility (beyond normal) of a joint indicates connective tissue disorders, ligament tears, and possible joint fractures (Table 14.3).

Table 14.3 Range-of-Motion Exercises

Body Part	Type of Joint	Type of Movement	Range (°)	Primary Muscles
Neck, cervical spine	Pivotal	*Flexion:* Bring chin to rest on chest.	45	Sternocleidomastoid
		Extension: Return head to erect position.	45	Trapezius
		Hyperextension: Bend head back as far as possible.	10	Trapezius
		Lateral flexion: Tilt head as far as possible toward each shoulder.	40–45	Sternocleidomastoid
		Rotation: Turn head as far as possible in circular movement.	180	Sternocleidomastoid, trapezius
Shoulder	Ball and socket	*Flexion:* Raise arm from side position forward to position above head.	180 45–60	Coracobrachialis, biceps brachii, deltoid, pectoralis major
		Extension: Return arm to position at side of body.	180	Latissimus dorsi, teres major, triceps brachii
		Hyperextension: Move arm behind body, keeping elbow straight.	45–60	Latissimus dorsi, teres major, deltoid
		Abduction: Raise arm to side to position above head with palm away from head.	180	Deltoid, supraspinatus
		Adduction: Lower arm sideways and across body as far as possible.	320	Pectoralis major
		Internal rotation: With elbow flexed, rotate shoulder by moving arm until thumb is turned inward and toward back.	90	Pectoralis major, latissimus dorsi, teres major, subscapularis
		External rotation: With elbow flexed, move arm until thumb is upward and lateral to head.	90	Infraspinatus, teres major, deltoid
		Circumduction: Move arm in full circle. (Circumduction is combination of all movements of ball-and-socket joint.)	360	Deltoid, coracobrachialis, latissimus dorsi, teres major
Elbow	Hinge	*Flexion:* Bend elbow so lower arm moves toward its shoulder joint and hand is level with shoulder.	150	Biceps brachii, brachialis, brachioradialis
		Extension: Straighten elbow by lowering hand.	150	Triceps brachii
Forearm	Pivotal	*Supination:* Turn lower arm and hand so palm is up.	70–90	Supinator, biceps brachii
		Pronation: Turn lower arm so palm is down.	70–90	Pronator teres, pronator quadratus
Wrist	Condyloid	*Flexion:* Move palm toward inner aspect of forearm.	80–90	Flexor carpi ulnaris, flexor carpi radialis
		Extension: Move fingers and hand posterior to midline.	80–90	Extensor carpi radialis brevis, extensor carpi radialis longus, extensor carpi ulnaris
		Hyperextension: Bring dorsal surface of hand back as far as possible.	80–90	Extensor carpi radialis brevis, extensor carpi radialis longus, extensor carpi ulnaris
		Abduction: Place hand with palm down and extend wrist laterally toward fifth finger.	Up to 30	Flexor carpi radialis, extensor carpi radialis brevis, extensor carpi radialis longus
		Adduction: Place hand with palm down and extend wrist medially toward thumb.	30–50	Flexor carpi ulnaris, extensor carpi ulnaris
Fingers	Condyloid hinge	*Flexion:* Make fist.	90	Lumbricals, interosseus volaris, interosseus dorsalis
		Extension: Straighten fingers.	90	Extensor digiti quinti proprius, extensor digitorum communis, extensor indicis proprius
		Hyperextension: Bend fingers back as far as possible.	30–60	Extensor digitorum
		Abduction: Spread fingers apart.	30	Interosseus dorsalis
		Adduction: Bring fingers together.	30	Interosseus volaris
Thumb	Saddle	*Flexion:* Move thumb across palmar surface of hand.	90	Flexor pollicis brevis
		Extension: Move thumb straight away from hand.	90	Extensor pollicis longus, extensor pollicis brevis
		Abduction: Extend thumb laterally (usually done when placing fingers in abduction and adduction).	30	Abductor pollicis brevis
		Adduction: Move thumb back toward hand.	30	Adductor pollicis obliquus, adductor pollicis transversus
		Opposition: Touch thumb to each finger of same hand.		Opponens pollicis, opponens digiti minimi
Hip	Ball and socket	*Flexion:* Move leg forward and up.	90–120	Psoas major, iliacus, sartorius
		Extension: Move back beside other leg.	90–120	Gluteus maximus, semitendinosus, semimembranosus
		Hyperextension: Move leg behind body.	30–50	Gluteus maximus, semitendinosus, semimembranosus
		Abduction: Move leg laterally away from body.	30–50	Gluteus medius, gluteus minimus
		Adduction: Move leg back toward medial position and beyond if possible.	30–50	Adductor longus, adductor brevis, adductor magnus
		Internal rotation: Turn foot and leg toward other leg.	90	Gluteus medius, gluteus minimus, tensor fasciae latae

Table 14.3 Range-of-Motion Exercises—cont'd

Body Part	Type of Joint	Type of Movement	Range (°)	Primary Muscles
		External rotation: Turn foot and leg away from other leg.	90	Obturatorius internus, obturatorius externus
		Circumduction: Move leg in circle.		Psoas major, gluteus maximus, gluteus medius, adductor magnus
Knee	Hinge	*Flexion:* Bring heel back toward back of thigh.	120–130	Biceps femoris, semitendinosus, semimembranosus, sartorius
		Extension: Return leg to floor.	120–130	Rectus femoris, vastus lateralis, vastus medialis, vastus intermedius
Ankle	Hinge	*Dorsal flexion:* Move foot so toes are pointed upward.	20–30	Tibialis anterior
		Plantar flexion: Move foot so toes are pointed downward.	45–50	Gastrocnemius, soleus
Foot	Gliding	*Inversion:* Turn sole of foot medially.	10 or less	Tibialis anterior, tibialis posterior
		Eversion: Turn sole of foot laterally.	10 or less	Peroneus longus, peroneus brevis
Toes	Condyloid	*Flexion:* Curl toes downward.	30–60	Flexor digitorum, lumbricalis pedis, flexor hallucis brevis
		Extension: Straighten toes.	30–60	Extensor digitorum longus, extensor digitorum brevis, extensor hallucis longus
		Abduction: Spread toes apart.	15 or less	Abductor hallucis, interosseus dorsalis
		Adduction: Bring toes together.	15 or less	Adductor hallucis, interosseus plantaris

Gait

Gait is the manner or style of walking including rhythm, cadence, length of stride, and speed. Assessing gait allows for conclusions about balance, posture, and the ability to walk without assistance (see Chapter 14). While a patient walks, look for conformity, a regular smooth rhythm and symmetry in the length of leg swing; smooth swaying related to the gait phase; and a smooth symmetrical arm swing (Ball et al., 2015). An abnormal gait is a common risk factor for patient falls.

Activity Tolerance

Activity tolerance is the type and amount of exercise or work that a person is able to perform without undue exertion or injury (Box 14.7). Observe patients after ambulation, self-bathing, or sitting in a chair for several hours, and assess their verbal report of fatigue and weakness. Do they exhibit difficulty breathing or report being short of breath after exercise? Assess heart rate and blood pressure response to activity by comparing with baseline rates at rest. Both heart rate and blood pressure should increase. When you care for a patient who is relatively healthy and able to exercise regularly, assess what the patient sets as his or her target heart rate during exercise. Use this finding to determine whether the patient has set an adequate target rate for exercise training (American Heart Association [AHA], 2015).

Older Adult Considerations

Older adults who experience a disease or debilitating illness often experience a decline in physical activity and changes in joints that predispose to problems with mobility and limit joint flexibility. In addition, chronic conditions increase in older adults, and certain medications (e.g., cardiovascular medication or diuretics, or changes in dosages of these medications) affect a person's activity and exercise tolerance. It is important for older adults to exercise and remain active. A program of exercise promotes health and improves illness, trauma, and rehabilitation outcomes (CDC, 2015). As people age, they lose lifelong partners and friends, and opportunities for exercise and activities lessen.

BOX 14.7 Factors Influencing Activity Tolerance

Physiological Factors

- Skeletal abnormalities
- Muscular impairments
- Endocrine or metabolic illnesses (e.g., diabetes mellitus, thyroid disease)
- Hypoxemia
- Decreased cardiopulmonary function
- Decreased endurance
- Impaired physical stability
- Pain
- Sleep pattern disturbance
- Prior exercise patterns
- Infectious processes and fever

Emotional Factors

- Anxiety
- Depression
- Chemical addictions
- Motivation

Developmental Factors

- Age
- Sex
- Pregnancy
- Physical growth and development of muscle and skeletal support

Nursing Diagnosis

Data from your nursing assessment including a patient's knowledge of or motivation to be active and alterations in body alignment, joint mobility, and neurological function are the defining characteristics or risk factors to support a nursing diagnosis.

A patient's assessment provides related clusters of risk factors or defining characteristics that lead to the identification of nursing diagnoses including the following examples:

- *Activity Intolerance*
- *Chronic Pain*
- *Fatigue*

- *Risk for Injury*
- *Impaired Physical Mobility*
- *Impaired Sitting*
- *Impaired Walking*
- *Sedentary Lifestyle*

If you select a problem-focused nursing diagnosis such as *Impaired Physical Mobility*, select a related factor that is relevant and will further aid you in intervention selection. For example, *Impaired Physical Mobility related to pain* will require different interventions than *Impaired Physical Mobility related to activity intolerance.*

The list of potential diagnoses is extensive because immobility affects multiple body systems. For example, an immobilized or partially immobilized patient can have one or more of the following nursing diagnoses:

- *Ineffective Airway Clearance*
- *Risk for Constipation*
- *Risk for Disuse Syndrome*
- *Risk for Falls*
- *Impaired Bed Mobility*
- *Impaired Physical Mobility*
- *Impaired Sitting*
- *Risk for Impaired Skin Integrity*

Planning

Use data gathered during assessment and critical thinking to develop an individualized plan of care based on the nursing diagnoses for your patients. The plan of care will include appropriate interventions that will allow you to maintain or optimize the patient's exercise and activity levels (Fig. 14.20).

Goals and Outcomes

Once you define appropriate nursing diagnoses, collaborate with the patient to set goals and expected outcomes that are relevant, appropriate, and timely. Each outcome provides a measure for later evaluating the success of your nursing interventions. For example, the goal of achieving optimum ROM in the right knee has the outcome of achieving 90° flexion in the right knee by discharge.

The plan of care considers risks for injury and preexisting health concerns. It is especially important to have knowledge of your patient's previous functional status and home environment.

Setting Priorities

Consider the patient's most immediate needs when selecting priorities of care. Determine the immediacy of any problem (e.g., pain, lack of knowledge about exercise, reduced ROM) by the effect the problem has on a patient's mental and physical health. For example, if a patient is in acute pain, relieving pain is a priority before you begin exercise therapy. Safety becomes a priority whenever you are assisting with the many skills associated with the care of patients with activity intolerance, improper body mechanics, or impaired mobility. For example, you must use caution to avoid a patient fall during transfer. Your priorities change from short-term to long-term when you plan for a patient's return to his or her home. For patients who remain disabled or limited in mobility, be sure that family caregivers are prepared to help with positioning and transfer techniques. When you perform skills that promote a patient's activity in the acute care setting, always be vigilant in monitoring your patients and supervising nursing assistive personnel in carrying out activities to prevent complications and potential injury.

Collaborative Care

Planning also involves an understanding of the resources necessary to maintain a patient's motor function and independence. Collaboration with other members of the health care team, such as physical or occupational therapists, is important in the provision of appropriate exercises and adaptive approaches to self-care. Long-term rehabilitation is sometimes necessary, and you begin discharge planning when a patient enters the health care system. In addition, always individualize a plan of care (see Care Plan given in the subsequent text).

Care Plan

Impaired Physical Mobility

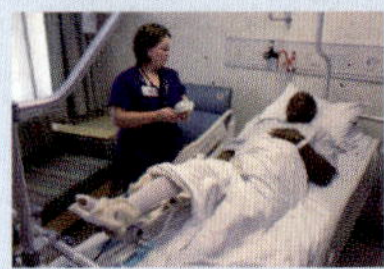

ASSESSMENT

Mr Girish Kumar is a 72-year-old man hospitalized for surgery on his right knee. Over the past 5 years, he has experienced pain and decreased mobility. He is now experiencing his first postoperative day following total right knee replacement using fast-track protocol. His incision is healing, and there is no edema or redness.

ASSESSMENT ACTIVITIES	FINDINGS[a]
Assess Mr Girish Kumar's pain level.	Mr Girish Kumar is **hesitant to ambulate** or participate in active exercises on his first postoperative day using the early mobility protocol. He rates his **pain as 6–7** on a scale of 0–10 and is using a patient-controlled analgesia (PCA) pump. He states, **"I can't put all my weight on my right leg. It's just too painful."**
Assess Mr Girish Kumar's baseline mobility and endurance.	His degree of knee flexion is now 70°. He is able to ambulate 10 feet with a walker but states, "I can't go any farther." In addition, he further describes his right leg as feeling weak and tired after walking a short distance.
Assess Mr Girish Kumar's knowledge about proper use of his walker.	The nurse observes Mr Girish Kumar using the walker incorrectly.

[a]**Defining characteristics/risk factors** are shown in **bold** type.

Care Plan—cont'd

Nursing diagnosis: Impaired Physical Mobility related to pain, muscle weakness, and limited joint motion.

PLANNING

GOALS	EXPECTED OUTCOMES (NOC)[b]
	Self-Care: Activities of Daily Living
Mr Girish Kumar will obtain a tolerable level of pain during self-care activities.	Mr Girish Kumar's pain is below 3 at rest and below 5 with activity on a scale of 0–10 with oral pain relief medication by discharge. Mr Girish Kumar is able to climb stairs, dress independently, and go to the toilet independently by discharge.
	Mobility
Mr Girish Kumar will gain optimal functioning of the right knee with independent, purposeful movement on discharge.	Mr Girish Kumar ambulates four times with aid of walker, each time increasing distance, without reports of increasing fatigue by discharge.
	Ambulation
Mr Girish Kumar will use walker properly while ambulating.	Mr Girish Kumar performs a return demonstration of proper use of walker.

[b]Outcome classification labels from Moorhead S, et al, editors: *Nursing outcomes classification (NOC)*, ed 5, St Louis, 2013, Mosby.

INTERVENTIONS (NIC)[c]	RATIONALE
Exercise Therapy: Ambulation	
Encourage Mr Girish Kumar to use PCA pump at least 20 min before ambulation.	Peak actions of analgesic occur as the patient begins activity (Schofield, 2014).
Advance the patient to multimodal analgesia for pain control by day 2 postoperatively. Practices will vary, but multimodal analgesics usually include oral acetaminophen, celecoxib, and oxycodone (OxyContin) at prescribed intervals.	There is mounting evidence that multimodal analgesia provides superior pain relief, while speeding up functional recovery, minimizing the adverse effects of traditional opioid-based analgesia, increasing patient satisfaction, and reducing length of hospital stay (Halawi et al., 2015).
Initiate early mobility protocol by having Mr Girish Kumar sit in bed or on side of bed (dangle) before standing to ambulate.	Allowing the patient to dangle before changing positions helps reduce or prevents orthostatic hypotension, maintains safety, and prevents injury to patient.
Have Mr Girish Kumar ambulate (marching in place, walking in halls), increasing time and distance each day of hospitalization.	Gradually increasing physical activity and setting realistic goals for ambulation encourage activity in older adults (Doherty-King et al., 2014).
Collaborate with physical therapist in instructing Mr Girish Kumar and family caregiver on proper use of walker and how to climb stairs. Provide written material that reinforces verbal instructions. Have the patient return demonstrate stair walking.	Providing instructions in a quiet environment and giving written instructions in large, easy-to-read print enhances learning for older adults (Touhy and Jett, 2014). Return demonstration ensures patient safety.
Self-Care Assistance	
Consult with occupational therapist to prepare the patient to learn how to dress self and use the toilet with minimal assistance.	Preserves the patient's sense of independence.

[c]Intervention classification labels from Bulecheck GM, et al, editors: *Nursing interventions classification (NIC)*, ed 6, St Louis, 2013, Mosby.

EVALUATION

Nursing Actions	Patient Response/Finding	Achievement of Outcome
Ask Mr Girish Kumar to rate the level of pain on a scale of 0–10.	Mr Girish Kumar rates his pain at a 3 and states, "I am able to walk now that my knee doesn't hurt so badly anymore."	Mr Girish Kumar's pain is under control, and he is able to ambulate with minimal discomfort.
Observe Mr Girish Kumar's range of motion (ROM).	Able to perform ROM.	Outcome met. Mr Girish Kumar expresses understanding of need for ROM.
Observe Mr Girish Kumar use toilet and dress self.	The patient is a bit hesitant to rotate correctly before sitting on toilet seat. Needs assistance with applying pants.	Continue therapy sessions.
Monitor distance Mr Girish Kumar ambulates.	Mr Girish Kumar ambulates within 12 h postoperatively 60 feet, then ambulates twice postoperative day 2 for a total of 140 feet using walling.	Ambulation is progressing. Continue ambulation sessions up to discharge. Demonstrates correct use of walker.

IMPLEMENTATION

Health Promotion and Acute Care

A goal of the Healthy People 2020 (HealthyPeople.gov, 2015) initiative is to improve health, fitness, and quality of life through daily physical activity. This goal is based on guidelines that suggest that regular physical activity can improve the health and quality of life of Americans of all ages, regardless of the presence of a chronic disease or disability (USDHHS, 2008a, 2008b). As a nurse, you may work in outpatient settings with the opportunity to plan health promotion activities. It is crucial to educate patients and family caregivers about the importance of regular physical activity and exercise and how these activities can be incorporated into daily routines (see Box 14.2 and Skill 14.1).

Evaluation

Patient Outcomes

You evaluate a patient's response to all nursing interventions by comparing a patient's actual response with the expected outcomes for each goal. You evaluate specific outcomes designed to demonstrate improved activity and exercise tolerance. You revise the plan if the patient does not achieve the expected outcomes. For example, a patient may achieve improved joint ROM as determined by measuring the ROM, but if exercise tolerance is still poor (accelerated heart rate, shortness of breath), there may be a need to increase duration of exercise. The success in meeting each outcome is based on the use of evaluative measures such as ROM, ability to ambulate, distance of ambulation, and activity/exercise tolerance. In many cases, evaluation will occur in the long-term (e.g., weeks or months) before patients regain full function.

Patient Expectations

To evaluate a patient's perception of whether expectations were met, ask the patient the extent to which the patient perceives he or she reached desired activity levels. Also, evaluate whether the patient perceives whether he or she is able to follow any activity restrictions and how to use any assistive devices at home, when applicable. What is acceptable or anticipated on your part is sometimes vastly different from what a patient and family members anticipate or accept. Ask patients to describe their satisfaction with the plan of care.

CARE OF PATIENT WITH CAST AND SPLINTS

Casting is a common procedure used for temporary immobilization for a client fracture. It provides opportunity for the client to carry out various ADLs while imparting enough immobilization to make sure stability to that particular body part. Cast could be prepared with natural material such as plaster of Paris (POP) and synthetic, fiberglass-free, latex-free polymer, or a hybrid of material.

Most commonly fractured patients are managed with casting in outpatient department and usually not required hospitalization or a short period of hospitalization. Therefore, it is responsibility of a nurse to teach the patient about care of cast and prevent complications. Box 14.8 summarized patient and family teaching regarding cast care.

BOX 14.8 **Patient Teaching Regarding Cast Care**

Do not

- Wet plaster cast
- Pull out padding
- Scratch or insert any foreign material inside the cast
- Cover the cast with plastic sheet or blanket for long duration
- Bear weight until 24–72 h (follow the instructions of health care provider)

Do

- Allow the cast to dry properly.
- Elevate the extremity above heart level
- Movement of joints below and above the cast routinely
- Know the signs and symptoms of potential problems and report to health care provider
  - Swelling or edema with pain and/or discoloration of any part
  - Increased pain at rest or pain during movement
  - Burning or tingling sensation, foul smell and ulcer under the plaster cast
- Take adequate rest and exercise per instruction of health care provider
- Maintain proper hydration
- Take balance diet
- Contact facility or health care provider per schedule or early in case of any complication

SAFETY GUIDELINES FOR NURSING SKILLS

Ensuring patient safety is an essential role of the professional nurse. To ensure patient safety, communicate clearly with members of the health care team, assess and incorporate the patient's priorities of care and preferences, and use the best evidence when making decisions about your patient's care. When performing the skills in this chapter, remember the following points to ensure safe, individualized patient care:

- Clear the immediate environment where a patient will walk of any obstacles or clutter.
- Monitor a patient's activity tolerance throughout any extended ambulation.
- Mentally review the steps of a transfer before beginning to ensure safety of both the patient and you.
- Assess the patient's mobility and strength to determine the assistance that the patient is able to offer during transfer. Stand on patient's weak side when assisting (Pierson and Fairchild, 2013).
- Determine the amount and type of assistance required for transfer including type of transfer equipment and the number of personnel it will take to safely transfer and prevent harm to the patient and health care providers.
- Raise the **side rail** on the side of the bed opposite of where you are standing to prevent the patient from falling out of bed on that side.
- Make sure all personnel understand how lift and transfer equipment functions before it is used.
- Educate patients about how equipment functions to reduce their anxiety and enlist their cooperation.
- Arrange equipment (e.g., intravenous [i.v.] lines, feeding tube, Foley catheter) so that it will not interfere with the transfer process.
- Evaluate the patient for correct body alignment and pressure risks after a transfer.

SKILL 14.1 Promoting Early Ambulation/Activity and Exercise

Equipment

- Inpatient
  - Pulse oximeter
  - Gait belt
  - Appropriate assistive devices (e.g., cane, walker)
- Outpatient
  - Appropriate devices, depending on type of exercise recommended (e.g., 2.2-kg [5-lb] weights, resistance bands)

STEP	RATIONALE
Assessment	
1. Identify the patient by using at least two identifiers (e.g., name and birthday or name and medical record number) according to agency policy.	Ensures correct patient. Complies with The Joint Commission standards and improves patient safety (TJC, 2018).
2. Perform hand hygiene. Gather baseline assessment of vital signs and oxygen saturation (if available).	Reduces transmission of microorganisms. Allows you to evaluate the patient's response to activity/exercise.
3. Assess the patient's pain level; ask the patient to rate pain on a scale of 0–10.	Determines whether there is need for an analgesic before mobilizing or ambulating inpatient. In outpatient settings, data will allow you to counsel the patient about the best time to try more strenuous exercise.
4. Assess the patient's beliefs, values, and perceptions regarding current health status and confidence in being capable of performing exercise.	Perceived self-efficacy is a judgment of capability. The outcomes that people anticipate depend largely on their judgments of how well they will be able to perform in given situations.
5. Review the patient's medical history for conditions that could influence or contraindicate mobility/exercise (e.g., dysrhythmias, recent myocardial infarction, stroke, paralyzed extremity, neuromuscular disease, peripheral neuropathy, current pregnancy). Review health care provider's order for early mobility or exercise program. Obtain physician clearance for outpatient exercise.	Examples of conditions that may contraindicate or require adjustments to activity. Patients should have medical clearance to begin activity/exercise program.
6. Implement Inpatient Early Mobility Protocol Screening—this example describes screening for a protocol to begin in intensive care unit (ICU) (AACN, 2013).	Protocol established for ICU patients; however, different screening criteria can be used based on the patient population (e.g., surgical ICU versus medical ICU). Also, different criteria are likely used when patients have been transferred out of an ICU.
Clinical decision point: Similar protocols to the one developed by AACN are being adopted on acute care inpatient units as well.	
7. Perform safety screening (MOVE) (AACN, 2013).	
M: Assess the patient's myocardial stability. ▪ No evidence of active myocardial ischemia has occurred over last 24 h. ▪ No dysrhythmia requiring new antidysrhythmic drug has occurred over last 24 h.	Ensures cardiac stability. Exercise can initiate ischemic attack or worsen dysrhythmias.
O: Assess oxygenation status; must be adequate on: ▪ FiO_2 0.6 or less. ▪ Positive end-expiratory pressure (on ventilator) less than 10 cm H_2O. ▪ *Option:* Heart rate less than 120 beats/min at rest, mean arterial blood pressure 60–110 mm Hg, respiratory rate less than 28 breaths/min.	Medical stability involves having sufficient perfusion to maintain normal organ function. Activity assessment criteria allow for early ambulation.
V: Minimal vasopressors: ▪ No increase of any vasopressor has occurred for last 2 h.	Change in vasopressor dose could lead to side effects such as tachycardia, dysrhythmias, and blood pressure changes such as orthostatic hypotension (Burchum and Rosenthal, 2016).
E: The patient engages to voice of caregiver. ▪ The patient responds appropriately to verbal stimulation/commands.	The patient must be alert and responsive, able to follow directions.
8. Outpatient assessment	
a. Identify the patient's activity/exercise history: ▪ Which type of regular daily exercise do you perform at home? ▪ Do you exercise or play a sport at least three times a week? ▪ On a scale of 0–5 with 0 being no daily exercise and 5 being strenuous regular exercise daily, how would you rate yourself? ▪ How long have you been exercising regularly?	Provides information about the patient's motivation or willingness to exercise regularly. Allows you to plan exercise that complements and advances the patient's activity level.

STEP	RATIONALE
b. Ask the patient to what extent he or she enjoys exercising and what his or her beliefs are about ability to exercise.	Factors positively associated with adult physical activity (HealthyPeople.gov, 2015).
c. Determine whether the patient has social support from peers, family, or spouse.	Factors positively associated with adult physical activity (HealthyPeople.gov, 2015).
d. Determine whether the patient has access to facility or area to exercise. Is neighborhood considered safe?	Absence of facility or sense of safety discourages activity/exercise.
e. Consider these factors in your assessment: patient's age, income level, time available to exercise, rural resident, overweight, being disabled.	Factors negatively associated with adult participation in activity (HealthyPeople.gov, 2015).
f. Have the patient rate level of quality of life based on current activity level.	Serves as baseline to measure long-term benefits of exercise.
Planning	
1. Inpatient: Consult with physical therapist (PT) regarding role in protocol to provide planned active resistance exercise for patients. If PT is available in home health care setting, consult on types of exercises suited for outpatient's mobility restrictions.	Progressive resistance exercise (PRE) is method of increasing ability of muscles to generate force.
2. All patients: Explain benefits and reasons for activity/exercise. Do so in a way that matches the patient's beliefs and values regarding recovery or maintaining health.	Exercise self-efficacy is an important predictor of the adoption and maintenance of exercise behaviors. Self-efficacy is the belief and conviction that one can perform a given activity successfully (Fletcher and Banasik, 2001; Shieh et al., 2015).
3. Inpatients: Explain precautions that will be taken to prevent falls during ambulation (gait belt, assisted walking, monitoring for dizziness).	Patients may have a fear of falling. Explanation may relieve anxiety.
4. Inpatients: As the patient progresses to ambulating, try to schedule ambulation around the patient's other activities.	Avoids overexertion of the patient. Organizes nursing care activities.
5. Perform hand hygiene. Prepare equipment and supplies.	Reduces transmission of microorganisms. Ensures organized procedure.
Implementation	
1. Inpatient Early Progressive Mobility Protocol (AACN, 2013) Each patient starts at a different level, depending on his or her medical status and ability to participate in mobility.	
Level 1 ▪ Initiate passive ROM exercises three times daily. Turn the patient every 2 h. ▪ Help patient to sitting position in bed (e.g., stretcher chair or elevating head of bed to 45 degrees) and maintain for 20 minutes 3 times daily. ▪ Obtain a PT consultation if patient is alert to determine if strengthening exercises are indicated.	This level is designed for patients who are medically unstable to tolerate activity and/or have bed rest orders because of a medical condition.
Level 2 ▪ Continue passive ROM exercises three times daily. ▪ Turn the patient every 2 h. ▪ Help the patient to sitting position in bed and maintain for 20 min three times daily. ▪ Initiate sitting the patient on edge of bed or lift patient to chair (using safe mobility techniques). ▪ Obtain PT consultation for mobility/strengthening program (e.g., active resistance exercise).	The patient begins to progress, he or she is starting to be able to sit independently on edge of bed or tolerate sitting up in a chair. Principles of active resistance exercise: (1) to perform small number of repetitions until fatigue, (2) to allow sufficient rest between exercises for recovery, and (3) to increase resistance as ability to generate force increases. There is some evidence that PRE improves endurance and ability to generate muscle force, which can carry over into an improved ability to do everyday tasks (Taylor et al., 2005).
Level 3 ▪ Continue passive ROM exercises three times daily. ▪ Turn the patient every 2 h. ▪ Help the patient to sitting position in bed and maintain for 20 min three times daily; sitting on edge of bed unsupported (but supervised). ▪ Active transfer to chair with the patient sitting up in chair 20 min three times daily. ▪ PT to continue with strengthening program as ordered.	The patient progresses to transfer training, prewalking activities.

STEP	RATIONALE
Level 4 ■ Continue passive ROM three times daily. ■ Turn the patient every 2 h. ■ Active transfer to chair with patient sitting up in chair 20 min three times daily sitting on edge of bed unsupported (but supervised). ■ PT to continue with strengthening program. ■ Initiate ambulation. Apply gait belt securely around the patient's waist. Have the patient ambulate (marching in place, walking in halls). **Note:** Ambulation time/distance should increase daily during hospitalization.	Patients can still be in ICU during this phase or out on general nursing unit. Progression of mobility (amount of help required and distance walked) should occur until hospital discharge.
2. Outpatient Exercise and Activity Promotion	
a. Initiate an exercise program that contains any of the following components: ■ Warm-up (5–10 min) ■ Strengthening exercises ■ Endurance exercises ■ Balance exercises ■ Flexibility exercises Consider consulting PT to help develop complete exercise program that would fit needs of your patient. A good overview of exercise programs can be found at http://health.gov/paguidelines/guidelines.	Warm-up directs needed blood flow to muscles and prepares body for exercise. Warming up is important for preventing injury. Flexibility exercises help prevent tightness of muscles and improve joint ROM. Loss of ROM or muscle tightness can impede a person's function. Cool downs help body recover from exercises.
b. Recommend strength training for adults in collaboration with PT.	Strength training has been shown to improve strength and bone density and can be beneficial for older adults.
c. AHA (2015) recommends aerobic exercise at least 150 min per week of moderate exercise or 75 min per week of vigorous exercise (or combination of moderate and vigorous activity). This includes activities (e.g., climbing stairs; playing sports; or aerobic activities such as walking, jogging, swimming, or biking).	Designed to improve overall cardiovascular health.
d. Recommend balance exercises for older adults to decrease risk of falls. Have the patient be sure to have something sturdy nearby to hold onto (wall or chair) if he or she becomes unsteady. ■ Perform exercises: standing on one foot, walking heel to toe, balance walking, back leg raises, side leg raises. Have the patient do strength exercises while holding back of chair (back leg raises, side leg raises) 2 or more days per week but not on any 2 days in a row (National Institute on Aging [NIA], 2016).	Helps to improve the patient's balance while standing or sitting and may decrease risk of falls.
e. Recommend the patient to perform cool down (5–10 min) after exercising: quadriceps stretch, hamstring/calf stretch, chest and arm stretch, neck, upper back, and shoulder stretch.	Exercises help muscles relax and become more flexible.
Evaluation	
1. Measure vital signs and oxygen saturation during activity/exercise and compare findings with baseline.	Determines the patient's exercise tolerance.
Clinical decision point. Terminate physical activity when (Adler and Malone, 2012): ■ Heart rate is more than a 20% decrease in resting value or less than 40 beats/min or more than 130 beats/min. ■ Oxygen saturation shows more than 4% drop from baseline or less than 88%–90%. ■ Blood pressure: Systolic pressure is more than 180 mm Hg or more than 20% decrease in systolic/diastolic or orthostatic hypotension. ■ Respirations: Less than 5 breaths/min or more than 40 breaths/min. ■ Terminate exercise if dizziness lasts 60 s or fainting or diaphoresis occurs; change in breathing pattern occurs with increase in accessory muscle use, extreme fatigue, or severe dyspnea with respiratory rate greater than baseline by more than 20 breaths/min (Myszenski, 2014).	
2. Evaluate the patient's pain severity by using 0–10 pain scale.	Exercises can increase muscle discomfort.
3. After the patient has reached level 4 of inpatient mobility protocol or after outpatient has been exercising more than 2–3 months, evaluate level of confidence in performing exercises.	Determines self-efficacy and likelihood of continued participation in exercise.
4. **Use teach back:** "We've talked about doing a warm-up and cool down as part of your exercise plan. Tell me why each is important." Revise your instruction now or develop plan for revised patient/family caregiver teaching if the patient/family caregiver is not able to teach back correctly.	Determines the patient's/family caregiver's level of understanding of instructional topic.

Recording and Reporting

- Record in the inpatient medical record or clinic record results of patient screening, type of exercise implemented, pre-exercise and postexercise assessments, and patient's tolerance in nurses' notes in electronic health record (EHR) or chart.
- Document your evaluation of patient learning.
- Report to health care provider any signs or symptoms indicative of exercise intolerance.

Unexpected Outcomes and Related Interventions

- The patient has abnormal vital sign response or decrease in oxygen saturation requiring termination of exercise. (In home setting, be sure that the patient or family caregiver knows patient's normal pulse range and when to terminate exercise.)
  - Return the patient to chair or bed immediately using safe patient-handling principles.
  - Notify health care provider.
  - Continue to monitor vital signs until the patient's condition stabilizes.
- The patient develops chest pain and/or discomfort during exercise.
  - Return the patient to chair or bed immediately using safe patient-handling principles.
  - Notify health care provider.
  - Prepare for possible electrocardiogram.
  - Continue to monitor vital signs until the patient's condition stabilizes.
  - In home setting, call caregiver.

SKILL 14.2 Moving and Positioning Patients in Bed

STEP	RATIONALE
Assessment	
1. Identify the patient by using two identifiers (e.g., name and birthday or name and medical record number), according to agency policy.	Ensures correct patient. Complies with The Joint Commission standards and improves patient safety (TJC, 2016).
2. Assess the patient's body alignment and comfort level while he or she is lying down.	Provides baseline data for later comparisons. Determines ways to improve position and alignment.
3. Assess for risk factors that contribute to complications of immobility:	Increased risk factors require more frequent repositioning.
a. Paralysis, hemiparesis resulting from a cerebrovascular accident (CVA); decreased sensation	Paralysis impairs movement; muscle tone changes; sensation is often affected. Because of difficulty in moving and poor awareness of involved body part, the patient is unable to protect and position body part for self (Lewis et al., 2013).
b. Impaired mobility from traction, arthritis, or other contributing disease processes	Traction or arthritic changes of affected extremity result in decreased range of motion (ROM).
c. Impaired circulation	Decreased circulation to skin and underlying tissue predisposes the patient to pressure ulcers.
d. *Age:* Very young, older adults	Premature and young infants require frequent turning because their skin is fragile. Normal physiological changes associated with aging predispose older adults to greater risks for developing complications of immobility (Drake et al., 2012).
e. *Sensation:* Decreased from CVA, paralysis, neuropathy.	Because of poor awareness of body part or reduced sensation, the patient is unable to protect and position body part from pressure.
f. Level of consciousness and mental status	Determines need for special aids or devices. Patients with altered levels of consciousness may not understand instructions or be able to help during positioning.
4. Assess the patient's physical ability to help with moving and positioning:	Enables nurse to use patient's mobility, coordination, and strength; determines need for additional help. Ensures patient's and nurse's safety (VISN8, 2015).
a. Age	Some older adults move more slowly with less strength.
b. Disease process	Cardiopulmonary disease requires the patient to have head of bed elevated.
c. Strength, coordination	Determines amount of assistance provided by the patient during position change.
d. ROM	Limited ROM contraindicates certain positions.
5. Assess the patient's height, weight, and body shape.	Devices used for safe patient handling have different weight restrictions; bariatric patients require special beds, lifts, wheelchairs, and toileting and bathing equipment (Pierson and Fairchild, 2013).

STEP	RATIONALE
6. Assess health care provider's orders before positioning. Clarify whether any positions are contraindicated because of patient's condition (e.g., spinal cord injury; respiratory difficulties; certain neurological conditions; presence of incisions, drains, and tubing).	Placing the patient in an inappropriate position causes injury.
7. Assess for presence of tubes, incisions, and equipment (e.g., traction).	Alters positioning procedure and affects patient's ability to independently change positions.
8. Assess condition of the patient's skin (see Chapter 17).	Provides baseline to determine effects of positioning.
9. Assess ability and motivation of the patient and family caregivers to participate in moving and positioning the patient in bed in anticipation of discharge to home.	Determines ability of the patient and caregivers to help with positioning.
Planning	
1. Collect appropriate equipment. Get extra help as needed. Close door to room or bedside curtains.	Having appropriate number of people to position the patient prevents patient and nurse injury. Provides for the patient privacy.
2. Perform hand hygiene.	Reduces transfer of microorganisms.
3. Raise level of bed to comfortable working height. Remove all pillows and devices used for positioning.	Raises work toward nurse's center of gravity. Reduces any interference during positioning.
4. Explain procedure to the patient.	Helps to relieve anxiety and allows the patient to participate more actively.
Implementation	
1. Assist the Patient in Moving Up in Bed a. ***Can the patient assist?*** (1) Fully able to assist, nurse assistance not needed; nurse stands by to assist. (2) Partially able to assist; the patient can assist with nurse using positioning cues or aids (e.g., drawsheet or friction-reducing device).	Determines the degree of risk in repositioning the patient and technique required to safely assist the patient.
Clinical decision point: ***Before lowering head of bed to flatten bed, account for all tubing, drains, and equipment to prevent dislodgement or tipping if caught in mattress or bedframe as bed is lowered.***	
b. ***Assist the patient moving up in bed, using a drawsheet (two or three nurses).***	This is not a one-person task. Helping a patient move up in bed without help from other coworkers or without the aid of an assistive device (i.e., friction-reducing pad) is not recommended or considered safe for the patient or nurse (ANA, 2010; CDC, 2009). If the patient is unable to fully assist, refer to Step 1c.
(1) Place the patient supine with head of bed flat. A nurse stands on each side of bed.	Enables the nurse to assess body alignment. Reduces pull of gravity on patient's upper body.
(2) Remove pillow from under head and shoulders and place it at head of bed.	Prevents striking the patient's head against head of bed.
(3) Turn the patient side to side to place drawsheet under him or her, extending from shoulders to thighs.	Supports the patient's body weight and reduces friction during movement.
(4) Return the patient to supine position.	Even distribution of the patient's weight makes lifting and positioning easier.
(5) Fanfold drawsheet on both sides, with each nurse grasping firmly near the patient.	Provides strong handles to grip drawsheet without slipping.
Clinical decision point: ***Protect the patient's heels from shearing force by having a third nurse lift heels while moving the patient up in bed.***	
(6) Nurses place their feet apart with forward–backward stance. Flex knees and hips. On the count of three, shift weight from front to back leg and move the patient and drawsheet to desired position in bed (see illustration).	Facing direction of movement ensures proper balance. Shifting weight reduces force needed to move load. Flexing knees lowers center of gravity and uses thigh muscles instead of back muscles.
c. ***Assist moving up in bed using a friction-reducing device (three nurses assist).***	Patients weighing less than 90.71 kg require at least three nurses; patients over 90.71 kg require mechanical assist device.
(1) Position patient as in Step 1b (1–3).	Prepares the patient for placement of friction-reducing device.
(2) With the patient already on side, place friction-reducing device under drawsheet and then have the patient turn over to other side.	Prevents friction from contact of skin with board.

STEP | RATIONALE

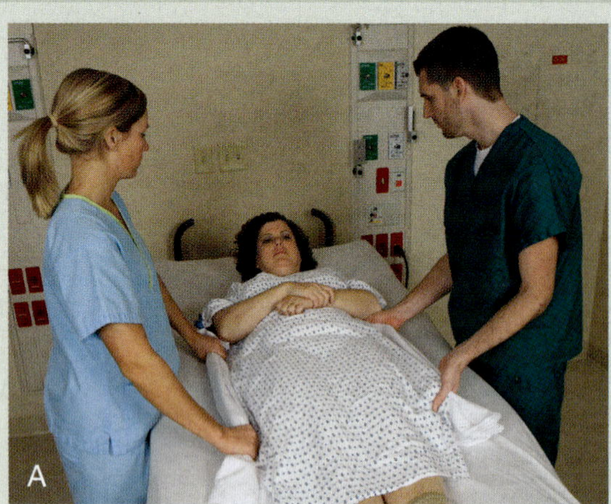

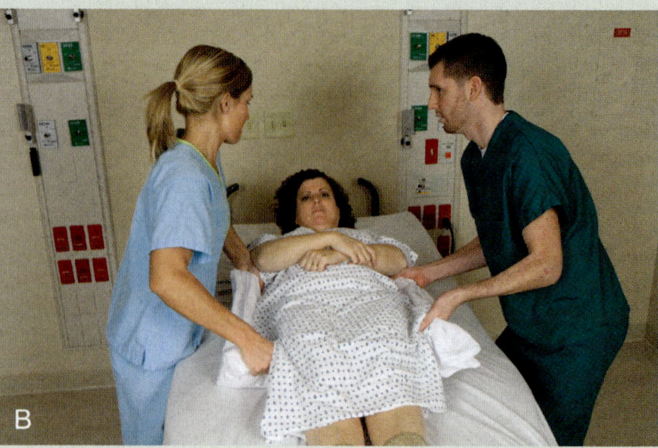

Step 1b(6) A and **B**, Moving immobile patient up in bed with drawsheet.

(3) Move the patient up in bed by having two nurses grasp drawsheet and one hold on to friction-reducing device. Follow Step 1b (5 and 6), moving patient up in bed.
— The slide board remains stationary, provides a slippery surface to reduce friction, and allows the patient to move easily up in bed.

2. Position the patient in one of the following positions using correct body alignment to protect pressure areas. Begin with the patient lying supine and move up in bed following either Step 1b or 1c.
— Prevents injury to the patient's musculoskeletal system.

a. ***Positioning the patient in supported Fowler's position (see illustration):***

(1) With the patient supine, elevate head of bed 45–60° if not contraindicated.
— Increases comfort, improves ventilation, and increases the patient's opportunity to socialize or relax.

(2) Rest head against mattress or on small pillow.
— Prevents flexion contractures of cervical vertebrae.

(3) Use pillows to support arms and hands if the patient does not have voluntary control or use of hands and arms.
— Prevents shoulder dislocation from effect of downward pull of unsupported arms, promotes circulation by preventing venous pooling, and prevents flexion contractures of arms and wrists.

(4) Position small pillow at lower back.
— Supports lumbar vertebrae and decreases flexion of vertebrae.

(5) Place small pillow under thigh. Support calves with pillows.
— Prevents hyperextension of knee and occlusion of popliteal artery from pressure from body weight. Heels should not be in contact with bed to prevent prolonged pressure of mattress on heels. This is sometimes referred to as "floating" heels.

(6) *Option:* Use a heel pressure–relieving device (pillow or heel boot).
— Pressure on the heels must be relieved by off-loading, which is done by regular repositioning or using a purpose-made pressure-relieving device. When pillows are used, they must be repositioned each time the patient moves (Bangova, 2013).

Clinical decision point: To keep feet in proper alignment and prevent footdrop, use foot support devices (check agency policy). In addition, a foot cradle is often used for patients with poor peripheral circulation as a means of reducing pressure on the tips of the patient's toes.

b. ***Positioning hemiplegic patient in supported Fowler's position:***

(1) Elevate head of bed 45–60°. Adjust head of bed according to the patient's condition. For example, those with increased risk of pressure ulcers remain at 30° angle (semi-Fowler's) (see Chapter 10).
— Increases comfort, improves ventilation, and increases the patient's opportunity to relax.

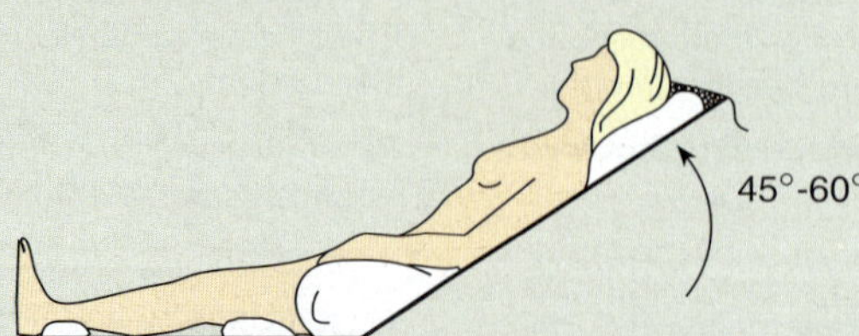

Step 2a Supported Fowler's position.

STEP	RATIONALE
(2) Position the patient in sitting position as straight as possible.	Counteracts tendency to slump toward affected side. Improves ventilation and cardiac output; decreases intracranial pressure. Improves the patient's ability to swallow and helps to prevent aspiration of food, liquids, and gastric secretions.
(3) Position head on small pillow with chin slightly forward. If the patient is totally unable to control head movement, avoid hyperextension of neck.	Prevents hyperextension of neck. Too many pillows under head cause or worsen neck flexion contracture.
(4) Provide support for involved arm and hand on overbed table in front of the patient. Place arm away from the patient's side and support elbow with pillow.	Paralyzed muscles do not automatically resist pull of gravity as they do normally. As a result, shoulder subluxation, pain, and edema may occur.

Clinical decision point:

- *Position flaccid hand in normal resting position with wrist slightly extended, arches of hand maintained, and fingers partially flexed; use section of rubber ball cut in half; clasp the patient's hands together.*
- *Position spastic hand with wrist in neutral position or slightly extended; extend fingers with palm down or leave them in relaxed position palm up. At times, it is difficult to position spastic hands without the use of specially made splints for the patient.*

STEP	RATIONALE
(5) Place trochanter rolls (rolled blanket) alongside of the patient's legs.	Reduces external rotation of hip.
(6) If needed, support feet in dorsiflexion with therapeutic boots or splints (check agency policy) (see illustration).	Maintains foot in dorsiflexion and prevents footdrop. Pillows prevent stimulation to ball of foot by hard surface, which has a tendency to increase muscle tone in the patient with extensor spasticity of lower extremity.
c. ***Positioning the patient in supported supine position:***	
(1) Be sure that the patient is comfortable on back with head of bed flat.	Some patients' physical conditions do not tolerate supine position.
(2) Place small rolled towel under lumbar area of back.	Provides support for lumbar spine.
(3) Place pillow under upper shoulders, neck, or head.	Maintains correct alignment and prevents flexion contractures of cervical vertebrae.
(4) Place trochanter rolls or sandbags parallel to lateral surface of the patient's thighs if the patient is immobile.	Reduces external rotation of hip.
(5) Position the patient's heels in heel boots or other heel pressure–relief device (check agency policy).	Heel pressure–relief devices are more effective than pillows for consistently reducing pressure from the mattress on the heels.
(6) If needed, support feet in dorsiflexion with foot support devices (check agency policy).	Maintains foot in dorsiflexion and prevents footdrop. Pillows prevent stimulation to ball of foot by hard surface, which has tendency to increase muscle tone in the patient with extensor spasticity of lower extremity.
(7) Place pillows under pronated forearms, keeping upper arms parallel to the patient's body (see illustration).	Reduces internal rotation of shoulder and prevents extension of elbows. Maintains correct body alignment.
(8) Place hand rolls in the patient's hands. Consider physical therapy referral for use of hand splints.	Reduces extension of fingers and abduction of thumb. Maintains thumb slightly adducted and in opposition to fingers.

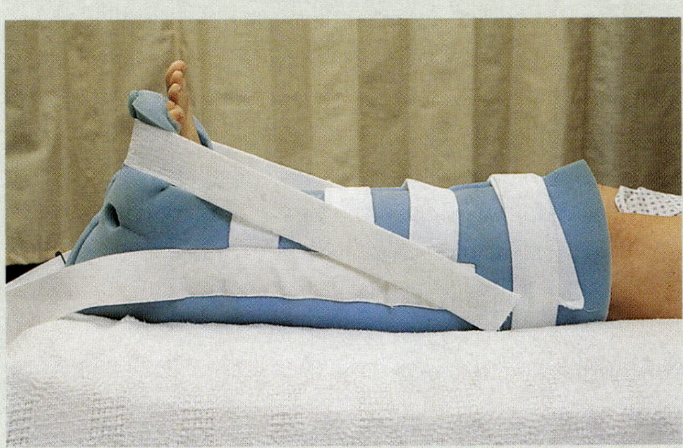

Step 2b(6) Foot boot with lower leg extension.

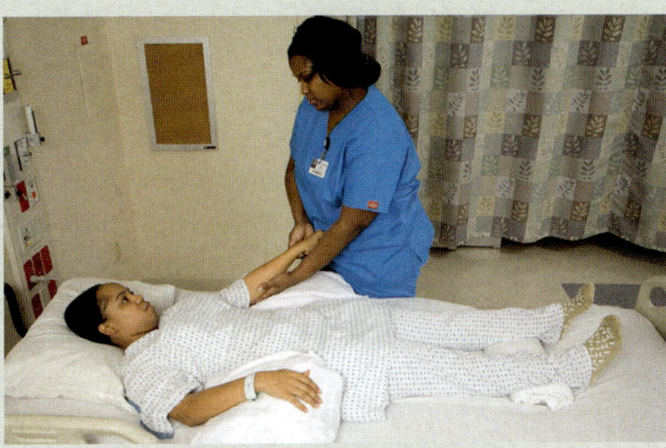

Step 2c(7) Supported supine position with pillows in place.

STEP	RATIONALE
d. ***Positioning hemiplegic patient in supine position:***	
(1) Be sure that the patient is comfortable on back with head of bed flat.	Some patients' physical conditions do not tolerate supine position.
(2) Place folded towel or small pillow under shoulder of affected side.	Decreases possibility of pain, joint contracture, and subluxation. Maintains mobility in muscles around shoulder to permit normal movement patterns.
(3) Keep affected arm away from body with elbow extended and palm up. (Alternate position is to place arm out to side, with elbow bent and hand toward head of bed.)	Maintains mobility in arm, joints, and shoulder to permit normal movement patterns. (Alternate position counteracts limitation of ability of arm to rotate outward at shoulder [external rotation]. Need external rotation to raise arm overhead without pain.)
Clinical decision point: *Position affected hand in one of the recommended positions for flaccid or spastic hand.*	
(4) Place folded towel under hip of involved side.	Diminishes effect of spasticity in entire leg by controlling hip position.
(5) Flex affected knee 30° by supporting it on pillow or folded blanket.	Slight flexion breaks up abnormal extension pattern of leg. Extensor spasticity is most severe when the patient is supine.
(6) If needed, support feet in dorsiflexion with foot support devices (check agency policy).	Maintains foot in dorsiflexion and prevents footdrop. Pillows prevent stimulation to ball of foot by hard surface, which has tendency to increase muscle tone in the patient with extensor spasticity of lower extremity.
e. ***Positioning the patient in prone position, with the help of two to three nurses:***	In certain patients with pulmonary conditions such as acute respiratory distress syndrome, the use of the prone position can help improve oxygenation.
(1) With head of bed flat and one nurse standing on each side of bed, roll the patient to one side while placing arm on side to be turned alongside of body.	Prepares the patient for positioning.
(2) Roll the patient over arm positioned close to body, with elbow straight and hand under hip. Position on abdomen in center of bed.	Positions the patient correctly so that alignment can be maintained.
(3) Turn the patient's head to one side and support it with small pillow (see illustration).	Reduces flexion or hyperextension of cervical vertebrae.
(4) Place small pillow under the patient's abdomen below level of diaphragm.	Reduces pressure on breasts of some female patients and decreases hyperextension of lumbar vertebrae and strain on lower back. Improves breathing by reducing mattress pressure on diaphragm.
(5) Support arms in flexed position level at shoulders.	Maintains proper body alignment. Support reduces risk of joint dislocation.
(6) Support lower legs with pillows to elevate toes.	Prevents footdrop. Reduces external rotation of hips. Eliminates mattress pressure on toes.
f. ***Positioning patient in 30° lateral (side-lying) position (one nurse):***	
(1) Lower head of bed completely or as low as the patient can tolerate.	Provides position of comfort for the patient and removes pressure from bony prominences on back.

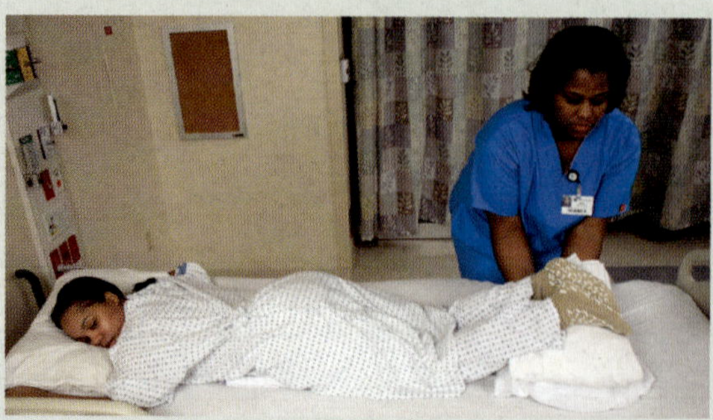

Step 2e(3) Prone position with pillows supporting lower legs.

STEP	RATIONALE
(2) Position the patient in supine position on side of bed opposite direction toward which the patient is to be turned. Move upper trunk, supporting shoulders first, followed by moving lower trunk, supporting hips. Raise side rails and move to opposite side of bed.	Provides room for the patient to turn to side. Use of safe patient-handling equipment reduces workload of caregivers and enhances safety (Burnfield et al., 2013; Griffis, 2012).
(3) Prepare to turn the patient onto side. Flex the patient's knee that will not be next to mattress. Place one hand on the patient's knee and one hand on the patient's shoulder.	Use of leverage makes turning to side easy.
(4) Roll the patient onto side toward you.	Rolling decreases trauma to tissues. In addition, the patient is positioned so leverage on hip makes turning easy.
(5) Place pillow under the patient's head and neck.	Maintains alignment. Reduces lateral neck flexion. Decreases strain on sternocleidomastoid muscle.
(6) Bring dependent shoulder blade forward.	Prevents the patient's weight from resting directly on shoulder joint.
(7) Position both arms in slightly flexed position. Support upper arm by pillow level with shoulder; support the other arm with mattress.	Decreases internal rotation and adduction of shoulder. Supporting both arms in slightly flexed position protects joint and improves ventilation because chest is able to expand more easily.
(8) Place your hands under the patient's hips and bring dependent hip slightly forward so angle from hip to mattress is approximately 30°.	The 30° lateral position reduces pressure on trochanter.
(9) Place small tuck-back pillow behind the patient's back. (Make by folding pillow lengthwise. Smooth area is slightly tucked under the patient's back.)	Provides support to maintain the patient on side.
(10) Place pillow under semiflexed upper leg level at hip from groin to foot (see illustration).	Flexion prevents hyperextension of leg. Maintains leg in correct alignment. Prevents pressure on bony prominences.
(11) Support feet in dorsiflexion with foot support devices (check agency policy).	Maintains foot in dorsiflexion and prevents footdrop. Pillows prevent stimulation to ball of foot by hard surface, which has tendency to increase muscle tone in the patient with extensor spasticity of lower extremity.
g. ***Positioning the patient in Sims' (semiprone) position (one nurse):***	
(1) Position the patient in supine position on side of bed opposite direction toward which the patient is to be turned. Move upper trunk, supporting shoulders first; move lower trunk, supporting hips. Raise side rails and move to opposite side of bed.	Prepares the patient for positioning.
(2) Move to other side of bed and turn the patient on side. Position in lateral position, lying partially on abdomen, with dependent shoulder lifted out and arm placed at the patient's side.	The patient is rolled only partially on abdomen.

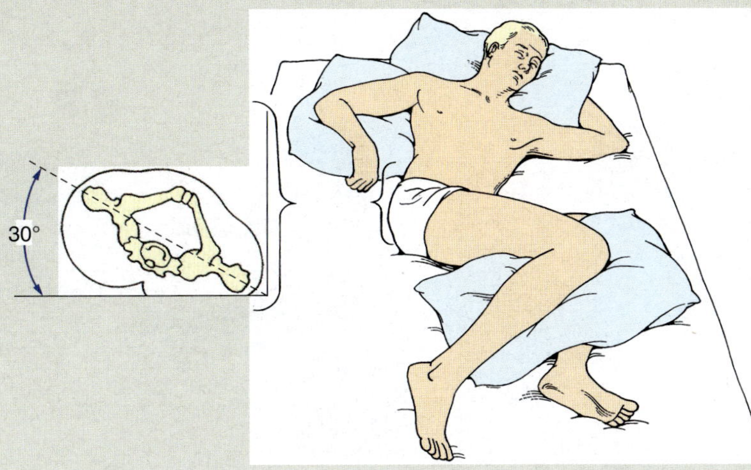

Step 2f(10) Thirty degree lateral position with pillows in place.

STEP	RATIONALE
(3) Place small pillow under the patient's head.	The patient is rolled only partially on abdomen.
(4) Place pillow under flexed upper arm, supporting arm level with shoulder.	Maintains proper alignment and prevents lateral neck flexion. Prevents internal rotation of shoulder.
(5) Place pillow under flexed upper leg, supporting leg level with hip.	Prevents internal rotation of hip and adduction of leg. Flexion prevents hyperextension of leg. Reduces mattress pressure on knees and ankles.
(6) Support feet in dorsiflexion with foot support devices (check agency policy).	Maintains foot in dorsiflexion and prevents footdrop. Pillows prevent stimulation to ball of foot by hard surface, which has tendency to increase muscle tone in the patient with extensor spasticity of lower extremity.

h. ***Logrolling patient (three nurses):***

Clinical decision point: *Supervise and assist NAP when there is a health care provider's order to logroll a patient. Patients who have suffered from spinal cord injury or are recovering from neck, back, or spinal surgery often need to keep the spinal column in straight alignment to prevent further injury.*

STEP	RATIONALE
(1) Place the patient in supine position on side of bed opposite direction to be turned.	Prepares the patient for turning onto side.
(2) Place small pillow between the patient's knees.	Prevents tension on spinal column and adduction of hip.
(3) Cross the patient's arms on chest.	Prevents injury to arms.
(4) Position two nurses or other staff members on side of bed to which the patient will be turned. Position third nurse or staff member on other side of bed (see illustration). If needed, four nurses are used; fourth nurse stands on same side as third nurse.	Distributes weight equally among nurses.
(5) Fanfold or roll drawsheet alongside of the patient.	Provides strong handles to grip the drawsheet or pull sheet without slipping.
(6) With one nurse grasping drawsheet at lower hips and thighs and the other nurse grasping drawsheet at the patient's shoulders and lower back, roll the patient as one unit in a smooth, continuous motion on the count of three (see illustration).	This maintains proper alignment by moving all body parts at the same time, preventing tension or twisting of the spinal column.
(7) Nurse on opposite side of bed places pillows along length of the patient (see illustration).	Pillows keep the patient aligned.
(8) Gently lean the patient as a unit back toward pillows for support (see illustration).	Ensures continued straight alignment of spinal column, preventing injury.
3. Perform hand hygiene.	Reduces transmission of microorganisms.

Evaluation

STEP	RATIONALE
1. Evaluate the patient's body alignment, position, and level of comfort (using pain scale). The patient's body should be supported by adequate mattress, and vertebral column is properly aligned.	Determines effectiveness of positioning. Patients who have adequate pain control and are comfortable maintain proper positioning.

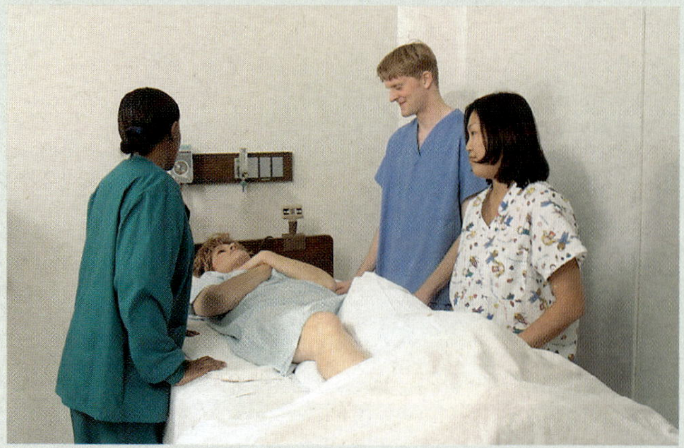

Step 2h(4) Preparing patient for logroll.

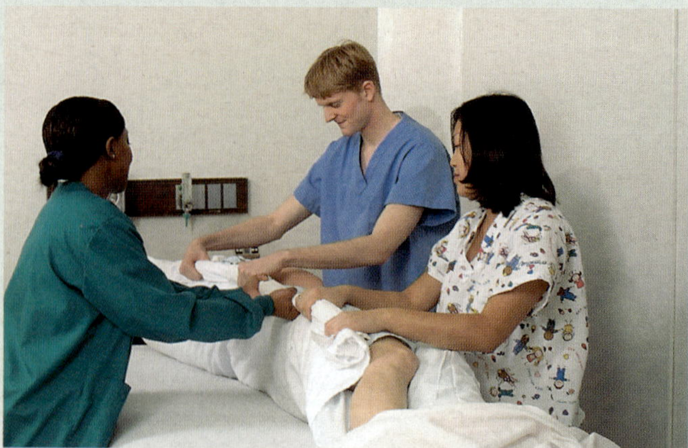

Step 2h(6) Move patient as a unit, logrolling onto side.

STEP	RATIONALE
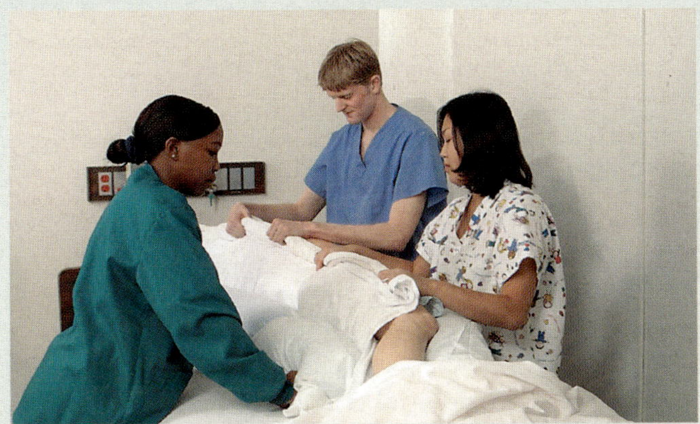 **Step 2h(7)** Place pillows along patient's back for support.	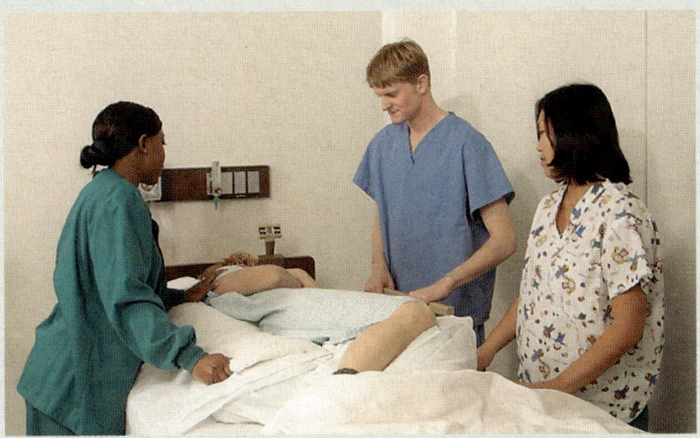 **Step 2h(8)** Gently lean patient as a unit against pillows.
2. Measure ROM.	Determines whether joint contracture is developing.
3. Observe skin for areas of erythema or breakdown, especially under bony prominences.	Indicates complications of immobility or improper positioning of body part. Determines whether need exists for increasing frequency of repositioning the patient.
4. Use ***teach back*** to determine patient and family understanding of moving and positioning. State, "I want to be sure I explained how proper moving and positioning prevents risk for injury while providing you safe care. Can you explain to me why it is important we move and position you often?" Revise your instruction now or develop plan for revised patient teaching if the patient is not able to teach back correctly.	Evaluates what the patient is able to explain or demonstrate.

Unexpected Outcomes and Related Interventions

1. Joint contractures develop or worsen.
   - Consult physical and/or occupational therapy.
   - Ensure that activity and ROM orders are implemented consistently.
2. Skin shows areas of erythema and breakdown.
   - Increase frequency of turning and repositioning.
   - Place turning schedule above the patient's bed.
   - Implement other activities per agency skin care policy or protocol (e.g., assess more frequently, consult dietitian, place the patient on pressure-relieving mattress).
3. The patient avoids moving.
   - Administer analgesia as ordered by a health care provider to ensure the patient's comfort before moving if he or she is in pain.
   - Allow pain medication to take effect before proceeding.
   - Provide the patient education about benefits of moving.

Recording and Reporting

- Document repositioning or turning and any relevant observations during procedure (e.g., condition of skin, joint movement, patient's ability to assist with positioning) in nurses' notes.
- Report observations at change of shift hand-off.
- Document your evaluation of patient learning.

Home Care Considerations

- Teach family how to use safe patient-handling equipment if necessary.
- Teach the patient and family about the signs of skin breakdown and the importance of safety during positioning for patients with decreased sensation.

SKILL 14.3 Using Safe and Effective Transfer Techniques

Equipment

- Gait belt, sling, or lapboard (as needed)
- Nonskid shoes, bath blankets, and pillows
- Wheelchair (position chair at 45–60° angle to bed, lock brakes, remove footrests, and lock bed brakes)
- Stretcher (position next to bed, lock brakes on stretcher, lock brakes on bed)
- Mechanical/hydraulic lift (use frame, canvas strips or chains, and hammock or canvas strips)
- Stand-assist lift device

STEP	RATIONALE
Assessment	
1. Identify the patient by using at least two identifiers (e.g., name and birthday or name and medical record number) according to agency policy.	Ensures correct patient. Complies with The Joint Commission standards and improves patient safety (TJC, 2018).
2. Refer to medical record for most recent recorded weight and height for the patient.	A factor used to determine whether a mechanical transfer device or a friction-reducing device is needed for transfer.
3. Review history and assess patient's specific risk for falling or being injured during transfer (e.g., neuromuscular deficit, visual loss, motor weakness or incoordination, fear of falling, bone loss).	Causes risk for tripping or losing balance.
4. Assess previous mode of transferring to bed or chair (if applicable).	Determines mode of transfer and assistance required to provide continuity.
5. Assess the patient's specific risk of falling or being injured when transferred (e.g., neuromuscular deficits, motor weakness, calcium loss from bone, cognitive and visual dysfunction, altered balance).	Certain conditions increase risk of falling or potential injury.
6. Perform hand hygiene.	Reduces transmission of microorganisms.
7. Assess the patient's mobility: including ability to sit up on side of bed or chair, and ability to stand. *Option:* Administer the Banner Mobility Assessment Tool (BMAT) (Boynton et al., 2014).	The BMAT is an assessment tool to guide a patient through a four-step functional task list to identify the level of mobility a patient can achieve. This assessment aids in determining the patient's level of mobility (e.g., Mobility Level 1) and recommends the equipment and tools needed to safely lift, transfer, and mobilize the patient.
a. **Sit and Shake:** From a semireclined position, ask the patient to sit upright and rotate to a seated position at the side of the bed; the patient may use bedrail. Note the patient's ability to maintain bedside position. Ask the patient to reach out and grab your hand and shake, making sure the patient reaches across his or her midline.	If the patient fails to Sit and Shake: Use total lift with sling and/or positioning sheet and/or straps, and/or use lateral transfer devices such as rollboard, friction-reducing device (slide sheets/tube), or air-assisted device.
b. **Stretch and Point:** With the patient in seated position at the side of the bed, have the patient place both feet on the floor (or stool) with knees no higher than hips. Ask the patient to stretch one leg and straighten the knee, then bend/flex the ankle and point the toes. If appropriate, repeat with the other leg.	If the patient fails Stretch and Point: Use total lift for the patient unable to bear weight on at least one leg; use sit-to-stand lift for the patient who can bear weight on at least one leg.
c. **Stand:** Ask the patient to elevate off the bed or chair (seated to standing) using an assistive device (cane, bedrail). The patient should be able to raise buttocks off bed and hold for a count of five. May repeat once.	If the patient fails to Stand: Use nonpowered raising/stand aid (default to powered sit-to-stand lift if no stand aid available), use total lift with ambulation accessories, or use assistive device (cane, walker, crutches).
d. **Walk** (march in place and advance step): Ask the patient to march in place at bedside, then ask the patient to advance step and return each foot. The patient should display stability while performing tasks. Assess for stability and safety awareness.	If the patient cannot Walk: Use nonpowered raising/stand aid (default to powered sit-to-stand lift if no stand aid available), use total lift with ambulation accessories, or use assistive device (cane, walker, crutches).
8. Assess for weakness, dizziness, or risk for orthostatic (postural) hypotension (e.g., previously on bed rest, first time arising from supine position after surgical procedure, history of dizziness when arising).	Determines risk of fainting or falling during transfer. Immobilized patients have decreased ability of autonomic nervous system to equalize blood supply, resulting in initial drop of 40 mm Hg systolic or more in blood pressure when rising from sitting position (Frith et al., 2014; Lewis et al., 2014; Mills et al., 2014).
9. Assess activity tolerance, noting for fatigue during sitting and standing.	Determines ability of the patient to help with transfer.
10. Assess proprioceptive function (awareness of posture and changes in equilibrium) including ability to maintain balance while sitting in bed or on side of bed and tendency to sway toward one side.	Determines stability of the patient's balance for transfer and risk for falls.
11. Assess sensory status including central and peripheral vision, adequacy of hearing, and presence of peripheral sensation loss.	Determines influence of sensory loss on ability to make transfer. Visual field loss decreases the patient's ability to see in direction of transfer. Peripheral sensation loss decreases proprioception. Patients with visual and hearing losses need transfer techniques adapted to deficits.

STEP	RATIONALE
Clinical decision point: Patients with hemiplegia may "neglect" one side of the body (inattention to or unawareness of one side of body or environment), which distorts perception of the visual field. If the patient experiences neglect of one side, instruct him or her to scan all visual fields when transferring.	
12. Assess level of comfort (e.g., joint discomfort, muscle spasm) and measure level of pain using a scale of 0–10. Offer prescribed analgesic 30 min before transfer. (**Note:** The patient will require assistance when analgesic has been given.)	Pain reduces the patient's motivation and ability to be mobile. Pain relief before transfer enhances the patient's ability to participate (Schofield, 2014).
13. Assess vital signs.	Vital sign changes, such as increased pulse and respiration and drop in blood pressure, indicate activity intolerance (see Chapter 6).
14. Assess the patient's cognitive status including ability to follow verbal instructions, short-term memory, and recognition of physical deficits and limitations to movement.	Determines the patient's ability to follow directions and learn transfer techniques.
Clinical decision point: Patients with head trauma or cerebrospinal fluid loss may have perceptual cognitive defects that create safety risks. If the patient has difficulty comprehending, simplify instructions by providing one step at a time and maintain consistency.	
15. Assess the patient's level of motivation such as eagerness versus unwillingness to be mobile and perception of value of exercise.	Altered physiological and psychological conditions reduce a patient's desire to engage in activity.
16. Assess special transfer equipment needed for home setting and previous mode of transfer (if applicable).	Prior teaching of family caregivers and support people, assessing home for safety risks and functionality, and providing applicable aids greatly enhance transfer ability at home.
Planning	
1. Perform hand hygiene. Gather appropriate equipment.	Reduces transmission of microorganisms. Ensures safe and organized procedure.
2. Determine number of people needed to assist with transfer by referring to proper algorithm. Do not start procedure until all caregivers are available.	Ensures safe patient transfer. Algorithms for safe patient handling and movement are available at https://cseany.org/wp-content/uploads/2014/02/SPHMALGORITHMS.PDF.
3. Verify that bed brakes are locked.	Provides for the patient and caregiver safety, preventing inadvertent movement of bed.
4. Explain procedure to the patient and family.	Increases patient participation and family caregiver knowledge of continued care of patient on discharge (Wrobleski et al., 2014).
Implementation	
1. Perform hand hygiene.	Reduces transmission of microorganisms.
2. Assist the patient from supine position to sitting position on edge of bed with bed positioned so that top of mattress is even with your elbows.	Reduces strain on your back.
3. Allow the patient to sit on the side of the bed for a few minutes. Have the patient alternately flex and extend feet, and move lower legs up and down. Ask whether the patient feels dizzy; if so, check blood pressure. Have the patient relax and take a few deep breaths until dizziness subsides and balance is gained. If dizziness lasts more than 60 s, return the patient to bed (Frith et al., 2014; Mills et al., 2014). Recheck blood pressure.	Allows patient's circulation to equilibrate to reduce chance of orthostatic hypotension.
Clinical decision point: Remain in front of patient until patient regains balance, and continue to provide physical support to weak or cognitively impaired patient.	
4. Transfer the patient from bed to chair:	
a. Have a chair in position at 45° angle with one side against bed, facing foot of bed.	Positions chair with easy access for transfer.
b. Place bed in low position or to point where the patient's feet are comfortably on the floor.	Provides the patient stability when transferring.
c. *If the patient has partial weight bearing with upper body strength or caregiver must lift more than 15.9 kg (35 lb), use mechanical lift or transfer aid with minimum of two or three caregivers* (see Fig. 14.18): Follow guidelines of lift manufacturer to apply.	The use of mechanical lift devices is strongly recommended to transfer a patient to reduce risk for musculoskeletal injury (Degelau et al., 2012; Occupational Safety and Health Administration [OSHA], 2014, n.d.).
Clinical decision point: If the patient demonstrates weakness or paralysis of one side of the body, place chair on the patient's strong side.	
d. *If the patient has partial weight bearing, is cooperative and able to stand, and has upper body strength, use stand-and-pivot technique with one caregiver* (VISN8, 2014):	

STEP	RATIONALE
(1) Apply gait belt. Be sure that it completely circles the waist. Place the belt low and be sure that it is snug. Avoid placing the belt over any i.v. lines, incisions, or drainage tubes.	Gait belt allows you to maintain stability of the patient during transfer and reduces risk for falling (Degelau et al., 2012; OSHA, 2014).
(2) If not already in place, help the patient apply stable, nonskid shoes or socks. Place the patient's weight-bearing or strong leg forward on floor, with weak foot back.	Nonskid soles decrease risk for slipping during transfer. Always have the patient wear nonskid shoes or socks during transfer; bare feet increase risk for falls. The patient will stand on stronger or weight-bearing leg.
(3) Spread your feet apart. Then flex hips and knees, aligning knees with the patient's knees.	Ensures balance with wide base of support. Flexing knees and hips lowers your center of gravity to object to be raised; aligning your knees with the patient's knees allows for stabilization of knees when the patient stands.
(4) Grasp gait belt, keeping your palms up, along the patient's sides (see illustration).	Gait belt allows you to move the patient at center of gravity. Patients should never be lifted by or under their arms.
(5) Rock the patient up to standing position on count of three while straightening hips and legs and keeping knees slightly flexed (see illustration). While rocking the patient in back-and-forth motion, make sure that your body weight is moving in the same direction as the patient's weight to ensure that you and the patient are moving in same direction simultaneously. Unless contraindicated, the patient may be instructed to use hands to push up if applicable.	Rocking motion gives the patient's body momentum and requires less muscular effort to lift him or her.
(6) Maintain stability of the patient's weakened leg with your knee.	Ability to stand can often be maintained in weak limb with support of knee to stabilize.
(7) Pivot on foot farthest from chair.	Maintains support of the patient while allowing adequate space for the patient to move.
(8) Instruct the patient to use armrests on chair for support and ease into chair (see illustration).	Increases the patient stability.
(9) Flex hips and knees while lowering the patient into chair.	Prevents injury from poor body mechanics.
(10) Assess the patient for proper alignment in sitting position. Provide support for weakened extremity. You can use a sling or lap board to support an injured or flaccid arm. Stabilize leg with bath blanket or pillow.	Prevents injury to the patient from poor body alignment.

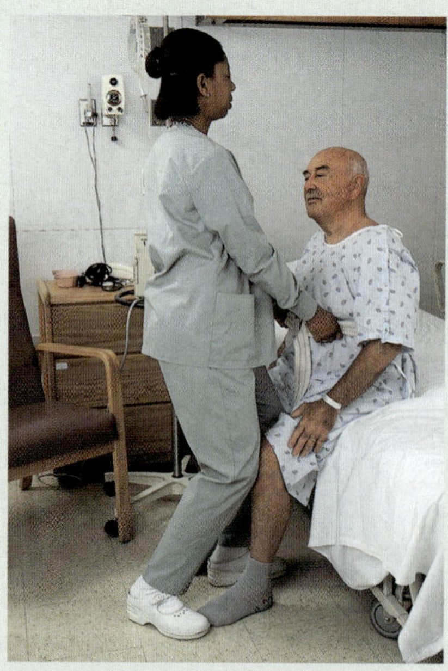

Step 4d(4) Nurse flexes hips and knees, aligns knees with patient's knee, and grasps gait belt palms up.

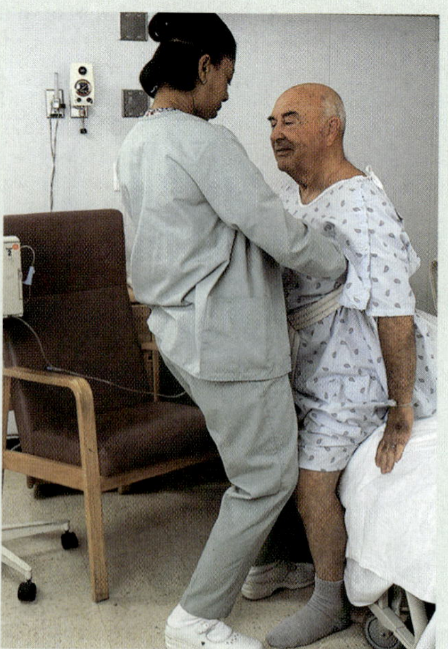

Step 4d(5) Nurse rocks patient (who is able to assist) to standing position.

STEP	RATIONALE

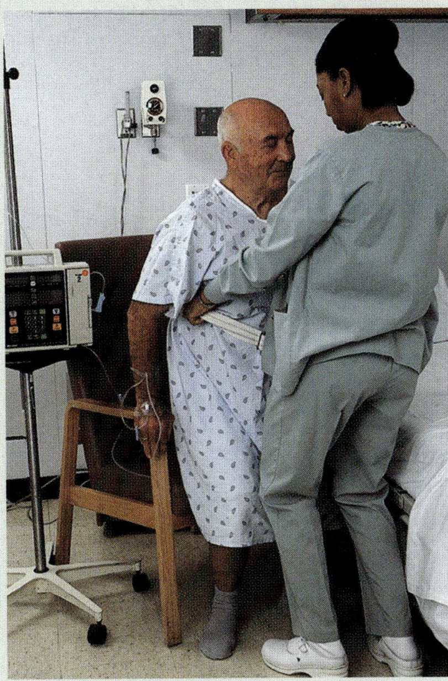

Step 4d(8) Patient uses armrests and is guided to sit in chair.

STEP	RATIONALE
(11) Proper alignment for sitting position: Head is erect, and vertebrae are in straight alignment. Body weight is evenly distributed on buttocks and thighs. Thighs are parallel and in horizontal plane. Both feet are supported on floor, and ankles are comfortably flexed. A 2.5- to 5-cm (1- to 2-inch) space is maintained between edge of seat and popliteal space on posterior surface of knee.	Prevents stress on intravertebral joints. Prevents increased pressure over bony prominences and reduces damage to underlying musculoskeletal system.
e. *If the patient is not able to cooperate (regardless of ability to bear weight) or has no upper body strength:* Use ceiling or floor hydraulic lift to transfer the patient from bed to chair (VISN8, 2014).	Research supports use of mechanical lifts to prevent musculoskeletal injuries (ANA, 2013a, 2013b). Use of ceiling-mounted lifts is a popular choice because of availability of lift in each patient's room (see illustration).
(1) Bring mechanical floor lift to bedside or lower ceiling lift and position properly.	Ensures safe elevation of the patient off the bed.
(2) Position chair near bed and allow adequate space to maneuver lift.	Prepares environment for safe use of lift and subsequent transfer.
(3) Raise bed to high position with mattress flat. Lower side rail on side near chair.	Allows you to use proper body mechanics.
(4) Have a second nurse positioned at opposite side of bed.	Maintains the patient safety, preventing fall from bed.
(5) Roll the patient on side away from you.	Positions the patient for placement of lift sling.
(6) Place hammock or canvas strips under the patient to form sling. With two canvas pieces, lower edge fits under the patient's knees (wide piece), and upper edge fits under the patient's shoulders (narrow piece).	Two types of seats are supplied with mechanical/hydraulic lift: Hammock style is better for patients who are flaccid, weak, and need support; canvas strips can be used for patients with normal muscle tone. Hooks should face away from the patient's skin. Place sling under the patient's center of gravity and greatest portion of body weight.
(7) Roll the patient back toward you as second nurse pulls hammock (straps) through.	Ensures sling is in proper position before lift.
(8) Return the patient to supine position. Be sure that hammock or straps are smooth over bed surface. Sling should extend from shoulders to knees (hammock) to support the patient's body weight equally.	Completes positioning of the patient on mechanical/hydraulic sling.
(9) Remove the patient's glasses if appropriate.	Swivel bar is close to the patient's head and could break eyeglasses.
(10) Place horseshoe base of a floor lift under the patient's bed (on side with chair).	Positions lift efficiently and promotes smooth transfer.

STEP	RATIONALE
(11) Lower horizontal bar to sling level by following manufacturer directions. Lock valve if required.	Positions hydraulic lift close to the patient. Locking valve prevents injury to the patient.
(12) Attach hooks on strap (chain) to holes in sling. Short chains or straps hook to top holes of sling; longer chains hook to bottom of sling (see manufacturer's directions).	Secures hydraulic lift to sling.
(13) Elevate head of bed to Fowler's position.	Positions the patient in sitting position.
(14) Have the patient fold arms over chest.	Prevents injury to the patient's arms during transfer.
(15) Either use power cord to turn on lift or pump hydraulic handle using long, slow, even strokes until the patient is raised off bed (see illustration). For ceiling lift, turn on control device to move the lift.	Ensures safe support of the patient during elevation.
(16) Use lift to raise the patient off bed and use steering handle to pull lift from bed as you and other nurse maneuver the patient to chair. Have second nurse alongside the patient.	Lifts the patient off bed safely, nurse's position reduces any risk of the patient falling from sling.
(17) Roll base of lift around chair. Release check valve slowly and lower the patient into chair (see manufacturer directions and see illustration).	Positions lift in front of chair in which the patient is to be transferred. Safely guides the patient into back of chair as seat descends.
(18) Close check valve as soon as the patient is down in chair and straps can be released.	If the valve is left open, boom may continue to lower and injure patient.
(19) Remove straps and roll mechanical/hydraulic lift out of the patient's path.	Prevents damage to skin and underlying tissues.
(20) Check the patient's sitting alignment and correct if necessary.	Prevents injury from poor posture.
5. Perform lateral transfer from bed to stretcher:	The three-person lift (using lift sheet) for horizontal transfer from bed to stretcher is no longer recommended and is discouraged (Anderson et al., 2014; OSHA, 2014). Physical stress can be decreased significantly by using slide board or friction-reducing board positioned under lift sheet beneath the patient. In addition, the patient is more comfortable using this method.
a. Can the patient assist?	
(1) If the patient can assist, caregiver needed only to stand by for safety, with stretcher and bed locked as the patient moves to stretcher (VISN8, 2014).	The patient's level of strength and weight determine level of assistance required for safe transfer. During any patient transferring task, if any caregiver is required to lift more than 15.9 kg (35 lb) of a patient's weight, the patient is considered fully dependent, and an assistive device is used (OSHA, 2014, n.d.).
(2) If the patient is partially able or not at all able and weighs less than 90.7 kg (200 lb), use friction-reducing device or lateral transfer board (VISN8, 2014).	

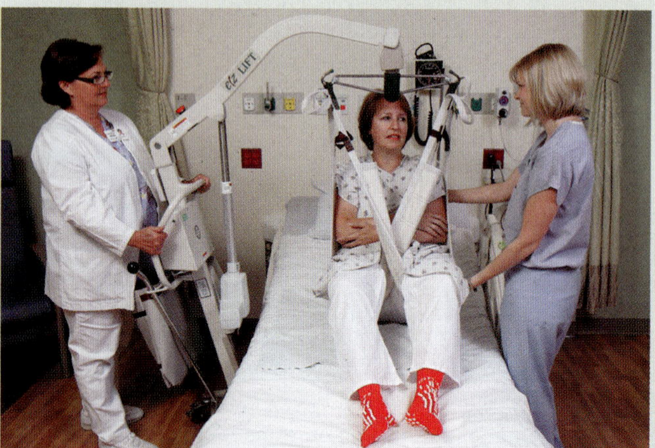

Step 4e(15) Patient lifted in hydraulic lift above bed.

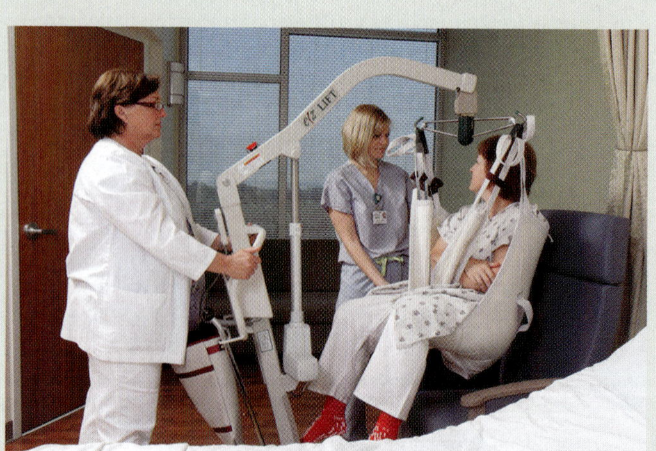

Step 4e(17) Use of hydraulic lift lowers patient into chair.

STEP	RATIONALE
(3) If the patient is partially able or not at all able and weighs more than 90.7 kg (200 lb), use a ceiling lift with supine sling or a mechanical lateral transfer device with three caregivers (VISN8, 2014).	
b. Lateral transfer with friction-reducing device—slide board (see illustration) or air-assisted device:	Maintains alignment of spinal column. Ensures that bed does not move inadvertently.
(1) Lower head of bed as much as the patient can tolerate. Be sure to lock bed brakes.	
(2) Cross the patient's arms on chest.	Prevents injury to arms during transfer.
(3) Lower side rails. To place slide board under the patient, position two nurses on side of bed toward which the patient will be turned. Position the third nurse on other side of the bed.	Distributes weight equally between nurses.
(4) Fanfold lift sheet on both sides.	Provides strong handles to grip lift sheet without slipping.
(5) On count of three, logroll the patient onto side toward the two nurses. Turn the patient as one unit with a smooth, continuous motion.	Maintains body in alignment, preventing stress on any part.
(6) Place slide board under lift sheet (see illustrations). Option: Apply air-assisted device.	Prevents friction from contact of skin with board.
(7) Gently roll the patient back onto slide board.	
(8) Line up stretcher so that surface is ½ inch lower than bed (VISN8, 2014). Lock brakes on stretcher. Instruct the patient not to move.	Ensures that stretcher does not move inadvertently during transfer.
(9) Two nurses position themselves on side of stretcher while the third nurse positions self on the side of bed without stretcher. All three nurses place feet widely apart with one foot slightly in front of the other and grasp friction-reducing device.	

Clinical decision point: A nurse may also be positioned at the head of patient's bed to protect and support his or her head and neck if the patient is weak or unable to assist.

STEP	RATIONALE
(10) Holding fanfolded lift sheet and one nurse counting to three, the two nurses pull lift sheet across slide board positioning the patient onto stretcher. The third nurse holds slide board in place (see illustrations). Option: Inflate air-assisted device and slide the patient across bed onto stretcher.	Slide board remains stationary and provides slippery surface to reduce friction and allows the patient to transfer easily to stretcher.
(11) Position the patient in center of stretcher. Raise head of stretcher if not contraindicated. Raise stretcher side rails. Cover the patient with blanket.	Provides for the patient comfort.
6. Perform hand hygiene.	Reduces transmission of microorganisms.

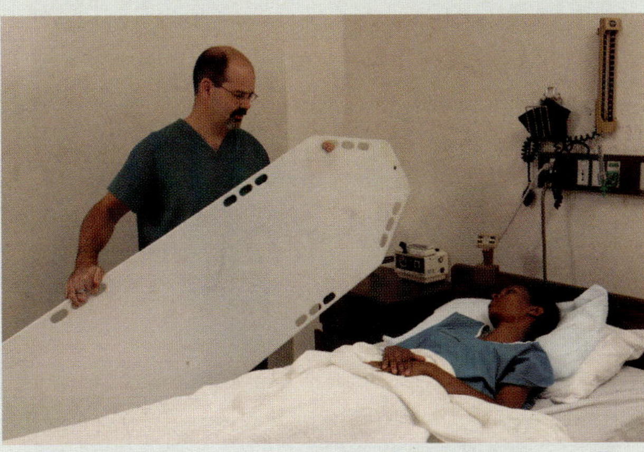

Step 5b Slide board.

STEP	RATIONALE

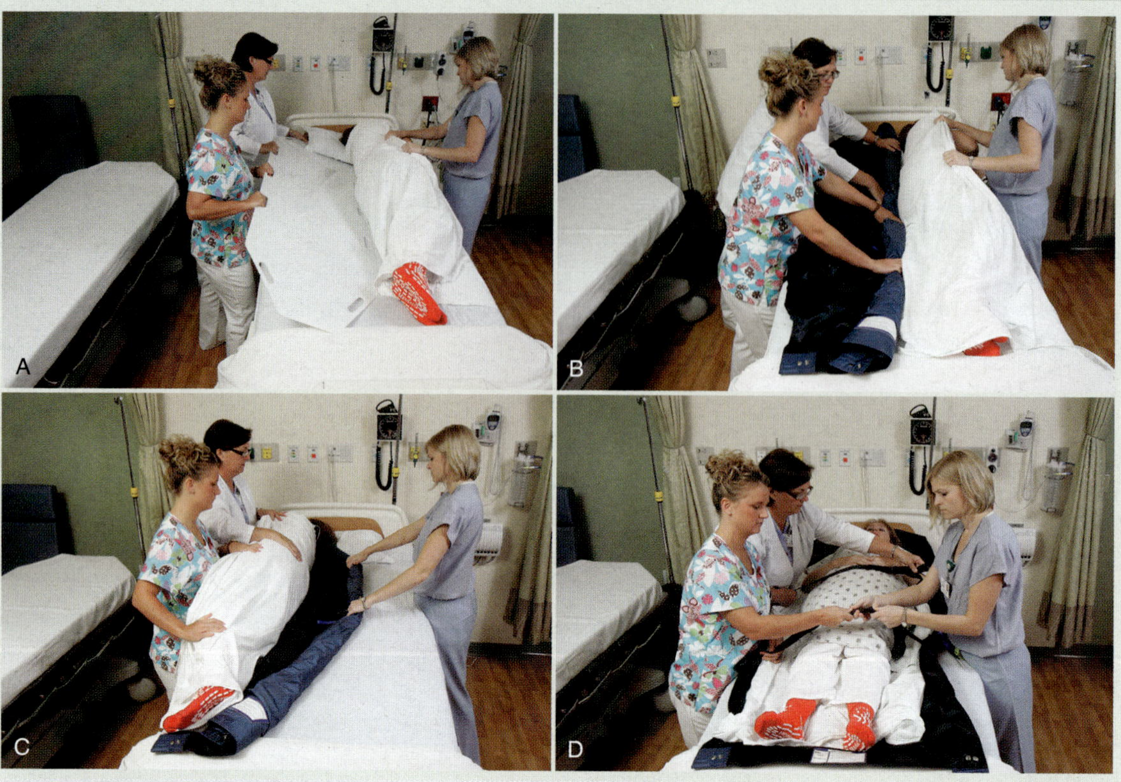

Step 5b(6) **A,** Two caregivers placing slide board under lift sheet. **B,** Two caregivers place air-assisted device under patient. **C,** Patient rolls to opposite side, while other caregiver unrolls air-assisted device. **D,** Secure safety straps.

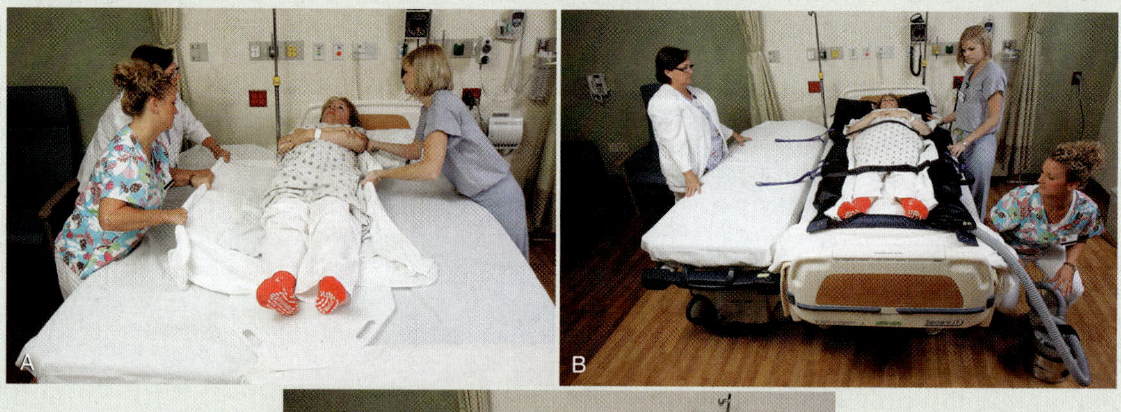

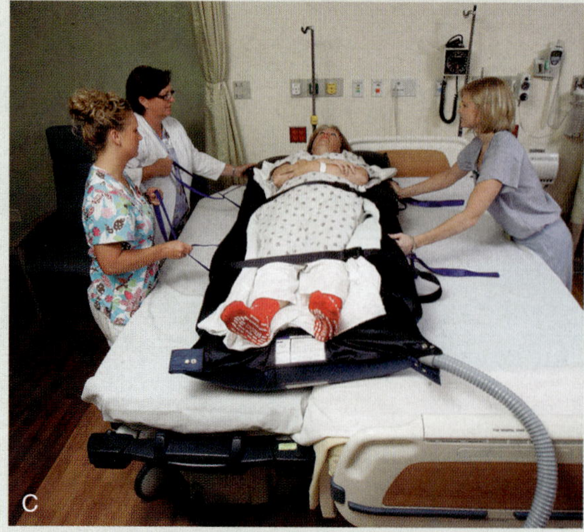

Step 5b(10) **A,** Transfer of patient to stretcher using slide board. **B,** Inflating air-assisted transfer device. **C,** Transfer of patient using air-assisted device.

STEP	RATIONALE
Evaluation	
1. Evaluate vital signs. Ask whether the patient feels tired or dizzy.	Evaluates the patient's response to postural changes and activity.
2. Observe for correct body alignment and presence of pressure points on skin.	Minimizes risk for immobility complications.
3. Ask whether the patient experienced pain during transfer; measure current pain level.	Determines need for additional pain control or alteration of technique of transferring.
4. **Use teach back:** "We have discussed how to transfer from the bed to the chair. Tell me the steps you take to move safely from the bed to a chair." Revise your instruction now or develop a plan for revised patient/family caregiver teaching if the patient/family caregiver is not able to teach back correctly.	Determines the patient's/family caregiver's level of understanding of instructional topic.

Recording and Reporting

- Record procedure including pertinent observations—weakness, ability to follow directions, weight-bearing ability, balance, ability to pivot, number of personnel needed to assist, assistive device used, amount of assistance (muscle strength) required, and the patient's response—in nurses' notes in electronic health record (EHR) or chart.
- Document your evaluation of the patient learning.
- Report transfer ability and assistance needed to next shift or other caregivers. Report progress or remission to rehabilitation staff (physical therapist, occupational therapist).

Unexpected Outcomes and Related Interventions

- The patient is unable to comprehend and follow directions for transfer.
  - Reassess continuity and simplicity of instructions.
- The patient sustains injury on transfer.
  - Evaluate the incident that caused injury (e.g., inadequate assessment, change in patient status, improper use of equipment).
  - Complete occurrence report according to agency policy.
- The patient is unable to stand for time required to transfer to chair.
  - Provide for adequate assistance during transfer.
  - Assess for orthostatic changes in blood pressure when transferring the patient.

KEY POINTS

- Muscles primarily associated with movement are located near the skeletal region, where movement results from leverage.
- Muscles primarily associated with posture are located in the lower extremities, trunk, neck, and back.
- Body alignment is the positioning of joints, tendons, ligaments, and muscles in various body positions.
- Body balance is achieved when there is a wide base of support, the center of gravity falls within the base of support, and a vertical line falls from the center of gravity through the base of support.
- Conditions that affect body alignment and mobility include postural abnormalities, altered bone formation or joint mobility, impaired muscle development, central nervous system damage, and musculoskeletal system trauma.
- Assessment of a patient's mobility enables you to determine the patient's coordination, balance, and ability to complete ADLs and makes it possible to evaluate or plan an exercise program.
- When implementing early mobility protocols, remember that each patient starts at a different level, depending on his or her medical status and ability to participate in mobility.
- Apply proper algorithms when you transfer and lift patients.
- Assistive devices such as canes, crutches, and walkers require specific techniques to walk safely.

REFERENCES

Adler J, Malone D. Early mobilization in the intensive care unit: a systematic review. Cardiopulm Phys Ther J 2012;23(1):5.

Agency for Healthcare Research and Quality (AHRQ): Pressure injury prevention and treatment, 2014. https://www.ahrq.gov/patient-safety/settings/hospital/resource/pressureulcer/tool/index.html Accessed September 2019.

American Academy of Orthopaedic Surgeons. How to use crutches, canes, and walkers. 2015. Available from: http://orthoinfo.aaos.org/topic.cfm?topic=A00181.

American Association of Critical-Care Nurses (AACN). Early progressive mobility protocol. 2013. Available from: https://www.aacn.org/docs/EventPlanning/WB0007/Mobility-Protocol-szh4mr5a.pdf.

American College of Foot and Ankle Surgeons (ACFAS). Instructions for using crutches. 2016. Available from: http://www.acfas.org/footankleinfo/crutches.htm.

American Heart Association (AHA). Target heart rates chart. 2015. Available from: http://www.heart.org/HEARTORG/HealthyLiving/PhysicalActivity/FitnessBasics/Target-Heart-Rates_UCM_434341_Article.jsp#.

American Nurses Association (ANA): *Statement of the American Nurses Association for the committee on Health, Education, Labor, and Pensions of the United States Senate subcommittee on Employment and Workplace Safety*, 2010. http://www.nursingworld.org/DocumentVault/GOVA/Federal/Testimonies/SPH-Testimony.pdf. Accessed September 2020.

American Nurses Association (ANA). Safe patient handling and mobility interprofessional standards. Silver Spring, MD: The American Nurses Association; 2013a.

American Nurses Association (ANA). ANA leads initiative to develop national safe patient handling standards. Silver Springs, MD: The American Nurses Association; 2013b.

Anderson MP, Carlisle S, Thomson C, Ross C, Reid HJ, Hart ND, et al. Safe moving and handling of patients: an interprofessional approach. Nurs Stand 2014;28(46):37.

Ball J, Dains J, Flynn J, Solomon B, Stewart R. Seidel's guide to physical examination. 8th ed. St. Louis: Mosby; 2015.

Bangova A: Prevention of pressure ulcers in nursing home residents, Nurs Stand 27 (24): 54, 2013.

Behrendt R, et al: Continuous bedside pressure mapping and rates of hospital-associated pressure ulcers in a medical intensive care unit, Am J Crit Care 23(2):127, 2014.

Boynton T, Kelly L, Perez A, Miller M, An Y, Trudgen C. Banner Mobility Assessment Tool for nurses: instrument validation. Am J SPHM 2014;4(3):86–92.

Burnfield J, et al: Comparative kinematic and electromagnetic assessment of clinician- and device-assisted sit-to-stand transfers in patients with stroke, PhysTher 93 (10): 1331, 2013.

Burchum JR, Rosenthal LD. Lehne's pharmacology for nursing care. 9th ed. St. Louis: Elsevier; 2016.

Centers for Disease Control and Prevention (CDC). How much physical activity do adults need? 2015. Available from: https://www.cdc.gov/physicalactivity/basics/adults/.

Centers for Disease Control and Prevention (CDC): *Safe patient handling training for schools of nursing: curricular materials*, 2009. http://www.cdc.gov/niosh/docs/2009-127/pdfs/2009-127.pdf. Accessed September 2019.

Chmelo EA, Crotts CI, Newman JC, Brinkley TE, Lyles MF, Leng X, et al. Heterogeneity of physical function responses to exercise training in older adults. J Am Geriatr Soc 2015;63(3):462.

Degelau J, Belz M, Bungum L, Flavin PL, Harper C, Leys K, et al. Institute for Clinical Systems Improvement (ICSI). Prevention of falls (acute care). Bloomington, MN: Institute for Clinical Systems Improvement (ICSI); 2012. Available from: https://pdfs.semanticscholar.org/59cb/ea99bce55e2928e58311a5ff8451508c2488.pdf.

Doherty-King B, Yoon JY, Pecanac K, Brown R, Mahoney J. Frequency and duration of nursing care related to older patient mobility. J Nurs Scholarsh 2014;46(1):20.

Drake J, et al: Pediatric skin care: what do nurses really know? J Spec PediatrNurs 17: 329, 2012.

Edelman C, Mandle CL, Kudzma EC. Health promotion throughout the life span. 8th ed. St. Louis: Mosby; 2014.

Fletcher JS, Banasik JL. Exercise self-efficacy. Clin Excell Nurse Pract 2001;5(3):134.

Frith J, Newton JL, Parry SW. Measuring and defining orthostatic hypotension in the older person. Age Ageing 2014;43(2):168.

Griffis H: Adverse risk: a dynamic interaction model of patient moving and handling, J NursManag 20 (6): 713, 2012.

Halawi MJ, Grant SA, Bolognesi MP. Multimodal analgesia for total joint arthroplasty. Orthopedics 2015;38(7):e616.

Healey F, Darowski A: Older patients and falls in hospitals, Clin Risk 18 (5): 170, 2012.

HealthyPeople.gov. Physical activity. 2015. Available from: http://www.healthypeople.gov/2020/topics-objectives/topic/physical-activity.

Henderson WR, et al: Does prone positioning improve oxygenation and reduce mortality in patients with acute respiratory distress syndrome?, Can Respir J 21(4):213, 2014.

Hockenberry MJ, Wilson D. Wong's nursing care of infants and children. 10th ed. St. Louis: Mosby; 2015.

Huether SE, McCance KL. Understanding pathophysiology. 6th ed. St Louis: Mosby; 2017.

Kim MK, Choi JH, Gim MA, Kim YH, Yoo KT. Effects of different types of exercise on muscle activity and balance control. J Phys Ther Sci 2015;27(6):1875.

Lewis SL, et al: *Medical-surgical nursing assessment and management of clinical problems*, ed 9, St Louis, 2013, Mosby.

Lewis S, et al. Medical-surgical nursing: assessment and management of clinical problems. 9th ed. St. Louis: Mosby; 2014.

Mills P, Gray D, Krassioukov . Five things to know about orthostatic hypotension in the older adult. J Am Geriatr Soc 2014;62(9):1822.

Myszenski A. The essential role of lab values and vital signs in clinical decision making and patient safety for the acutely ill patient. 2014. Available from: https://www.physicaltherapy.com/articles/essential-role-lab-values-and-3637.

National Institute for Occupational Safety and Health (NIOSH). Safe patient handling and mobility (SPHM). 2016. Available from: http://www.cdc.gov/niosh/topics/safepatient/.

National Institute on Aging (NIA). Exercise and physical activity. 2016. Available from: https://www.cdc.gov/niosh/topics/safepatient/default.html.

Occupational Safety and Health Administration (OSHA). Safe patient handling: preventing musculoskeletal disorders in nursing homes. 2014. Available from: https://www.osha.gov/Publications/OSHA3708.pdf.

Occupational Safety and Health Administration (OSHA). Worker safety in hospitals. n.d. Available from: https://www.osha.gov/dsg/hospitals/.

Parreira RB, de Oliveira MR, Amorim CF, Teixeira And DC, da Silva RA. Older adults present better back endurance than young adults during a dynamic trunk extension exercise. J Back Musculoskelet Rehabil 2014;27(2):153.

Pashikanti L, Von Ah D. Impact of early mobilization protocol on the medical-surgical inpatient population: an integrated review of literature. Clin Nurse Spec 2012;26(2):87.

Patton KT, Thibodeau GA. Anatomy and physiology. 9th ed. St. Louis: Mosby; 2016.

Perry AG, et al: Clinical nursing skills and techniques, ed 9, St Louis, 2017, Elsevier.

Pierson F, Fairchild S. Principles and techniques of patient care. 5th ed. St. Louis: Saunders; 2013.

Schofield PA. The assessment and management of peri-operative pain in older adults. Anaesthesia 2014;6(1):54.

Shieh C, Weaver MT, Hanna KM, Newsome K, Mogos M. Association of self-efficacy and self-regulation with nutrition and exercise behaviors in a community sample of adults. J Community Health Nurs 2015;32(4):199.

Stevenson JM. Looking forward by looking back: helping to reduce work-related musculoskeletal disorders. Work 2014;47(1):137.

Swafford K, et al: Use of a comprehensive program to reduce the incidence of hospital-acquired pressure ulcers in an intensive care unit, Am J Crit Care 25(2):152, 2016.

Taylor NF, Dodd KJ, Damiano DL. Progressive resistance exercise in physical therapy: a summary of systematic reviews. PhysTher 2005;85(11):1208.

The Joint Commission (TJC): *2016 National Patient Safety Goals*, Oakbrook Terrace, IL, 2016, The Commission, Available at https://www.jointcommission.org/-/media/deprecated-unorganized/imported-assets/tjc/system-folders/topics-library/old---to-delete/2016_npsg_happdf.pdf?db=web&hash=23105C3839C69F741F877120E8183F51 Accessed November 2019.

The Joint Commission (TJC). 2018 National Patient Safety Goals. Oakbrook Terrace, IL: The Joint Commission; 2018. Available from: http://www.jointcommission.org/standards_information/npsgs.aspx.

Touhy T, Jett K. Ebersole and Hess'gerontological nursing and healthy aging. 4th ed. St. Louis: Mosby; 2014.

U.S. Department of Health and Human Services (USDHHS). Physical activity guidelines for Americans. Washington: HHS; 2008a.

U.S. Department of Health and Human Services (USDHHS). Physical activity guidelines advisory committee report. Washington: HHS; 2008b.

VISN8 Patient Safety Center (VISN8): *Algorithms for safe patient handling and movement*, 2015. http://www.visn8.va.gov/patientsafetycenter/safepthandling/. Accessed March 2020.

Wallace R, Lees C, Minou M, Singleton D, Stratton G. Effects of a 12-week community exercise programme on older people. Nurs Older People. 2014 Feb;26(1):20-6. doi: 10.7748/nop2014.02.26.1.20.e508. PMID: 24471550.

Wong H, et al: Efficacy of a pressure-sensing mattress cover system for reducing interface pressure: study protocol for a randomized controlled trial, Trials 16:434, 2015.

Wrobleski DM, Joswiak ME, Dunn DF, Maxson PM, Holland DE. Discharge planning rounds to the bedside: a patient- and family-centered approach. Medsurg Nurs 2014;23(2):111.

15 Patient Education

OBJECTIVES

After reading this chapter, the student should be able to:

- Describe standard for patient education.
- Identify common topics for a patient's health education needs.
- Describe the concepts of teaching and learning.
- Identify a nurse's role in teaching and learning
- Describe the domains of learning—cognitive, affective, and psychomotor learning.
- Identify the principles of effective teaching and learning.
- Discuss ways to adapt teaching approaches for patients with low health literacy and special needs of children.
- Describe ways to incorporate teaching with routine nursing care.
- Identify methods for evaluating learning.
- Apply the nursing process to the process of teaching.
- Describe how to use the teaching approaches.
- Describe appropriate documentation of teaching and learning.

KEY TERMS

affective learning, p. 321
analogies, p. 330
attentional set, p. 322
cognitive learning, p. 321
health literacy, p. 326
learning, p. 321
learning objective, p. 321
motivation, p. 322
psychomotor learning, p. 321
reinforcement, p. 328
return demonstration, p. 330
teach back, p. 331
teaching, p. 321

INTRODUCTION

Being a patient educator is one of the most important professional nursing roles because education is essential to patient safety, health, and well-being. Factors such as shorter hospital stays, the focus on reducing hospital readmissions within 30 days, and the increased demand on nurses' time support the importance of providing timely quality patient education. Nurses need to find the most effective way to educate patients because health care consumers continue to be more assertive in seeking information, understanding their health needs, and finding resources available within the health care system. Patient education is important because the patient must be informed to consent to treatment. In particular, a patient has the right to know and be informed of diagnosis and prognosis of illness, treatment options, how to perform care activities in the home, and risks associated with treatment. A well-designed, comprehensive teaching plan that fits a patient's unique learning needs improves quality of care, reduces health care costs, helps patients make informed decisions about their health care, and allows them to become healthier and more independent.

STANDARDS FOR PATIENT EDUCATION

Education has been a part of the nurse's role since the days of Florence Nightingale (Miller and Stoeckel, 2016). Patient education is considered a basic nursing competency by the American Association of Colleges of Nursing (AACN), National League for Nursing (NLN), Quality and Safety Education for Nurses (QSEN) Institute, and National Academy of Medicine (NAM) (formerly the Institute of Medicine [IOM]). The American Hospital Association (AHA) created the Patient's Bill of Rights. One of the rights is the right to information about one's diagnosis, treatment, and prognosis that is understandable, current, and relevant (Miller and Stoeckel, 2016). The American Nurses Association (ANA) (2015) specifically addresses a patient's right to self-determination and the nurse's obligation to assess the patient's understanding in Provision 1.4 of the *Code of Ethics for Nurses*. A nurse's role in patient education is becoming increasingly important because patients receive health care from several providers and specialties (Choi, 2015). Nurses provide information about illnesses and health and facilitate communication between a patient and the health care team to promote continuity of care. As a nurse, you need to ensure that patient and family education takes place, evaluate whether learning occurred, and document all steps of the process.

IMPORTANCE AND PURPOSES OF PATIENT EDUCATION

Patient education is a key intervention to improve health behaviors. The goal of patient education is to promote, retain, and restore health (Miller and Stoeckel, 2016).

Maintenance and Promotion of Health and Illness Prevention

By providing health education to patients, you promote positive, informed changes in habits and encourage patients to adapt habits that not only prevent disease and disability but also promote optimal health (Miller and Stoeckel, 2016). Nurses are in a unique position to act as educators because they have the most contact with patients. Patient education takes place in many settings in which nurses actively engage patients in learning how to manage their health, such as schools, hospitals, home, and the workplace (Box 15.1). Self-management is associated with improvements of health outcomes, especially for patients with chronic medical conditions such as diabetes or cardiovascular disease (Panagioti et al., 2014). For example, in childbearing classes, expectant parents learn about physical and psychological changes in the woman and about fetal development. After learning about normal childbearing, the mother is more likely to engage in physical exercise, and the father is more likely to support the mother during her pregnancy.

Restoration of Health

Patients who are injured or ill need information or skills to improve or restore their level of health (see Box 15.1). Patients who are recovering from illness or adapting to chronic illness are often receptive to health education and usually motivated to learn whatever is necessary to resume their normal life (Miller and Stoeckel, 2016). However, patients who are acutely ill benefit from information that focuses on their immediate problems. As a nurse, you need to identify a patient's current health state and readiness to learn to motivate him or her to learn (Bastable, 2014). Family caregivers and friends frequently contribute to a patient's return to health and need to know as much as the patient. However, do not assume that you should involve them. Assess a patient's relationships and level of involvement with others before including family members or friends in patient education.

Coping With Impaired Functioning

Not all patients fully recover from illness or injury. Patients who need to learn to cope with permanent health changes need new knowledge and skills to continue activities of daily living (see Box 15.1). For example, a patient who loses the ability to move the left arm after a stroke needs to learn how to carry out activities of daily living with the right hand. You must also consider chronic illness when planning patient education. Patients who are chronically ill often experience fluctuations in receptiveness to learning over time that are due to their perception that their illness is controlling them (Bastable, 2014).

In the case of serious illness or injury such as a heart attack or spinal cord injury, a patient's family caregiver often partners with the patient and learns how to help him or her

BOX 15.1 Topics for Health Education

Health Maintenance and Promotion and Illness Prevention

- First aid
- Avoidance of risk factors (e.g., smoking, alcohol)
- Growth and development
- Hygiene
- Immunizations
- Prenatal care and normal childbearing
- Nutrition
- Exercise
- Safety (e.g., in home, car, workplace, hospital)
- Screening (e.g., blood pressure, vision, cholesterol level)
- Lifestyle changes to reduce risk factors (e.g., smoking cessation, substance abuse treatment)

Restoration of Health

- Patient's disease or condition
  - Anatomy and physiology of body system affected
  - Cause of disease
  - Origin of symptoms
  - Expected effects on other body systems
  - Prognosis
  - Limitations on function
  - Rationale for treatment
  - Expected duration of care
- Medications
- Tests and therapies
- Nursing measures
- Surgical intervention
- Hospital or clinic environment
- Hospital or clinic staff
- Long-term care
- How patient can participate in care

Coping With Impaired Function

- Home care
  - Medications
  - Diet
  - Activity
  - Self-help devices
- Rehabilitation of remaining function
  - Physical therapy
  - Occupational therapy
  - Speech therapy
- Prevention of complications
  - Knowledge of risk factors
  - Implications of noncompliance with therapy
  - Environmental alterations

manage health care needs (Bastable, 2014). Begin teaching as soon as you identify a patient's needs and determine that the family caregiver is willing to help. Provide information to help families cope with and adapt to emotional effects when your patients have long-term functional limitations.

TEACHING AND LEARNING

Teaching occurs when you deliberately communicate information to a learner to enable him or her to meet identified learning needs. In the case of patients, teaching enables patients to acquire the knowledge and skills for improving health behaviors. The objective of patient teaching is to help a learner adopt desired behaviors to achieve healthy outcomes (Bastable, 2014). Nurses often provide education during teachable moments as they administer nursing care. Examples of teachable moments include during medication administration, after medical appointments, before procedures, and during patient transportation.

As a nurse, you are the sender who wants to communicate a message to the receiver, your patient. Many intrapersonal variables influence your style and approach. Attitudes, values, cultural preferences, emotions, and knowledge influence the way you send messages. Evaluating past experiences with teaching helps you choose the best way to present information with each new patient (Bastable, 2014).

The receiver in the teaching-learning process is the learner. Intrapersonal variables affect a patient's readiness and ability to learn. Language, attitudes, literacy level, cultural background, and values influence the ability to understand a message. The ability to learn also depends on emotional and physical health, stage of development, and previous knowledge.

Learning is the purposeful acquisition of new knowledge, attitudes, behaviors, or skills (Bastable, 2014). It is a complex process, especially if a patient is learning new skills, changing existing attitudes, transferring knowledge to new situations, or solving problems. Generally, teaching and learning begin when a person identifies a need for knowing or acquiring an ability to do something. Teaching is most effective when it responds to a learner's immediate needs. The teacher identifies these needs by asking questions and determining the learner's interests. After you identify what you need to teach, consider developing specific learning objectives. A **learning objective** describes what a patient will be able to do after successful instruction. Learning objectives clearly state the purpose of the teaching and the expectations of the teaching sessions. Both the patient and the nurse need to work together to create the learning objectives so that they are relevant and meaningful. The patient should believe that the learning objectives are achievable and realistic.

ROLE OF A NURSE IN TEACHING AND LEARNING

All nurses act as educators. This responsibility is outlined in the *Code of Ethics for Nurses*. Education about their health is the patients' rights, which is essential to make informed decisions about their care, which requires accurate, complete, and relevant information. Furthermore, it helps patients become more involved in their care and more aware of their right to know about the care they will receive in a language they can understand. You enhance patient safety by teaching patients their role in preventing medical errors.

Your responsibility is to provide information that your patients and their families need. To increase the effectiveness of education, you present information by engaging patients enthusiastically, including the use of appropriate humor, problem-solving activities, and role modeling, and by using examples and technology (Bastable, 2014).

To be an effective educator, engage your patients as partners in learning. Do not merely pass on facts.

Carefully determine what your patients need to know and provide education when they are ready to learn. Then evaluate the outcomes of teaching; for example: Can patients plan a medication schedule over 24 hours? Do patients prepare the right foods for their prescribed diet? Do patients know their activity restrictions?

DOMAINS OF LEARNING

Learning occurs in three domains: (1) cognitive (understanding), (2) affective (attitudes), and (3) psychomotor (motor skills).

Cognitive learning includes what a patient needs to know and understand. All intellectual behaviors are in the cognitive domain, including:

- Acquisition of knowledge
- Comprehension (ability to understand)
- Application (using abstract ideas in concrete situations)
- Analysis (relating ideas in an organized way)
- Synthesis (recognizing parts of information as a whole)
- Evaluation (judging the worth of a body of information)

Affective learning includes a patient's feelings, attitudes, opinions, and values. Research shows that you need to include the affective domain in teaching because it includes a patient's personal attitudes, beliefs, behaviors, and emotions (Miller and Stoeckel, 2016). Learning objectives in the affective domain include influencing attitudes and motivating the learner.

Psychomotor learning occurs when patients acquire skills that require the integration of knowledge and physical skills. Examples of psychomotor learning are learning how to administer insulin injections, use inhalers, and swipe a magnet across a vagal nerve stimulator (VNS). As patients begin to complete psychomotor skills with more confidence, they are able to perform the behaviors in more complex or different situations (e.g., using a walker to walk across a street curb). Adaptation occurs when a patient changes a response as a result of unexpected problems. This results in originating behavior, which involves creating new patterns of behavior.

BASIC LEARNING PRINCIPLES

To teach effectively and efficiently, you first need to understand how people learn. Learning depends on the motivation to learn, the ability to learn, learning styles, and the learning environment. The ability to learn depends on a patient's physical and cognitive characteristics, developmental level, physical wellness, and intellectual thought processes. Remember that people have different preferences for learning and that they learn information in different ways and at different speeds.

Motivation to Learn

Motivation is an internal state that helps arouse, direct, and sustain human behavior (Miller and Stoeckel, 2016). A patient's motivation to learn is influenced by the patient's belief of the need to know something. Patients who need knowledge for survival have a stronger motivation to learn than patients who need it for promoting health (Bastable, 2014). Patients who are motivated to learn are often actively involved in decisions about their care and thus are better able to manage their health care. If a person does not want to learn, it is unlikely that learning will occur.

An **attentional set** is the mental state that allows a learner to focus on and understand the information being taught. Before learning anything, patients must be able to pay attention to or concentrate on the information they will learn. Physical discomfort, anxiety, fatigue, nausea, and environmental distractions make it more difficult for patients to concentrate and thus interfere with learning. You determine a patient's level of comfort by assessing verbal and nonverbal cues and by using objective symptom assessment tools (e.g., pain scale) before beginning a teaching plan. Teach only when your patient can focus on the information.

Anxiety, an uneasiness or uncertainty resulting from anticipating a threat or danger, decreases a patient's ability to attend. Learning requires a change in behavior, often leading to anxiety. A mild level of anxiety motivates learning as abstract thinking and enhances information processing (Bastable, 2014). However, high levels of anxiety disable a person, creating an inability to attend to anything other than relieving the anxiety. If a patient is highly anxious, you can help decrease anxiety before education by using techniques such as guided imagery or using appropriate humor (Bastable, 2014) (see Chapter 4).

Health education often involves changing attitudes and values that are not easy to change simply by teaching facts. You enhance learning by actively involving patients and allowing them to make decisions during an educational session (Edelman and Mandle, 2014). Help patients learn what they need to adapt to their day-to-day lifestyle. For example, to help a patient with diabetes learn to monitor blood glucose levels, have the patient choose a blood glucose meter that is easy to use and affordable, and then observe the patient use it. You also attempt to incorporate the patient's lifestyle into a schedule for blood glucose testing (Fig. 15.1). In addition, knowing your patient's culture (see Chapter 33) and health beliefs helps you develop patient-centered interventions to motivate your patients to learn. Using a model such as the ACCESS model helps you to focus on cultural factors that influence patient education. The six aspects of the model are as follows:

1. **Assessment** of a patient's lifestyle, health beliefs, cultural traditions, and health practices
2. **Communication** with awareness of the many variations in verbal and nonverbal responses

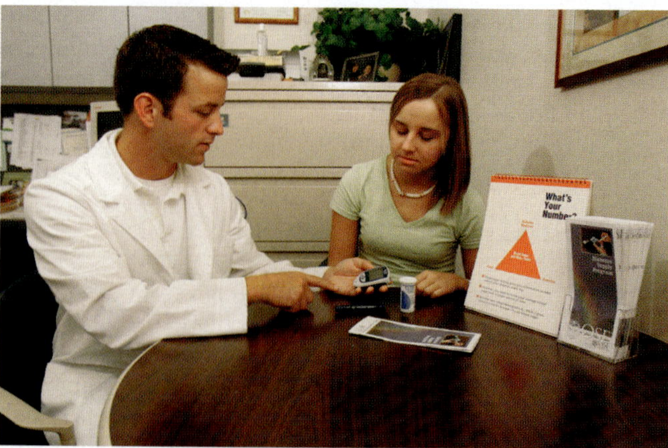

Fig. 15.1 Nurse instructing the patient with a glucose meter.

3. ***C*ultural negotiation and compromise** that encourages awareness of various characteristics of a patient's culture and one's own biases
4. ***E*stablishment** of respect for a patient's cultural beliefs and values; establishment of a caring rapport as the basis for a therapeutic relationship
5. ***S*ensitivity** to how patients from diverse backgrounds perceive their care needs and the various patterns of communications (terms, concepts, tone, and style of communication) they use.
6. ***S*afety** that enables patients to feel culturally secure and avoids disempowerment of their cultural identity; respecting and nurturing the unique cultural identity of the individuals is necessary (Purnell, 2014).

Readiness to Learn

Readiness to learn is based on a patient's willingness and ability to engage in learning (Miller and Stoeckel, 2016). Assess a patient's readiness to learn through discussion with the patient. Many factors affect readiness to learn. For example, patients cannot learn when they are unwilling or unable to accept the reality of illness. A loss of health is usually very difficult for patients to accept. Grief is a complex process that patients experience during illness (see Chapter 28). People experience the stages of grief at different rates. It is important to properly time patient teaching to ease a grieving patient's adjustment to illness or disability (Table 15.1). Introduce a teaching plan when your patient enters the stage of acceptance, which is most compatible with learning. Continue to teach as long as the patient remains in a stage conducive to learning. For example, a patient is recently diagnosed with seizures after a motor vehicle accident and you overhear the patient telling his wife that the result of his electroencephalogram (EEG) is wrong. It is inappropriate to initiate teaching with the patient regarding his new prescription for an antiseizure medication. Instead, you need to educate the patient about his testing and results.

A patient's health status also affects the readiness for education. Patients move along a continuum of health. As the patient moves along the continuum, his or her willingness to learn changes as well (Miller and Stoeckel, 2016). A patient who is acutely ill is concerned with survival. Conditions such as delirium, anxiety, fatigue, or pain interfere

Table 15.1 Relationship Between Psychosocial Adaptation to Illness and Learning

Stage	Patient's Behavior	Learning Implications	Rationale
Denial or disbelief	The patient avoids discussion of illness ("There's nothing wrong with me") and disregards physical restrictions. The patient suppresses and distorts information that has not been presented clearly.	Provide support, empathy, and careful explanations of all procedures while they are being performed. Let the patient know that you are available for discussion. Explain situation to the family. Teach in present tense (explain current therapy).	The patient is not prepared to deal with problem. Any attempt to convince or tell the patient about illness results in further anger or withdrawal. Provide only information the patient pursues or absolutely requires.
Anger	The patient blames and complains and often directs anger at nurse.	Do not argue with the patient but listen to concerns. Teach in present tense. Reassure the family of the patient's normality.	The patient needs opportunity to express feelings and anger. The patient is still not prepared to face future.
Bargaining	The patient offers to live better life in exchange for promise of better health. ("If God lets me live, I promise to be more careful.")	Continue to introduce only reality. Teach only in present tense.	The patient is still unwilling to accept limitations.
Resolution	The patient begins to express emotions openly, realizes that illness has created changes, and begins to ask questions.	Encourage expression of feelings. Begin to share information needed for future and set aside formal times for discussion.	The patient begins to perceive need for assistance and is ready to accept responsibility for learning.
Acceptance	The patient recognizes reality of condition, actively pursues information, and strives for independence.	Focus teaching on future skills and knowledge required. Continue to teach about present occurrences. Involve the family in teaching information for discharge.	The patient is more easily motivated to learn. Acceptance of illness reflects willingness to deal with its implications.

with thinking. At these times, the family caregiver often becomes the recipient of the education. Simple facts addressing immediate needs are most important. For example, a patient in pain is receptive to education about the use of a patient-controlled analgesia (PCA) pump but not how to use crutches.

Ability to Learn

A patient's developmental level and cognitive and physical capabilities influence the ability to learn. Consider the following important factors while developing a teaching plan.

Developmental Capability

Learning, similar to developmental growth, is an evolving process. Therefore, consider your patient's stage of development and intellectual abilities so that your teaching will be successful. Learning occurs more readily when new information complements existing knowledge. Assess a patient's level of knowledge, intellectual skills, and literacy level before beginning a teaching plan. For example, before reviewing a teaching booklet about healthy food choices, determine your patient's understanding of nutrition and his or her reading and comprehension skills.

Age Group

Age often reflects the developmental capability for learning and learning behaviors that a patient can acquire. Without proper biological, motor, language, and personal-social development, many types of learning cannot take place. Adapt your teaching approach based on a patient's developmental level (Box 15.2). When teaching a child, it is very important to match the information you provide with the child's developmental stage. As people mature into adulthood, they often become more self-directed and able to identify their own learning needs. Enhance learning by encouraging an adult learner to reflect on personal and life experiences. Consider generational differences as well. For example, many older patients prefer visual aids and focusing on one topic at a time, whereas younger patients prefer using technology.

Physical Capability

The ability to learn depends on a person's level of physical development and overall physical health. To learn a psychomotor skill, your patient needs to have the necessary level of strength, coordination, and sensory acuity. For example, it is unrealistic for you to teach your patient to transfer from a bed to a wheelchair if he or she has insufficient upper body strength. To learn psychomotor skills, your patient requires the following characteristics:

- Size (height and weight sufficient for the task to be performed or the equipment to be used [e.g., crutch walking])
- Strength (ability of the patient to follow strenuous exercise program)
- Coordination (ability to maintain balance or having the dexterity needed for complicated motor skills such as using utensils or changing a bandage)
- Sensory acuity (visual, auditory, tactile, gustatory, and olfactory—sensory resources needed to receive and respond to messages taught)

Any condition (e.g., fatigue, breathing difficulty, depression) that drains a person's energy impairs the ability to learn. Medications such as pain medications often influence the ability to learn. Postpone teaching when an illness becomes aggravated by complications such as pain, fever, or

BOX 15.2 Teaching Methods Based on Patient's Developmental Capacity

Infant

- Repetition and continuity are essential; keep routines (e.g., feeding, bathing) consistent.
- Hold infant firmly while smiling and speaking softly to convey sense of trust.
- Have infant touch different textures (e.g., soft fabric, hard plastic).

Toddler

- Use play to teach a procedure or activity (e.g., handling examination equipment, applying bandage to doll).
- Offer picture books that describe story of children in hospital or clinic.
- Use simple words such as *cut* instead of *laceration* to promote understanding.

Preschooler

- Use role playing, imitation, and play to make it fun for preschoolers to learn.
- Encourage questions and offer simple explanations and demonstrations.
- Encourage children to learn together through pictures and short stories about how to perform hygiene.

School-Aged Child

- Teach psychomotor skills needed to maintain health. (Complicated skills such as learning to use a syringe take considerable practice.)
- Offer opportunities to discuss health problems and answer questions.

Adolescent

- Help an adolescent learn about feelings and need for self-expression.
- Use teaching as collaborative activity.
- Allow adolescents to make decisions about health and health promotion (safety, sex education, substance abuse).
- Use problem-solving to help adolescents make choices.

Young or Middle-Aged Adult

- Encourage participation in teaching plan by setting mutual goals.
- Encourage independent learning.
- Offer information so that the patient understands effects of health problem.

Older Adult

- Teach when the patient is alert and rested.
- Involve the patient in discussion or activity.
- Focus on wellness and the patient's strength.
- Use approaches that enhance reception of stimuli for patients with sensory alterations (see Chapter 27).
- Keep teaching sessions short.

respiratory difficulty. While providing care, assess a patient's energy level by noting his or her willingness to communicate, amount of activity initiated, and responsiveness to questions. Stop teaching if a patient tires; resume teaching when the patient feels rested. Offer several short teaching sessions rather than one long session.

Learning Environment

Learning takes place in a variety of environments. Always assess the physical environment and ensure it is as conducive to learning as possible (Miller and Stoeckel, 2016). Choose settings (e.g., small classroom, office) that help patients focus attention on their learning task.

The ideal environment that promotes learning is a room that has good lighting and ventilation, appropriate furniture, and a comfortable temperature (Fig. 15.2). A room that is too cold, hot, stuffy, or crowded makes patients too uncomfortable to pay attention. Comfortable furniture eliminates distractions such as the need to change position or shift body weight. It is also important to choose a quiet setting that offers privacy and few interruptions. If a patient desires, include family members (especially the primary family caregiver) in discussions. However, remember that some patients are reluctant to engage in discussions about their illness when family members are present. Ask patients for permission to have family caregivers participate.

Teaching a group of patients requires a room that is an appropriate size and allows everyone to be seated comfortably and within hearing distance of the teacher. If the room is too large, participants are often tempted to sit outside the group along the perimeter. Arranging the group to allow participants to observe one another (e.g., in a circle) further enhances learning. More effective communication occurs as learners observe the verbal and nonverbal interactions of others.

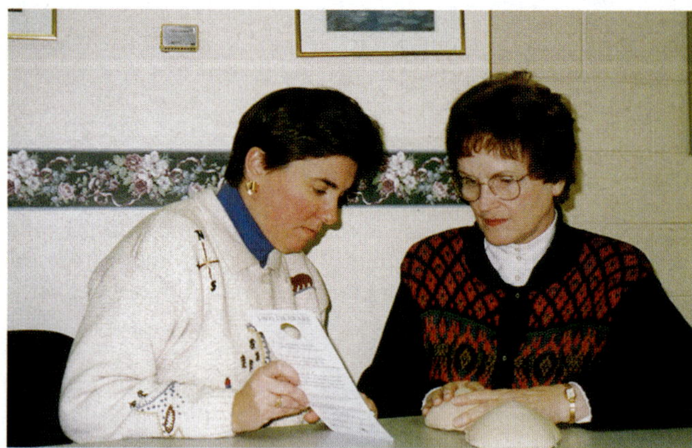

Fig. 15.2 Choosing a comfortable, pleasant environment enhances the learning experience. Nurse is explaining breast self-examination procedure to the patient.

INTEGRATING NURSING AND TEACHING PROCESSES

The teaching process parallels the nursing process (see Chapter 19). Both processes use the same steps (Table 15.2). Both processes require critical thinking. The two processes

Table 15.2 Comparison of Nursing and Teaching Processes

Basic Steps	Nursing Process	Teaching Process
Assessment	Collect data about patient's physical, psychological, social, cultural, developmental, and spiritual needs from the patient, family, all databases, medical record, nursing history, and literature.	Gather data about patient's learning needs, literacy level, cultural background, motivation, ability to learn, and teaching resources from the patient, family, learning environment, and all databases.
Nursing diagnosis	Identify appropriate nursing diagnoses.	Identify the patient's learning needs on the basis of three domains of learning.
Planning	Develop individualized care plan. Set diagnosis priorities based on the patient's immediate needs.	Establish learning objectives stated in behavioral terms. Identify priorities regarding learning needs. Collaborate with the patient on teaching plan.
Implementation	Collaborate with the patient on care plan. Perform nursing care therapies. Include the patient as active participant in care. Involve the family caregiver in care as appropriate.	Identify type of teaching method to use. Implement teaching methods. Actively involve the patient in learning activities. Include the family caregiver participation as appropriate.
Evaluation	Identify success in meeting desired outcomes and goals of nursing care.	Determine outcomes of teaching-learning process. Measure the patient's ability to achieve learning objectives. Reteach as needed.

Table 15.3 Focused Patient Assessment

Factors to Assess	Questions	Physical Assessment
Learning needs	Tell me what you know about your illness and its treatment. What would you like to know that would help you better manage your disease at home?	Observe expression on the patient's face (e.g., puzzled, attentive, distracted).
Resources for learning	Who is the primary person who can help you at home? Will you have any trouble getting to the local health department to obtain teaching materials?	Observe for signs of anxiety when discussing home and transportation issues.
Ability to learn	Do you wear glasses or contacts? Do you have trouble seeing words printed in the newspaper?	Observe where the patient holds reading material and for squinting of eyes when reading.
	Do you have any difficulties hearing when someone speaks to you?	Observe whether the patient turns head when attempting to listen.

differ in that the nursing process focuses on providing care, whereas the education process focuses on teaching (Bastable, 2014). Also, the outcomes of the processes are different. The outcomes of the nursing process include physical and psychosocial needs of the patient being met. The outcomes of the teaching process include changes in knowledge and skills. There are many models for patient education that you can use when developing education, including the ASSURE model. The acronym *ASSURE* stands for *a*nalyze the learner, *s*tate the objectives, *s*elect the instructional methods and materials, *u*se the instructional methods and materials, *r*equire learner performance, and *e*valuate the teaching plan (Bastable, 2014).

Assessment

An effective assessment for teaching provides the basis for individualized patient instruction. Apply critical thinking and consider what you know from your general nursing assessment (e.g., patient's condition, medications, physical status) to further explore and assess the patient's learning needs.

Ability to Learn

Begin your approach to teaching with an assessment of a patient's learning needs, readiness to learn, and preferred learning styles (Bastable, 2014). An individualized assessment ensures a more relevant and accurate approach to patient education (Table 15.3).

Patient Expectations

Because you need to focus education on the individual needs of a patient, gather information from the patient, analyze the information, and incorporate the information into a plan for patient education. It is also essential to understand what your patient expects to learn. Learning needs change, depending on your patient's health status. Assessment of learning needs is an ongoing activity. Examples of key areas of assessment are (1) questions raised by a patient or family about health issues; (2) a patient's understanding of current health status, implications of illness, types of therapy, and prognosis; (3) information or skills needed to perform self-care; (4) experiences that influence a patient's need to learn; and (5) information necessary for family caregivers to meet a patient's needs.

Motivation to Learn

Assess a patient's motivation to learn: Is the patient prepared and willing to learn based on the acuity and severity of his or her health risks or problems? Ask questions that relate to a patient's learning behaviors, health beliefs, cultural attitudes about health care providers, knowledge of health problems, and information to be learned. Other factors to assess include a patient's socioeconomic background, perception of the health problem, and perceived ability to perform health behaviors.

Teaching Environment

Ensure the environment is favorable to learning. Assess for distractions, noise, a patient's comfort level (e.g., sitting or lying, the need to use the toilet), and the availability of rooms and equipment. In the home setting, you need to assess lighting, space, and the availability of equipment.

Learning Styles

Learning styles are the ways in which learners most efficiently and effectively perceive, process, store, and recall information (Bastable, 2014). You assess learning styles by observation, interviews, and administering learning style assessments. An example of a learning style assessment is the VARK questionnaire (Bastable, 2014).

Resources for Learning

Identify resources for learning, which often include the support of family caregivers or significant others. Determine who the patient's primary caregiver is in the home and whether the patient wishes to include the person in instruction.

The family influences the health and health behavior of the patient. For example, you provide a male patient with information regarding dietary changes required because of a medication such as avoiding foods rich in vitamin K while taking warfarin (Coumadin). If you give the education regarding dietary changes to the patient, it may not be successful if his wife is the primary cook at home. Thus, you need to assess the readiness of family caregivers (as there may be more than one) to learn, when appropriate, to help care for a patient. Determine family caregivers' perceptions of a patient's illness and their willingness to help provide care. Determine the resources available in the home (e.g., running water, heating, access to transportation) and the teaching tools needed based on the patient's needs and ability to learn.

Language and Cultural Factors

Assess the language a patient most commonly uses. Sometimes you will need a translator to complete your assessment (see Chapter 33). TJC requires hospitals to provide qualified professional translators, whether the translator is physically present or available via telephone or interpreter care. Do not use family members as translators because they may not be able to translate important terms needed in obtaining informed consent or education, and many concepts are not easily translated.

Taking a patient's culture into account is essential in the educational assessment of a patient. Culture is a reflection of the whole of human behavior, including ideas, beliefs, and values; ways of relating to one another; language and manners of speaking; and work and lifestyle practices (Ball et al., 2015) (see Chapter 33). In terms of illness, patients often feel a loss of control, which often makes them hold on tighter to their cultural and family beliefs. You need to assess a patient's perception of health and illness, the use of traditional remedies and folk practitioners, the patient's perceptions of western medicine, the role of the family and family member relationships, and lastly the perception of emotional support (Bastable, 2014). For example, explore the significance prescribed medications and therapies have for a patient and consider alternative therapies he or she may use.

Health Literacy

Current evidence shows that health literacy is a key component that affects a patient's health care experience (National Institutes of Health [NIH], 2017). Therefore, you need to assess your patients' health literacy before providing instruction. **Health literacy** is defined by NAM (formerly IOM) as an individual's ability to obtain, process, and understand basic health information and services to make appropriate and informed health decisions (Toronto and Weatherford, 2016). Individuals with low health literacy are at greater risk for adverse health outcomes and are less likely to adhere to medical recommendations. People with low health literacy come from all age ranges, races, and socioeconomic and educational backgrounds (Miller and Stoeckel, 2016). Low health literacy is not always easy for nurses to recognize. Simply asking patients whether they can read often does not work because they do not feel comfortable admitting that they cannot read.

Current evidence supports using evidence-based assessment tools such as the Single-Item Literacy Screener (SILS). This tool asks questions such as "How often do you have to have someone help you read instructions, pamphlets, or other written material from your doctor or pharmacy?" and "How confident do you feel in filling out medical forms by yourself?" (Brice et al., 2014). Another assessment tool, the Newest Vital Sign (NVS) (http://www.pfizer.com/health/literacy/public_policy_researchers/nvs_toolkit), is available in English or Spanish; takes 3 minutes to complete; and screens a patient's general literacy level, numeracy skills, and comprehension of health-related written materials. Other assessment data that indicate low health literacy include a patient's inability to complete forms, read a prescription label, or adhere to a treatment plan or a displaying uncooperative behavior, asking no questions, or asking for help from the family (Driessnack et al., 2014).

Special Needs of Children

Children pass through several developmental stages. You need to assess a child's cognitive and psychomotor abilities, physical strength, coordination, and reading level (see Box 15.2). Involve the parents during your assessment to better understand a child's needs, especially when children are very young and unable to care for themselves.

Middle Age Considerations

Middle age is a time in which it becomes important for adults to begin to build positive health habits (e.g., diet, exercise, lifestyle practices) to be better prepared for the older adult stage of life. Middle-aged adults must adapt their physical and psychological changes with their social roles. For example, does their tolerance to exercise enable them to participate in sports activities? Is there a need to select friends who are less involved in risky social behaviors? Assess a patient's understanding of what healthy behaviors involve and whether he or she accepts what changes may be necessary to adopt those behaviors.

Older Adult Considerations

The population of older adults continues to increase, and their care is becoming more complex. Thus, use the best evidence when assessing an older adult's learning needs. Older adults experience numerous physical and psychological changes as they age. Assess each patient for sensory changes that require modification of teaching methods (Miller and Stoeckel, 2016). For example, if you assess decreased visual acuity in your patient, use large-print materials to provide and reinforce patient teaching.

Nursing Diagnosis

After assessing information related to your patient's ability and need to learn, interpret data and cluster defining characteristics to form nursing diagnoses that reflect the patient's specific learning needs. If a patient has several learning needs, the nursing diagnoses guide priority setting.

Several North American Nursing Diagnosis Association International (NANDA-I) nursing diagnoses apply to learning needs. When the diagnosis is *Deficient Knowledge*, the diagnostic statement describes the specific type of learning need and related factor (e.g., *Deficient Knowledge regarding psychomotor learning related to newly ordered injectable medication*). Some diagnoses are very similar to one another. Thus, to identify the correct problem-focused diagnosis, you must analyze the patient's defining characteristics carefully. For example, when you care for a patient who is not physically active because the patient does not understand the importance of physical activity, the nursing diagnosis is *Sedentary Lifestyle related to deficient knowledge of health benefits of physical exercise.* However, if this same patient is having difficulty completing activities of daily living because of increased weight and the patient needs to know how to adapt activities to meet health needs, the nursing diagnosis is *Activity Intolerance related to generalized weakness*, and your plan of care would include patient education regarding how to improve endurance.

Other examples of nursing diagnoses that indicate learning needs include the following:

- *Ineffective Denial*
- *Ineffective Health Maintenance*
- *Ineffective Health Management*
- *Risk-Prone Health Behavior*
- *Ineffective Family Health Management*

Planning

After determining nursing diagnoses, identify your patient's learning needs and develop a teaching care plan. When helping a patient change a health behavior, remember that knowledge alone does not change behavior. Discuss factors that facilitate and inhibit learning with your patient during planning. For the plan to be effective, collaborate with the patient, family caregiver(s), and other members of the health care team. The plan needs to include topics for instruction, teaching resources (e.g., equipment or booklets), recommendations for involving the family caregiver(s), and teaching objectives.

Goals and Outcomes

It is very important to set clear goals and measurable outcomes so that you can effectively establish and later evaluate and revise a teaching plan as needed. Include the patient if possible when establishing learning goals and outcomes. Expected outcomes guide the choice of teaching strategies and who is involved in the plan. Learning objectives are either short term (relating to immediate learning needs) or long term (relating to permanent adaptation to a health problem). Each objective is a statement of a single behavior that identifies a patient's ability to do something after a learning experience.

In some health care settings, you develop written teaching plans. Include topics for instruction and resources, recommendations for involving family, and objectives of the teaching plan in these cases. Some plans are very detailed, whereas others are in an outline format. Remember that the more specific your plan is, the easier it is to follow.

Setting Priorities

Learning objectives identify the expected outcomes of a planned learning experience, which help establish priorities for learning. Focus on what the patient needs to know, his or her nursing diagnoses, and previous knowledge. As a nurse, you are ultimately responsible for ensuring that all teaching needs have been met. Usually, patient safety is a teaching need that is most important. For example, a patient with newly diagnosed hypertension and angina needs to learn about newly prescribed medications, which typically include nitroglycerin for angina and an antihypertensive medication, such as an angiotensin-converting enzyme (ACE) inhibitor. In this situation, knowledge regarding the early identification of chest pain and appropriate use of nitroglycerin are the learning priorities.

Timing

When is the right time to teach? When a patient first enters a clinic or hospital? At discharge? At home? Each time point is appropriate because patients have learning needs as long as they stay in the health care system. There are times in which it is not appropriate to provide teaching such as when a patient receives bad results from a diagnostic test. Plan to teach when a patient is most attentive, receptive, and alert. The frequency of sessions depends on each patient's abilities and the complexity of the information that is being taught.

The length of teaching sessions also affects learning. Prolonged sessions cause patients to lose concentration and attentiveness, especially older adult patients. It is easier to maintain patients' interests when educational sessions are shorter (e.g., lasting 10−15 minutes) and more frequent. Nonverbal cues such as poor eye contact or slumped posture indicate that a patient has lost concentration. If you note a loss of concentration, stop the session.

Organizing Teaching Material

Consider the order of information presented. Organize material so that it progresses from simple to complex because a person learns simple facts and concepts before learning how to make associations or complex interpretations of ideas. For example, to teach a woman how to feed her husband who has a gastric tube (see Chapter 20), first teach her how to measure the tube feeding and manipulate the equipment. Once you accomplish this, teach her how to administer the feeding.

Because patients are more likely to remember information taught in the beginning of a teaching session, present essential information first. Informative but less critical content follows the essential information. Use repetition and summarize key points to reinforce learning.

Collaborative Care

Although you are the primary member of the health care team responsible for patient education, your patients' educational needs are often highly complex. Collaboration with other health care professionals is required to successfully meet patient needs. For example, refer a patient with a new diagnosis of chronic renal failure to a dietitian for dietary teaching. Patients in acute care settings often require assistance from discharge planners, case managers, and community agencies to be successfully discharged to home. It is your responsibility to collaborate with and include these interdisciplinary health care team members in the teaching plan. A variety of educational resources is available in the community including diabetes education clinics, prenatal classes, and support groups. Encourage your patients to use these resources and reinforce information provided.

Implementation

Implementation of a teaching plan requires you to use critical thinking while you analyze assessment data and nursing diagnoses and apply teaching and learning principles. Remember that each interaction with a patient is an opportunity to teach. You implement teaching strategies that integrate all styles of learning to fully engage the patient and enhance learning. Use evidence-based interventions to create an effective and active learning environment and maximize opportunities for learning. Because learning situations vary, there is no single correct way to teach.

Teaching Approaches

Teaching may be provided in a variety of ways, but it is important to choose a teaching approach that matches your patient's needs and learning style. A patient's learning needs change over time. Modify your teaching approach as you care for a patient over time.

Telling

Use the telling approach when teaching limited information such as when you are preparing a patient for an emergent diagnostic procedure. Outline the task a patient needs to do and give explicit instructions. There is no time for feedback with this method.

Participating

When using the participating approach, you and the patient participate in the learning process together. The patient helps decide content and how best to present it, and you guide and counsel the patient. For example, a parent with a child diagnosed with sickle cell disease works with you to manage the child's pain. You select pain management approaches that will likely be effective at times when the child's pain is the worst. At the end of each teaching session, you review the objectives with the parent and child and plan or revise what you will cover the next time you meet.

Entrusting

The entrusting approach gives patients the opportunity to manage their self-care. A patient accepts responsibilities and correctly performs a task while you observe the patient's progress and remain available for assistance. For example, a patient who is receiving continuous intravenous pain medication at home for end-stage cancer requires a higher dose of pain medication. The patient understands the dosage of the medication and how the medication pump works. You help the patient determine an appropriate new pain medication dosage and allow him or her to adjust the settings on the medication pump.

Reinforcing

Reinforcement is using a stimulus that increases the probability of a response. A learner who receives reinforcement before or after a desired learning behavior will likely repeat the behavior. Feedback is a common form of reinforcement. Reinforcers are positive or negative. Positive reinforcement such as a smile or praise and support produces the desired responses. Although negative reinforcement (e.g., frowning) may work, people usually respond better to positive reinforcement.

Three types of reinforcers are social, material, and activity. Use social reinforcers (e.g., smiles, compliments, words of encouragement, or physical contact) to acknowledge a learned behavior. Examples of material reinforcers are food, toys, and music. They work best with young children. Activity reinforcers (e.g., physical therapy) rely on the principle that a person is motivated to engage in an activity if there is an opportunity to participate in more desirable activity on completion of this first activity. Choosing an appropriate reinforcer involves careful thought and attention to individual preferences. Never use reinforcers as threats. Reinforcement is not effective with every patient.

Incorporating Teaching With Nursing Care

As you gain confidence in your knowledge and clinical skills, you find that you are able to teach more effectively while you provide care to your patients. For example, you educate your patient on the actions of medications while you administer them. When you follow a teaching plan informally, your patient feels less pressure to perform, and learning becomes more of a shared activity. Teaching during routine care is efficient and cost-effective and makes the information more relevant.

Teaching Methods

Active participation enhances learning. By actively experiencing a learning event, your patient is more likely to retain knowledge. A teaching method is the way you deliver information and is based on a patient's learning needs and preferences (Box 15.3). For example, older adults learn and remember more if the material is relevant to their needs and abilities and is provided at an appropriate pace (Box 15.4) (Miller and Stoeckel, 2016). The instructional method you choose depends on the time available for teaching, the setting, the resources available, and your comfort level with teaching.

One-on-One Discussion

Whenever you teach a patient at the bedside, in a health care provider's office, or in the home, you share information through one-on-one discussion. You provide information informally, allowing the patient to ask questions or share concerns. Use various teaching aids during the discussion, depending on the patient's learning needs.

BOX 15.3 Teaching Methods Based on Patient's Learning Needs

Cognitive

Discussion (One-on-One or Group)

- Involves nurse and patient or nurse with several patients
- Promotes active participation and focuses on topics of interest to patient
- Allows peer support
- Enhances application and analysis of new information

Lecture

- More formal method of instruction because teacher controls it
- Helps learner acquire new knowledge and gain comprehension

Question and Answer Session

- Designed specifically to address patient's concerns
- Helps the patient apply knowledge

Role Play, Discovery

- Allows the patient to actively apply knowledge in controlled situation
- Promotes synthesis of information and problem-solving

Independent Project (Computer-Assisted Instruction), Field Experience

- Allows the patient to assume responsibility for completing learning activities at own pace
- Promotes analysis, synthesis, and evaluation of new information and skills

Affective

Role Play

- Allows expression of values, feelings, and attitudes

Discussion (Group)

- Allows the patient to acquire support from others in group
- Permits the patient to learn from others' experiences
- Promotes responding, valuing, and organization

Discussion (One-on-One)

- Allows discussion of personal, sensitive topics of interest or concern

Psychomotor

Demonstration

- Provides presentation of procedures or skills by nurse
- Permits the patient to incorporate modeling of nurse's behavior
- Allows the nurse to control questioning during demonstration

Practice

- Gives the patient opportunity to perform skills using equipment
- Provides repetition

Return Demonstration

- Permits the patient to perform skills as nurse observes
- Is excellent source of feedback and reinforcement

Independent Project, Game

- Requires teaching method that promotes adaptation and origination of psychomotor learning
- Permits learner to use new skills

BOX 15.4 Care of an Older Adult

Effective Teaching Strategies for an Older Adult

- Provide individualized information that is based on what the patient needs to know.
- Present information slowly in frequent sessions.
- Include family caregivers when necessary.
- Repeat information frequently.
- Reinforce teaching with audiovisual material, written exercises, and practice.
- Emphasize the older adult's current concerns and past positive coping strategies (Touhy and Jett, 2016).
- Allow more time for learner to express himself or herself, demonstrate learning, and ask questions (Edelman and Mandle, 2014).
- Establish measurable and realistic short-term goals.
- Establish follow-up sessions.
- Base new information on patient's previous level of learning.

Group Instruction

Group instruction offers an economical way to teach several patients at one time and allows patients to develop a network of social support (Miller and Stoeckel, 2016). Group instruction often involves both lecture and discussion. Lectures are efficient in helping groups of patients learn about a subject. After hearing information from a lecture, learners need the opportunity to share ideas and seek clarification. Group discussions allow patients and families to learn from one another as they share common experiences.

Preparatory Instruction

Patients frequently face unfamiliar tests or procedures that create anxiety. Providing information about procedures helps them feel less anxious because they understand what to expect during a procedure. When preparatory instructions accurately describe actual experiences, patients usually cope more effectively with the stress from the procedure and therapies. The following are guidelines for giving preparatory explanations:

1. Describe physical sensations during the procedure but do not evaluate them. For example, when drawing a blood specimen, explain that the patient will feel a sticking sensation as the needle punctures the skin.
2. Describe the cause of the sensation, preventing false impressions of the experience. For example, explain that a needle insertion burns because alcohol used to cleanse the skin enters the puncture site.
3. Prepare patients only for aspects of the experience that have commonly been noticed by other patients. For example, explain that it is normal for a tight tourniquet (applied during an intravenous needle insertion) to cause a person's hand to tingle and feel numb.

Demonstrations

Use demonstrations when teaching psychomotor skills. An effective demonstration requires planning. Include the following steps in a demonstration:

1. Assemble and organize equipment.
2. Perform each step in sequence while analyzing the knowledge and skills involved.
3. Determine when to give explanations, considering the patient's learning needs.
4. Judge the proper speed and timing of the demonstration based on the patient's cognitive abilities and anxiety level.

Demonstrate the procedure or skill under the same conditions that the patient will experience at home and in the same order in which the patient will perform it. Encourage the patient to ask questions so that he or she clearly understands each step. To enable the patient to easily observe each step, perform demonstrations slowly and avoid rushing. Give the patient the opportunity to practice the procedure under supervision. At the end of the session, have the patient perform a **return demonstration,** allowing the patient to complete the procedure independently to show competence. When appropriate, also have family caregivers perform return demonstrations, especially when they are likely the ones who will provide the skill at home.

Analogies

Learning occurs when a teacher translates complex language or ideas into words or concepts that a patient understands. **Analogies** add to verbal instruction by providing familiar images that make complex information more real and understandable (Miller and Stoeckel, 2016). For example, comparing arterial blood pressure to the flow of water through a hose is an analogy that is useful when explaining hypertension to a patient. When using analogies, know the concept; keep the analogy simple and clear; and be aware of the patient's background, experience, and culture. Analogies work only if the other person understands the comparison.

Role Play

During role play, your patients play themselves or someone else in a situation. Patients learn required skills and feel more confident in performing them independently following the role play. For example, you are teaching a family caregiver effective communication strategies to use with an older, confused parent. You pretend to be the parent who is having difficulty getting dressed. The caregiver responds to you in this situation. At the end of the session, you help the caregiver evaluate the response and determine if an alternative approach would have been more effective.

Simulation

Simulation is a useful technique for teaching problem-solving, application, and independent thinking. During individual or group discussion, you present a problem or situation for patients to solve. For example, you ask patients with heart disease to plan a meal low in cholesterol.

Use of Technology

Communication and patient teaching do not happen only in person; it also occurs electronically. Most Americans have access to the internet, and about 56% of people own a smartphone (Miller and Stoeckel, 2016). As technology continues to improve, more people are online and use online resources to enhance their health. For example, some hospitals use Twitter to improve communication to share news and health information with the community (Gomes and Coustasse, 2015). A trend in the hospital setting is to use technology through TV networks and tablets to provide self-paced and self-directed learning (Sawyer et al., 2016). The patient completes surveys on admission, and then the nurse launches education modules for the patient; the program is evaluated using review questions at the end of each topic segment. Another technology platform called the GetWellNetwork uses the television in a patient's room (Kompany et al., 2016). The GetWellNetwork delivers age-appropriate education, including interactive education for children. Technology is also used in the outpatient setting to provide education. Placing education materials in waiting rooms using tablets helps improve patient satisfaction, which increases compliance with treatment plans and future appointments (Stribling and Richardson, 2016).

Maintaining Attention and Participation

All the senses are channels for presenting information. Patients learn best when you use multiple senses while you teach. In addition, your actions can increase learner attention and participation. When conducting a discussion with a patient, change the tone and intensity of your voice, make eye contact, and use gestures that accentuate key points of discussion.

Illiteracy and Other Disabilities

Medical terms are very confusing. Thus, you need to provide information in words that your patients are able to understand. People who have problems with illiteracy or other learning disabilities often have difficulty analyzing instructions and synthesizing information. Use a variety of resources (e.g., audiotapes, videos, drawing pictures) with patients who have low health literacy or other difficulties learning (Box 15.5).

Sometimes, you provide education to patients who have sensory alterations (see Chapter 27). When caring for patients who are hearing impaired, you may need to include a sign language interpreter to help implement your interventions or use a white board to write messages to each other. Visual impairments also affect the teaching strategy you use. Patients who are blind or have reduced vision often have acute listening skills. To enhance communication and decrease anxiety, tell the patient that you are there, and do not shout during teaching sessions.

Cultural Awareness

Health education materials often fail to address a patient's cultural beliefs, values, language, perceptions, and attitudes. Be aware of a patient's cultural background, beliefs, and ability to understand instructions. In some cases, you need to provide information written in the patient's native language.

Cultural awareness helps you provide culturally sensitive health care and patient education. For example, how you explain guidelines for safe sex varies if a patient is

BOX 15.5 Patient Teaching Strategies for Patients With Limited Health Literacy

- Make time for one-on-one educational sessions. Speak clearly and listen carefully.
- Individualize teaching materials (e.g., reading level, use of graphics, photographs) to meet a patient's needs and match his or her reading level; if you do not know a patient's reading level, provide information at a fifth-grade or lower level.
- Keep a lesson simple. In general, introduce no more than four topics (USDHHS, n.d.).
- Provide information in a variety of ways (e.g., written, on a computer, videotape, audiotape).
- Make teaching materials visually appealing. For written materials, use at least 12-point font and avoid using all capital letters, italics, and fancy script (USDHHS, n.d.).
- Use simple words that a patient can understand (e.g., shot instead of injection, walk instead of ambulate, medicine instead of medication). Avoid long or run-on sentences (USDHHS, n.d.).
- Use the active voice when providing instructions (e.g., tell patient to "take medicine before bedtime" instead of "medicine should be taken at bedtime").
- Use examples (e.g., what to do when feeling bad, how to set up a pill counter at home) to keep a patient an active participant in learning.
- Present the most important information first, and summarize it at the end of the session.
- Space out information to decrease intimidation.
- Use pictures or illustrations when possible.
- Encourage patients to ask questions during the teaching session.
- Ask specific questions (e.g., "When will you take this medicine each day?") and ask the patient to "teach back" or "show back" what you have taught to evaluate learning. Examples are "We discussed the problems you need to call your doctor about; tell me what those are" and "I explained the type of foods that are high in salt; give me three examples."
- Observe the patient's ability to perform any desired behaviors or self-care activities.

heterosexual versus homosexual. A patient from a lower socioeconomic background will require nutritional education with a different focus on foods than a patient who has unlimited financial resources and is able to purchase any type of food.

Effective educational strategies often require the use of different patterns of communication. When educating patients of different ethnic groups, do the following:

- Become aware of the distinctive aspects of each culture (Mott-Coles, 2014).
- If an interpreter is necessary, determine your patient's beliefs about using an interpreter. First, in some cultures, it is inappropriate to discuss private health-related issues with people of the opposite sex or people who are younger. Always use a professional interpreter who understands medical terminology.
- Demonstrate respect for your patient and the family, address them using their appropriate titles, and pronounce their names correctly.
- Use culturally relevant teaching resources and approaches (Mott-Coles, 2014).

BOX 15.6 Teach Back Method of Evaluation

Use the following questions to evaluate patient understanding of education. Ask the questions in an open-ended, respectful manner and modify them as needed (AHRQ, 2015).

- "I want to be sure that I explained this clearly. How should you take this medication?"
- "Let's review the main side effects of (insert name of medication). What two things do you need to watch for?"
- "We've talked a lot today about (insert appropriate topic). I want to be sure that I've explained everything clearly. What changes in (insert appropriate topic/condition/routine/person) will you call the health care provider about?"
- "On days when you and your wife (or husband) go out, what will you do about taking your (insert name of medication)?"
- "After talking today, what will your daily routine look like?"
- "Please use this model to show me how you'll do (procedure)."

Evaluation

Patient Outcomes

Patient education is not complete until you evaluate the outcomes of the teaching-learning process. Studies show that patients forget about 40%–80% and misunderstand about 50% of information taught during office visits (Agency for Healthcare Research and Quality [AHRQ], 2015).In addition, the IOM Committee of Health Literacy reported that many patients are hesitant to admit they do not understand what was taught to them (Caplin and Saunders, 2015). Thus, it is important to determine whether your patient achieved learning objectives set during the planning stage. Regardless of information you provide to patients, use the **teach back** method (Box 15.6) because it enables you to immediately confirm patient understanding, which improves compliance (Caplin and Saunders, 2015). Many health care organizations such as AHQR, National Quality Forum, TJC, and Institute for Healthcare Improvement encourage nurses to use the teach back method.

Modify the teaching plan if evaluation indicates that a knowledge or skill deficit still exists. Alternative teaching methods often help to clarify information or strengthen skills that the patient was unable to comprehend or perform originally. Evaluation reveals new learning needs or new factors that may interfere with the patient's ability to learn. Similar to the nursing process, the teaching process is continuous and ever changing.

Patient Expectations

After receiving education to manage health promotion activities, disease processes, and physical and functional limitations, patients return to their homes and communities. It is important to have a method to evaluate a patient's expectations regarding patient education. Ask patients whether they believe they have learned what is needed to manage their health care in the home. Have patients' describe how they have adapted any instructions you have provided and whether they feel satisfied with the information. If patients' expectations are not met, it is more likely that they will not continue to follow the prescribed treatment plan, will be less independent, and perhaps will ignore signs and/or symptoms indicating a need to make an appointment with their health care provider.

DOCUMENTATION OF PATIENT TEACHING

Because patient teaching often occurs informally (e.g., during medication administration or physical examination), it is difficult to document it consistently. However, because nurses are professionally and legally responsible for providing accurate and timely information to patients, quality documentation is essential. Documentation also helps members of the health care team coordinate patient education. Document the following information about patient education:

1. *Assessment data and related nursing diagnoses:* Provide information and support for goals and outcomes.
2. *Interventions planned and used:* Planned education provides continuity of care. Specifically describe subject matter and what has been presented so that other nurses can follow up and reinforce teaching (e.g., "verbalized side effects of digoxin").
3. *Evaluation of learning:* Document evidence of learning (e.g., a return demonstration of coughing and deep breathing). This informs staff about the patient's progress and determines material that you still need to teach. Always use the teach back method.
4. *Ability of patient and/or family caregiver to manage care:* Identify needs for outpatient or home care follow-up after discharge. Appropriate referrals meet the patient's needs better.

KEY POINTS

- Health education is aimed at the promotion, restoration, and maintenance of health.
- Teaching is most effective when it is responsive to a learner's needs and requires the learner's active involvement.
- Teaching is a form of interpersonal communication, with teacher and student actively involved in a process that increases the student's knowledge and skills.
- Teaching a patient a specific behavior involves incorporation of behaviors from all three learning domains.
- A person's health beliefs influence the willingness to gain the knowledge and skills necessary to maintain health.
- Patients of different age groups require different teaching strategies because of developmental capabilities.
- Presentation of teaching content progresses from simple to more complex ideas.
- Assess the reading ability and the ability of the patient to understand health information before providing patient education.
- Patient teaching is culturally sensitive and individualized to meet the needs of each patient.
- A patient is an active participant in a teaching plan, agreeing to the plan, helping to choose instructional methods, and recommending times for instruction.
- A combination of teaching methods improves a learner's attentiveness and involvement.
- Match teaching methodologies to a patient's learning needs.
- Learning objectives describe what a person is to learn in behavioral terms.
- Evaluate a patient's learning by using the teach back method and observing the performance of expected learning behaviors under desired conditions.

REFERENCES

Agency for Healthcare Research and Quality (AHRQ). Health literacy universal precautions toolkit. 2nd ed. 2015. Available from: https://www.ahrq.gov/professionals/quality-patient-safety/quality-resources/tools/literacy-toolkit/healthlittoolkit2-tool5.html.

American Nurses Association (ANA). Code of ethics for nurses with interpretive statements, 2015. Available from: http://nursingworld.org/DocumentVault/Ethics-1/Code-of-Ethics-for-Nurses.html.

Ball JW, Dains J, Flynn J, Solomon B, Stewart R. Seidel's guide to physical examination. 8th ed. St. Louis: Elsevier; 2015.

Bastable S. Nurse as educator: principles of teaching and learning for nursing practice. 4th ed. Sudbury, MA: Jones & Bartlett; 2014.

Brice JH, Foster MB, Principe S, Moss C, Shofer FS, Falk RJ, et al. Single-item or two-item literacy screener to predict the S-TOFHLA among adult hemodialysis patients. Patient Educ Couns 2014;94(1):71.

Caplin M, Saunders T. Utilizing Teach-Back to reinforce patient education: a step-by-step approach. Orthop Nurs 2015;34(6):365.

Choi PP. Patient advocacy: the role of the nurse. Nurs Stand 2015;29(41):52.

Driessnack M, Chung S, Perkhounkova E, Hein M. Using the "Newest Vital Sign" to assess health literacy in children. J Pediatr Health Care 2014;28(2):165.

Edelman CL, Mandle CL. Health promotion throughout the life span. 7th ed. St. Louis: Mosby; 2014.

Gomes C, Coustasse A. Tweeting and treating: how hospitals use twitter to improve care. Health Care Manag (Frederick) 2015;34(3):203.

Kompany L, Luis K, Manganaro J, Motacki K, Mustacchio E, Provenzano D. Children's Specialized Hospital and GetWellNetwork collaborate to improve patient education and outcomes using an innovative approach. Pediatr Nurs 2016;42(2):95.

Miller MA, Stoeckel PR. Client education: theory and practice. Sudbury, MA: Jones & Bartlett; 2016.

Mott-Coles S. Patients' cultural beliefs in patient-provider communication with African American women and Latinas diagnosed with breast cancer. Clin J Oncol Nurs 2014;18(4):443.

National Institutes of Health (NIH). Health literacy. 2017. Available from: https://www.nih.gov/institutes-nih/nih-office-director/office-communications-public-liaison/clear-communication/health-literacy.

Panagioti M, ichardson G, Small N, Murray E, Rogers A, Kennedy A, et al. Self-management support interventions to reduce health care utilization without compromising outcomes: a systematic review and meta-analysis. BMC Health Serv Res 2014;14(1):356.

Purnell LD. Guide to culturally competent health care. Philadelphia: FA Davis; 2014.

Sawyer T, Nelson MJ, McKee V, Bowers MT, Meggitt C, Baxt SK, et al. Implementing electronic tablet-based education of acute care patients. Crit Care Nurse 2016;36(1):60.

Stribling JC, Richardson JE. Placing wireless tablets in clinical settings for patient education. J Med Libr Assoc 2016;104(2):159.

Toronto CE, Weatherford B. Registered nurses' experiences with individuals with low health literacy: a qualitative descriptive study. J Nurses Prof Dev 2016;32(1):8.

Touhy TA, Jett K. Ebersole and Hess' toward healthy aging: human needs and nursing response. 9th ed. St. Louis: Mosby; 2016.

U.S. Department of Health and Human Services (USDHHS). Quick guide to health literacy. n.d. Available from: https://healthliteracycentre.eu/wp-content/uploads/2015/11/Quick-guide-to-health-literacy.pdf.

16 Hygiene

OBJECTIVES

After reading this chapter, the student should be able to:

- Describe health and factors that influence personal hygiene practices.
- Explain purposes of hygienic care including health, social, and psychological purposes.
- Perform a comprehensive assessment of a patient's hygiene needs.
- Discuss factors that affect the condition of the skin, mouth, hair, scalp, nails, and feet.
- Identify common problems involving the skin, feet, nails, hair, and scalp if hygienic care is neglected.
- Discuss appropriate interventions for hygiene problems.
- Understand and perform hygiene procedures for care of a patient's skin, perineum, feet, nails, mouth, eyes, ears, and nose.
- Discuss care plan and nursing intervention for patients with hygienic needs.
- Describe how hygiene for older adults differs from hygiene for younger patients.
- Understand the importance of patients' room environment and how it needs to be managed.
- Identify ways to foster patient-centered care when providing hygiene care.
- Incorporate safety measures and guidelines for nursing skills into hygiene care activities.

KEY TERMS

bathing, p. 338
back rub, p. 339
denture stomatitis, p. 347
effleurage, p. 339
hair care, p. 339
maceration, p. 352
perineal care, p. 342

INTRODUCTION

Personal hygiene influences your patients' comfort, safety, and well-being. Hygiene includes cleaning and grooming activities that maintain personal body cleanliness and appearance. A variety of personal, social, and cultural factors influence hygiene practices.

Because hygiene care requires close contact with your patients, use communication skills (e.g., listening, reflecting, focusing) to promote caring therapeutic relationships (see Chapter 4). When providing hygiene, you can integrate other nursing activities including patient assessment and interventions such as range-of-motion (ROM) exercises, application of dressings, or inspection and care of i.v. sites. Assess each patient's ability to perform hygiene care; ensure privacy; convey respect; and foster a patient's independence, safety, and comfort.

Providing hygiene for patients requires an understanding of the anatomy and physiology of the skin, nails, oral cavity, eyes, ears, and nose. Whether patients perform their own hygiene or you help them, effective hygiene techniques promote the normal structure and function of body tissues.

FACTORS INFLUENCING HYGIENIC PRACTICE

Social Practices

Social groups influence hygiene preferences and practices, including the type of hygiene products used and the nature and frequency of personal care practices. An example is the choice by adolescent girls of the type of sanitary pads used during menstruation (Kamaljit et al., 2012). Parents and caregivers perform hygiene care for infants and young children. Family customs play a major role during childhood in determining hygiene practices such as the frequency of bathing, the time of day bathing is performed, and even whether certain hygiene practices such as brushing the teeth or flossing are performed. As children enter adolescence, peer groups and media often influence hygiene practices. For example, some young girls become more interested in their personal appearance and begin to wear makeup. During the adult years, involvement with friends and work groups shapes the expectations that people have about personal appearance. Some older adults' hygiene practices change because of changes in living conditions and available resources.

Personal Preferences

Patients have individual preferences about when to perform hygiene and grooming care. Some patients prefer to shower, whereas others prefer to bathe. Patients select different hygiene and grooming products according to personal preferences. Knowing patients' personal preferences promotes individualized care. Culture plays a role in sensitivity to personal space and gender. Help a patient develop new hygiene practices when indicated by an illness or condition. For example, you may need to teach a patient with diabetes proper foot hygiene or a bariatric patient adaptive bathing methods. Safe and effective patient-centered nursing care improves patient satisfaction and health and reduces costs (Burman et al., 2013).

Body Image

Body image is a person's subjective concept of his or her body, including physical appearance, structure, or function. It affects the way in which individuals maintain personal hygiene. If a patient maintains a neatly groomed appearance, be sure to consider the details of grooming when planning care and consult with the patient before making decisions about how to provide hygiene. Patients who appear unkempt or uninterested in hygiene sometimes need education about its importance or further assessment regarding their ability to participate with daily hygiene.

Surgery, illness, or a change in emotional or functional status often affects a patient's body image. Discomfort and pain, emotional stress, or fatigue diminishes the ability or desire to perform hygiene self-care and requires extra effort to promote hygiene and grooming.

Socioeconomic Status

A person's economic resources influence the type and extent of hygiene practices used. Be sensitive in considering that a patient's economic status influences the ability to regularly maintain hygiene. He or she may not be able to afford desired basic supplies such as deodorant, shampoo, and toothpaste. A patient may need to modify the home environment by adding safety devices such as nonskid surfaces and grab bars in the bath to perform hygiene self-care safely. When patients lack socioeconomic resources, it becomes difficult for them to participate and take responsible roles in health promotion activities such as basic hygiene.

Health Beliefs and Motivation

Knowledge about the importance of hygiene and its implications for well-being influences hygiene practices. However, knowledge alone is not enough. Motivation also plays a key role in a patient's hygiene practices. Patient teaching is often needed to foster hygiene self-care. Provide information that focuses on a patient's personal health-related issues relevant to the desired hygiene care behaviors. Patient perceptions of the benefits of hygiene care and the susceptibility to and seriousness of developing a problem affect the motivation to change behavior (Pender et al., 2011). For example, do patients perceive that they are at risk for dental disease, or that dental disease is serious, and that brushing and flossing are effective in reducing risk? When they recognize that there is a risk and that they can take reasonable action without negative consequences, they are more likely to be receptive to nurses' counseling and teaching efforts.

Cultural Variables

Cultural beliefs and personal values influence hygiene care. People from diverse cultural backgrounds (e.g., level of education, gender preference, geographic location) frequently follow different self-care practices. For example, maintaining cleanliness does not hold the same importance for some ethnic or social groups as it does for others (Giger, 2013). In North America, many are fortunate to be able to bathe or shower daily and use deodorant to prevent body odors. However, people from some socioeconomic or cultural groups are not sensitive to body odors, prefer to bathe less frequently, and do not use deodorant. Do not express disapproval when caring for patients whose hygiene practices differ from yours. Avoid forcing changes in hygiene practices unless the practices affect a patient's health. In these situations, use tact, provide information, and allow choices. Some homeless people may be reluctant to remove shoes for bathing or to check for skin breakdown. Their feet may be edematous or have neuropathic symptoms (Chen et al., 2013).

Religious beliefs associated with culture sometimes influence hygiene practices. Middle Eastern practices encourage one hand to be kept clean at all times. Muslim patients often remove their shoes and assume different positions for prayer. This increases the risk of developing foot pathology such as calluses on the toes and lateral ankles. When caring for Muslim patients who have diabetes mellitus, you need to be supportive of religious practices while also stressing the need to be diligent in inspecting the feet after prayer sessions for any blisters or calluses.

Developmental Stage

The normal process of aging affects the condition of body tissues and structures. A patient's developmental stage affects the ability of a patient to perform hygiene care and the type of care needed.

Physical Condition

Patients with certain types of physical limitations or disabilities associated with disease and injury lack the physical energy and dexterity to perform hygiene self-care safely. A patient whose arm is in a cast or who has an i.v. line needs help with hygiene care. A weakened grasp resulting from arthritis, stroke, or muscular disorders makes using a toothbrush, washcloth, or hairbrush difficult or ineffective. Sensory deficits not only alter a patient's ability to perform care but also place the patient at risk for injury. Safety is a priority for a patient with a sensory deficit. For example, the inability to feel that the water is too hot can lead to a burn injury during bathing.

Chronic illnesses such as cardiac, pulmonary, and neurological diseases; cancer; dementia; and some mental health illnesses often exhaust or incapacitate patients. Patients who become tired or short of breath frequently need to have complete hygiene care provided. Include periods of rest during care to allow patients who are tired the opportunity to participate in their care. Pain often accompanies illness and injury, limiting a patient's ability to tolerate hygiene and grooming activities or perform self-care. Pain frequently limits ROM, resulting in impaired use of the arms or hands or limited ability to move about in the environment, impairing the ability to perform hygiene self-care. Sedation and drowsiness associated with analgesics used for pain management also limit a patient's ability to safely participate in care.

Limited mobility caused by a variety of factors (e.g., obesity, physical injury, weakness, surgery, pain, prolonged inactivity, medication effect, and presence of medical devices [e.g., indwelling catheter, feeding tube, or i.v. line]) decreases a patient's ability to perform hygiene self-care activities safely. Individualized care considers a patient's ability to perform care, the amount of assistance needed, and the need for assistive and safety devices to facilitate safe hygiene care.

Acute and chronic cognitive impairments such as stroke, brain injury, psychoses, and dementia often result in the inability to perform self-care independently. When people with cognitive impairments are unaware of their hygiene and grooming needs, they become fearful and agitated during hygiene care, resulting in aggressive behavior (Zimmerman et al., 2014). Safe, effective patient care takes the effect of cognitive impairment on hygiene care into consideration and allows for appropriate modifications.

PURPOSES OF HYGIENIC CARE

The main purpose of practicing good hygiene is to maintain an optimum level of health and prevention of the development and spread of infection and diseases. Practicing good personal hygiene is indicated and needed for many purposes, which include personal, health, social, and psychological.

Health Purposes

- To promote and maintain optimum level of health
- To prevent the spread of infections
- To prevent the development of diseases
- To promote the relaxation
- To eliminate the odors
- To enhance the interpersonal relationship between patients and health care team members

Social Purposes

- To enhance personality
- To care for one's appearance
- To maintain and enhance self-discipline
- To maintain the society clean and free from various diseases

Psychological Purposes

- To maintain and improve the mental health
- To enhance self-esteem
- To develop confidence
- To enhance the sense of feel good in a patient

EFFECTS OF NEGLECTED HYGIENIC CARE

Some patients present risks that require more attentive and rigorous hygiene care. These risks result from side effects of medications or other medical therapy; lack of knowledge; immobilization; inability to perform hygiene; or a physical condition that potentially injures the skin (Table 16.1), feet and nails (Table 16.2), hair (Table 16.3), or oral cavity structures (Box 16.1).

Table 16.1 Common Skin Problems

Problem	Characteristics	Implications	Interventions
Dry skin	Flaky, rough texture caused by lack of moisture in outer stratum corneum, resulting in less pliable epidermis; most common on anterior surfaces of lower legs, knees, elbows, and backs of hands	Skin may crack, bleed, and become inflamed. As a result, redness, pruritus, and discomfort may develop. Skin may become infected if epidermal layer cracks.	Effective treatment of dry skin does not include limiting frequency of bathing but lies in bathing with warm, not hot, water and using moisturizers (nonpetroleum). Use superfatted soap (e.g., Dove) for cleansing. Rinse body of all soap well because residue left can cause irritation and breakdown. Add moisture to air through use of humidifier. Increase fluid intake when skin is dry. Use moisturizing lotion to aid healing process; lotion forms protective barrier and helps maintain fluid within skin.
Hirsutism	Excessive growth of body and facial hair, especially in women	Hair may cause negative body image by giving a woman a male appearance.	Shaving is safest method to remove hair. Electrolysis and laser permanently remove hair. Tweezing and bleaching are temporary.
Skin rashes	Skin eruption that may result from overexposure to sun or moisture or from allergic reaction; appears flat or raised, localized or systemic, pruritic or nonpruritic	If the patient scratches skin, inflammation and infection occur. Rashes also cause discomfort.	Wash area thoroughly and apply antiseptic spray or lotion to prevent further itching and aid healing process. Warm or cold soaks may relieve inflammation and promote comfort.

Continued

Table 16.1 Common Skin Problems—cont'd

Problem	Characteristics	Implications	Interventions
Contact dermatitis 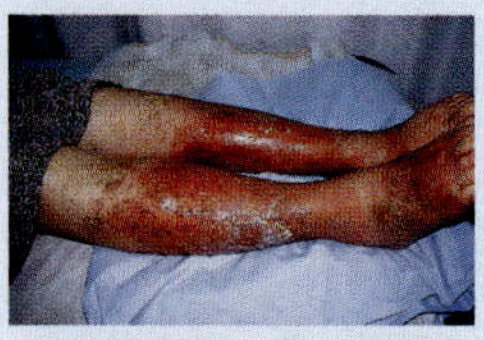 (From Morison MJ: *Nursing management of chronic wounds*, Edinburgh, 2001, Mosby.)	Inflammation of skin characterized by abrupt onset with erythema, pruritus, pain, and appearance of scaly, oozing lesions; seen on face, neck, hands, forearms, trunk, and genitalia	Dermatitis is often difficult to eliminate because the person is usually in continual contact with substance causing skin reaction. Substance is sometimes hard to identify.	Identify and avoid contributing agents (e.g., cleansers, cosmetics, latex, poison ivy or oak). Treatment consists of removing contributing agent and applying over-the-counter topical steroids or calamine lotion. In some cases, prescription steroids may be ordered. Patients may find that tepid baths provide comfort.
Abrasion 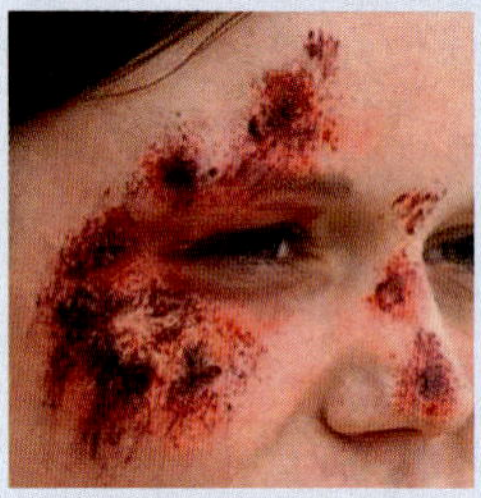 (From Lanzi GL: Facial injuries in sports, soft tissue injuries [abrasions, contusions, lacerations], *Clin Sports Med* 36[2]:287, 2017.)	Scraping or rubbing away of epidermis; results in localized bleeding and later weeping of serous fluid	Infection occurs easily as a result of loss of protective skin layer.	Wash abrasions with mild soap and water. Dressing or bandage could increase risk for infection because of retained moisture.

Table 16.2 Common Foot and Nail Problems

Problem	Characteristics	Implications	Interventions
Callus 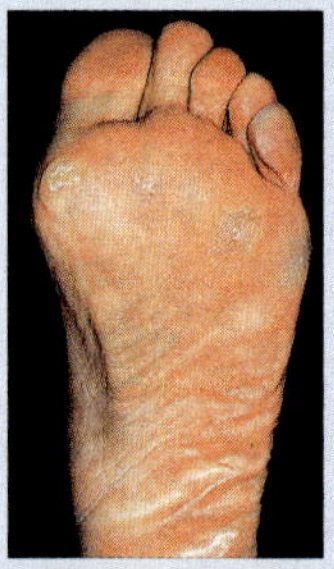	Thickened portion of epidermis consisting of mass of horny, keratotic cells; usually flat and painless; found on undersurface of foot or on palm of hand; caused by local friction or pressure	Foot calluses often cause discomfort when wearing tight-fitting shoes.	Refer the patient to podiatrist; do not self-treat. Use of orthotic devices cushions and redistributes weight and pressure off calluses.
Corns 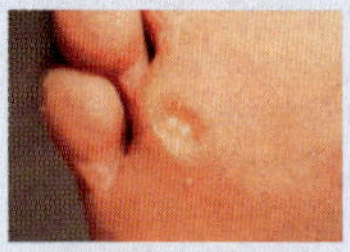	Keratosis caused by friction and pressure from shoes; mainly on toes, over bony prominence; usually cone shaped, round, and raised; calluses with painful core	Conical shape compresses underlying dermis, making it thin and tender. Tight shoes aggravate pain. Tissue attaches to bone if allowed to grow. The patient may have alteration in gait because of pain.	Refer the patient to podiatrist. Avoid use of oval corn pads, which increase pressure on toes. Use wider, softer shoes.
Plantar warts 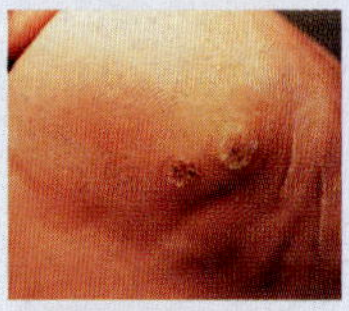	Fungating lesion that appears on sole of foot; caused by papillomavirus	Warts are sometimes contagious, are painful, and make walking difficult.	Refer the patient to podiatrist.
Athlete's foot (tinea pedis) 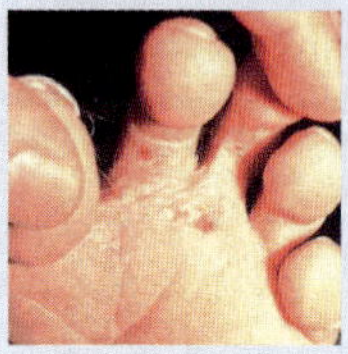	Fungal infection of foot; scaliness and cracking of skin between toes and on soles of feet; small blisters containing fluid appear, apparently induced by constricting footwear (e.g., sneakers)	Athlete's foot can spread to other body parts, especially hands. It is contagious and often recurs.	Feet should be well ventilated. Drying feet well after bathing and applying powder help prevent infection. Wearing clean socks or stockings reduces incidence. Health care provider orders application of griseofulvin, miconazole nitrate, or tolnaftate.

Table 16.2 Common Foot and Nail Problems—cont'd

Problem	Characteristics	Implications	Interventions
Ingrown nails	Toenail or fingernail growing inward into soft tissue around nail; results from improper nail trimming, poor shoe fit, or heredity	Ingrown nails cause localized pain in the presence of pressure; some become infected.	Treatment is frequent warm soaks (*exception:* a patient with diabetes or other vascular diseases such as Berger disease) in antiseptic solution and removal of part of nail that has grown into skin. Teach the patient proper nail-trimming techniques. Refer to podiatrist.
Paronychia	Inflammation of tissue surrounding nail after hangnail or other injury; occurs in people who frequently have their hands in water; common in patients with diabetes	Area sometimes becomes infected.	Treatment is warm compresses or soaks (*exception:* a patient with diabetes) and local application of antibiotic ointments. Paronychia can be prevented by careful manicuring.
Foot odors	Result of excess perspiration promoting microorganism growth; faulty foot hygiene or improper footwear causes foot odor	Odor frequently embarrasses the patient.	Frequent washing, use of foot deodorants and powders, and clean footwear prevent or reduce this problem.

Table 16.3 Hair and Scalp Problems

Problem	Characteristics	Implications	Interventions
Dandruff	Scaling of the scalp accompanied by itching; in severe cases dandruff on eyebrows	Dandruff may cause embarrassment; if it enters the eyes, conjunctivitis often develops.	Shampoo regularly (preferably daily) with over-the-counter dandruff shampoo or medicated shampoo. Make an appointment with health care provider if symptoms do not respond to over-the-counter treatments.
Ticks	Small gray-brown parasites that burrow into skin and suck blood	Ticks sometimes transmit Rocky Mountain spotted fever, Lyme disease, and tularemia.	Removal of tick (CDC, 2015): Use fine-tipped tweezers to grasp tick as close to the skin's surface as possible. Pull upward with steady, even pressure. Do not twist or jerk tick; this can cause the mouth parts to break off and remain in the skin. If this happens, remove the mouth parts with tweezers. If you are unable to remove mouth parts easily with clean tweezers, leave them alone and let the skin heal. After removing the tick, thoroughly clean the bite areas and your hands with rubbing alcohol and iodine scrub or soap and water. Save tick in plastic bag and store in freezer if it is necessary to identify the type of tick. If you develop a rash or fever within several weeks of removing a tick, see your health care provider.
Pediculosis capitis (head lice)	Tiny grayish-white parasitic insects that attach to hair strands; eggs look like oval particles, resemble dandruff; bites or pustules may be found behind ears and at hairline	Head lice are difficult to remove and if not treated spread to furniture and other people. They do not carry disease, cannot jump or fly, and are carried by animals.	Wearing gloves, check entire scalp with tongue depressor or special lice comb. *Caution against use of products containing lindane because the ingredient is a neurotoxin known to cause adverse reactions* (CDC, 2016). Check hair for nits and comb with a nit comb for 2–3 days until all lice and nits have been removed. Vacuum infested areas of home and car upholstery.
Pediculosis corporis (body lice)	Tend to cling to clothing, making them difficult to see; body lice suck blood and lay eggs on clothing and furniture	The patient itches constantly; scratches on skin become infected; hemorrhagic spots appear on skin where lice are sucking blood.	Have the patient bathe or shower thoroughly; after drying skin, apply lotion for eliminating lice; after 12–24 h, have the patient take another bath or shower; bag infested clothing or linen until laundered.
Pediculosis pubis (crab lice)	Found in pubic hair; grayish-white with red legs	Lice spread through bed linen, clothing, furniture, or sexual contact.	Shave hair off affected areas; cleanse as for body lice; if lice were sexually transmitted, the patient needs to notify partner.
Alopecia	Balding patches; hair becomes brittle and broken; caused by improper use of hair curlers and picks, tight braiding, hot styling tools, genetics, and certain diseases	Patches of uneven hair growth and loss alter the patient's appearance.	Stop hair-care practices that damage hair (e.g., teasing hair, hair picks, tight braiding, excessive heat when blow-drying).

BOX 16.1 Common Oral Problems

Dental Caries (Cavities)

- Most common among young people
- Buildup of plaque causes acid destruction of tooth enamel; initially appears as chalky, white discoloration of the tooth

Periodontal Disease (Pyorrhea)

- Most common after age 35
- Involves destruction of gingiva (gums) and other supporting structures with bleeding gums, inflammation, and receding gum lines, which may lead to tooth loss

Other Problems

- Oral mucositis (oral erythema, ulceration, and pain)
- Glossitis (inflammation of the tongue)
- Gingivitis (inflammation of the gums)
- Halitosis (bad breath)
- Cheilitis (cracked lips)
- Oral malignancy (mouth lumps or ulcers)

BOX 16.2 Types of Baths

- **Complete bed bath:** It refers to bath administered to a totally dependent patient in bed (see Skill 16.1).
- **Partial bed bath:** It refers to bed bath that consists of bathing only those body parts that would cause discomfort if left unbathed such as the hands, face, axillae, and perineal area. Partial bath also includes washing the back and providing a back rub. Give a partial bath to patients who are dependent and need partial hygiene or patients who are bedridden and cannot reach all body parts.
- **Sponge bath at the sink:** It involves bathing from a bath basin or sink with the patient sitting in a chair. The patient can perform part of the bath independently. You help the patient with hard-to-reach areas.
- **Tub bath:** It involves immersion in a tub of water that allows more thorough washing and rinsing than a bed bath. The patient may still require assistance. Some institutions have tubs equipped with lifting devices to help move patients in and out of the tub when necessary.
- **Shower:** The patient sits or stands under a continuous stream of water. The shower provides more thorough cleansing than a bed bath but can be fatiguing.
- **Bag bath/travel bath:** It contains several soft, nonwoven cotton cloths that are premoistened in a solution of no-rinse surfactant cleanser and emollient. The bag bath offers ease of use, reduced bathing time, and patient comfort.
- **Chlorhexidine gluconate (CHG) bath:** An antimicrobial agent is used to reduce incidence of hospital-acquired infections on skin, invasive lines, and catheters (Boonyasiri et al., 2016; Cassir et al., 2015; Shah et al., 2016).

BATHING AND SKIN CARE

Assess the skin, noting color, texture, thickness, turgor, temperature, and hydration. Pay special attention to characteristics of any lesions. Note dryness of the skin indicated by flaking, redness, scaling, and cracking. Discovering common skin problems influences how you administer hygiene care (Table 16.1).

Consider a patient's normal grooming routines including preferred hygiene products and preferred time of day for hygiene care. The extent, type, and timing or frequency of bathing and the methods used depend on the patient's physical abilities, health problems, and degree of hygiene needed.

Use the tub bath or shower to give a more thorough bath than a bed bath (see Skill 16.1). Cleanse the skin at the time of any soiling and at routine intervals. Problems such as incontinence, wound drainage, or excessive diaphoresis require more frequent cleansing to promote comfort and prevent skin breakdown and infection.

A patient with overly dry skin is predisposed to skin impairment. Use soap and lotions that contain emollients to hydrate dry skin. Use the opportunity of a complete bath to reassess a patient's skin and help with joint ROM exercises. Regardless of the type of bath (Box 16.2), use the following guidelines when **bathing** a patient:

- *Provide privacy:* Close the door and/or pull room curtains around the bathing area. Expose only the areas being bathed by using proper draping.
- *Maintain safety:* Keep side rails up and the bed in a low position when away from the bedside. **Note:** You need a health care provider's order (see agency-specific policy) for restraint use when side rails serve as a restraint (see Chapter 12). Be sure nurse call system is in an accessible location within the patient's reach if leaving the bedside even temporarily. Protect patients from injury by assessing and controlling the bath water temperature. This is especially important for older adult patients and patients with reduced sensation such as patients with diabetes, peripheral neuropathy, or spinal cord injuries. Use assistive devices such as bath chairs when indicated. Place a chair in the shower for a patient with weakness or poor balance. Both tubs and showers must have grab bars for patients to hold during entry and exit and for maneuvering during the bath or shower.
- *Maintain warmth:* Keep the room warm to prevent chilling. Prevent drafts and keep windows closed. Cover your patient, exposing only the body part being washed. Moisture on the skin causes excessive heat loss through evaporation.
- *Promote independence:* Encourage your patient to participate with bathing as much as possible. Offer assistance as needed, but assess carefully for activity intolerance.
- *Anticipate needs:* Implement actions to address the patient's need to use the bedpan or urinal and to receive relief from pain or nausea before hygiene care. Bring all needed items including linen, hygiene products, and new gown before initiating bath.

A complete bed bath, tub bath, or shower (see Skill 16.1) may exhaust a patient. Be alert for the patient's activity intolerance during hygiene care. Observe respirations, noting changes in rate and depth or any shortness of breath. Observe for changes in skin color. Palpate the pulse to detect changes in rate and regularity and question the patient about dizziness, weakness, or fatigue. If the patient experiences activity intolerance (e.g., rapid, irregular heart rate) during care, seek assistance, return him or her to bed, and observe carefully for improvement with rest. Provide a partial bed bath to a patient who needs only partial hygiene, who is too debilitated or unable to tolerate a complete bed bath, or who can perform self-care but needs help with completing the bath.

The use of bath basins with soap and water became an issue after a recent study conducted in intensive care units. Researchers found that when baths were given with regular soap and water, bath basins become a reservoir for bacteria, which possibly leads to transmission of hospital-acquired infections. Research shows a link between waterborne pathogens and the development of biofilm (multiple colonies of microorganisms attached to a surface such as a bath basin). The formation of a biofilm combined with the transmission of organisms through patient contact with a nurse's unwashed hands can create a reservoir of bacteria that can be transferred to and maintained in a patient's bath basin (Strouse, 2015).

In contrast, researchers found that using chlorhexidine gluconate (CHG) 4% solution in place of standard soap and water in washbasins reduces bacterial growth in basins (Powers et al., 2012; Shah et al., 2016) and reduces critical care–acquired methicillin-resistant *Staphylococcus aureus* (MRSA) (Petlin et al., 2014). Be sure to air-dry bath basins completely, and do not use the basin to store supplies.

Another alternative to using CHG in bath basins is the use of CHG 2%–impregnated disposable washcloths. The CHG in the washcloth acts quickly, has broad-spectrum microorganism coverage, continues antimicrobial activity up to 24 hours after application, and is rinse free and disposable (Agency for Healthcare Research and Quality [AHRQ], 2013). Research shows that compared with the use of antimicrobial washcloths, daily bathing with CHG 2%–impregnated cloths reduces a patient's risk of becoming infected with multidrug-resistant organisms (Cassir et al., 2015; Climo et al., 2013). Some reports show a risk of skin irritation after repeated use; thus, bathing the patient with the cloths every other day may be an option. Another option is the bag bath. The bag bath contains a no-rinse surfactant, a humectant to trap moisture, and an emollient. The bag bath does not contain CHG. When using cloths or the bag bath, no bath basin is needed.

Health care–associated infections (HAIs) are one of the most common adverse events that occur during hospitalization. HAIs cause prolonged hospitalization and a high rate of fatalities resulting in a large financial burden. Several studies have tested the effect of interventions to reduce these central line infections. Among the interventions tested is daily bathing with chlorhexidine-impregnated cloths or chlorhexidine liquid soap (e.g., Hibiclens). Findings consistently validate significant reductions in colonization and infection after use of chlorhexidine for bathing (Climo et al., 2013; Munoz-Price et al., 2012).

Patients with dementia require special considerations in bathing. Assess patients entering long-term care facilities for cognitive and functional status (Hall et al., 2013). Patients with cognitive impairments sometimes become more confused and combative as a result of pain, fatigue, weakness, anxiety from exposure during a bath, and discomfort from a cold or drafty bathing area. Calmly speaking to the patient in a conversational but informative voice and using a calm, organized approach to bathing has been shown to be effective (Hall et al., 2013).

A thermal towel bath reduces agitation compared with tub baths. This is a person-centered, in-bed approach in which a nurse uses a large towel, one or two regular-size towels, washcloths, a bath blanket, and no-rinse soap and water (Hall et al., 2013).

BACK RUB

A **back rub** usually follows the bath. It promotes relaxation, relieves muscular tension, and reduces pain perception. Evidence shows that **effleurage** (long, light, gliding strokes used in a massage) may reduce anxiety, heart rate, and respiratory rate (Zullino et al., 2005). Research shows that slow-stroke back massages of 3 minutes' duration and hand massages of 10 minutes' duration significantly improve both physiological and psychological indicators of relaxation in older adults (Harris and Richards, 2010).

Always ask whether a patient would like a back rub or whether he or she prefers gentle instead of deep massage because some patients dislike physical contact. In addition, review the patient's record for any contraindications to a massage such as spinal cord injury, rib fracture, and other painful conditions.

NAIL AND FOOT CARE

A variety of common foot and nail problems can be caused by inadequate hygiene and are often detected during hygiene care (Table 16.2). Routine nail and foot care includes soaking to soften cuticles and layers of horny cells, thorough cleaning, drying, and proper nail trimming. In some settings or with some patients, such as a patient with diabetes mellitus or peripheral vascular disease, you need a health care provider's order to trim toenails. Sit patients in a chair if possible when providing foot and nail care. When patients are immobilized, you perform care while they are in bed (Box 16.3).

Recognize conditions that place a patient at an increased risk for amputation such as uncontrolled diabetes, peripheral neuropathy, limited joint mobility, bony deformity, peripheral vascular disease, and a history of skin ulcers or previous amputation. Observe for changes that indicate peripheral neuropathy or vascular insufficiency.

HAIR CARE

Routine assessment of the condition of the hair and scalp reveals problems and determines the frequency and type of care needed (Table 16.3). Observe your patient's ability to perform **hair care**. Patients appreciate the opportunity to have their hair brushed and combed before others visit them. Long hair easily becomes matted when a patient is confined to bed, even for a short period. Blood and topical medications also cause tangling when lacerations or incisions involve the scalp. Frequent brushing and

BOX 16.3 Procedural Guidelines

Performing Nail and Foot Care

Equipment

Washbasin, emesis basin, washcloth, towels, nail clippers (check agency policy), soft nail or cuticle brush, plastic applicator stick, emery board or nail file, lotion, disposable bath mat, paper towels, linen bag, clean gloves if drainage is present.

Steps

1. Identify the patient by using at least two identifiers (e.g., name and birthday or name and medical record number) according to agency policy.
2. Verify health care provider's order for cutting nails.
3. Determine the patient's knowledge of nail and foot care.
4. Explain procedure to the patient. Inform the patient that proper soaking requires several minutes.
5. Pull curtain around bed or close room door to provide privacy.
6. Help the patient who is ambulatory sit in chair and place disposable bath mat on floor under the patient's feet. Help the patient who must stay in bed to supine position with head of bed elevated 45° and place waterproof pad on mattress (keep side rail up until ready to begin).
7. Perform hand hygiene and apply clean gloves. Inspect all surfaces of fingers, toes, feet, and nails. **Note:** You can do this inspection during the bath. Pay close attention to areas of dryness, inflammation, or cracking. Also, inspect areas between toes, heels, and soles of feet. Inspect socks for stains. Remove gloves.
8. Fill washbasin with warm water. Test water temperature. Place basin on floor or lower side rail and place basin on pad on mattress. Have the patient immerse feet. If the patient has diabetes mellitus, peripheral neuropathy, or peripheral vascular disease, go to Step 12 to begin foot care.
9. Fill emesis basin with warm water and place basin on towel on overbed table. Test water temperature.
10. Have the patient place fingers in emesis basin and arms in comfortable position.
11. Allow feet and fingernails to soak for 5–10 min.

Clinical decision point: If the patient has diabetes mellitus, peripheral neuropathy, or peripheral vascular disease, skip this step and go straight to Step 12.

12. Clean gently under fingernails with end of plastic applicator stick. Do this while fingers are immersed unless the patient has diabetes (see illustration).
13. Trim nails straight across at level of finger or follow curve of finger, ensuring that you do not cut down into nail grooves (see illustration). Use disposable emery board and file nail to ensure that there are no sharp corners. (Verify agency policy on nail care regarding filing and trimming.)
14. Use a soft cuticle brush or nailbrush to clean around cuticles. Remove hands from basin and dry completely.
15. Move overbed table away from the patient. Begin foot care by scrubbing callused areas of feet with washcloth.
16. Scrub callused areas of feet and clean between toes with washcloth.
17. Dry feet thoroughly and trim or cut toenails (see Step 13).
18. Apply lotion to feet and hands. Rub in thoroughly. Do not leave excess lotion between toes.
19. Help the patient back to bed and into comfortable, safe position. Be sure nurse call system is in an accessible location within the patient's reach.
20. Sanitize equipment according to organizational policy and return equipment to proper place. Emery boards should be disposable. Dispose of soiled linen in dirty laundry bag. Remove and dispose of gloves. Perform hand hygiene.
21. During evaluation, inspect nails, areas between fingers and toes, and surrounding skin surfaces.
22. **Use teach back:** "We discussed how to prevent infection in the skin around your nails. Tell me the tips you should follow to protect your feet from infection." Revise your instruction now or develop a plan for revised patient/family caregiver teaching if the patient/family caregiver is not able to teach back correctly.
23. Record condition and appearance of nails and feet, condition of circulation, and care and instructions provided.
24. Document your evaluation of patient/family caregiver learning.
25. Report any breaks in the skin, reddened or tender areas, or any discomfort.

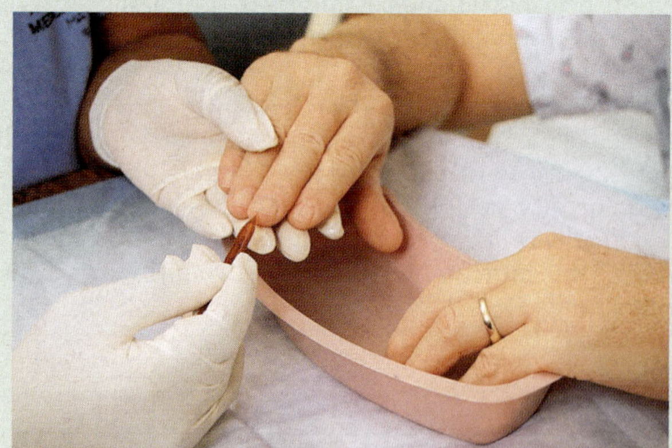

Step 12 Clean under fingernails.

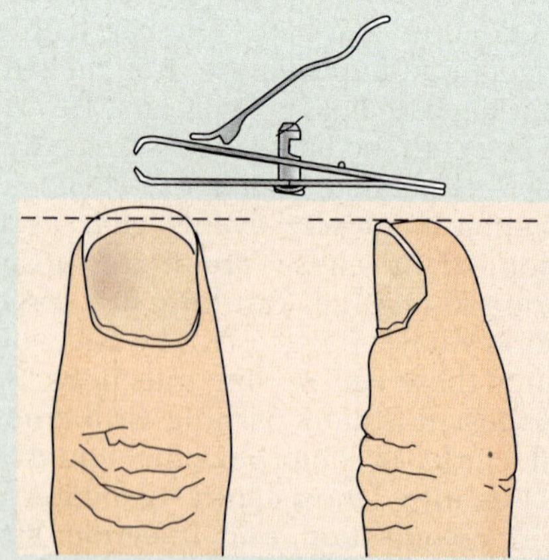

Step 13 Trim nails straight across when using nail clipper.

combing keep long hair neatly groomed. Braiding helps to avoid repeated tangles. Ask permission before braiding a patient's hair.

To brush hair, part it into two sections and separate each into two more sections. It is easier to brush smaller sections of hair. Brushing from the tip of the hair ends and moving to the scalp minimizes pulling. Moistening the hair with water or an alcohol-free detangle product makes the hair easier to comb. Do not cut a patient's hair without consent.

The frequency of shampooing depends on a patient's preferences and the condition of the hair. Remind patients they may need more frequent shampooing if they are on constant bed rest or have excess perspiration or treatments that leave blood or solutions in their hair. A patient who can take a shower or bath usually shampoos the hair independently. Use a shower chair for a patient who is ambulatory but becomes tired or faint. Handheld shower nozzles allow patients to wash the hair during a tub bath or shower.

If a patient can sit in a chair, you usually shampoo the hair in front of a sink. If a patient sits at the bedside, shampoo the hair as the patient leans forward over a washbasin. If bending is limited or contraindicated (e.g., after eye surgery or neck injury), teach the patient and family caregivers the degree of bending allowed.

Transfer patients who cannot sit but can be moved to a stretcher for transportation to a sink or shower equipped with a handheld nozzle. Place a towel or small pillow under the patient's head and neck, allowing the head to hang slightly over the edge of the stretcher. Use caution when shampooing patients with neck injuries because hyperextension of the neck can cause further injury. You need a health care provider's order to shampoo the hair of patients with neck injuries. Another option is to wash the patient's hair in the bed (Box 16.4).

When patients are unable to move, sit in a chair, be transferred to a stretcher, or tolerate a wet hair-washing

BOX 16.4 Procedural Guidelines

Shampooing Hair of Bed-Bound Patient

Equipment

Bath towels, clean gloves, clean gown *(optional)* (if the patient has known head lice), clean comb and brush

Regular shampoo: Washcloth, shampoo, hair conditioner *(optional)*, hydrogen peroxide *(optional)*, water pitcher with warm water, plastic shampoo board, washbasin, waterproof pad, saline *(optional)*

Disposable shampoo: Disposable shampoo cap product

Steps

1. Identify the patient by using at least two identifiers (e.g., name and birthday or name and medical record number) according to agency policy.
2. Review medical record to determine that there are no contraindications to procedure. Check agency policy for health care provider order as needed. Certain medical conditions such as head and neck injuries and spinal cord injuries place the patient at risk for injury because of positioning and manipulation of the patient's head and neck.
3. Make sure that bed is in locked, low position (QSEN, 2014).
4. Perform hand hygiene and apply gloves. Inspect condition of hair and scalp. This determines whether special shampoos or treatments are necessary (e.g., dandruff, lice, removal of blood). If draining head wounds are suspected, apply clean gloves. If lice are present, wear disposable gown and gloves. Remove gloves and perform hand hygiene.
5. Explain procedure to the patient, using simple language.
6. Assemble equipment at bedside including pitcher with warm water.
7. Provide privacy by closing room door or curtain dividers. Raise bed to comfortable working height and lower side rail on side on which you will stand.
8. **Shampooing bed-bound patient with shampoo board:**
   a. Apply clean gloves. Place waterproof pad under the patient's shoulders, neck, and head.
   b. Position the patient supine with head and shoulders at top edge of bed. Place shampoo board under the patient's head and washbasin under end of trough spout (see illustration). Be sure that trough spout extends beyond edge of mattress.
   c. Place rolled towel under the patient's neck and bath towel over the patient's shoulders.
   d. Brush and comb the patient's hair.
   e. Ask the patient to hold towel or washcloth over eyes.
   f. Test water temperature. Slowly pour water from pitcher over hair until it is completely wet (see illustration). If hair contains matted blood, apply hydrogen peroxide to dissolve clots and rinse with saline. Apply small amount of shampoo.
   g. Work up lather with both hands. Start at hairline and work toward back of neck. Lift head slightly with one hand to wash back of head. Shampoo sides of head. Massage scalp by applying pressure with fingertips.
   h. Rinse hair with water. Make sure that water drains into basin. Repeat rinsing until hair is free of soap. (If you need to refill pitcher, raise side rail when leaving bedside.)
   i. Apply conditioner or cream rinse if requested and rinse hair thoroughly.
   j. Wrap the patient's head in bath towel. Dry face with cloth used to protect eyes. Dry off any moisture along neck or shoulders.

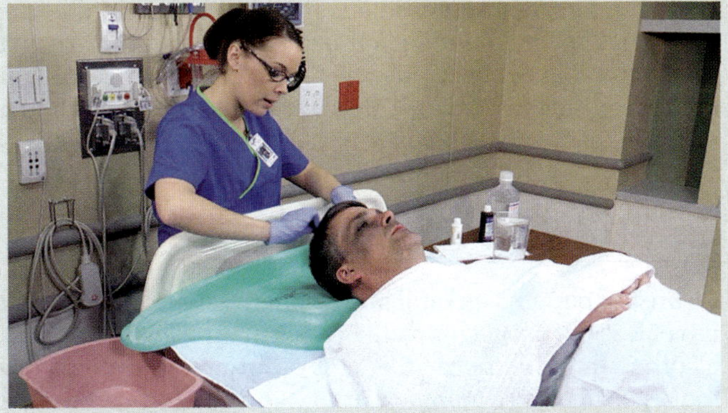

Step 8b Patient positioned over shampoo board.

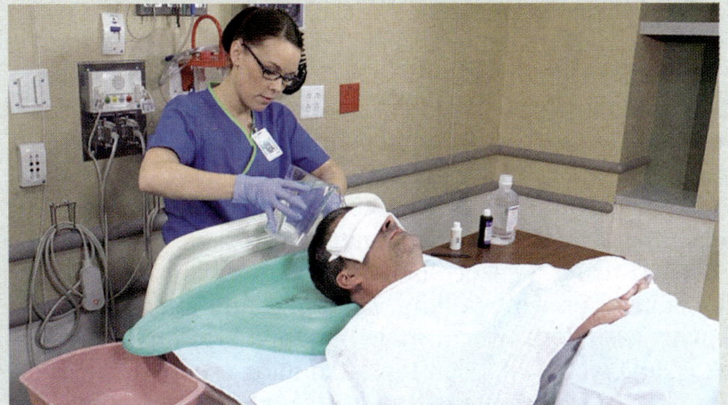

Step 8f Nurse pouring water over patient's hair.

Continued

BOX 16.4 **Procedural Guidelines—cont'd**

k. Dry the patient's hair and scalp. Use second towel if first one becomes saturated.
l. Comb hair to remove tangles and dry with dryer if desired.
m. Apply oil preparation or conditioning product to hair if desired by the patient.
n. Variation for patients with coarse, curly hair: Condition hair after washing. To untangle hair, use wide teeth of comb. Beginning at nape of neck, comb small subsections of hair, starting at hair ends. Continue to work through small sections until hair is free of tangles.
o. Help the patient to comfortable position and complete styling of hair. Be sure nurse call system is in an accessible location within the patient's reach.
p. Dispose of supplies. Store reusable supplies. Remove gloves and perform hand hygiene.

9. **Shampooing with disposable shampoo product:**
   a. The patient can be sitting on chair or in bed. Apply clean gloves.
   b. Comb hair to remove any tangles or debris.
   c. Open package, apply cap, and secure all hair beneath cap (see illustration).
   d. Massage head through cap. Check fitting around head to maintain correct fit.
   e. Massage 2–4 min according to directions on package; additional time may be required for longer hair or hair matted with blood.
   f. Discard cap in trash; do not dispose of in toilet because it may clog plumbing.
   g. If the patient desires, towel dry hair. Brush or comb the patient's hair.
   h. Remove gloves. Perform hand hygiene.
   i. Help the patient to comfortable position, and be sure nurse call system is in an accessible location within the patient's reach.

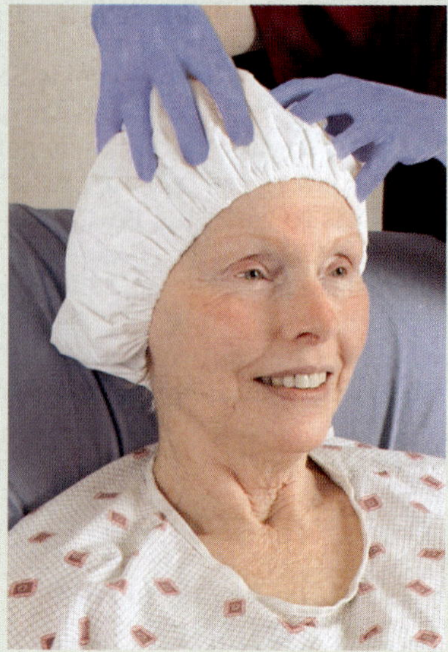

Step 9c Patient wearing disposable shampoo cap.

10. Inspect condition of hair and scalp.
11. **Use teach back:** "During the shampoo we discussed ways to reduce the risk of getting exposed to lice in your home. Tell me three ways to reduce the chance of exposing yourself and others to lice." Revise your instruction now or develop a plan for revised patient/family caregiver teaching if the patient/family caregiver is not able to teach back correctly.
12. Record relevant observations (objective and subjective), condition of scalp and skin, and patient comfort.
13. Document your evaluation of patient/family caregiver learning.

procedure, you can use various dry shampoo products. Read manufacturer guidelines carefully. In general, you massage these products into the patient's hair and scalp. Some products require you to apply a towel to remove excess oil and dirt, whereas others require you to brush the product through the patient's hair.

SHAVING

Shave facial hair after a bath or shampoo. Some women prefer to shave their legs or axillae while bathing. Use caution when helping a patient shave to avoid cutting the patient with the razor blade. Patients prone to bleeding (e.g., patients receiving anticoagulants or high doses of aspirin, patients with bleeding disorders such as thrombocytopenia and leukemia) must use an electric razor. Before you use an electric razor, check it for electrical hazards. Use an electric razor on only one patient to eliminate the risk of infection transmission.

When using a razor blade for shaving, you must soften the skin to prevent pulling, scraping, and cuts. Placing a warm washcloth over a male patient's face for a few seconds, followed by application of shaving cream or a lathering of mild soap, softens the skin. You must shave patients who cannot shave themselves independently. To avoid causing discomfort or razor cuts, gently pull the skin taut and use short, firm razor strokes in the direction the hair grows. Short downward strokes work best to remove hair over the upper lip. The patient usually can explain the best way to move the razor across the skin. Facial hair of African Americans tends to be curly and becomes ingrown unless shaved close to the skin.

MUSTACHE AND BEARD CARE

Mustaches or beards require daily grooming. Grooming keeps food particles and mucus from collecting in the hair. You must groom a patient's mustache and beard if the patient is unable to carry out self-care. Comb out beards gently, and obtain a patient's permission before trimming or shaving off a mustache or beard.

PERINEAL CARE

Cleansing patients' genital and anal areas is called **perineal care**. It is part of a complete bed bath but also is performed at other times as needed. Factors that create the need for more perineal care include urinary and bowel incontinence, presence of indwelling urinary catheters, menstruation, vaginal drainage or draining wounds, and obesity.

Prolonged contact of urine on the skin can alter the normal protective skin flora by raising the pH of the skin. Contact with moisture from incontinence weakens the skin, making it more prone to damage from friction (Voegeli, 2016). Stool remaining on the skin contains active fecal enzymes that damage the skin. Bacteria in the feces also can penetrate the skin and contribute to secondary infections. Incontinence-related dermatitis increases the risk for pressure injuries (Beeckman et al., 2014).

Encourage patients to perform their own perineal care if they are able. You may feel embarrassed about providing perineal care, particularly to a patient of the opposite gender. Similarly, a patient may feel embarrassed. Do not let these feelings cause you to overlook a patient's perineal hygiene needs. When staffing permits, use a gender-congruent caregiver. A professional, dignified, and sensitive approach reduces embarrassment and helps put the patient at ease.

If the patient performs perineal care without assistance, various issues such as vaginal or urethral discharge, perineal irritation, and unpleasant odors may go undetected. Emphasize the importance of perineal care in preventing skin breakdown and infection. Be alert for complaints of burning during urination or localized soreness, excoriation, or pain in the perineum. Inspect vaginal and perineal areas and the bed linen for evidence of discharge and use your sense of smell to detect abnormal odors.

ORAL CARE

Assess the mouth carefully for color, hydration, texture, and lesions. Patients may develop oral problems as a result of inadequate oral care or disease (e.g., oral malignancy) or as a side effect of medications, radiation, and chemotherapy. Localized pain or tenderness and infection accompany many common oral problems (Box 16.1).

When patients become ill, many factors influence their need for oral hygiene. Base the frequency of care on the condition of the oral cavity and a patient's level of comfort (Box 16.5). Some patients require oral hygiene every 1–2 hours.

BOX 16.5 Procedural Guidelines

Performing Oral Hygiene

Equipment

Soft-bristle toothbrush; nonabrasive fluoride toothpaste; dental floss; chlorhexidine gluconate (CHG) 0.12% (*optional*; see agency policy); tongue depressor; glass with cool water, normal saline, or antiseptic mouth rinse (*optional* depending on patient preference); moisturizing lubricant for lips *(optional)*; dental floss; emesis basin; face towel; paper towels; clean gloves; penlight; linen bag or hamper

Steps

1. Identify the patient by using at least two identifiers (e.g., name and birthday or name and medical record number) according to agency policy.
2. Review medical record and identify presence of common oral cavity problems: dental caries, chalky white discoloration of tooth or presence of brown or black discoloration; gingivitis, inflammation of gums; periodontitis, receding gum lines, inflammation, gaps between teeth; halitosis, bad breath; cheilitis, cracked lips; dry, cracked, and coated tongue.
3. Determine the patient's oral hygiene practices such as frequency of brushing and flossing, type of toothpaste and mouthwash used, last dental visit, and frequency of dental visits.
4. Perform hand hygiene and apply clean gloves.
5. Using tongue depressor and penlight, inspect integrity of lips, teeth, buccal mucosa, gums, palate, and tongue; also, assess for gag reflex and ability to swallow.
6. Confirm presence of common oral problems.
7. Remove gloves and perform hand hygiene.
8. Explain procedure to the patient, discussing the patient's preferences and willingness to help with oral care.
9. Assess the patient's ability to grasp and manipulate toothbrush.
10. Place paper towels on overbed table and arrange other equipment within easy reach.
11. Provide privacy by closing room doors and drawing room divider curtain. Raise bed to comfortable working position. Raise head of bed (if allowed) and lower near side rail. Move the patient or help him or her move closer to side. Place the patient in side-lying position if needed (if aspiration risk). Place towel over the patient's chest.
12. Apply clean gloves.
13. Apply enough toothpaste to brush to cover extent of bristles. Hold brush over emesis basin. Pour small amount of water over toothpaste.
14. The patient may help with brushing. Hold toothbrush bristles at a 45° angle to gum line (see illustration A). Be sure that tips of bristles rest against and penetrate under gum line. Brush inner and outer surfaces of upper and lower teeth by brushing from gum to crown of each tooth. Clean biting surfaces of teeth by holding top of bristles parallel with teeth and brushing gently back and forth (see illustration B). Brush sides of teeth by moving bristles back and forth (see illustration C).
15. Have the patient hold brush at a 45° angle and lightly brush over surface and sides of tongue (see illustration). Avoid initiating gag reflex.

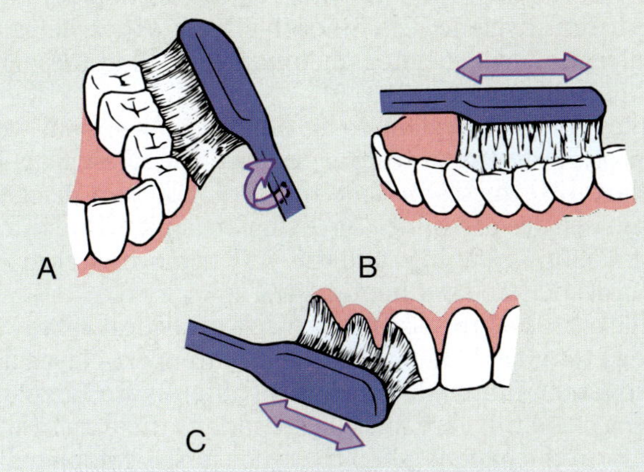

Step 14 A–C, Directions of brush for toothbrushing.

Continued

BOX 16.5 Procedural Guidelines—cont'd

16. Allow the patient to rinse mouth thoroughly by taking several sips of cool water, swishing water across all tooth surfaces, and spitting into emesis basin. Use this time to observe the patient's brushing technique and teach importance of regular hygiene.
17. Have the patient rinse mouth with antiseptic rinse for 30 s. Then have the patient spit rinse into emesis basin. Help wipe the patient's mouth.

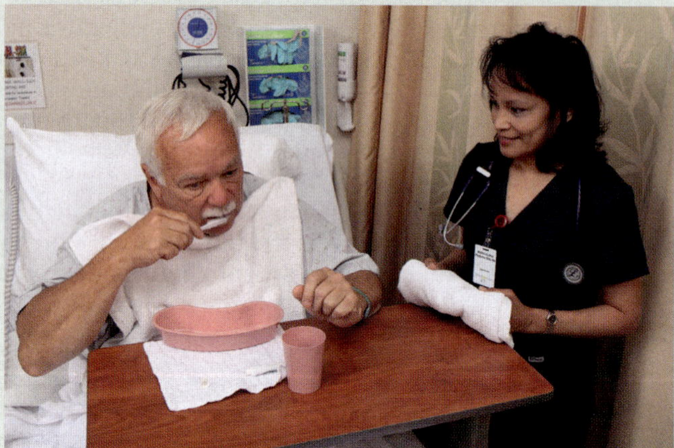

Step 15 Nurse observes patient's toothbrushing technique including brushing of tongue.

18. *Option:* Floss or allow the patient to floss between all teeth (see illustration).
19. Allow the patient to rinse mouth thoroughly with cool water and spit into emesis basin. Help wipe the patient's mouth.
20. Inspect oral cavity to determine effectiveness of oral hygiene and rinsing. Ask the patient whether mouth feels clean or whether there are any sore or tender areas. Remove towel and place in linen bag.
21. **Use teach back:** "I want to be sure you know how often to brush your teeth and floss. Tell me how often you should floss your teeth." Revise your instruction now or develop a plan for revised patient/family caregiver teaching if the patient/family caregiver is not able to teach back correctly.
22. Help the patient to comfortable position, raise side rail, and lower bed to original position.
23. Clean and dry basin before returning basin and nondisposable supplies.
24. Remove gloves and perform hand hygiene.
25. Record relevant observations, condition of oral cavity, amount of care the patient could perform, and whether additional instruction is needed.
26. Document your evaluation of patient/family caregiver learning.
27. Report bleeding, pain, or presence of lesions to nurse in charge or health care provider.

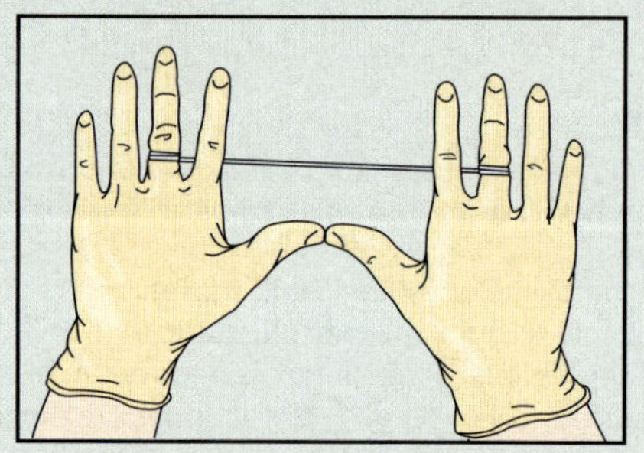

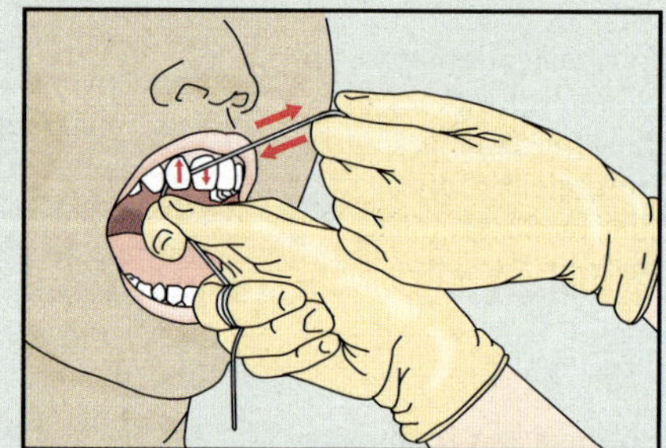

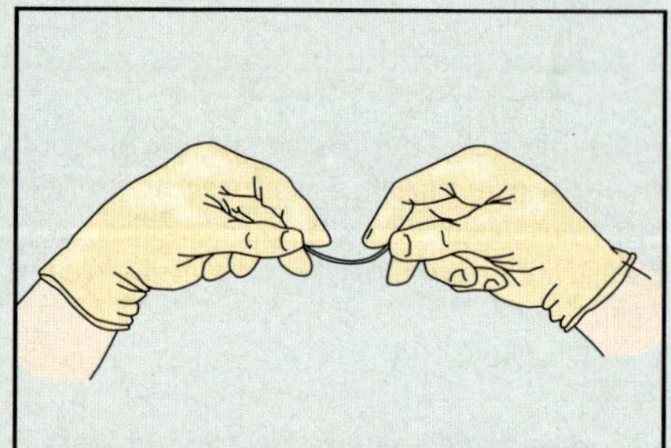

Step 18 Flossing. **A,** Dental floss is held between middle fingers to floss upper teeth. **B,** Floss is moved in up-and-down motion between teeth. Floss is moved up and down from crown to gum line. **C,** Floss is held with index fingers to floss lower teeth.

Patients who are unconscious or have artificial airways (e.g., endotracheal or tracheal tubes) need special precautions with oral care because they often do not have a gag reflex (Box 16.6). These patients require meticulous and frequent oral hygiene. CHG mouth rinse further helps to reduce ventilator-associated pneumonia (VAP) in these patients (El-Rabbany et al., 2015).

While providing hygiene to an unconscious patient, you must protect the airway from aspiration. The safest practice is to have two nurses provide the care. You can delegate nursing assistive personnel (NAP) to participate. One nurse does the actual cleaning, and the NAP removes secretions using oral suction (see Chapter 24).

While cleansing the oral cavity, use a small oral airway or a padded tongue blade to hold the mouth open. Never use your fingers. A human bite is highly contaminated. Explain the steps of mouth care and the sensations the patient will feel. Inform the patient when the procedure is completed.

Proper oral hygiene requires keeping the mucosa moist and removing secretions that can lead to infection. Researchers have found that foam stick applicators stimulate the mucosal tissues but are ineffective in removing debris from the teeth. Limit the use of foam swabs to situations in which gentle cleansing is required. Examples include patients who have bleeding tendencies or sustained trauma to the oral cavity (Kiyoshi-Teo and Blegen, 2015). A child-size toothbrush fits more easily around an endotracheal tube than an adult-size toothbrush.

DENTURE CARE

When patients become disabled, someone must assume responsibility for denture care (Box 16.7). Dentures are a patient's personal property and must be handled with care because they break easily. To prevent warping, keep them covered in water when they are not being worn, and always store them in an enclosed, labeled cup with the cup placed in a drawer in the patient's bedside stand. Discourage patients from removing their dentures and placing them on a

BOX 16.6 Procedural Guidelines

Performing Oral Hygiene for a Patient Who Is Unconscious or a Debilitated Patient

Equipment

Small pediatric, soft-bristled toothbrush; toothette sponges or suction toothbrushes for patients for whom brushing is contraindicated; antibacterial solution per agency protocol (e.g., chlorhexidine gluconate [CHG]); fluoride toothpaste; water-based mouth moisturizer; tongue blade; penlight; oral suction equipment; oral airway (uncooperative patient or patient who shows bite reflex); water-soluble lip lubricant; glass with cool water; face and bath towel; emesis basin; clean gloves

Steps

1. Identify the patient by using at least two identifiers (e.g., name and birthday or name and medical record number) according to agency policy.
2. Review medical record for presence of oral cavity problems.
3. Perform hand hygiene and apply clean gloves.
4. Assess for presence of gag reflex by placing tongue blade on back half of tongue.

Clinical decision point: Patients with impaired gag reflex still require oral care but have a higher risk for aspiration. Keep suction equipment available when caring for patients who are at risk for aspiration.

5. Inspect condition of oral cavity. Confirm presence of oral problems.
6. Remove gloves. Perform hand hygiene.
7. Explain procedure to the patient, even if the patient is unconscious.
8. Pull curtain around bed or close room door.
9. Place towel on overbed table and arrange equipment. If needed, turn on suction machine and connect tubing to suction catheter.
10. Raise bed to appropriate working height. Unless contraindicated (e.g., head injury, neck trauma), position the patient in Sims' or side-lying position. Turn the patient's side of face toward mattress in dependent position with head of bed elevated at least 30°.
11. Apply gloves.
12. Lower side rail. Place towel under the patient's head and one across chest. Place emesis basin under the patient's chin.
13. If the patient is uncooperative or having difficulty keeping mouth open, insert an oral airway. Insert upside down and turn airway sideways and over tongue to keep teeth apart. Insert when the patient is relaxed if possible. Do not use force.

Clinical decision point: Never place fingers into the mouth of a patient who is unconscious or debilitated. This could occlude the airway. In addition, the normal response is to bite down.

14. Clean mouth using brush moistened in water. Apply toothpaste or use antibacterial solution first to loosen crusts. Hold toothbrush bristles at a 45° angle to gum line. Be sure that tips of bristles rest against and penetrate under gum line. Brush inner and outer surfaces of upper and lower teeth by brushing from gum to crown of each tooth, and then clean biting surfaces of teeth by holding top of bristles parallel with teeth and brushing gently back and forth. Brush sides of teeth by moving bristles back and forth. Use a toothette sponge if the patient has a bleeding tendency or use of toothbrush is contraindicated. Suction any accumulated secretions. Moisten brush with clear water or CHG solution to rinse. Use brush or toothette to clean roof of mouth, gums, and inside cheeks. Gently brush tongue, but avoid stimulating gag reflex (if present). Repeat rinsing several times, and use suction to remove secretions. Use towel to dry off lips (see illustration).
15. Apply thin layer of water-soluble moisturizer to lips (see illustration).
16. Inform the patient that procedure is complete. Return the patient to comfortable and safe position.
17. Raise side rails as appropriate and return bed to locked, low position. Be sure nurse call system is in an accessible location within the patient's reach.
18. Clean equipment and return to its proper place. Place soiled linen in dirty laundry bag.
19. Remove and dispose of gloves in proper receptacle and perform hand hygiene.
20. To evaluate condition of oral cavity, apply clean gloves and use tongue blade and penlight to inspect oral cavity.
21. Ask a debilitated patient whether mouth feels clean.
22. **Use teach back:** "I explained what is needed to reduce your husband's risk of choking on secretions in his throat. Tell me the ways you will prevent him from choking when you give mouth care at home." Revise your instruction now or develop a plan for revised patient/family caregiver teaching if the patient/family caregiver is not able to teach back correctly.
23. Record relevant observations (objective and subjective), relevant details of procedure, and information about specific equipment uses and patient response as related to specific skill.
24. Document your evaluation of patient/family caregiver learning.
25. Report unexpected responses (e.g., ulceration, bleeding, choking) to nurse or health care provider.

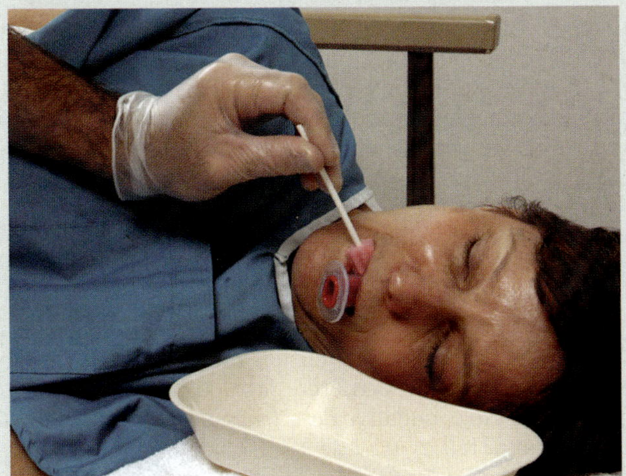

Step 14 Cleaning lips and mucosa around oral airway with toothette.

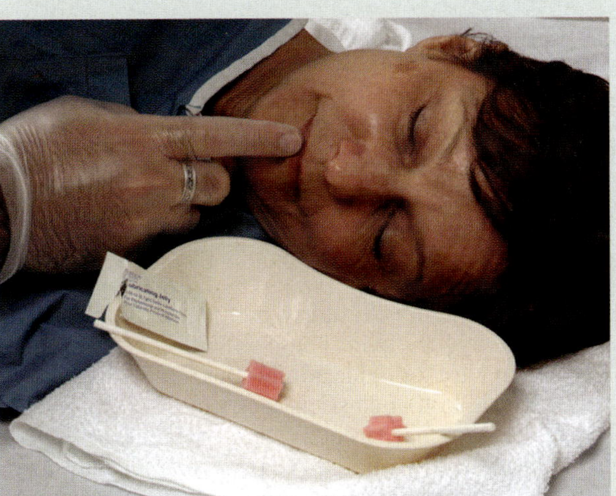

Step 15 Application of water-soluble moisturizer to lips.

BOX 16.7 Procedural Guidelines

Cleaning Dentures

Equipment

Soft-bristle toothbrush or denture toothbrush, denture-cleaning agent or toothpaste, denture adhesive *(optional)*, glass of water, emesis basin or sink, washcloth, gauze (4 × 4–inch), clean gloves, denture cup (for storage)

Steps

1. Identify the patient by using at least two identifiers (e.g., name and birthday or name and medical record number) according to agency policy.
2. Assess environment for safety (e.g., check room for spills, make sure that equipment is working properly and that bed is in locked, low position).
3. Perform hand hygiene.
4. Ask the patient whether dentures fit and whether there is any gum or mucous membrane tenderness or irritation. Ask the patient about denture care and product preferences.
5. Determine whether the patient has necessary dexterity to clean dentures independently or requires assistance.
6. Position the patient comfortably sitting up in bed or assist the patient to walk from bed to a chair placed in front of sink.
7. Fill emesis basin with tepid water. (If using sink, place washcloth in bottom of sink and fill sink with approximately 2.5 cm [1 inch] of water.)
8. Apply clean gloves.
9. Ask the patient to remove dentures. If the patient is unable to do this independently, grasp upper plate at front with thumb and index finger wrapped in gauze and pull downward. Gently lift lower denture from jaw and rotate one side downward to remove from the patient's mouth. Place dentures in emesis basin or sink lined with washcloth and filled with 2.5 cm (1 inch) of water.
10. Apply cleaning agent to brush and brush surfaces of dentures (see illustration). Hold dentures close to water. Hold brush horizontally and use back-and-forth motion to clean biting surfaces. Use short strokes from top of denture to biting surfaces to clean outer teeth surfaces. Hold brush vertically and use short strokes to clean inner teeth surfaces. Hold brush horizontally and use back-and-forth motion to clean undersurface of dentures.
11. Rinse dentures thoroughly in tepid water. If water is too cold, dentures can crack. If water is too hot, dentures can become warped and no longer fit.

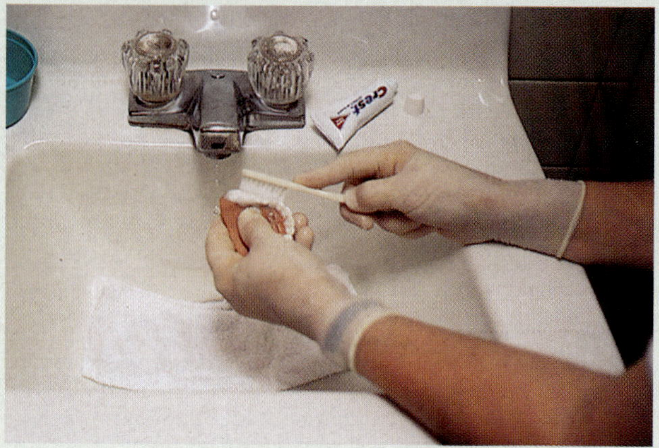

Step 10 Brushing surface of dentures.

12. Some patients use an adhesive to seal dentures in place. Apply a thin layer to undersurface before inserting.
13. If the patient needs help with inserting dentures, moisten upper denture and press firmly to seal it in place. Insert moistened lower denture (if applicable). Ask whether dentures feel comfortable.
14. **Use teach back:** "I explained the importance of regular cleansing of your dentures. Tell me why it is important to clean your dentures daily." Revise your instruction now or develop a plan for revised patient/family caregiver teaching if the patient/family caregiver is not able to teach back correctly.
15. Some patients prefer to store their dentures to give gums a rest and reduce risk for infection. Store in tepid water in an enclosed, labeled denture cup. Keep denture cup in a secure place labeled with the patient's name to prevent loss when not worn (e.g., at night, during surgery).
16. Dispose of supplies. Remove and discard gloves and perform hand hygiene.
17. Return the patient to a comfortable position. Be sure nurse call system is in an accessible location within the patient's reach.

napkin or tissue, on the bed, or in a chair because they could easily be thrown away.

SPECIAL CONSIDERATIONS FOR CARE OF OLDER PEOPLE

Bathing and Skin Care

Changes associated with aging include thinning, dryness, and roughness of the skin. These changes result in the need to adapt skin care for older adults (Box 16.8). The thinning of the skin and loss of elasticity associated with aging contribute to the increased frequency of skin tears, which often occur where an age-related purpura has already formed. Ayello and Fulmer (2012) recommend the following interventions to reduce the risk of skin tears: Use a standardized assessment tool to determine skin tear risk; use a no-rinse, one-step bath product instead of the traditional washcloth, soap, and water bathing method; implement measures to limit trauma, such as wearing long sleeves and pants, providing adequate light to reduce the chance of bumping into items, and making the environment safe for patients who wander; and educate all staff and family caregivers on the risk for skin tears and ways to prevent them.

Bathing often creates discomfort for patients with dementia. Confusion makes people feel vulnerable during bathing, resulting in screaming, crying, and even aggressively lashing out at caregivers. Research shows that using nontraditional bathing techniques and educating caregivers to provide person-centered care ease the conflict and reduce aggressive, negative behaviors associated with bathing activities (Hall et al., 2013). Use person-centered techniques such as covering the patient with towels as much as possible, avoiding rushing, using favorite soaps and no-rinse products, and padding the shower chair for comfort.

BOX 16.8 Care of an Older Adult

Skin Changes With Aging

- Skin changes associated with aging include thinning, dryness, and roughness. Epithelial renewal may take 30%–50% longer in older adults because keratinocytes become smaller and regeneration slows (Touhy and Jett, 2014).
- The dermis loses approximately 20% of its thickness with aging (Meiner, 2015).
- The American Academy of Dermatology (2016) recommendations for care of aging skin include the following:
  - Bathing daily using warm (not hot) water, limiting bath or shower time to 5–10 min
  - Closing bathroom door to maximize humidity
  - Using only mild cleansers; avoiding deodorant bars, perfumed soaps, and any products with alcohol
  - Gently patting skin dry
  - Applying moisturizer within 3 min of getting out of bath or shower; this maximizes trapping of moisture in skin
  - Moisturizing more frequently throughout the day as needed
  - Selecting correct type of moisturizer: Ointments and creams are better suited for dry skin than lotions
  - Using moisturizers with hyaluronic acid, which helps skin hold water; dimethicone and glycerin can draw water to skin and keep it there; mineral oil, lanolin, and petrolatum work well to trap moisture in skin
  - Checking any antiaging products for presence of retinoids or an alpha hydroxy acid, which can irritate and dry the skin
  - Protecting hands by wearing gloves when out in cold, dry air; applying hand cream after each handwashing; and wearing waterproof gloves if hands are frequently in water
  - Wearing sunscreen with a sun protection factor (SPF) of 30 or higher on all exposed skin daily, even in winter
  - Using lip balm with an SPF of at least 30
  - Seeing a dermatologist

Oral Care

Implement measures to prevent **denture stomatitis**, also called *denture sore mouth*. Denture stomatitis is a disease of the mouth and gums caused by ill-fitting dentures and poor dental hygiene habits (Tay et al., 2014). Measures to prevent denture stomatitis include rinsing the dentures after meals, cleaning them carefully, soaking them overnight, brushing and flossing remaining teeth, and teaching patients and family caregivers how to prevent this complication.

Hearing Aid Care

Hearing aids amplify sound in a controlled manner; the hearing aid receives normal low-intensity sound inputs and delivers them to the patient's ear as louder outputs. Hearing aids come in a variety of types (see Chapter 27). Box 16.9 outlines care for a patient with a hearing aid including patient teaching.

Patient's Room Environment

A patient's room should be safe and large enough to allow patients and their visitors to move about freely. Control room temperature, ventilation, noise, and odors.

BOX 16.9 Care and Use of Hearing Aids

Follow these guidelines when caring for a patient's hearing aids and when teaching patients about care of hearing aids:

- Perform hand hygiene before handling the hearing aid.
- Check battery by holding hearing aid in your hand and turning up volume. If battery is working, you hear a "whistle." This is feedback noise.
- After inserting or applying the hearing aid, slowly turn up volume to one-third to one-half volume to obtain a comfortable hearing level for talking at 3-feet or 36 inches.
- A whistling sound while the patient is wearing hearing aid indicates incorrect earmold insertion, improper fit of hearing aid, or buildup of earwax or fluid.
- Do not wear hearing aid under heat lamp or hair dryer or in very wet, cold weather.
- Do not store hearing aid in warm place such as a windowsill or in a car. Heat can change the shape of the earmold, causing hearing aid to not fit properly.
- Remove battery from hearing aid when hearing aid is not being used for a day or longer.
- Avoid dropping hearing aid or twisting cord.
- Remove hearing aid before radiological examination or radiation therapy to avoid damage.
- Protect hearing aid from water, alcohol, aerosol sprays, perspiration, and cologne.
- Use manufacturer-recommended cleaning solution and soft, lint-free cotton cloth to clean earmold. Regularly remove earwax from hearing aid with a wax loop or device supplied with aid.

Data from National Institute on Deafness and Other Communication Disorders (NIDCD): *Hearing aids*, 2016, https://www.nidcd.nih.gov/health/hearing-aids.

Maintaining Comfort

Depending on a patient's age and physical condition, maintain the room temperature between 20°C and 23°C (68°F and 73.4°F). Infants, older adults, and acutely ill patients often need a warmer room. However, patients with certain illnesses benefit from cooler room temperatures to help reduce the body's metabolic demands. Protect acutely ill patients, infants, and older adults from drafts by ensuring that they are adequately dressed and covered with a lightweight blanket.

An effective ventilation system prevents stale air and odors from lingering in the room. Good ventilation reduces lingering odors caused by draining wounds, emesis, bowel movements, and used bedpans and urinals. Always empty and cleanse bedpans and urinals promptly. Room deodorizers help remove many unpleasant odors; however, be sure that your patient is not allergic or sensitive to the deodorizer itself.

Make every effort to limit the noise level, especially when patients are trying to sleep. Explain the source of unfamiliar noises such as an i.v. pump or a pulse oximeter alarm.

Proper lighting helps ensure safety and comfort. A brightly lit room usually stimulates the patient, whereas a darkened room promotes rest and sleep. Adjust room lighting by closing or opening drapes, regulating overbed and floor lights, and closing or opening room doors. When entering a patient's room at night, avoid abruptly turning on the overhead light unless necessary.

Room Equipment

Although rooms can vary across health care settings, the typical room contains a bed, overbed table, bedside stand, and chairs (Fig. 16.1). An overbed table rolls on wheels and adjusts to various heights over the bed or a chair. The overbed table is an ideal working space for performing procedures. It also serves as a surface for meal trays, toiletry items, and objects that a patient often uses. Clean the top of the overbed table with an antiseptic cleaner before using it for meals. Do not place a bedpan or urinal on the table. Use the bedside stand to store a patient's personal possessions and hygiene equipment. Patients often use bedside stands for their telephone, water pitcher, and drinking cup.

Most patient rooms contain a straight-backed chair or an upholstered lounge chair with arms. Armless straight-backed chairs are convenient when temporarily transferring a patient from the bed such as during bed making. Upholstered lounge chairs or recliners tend to be more comfortable for patients who can sit for longer times.

Each room usually has an overbed light and floor-level night lighting. Patients often have access to lighting controls via their nurse call system. Additional portable or built-in examination lighting provides extra light during bedside procedures.

Other equipment usually found in a patient's room includes a nurse call system, a television set, a wall-mounted blood pressure gauge, oxygen and vacuum wall outlets, and personal care items. Special equipment designed for promoting comfort or positioning patients includes footboards and foot boots, special mattresses, and bed boards.

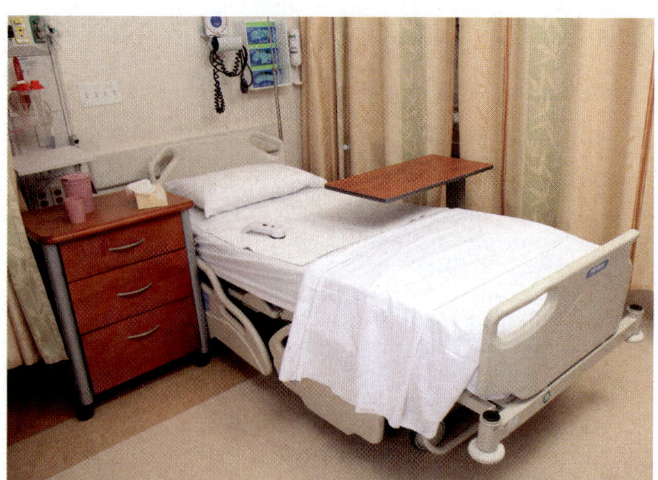

Fig. 16.1 Room furniture.

SAFETY GUIDELINES FOR NURSING SKILLS

Safety Considerations

To ensure patient safety, communicate clearly with members of the health care team, assess and incorporate a patient's priorities of care and preferences, and use the best evidence when making decisions about your patient's care. When performing the skills in this chapter, remember the following points to ensure safe, individualized patient care:

- Patients who are totally dependent on a caregiver require help with personal hygiene measures. Always perform hygiene measures while moving from cleanest to less clean or dirty areas. This often requires you to change gloves and perform hand hygiene during care activities.
- Use clean gloves when you anticipate contact with nonintact skin or mucous membranes or when there is or may likely be contact with drainage, secretions, excretions, or blood during hygiene care.
- When using water or solutions for hygiene care, be sure to test the temperature to prevent burn injury.
- Use principles of body mechanics and safe patient handling to avoid injury to patient or self when performing hygiene care (Quality and Safety Education for Nurses [QSEN], 2014).
- You are responsible and accountable for the care provided. Give proper direction to NAP when delegating hygiene measures.

SKILL 16.1 Bathing and Perineal Care

Equipment

- Bar soap and soap dish or chlorhexidine 4% liquid soap (e.g., Hibiclens)
  - *Option:* CHG cloths or disposable bag bath cloths.
- Four to six washcloths
- Bath towels
- Bath blanket
- Toiletry items (deodorant, powder)
- Body lotion (**Note:** if using CHG soap, use a lotion that is hospital approved such as Aloe Vesta)
- Toilet tissue or hygiene wipes
- Warm water
- Clean hospital gown or patient's own pajamas or gown
- Laundry bag
- Clean gloves (when risk for contacting body fluids)
- Washbasin (used for bath water only)

STEP	RATIONALE
Assessment	
1. Identify the patient by using at least two identifiers (e.g., name and birthday or name and medical record number) according to agency policy.	Ensures correct patient. Complies with The Joint Commission standards and improves patient safety (TJC, 2018).

STEP	RATIONALE
2. Review medical record for orders for specific precautions concerning the patient's movement or positioning and whether there is an order for a therapeutic bath. Note and confirm with the patient any allergies or sensitivities to bath products.	Prevents accidental injury to the patient during bathing activities. Determines level of assistance required by the patient. Prevents allergic reactions to hygiene products during bathing.
3. Check for health care provider's therapeutic bath order; if there is an order, note type of solution, length of time for bath, and body part to be attended.	Therapeutic baths are ordered for specific physical effect, which usually includes promotion of healing or soothing effects.
4. Perform hand hygiene. Assess room environment for safety (e.g., check room for spills, make sure that equipment is working properly and that bed is in locked, low position).	Reduces transmission of microorganisms. Identifies safety hazards in the patient environment that could cause or potentially lead to harm (QSEN, 2014).
5. Assess the patient's fall risk status (if partial bathing out of bed or self-bath is to be performed).	Allows you to anticipate needed precautions such as having the patient sit on a chair in front of a basin.
6. Assess the patient's tolerance for bathing: activity tolerance, comfort level during movement, cognitive ability, musculoskeletal function, and presence of shortness of breath.	Determines the patient's ability to perform or tolerate bathing and level of assistance required (e.g., tub bath, partial bed bath).
7. Assess the patient's cognitive (Mini-Mental State Examination) and functional (e.g., Barthel Index of Activities of Daily Living [Hall et al., 2013] to measure self-care ability) status. For patients with suspected dementia, observe behavior especially after telling the patient it is bath time; does the patient become agitated?	Every person entering a long-term care setting needs to be formally assessed for cognitive and functional status (Hall et al., 2013). Functional status assesses a patient's capacity for self-bathing and/or the amount of supervision/assistance needed to accomplish ADL tasks. Every attempt should be made to avoid bathing people against their will (Hall et al., 2013).
Clinical decision point: Patients with dementia may become agitated and aggressive during bathing. Consider using alternative bathing procedures such as bag wipes. Maintain a calm, nonthreatening, quiet environment using therapeutic communication.	
8. Assess the patient's visual status, ability to sit without support, hand grasp, and ROM of extremities.	Determines degree of assistance the patient needs for bathing. ROM may be delegated to assistive personnel.
9. Assess for presence of equipment (e.g., i.v. line, oxygen tubing, indwelling urinary catheter).	Affects how you plan bathing activities and positioning. Helps determine how to set up supplies.
10. Assess for allergy or sensitivity to CHG.	If allergy exists, select another cleansing solution.
11. Assess the patient's comfort on a 0–10 pain scale.	Bathing can soothe and comfort the patient. Provides baseline measure.
12. Assess the patient's bathing preferences: frequency and time of day preferred, type of hygiene products used, and other factors related to the patient's preferences.	The patient participates in plan of care. Promotes the patient's comfort and willingness to cooperate. Includes cultural or personal hygiene preferences into care.
13. Ask whether the patient has noticed any problems related to condition of skin and genitalia: excess moisture, inflammation, drainage or excretions from lesions or body cavities, rashes, or other skin lesions.	Provides you with information to direct physical assessment of skin and genitalia during bathing and influences selection of skin care products.
14. Before or during bath, assess condition of patient's skin. Note presence of dryness, indicated by flaking, redness, scaling, and cracking.	Provides a baseline for comparison over time in determining whether bathing improves condition of skin.
15. Identify risks for skin impairment: older age, immobilization, reduced sensation, nutrition and hydration, excess skin moisture or drainage, shear or friction on skin, vascular insufficiencies, and presence of external devices. *Option:* Use a pressure injury assessment tool (e.g., Braden Scale).	Prompt identification of risk factors reduces the likelihood of injury to the skin resulting from pressure, impaired tissue synthesis, softening of or friction on tissues, and impaired circulation (AHRQ, 2014).
16. Assess the patient's knowledge of and perceptions of importance of skin hygiene, preventive measures to take, and common skin problems encountered (see Table 16.1).	Determines the patient's willingness to learn and type of instruction required.
17. Assess the patient's or family caregiver's knowledge of skin hygiene in terms of its importance, preventive measures to take, and common problems.	Determines the patient's learning needs.
Planning	
1. Provide privacy and prepare bedside environment for patient safety.	Helps the student/nurse think about the steps needed to remove clutter from overbed or bedside table, removing barriers.
2. Prepare and organize equipment and supplies. If it is necessary to leave room, be sure nurse call system is in an accessible location within the patient's reach.	Avoids interrupting the procedure or leaving the patient unattended to retrieve missing equipment.

STEP	RATIONALE
3. Explain procedure and ask the patient for suggestions on how to prepare supplies. If partial bath, ask how much of bath the patient wishes to complete. If using CHG, explain benefit of reducing infection and that solution leaves a sticky feeling.	Promotes the patient's cooperation and participation. Patients who prefer using their own bathing supplies may need to discuss benefits of CHG.
Implementation	
1. Perform hand hygiene and apply clean gloves. Offer the patient bedpan or urinal. Provide toilet tissue and dispose of any excrement properly. Provide the patient a towel and moist washcloth.	The patient will feel more comfortable after voiding. Prevents interruption of bath.
a. Remove bedpan or urinal, dispose of contents, remove gloves, and perform hand hygiene.	
2. If the patient has nonintact skin or skin is soiled with drainage, excretions, or body secretions, apply new pair of clean gloves before beginning bath.	Reduces transmission of microorganisms.
3. Raise bed to comfortable working height. Verify that bed is in locked position.	Reduces strain on back. Prevents bed from moving.
4. Lower side rail closest to you. Bring the patient toward you and help the patient assume a comfortable supine position, maintaining body alignment.	Maintains the patient's comfort throughout the bath. Safe patient handling minimizes strain on the care provider's muscles. If the patient is overweight or unable to assist with positioning, use another caregiver or lift device (see Chapter 14).
5. Complete or partial bed bath:	
a. Verify that the patient is not allergic to latex.	Prevents allergic reaction if latex gloves are used.
b. Place bath blanket over the patient and loosen and remove top covers without exposing him or her. If possible, have the patient hold top of bath blanket while you remove linen. Place soiled linen in laundry bag. Take care to not allow linen to touch your uniform. *Optional:* Use top sheet when bath blanket is not available or if the patient prefers top sheet.	Bath blanket provides warmth and privacy during bath.
c. Remove the patient's gown or pajamas.	Provides full exposure of body parts during bathing.
(1) If using gown with ties or snaps on sleeves for a patient with i.v. line, upper extremity injury, or limited ROM, unsnap or untie and remove gown.	
(2) If regular gown is used and the patient has limited upper extremity ROM or i.v. access, remove gown from *unaffected side first*.	Undressing unaffected side first allows easier manipulation of gown over body part with reduced ROM.
(3) Remove gown from arm with i.v. line (see illustrations A–C). Remove i.v. bag and tubing from pole, and slide i.v. container and tubing through arm of the patient's gown. Rehang i.v. container and check flow rate (see illustration D). Regulate if necessary.	Manipulation of i.v. tubing and container may disrupt flow rate. Do *not* delegate regulation of i.v. flow rate to NAP.
(4) If i.v. pump is in use, turn pump off, clamp tubing, remove tubing from pump, and proceed as in Step (3). Reinsert tubing into pump, unclamp tubing, and turn pump on at correct rate. Observe flow rate and regulate if necessary. *Do not disconnect tubing.*	Regulation is necessary to prevent improper infusion of fluids. Do *not* delegate regulation of i.v. pump to NAP. Disconnecting i.v. tubing places patient at risk of introduction of microorganisms into i.v. line.
d. Raise side rail. Lower bed temporarily to lowest position and raise to comfortable working height on return. Place basin and supplies on overbed table. Check water temperature and have the patient place fingers in water to test temperature tolerance. Place plastic container of bath lotion in bath water to warm if desired.	Maintains the patient's safety while you leave bedside. Keeping bed at working height during bath prevents back strain. Warm water promotes comfort, relaxes muscles, and prevents unnecessary chilling. CHG is most effective at full strength. Testing temperature prevents accidental burns. Bath water warms lotion for application to the patient's skin.
e. Lower side rail, remove pillow if tolerated, and raise head of bed 30–45° if allowed. Place bath towel under the patient's head. Place second bath towel over the patient's chest.	Helps your access to the patient. You do not have to reach across bed, minimizing strain on back muscles. Removal of pillow makes it easier to wash the patient's ears and neck. Placing towels prevents bed linen and bath blanket from getting soiled or wet.
f. Wash face.	

Clinical decision point: If using CHG solution in bath water, do not use to wash the face. Use clear water only or mild soap and water on the face.

STEP	RATIONALE

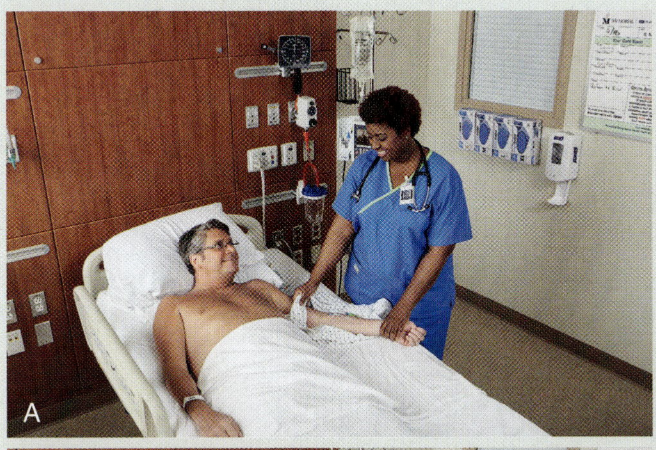
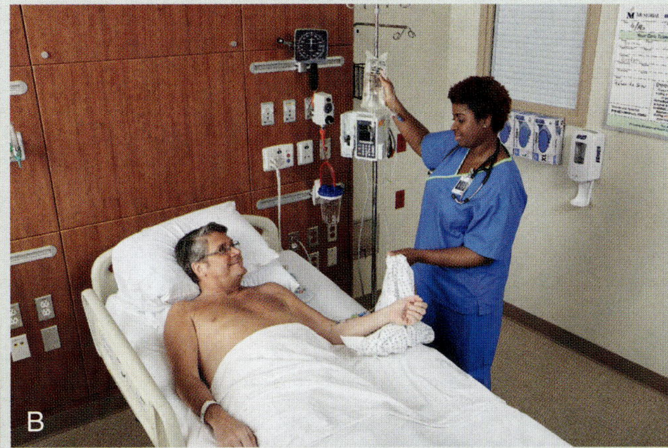
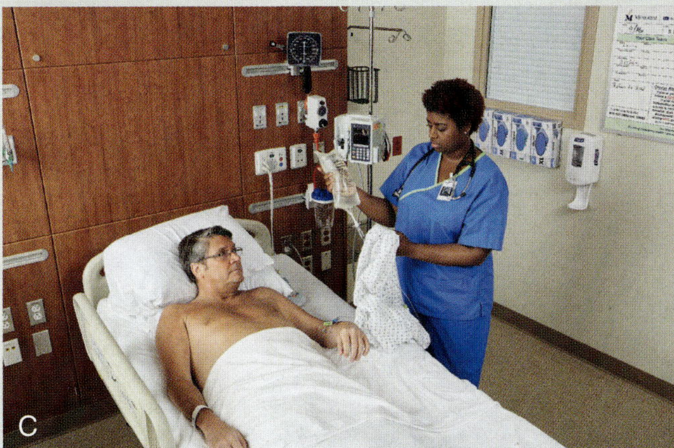
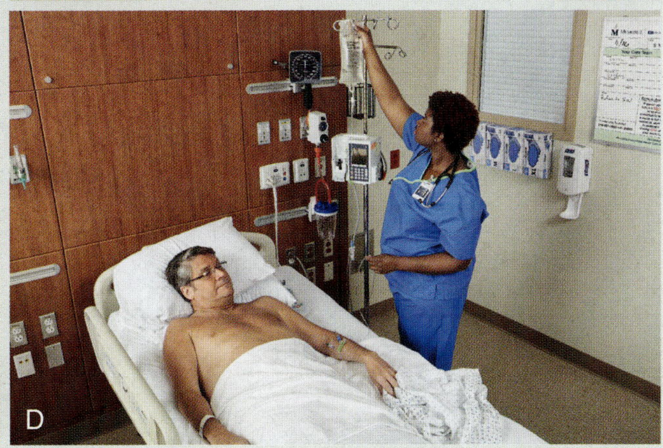

Step 5c(3) **A,** Remove patient's gown. **B,** Remove i.v. bag from pole. **C,** Slide i.v. tubing and bag through arm of patient's gown. **D,** Rehang i.v. bag.

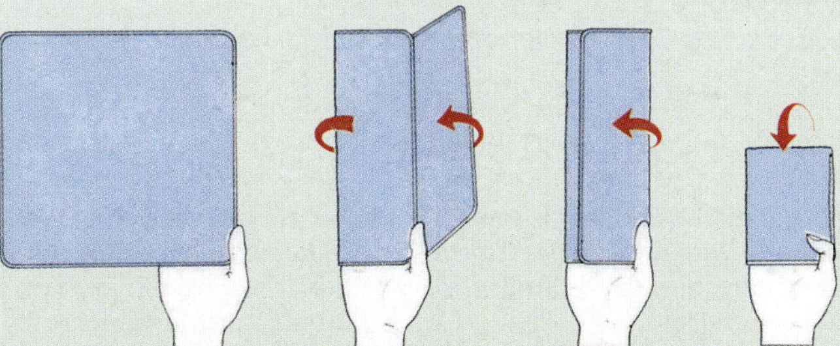

Step 5f(2) Steps for folding washcloth to form a mitt.

STEP	RATIONALE
(1) Ask whether the patient is wearing contact lenses.	Prevents accidental injury to eyes.
(2) Fold washcloth around fingers of your hand to form a mitt (see illustration). Immerse mitt in water and wring thoroughly.	Mitt retains water and heat better than loosely held washcloth; keeps cold edges from brushing against the patient, and prevents splashing.
(3) Wash the patient's eyes with plain warm water. Use different section of mitt for each eye. Move mitt from inner to outer canthus (see illustrations). Soak any crusts on eyelid for 2–3 min with damp cloth before attempting removal. Dry eyes thoroughly but gently.	Soap irritates eyes. Use of separate sections of mitt reduces infection transmission. Bathing eye from inner to outer canthus prevents secretions from entering nasolacrimal duct. Pressure can cause internal injury.
(4) When using soap and water, ask whether the patient prefers to use soap on face. Otherwise wash, rinse, and dry forehead, cheeks, nose, neck, and ears without using soap. (Men may wish to shave at this point or wait until after bath.)	Soap tends to dry face, which is exposed to air more than other body parts.

STEP	RATIONALE

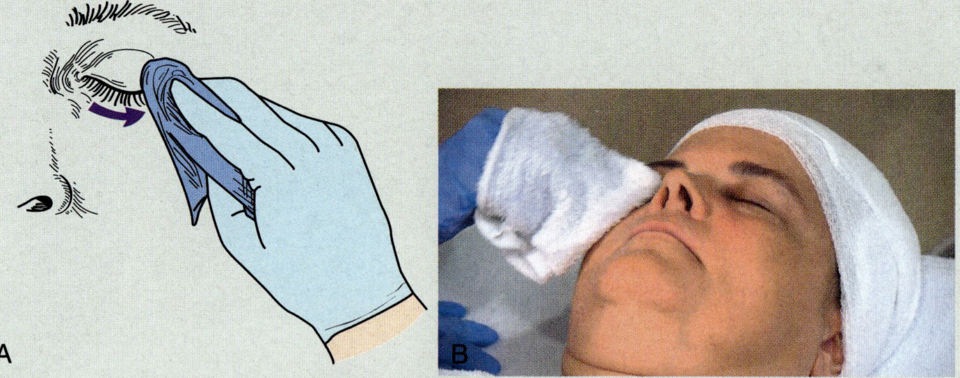

Step 5f(3) Wash eye from inner to outer canthus. **A,** Direction for cleansing eye. **B,** Washing eye from inner to outer canthus.

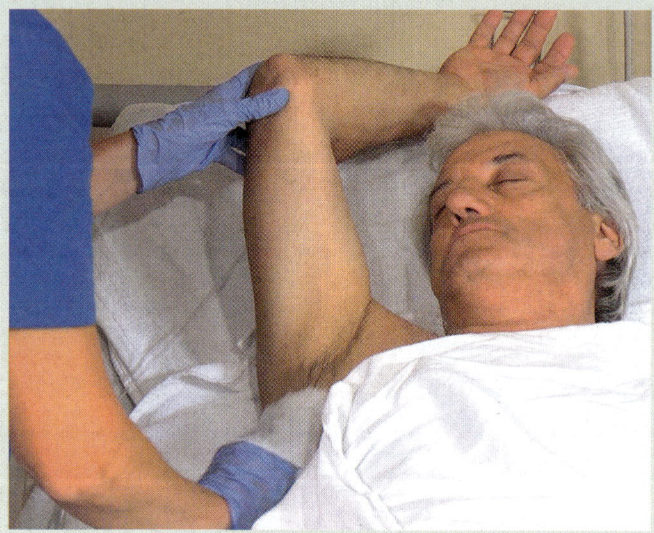

Step 5g(2) Position of patient's arm for washing axilla.

g. Wash trunk and upper extremities.

(1) Remove bath blanket from the patient's arm that is closest to you. Place bath towel lengthwise under arm. Bathe arm with soap and water using long, firm strokes from distal to proximal areas (fingers to axilla).

Towel prevents soiling of bed. Soap lowers surface tension and facilitates removal of debris and bacteria when friction is applied during washing. Long, firm strokes stimulate circulation; moving distal to proximal promotes venous return.

(2) Raise and support arm above head (if possible) to wash, rinse, and dry axilla thoroughly (see illustration). Apply deodorant or powder to underarms if desired or needed.

Movement of arm exposes axilla and exercises normal ROM of joint. Rinsing removes alkaline residue from soap. Drying prevents excess moisture, which can cause skin **maceration** or softening.

(3) Move to other side of bed and repeat Steps (1) and (2) with other arm.

Provides for better access to the patient and helps prevent back strain.

(4) Place bath towel across the patient's chest so that it covers chest and arms, and fold bath blanket down to umbilicus. While lifting edge of towel away from chest with one hand, bathe chest with mitted washcloth on other hand using long, firm strokes. Take special care to wash skinfolds under the breasts of a female patient. It is often necessary to lift breast upward while bathing underneath it. Keep the patient's chest covered between wash and rinse. Rinse and dry well.

Draping prevents unnecessary exposure of body parts. Towel maintains warmth and privacy. Secretions and dirt collect easily in areas of tight skinfolds. Skin under breasts is vulnerable to excoriation if not kept clean and dry.

h. Wash hands and nails (see Box 16.3).

i. Check temperature of bath water and change water when cool or soapy. (See agency policy regarding changing water when using CHG solution.)

Warm water maintains the patient's comfort. Alkaline soap residue is irritating to skin and can decrease normal protectiveness of acid pH.

STEP	RATIONALE
Clinical decision point: If the patient is at risk for falling, be sure that two side rails are up before obtaining fresh water. Lower bed when it is necessary to leave bedside. **Note:** Having all side rails raised is considered a restraint. Check agency policy.	
j. Wash abdomen.	
(1) Place bath towel lengthwise over chest and abdomen. (Two towels may be needed.) Fold bath blanket down to just above pubic region. With one hand, lift bath towel. With mitted hand, bathe and rinse abdomen, giving special attention to umbilicus and skinfolds of abdomen and groin. Stroke from side to side. Keep abdomen covered between washing and rinsing. Rinse and dry well.	Draping prevents unnecessary exposure of body parts. Towel maintains warmth and privacy. Keeping skinfolds clean and dry helps prevent odor and skin irritation. Moisture and sediment that collect in skinfolds predispose skin to maceration.
(2) Apply clean gown or pajama top. If an extremity is injured or immobilized, dress affected side first. (This step may be omitted until completion of bath; gown should not become soiled during remainder of bath.)	Maintains the patient's warmth and comfort. Dressing affected side first allows easier manipulation of gown over body part with reduced ROM.
k. Wash lower extremities.	
(1) Cover chest and abdomen with top of bath blanket. Cover legs with bottom of blanket. Expose near leg by folding blanket toward midline. Be sure to keep other leg and perineum draped.	Prevents unnecessary exposure.
(2) Place bath towel under leg, supporting leg at knee and ankle. If appropriate, place the patient's foot in bath basin to soak while washing and rinsing. (Bend the patient's leg at knee; while grasping the patient's heel, elevate leg from mattress slightly and place bath basin on towel.) If the patient is unable to support leg, you can wash feet thoroughly with washcloth.	Towel prevents soiling of bed linen. Support of joint and extremity during lifting prevents strain on musculoskeletal structures. Sudden movement by the patient could spill bath water. Soaking softens calluses and rough skin.
Clinical decision point: If the patient has diabetes or peripheral vascular disease with impaired circulation and/or sensation, do not soak feet. Maceration of skin may predispose to infection.	
(3) Wash leg using long, firm strokes from ankle to knee and from knee to thigh (see illustration). Do not rub or massage back of calf. Rinse and dry well. Clean foot, making sure to bathe between toes. Rinse and dry toes and feet completely. Clean and clip nails as needed (see Box 16.3). Remove and discard towel.	Promotes circulation and venous return. Excess massage of calf could loosen deep vein thrombus. Secretions and moisture may be present between toes, predisposing the patient to maceration and breakdown. Avoid cutting nails of the patient with diabetes. See agency policy for podiatric care.
(4) Raise side rail, move to opposite side of bed, lower side rail, and repeat Steps (2) and (3) for other leg and foot. If skin is dry, apply moisturizer. When finished, cover the patient with bath blanket.	

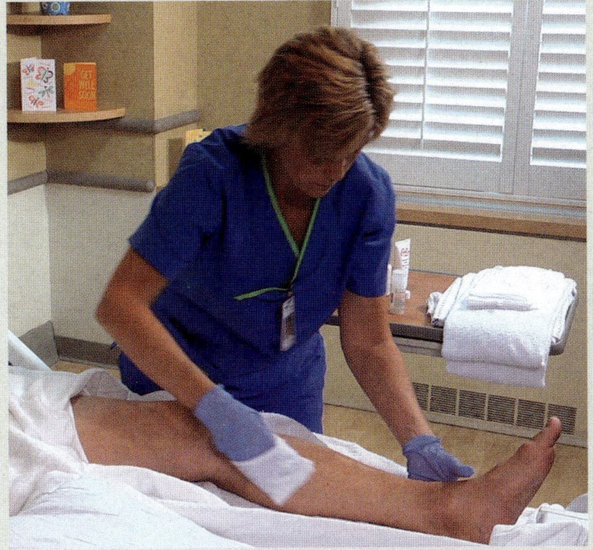

Step 5k(3) Washing patient's leg.

STEP	RATIONALE
Clinical decision point: Do not use long, firm strokes to wash lower extremities of patients with history of deep vein thrombosis or blood clotting disorders. Use short, light strokes instead.	
l. Cover the patient with bath blanket, raise side rail for the patient's safety, remove soiled gloves, and perform hand hygiene. Change bath water.	Cooler bath water causes chilling. Clean water reduces microorganism transmission to perineal structures.
m. Provide perineal hygiene.	
(1) If the patient is able to maneuver and handle washcloth, allow him or her to clean perineum on own.	Maintains the patient's dignity and self-care ability.
Clinical decision point: CHG is safe to use on the perineum and external mucosa (AHRQ, 2013).	
(2) Female patients	
(a) Apply pair of clean gloves. Lower side rail. Help the patient into dorsal recumbent position. Note restrictions or limitations in the patient's positioning. Place waterproof pad under the patient's buttocks. Drape the patient with bath blanket placed in shape of a diamond. Lift lower edge of bath blanket to expose perineum (see illustration).	Provides full exposure of female genitalia. If the patient is totally dependent, provide assistance to support her in side-lying position and raise leg as perineum is bathed. If position causes the patient discomfort, reduce degree of abduction in her hips.
(b) Fold lower corner of bath blanket up between the patient's legs onto abdomen. Wash and dry the patient's upper thighs.	Keeping the patient draped until procedure begins minimizes anxiety. Buildup of perineal secretions soils surrounding skin surfaces.
(c) Wash labia majora. Use nondominant hand to gently retract labia from thigh; with dominant hand, wash carefully in skinfolds. Wipe in direction from perineum to rectum. Repeat on opposite side with separate section of washcloth. Rinse and dry area thoroughly.	Perineal care includes thorough cleaning of the patient's external genitalia and surrounding skin. Skinfolds may contain body secretions that harbor microorganisms. Wiping front to back reduces chance of transmitting fecal organisms to urinary meatus.
(d) Gently separate labia with nondominant hand to expose urethral meatus and vaginal orifice. With dominant hand, wash downward from pubic area toward rectum in one smooth stroke (see illustration). Wash middle and both sides of perineum. Use separate section of cloth for each stroke. Clean thoroughly around labia minora, clitoris, and vaginal orifice. Avoid placing tension on indwelling catheter if present, and clean area around it thoroughly.	Cleansing method reduces transfer of microorganisms to urinary meatus. (For menstruating women or patients with indwelling catheters, clean with cotton balls.)
(e) Provide catheter care using a CHG wipe or a clean washcloth to clean down along catheter from exit site (check agency policy) (see Chapter 21).	Reduces incidence of health care–associated urinary tract infection (Strouse, 2015).
(f) Rinse perineal area thoroughly. May use bedpan and pour warm water over perineal area. Dry thoroughly from front to back.	Rinsing removes soap and microorganisms more effectively than wiping. Retained moisture harbors microorganisms.
(g) Fold lower corner of bath blanket back between the patient's legs and over perineum. Ask the patient to lower legs and assume comfortable position.	
(3) Male patients	
(a) Apply pair of clean gloves. Lower side rail. Help the patient to supine position. Note any restriction in mobility.	Provides full exposure of male genitalia. Position patients who are unable to lie supine on their side.

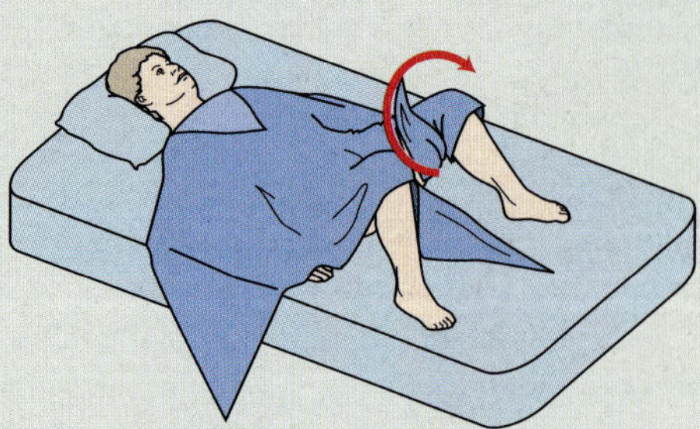

Step 5m(2)(a) Drape patient for perineal care.

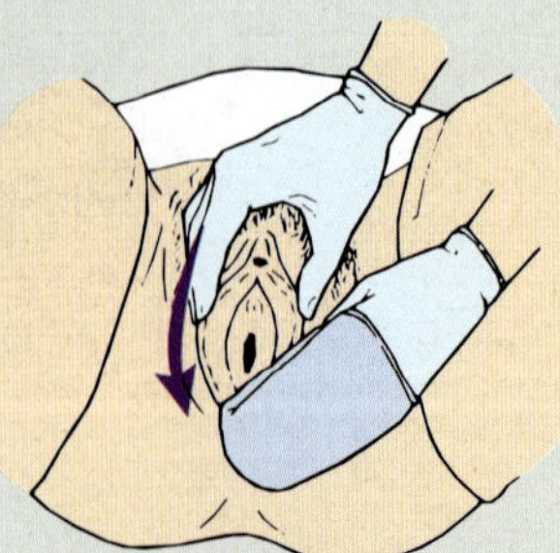

Step 5m(2)(d) Clean from perineum to rectum (front to back).

STEP	RATIONALE
(b) Fold lower half of bath blanket up to expose upper thighs. Wash and dry thighs.	Buildup of perineal secretions soils surrounding skin surfaces.
(c) Cover thighs with bath towels. Raise bath blanket up to expose genitalia. Gently raise penis and place bath towel underneath. Gently grasp shaft of penis. If the patient is uncircumcised, retract foreskin (see illustration). If the patient has an erection, defer procedure until later.	Draping minimizes patient anxiety. Towel prevents moisture from collecting in inguinal area. Gentle but firm handling of penis reduces chance of an erection. Secretions capable of harboring microorganisms collect underneath foreskin.
(d) Wash tip of penis at urethral meatus first. Using circular motion, clean from meatus outward (see illustration). Discard washcloth and repeat with clean cloth until penis is clean. Rinse and dry gently.	Direction of cleaning moves from area of least contamination to area of most contamination to prevent microorganisms from entering urethra.
(e) Return foreskin to its natural position. This is extremely important in patients with decreased sensation in the lower extremities.	Tightening of foreskin around shaft of penis causes local edema and discomfort. Patients with reduced sensation do not feel tightening of foreskin.
(f) Gently clean shaft of penis and scrotum by having the patient abduct legs. Pay special attention to underlying surface of penis. Lift scrotum carefully and wash underlying skinfolds. Rinse and dry thoroughly.	Vigorous massage of penis may cause an erection. Underlying surface of penis is an area where secretions accumulate. Abduction of legs provides easier access to scrotal tissues. Secretions collect easily between skinfolds.
(g) Provide catheter care as needed (see Step m(2)(e)). Avoid placing tension on indwelling catheter and clean area around it thoroughly. Provide catheter care (see Chapter 21).	Cleaning along catheter from exit site reduces incidence of nosocomial urinary tract infection.
n. Remove soiled gloves and discard in trash; raise side rail before leaving bedside to dispose of water and obtain fresh water.	Prevents transmission of infection. Protects the patient from injury.
o. Wash back. (This follows both female and male perineal care.)	
(1) Perform hand hygiene and apply clean pair of gloves. Lower side rail. Help the patient into prone or side-lying position (as applicable). Place towel lengthwise along the patient's side and keep him or her covered with bath blanket.	Exposes back and buttocks for bathing while limiting exposure.
(2) Keep the patient draped by sliding bath blanket over shoulders and thighs during bathing. Wash, rinse, and dry back from neck to buttocks using long, firm strokes.	Cleaning back before buttocks and anus prevents contamination of water.
(3) Move from back to buttocks and anus. Have the patient remain in prone or side-lying position and keep covered to avoid chilling. Clean anus and buttocks area.	Exposes back and buttocks for bathing while limiting exposure.
(4) If fecal material is present, enclose in fold of underpad or toilet tissue and remove with disposable wipes.	Skinfolds near buttocks and anus may contain fecal secretions that harbor microorganisms.
(5) Clean buttocks and anus, washing front to back (see illustration). Clean, rinse, and dry area thoroughly. If needed, place a clean absorbent pad under the patient's buttocks. Remove contaminated gloves. Raise side rail and perform hand hygiene.	Cleaning motion prevents contaminating perineal area with fecal material or microorganisms.
(6) Return to bed and lower side rail; give a back rub if appropriate or desired by the patient.	Promotes patient relaxation. Back rubs are contraindicated in some cardiac patients.

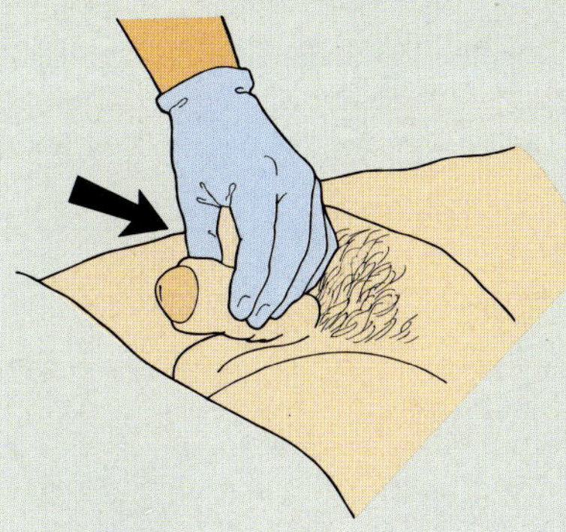

Step 5m(3)(c) Retract foreskin.

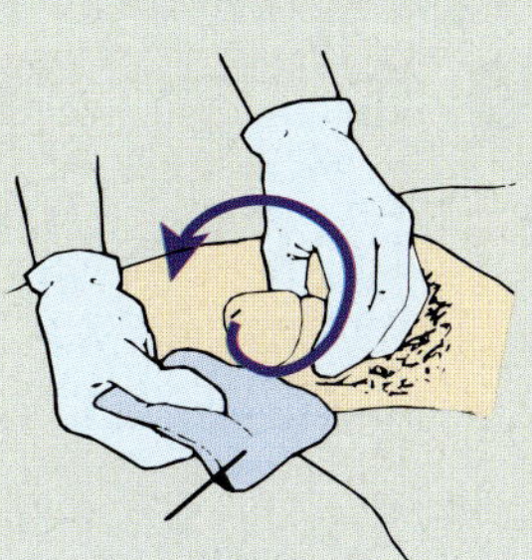

Step 5m(3)(d) Use circular motion to clean tip of penis.

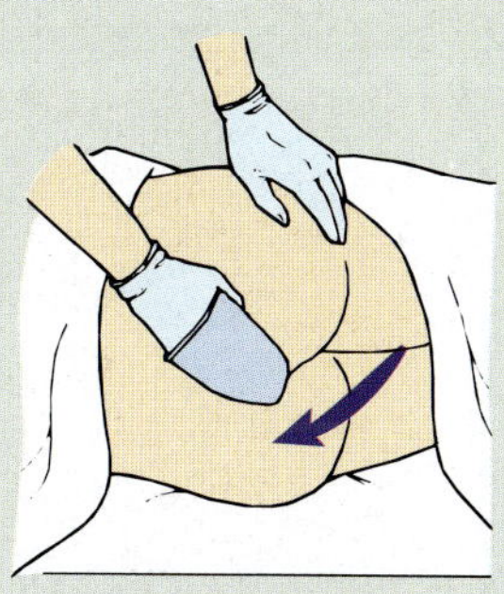

Step 5o(5) Clean buttocks and anus, washing front to back.

STEP	RATIONALE
p. Apply additional body lotion or oil to the patient's skin as needed.	Moisturizing lotion prevents dry, chapped skin.
q. Remove soiled linen and place in dirty-linen bag. Clean and replace bathing equipment. Wash hands.	Reduces transmission of microorganisms.
r. Help the patient dress. Comb the patient's hair. Women may want to apply makeup. Help as needed.	Promotes the patient's body image.
s. Make the patient's bed.	Provides clean, comfortable environment.
t. Check function and position of external devices (e.g., indwelling urethral catheters, nasogastric tubes, i.v. lines).	Ensures that systems remain functional after bathing activities.
u. Place bed in lowest position.	Maintains the patient's safety by decreasing height of bedframe from floor.
v. Place nurse call system and personal possessions in an accessible location. Leave room as clean and comfortable as possible.	Prevents transmission of infection. Clean environment promotes the patient's comfort. Promotes the patient's safety.
w. Perform hand hygiene.	Reduces transmission of microorganisms.
6. Commercial bag bath or CHG cleansing pack:	
a. A cleansing pack contains six to eight premoistened towels for cleaning. Warm package contents in microwave following package directions. If you are bathing the patient using warm commercial or CHG cloth, check temperature of cloth before use. Gloves diminish sense of heat.	Provides warm, soothing heat. CHG reduces bacteria for up to 24 h and prevents infection (AHRQ, 2013). Prevents burn to skin.
b. Use all six CHG cloths in the following order (see illustration): ▪ Cloth 1: Neck, shoulders, and chest ▪ Cloth 2: Both arms, both hands, web spaces, and axilla ▪ Cloth 3: Abdomen and groin/perineum ▪ Cloth 4: Right leg, right foot, and web spaces ▪ Cloth 5: Left leg, left foot, and web spaces ▪ Cloth 6: Back of neck, back, and buttocks	Reduces transmission of microorganisms.
c. Firmly massage skin when using cloth. Allow skin to air dry for 30 s. Do not rinse. It is permissible to lightly cover the patient with bath towel to prevent chilling. **Note:** If there is excessive soiling (e.g., in perineal region), use an extra cloth or conventional washcloths, soap, water, and towels.	Drying skin with towel removes emollient that is left behind after water/cleaner solution evaporates.

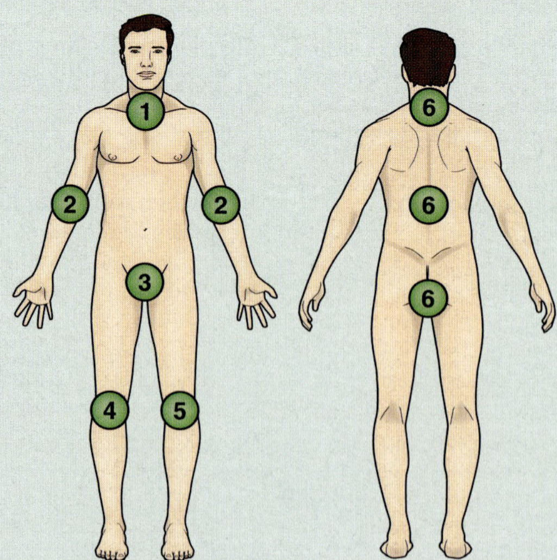

Step 6b Using CHG bathing cloths. (From Agency for Healthcare Research and Quality [AHRQ]: *Appendix E. Training and educational materials: daily chlorhexidine bathing patient information,* 2013, Agency for Healthcare Research and Quality, Rockville, MD. http://www.ahrq.gov/professionals/systems/hospital/universal_icu_decolonization/universal-icu-ape.html.)

STEP	RATIONALE
7. Tub bath or shower:	
a. Consider the patient's condition and review orders for precautions concerning movement or positioning of the patient.	Prevents accidental injury to the patient during bathing.
b. Schedule use of shower or tub.	Prevents unnecessary waiting, which causes fatigue.
c. Check tub or shower for cleanliness. Use cleaning techniques outlined in agency policy. Place rubber mat on tub or shower bottom. Place disposable bath mat or towel on floor in front of tub or shower.	Cleaning prevents transmission of microorganisms. Mats prevent slipping and falling.
d. Collect all hygienic aids, toiletry items, and linens requested by the patient. Place within easy reach of tub or shower.	Placing items close at hand prevents possible falls when the patient reaches for items.
e. Help the patient move to bathroom if necessary. Have the patient wear robe and nonskid slippers.	Assistance prevents accidental falls. Wearing robe and slippers prevents chilling.
f. Demonstrate how to use call signal for assistance.	Bathrooms are equipped with signaling devices in case the patient feels faint or weak or needs immediate assistance. Patients prefer privacy during bath if safety is not jeopardized.
g. Place "occupied" sign on bathroom door.	Maintains the patient's privacy.
h. Fill bath tub halfway with warm water. Check temperature of bath water, have the patient test water, and adjust temperature if water is too warm. Explain which faucet controls hot water. If the patient is taking shower, turn shower on and adjust water temperature before the patient enters shower stall. Use shower seat or tub chair if needed (see illustration).	Adjusting water temperature prevents accidental burns. Older adults and patients with neurological alterations (e.g., diabetes, spinal cord injury) are at high risk for burn because of reduced sensation. Use of assistive devices facilitates bathing and minimizes physical exertion.
i. Instruct the patient to use safety bars when getting in and out of tub or shower, and to pull cord to summon assistance (if available). Caution the patient against use of bath oil in tub water.	Prevents slipping and falling. Oil causes tub surfaces to become slippery.
j. Instruct the patient not to remain in tub longer than 10 or 15 min. Check on the patient every 5 min.	Prolonged exposure to warm water causes vasodilation and pooling of blood in some patients, leading to light-headedness or dizziness.
k. Return to bathroom when the patient signals and knock before entering.	Provides privacy.
l. For a patient who is unsteady, drain tub of water before he or she tries to get out. Place bath towel over the patient's shoulders. Help the patient out of tub as needed and help with drying.	Prevents accidental falls. The patient may become chilled as water drains.

Clinical decision point: Weak or unstable patients need extra assistance in getting out of a tub. Planning for additional personnel is essential before attempting to help the patient. Lift equipment may be used for transfer in some cases. See agency policy.

STEP	RATIONALE
m. Help the patient as needed with getting dressed in clean gown or pajamas, slippers, and robe. (In home setting, the patient may put on regular clothing.)	Maintains warmth to prevent chilling.
n. Help the patient to room and comfortable position in bed or chair.	Maintains relaxation gained from bathing.

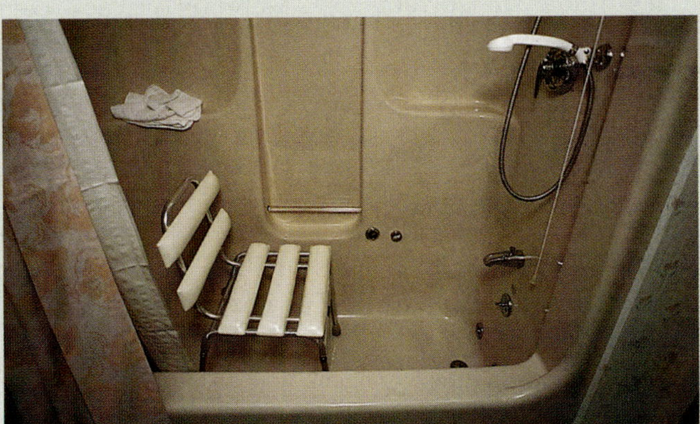

Step 7h Shower seat for patient safety.

STEP	RATIONALE
o. Clean tub or shower according to agency policy. Remove soiled linen and place in dirty-linen bag. Discard disposable equipment in proper receptacle. Place "unoccupied" sign on bathroom door. Return supplies to storage area.	Prevents transmission of infection through soiled linen and moisture.
p. Perform hand hygiene.	Reduces transfer of microorganisms.
Evaluation	
1. Observe skin, paying particular attention to areas previously soiled, reddened, dry, or showing early signs of breakdown.	Techniques used during bathing leave skin clean and clear. Over time, dryness of skin diminishes. If the patient shows areas of redness, use Braden Scale to measure risk for pressure injuries (see Chapter 17).
2. Observe ROM during bath.	Measures joint mobility.
3. Ask the patient to rate level of comfort.	Determines the patient's tolerance of bathing activities.
4. Ask the patient to rate level of fatigue.	Determines the patient's tolerance of bathing activities.
5. **Use teach back:** "We talked about why it is important for you to have a daily bath while in the hospital. Please tell me why we are using bathing cloths for your bath. How will you be sure the area around your wound is bathed correctly once you get home?" Revise your instruction now or develop a plan for revised patient teaching if the patient/family caregiver is not able to teach back correctly.	Determines the patient's/family caregiver's level of understanding of instructional topic.

Recording and Reporting

- Record in nurses' notes in electronic health record (EHR), chart, or flow sheets the amount of assistance provided, patient's participation in care, condition of skin, and any significant findings (e.g., reddened areas, breaks in skin, inflammation, ulcerations).
- Document your evaluation of patient/family caregiver learning.
- Report any skin irritations, breaks in skin, or ulcerations or patient's intolerance to activity to the nurse in charge or health care provider.

Unexpected Outcomes and Related Interventions

- Areas of excessive dryness, rashes, or pressure injuries appear on the skin.
  - Complete pressure injury assessment (see Chapter 17).
  - Apply moisturizing lotions or topical skin applications per agency policy.
  - Limit frequency of complete baths. It may become necessary (if the patient has a sensitivity to CHG) to switch to plain soap and water.
  - Obtain special bed surface.
- The patient becomes excessively tired or unable to cooperate or participate in bathing.
  - Reschedule bathing time when the patient is more rested.
  - Provide a pillow or elevate the head of the bed during bath for a patient with breathing difficulties.
  - Notify the health care provider if there is a change in the patient's fatigue level.
  - Perform hygiene measures in stages between scheduled rest periods.
- The rectum, perineum, or genital area is inflamed or swollen or has foul-smelling odor.
  - Bathe the perineal area frequently enough to keep it clean and dry.
  - Obtain an order for a sitz bath.
  - Apply protective barrier ointment or anti-inflammatory cream.
  - Report findings to the health care provider.

KEY POINTS

- Various personal, social, cultural, and developmental factors influence the patients' hygiene practices.
- Assess a patient's physical and cognitive ability to perform hygiene self-care and provide care according to the patient's needs and preferences.
- Incorporate knowledge of the factors influencing an individual patient's hygiene practices into hygiene care.
- Integrate physical assessment, wound care, teaching, and range-of-motion (ROM) exercises into hygiene care.
- Use communication skills and teaching to develop a caring relationship with the patient.
- Maintain privacy, comfort, and patient safety when providing hygiene care.
- Provide oral care for patients who are debilitated or unconscious; take precautions to reduce risk for ventilator-associated pneumonia (VAP) and aspiration.
- Patients who are immobilized and poorly nourished and who have reduced sensation or peripheral circulation are at risk for altered skin integrity; these patients require special nail, foot, and skin care.
- Patients with diabetes mellitus or other peripheral vascular diseases require special foot care practices.
- Maintain the patient's environment clean and free of clutter.
- Base evaluation of hygiene care on the patient's sense of comfort, relaxation, well-being, and understanding of hygiene techniques.

REFERENCES

Agency for Healthcare Research and Quality (AHRQ). Appendix E. Training and educational materials: daily chlorhexidine bathing patient information. Rockville, MD: Agency for Healthcare Research and Quality; 2013. Available from: http://www.ahrq.gov/professionals/systems/hospital/universal_icu_decolonization/universal-icu-ape.html.

Agency for Healthcare Research and Quality (AHRQ). Preventing pressure ulcers in hospitals. 2014. Available from: https://www.ahrq.gov/sites/default/files/publications/files/putoolkit.pdf.

American Academy of Dermatology (AAD). Dermatologists' top tips for relieving dry skin. 2016. Available from: https://www.aad.org/public/skin-hair-nails/skin-care/dry-skin.

American Diabetes Association. Diabetes statistics. 2018. Available from: http://www.diabetes.org/diabetes-basics/statistics/.

Ayello EA, Fulmer T. Hartford Institute for Geriatric Nursing Preventing pressure ulcers and skin tears. In: Boltz M, et al., editors: Evidence-based geriatric protocols for best practice. 4th ed. New York: Springer; 2012. p. 298.

Beeckman D, Van Lancker A, Van Hecke A, Verhaeghe S. A systematic review and meta-analysis of incontinence-associated dermatitis, incontinence, and moisture as risk factors for pressure ulcer development. Res Nurs Health 2014;37:204.

Boonyasiri A, Thaisiam P, Permpikul C, Judaeng T, Suiwongsa B, Apiradeewajeset N, et al. Effectiveness of chlorhexidine wipes for the prevention of multidrug-resistant bacterial colonization and hospital-acquired infections in intensive care unit patients: a randomized trial in Thailand. Infect Control Hosp Epidemiol 2016;36(3):245.

Burman ME, Robinson B, Hart AM. Linking evidence-based nursing practice and patient-centered care through patient preferences. Nurs Adm Q 2013;37(3):231.

Cassir N, Thomas G, Hraiech S, Brunet J, Fournier PE, La Scola B, et al. Chlorhexidine daily bathing: impact on health care-associated infections caused by gram-negative bacteria. Am J Infect Control 2015;43:640.

Centers for Disease Control and Prevention (CDC). Tick removal and testing. 2015. Available from: http://www.cdc.gov/lyme/removal/index.html.

Centers for Disease Control and Prevention (CDC). Head lice: treatment. 2016. Available from: https://www.cdc.gov/parasites/lice/head/treatment.html.

Chen W, Li S, Li L, Wu X, Zhang W. Effects of daily bathing with chlorhexidine and acquired infection of methicillin-resistant *Staphylococcus aureus* and vancomycin-resistant *Enterococcus*: a meta-analysis. J Thorac Dis 2013;5(4):518.

Climo MW, Yokoe DS, Warren DK, Perl TM, Bolon M, Herwaldt LA, et al. Effect of daily chlorhexidine bathing on hospital-acquired infection. N Engl J Med 2013;368(6):533.

El-Rabbany M, Zaghlol N, Bhandari M, Azarpazhooh A. Prophylactic oral health procedures to prevent hospital-acquired and ventilator-associated pneumonia: a systematic review. Int J Nurs Stud 2015;52(1):452.

Giger JN, editor. Transcultural nursing: assessment and intervention. 6th ed. St. Louis: Mosby; 2013.

Hall GR, Gallagher M, Hoffmann-Snyder C. Bathing persons with dementia. Iowa City (IA): University of Iowa College of Nursing, John A. Hartford Foundation Center of Geriatric Nursing Excellence; 2013. 58 p. Available from: https://jesse.tg/ngc-archive/summary/9791

Harris M, Richards KC. The physiological and psychological effects of slow-stroke back massage and hand massage on relaxation in older people. J Clin Nurs 2010;19(7):917.

Kamaljit K, et al: Social beliefs and practices associated with menstrual hygiene among adolescent girls of Amritsar, Punjab, India, *JIMSA* 25 (2): 69, 2012.

Kiyoshi-Teo H, Blegen M. Institutional guidelines on oral hygiene practices in intensive care units. Am J Crit Care 2015;24(4):309.

Meiner SE. Gerontologic nursing. 5th ed. St. Louis: Mosby; 2015.

Munoz-Price LS, Dezfulian C, Wyckoff M, Lenchus JD, Rosalsky M, Birnbach DJ, et al. Effectiveness of stepwise interventions targeted to decrease central catheter-associated bloodstream infections. Crit Care Med 2012;40(5):1464.

Pender N, et al: *Health promotion in nursing practice*, Upper Saddle River, NJ, 2011, Pearson Education.

Petlin A, Schallom M, Prentice D, Sona C, Mantia P, McMullen K, et al. Chlorhexidine gluconate bathing to reduce methicillin-resistant *Staphylococcus aureus* acquisition. Crit Care Nurse 2014;34(5):17.

Powers J, Peed J, Burns L, Ziemba-Davis M. Chlorhexidine bathing and microbial contamination in patients' bath 186 basins. Am J Crit Care 2012;21(5):338.

Quality and Safety Education for Nurses (QSEN). Pre-licensure KSAs. 2014. Available from: http://qsen.org/competencies/pre-licensure-ksas/.

Shah HN, Schwartz JL, Luna G, Cullen DL. Bathing with 2% chlorhexidine gluconate. Crit Care Nurs Q 2016;39:42.

Strouse AC. Appraising the literature on bathing practices and catheter-associated urinary tract infection preventions. Urol Nurs 2015; 35(1):11.

Tay LY, Jorge JH, Herrera DR, Campanha NH, Gomes BP, Andre Dos Santos F. Evaluation of different treatment methods against denture stomatitis: a randomized clinical study. Oral Surg Oral Med Oral Pathol Oral Radiol 2014;118:72.

The Joint Commission (TJC): 2018 National Patient Safety Goals. Oakbrook Terrace, IL: The Joint Commission; 2018. Available from: https://www.jointcommission.org/standards/national-patient-safety-goals/.

Touhy TA, Jett K. Ebersole and Hess'gerontological nursing and healthy aging. 4th ed. St. Louis: Mosby; 2014.

Voegeli D. Incontinence-associated dermatitis: new insights into an old problem. Br J Nurs 2016;25(5):256.

Zimmerman S, Sloane PD, Cohen LW, Barrick AL. Changing the culture of mouth care: mouth care without a battle. Gerontologist 2014; 54(Suppl. 1):S25.

Zullino DF, Krenz S, Frésard E, Cancela E, Khazaal Y. Local back massage with an automated massage chair: general muscle and psychophysiologic relaxing properties. J Altern Complement Med 2005;11(6):1103.

17 Skin Integrity: Prevention and Care of Pressure Ulcers

OBJECTIVES

- To define pressure injuries/pressure ulcers.
- To explain causes and risk factors for pressure ulcer development.
- To enlist the pathogenesis of pressure ulcers.
- To describe classification of pressure injury.
- To discuss the response of the body during each phase of the wound-healing process.
- To differentiate healing by primary, secondary, and tertiary intention.
- To describe common complications of wound healing.
- To discuss the use of risk assessment tools in the assessment of pressure injuries.
- To describe wound assessment criteria: anatomical location, size, type and percentage of wound tissue, volume and color of wound drainage, and condition of surrounding skin.
- To describe the purposes of and precautions taken with applying dressings and binders.
- To describe the mechanism of action of wound care dressings.
- To describe the differences in therapeutic effects of heat and cold.
- To complete an assessment for a patient with risk for or actual impaired skin integrity.
- To list nursing diagnoses associated with risk for or actual impaired skin integrity.
- To develop a nursing care plan and evaluate outcomes for a patient with risk for or actual impaired skin integrity.

KEY TERMS

abrasion, p. 361
binders, p. 388
blanchable hyperemia, p. 362
compress, p. 383
debride, p. 374
dehiscence, p. 369
eschar, p. 363
evisceration, p. 369
friction, p. 361
granulation tissue, p. 367
hematoma, p. 368
hemostasis, p. 368
induration, p. 362
intertriginous dermatitis (ITD), p. 363
laceration, p. 367
maceration, p. 372
nonblanchable hyperemia, p. 364
pressure injury, p. 362
primary intention, p. 367
reactive hyperemia, p. 364
secondary intention, p. 367
shear, p. 361
sitz bath, p. 383
slough, p. 363
tertiary intention, p. 367
tissue ischemia, p. 362

PRESSURE ULCERS

Pressure ulcer (formerly called pressure sore, *pressure ulcer, decubitus ulcer,* or *bedsore*) is localized damage to the skin and underlying soft tissue usually over a bony prominence or related to a medical or other device (Fig. 17.1). The injury can appear as intact skin or an open ulcer and may be painful. The injury occurs as a result of intense and/or prolonged pressure or pressure in combination with shear. The tolerance of soft tissue for pressure and shear may also be affected by microclimate, nutrition, perfusion, comorbid conditions, and condition of the soft tissue (Edsberg et al., 2016). The term *pressure injury* replaces *pressure ulcer* in the National Pressure Ulcer Advisory Injury Staging System (National Pressure Ulcer Advisory Panel [NPUAP], 2016). The updated staging definitions and change in terminology more accurately describe pressure injuries to both intact and ulcerated skin. In the previous staging system, Stage 1 and deep tissue injury described injured intact skin, whereas the other stages described open ulcers. This led to confusion because the definitions for each of the stages referred to the injuries as "pressure ulcers." In addition to the change in

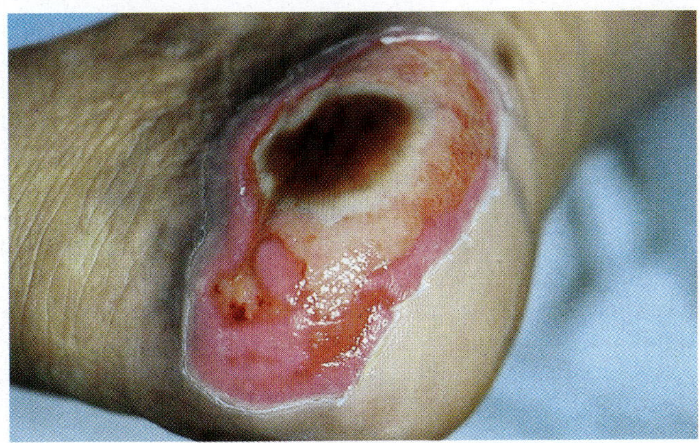

Fig. 17.1 Pressure injury with tissue necrosis.

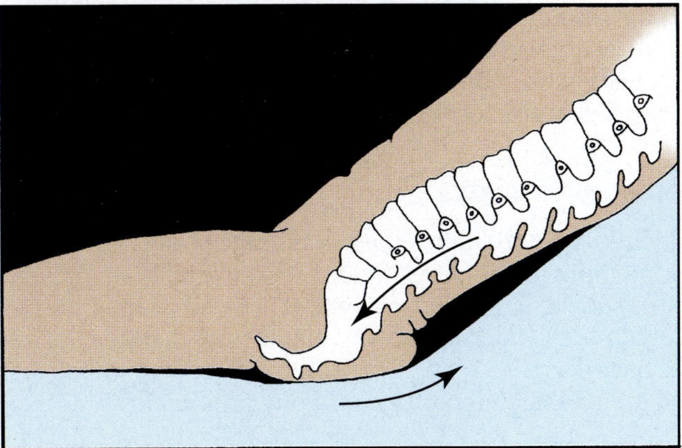

Fig. 17.2 Shearing force.

terminology, Arabic numbers are now used in the names of the stages instead of Roman numerals. The term *suspected* has been removed from the deep tissue injury diagnostic label. The definitions from the 2016 NPUAP staging system follow (Edsberg et al., 2016).

CAUSES AND RISK FACTORS FOR PRESSURE ULCER DEVELOPMENT

Many factors contribute to the formation of a pressure ulcer. Pressure is the major cause. Tissue receives oxygen and nutrients and eliminates metabolic wastes via the blood. Any factor that interferes with blood flow in turn interferes with cellular metabolism and the function or life of the cells. Prolonged, intense pressure affects cellular metabolism by decreasing or obliterating blood flow, resulting in tissue ischemia and ultimately tissue death.

A variety of factors predispose a patient to pressure ulcer formation. These factors are often directly related to disease such as decreased level of consciousness, the presence of a cast, or secondary to an illness (e.g., decreased sensation following a cerebrovascular accident).

Shear

The force exerted against the skin while the skin remains stationary and the bony structures move is called **shear.** For example, when the head of the bed is elevated, gravity causes the bony skeleton to pull toward the foot of the bed while the skin remains against the sheets (Fig. 17.2). The underlying tissue blood vessels become stretched and bent, impeding blood flow to the deep tissue. Injuries occur with large areas of undermining and less damage at the skin surface and may not be immediately visible at the skin surface because the injury occurs in deeper tissue (Maklebust and Magnan, 2016).

Friction

Friction is surface damage caused by the skin rubbing against another surface that often results in an abrasion. An **abrasion** is the loss of the epidermis, the top layer of the skin. The body surfaces most at risk for friction are the elbows and heels because abrasion of these surfaces occurs when they are rubbed against the sheets during repositioning. This type of damage alone should not be confused with or classified as a pressure injury, as friction alone is not an etiological factor for pressure injuries (Doughty and McNichol, 2016).

Moisture

Skin moisture increases the risk for injury formation. Moisture softens the skin and reduces its resistance to other physical factors such as pressure or shear. Moisture comes from many sources such as wound drainage, perspiration, and fecal and urinary incontinence. Skin moisture and wetness from incontinence frequently cause skin breakdown (Bryant, 2016).

Nutrition

Poor nutrition, specifically severe protein deficiency, increases the risk of the breakdown of soft tissue and alters fluid and electrolyte balance. Patients with protein loss have hypoalbuminemia. Low protein levels cause edema or swelling, which contributes to problems with the transportation of oxygen and nutrients (Pieper, 2016). When serum albumin levels fall drastically (e.g., to less than 3 g/100 mL), patients experience a shift of fluid from the extracellular fluid volume to the tissues, resulting in edema (Pieper, 2016).

Age

The dermis is thin in neonates and becomes thin in older adults. This makes the skin appear nearly transparent and increases the risk for skin tears. Thus, neonates and young children (i.e., younger than 5 years) are at higher risk for pressure injury occurrence (Nix et al., 2016). An older patient's skin is more vulnerable to pressure, shear, and friction (Pieper, 2016).

Impaired Sensory Perception

Patients with altered sensory perception for pain and pressure are more at risk for impaired skin integrity than those with normal sensation. Patients with impaired sensory perception of pain and pressure are unable to feel when a part of their body undergoes increased, prolonged pressure or pain. Thus, a patient who cannot feel or sense that there is pain or pressure is at risk for the development of pressure ulcers.

Impaired Mobility

Patients unable to independently change positions are at risk for pressure ulcer development. For example, a morbidly obese patient who is seriously ill will be weakened and less likely to turn independently. Patients with spinal cord injuries have decreased or absent motor and sensory impairment and are unable to reposition off bony prominences.

Alteration in Level of Consciousness

Patients who are confused or disoriented, those who have expressive aphasia or the inability to verbalize, or those with changing levels of consciousness are unable to protect themselves from pressure ulcer development. Patients who are confused or disoriented are sometimes able to feel pressure but are not always able to understand how to relieve it or communicate their discomfort. A patient in a coma cannot perceive pressure and is unable to move voluntarily to relieve pressure.

PATHOGENESIS OF PRESSURE ULCERS

Pressure is the major element in the cause of pressure ulcers. Three pressure-related factors contribute to pressure ulcer development: (1) pressure intensity, (2) pressure duration, and (3) tissue tolerance.

Pressure Intensity

A classic research study identified capillary closing pressure as the minimal amount of pressure required to collapse a capillary (e.g., when the pressure exceeds the normal capillary pressure range of 15−32 mm Hg) (Burton and Yamada, 1951). Therefore, if the pressure applied over a capillary exceeds the normal capillary pressure and the vessel is occluded for a prolonged period of time, **tissue ischemia** can occur. If the patient has reduced sensation and cannot respond to the discomfort of the ischemia, tissue ischemia and tissue death result.

The clinical presentation of obstructed blood flow occurs when evaluating areas of pressure. After a period of tissue ischemia, if the pressure is relieved and the blood flow returns, the skin turns red. The effect of this redness is vasodilation (blood vessel expansion), called *hyperemia* (redness). You assess an area of hyperemia by pressing a finger over the affected area. If it blanches (turns lighter in color) and the erythema returns when you remove your finger, the hyperemia is transient and is an attempt to overcome the ischemic episode, thus called **blanchable hyperemia**. However, if the erythematous area does not blanch (**nonblanchable erythema**) when you apply pressure, deep tissue damage is probable.

Blanching occurs when the normal red tones of the light-skinned patient are absent. When checking for pressure ulcers in dark-skinned patients, dark skin may not show the blanch response. Instead, after applying light pressure, look for an area darker than the surrounding skin or one that is taut, shiny, or indurated (hardened). The light from a camera flash can be used to enhance visualization of dark skin. Check for localized changes in skin texture and temperature. Early signs of skin damage include **induration**, bogginess (less-than-normal stiffness), and increased warmth at the injury site compared with nearby areas. Over time, as tissues become more damaged, the area becomes cooler to the touch (Sommers, 2011). There are characteristics of intact dark skin that alert nurses to the potential for pressure ulcers.

Pressure Duration

Low pressure over a prolonged period and high-intensity pressure over a short period are two concerns related to duration of pressure. Both types of pressure cause tissue damage. Extended pressure occludes blood flow and nutrients and contributes to cell death (Pieper, 2016). Clinical implications of pressure duration include evaluating the amount of pressure (checking skin for nonblanching hyperemia) and determining the amount of time that a patient tolerates pressure (checking to be sure after relieving pressure that the affected area blanches).

Tissue Tolerance

The ability of tissue to endure pressure depends on the integrity of the tissue and the supporting structures. The extrinsic factors of shear, friction, and moisture affect the ability of the skin to tolerate pressure: the greater the degree to which the factors of shear, friction, and moisture are present, the more susceptible the skin will be to damage from pressure. The second factor related to tissue tolerance is the ability of the underlying skin structures (blood vessels, collagen) to help redistribute pressure. Systemic factors such as poor nutrition, increased aging, hydration status, and low blood pressure affect the tolerance of the tissue to externally applied pressure.

STAGES OF PRESSURE ULCERS

- **Stage 1 pressure injury:** Intact skin with a localized area of nonblanchable erythema, which may appear differently in darkly pigmented skin. The presence of blanchable erythema or changes in sensation, temperature, or firmness may precede visual changes. Color changes do not include purple or maroon discoloration; these may indicate deep tissue pressure injury (DTPI).
  Teaching points:
  - Stage 1 pressure injuries are often the first visible changes in the skin and have been historically referred to as the "heralding sign."
  - It is important that scar tissue and DTPI not be classified as a Stage 1 pressure injury.
  - The skin's blanching response can be assessed by pressing the skin with a finger to close the capillary bed. On release of pressure, the skin should

immediately return to the native skin color. Diascopy, examination of the skin's blanch response through a color disc pressed on the skin, also may be used to assess the cutaneous blanche response.

- **Stage 2 pressure injury:** Partial-thickness skin loss with exposed dermis. The wound bed is viable, pink or red, and moist, or injury may manifest as an intact or ruptured serum-filled blister. Adipose (fat) is not visible, and deeper tissue is not visible. Granulation tissue, **slough** (soft, moist, devitalized tissue that may be yellow, tan, or green and either loose or firmly adherent), and **eschar** are not present. These injuries commonly result from adverse microclimate and shear in the skin over the pelvis and shear in the heel.

  Teaching points:
  - This stage should not be used to describe moisture-associated skin damage (MASD) including incontinence-associated dermatitis (IAD) and **intertriginous dermatitis (ITD)** (inflammation of skin where two surfaces rub such as groin, beneath breasts, and underarm area).
  - This stage should not be used to describe medical adhesive–related skin injury (MARSI) or traumatic wounds (skin tears, burns, abrasions).
  - It is especially important if an injury is suspected of being a Stage 2 pressure injury that the presence or history of pressure and/or shear be confirmed.
- **Stage 3 pressure injury:** Full-thickness loss of skin, in which adipose (fat) is visible in the ulcer, and granulation tissue and epibole (rolled wound edges) are often present. Slough and/or eschar may be visible. The depth of tissue damage varies by anatomical location; areas of significant adiposity can develop deep wounds. Undermining (skin separates from the underlying tissue at the wound margins creating areas of tissue damage below the skin surface and less damage at the surface) and tunneling may occur. Fascia, muscle, tendon, ligament, cartilage, or bone is not exposed. If slough or eschar obscures the extent of tissue loss, this is an unstageable pressure injury.

  Teaching points:
  - Anatomical differences in body areas such as the buttocks versus the sacrum can result in very different depths of injury. Accurate staging is based on assessment of the extent of damage and visible tissue layer.
  - For many years, slough was considered a nonviable tissue. However, research on biofilm has improved our understanding of the role of inflammation in chronic wounds. Slough is now recognized as an inflammatory exudate composed of proteinaceous tissue, fibrin, neutrophils, and bacteria, rather than nonviable tissues. The inflammatory exudate is often produced in response to biofilm. If the biofilm is not controlled, the slough will recur following debridement. Slough is usually light yellow/cream colored and moist and soft. Eschar is black/brown, dry, thick, and leathery.
  - With full-thickness skin loss, adipose (fat) is visible in the ulcer, and granulation tissue and epibole (rolled wound edges) are often present. Slough and/or eschar may be visible. The depth of tissue damage varies by anatomical location; areas of significant adiposity can develop deep wounds. Undermining and tunneling may occur.
  - Fascia, muscle, tendon, ligament, cartilage, or bone is not exposed. If slough or eschar obscures the extend of tissue loss, that is an unstageable pressure injury.
- **Stage 4 pressure injury:** Full-thickness skin and tissue loss with exposed or directly palpable fascia, muscle, tendon, ligament, cartilage, or bone in the ulcer. Slough and/or eschar may be visible. Epibole (rolled edges), undermining, and tunneling often occur. Depth varies by anatomical location. If slough or eschar obscures the extent of tissue loss, this is an unstageable pressure injury.

  Teaching point:
  - Clinicians should assess for osteomyelitis, which may be present in Stage 4 pressure injuries.
- **DTPI:** Intact or nonintact skin with localized area of persistent nonblanchable deep red, maroon, or purple discoloration or epidermal separation revealing a dark wound bed or blood-filled blister. Pain and temperature change often precede skin color changes. Discoloration may appear differently in darkly pigmented skin. This injury results from intense and/or prolonged pressure and shear forces at the bone–muscle interface. The wound may evolve rapidly to reveal the actual extent of tissue injury or may resolve without tissue loss. If necrotic tissue, subcutaneous tissue, granulation tissue, fascia, muscle, or other underlying structures are visible, this indicates a full-thickness pressure injury (unstageable, Stage 3, or Stage 4). Do not use DTPI to describe vascular, traumatic, neuropathic, or dermatological conditions.

  Teaching points:
  - Confirm purple skin (appearing as ecchymosis or bruising) is due to pressure or shear and not a response to medication or trauma.
  - Attempt to identify the timing and setting of the pressure and shear that lead to DTPI for root cause analysis.
  - Document the evolution of DTPI following discovery (e.g., sloughing of epidermis to reveal deeper tissue damage and ultimately, if injury becomes full thickness, the stage of the resultant injury).
- **Unstageable pressure injury:** Full-thickness skin and tissue loss in which extent of tissue damage within the ulcer cannot be confirmed because it is obscured by slough or eschar. If slough or eschar is removed, a Stage 3 or Stage 4 pressure injury will be revealed. Stable eschar (i.e., dry, adherent, intact without erythema or fluctuance) on ischemic limb or heels should not be softened or removed.

  Teaching points:
  - When teaching others about unstageable pressure injury, clarify that this stage is unstageable because of the inability to visualize the wound base rather than the clinician's inability to determine the injury stage.
  - Describe the role of eschar as the body's natural (biological) cover. Removing stable eschar in the poorly perfused area results in an open wound that may expose the limb to infection and tax the ability to heal.

- Treat stable eschar as dry gangrene, do not moisten or soften it. The most important intervention when managing an unstable pressure injury is pressure redistribution rather than eschar removal. As eschar loosens from the wound bed, trim the edges to avoid inadvertent removal.

Although a number of contributing or confounding factors are associated with pressure injuries, the significance of these factors is not fully understood. A patient with decreased mobility, inadequate nutrition, excessive skin moisture, decreased sensory perception, or decreased activity is at risk for development of pressure injury. Statistics vary, but in the United States, pressure injury prevalence in acute care settings ranges from 0% to 15.8% (Pieper, 2016). Because pressure injuries often develop quickly when a patient becomes ill, it is important to identify patients who are at high risk to implement prevention interventions.

Tissue ischemia (i.e., decreased blood flow to tissues) usually results in tissue death and occurs when capillary blood flow is obstructed, as in the case of pressure. When pressure is relieved in a relatively short time, reactive hyperemia occurs in an attempt to overcome the ischemic episode. **Reactive hyperemia** is a redness of the skin resulting from dilation of the superficial capillaries (Pieper, 2016). Reactive hyperemia blanches (turns light in color). Blanching erythema is an area of erythema that becomes white (blanches) when compressed by a finger (Fig. 17.3). This hyperemia usually resolves without tissue loss if pressure is reduced or eliminated. **Blanchable hyperemia** is more difficult to assess in patients with dark skin. The discoloration or redness is warm to touch and is often purple/blue or violet instead of red in darkly pigmented skin (Nix, 2016).

Nonblanchable hyperemia is redness that persists after palpation and indicates tissue damage (Fig. 17.4). When you press a finger against the red or purple area, it does not turn lighter in color. This indicates deep tissue damage and is commonly the first stage of pressure injury development. This stage of skin injury is sometimes reversible if the pressure is relieved and the tissue is protected.

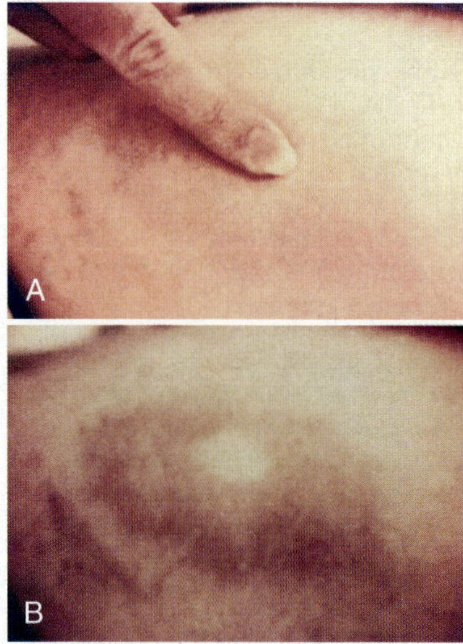

Fig. 17.3 **A,** Check for blanching by applying fingertip pressure. **B,** Area of blanchable hyperemia.

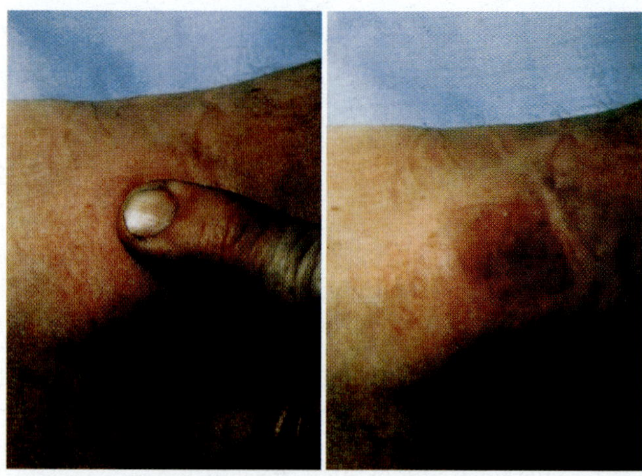
Fig. 17.4 Nonblanchable hyperemia is darker than the surrounding skin and does not blanch with fingertip pressure.

Deeper tissue destruction occurs in some injuries. The skin separates from the underlying granulation tissue at the wound margins causing undermining. Undermining creates large areas of tissue damage below the surface of the skin and less damage at the surface. With continuous pressure over the area, deep tissue destruction continues, which often results in a larger pocket of necrotic tissue beneath the opening of the main wound that resembles a tunnel; this is referred to as *tunneling*. Some wounds have more than one tunnel.

PREDICTION AND PREVENTION OF PRESSURE ULCERS

Guidelines for Prevention and Management of Pressure Ulcers from the Wound, Ostomy and Continence Nurses (WOCN) Society were recently reviewed and updated by nurse experts who performed extensive searches on the most up-to-date literature on pressure injuries (WOCN Society, 2016). The new guidelines provide the best available evidence in the prevention and management of pressure injuries (Box 17.1). These guidelines were accepted by the Agency for Healthcare Research and Quality (AHRQ). They include predictive tools that identify patients at highest risk for pressure injury development (WOCN Society, 2016). Patients identified to be at risk need a care plan to address and reduce identified risk factors.

The Braden Pressure Ulcer Risk Assessment Scale is one highly reliable tool that identifies patients at greatest risk for pressure injuries (Bergstrom et al., 1987a, 1987b, 1998). It is composed of six subscales: sensory perception, moisture, activity, mobility, nutrition, and friction and shear (Table 17.1). An adult in the hospital with a score of 16 or less or an older adult with a score of 18 or less is at risk for pressure injury development (Bergstrom et al., 1998; Ayello and Braden, 2002). **The Norton Pressure Sore Risk Assessment Scale** is also used for pressure ulcer risk assessment.

BOX 17.1 Pressure Injury Prevention Points

Assessment

- Assess individual risk for developing pressure injuries.
- Perform pressure injury risk assessment using a validated tool such as the Braden Scale on all patients who have one or more risk factors when admitted to an acute care facility, home care, hospice, or extended care facility (NPUAP, EPUAP, and PPPIA, 2014; WOCN Society, 2016).
- Assess for intrinsic and extrinsic risk factors such as general medical conditions (e.g., diabetes, stroke, cardiopulmonary disease, other peripheral vascular diseases), significant weight loss, poor nutrition, increased length of stay in a health care agency, and stay in the intensive care unit because of critical illness.
- Inspect skin and bony prominences at least daily.
- Assess for history of prior pressure injury and/or presence of current injury because this places patient at increased risk for additional pressure injuries.

Skin Care and Early Treatment

- Continue preventive measures even when a patient has a pressure injury to prevent pressure injury stage from advancing or additional pressure areas from developing.
- Clean and dry skin after each incontinent episode, using skin barriers such as cream, ointment, or paste to protect and maintain intact skin. Risk for skin injury is increased by prolonged skin moisture and wetness from urinary and fecal incontinence (Thayer et al., 2016).
- Minimize or eliminate pressure from medical devices such as oxygen tubing, catheters, cervical collars, casts, and restraints. Heat and humidity develop between the device and the skin, changing the microclimate of the skin. Prompt routine assessment of the skin under and surrounding the device reduces the risk for pressure injuries (Pittman et al., 2015).
- Turn and reposition a patient often to redistribute pressure from the superficial capillaries and allow tissues to compensate for temporary ischemia. Use safe patient-handling measures to turn and reposition patients every 1–2 h as their condition allows. Proper positioning helps minimize formation of pressure injury.
- Use approaches to minimize friction and shear. Use lift sheets and devices when repositioning patients to reduce rubbing skin against the sheets. Raise head of bed no more than 30° or at the lowest level of elevation consistent with patient's medical condition to prevent sliding and shear injury (WOCN Society, 2016).
- Avoid vigorous massage over bony prominences.

Support Surfaces and Pressure Redistribution

- Place patients at risk on a pressure-redistribution surface (McNichol et al., 2015; WOCN Society, 2016).
- Schedule regular and frequent turning and repositioning for patients who are bed-bound or chair-bound, taking into consideration the condition of the patient and the pressure redistribution support surface in determining repositioning strategy.
- Position sitting patients with special attention to the individual's anatomy, postural alignment, distribution of weight, and support of the feet.

Nutrition

- Offer patients with nutritional and pressure injury risks a minimum of 30–35 kcal/kg body weight of protein per day with 1.25–1.5 g/kg/day protein and 1 mL of fluid intake per kcal per day (Stotts, 2016b).
- Provide prescribed doses of vitamin A (1000–2000 retinol equivalents), vitamin C (100–100 mcg), vitamin B (200% recommended dietary allowance), zinc (15–30 mg), iron (20–30 mg), and glutamine (0.3–0.4 g) and a daily multivitamin (Stotts, 2016b).
- Refer patients with nutritional and pressure injury risks to a registered dietitian.

Patient and Family Caregiver Education

- Educate the patient and family caregiver about causes and risk factors for developing pressure injuries and ways to minimize risk.
- Include information about the following:
  - Etiology of and risk factors for pressure injuries
  - Importance of performing regular inspection of the skin, especially over bony prominences
  - Keeping the skin clean and dry
  - Selection and use of support surfaces
  - Measures to reduce friction from the sheet such as lifting rather than dragging across the bed
  - Demonstration of positioning to decrease risk for tissue breakdown
  - Promptly reporting health care changes and nutritional problems to health care providers

Data adapted from Wound, Ostomy and Continence Nurses (WOCN) Society: *Guideline for prevention and management of pressure ulcers*, WOCN Clinical Practice Guidelines Series, Mount Laurel, NJ, 2016, The Society.

Table 17.1 Braden Scale for Predicting Pressure Sore Risk

SENSORY PERCEPTION				
Ability to respond appropriately to pressure-related discomfort	1. **Completely limited:** Unresponsive (does not moan, flinch, or grasp) to painful stimuli as a result of diminished level of consciousness or sedation *or* Limited ability to feel pain over most of body	2. **Very limited:** Responds only to painful stimuli Cannot communicate discomfort except by moaning or restlessness *or* Has sensory impairment that limits ability to feel pain or discomfort over half of body	3. **Slightly limited:** Responds to verbal commands but cannot always communicate discomfort or need to be turned *or* Has some sensory impairment, which limits ability to feel pain or discomfort in one or two extremities	4. **No impairment:** Responds to verbal commands Has no sensory deficit that limits ability to feel or voice pain or discomfort

Continued

Table 17.1 Braden Scale for Predicting Pressure Sore Risk—cont'd

MOISTURE				
Degree to which skin is exposed to moisture	1. **Constantly moist:** Skin kept moist almost constantly (e.g., by perspiration, urine) Dampness detected every time patient is moved or turned	2. **Very moist:** Skin often but not always moist Linen must be changed at least once a shift	3. **Occasionally moist:** Skin occasionally moist, requiring an extra linen change approximately once per day	4. **Rarely moist:** Skin usually dry; linen change only required at routine intervals
ACTIVITY				
Degree of physical activity	1. **Bedfast:** Confined to bed	2. **Chairfast:** Ability to walk severely limited or nonexistent Cannot bear own weight and/or must be assisted into chair or wheelchair	3. **Walks occasionally:** Walks occasionally during day, but for very short distances, with or without assistance Spends majority of each shift in bed or chair	4. **Walks frequently:** Walks outside room at least twice a day and inside room at least once every 2 h during waking hours
MOBILITY				
Ability to change and control body position	1. **Completely immobile:** Does not make even slight changes in body or extremity position without assistance	2. **Very limited:** Makes occasional slight changes in body or extremity position but unable to make frequent or significant changes independently	3. **Slightly limited:** Makes frequent though slight changes in body or extremity position independently	4. **No limitations:** Makes major and frequent changes in position without assistance
NUTRITION				
Usual food intake pattern	1. **Very poor:** Never eats a complete meal Rarely eats more than one-third of any food offered Eats two servings or less of protein (meat or dairy products) per day Takes fluids poorly Does not take a liquid dietary supplement *or* Is NPO and/or maintained on clear liquids or i.v. feeding for more than 5 days	2. **Probably inadequate:** Rarely eats a complete meal and generally eats only about half of any food offered Protein intake includes only three servings of meat or dairy products per day Occasionally takes a dietary supplement *or* Receives less than optimal amount of liquid diet or tube feeding	3. **Adequate:** Eats over half of most meals Eats a total of four servings of protein (meat, dairy products) each day Occasionally refuses a meal but usually takes a supplement if offered *or* Is on a tube-feeding or TPN regimen that probably meets most nutritional needs	4. **Excellent:** Eats most of every meal Never refuses a meal Usually eats a total of four or more servings of meat and dairy products Occasionally eats between meals Does not require supplementation
FRICTION AND SHEAR				
	1. **Problem:** Requires moderate to maximal assistance in moving Complete lifting without sliding against sheets impossible Frequently slides down in bed or chair, requiring frequent repositioning with maximal assistance	2. **Potential problem:** Spasticity, contractions, or agitation leads to almost constant friction Moves feebly or requires minimal assistance During a move, skin probably slides to some extent against sheets, chair, restraints, or other devices Maintains relatively good position in chair or bed most of the time but occasionally slides down	3. **No apparent problem:** Moves in bed and chair independently and has sufficient muscle strength to sit up completely during move Maintains good position in bed or chair at all times	

I.v., intravenous; *NPO,* nothing by mouth; *TPN,* total parenteral nutrition.

Instructions: Score patient in each of the six subscales; add all subscales for overall score. Level of risk: not at risk, greater than 18; mild risk, 15–18; moderate risk, 13–14; high risk, 10–12; and very high risk, less than 9.

WOUND-HEALING PROCESS

All wounds heal through an orderly series of integrated physiological responses. Multiple factors promote or impede wound healing (Box 17.2). A wound with little or no tissue loss such as a clean surgical incision heals by **primary intention.** The skin edges approximate, or close together, and the risk for infection is minimal.

In contrast, a wound involving loss of tissue such as a severe **laceration** or a chronic wound such as a pressure injury heals by **secondary intention.** The skin edges cannot come together because of the extensive tissue loss, and healing occurs gradually. A layer of **granulation tissue,** which is red, moist tissue consisting of blood vessels and connective tissue, covers the wound base; wound contraction brings the wound edges together; and the wound closes with scar formation.

There are also instances in which a surgical wound is initially closed in the deep tissue layers; however, the subcutaneous fat and skin layers are left open. This method of wound closure is called **tertiary intention** or delayed primary closure. The wound heals with a layer of granulation tissue at the edges and base, and several days after the initial wounding, the health care provider brings the wound edges together with sutures or adhesive closures. An example of wound closure by delayed primary closure occurs when a patient has a ruptured appendix. In some cases, the surgeon is unsure whether the appendix had microperforations that caused subsequent spilling of the intestinal contents into the abdomen and wound. Thus, the surgeon leaves the incision open for 4–5 days following surgery and then evaluates the wound. If after 4–5 days there are no clinical signs of infection, the surgeon closes the wound with either adhesive strips or sutures (Doughty and Sparks, 2016).

Wounds heal by one of two mechanisms: partial-thickness wound repair or full-thickness wound repair. Partial-thickness wound repair is necessary when there is loss of only the epidermis and/or part of the dermis such as wound healing by primary intention. Full-thickness wound repair is necessary when there is loss of the epidermis; loss of the dermis; and possible extension into subcutaneous layers, bone, and muscle.

Partial-Thickness Wound Repair

By resurfacing the wound with new epidermal cells, the body repairs wounds that heal by primary intention, shallow wounds that involve loss of only the epidermis and

BOX 17.2 Factors Influencing Wound Healing

Age

- Blood circulation and oxygen delivery to the wound, clotting, and the inflammatory response are sometimes impaired in very young patients and older adult patients. Risk for infection is greater in these populations.
- Cell growth and differentiation in reconstruction are slower with advancing age.
- Scar tissue increases the risk for altered body part function in older adults.
- Age affects all phases of wound healing. A decline in the number of white blood cells places older adults at greater risk for a wound infection. A slowdown in the deposition of collagen in reepithelialization is common.

Scar Tissue

- Scar tissue never regains the tensile strength of noninjured skin, increasing the risk for further tissue injury and altered body part function.

Nutrition Status

- Adequate nutrition status is critical for collagen synthesis, tensile strength, and immune function.
- Tissue repair and infection resistance depend on a balanced diet. Surgery, severe wounds, serious infections, and preoperative nutrition deficits increase nutritional requirements.

Immunosuppression

- The repair process is more susceptible to infection.
- The body's ability to manifest signs of infection is compromised.

Obesity

- Adipose tissue has a poor blood supply.
- Large volume of adipose tissue puts additional stress on incisional lines increasing the risk for dehiscence.
- Risk for infection is increased.

Extent of Wound

- Wounds with extensive tissue loss heal by secondary intention and remain open for a prolonged period of time.
- Sustained wound stress (e.g., vomiting, abdominal distention, coughing) disrupts wound layers and tissue repair.

Tissue Perfusion

- Chronic tissue hypoxia impairs collagen synthesis and reduces tissue resistance to infection.
- Oxygen fuels cellular function needed for tissue repair.
- Smoking reduces oxygenation and thus reduces fibroblast activity.

Diabetes Mellitus and Peripheral Vascular Diseases

- Patients with diabetes mellitus have small-vessel disease that impairs tissue perfusion; thus, oxygen delivery is poor.
- An elevated blood glucose level (hyperglycemia) impairs macrophage function. Risk for infection is increased because of hyperglycemia and poor wound healing.
- Patients with diabetes demonstrate the following problems with wound healing: reduced collagen synthesis, decreased wound strength, and impaired white blood cell functioning. These adverse effects are at least in part caused by poor glycemic control.

Radiation

- Radiation therapy, which eventually results in fibrosis and vascular scarring, interferes with postoperative wound healing when surgery is delayed more than 4–6 weeks and irradiated tissues become fragile and poorly perfused.

Stress

- Stress increases production of corticosteroids, which impedes wound healing.
- The body's ability to show signs of infection is compromised.

Modified from Doughty DB, Sparks B: Wound healing physiology and factors that affect the repair process. In Bryant RA, Nix DP, editors: *Acute and chronic wounds: current management concepts*, ed 5, St Louis, 2016, Mosby.

perhaps some of the dermis. The wounds go through several phases of wound healing, which are described next.

Inflammatory Response

Erythema and edema are the first response, bringing white blood cells (WBCs) to the site. The wounded area appears red and swollen. If the exudate, or discharge, that brings the WBCs to the area is allowed to dry, a scab forms. This response is brief and usually subsides in less than 24 hours (Doughty and Sparks, 2016).

Epidermal Repair

Epidermal cells begin migration across the wound, originating from the epidermal cells at the wound edges or the epidermal appendages. Peak epithelial proliferation occurs 24–72 hours after injury. Wounds kept in a moist environment heal in approximately 4 days, as opposed to 7 days when kept dry because new epithelial cells migrate across a moist surface. If a wound is dry, the cells need to find moisture below the skin surface (Doughty and Sparks, 2016).

Dermal Repair

The epidermis thickens, anchors to adjacent cells, and resumes normal function. The new epidermis is pink, dry, and fragile. If dermal repair is necessary, it occurs concurrently with epidermal repair.

Full-Thickness Wound Repair

Full-thickness wounds involve total loss of the skin layers (epidermis and dermis) and frequently involve the deeper tissue layers as well (subcutaneous tissue, muscle, and bone). A full-thickness wound is either acute (a surgical wound) or chronic (a pressure injury). Healing of a full-thickness acute wound such as a surgical incision proceeds by primary intention; healing of a full-thickness chronic wound such as a pressure injury proceeds by secondary intention. The key events differ between a chronic wound healing by secondary intention and an acute wound healing by primary intention.

Hemostasis Phase

A full-thickness wound healing by primary intention first goes through the hemostasis phase, which controls bleeding. Platelets cause coagulation and vasoconstriction. The platelets break down and release growth factors, which appear to initiate the entire wound-healing process (Beitz, 2016). Bleeding and hemostasis do not occur in wounds healing by secondary intention, thus compromising the repair process (Doughty and Sparks, 2016).

Inflammation Phase

The goal of this phase is to establish a clean wound bed and obtain bacterial balance. The inflammatory response brings WBCs to the area, cleaning up the site and releasing additional growth factors. This phase lasts approximately 3 days in an acute clean wound such as a surgical incision. However, in a chronic wound healing by secondary intention, this phase is prolonged and often lasts longer than 3 days.

Proliferative Phase

The key events in the proliferative phase are production of new tissue, epithelialization, and contraction. In wound healing by primary intention new capillary networks form to provide oxygen and nutrients for new tissue and contribute to the synthesis of collagen. As collagen fibers and capillary networks continue to synthesize and increase in size, the wound begins to contract. The last component of this phase is epithelialization, in which the epithelial cells migrate and cover the defect. Epithelialization occurs faster in a moist environment, supporting the role of moist wound dressings in wound care. In healing by secondary intention in a chronic wound such as a pressure injury, the proliferative phase is prolonged. As granulation tissue forms to fill in the wound bed, it is followed by contraction and epithelialization, the final phase. Contraction is much more important in secondary intention wounds because it reduces the amount of granulation tissue needed to fill the wound bed (Doughty and Sparks, 2016).

Remodeling Phase

The remodeling phase, which lasts up to 1 year, reorganizes the collagen to produce a more elastic, stronger collagen for the scar tissue. The tensile strength of the scar tissue is never more than 80% of the tensile strength in nonwounded tissue (Doughty and Sparks, 2016). The remodeling process is the same for wounds healing by primary intention and secondary intention.

COMPLICATIONS OF WOUND HEALING

Wound healing frequently has complications. When caring for patients with wounds, you need to assess a patient's wound-healing process while observing for complications.

Hemorrhage

Bleeding from an acute wound is normal during and immediately after initial trauma, but **hemostasis,** which is cessation of bleeding by vasoconstriction and coagulation, usually occurs within several minutes. Hemorrhage occurring later possibly indicates a slipped surgical suture, a dislodged clot, infection, or the erosion of a blood vessel by a foreign object (e.g., a drain). Hemorrhage is external or internal. Severe symptoms of internal hemorrhage are hypovolemic shock and swelling of the affected body part. Less severe internal hemorrhage symptoms include a **hematoma,** which is a localized collection of blood under the tissue, often appearing as a bluish swelling or mass. External hemorrhaging is obvious because dressings covering the wound quickly become saturated with blood.

Infection

Bacterial wound infection prevents healing by increasing tissue damage and altering the healing process. The chances of wound infection are greater when the wound contains dead or necrotic tissue, when foreign bodies are in or near the wound, and when the blood supply and local tissue defenses are lower than normal.

A contaminated or traumatic wound infection develops within 2–3 days; a surgical wound infection develops within 4–5 days. Locally, drainage is often yellow, green, or brown and may be odorous, depending on the causative organism. The wound edges appear tense, swollen, and painful, with redness extending beyond the immediate wound edge. Systemic signs include fever, general malaise, and an elevated WBC count.

Dehiscence

When an acute wound fails to heal properly, the layers of skin and tissue separate. This most commonly occurs before collagen formation (3–11 days after injury). **Dehiscence** is the partial or total separation of layers of skin and tissue above the fascia in a wound that is not healing properly. Patients who are obese have a high risk for dehiscence because of constant strain on their wounds and the poor vascularity of fatty tissue. It occurs most often in abdominal surgical wounds after a sudden strain such as coughing, vomiting, or sitting up in bed. Patients often report feeling as though something has given way. When serosanguineous drainage increases from a wound, be alert for dehiscence.

Evisceration

Evisceration occurs when wound layers separate below the fascial layer and visceral organs protrude through the wound opening. It is a medical emergency requiring placement of sterile towels soaked in sterile saline over the extruding tissues to reduce chances of bacterial invasion and drying before surgical repair occurs.

CARE FOR PRESSURE ULCERS

Assessment

Baseline Assessment

Baseline and continual focused assessment data provide critical information about a patient's skin integrity and the increased risk for pressure injury development or impaired wound healing (Table 17.2). Although multiple factors affect skin integrity, it is important that you identify and assess the factors relevant for your patients.

Pressure Ulcer Risk Assessment

Pressure ulcer risk assessment must be done using agency-approved skin assessment tools (Table 17.1) and perform assessment of a patient for risk of development of pressure injuries on admission to the hospital, 24–48 hours after admission, at regular intervals, and when there is a significant change in a patient's condition.

Skin Assessment

Assessment for tissue pressure damage includes visual and tactile inspection of the skin. Baseline assessment determines a patient's normal skin characteristics and any actual or potential areas of breakdown. This is especially important with high-risk patients such as patients with diabetes, stroke, or serious malnutrition. Note the presence of medical devices such as a nasogastric (NG) tube, oxygen equipment, and artificial airways and areas exposed to casts, traction, or splints (Pittman et al., 2015). In addition, the skin of an older adult patient is more fragile and has an increased risk for skin breakdown (Box 17.3).

Assess all areas of the skin from head to toe, paying attention to any reddened areas or breaks in skin integrity. Document the assessment. When you notice hyperemia, document location, size, and color, and reassess the area after 1 hour. If you suspect nonblanchable hyperemia, outline the affected area with a marker to make reassessment easier. Nonblanchable hyperemia is an early indicator of impaired skin integrity, but damage to the underlying tissue is sometimes more progressive. Palpate the tissues next to the observed area to gather further data about **induration** (hardening of tissue caused by edema or inflammation) and damage to the skin and underlying tissues.

Table 17.2 Focused Patient Assessment

Factors to Assess	Questions	Physical Assessment
Adequacy of patient's sensory perception	Do you feel me pinching the skin on your left hip? Can you feel me rubbing your left lower leg?	Apply painful stimuli to various body locations. If the patient is unable to respond by affirming that he or she feels the stimuli, the patient has limited sensory perception.
Moisture	Does the bed sheet under your buttocks feel moist?	Routinely observe the patient's bed linens for moisture. Observe the patient's skin, noting whether it is dry (rarely moist) or seldom damp (occasionally moist) or whether the skin is often but not always wet (moist). Observe for wound drainage.
Activity	Can you get out of bed by yourself to use the toilet? Are you able to get out of the bed or chair by yourself? Are you able to change your position in bed by yourself?	Check whether the patient is incontinent of urine and stool. Assess the patient's ability to walk at least once every 2 h while awake (walks frequently) or whether the patient is able to ambulate only short distances and whether assistance is needed. Observe whether the patient is able to independently change positions in bed.
Nutrition	Were you able to eat the entire tray of food at mealtime? Assess last two meals. Are you hungry at mealtime?	Observe patient eating: Does the patient need assistance? Assess amount of food the patient eats at meals for adequate nutrition, such as whether the patient finishes over half of meals or is on tube feedings or TPN.
Friction and shear	When you are sitting up in the bed, do you find that you slide down toward the foot of the bed? Do you need assistance in moving up in bed or chair?	Assess whether the patient moves in bed and chair independently and maintains a good position at all times. Determine whether the patient requires any assistance in moving up in bed and/or chair.

TPN, total parenteral nutrition.

BOX 17.3 Care of an Older Adult

Issues Related to Skin Integrity

- There is decreased barrier function and less protection from excessive moisture, shear, friction, and pressure.
- Aging skin experiences decreased epidermal turnover; thus, healing requires more time.
- The dermis is not as thick and the skin over the legs and arms is especially thin. This predisposes an older adult's skin to tearing.
- Decreased subcutaneous tissue reduces padding protection over bony prominences.
- There is decreased inflammatory reaction and more susceptibility to infection.
- Sensory perception is reduced; thus, ability to detect pain on initial injury is lessened.

Data from Wysocki A: Anatomy and physiology of skin and soft tissue. In Bryant RA, Nix DP, editors: *Acute and chronic wounds: current management concepts,* ed 5, St Louis, 2016, Mosby.

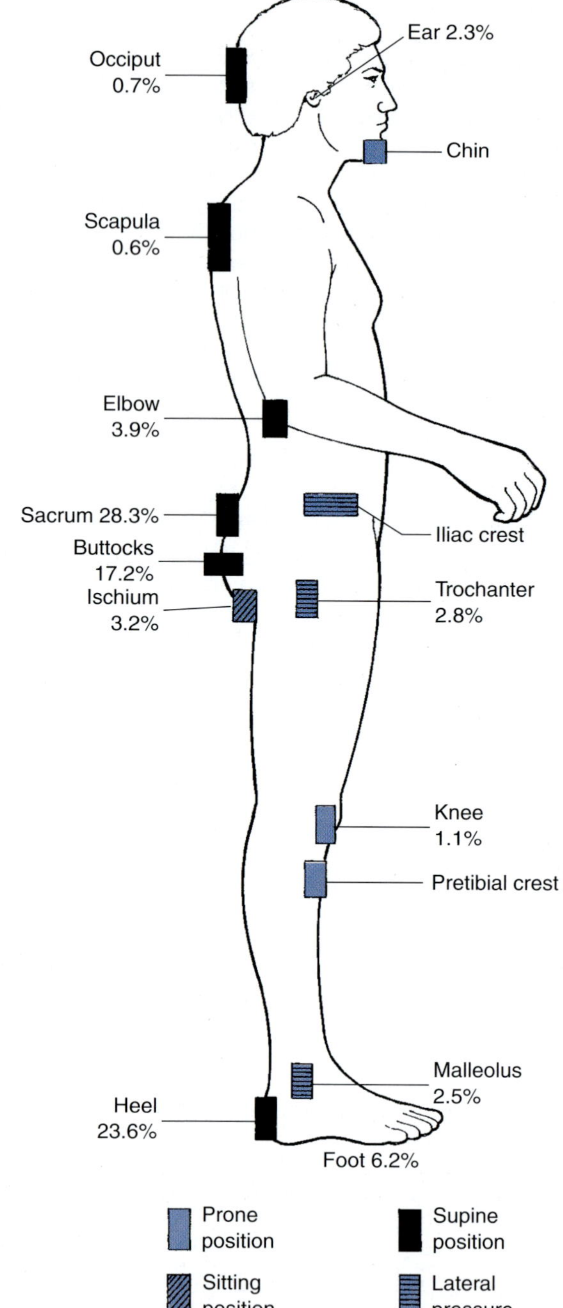

Fig. 17.5 Sites for pressure injuries and frequency of ulceration per site. Note that sites for device-related pressure injuries, which may not involve bony prominences, are not included. (Data from VanGilder C, et al: Results of the 2008–2009 International Pressure Ulcer Prevalence Survey and a 3-year, acute care, unit specific analysis, *Ostomy Wound Manage* 55(11):39, 2009. In Bryant RA, Nix DP: *Acute and chronic wounds: current management concepts,* ed 5, St Louis, 2016, Elsevier.)

Assess patients with lightly pigmented skin for blanching with return to normal skin tones. Also note changes in color, temperature, and hardness of the surrounding skin and tissues. Use visual and tactile inspection over the body areas most frequently at risk for pressure injury development. Pressure injuries occur most commonly over bony prominences such as the sacrum, ischial tuberosity, and trochanter. In addition, the skin under medical devices, such as endotracheal tubes, oxygen tubing, casts, traction, and splints, is also at risk. When a patient lies in bed or sits in a chair, pressure occurs over bony prominences. Body surfaces subjected to the greatest weight or pressure such as the sacrum or ischium are at increased risk for pressure injury formation (Fig. 17.5).

Mobility Assessment

Assessment includes documenting level of mobility, the potential effects of impaired mobility on skin integrity, and data regarding the quality of muscle tone and strength. For example, determine whether a patient is able to lift the weight off the ischial tuberosities and roll to a side-lying position. Some patients have adequate range of motion to independently move into a more protective position, but others do not. Finally, assess the patient's activity tolerance (see Chapter 14).

Nutrition Status Assessment

Malnutrition is associated with overall morbidity and mortality. Perform a nutrition assessment when a patient enters a new health care setting and whenever there is a change in the patient's condition (Box 17.4) (see Chapter 20) (WOCN Society, 2016). Inadequate caloric intake causes weight loss and a decrease in subcutaneous tissue, allowing bony prominences to compress and restrict circulation. Assess nutrition status using a variety of approaches (e.g., monitoring intake and output, completing a 3-day calorie count, assessing serum albumin) to identify patients who need nutrition support.

Assessment of Wounds

Assessment of a patient's wound varies from one health care setting to another. Consistent wound assessment over time reveals patterns and trends that indicate improvement or deterioration in a wound (Nix, 2016).

Health Promotion

Early identification of patients' risk factors helps prevent pressure injuries. Prevention minimizes the effect of risk factors and contributing factors on pressure injury development

BOX 17.4 Nutrition Assessment and Management of Pressure Injuries: Wound, Ostomy and Continence Nurses (WOCN) Society Recommendations

Screen for nutritional deficiencies at admission to care setting and whether the patient's condition changes (see Chapter 20). Include the following parameters in assessment:

- Current and usual weight
- History of unintentional weight loss or gain: 5% or more in 30 days or 10% or more in 180 days
- Nutritional intake versus needs, incorporating protein, calorie, and fluid needs
- Adequacy of nutritional intake (i.e., calories, protein, and fluid)
- Signs of dehydration (i.e., skin turgor, urine output, elevated sodium)
- Medical/surgical history or interventions that influence nutritional intake or absorption of nutrients
- Psychosocial factors affecting food intake: ability to obtain and pay for food, facilities for cooking and environment for eating, and food preferences

Data from Wound, Ostomy and Continence Nurses (WOCN) Society: *Guideline for prevention and management of pressure ulcers,* WOCN Clinical Practice Guidelines Series, Mount Laurel, NJ, 2016, The Society.

(see Box 17.1). Nursing interventions for prevention of pressure injuries include positioning, topical skin care, nutrition support, and the use of support surfaces.

Positioning

Repositioning is moving a patient to another position to relieve pressure off a particular part of the body or to redistribute the pressure on a body part (Maklebust and Magnan, 2016). Positioning interventions reduce pressure (Box 17.5). Repositioning frequency is determined by tissue tolerance, level of activity and mobility, general medical condition, overall treatment objectives, and support surface (European Pressure Ulcer Advisory Panel [EPUAP] and National Pressure Ulcer Advisory Panel [NPUAP], 2014). Therefore, a standard turning interval of 1–2 hours does not prevent pressure injury development in some patients. The WOCN Society (2016) recommends reducing shear by maintaining the elevation of the head of the bed at 30° or less for the supine position, using assistive devices when turning or transferring patients, and using the 30° lateral position (Fig. 17.6).

When a patient can sit in a chair, reposition the patient every hour and limit sitting to 2 hours (EPUAP and NPUAP, 2014). In the sitting position, the pressure on the ischial tuberosities is greater than when in the supine position. In addition, assist or teach patients with the ability to shift weight to reposition every 15 minutes. The patient should sit on gel or an air cushion to redistribute weight, decreasing the amount of weight on the ischial tuberosities.

A patient's heels are an area of concern because of the small surface area (Fig. 17.7). Keep heels off the bed by using a pillow, support surfaces, and heel suspension devices to float the heels. When using pillows, position them under the calf muscle with slight knee flexion while preventing the heels from contacting the bed surface (Bryant and Nix, 2016a).

BOX 17.5 Wound, Ostomy and Continence Nurses (WOCN) Society Recommendations for Pressure Reduction and Relief

- Use turn sheets, trapeze bars, and lift equipment to help with mobility.
- Maintain elevation of the head of the bed to 30° or less for the supine position to prevent shear and subsequent tissue injury.
- Reposition and turn regularly and frequently.
- Use positioning devices to avoid placing the patient on the pressure injury or other areas at risk for pressure injury.
- When side lying, use a 30° laterally inclined position to relieve pressure over the trochanter.
- Continue to turn and reposition the patient when support surfaces are in use.

Data adapted from Wound, Ostomy and Continence Nurses Society: *Guideline for prevention and management of pressure ulcers,* WOCN Clinical Practice Guidelines Series, Mount Laurel, NJ, 2016, The Society.

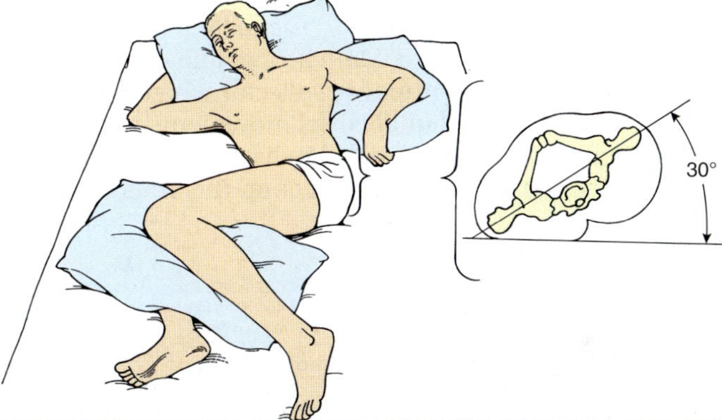

Fig. 17.6 Thirty-degree lateral position. (Adapted from Bryant RA, Nix DP: *Acute and chronic wounds: current management concepts,* ed 5, St Louis, 2016, Elsevier.)

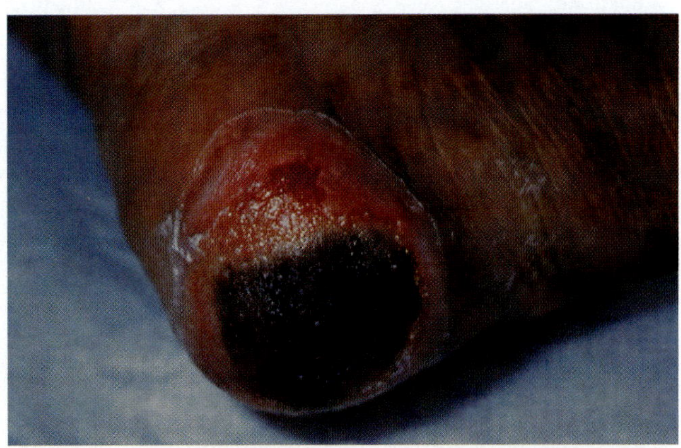

Fig. 17.7 Formation of pressure injury on heel resulting from external pressure from mattress of bed. (Courtesy Janice Colwell, RN, MS, CWOCN, FAAN, Clinical Nurse Specialist, University of Chicago Medicine.)

Topical Skin Care

Assess the skin daily, paying special attention to bony prominences. Do not massage reddened areas because reddened areas indicate tissue injury. Massage to these areas further injures the tissue by causing damage to the tissue capillaries. Examine your patient's skin for signs of dryness, cracking, edema, or excessive moisture.

Use a mild cleansing agent when cleansing intact skin. Soap causes dryness, which increases the risk for skin infection. Skin lubrication helps keep the skin intact; consider using a moisturizer on a routine basis (WOCN Society, 2016). Because intact skin is the initial defense for preventing skin breakdown, keep your patient's skin clean and dry. Many types of products are available for skin care; match their uses to the specific needs of your patient.

Use an incontinence cleanser for a patient who is incontinent of stool or urine. To protect the skin, apply a moisture-barrier product (generally petrolatum or dimethicone based) liberally to the exposed area. The moisture barrier provides skin protection from the irritating effects of stool or urine and allows you to clean the next incontinent episode easily. Apply the moisture-barrier ointment after each cleansing. For skin that has become exposed or stripped from incontinence, use a barrier paste that adheres to the irritated area and will not be removed with each cleansing. Offer a patient frequent access to the toilet to prevent fecal and urinary incontinence. You can contain fecal incontinence with a fecal incontinence collector when a patient is experiencing frequent liquid bowel movements and has intact perianal skin. An adhesive skin barrier is attached to a drainable pouch that is applied around the anus to collect liquid stool. Other external collection devices include male external catheters applied to the shaft of the penis to collect urine.

When providing skin care to a patient who is incontinent, the health care team first assesses and treats the cause of the incontinence and then decides on protection and/or collection interventions. Underpads and diapers can protect skin in patients incontinent of stool and urine. Avoid using underpads and diapers with a plastic outer lining that holds moisture against the skin, which causes **maceration** (softening of the skin caused by moisture) (WOCN Society, 2016). Instead, select underpads or diapers that are absorbent and wick incontinence moisture away from the skin rather than trap it against the skin.

Support Surfaces

Support surfaces redistribute pressure exerted over bony prominences by maximizing contact (allowing the body to touch the entire surface) and redistributing weight over a large area. They also often reduce shear, friction, and moisture. Support surfaces include mattresses, overlays, framed specialty beds, chair pads, table pads, and crib mattresses or pads (Table 17.3).

Use the WOCN Society's evidence- and consensus-based support surface algorithm (Fig. 17.8) to help you select the best support system for your patients (McNichol et al., 2015). Make sure that there are minimal layers of bed linens between your patient and the support surface to keep your patient as close as possible to the surface for it to be effective. Remember, even when using a support surface, you still need to reposition your patient. Once a support surface is in use, reevaluate patients on a frequent

Table 17.3 Support Surfaces

Category and Mechanism of Action	Indications for Use	Advantages	Disadvantages
SUPPORT SURFACES AND OVERLAYS			
Foam Overlay (Available as an Overlay or in a Full Mattress)			
Reduces pressure; the cover (top) can reduce friction and shear. Base height of 7.5–10 cm (3–4 inches); see manufacturer guidelines regarding amount of body weight supported.	Use for patients with moderate-to-high risk.	One-time charge No setup fee Cannot be punctured Available in various sizes (e.g., bed, chair, operating room table) Little maintenance Does not need electricity	Elevated body temperature Hot and may trap moisture Limited life span Plastic protective sheet needed for incontinent patients or patients with draining wounds Not indicated for patients with existing Stage 3 or Stage 4 pressure injuries
Water Overlay (Available as an Overlay or in a Full Mattress)			
Reduces pressure and pressure points because surface provides flotation with pressure reduction by redistributing patient's weight evenly over entire support surface.	Use for patients with high risk.	Readily available Some control over motion sensations Easy to clean	Easily punctured Heavy Fluid motion may make procedures (e.g., dressing changes, CPR) difficult Maintenance needed to prevent microorganism growth Patient transfers out of bed are difficult Difficult to raise and lower head of bed
Gel Overlay			
Reduces pressure and pressure points because surface provides flotation by redistributing patient's weight evenly over entire support surface.	Use for patients with moderate-to-high risk. Use for patients who are wheelchair dependent.	Low maintenance Easy to clean Multiple-patient use Impermeable to needle punctures	Heavy Expensive Lacks airflow for moisture control Variable friction control

Table 17.3 Support Surfaces—cont'd

Category and Mechanism of Action	Indications for Use	Advantages	Disadvantages
Nonpowered Support Surface			
Reduces pressure by lowering mean interface pressure between patient's tissue and mattress.	Use for patients with moderate-to-high risk. Use for patients who can reposition themselves.	Easy to clean Multiple-patient use Low maintenance Potential repair of some air-filled products Durable	Damaged by punctures from needles and sharps Requires routine monitoring to determine adequate inflation pressure Patient transfers out of bed are difficult
Low-Air-Loss Overlay (Available as an Overlay or in a Full Mattress)			
Maintains constant and slight air movement against patient's skin, also assists in managing heat and humidity (microclimate) of the skin.	Use for patients with moderate-to-high risk.	Easy to clean Maintains constant inflation Deflates to facilitate transfer and CPR Moisture control Fabric covering overlay is air permeable, bacteria impermeable, and waterproof Reduces shear and friction Setup provided by manufacturer	Damaged by needles and sharps Noisy Requires electricity, but some are available with short backup battery In home, may need to purchase backup generator in case of loss of electrical power
SPECIALTY BEDS			
Air-Fluidized Bed			
Bed frame contains silicone-coated beads and provides pressure redistribution by the fluidlike medium that is created by forcing air through beads resulting in immersion and envelopment of patient.	Use for patients at high risk. Use for patients with Stage 3 or Stage 4 pressure injuries or burns.	Less frequent turning or repositioning Improved patient comfort Quickly becomes firm for CPR or other treatments when device is turned "off" Reduces shear, friction, and edema to site May facilitate management of copious wound drainage or incontinence Setup provided by manufacturer	Continuous circulation of warm, dry air may increase patient risk for dehydration Possible increase in room temperature Patient may experience disorientation Patient transfer difficult Heavy Expensive May not be wide enough for use with obese patients or patients with contractures Patient cannot lie prone because of risk of suffocation
Low-Air-Loss Bed			
Bed frame with series of connected air-filled pillows. Flow of air controls the amount of pressure in each pillow and assists in managing heat and humidity (microclimate) of the patient's skin.	Use for patients who need pressure relief, who cannot be repositioned frequently, or who have skin breakdown on more than one surface. Contraindicated in patients with unstable spinal column.	Can raise and lower head and foot of bed Easy transfer in and out of bed Less frequent turning schedule Pillows can be transferred to stretcher with patient Setup provided by manufacturer	Portable motor is noisy Bed surface material is slippery; patients can easily slide down mattress or out of bed when being transferred
Kinetic Therapy			
Provides continuous passive motion to promote mobilization of pulmonary secretions and low air loss, which provides pressure relief.	Use primarily for patients needing spinal stabilization. Should not be used when the patient is hemodynamically unstable.	Reduces pulmonary complications associated with restricted mobility Reduces risk for urinary stasis and urinary tract infections Reduces venous stasis	Does not reduce shear or moisture Cannot be used with cervical or skeletal traction Possible motion sickness initially Possible sensations of claustrophobia

CPR, cardiopulmonary resuscitation.
Data from Doughty D, McNichol L: *Wound, Ostomy, and Continence Nurses Society core curriculum: wound management,* Philadelphia, PA 2016, Wolters Kluwer; and Wound Ostomy and Continence Nurses (WOCN) Society: *Guideline for prevention and management of pressure ulcers,* WOCN Clinical Practice Guidelines Series, Mount Laurel, NJ, 2016, The Society.

basis to determine the continued need and the effectiveness of the product. Patient and caregiver education on the importance and use of the support product is essential (Box 17.6).

Nutrition

Nutrition is fundamental to normal cell activity and tissue repair and regeneration. Although nutrition is important for all patients, it is of particular importance for a patient with a wound to prevent severe or prolonged depletion of nutrients that can impact healing (Stotts, 2016b). Complete a nutrition assessment on a patient who has a wound, collecting important data such as relevant patient history and laboratory data. Normal wound healing requires adequate intake of protein, fat, and carbohydrates. Consider consulting with a registered dietitian to obtain a thorough evaluation of a patient's nutrition status and identify related interventions to improve nutritional intake. The nutritional assessment and management of pressure injures provided by WOCN may also be referred (Box 17.4).

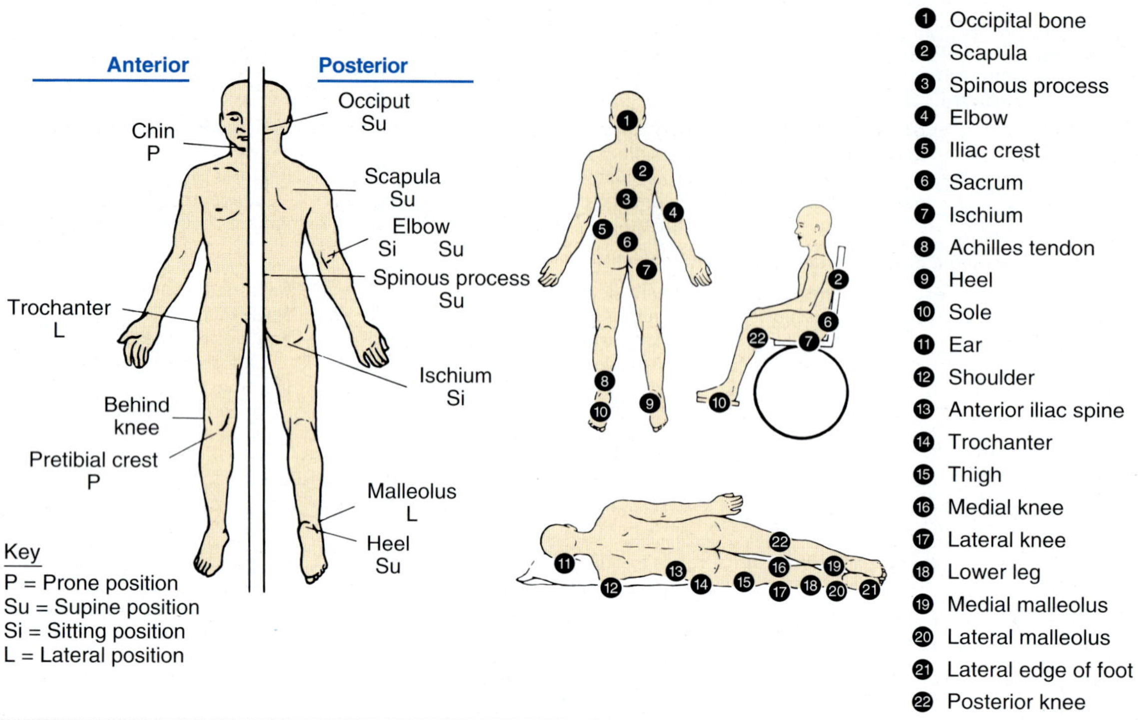

Fig. 17.8 Wound, Ostomy and Continence Nurses (WOCN) Society evidence- and consensus-based support surface algorithm. (From Trelease CC: Developing standards for wound care, *Ostomy Wound Manage* 20:46, 1988.)

BOX 17.6 Guidelines for Patient Education Regarding Therapeutic Surfaces

- Explain the rationale for use of support surfaces. Be sure that the patient and family caregiver know that this reduces pressure on the bony prominences by redistributing pressure between the surface and patient's skin.
- Teach the patient and family caregiver the importance of using minimal layers of linen or absorbent pads between patient and surface.
- Explain the importance of frequent position changes even while on the support surfaces.
- Demonstrate to the patient and family caregiver how to shift weight while on support surface.
- Demonstrate to the patient and family caregiver how to use the 30° angle lateral position and pillows to support various positions.

Management of Pressure Ulcers

Address wound-management principles in an orderly fashion (Box 17.7). Provide appropriate wound management including managing pressure, shear, friction, and moisture (see Skill 17.1). Provide systemic support to enhance your patient's wound healing. Comorbidities such as cardiovascular or pulmonary disease decrease the amount of oxygen-rich hemoglobin available for delivery to injured tissue. Oxygen is necessary for wound healing and resistance to infection. Interventions that maximize oxygen levels include pulmonary hygiene interventions and administering low-flow supplemental oxygen (see Chapter 24).

BOX 17.7 Wound-Healing Principles

- Control or eliminate causative factors.
  - Offload pressure.
  - Reduce friction and shear.
  - Protect from moisture.
- Provide systemic support to reduce existing and potential cofactors.
  - Optimize nutrition.
  - Provide adequate hydration.
  - Reduce edema.
  - Control blood glucose levels.
- Maintain physiological wound environment.
  - Prevent and manage infection.
  - Cleanse wound.
  - Remove nonviable tissue (debridement).
  - Maintain appropriate level of moisture.
  - Eliminate dead space.
  - Control odor.
  - Eliminate or minimize pain.
  - Protect periwound skin

From Bryant RA, Nix DP: Topical management. In Bryant RA, Nix, DP, editors: *Acute and chronic wounds: current management concepts,* ed 5, St Louis, 2016, Elsevier.

Wound healing also depends on adequate nutrition. Protein intake is necessary to support the development of new blood vessels and collagen synthesis. Carbohydrates, fats, and vitamins provide energy for cellular function. Interventions to support adequate nutrition intake include a nutrition referral and appropriate dietary supplements.

Certain medications (e.g., steroids) and medical conditions (e.g., diabetes) negatively influence wound healing.

Because hyperglycemia impairs wound healing, blood glucose control is essential.

A stable wound environment and appropriate treatment are necessary to promote healing (Table 17.4). To maintain an environment to support healing, it is important to control infection, **debride** (remove) necrotic tissue, provide exudate management, control dead space, and provide wound protection. Assess a patient with a pressure injury for signs and symptoms of a wound infection such as redness, warmth of surrounding tissue, odor, and the presence of exudate. If any of these signs is present, consult with the health care team to determine whether you need to culture the wound and whether systemic or topical antibiotics are indicated.

Cleanse pressure injuries at each dressing change to remove wound debris from the wound surface (WOCN Society, 2016). Cleanse dirty wounds by irrigation. Clean wounds require gentle flushing with normal saline solution.

Necrotic tissue slows wound healing because it is a source for infection and a barrier for epithelialization. After consulting with a health care provider or wound care specialist, plan a method of debridement. Types of debridement include mechanical, chemical, sharp, and autolytic (Ramundo, 2016).

A moist wound environment supports wound healing; however, excessive wound moisture macerates the wound edges, which puts the wound at risk for increasing in size and interferes with wound healing. Select a dressing that absorbs excessive moisture while providing the wound with necessary hydration. Eliminate dead space by loosely filling all cavities with dressings. Lightly fill wound cavities to support the growth of granulation tissue and discourage infection. Overfilling a wound with gauze places pressure within the wound bed and prevents development of granulation tissue.

Involve a patient's family or caregiver in management of pressure injuries and their treatment. Frequently patients require dressing changes after discharge. A patient's family or caregiver is an excellent source for dressing support and identification of possible wound-healing complications (Box 17.8).

Table 17.4 Treatment Options by Pressure Injury Stage

Injury Stage	Injury Status	Dressing	Comments[a]	Expected Change	Treatments
1	Intact	None	Allows visual assessment.	Resolves slowly without epidermal loss over 7–14 days.	Turning schedule. Support hydration. Nutrition support. Pressure redistribution mattress or chair cushion.
		Transparent dressing	Protects from shear. Do not use in the presence of excessive moisture.		
		Hydrocolloid	Does not allow visual assessment.		
2	Clean, granular base	Composite film	Limits shear.	Heals through reepithelialization.	See previous stage. Manage incontinence.
		Hydrocolloid	Change when seal of dressing breaks, maximal wear time 7 days.		
		Hydrogel	Provides moist environment.		
3	Clean, granular base	Hydrocolloid	Change when seal of dressing breaks, maximum wear time 7 days. Apply over wound to protect and absorb moisture.	Heals through granulation and reepithelialization.	See previous stages. Evaluate pressure redistribution needs.
		Hydrogel covered with foam	Apply over wound to protect and absorb moisture.		
		Calcium alginate	Use when there is significant exudate. Cover with secondary dressing.		
		Gauze	Use with normal saline or other prescribed solution. Wring out excess solution; unfold to make contact with wound.		
		Growth factors	Used with gauze per manufacturer instructions		
4	Clean	Hydrogel covered with foam dressing	See Stage 3, clean.	Heals through granulation and reepithelialization.	Surgical consultation often necessary for closure. See Stages 1, 2, and 3.
		Calcium alginate	Used with significant exudate; must cover with secondary dressing.		
		Gauze	See Stage 3, clean.		
Unstageable	Wound covered with eschar	Adherent film	Facilitates softening of eschar.	Eschar lifts at edges as healing progresses.	See previous stages. Surgical consultation may be considered for debridement.
		Gauze plus ordered solution	Delivers solution and wicks wound drainage.	Eschar softens.	
		Enzymes	Breaks down eschar, providing debridement.	Eschar loosens over time.	
		None	Rarely, if eschar is dry and intact, no dressing is used, allowing eschar to act as physiological cover.		

[a]As with *all* occlusive dressings, wounds should *not* be clinically infected.

BOX 17.8 Patient Teaching

Pressure Injury Dressing Change

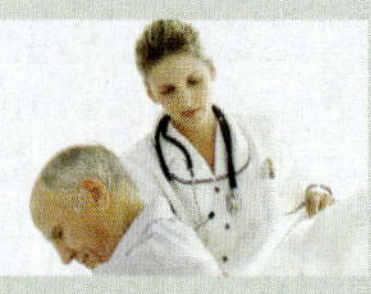

In preparation for Mr Manoj's discharge, RN Sangeetha develops a teaching plan for Mrs Manoj to teach her how to change Mr Manoj's pressure injury dressing.

Outcome

At the end of the teaching session, Mrs Manoj changes Mr Manoj's dressing correctly.

Teaching Strategies

- Avoid using words and medical terminology that Mrs Manoj will not understand.
- Provide a brief description of what you will teach. Include Mr Manoj in all the teaching, even though he is unable to see the wound.
- Bring an extra dressing to the bedside to show Mr and Mrs Manoj what the dressing looks like; explain how it works and how to apply it.
- Use pictures of a pressure injury to help Mrs Manoj understand what the wound looks like and how it will change in appearance as it heals or worsens.
- Allow Mrs Manoj to watch at least one demonstration of you cleansing the wound and applying the dressing.
- Have Mrs Manoj change the dressing with your supervision, allowing for return demonstrations.

Evaluation

- Use the principles of teach back to evaluate the patient/family caregiver leaning:
  - While observing Mrs Manoj changing the dressing, ask her, "Explain the steps you are taking to clean the wound and change the dressing."
  - "Tell me what information about the wound you need to report to the home health nurse."

MANAGEMENT OF WOUNDS

First Aid for Wounds

When a patient sustains a traumatic wound, first-aid interventions include promoting hemostasis, cleansing the wound, and protecting the wound from further injury.

Hemostasis

After assessing the type and extent of the wound, control bleeding from a laceration by applying direct pressure to the wound with a sterile or clean dressing. After bleeding subsides, an adhesive dressing strip or gauze dressing taped over the laceration allows skin edges to close and a blood clot to form. If a dressing becomes saturated with blood, add another layer of dressing, continue to apply pressure, and elevate the affected part. A health care provider sutures serious lacerations in an emergency clinic or hospital.

If a penetrating object such as a knife blade is in a patient's body, do not remove the object. Removal causes massive, uncontrolled bleeding. Apply pressure by rolling sterile gauze taped in place around the object but not on it or on surrounding tissues.

Cleansing

Gentle cleansing of a wound removes contaminants that serve as sources of infection. However, vigorous cleaning causes bleeding or further injury. For abrasions, minor lacerations, and small puncture wounds, rinse the wound in running water, gently cleanse with mild soap and water, rinse, and apply an over-the-counter antiseptic. When a laceration is bleeding profusely, only brush away surface contaminants and concentrate on hemostasis until the patient reaches a clinic or hospital.

Protection

Protect a wound by applying a sterile or clean dressing and immobilize the body part. A light dressing applied over minor wounds prevents entrance of microorganisms. In the case of small abrasions, it is acceptable to leave the wound open to air so that a scab forms.

The more extensive the wound, the larger the dressing required. In a home emergency, a clean towel or diaper is often the best dressing. A bulky dressing applied with pressure minimizes movement of underlying tissues and helps to immobilize the entire body part. A dressing or cloth wrapped around a penetrating object immobilizes it adequately.

Dressings

The use of dressings requires an understanding of wound healing and factors influencing healing. A variety of dressing materials are available commercially. The choice of dressing and how it is applied influence wound healing. The proper dressing does not allow a full-thickness wound to become dry with scab formation. When this occurs, the dermis dehydrates and crusts. As a result, a barrier forms against normal epidermal cell growth, slowing wound healing. Furthermore, dryness increases discomfort. Ideally, a dressing provides a moist environment to promote normal epidermal cell migration. The proper dressing also absorbs drainage to prevent bacterial growth and wound drainage from coming in contact with intact skin.

For surgical wounds that heal by primary intention, dressings are commonly removed as soon as drainage stops. Frequently, the health care provider removes the dressing 24–48 hours after surgery, which coincides with initial epithelialization.

Purposes of Dressing

A dressing serves several purposes. It minimizes exposure to microorganisms. In wounds with minimal drainage, the natural formation of a fibrin seal eliminates the need for a dressing. A pressure dressing promotes hemostasis by exerting localized, downward pressure over an actual or potential bleeding site. A moist dressing lightly packed into the wound fosters normal healing by eliminating dead space in underlying tissues. Assess skin color, temperature, pulses in distal extremities, patient comfort, and any changes in sensation to ensure that dressings do not interfere with circulation.

A dry dressing promotes healing by allowing the wound to heal by primary intention and absorbing minimal oozing of wound drainage. When a wound is healing by secondary intention, use a dressing to provide a moist environment. Moisten the gauze with a solution, usually normal saline, wring it out, and unfold and lightly pack it into the wound. The purpose of a moist gauze dressing is to act as a sponge, absorbing excessive wound drainage while providing a moist environment. Change the dressing when it is saturated or if it begins to dry out. Always cover a moist dressing with a dry, secondary dressing.

A firmly taped or wrapped dressing supports or immobilizes a body part, minimizing movement of the underlying incision and traumatized tissues. Finally, a dressing promotes thermal insulation to the wound surface and protects it from the dehydrating effects of air.

Type of Dressing

Dressings vary by type of material and mode of application (dry or moist). Gauze is the most common dressing type. It does not interact with wound tissue and thus causes little wound irritation. It is available in different textures and shapes such as square, rectangle, and rolls of various lengths and widths. Moist or dry gauze dressings are best for wounds with moderate drainage, deep wounds, undermining, and tunnels. Saturate a moist gauze dressing with the prescribed solution, wring it out, then open and place it onto the wound tissue. The moistened gauze increases the ability of the dressing to absorb exudate. Cover the moist gauze with a secondary layer of dry gauze. Be sure that the moist gauze does not cover normal skin to prevent maceration. The moist dressing is changed on a scheduled basis to prevent drying of the gauze.

Transparent film dressings are clear sheets coated on one side with an adhesive. The adhesive side does not stick to the wound because of the moisture and traps moisture over the wound bed, providing a moist environment. The film is impermeable to fluid but semipermeable to oxygen. This type of dressing is used as a primary dressing in wounds with minimal tissue loss that have very little wound drainage. The dressing is applied to extend approximately 1½ inches beyond the wound to allow for adherence. Change the dressing when the seal is broken.

Hydrocolloid dressings are made of gelling agents and have an adhesive wound surface. They come in a variety of sizes and shapes and are used to cover wounds, extending the hydrocolloid dressing at least 1½ inches beyond the wound margin. Hydrocolloids form a gel as they interact with the wound surface. Because they are occlusive, they protect the wound from surface contaminants, and you can leave them over a wound for several days. When removed, you will note a gel over the wound base; the gel maintains a moist environment to support healing and washes away during wound cleansing.

Hydrogel dressings are available in sheets, spray bottles, or a gel in a tube (amorphous). They contain a high percentage of water and are used when wounds require moisture—either a wound with granulation (maintaining the moist wound environment needed for healing) or a wound that has a high percentage of necrotic tissue (the hydrogel facilitates debridement by softening the dead tissue). Hydrogels maintain moisture in some wounds for 1–3 days.

Alginate dressings are highly absorptive dressings made of spun fibers of seaweed. They absorb and hold exudate, maintain a moist environment, and are available in sheets or ropes. They are indicated for moderately to highly exudative wounds (Bryant and Nix, 2016b).

Negative-pressure wound therapy (NPWT) uses a combination dressing (foam and transparent film) with negative pressure via suction to help wound healing (Fig. 17.9). NPWT supports wound healing by evacuating wound fluids, stimulating granulation tissue formation, reducing the bacterial burden of a wound, and maintaining a moist wound environment (Netsch et al., 2016). Before applying NPWT, assess your patient's level of comfort. Some patients may require analgesia.

Apply NPWT by fitting the foam or dressing to the shape of the wound and placing a drainage/suction tube in the interior or on top of the dressing. Seal the dressing and the tube with a transparent dressing and connect the tube to a prescribed amount of negative pressure, which creates suction. The suction pulls all air out of the wound and creates an airtight seal. This therapy provides removal of excess wound fluid to stimulate granulation tissue and decrease wound bacteria (see Skill 17.2). Connect the suction tubing to a container that collects the wound fluid. NPWT is changed on a scheduled basis, usually every 48 hours. Current evidence shows that this therapy often reduces healing time in chronic wounds and results in early grafting of wounds (Netsch et al., 2016).

Changing Dressings

To prepare to change a dressing, you need to know the type of dressing, any underlying drains used, and the type of supplies needed for wound care. You adjust the type and amount of dressings if the amount of drainage changes or a wound becomes deeper. Notifying the health care provider of any change is essential.

The order for changing a dressing usually indicates the dressing type, frequency of changing, and solution or ointment you will apply. An order to "reinforce dressing prn" (add dressings without removing existing ones as needed) is

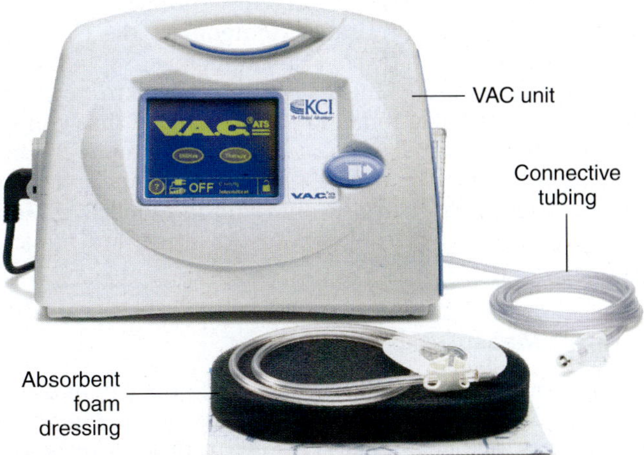

Fig. 17.9 The vacuum-assisted closure (VAC) ATS negative-pressure wound therapy system. *(Top to bottom)* VAC system, connective tubing to go between VAC system and dressing, absorbent foam dressing. (Courtesy KCI Licensing, San Antonio, TX.)

common immediately after surgery when a health care provider does not want accidental disruption of the suture line or loss of hemostasis. A patient's medical or operating room record usually reveals whether drains are present. After the initial dressing change, communicate on the care plan the type of dressing materials and solutions to use and the type and location of drains. Skill 17.3 outlines the steps for applying moist saline dressings.

Use aseptic technique during dressing change procedures (see Chapter 9). It is also essential for a patient to understand the steps of the procedure beforehand to reduce anxiety. Describe normal signs of the healing process and answer questions about the procedure or wound.

If a patient needs to care for a wound at home, demonstrate dressing changes and provide an opportunity for the patient and family caregiver to practice. In the home, patients and family caregivers usually need to learn clean technique. Make sure that the patient is able to change a dressing independently or with assistance from a family caregiver before discharge unless home care will be provided.

Securing Dressings

Use tape, ties, or cloth binders to secure a dressing over a wound site. **Binders** are dressings made of large pieces of material to fit a specific body part. An arm sling is an example of a binder. A binder reduces stress on a wound.

The choice of anchoring depends on wound size, location, drainage, frequency of dressing changes, and patient's level of activity. You most often use tape to secure dressings if a patient does not react to tape. Hypoallergenic paper, plastic, and woven fabric tapes minimize skin reactions.

Tape comes in various widths. Choose a size that secures the dressing sufficiently. Make sure that the tape crosses the dressing and adheres to several inches of skin on each side. When securing the dressing, gently press the tape, exerting pressure away from the wound. Never apply tape over irritated skin. Apply a skin barrier to the skin around the wound to secure the tape to the skin barrier rather than to sensitive skin. To remove tape safely, loosen the end and gently release the tape from the patient's skin by pressing the skin away from the tape.

To avoid repeated removal of tape from sensitive skin, secure dressings with reusable Montgomery ties (see Skill 17.3, Step 13b). Each tie consists of a long strip; half contains an adhesive backing to apply to the skin, and the other half folds back and contains a cloth tie that you tie across a dressing and untie at dressing changes. A long dressing requires two or more sets of Montgomery ties. To provide even support to a wound and immobilize a body part, apply elastic gauze or cloth dressings and binders over a dressing.

Comfort Measures

Any wound can be painful, depending on the extent of tissue injury. Interventions for pain reduction during dressing changes include analgesia before the procedure, allowing "time-outs" during painful procedures, soaking dried dressings before removal, avoiding aggressive packing, positioning and supporting the wound area for comfort, and considering using low adhesive or nonadhesive dressings (Hopf et al., 2016).

Wound Cleansing

Wound cleansing removes surface bacteria, preventing the invasion of healthy tissue. Normal saline effectively cleans when delivered to the wound site with adequate force to agitate and wash away bacteria (Bryant and Nix, 2016b). Do not use povidone-iodine (Betadine), hydrogen peroxide, and acetic acid to irrigate a clean, granular wound. These solutions are toxic to fibroblasts, a key cellular component in wound healing. Apply the following concepts when cleaning wounds:

1. Cleanse in a direction from the least contaminated area to the most contaminated such as from the wound or incision to the surrounding skin or from an isolated drain site to the surrounding skin (see Skill 17.3, Steps 9b and 9c).
2. Use light friction when applying antiseptics locally to the skin.
3. When irrigating, allow the solution to flow from the least contaminated to the most contaminated area.

Wound Irrigation

Irrigation is a way of cleansing wounds of exudate and debris. You use an irrigating syringe to flush the area with a constant flow of solution. Irrigations clean open, deep wounds and sensitive or inaccessible body parts. Administer the prescribed solution (usually normal saline) at body temperature to enhance comfort and provide local cleansing application.

When irrigating a clean wound, use sterile technique and an irrigation system with a safe level of pressure (4−15 psi) to prevent trauma to the newly formed granulation tissue (WOCN Society, 2016). This method provides an ideal solution pressure for cleansing wounds while minimizing tissue trauma (Fig. 17.10). Make sure that the syringe tip is over but not sticking into the wound. Skill 17.4 lists the steps for wound irrigation.

Suture Care

A health care provider closes a wound by bringing the edges as close together as possible to reduce the formation of scar tissue while minimizing trauma and tension and controlling bleeding. Sutures are threads or wires made of silk,

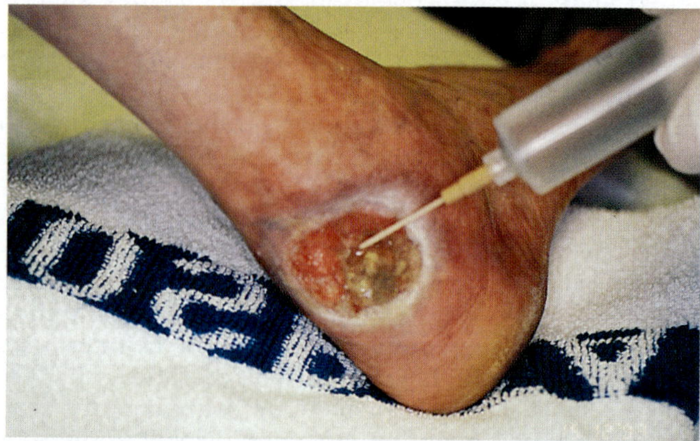

Fig. 17.10 Wound irrigation using 35-mL syringe to facilitate removal of necrotic tissue.

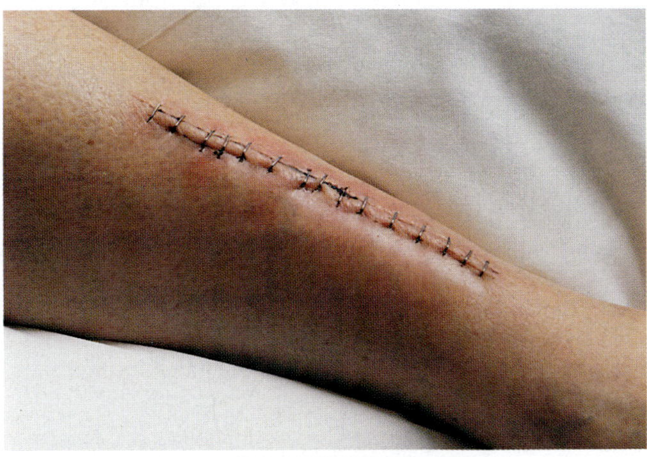

Fig. 17.11 Wound closed with staples.

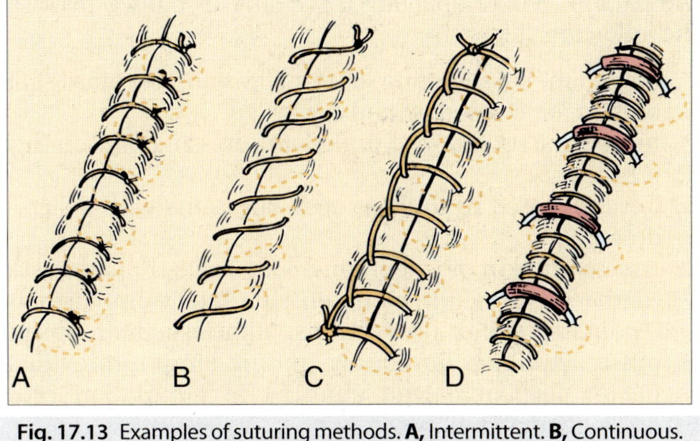

Fig. 17.13 Examples of suturing methods. **A,** Intermittent. **B,** Continuous. **C,** Blanket continuous. **D,** Retention.

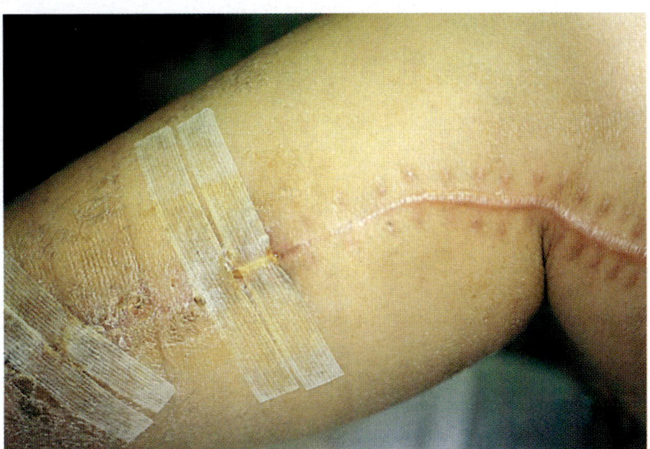

Fig. 17.12 Steri-Strips placed over incision for closure.

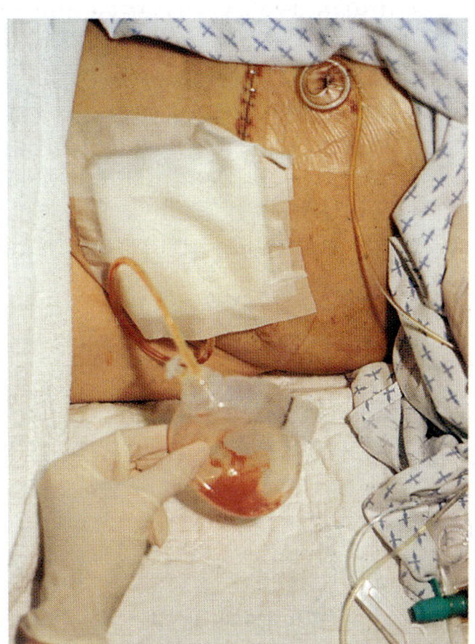

Fig. 17.14 Jackson-Pratt drain and reservoir.

steel, cotton, nylon, and polyester (Dacron) and are used to sew body tissues together. Dacron sutures minimize scar formation. Surgeons frequently use steel staples, a type of outer skin closure, because they result in less tissue trauma while providing extra strength (Fig. 17.11). Wounds can also be closed with Steri-Strips, a sterile tape applied along both sides of a wound to keep the edges closed (Fig. 17.12).

Be familiar with the types of suture methods (Fig. 17.13). Policies vary among institutions as to who removes sutures. If you remove sutures, a health care provider's order is necessary.

Drainage Evacuation

When drainage interferes with healing, drainage evacuation is achieved by using a drain or a drainage tube with continuous suction. Drainage evacuators are convenient, portable units that connect to tubular drains within a wound bed and exert a safe, constant, low-pressure vacuum to remove and collect drainage (Fig. 17.14). Ensure that suction is exerted and that all connection points between the evacuator and tubing are intact. The evacuator collects drainage that is assessed for volume and character. When the evacuator fills, measure output by emptying the contents into a graduated cylinder and immediately reset the evacuator to apply suction.

BANDAGES AND BINDERS

A simple gauze dressing is often not enough to immobilize or provide support to a wound. Bandages and binders applied over or around dressings provide extra protection and therapeutic benefits by creating pressure over a body part, immobilizing a body part, supporting a wound, reducing or preventing edema, securing a splint, or securing dressings.

Dressings are available in rolls of various widths and materials including gauze, elasticized knit, and elastic webbing. Gauze dressings are lightweight, mold easily around contours of the body, and permit air circulation to underlying skin to prevent maceration. Elastic dressings conform well to body parts but are also used to exert pressure over a body part.

Principles for Application of Bandages and Binders

Correctly applied dressings and binders do not cause injury to underlying or nearby body parts or create discomfort for the patient. Before applying a dressing or binder, perform the following steps:

1. Inspect the surrounding skin for abrasions, edema, discoloration, or exposed wound edges.
2. Inspect the condition of underlying dressings and change if soiled.
3. Cover exposed wounds or open abrasions with a sterile dressing.
4. Assess the skin of underlying body parts that are distal to the dressing for signs of circulatory impairment (coolness, pallor or cyanosis, diminished or absent pulses, swelling, numbness, and tingling) to provide a means for comparing changes in circulation after dressing application.

Table 17.5 outlines the principles of dressing and binder application. After you apply a dressing, assess, document, and immediately report any changes in circulation, comfort level, body function such as ventilation, and skin integrity. Explain to the patient that any dressing or binder will feel relatively firm or tight; assess the dressing carefully to be sure that it is applied properly and is providing therapeutic benefit, readjust it as necessary, and replace dressings when they become soiled. Seek an order before loosening or removing a dressing applied by a health care provider.

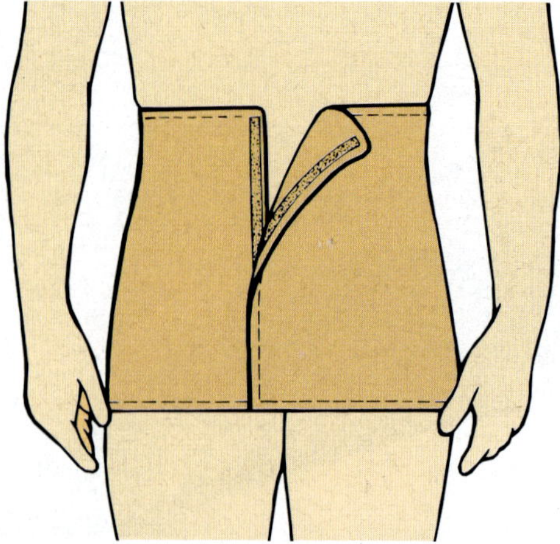

Fig. 17.15 Abdominal binder secured with Velcro.

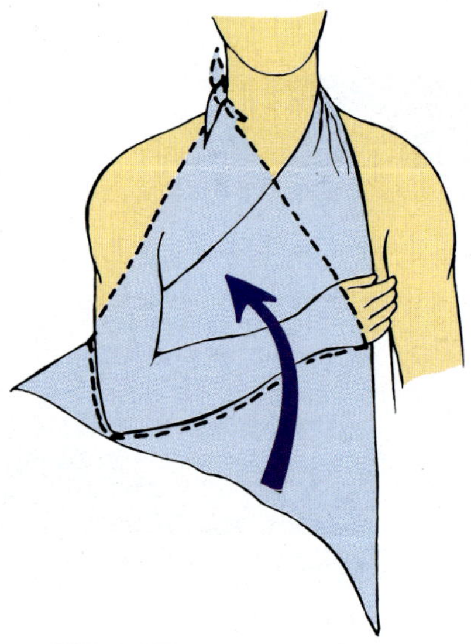

Fig. 17.16 Application of a sling.

Binder Application

Binders are especially designed for the body part to be supported. The most common types of binders are an abdominal binder and sling.

Abdominal Binder

An abdominal binder supports large incisions that are vulnerable to stress when the patient moves or coughs. It is a rectangular piece of cotton or elasticized material with many tails attached to the two longer sides or long extensions on each side to surround the abdomen (Fig. 17.15).

Slings

Slings support arms with muscular sprains or fractures. Commercially made slings have a long sleeve that extends to the elbow and a strap that fits around the neck. In the home, patients can use a large triangular piece of cloth as a sling. The patient sits or lies supine for a sling application (Fig. 17.16). Instruct the patient to bend the affected arm, bringing the forearm straight across the chest. The open sling fits under the patient's arm and over the chest, with the base of the triangle under the wrist and the point of the triangle at the

Table 17.5 Principles for Bandage and Binder Application

Principle	Rationale
Position body part you will be dressing in comfortable position of normal anatomical alignment.	Dressings cause restriction in movement. Immobilization in normal functioning position reduces risks of deformity or injury.
Prevent friction between and against skin surfaces by applying gauze or cotton padding.	Skin surfaces in contact with one another (e.g., between toes, under breasts) rub against one another to cause abrasion or chafing. Dressings over bony prominences rub against skin to cause breakdown.
Apply dressings securely to prevent slippage during movement.	Friction between dressing and skin causes skin breakdown.
When bandaging extremities, apply dressing first at distal end and progress toward trunk.	Gradual application of pressure from distal toward proximal portion of extremity promotes venous return and minimizes risk for edema or circulatory impairment.
Apply dressings firmly, with equal tension exerted over each turn or layer. Avoid excessive overlapping of dressing layers.	Equal tension prevents unequal pressure distribution over dressing body part. Localized pressure causes circulatory impairment.
Position pins, knots, or ties away from wound or sensitive skin areas.	Pins and ties used to secure dressings and binders exert localized pressure and irritation.

elbow. One end of the sling fits around the back of the neck. Bring the other end up over the affected arm while supporting the extremity. Tie the two ends at the side of the neck so that the knot does not press against the cervical spine. You can fold the loose fold at the elbow evenly around the elbow and pin it. To prevent the formation of dependent edema, make sure that the lower arm is always supported at a level above the elbow.

Bandage Application

Rolls of dressing secure or support dressings over irregularly shaped body parts. Each roll has a free outer end and a terminal end at the center. The rolled portion of the dressing is its body, and you place its outer surface against the patient's skin or dressing.

HEAT AND COLD THERAPY

Locally applying heat and cold to an injured body part provides therapeutic benefits. However, before using these therapies, understand normal body responses to local temperature variations, assess the integrity of the body part, determine the patient's ability to sense temperature variations, and ensure proper operation of equipment. You are legally responsible for the safe administration of all heat and cold applications.

Body Responses to Heat and Cold

Exposure to heat and cold causes systemic and local responses. Systemic responses occur through heat-loss mechanisms (sweating or vasodilation) or mechanisms promoting heat conservation (vasoconstriction or piloerection) and heat production (shivering) (see Chapter 6). Local responses to heat and cold occur through stimulation of temperature-sensitive nerve endings within the skin.

The adaptive ability of the body creates the major problem in protecting patients from injury resulting from temperature extremes. A person initially feels an extreme change in temperature but within a short time hardly notices the temperature variation. This phenomenon is dangerous because a person insensitive to heat and cold extremes is at risk for serious tissue injury. Recognize patients most at risk for injuries from heat and cold applications (Table 17.6).

Local Effects of Heat and Cold

Heat and cold stimuli create different physiological responses. The choice of heat or cold therapy depends on the local responses desired for wound healing (Table 17.6).

Heat, especially moist heat, is generally therapeutic. However, prolonged heat application (e.g., for 1 hour or more) causes reflex vasoconstriction and reduces blood flow as the body attempts to control heat loss from the area. The periodic removal and reapplication of local heat restores vasodilation. Continuous exposure to heat damages epithelial cells, causing redness, localized tenderness, and even blistering of the skin.

Prolonged exposure of the skin to cold results in a reflex vasodilation. The inability of the cell to receive adequate blood flow and nutrients results in tissue ischemia. The skin initially takes on a reddened appearance, followed by a bluish-purple mottling with numbness and a burning type of pain. Tissues actually freeze from exposure to extreme cold.

Factors Influencing Heat and Cold Tolerance

The response of the body to heat and cold therapies depends on the following factors:

1. *Duration of application:* A person is better able to tolerate short exposures to heat or cold treatments.
2. *Body part:* The neck, inner aspect of the wrist and forearm, and perineal regions are more sensitive to temperature variations. The foot and the palm of the hand are less sensitive.
3. *Damage to body surface:* Exposed skin layers are more sensitive to temperature variations. Protect the skin when applying heat or cold therapies. Burns and skin injuries sustained from hot or cold therapies are serious reportable events and are preventable (National Quality Forum [NQF], 2016). Injuries from these therapies have functional applications; because they are viewed as preventable events, there is a potential that the related treatment health care costs are not reimbursable.
4. *Prior skin temperature:* The body responds best to minor temperature adjustments.
5. *Body surface area:* A person is less tolerant of temperature changes over a large area of the body.
6. *Age and physical condition:* Very young children and older adults are most sensitive to heat and cold. If a patient's physical condition reduces the reception or perception of sensory stimuli, the tolerance to temperature extremes is high, but the risk for injury is also high.

Table 17.6 Conditions That Increase Risk for Injury From Heat and Cold Application

Condition	Risk Factors
Very young; older adults	Thinner skin layers in children and older adults increase risk for burns; damage from cold; older adults have reduced sensitivity to pain.
Open wounds, broken skin	Subcutaneous tissue is more sensitive to temperature variations.
Areas of edema or scar formation	Scar tissue and edema have reduced sensation to temperature.
Peripheral vascular disease (e.g., diabetes, arteriosclerosis)	Body extremities are less sensitive to temperature and pain stimuli because of decreased peripheral circulation and/or local tissue injury. Cold applications further compromise blood flow.
Confusion or unconsciousness	There is reduced perception of sensory or painful stimuli. Patient may be unable to move away from or indicate discomfort from the heat or cold application.
Spinal cord injury	Alterations in nerve pathways prevent reception of sensory or painful stimuli.

Table 17.7 Strategies to Prevent Medical and Immobilization Device–Related Pressure Injury

Device	Pressure Areas	Prevention Strategies[a]
Nasogastric tubes	Nares Skin on nasal bridge	Secure tube using pressure-relieving techniques, which direct pressure from tube away from nares (see Chapters 20). Reposition tube.
Endotracheal tubes	Lips Tongue	Remove securing device daily and inspect for pressure injury (Branson et al., 2014). Rotate tube every shift or more often.
Nasotracheal tube	Nose/nasal bridge Nares	Remove securing device daily and inspect for pressure injury (Branson et al., 2014). Reposition.
Tracheostomy tubes	Front of neck and stoma site Back of neck	Remove securing device daily. Increase stoma care. Apply dressing to back of neck.
Oxygen cannula and tubing	Ears Nose	Apply dressing to external ear. Periodically remove cannula to relieve pressure and inspect for pressure injury (Schallom et al., 2015).
NIPPV/BiPAP	Forehead Nose/nasal bridge	Pretreat bridge of nose with dressing before application of mask. If possible, remove mask for a few minutes.
Drainage tubing	Area immediately next to drainage tube Adjacent area during patient position changes	Apply appropriate dressing around drainage tube. Check tubing placement with each position change. Instruct the patient not to lie on tubing (Pittman et al., 2015).
Indwelling catheter	Thighs Female: urethra, labia Male: tip of penis	Provide meticulous perineal care. Anchor and secure catheter to reduce pressure.
Orthopedic devices	All areas where device comes in contact with patient's skin and tissues	When possible and not contraindicated, inspect under device.
Neck collar	Neck and occipital region Scalp	Remove hard collar as soon as possible and replace with softer collar (Black et al., 2015). Inspect scalp daily.
Compression stockings	Calf Behind knee Heel Toes	Verify proper fit. To reduce pressure and risk of injury to skin and underlying tissues remove stockings twice daily for at least 1 hour (Black et al., 2015).
Immobilization devices	Wrists Ankles	Apply dressing between patient's skin and immobilizer (Black et al., 2015). Verify space between immobilizer and patient's skin. With assistive personnel present remove restraint one at a time to inspect skin.

BiPAP, bilevel positive airway pressure; *NIPPV*, noninvasive positive pressure ventilation.
[a]In addition to routine inspection and cleansing of skin under and around medical device.

Assessment for Temperature Tolerance

Before applying heat or cold therapies, first observe the area that you will treat. This observation provides baseline information so that you can evaluate therapy-related skin changes. Alterations in skin integrity such as abrasions, open wounds, edema, bruising, bleeding, or localized areas of inflammation increase the risk for thermal injury. Identify conditions that contraindicate heat or cold therapy. *Do not* apply heat over an active area of bleeding (risk for continued bleeding) or an acute localized inflammation such as appendicitis (risk for rupture). Cold is contraindicated if the site of injury is edematous or the patient has impaired circulation or is shivering (may intensify shivering and reduce blood flow).

Assess the patient's sensory function and ability to recognize when heat or cold becomes excessive. If a patient has paralysis or peripheral vascular disease, observe circulation to the extremities. If a patient is confused or unresponsive, observe skin temperature, circulation, and integrity frequently after therapy begins. Finally, assess the condition of all equipment used, checking for cracked cords, frayed wires, damaged insulation, exposed heating components, leaks, and evenness of temperature distribution.

Patient Education and Safety

Before applying heat or cold therapy, make sure that the patient and family caregiver understand its purpose, the symptoms of temperature exposure, and the precautions taken to prevent injury. Box 17.9 provides safety guidelines for applying heat and cold therapy.

Applying Heat and Cold

A prerequisite to using heat or cold application is a health care provider's order, which includes the body site to be treated and the type, frequency, and duration of application. The correct temperature to use for heat and cold applications varies according to agency policy.

Choice of Moist or Dry

You administer heat and cold applications in dry or moist forms. Consider the type of wound or injury, location of the body part, and presence of drainage or inflammation when selecting dry or moist applications.

BOX 17.9 Safety Guidelines for Applying Heat or Cold Therapy

- Explain the sensations that the patient will feel during the procedure.
- Instruct the patient and/or family caregiver to report changes in sensation or discomfort immediately.
- Provide a timer, clock, or watch so that the patient can help you time the application.
- Be sure nurse call system is in an accessible location within patient's reach.
- Refer to institution policy and procedure manual for safe temperatures and duration of therapy.
- Do not allow the patient to adjust temperature settings.
- Do not allow the patient to move an application or place his or her hands on the wound site.
- Do not place the patient in a position that prevents movement away from the temperature source.
- Do not leave the patient who is unable to sense temperature changes or move from the temperature source unattended.

Warm Moist Compresses

A warm, moist compress improves circulation, relieves edema, and promotes concentration of pus and drainage. Moist heat is also beneficial in increasing muscle and ligament flexibility, relaxation, and healing and relieving muscle spasm and joint stiffness following the acute phase of a musculoskeletal injury (Petrofsky et al., 2013). A **compress** is a piece of gauze dressing moistened in a prescribed warmed solution. A pack is a larger cloth or dressing applied to a larger body area.

Heat from warm compresses evaporates quickly. To maintain a constant temperature, change the compress frequently or apply a waterproof heating pad over the compress. Because moisture conducts heat, make sure that the temperature setting of the device is lower for a moist compress than for a dry application. A layer of plastic wrap or a dry towel insulates the compress and retains heat. Moist heat promotes vasodilation and evaporation of heat from the surface of the skin. For this reason, a patient feels chilly. Control drafts and keep the patient covered with a blanket or robe.

Warm Soaks

Immersion of a body part in a warmed solution promotes circulation, lessens edema, increases muscle relaxation, and allows application of medicated solution. You also administer a soak by wrapping the body part in dressings and saturating them with the warmed solution.

Position the patient comfortably, place waterproof pads under the area you plan to treat, and heat the solution to the patient's tolerance. Check the temperature by placing a small amount of solution on the inside of your forearm. Adjust the temperature if the solution is too warm or not warm enough before applying it to a patient. After immersing the body part, cover the container and extremity with a towel to reduce heat loss. It is usually necessary to remove the cooled solution and the body part and add heated solution after about 10 minutes. The challenge is to keep the solution at a constant temperature. Never add a hotter solution while the body part remains immersed. After any soak, dry the body part thoroughly to prevent maceration.

Sitz Bath

The patient who has had rectal surgery or an episiotomy during childbirth or who has painful hemorrhoids or vaginal inflammation benefits from a **sitz bath,** a bath in which only the pelvic area is immersed in warm fluid. The patient sits in a special tub or chair or in a basin that fits on the toilet so the legs and feet remain out of the water. Immersing the entire body causes widespread vasodilation and negates the effect of local heat to the pelvic area.

The desired temperature for a sitz bath depends on whether the purpose is to promote relaxation or clean a wound. It is often necessary to carefully add warm water during the procedure, which usually lasts 20 minutes. A disposable basin contains an attachment that resembles an enema bag and allows the gradual introduction of warmer water.

Prevent overexposure by draping bath blankets around the patient's shoulders and thighs and controlling drafts. Make sure that the patient is able to sit in the basin or tub with feet flat on the floor and without pressure on the sacrum or thighs. Because exposure of a large portion of the body to heat causes extensive vasodilation, assess the patient's pulse and facial color and ask whether he or she feels light-headed or nauseated.

Commercial Hot Packs

Commercially prepared, disposable hot packs apply warm, dry heat to an injured area. Striking, kneading, or squeezing the pack mixes chemicals that release heat. Package directions recommend the time for heat application.

Aquathermia and Dry Heat

A water-flow pad such as an aquathermia pad, electric heating pads, and commercial heat packs are common forms of dry heat therapy. A new product, an air-activated wearable heat wrap, maintains a temperature of 40°C (104°F) and can be worn for 8–10 hours. The aquathermia pad (water-flow pad) used in health care settings consists of a waterproof rubber or plastic pad connected by two hoses to an electrical control unit that has a heating element and motor. Distilled water circulates through hollowed channels in the pad to the control unit where water is heated (or cooled).

Hot-Water Bottles

The hot-water bottle is an economical means of applying heat to an injured body part. Many patients still use them in the home. Provide the following instructions about the safe use of water bottles:

1. Ensure that there are no leaks. Fill the bottle with warm tap water, secure the cap, and turn the bottle upside down.
2. Fill the bag only two-thirds full, expel air at the top, and secure the cap. The bag is then easier to mold over a body part.
3. Wipe off moisture on the outside of the bag.

4. Never apply a water bottle directly to the skin surface. Cover it with a towel or pillowcase.
5. Keep the bottle in place for 20–30 minutes.

Electric Heating Pads

Another conventional form of heat therapy is the heating pad, an electric coil enclosed within a waterproof pad covered with cotton or flannel cloth. The pad is connected to an electric cord that has a temperature-regulating unit for a high, medium, or low setting. Instruct patients to cover the pad with a flannel cover, towel, or pillowcase and to never apply pad directly to the skin. Remind patients to never use the high setting and to never lie on the pad. Last, advise the patient not to insert a safety pin through a heating pad to avoid electrical shock.

Cold Moist Compresses

The procedure for applying cold moist compresses is the same as that for warm compresses. Apply cold compresses for 20 minutes at a temperature of 15°C (59°F) to relieve inflammation and swelling. Compresses are clean or sterile. Observe for adverse reactions such as burning or numbness, mottling of the skin, redness, extreme paleness, or a bluish skin discoloration.

Cold Soaks

The procedure for preparing cold soaks and immersing a body part is the same as for warm soaks. The desired temperature for a 20-minute soak is 15°C (59°F). Take precautions to protect the patient from chilling.

Ice Bag or Collar

For a patient who has a muscle sprain, localized hemorrhage, or hematoma or has undergone dental surgery, an ice bag is ideal to prevent edema formation, control bleeding, and anesthetize the body part. Use the bag correctly as follows:

1. Fill the bag with water, secure the cap, invert to check for leaks, and pour out the water.
2. Fill the bag two-thirds full with crushed ice so that it molds easily over a body part.
3. Release air from the bag by squeezing its sides before securing the cap (because excess air interferes with conduction of cold).
4. Wipe off excess moisture.
5. Cover the bag with a flannel cover, towel, or pillowcase.
6. Apply the bag to the injury site for 20–30 minutes; you may reapply it in an hour.

Commercial Cold Packs

Commercially prepared, single-use ice packs come in various sizes and shapes. When you squeeze or knead the pack, an alcohol-based solution is released inside to create the cold temperature. The soft outer coverings are usually safe to apply directly to the skin surface.

SKILL 17.1 Assessment of Patient for Pressure Injury: Risk and Skin Assessment

Delegation Considerations

The skill of pressure injury risk assessment cannot be delegated to nursing assistive personnel (NAP). The nurse instructs the NAP to:

- Report any changes to patient's skin such as redness, blistering, abrasion, or cuts to the nurse for further assessment.
- Keep patient's skin dry and provide hygiene after fecal or urinary incontinence.
- Frequently change patient's position according to patient's nursing care plan.
- Avoid trauma to patient's skin from tape, medical devices, pressure, friction, or shear. Report to the nurse any blistering, redness, or break in patient's skin.
- Report any abrasion from medical devices.

Equipment

- Risk assessment tool (use agency approved tool; see agency policy)
- Documentation record
- Pressure-redistribution mattress, bed, or chair cushion as needed
- Positioning aids
- Clean gloves

STEP	RATIONALE
Assessment	
1. Identify patient using at least two identifiers (e.g., name and birthday or name and medical record number) according to agency policy.	Ensures correct patient. Complies with The Joint Commission standards and improves patient safety (TJC, 2018).
2. Review medical record to assess patient's risk for pressure injury formation:	Determines need to administer preventive care and identifies specific factors that place patient at risk (NPUAP, EPUAP, and PPPIA, 2014).
a. Paralysis or immobilization	Patient is unable to turn or reposition independently to relieve pressure.

STEP	RATIONALE
b. Presence of medical device such as nasogastric (NG) tube, oxygen equipment, artificial airway, drainage tubing, or mechanical devices (Doughty and McNichol, 2016)	Medical devices have the potential to exert pressure on the patient's nares or ears or on tissue adjacent to artificial airways or drainage tubes (Pittman et al., 2015).
c. Sensory loss (e.g., hemiplegia, spinal cord injury)	Patient is unable to feel discomfort from pressure and does not independently change position.
d. Circulatory disorders (e.g., peripheral vascular diseases, vascular changes from diabetes mellitus, neuropathy)	Reduce perfusion of tissue layers of skin.
e. Fever	Increases metabolic demands of tissues. Accompanying diaphoresis leaves skin moist.
f. Anemia	Decreased hemoglobin level reduces oxygen-carrying capacity of blood and amount of oxygen available to tissues.
g. Malnutrition	Inadequate nutrition leads to weight loss, muscle atrophy, and reduced tissue mass. Nutrient deficiencies result in impaired or delayed healing (Stotts, 2016b).
h. Fecal or urinary incontinence	Skin becomes exposed to moist environment that contains bacteria. Excessive moisture macerates skin (Bryant, 2016).
i. Heavy sedation and anesthesia	Patient is not mentally alert and does not turn or change position independently. Sedation alters sensory perception.
j. Age	Neonates and very young children are at high risk with the head being most common site of pressure injury occurrence (WOCN Society, 2016). There is a loss of dermal thickness in older adults, impairing ability to distribute pressure (Pieper, 2016).
k. Dehydration	Results in decreased skin elasticity and turgor.
l. Edema	Edematous tissues are less tolerant of pressure, friction, and shear.
m. Existing pressure injuries	Limit surfaces available for position changes, placing available tissues at increased risk.
n. History of pressure injury	Tensile strength of skin from previously healed pressure injury is 80% or less; therefore this area cannot tolerate pressure as much as undamaged skin (Doughty and Sparks, 2016).
3. Select agency-approved risk assessment tool such as the Braden Scale or Norton Scale. Perform risk assessment when patient enters health care agency and repeat on regularly scheduled basis or when there is a significant change in patient's condition (WOCN Society, 2016).	Valid and reliable risk assessment tools evaluate patient's risk for developing a pressure injury (WOCN Society, 2016). Identifying risk factors that contribute to potential for skin breakdown allows you to target specific interventions for decreasing risk for skin breakdown.
4. Review assessment tool and levels of risk scores.	Risk cutoff score depends on instrument used. The score i nvolves identifying risk factors that contributed to it and minimizing those specific deficits (Ayello and Braden, 2002; Ayello, 2012).
5. Perform hand hygiene. Assess condition of patient's skin over regions of pressure (see Fig. 38.11). Apply gloves as needed with open and/or draining wounds. Also assess tissue adjacent to medical devices, drainage tubes, and artificial airways.	Body weight against bony prominences places underlying skin at risk for breakdown. Medical devices exert pressure directly on the skin or underlying tissue (Black et al., 2010, 2015).
a. Inspect for skin discoloration (redness in light-toned skin; purplish or bluish in darkly pigmented skin) and tissue consistency (firm or boggy feel) and/or palpate for abnormal sensations (Nix, 2016).	Indicates that tissue is under pressure; hyperemia is a normal physiological response to hypoxemia in tissues.
b. Palpate discolored area on skin and under and around medical devices, release your fingertip, and look for blanching.	If on palpation an area of redness blanches (lightens in color), this indicates normal reactive hyperemia; the tissue is not at risk for skin breakdown. Tissue that does not blanch when palpated indicates abnormal reactive hyperemia, an indication of possible ischemic injury.

STEP	RATIONALE
c. Inspect for pallor and mottling.	Persistent hypoxia in tissues that were under pressure; an abnormal physiological response.
d. Inspect for absence of superficial skin layers.	Represents early pressure injury formation, usually a partial-thickness wound that may have resulted from friction and/or shear.
e. Inspect for localized heat, edema, or induration, especially in individuals with darkly pigmented skin.	Localized heat, edema, and induration have been identified as warning signs for pressure injury development. As it is not always possible to see signs of redness on darkly pigmented skin, these additional signs should be considered in assessment (NPUAP, EPUAP, and PPPIA, 2014).
6. Assess skin around and beneath medical devices every nursing shift for additional areas of potential pressure injury caused by medical devices (Black et al., 2015).	Patients at high risk have multiple sites for pressure necrosis from medical devices in areas other than bony prominences (Coyer et al., 2014; Makic, 2015). Pressure points around medical devices (e.g., nares, oxygen cannula and masks, drainage tubing) can cause pressure injury to underlying tissue, which can become full-thickness pressure injuries (Black et al., 2015; Pittman et al., 2015; Stechmiller et al., 2016).
a. Nares: NG tube, oxygen cannula	Pressure to nares occurs from tape and other materials used to secure NG tube. Patients' ears and tips of nares are at risk for pressure from nasal cannula (Black et al., 2015; Schallom et al., 2015).
b. Tongue and lips: oral airway, endotracheal (ET) tube	Pressure results from artificial airway and materials used to secure airway (Black et al., 2015).
c. Ears: oxygen cannula, pillow	
d. Drainage or other tubing	Stress and pressure against tissue at exit site or from tubing lying under any part of patient's body (Black et al., 2015).
e. Wound drainage	Wound drainage increases risk for skin breakdown because it is caustic to skin and underlying tissues. Tubing from drainage devices (e.g., Jackson-Pratt, Hemovac) causes pressure under device and on adjacent skin (Black et al., 2015).
f. Indwelling urethral (Foley) catheter	For female patients the catheter can put pressure on the labia, especially when edematous. For male patients pressure from a catheter not properly anchored can put pressure on the tip of the penis and urethra (Black et al., 2015).
g. Orthopedic and positioning devices such as casts, neck collars, or splints	Applied devices have the potential to cause pressure to underlying and adjacent skin and tissue (Black et al., 2015).
h. Compression stockings	Compression stockings have the potential to cause pressure, especially if they are poorly fitting or rolled down (Black et al., 2015).
i. Immobilization device and restraints	If device is too tight or poorly placed or patient strains, pressure points occur under device.
7. Remove and dispose of gloves and perform hand hygiene.	Reduces transmission of organisms.
8. Observe patient for preferred positions when in bed or chair.	Preferred positions result in weight of body being placed on certain bony prominences. Presence of contractures may result in pressure exerted in unexpected places.
9. Observe ability of patient to initiate and help with position changes.	Potential for friction and shear increases when patient is completely dependent on others for position changes.
10. Assess patient and family caregiver understanding of risks for development of pressure injuries.	Determines baseline knowledge for pressure injury risk and identifies areas for patient teaching.
Planning	
1. Provide privacy and prepare bedside environment for patient safety.	Providing privacy and preparing environment before the procedure helps to ensure a clean and distraction-free area for organizing procedure-related equipment.
2. Prepare and organize equipment. Be sure you have correct risk assessment tool at patient's bedside.	Facilitates smooth completion of assessment.

STEP	RATIONALE
3. Explain procedure and purpose to patient and family caregiver.	Relieves anxiety and provides opportunity for education.
Implementation	
1. Implement prevention guidelines adapted from *Guideline for Prevention and Management of Pressure Ulcers* (WOCN Society, 2016).	Reduces patient's risk for developing a pressure injury.
2. Perform hand hygiene and apply clean gloves if patient has open, draining wounds.	Use of standard precautions prevents accidental exposure to body fluids.
3. Inspect skin at least once a day.	
a. Observe patient's skin; pay particular attention to bony prominences and areas around and under medical devices and tubes. If you find a reddened area, gently press the area with a gloved finger to check for blanching. If the area does not blanch, suspect tissue injury and recheck in 1 hour. Discoloration may vary from pink to a deep red.	Monitoring the skin on a routine basis provides a "watch" for changes that deviate from baseline data (Nix, 2016). Persistent redness when lightly pigmented skin is pressed can indicate tissue injury. If an area of redness blanches (lightens in color), this indicates that skin is not at risk for breakdown.
Clinical Decision Point: Do not massage reddened areas because doing so may cause additional tissue trauma. Reddened areas indicate blood vessel damage, and massaging can further damage the vessel (Bryant and Nix, 2016a).	
b. If patient has darkly pigmented skin, look for color changes that differ from patient's normal skin color such as red, blue, or purple tones.	Darkly pigmented skin may not blanch. Although the skin may not show direct changes in color, the color may differ from the surrounding area (see Box 38.4) (NPUAP, EPUAP, and PPPIA, 2014).
4. Each shift, check all treatment and assistive devices (e.g., catheters, feeding tubes, casts, braces) for potential pressure points (see Table 38.8). Remove gloves and perform hand hygiene.	Pressure from these devices increases the risk on bony prominences and other areas.
a. Verify that device is correctly sized, positioned, and secured.	Incorrect size, placement, and securing of a medical device can cause excessive pressure and rubbing by the device on the underlying skin (Makic, 2015).
b. Consider shielding the underlying at-risk skin with protective dressing (silicone, hydrocolloid).	These dressings absorb moisture from the body and reduce pressure to the underlying skin (Black et al., 2015; Makic, 2015).
Clinical Decision Point: Inspect skin around and beneath orthopedic devices (e.g., cervical collar, braces, cast). Note any abrasions or warmth in areas where devices can rub against the skin (Pittman et al., 2015; Schallom et al., 2015).	
5. Review patient's pressure injury risk assessment score.	Risk scores aid in identifying interventions to lessen or eliminate present risk factors.
6. If immobility, inactivity, or poor sensory perception is a risk factor for patient, consider one of the following interventions:	Immobility and inactivity reduce patient's ability or desire to independently change position. Poor sensory perception decreases patient's ability to feel the sensation of pressure or discomfort.
a. Reposition patient on a scheduled basis, and frequently assess the skin condition to help to identify early signs of pressure damage. If skin changes occur, reevaluate plan.	Reduces duration and intensity of pressure. Some patients may require more frequent repositioning (NPUAP, EPUAP, and PPPIA, 2014).
b. When patient is in side-lying position in bed, use 30-degree lateral position (see illustration). Avoid a 90-degree lateral position.	Reduces direct contact of trochanter with support surface.
c. When needed use pillow bridging (see illustration).	Use of pillows prevents direct contact between bony prominences.
d. Place patient (when lying in bed) on a pressure redistribution surface.	Reduces amount of pressure exerted on tissues.
e. Place patient (when in a chair) on a pressure redistribution device and shift the points under pressure at least every hour (WOCN Society, 2016).	Reduces amount of pressure on sacral and ischial areas.
7. If friction and shear are identified as risk factors, consider the following interventions:	Friction and shear damage underlying skin.
a. Use two nurses and a pull sheet to reposition patient. Use a slide board to transfer patient from bed to stretcher.	Proper repositioning of patient prevents dragging along the sheets. Slide board provides slippery surface to reduce friction.

STEP	RATIONALE

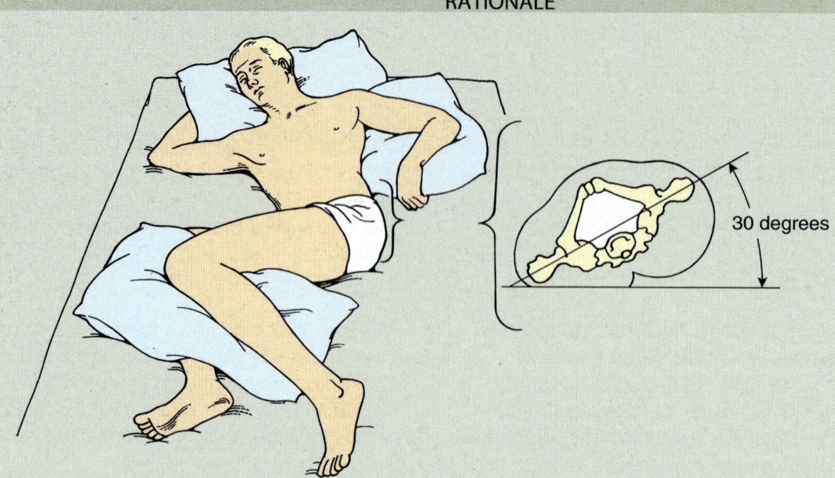

Step 6b Thirty-degree lateral position with pillow placement.

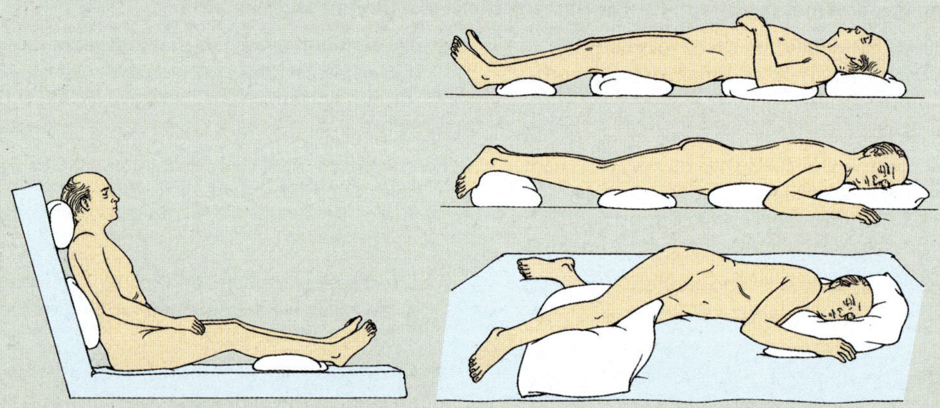

Step 6c Pillow bridging.

STEP	RATIONALE
b. Ensure that heels are free from the surface of the bed by using a pillow under the calves to elevate the heels or use a heel suspension device; knees should be in 5- to 10-degree flexion (Baath et al., 2016; WOCN Society, 2016).	"Floating" the heels from the bed surface offload the heel completely and redistribute the weight of the leg along the calf without applying pressure on the Achilles tendon (Baath et al., 2016).
c. Maintain head of bed at 30 degrees or lower or at lowest elevation consistent with patient's condition (do not lower head of bed if patient is at risk for aspiration) (WOCN Society, 2016).	Decreases potential for patient to slide toward foot of bed and incur shear injury.
8. If patient receives a low score on a moisture subscale, consider one of the following interventions:	Continual exposure of body fluids on patient's skin increases risk for skin breakdown and pressure injury development.
a. Apply clean gloves. Clean and dry the skin after each incontinent episode. Apply moisture-barrier ointment to perineum and surrounding skin after each incontinent episode (WOCN Society, 2016).	Protects the skin from fecal or urinary incontinence.
b. If skin is denuded, use a protective barrier paste after each incontinent episode.	Provides a barrier between the skin and stool and/or urine, allowing for healing.
c. If moisture source is from wound drainage, consider frequent dressing changes, protective barriers for skin, or collection devices.	Frequent exposure of skin to wound drainage is avoided.
9. If friction and shear are risk factors and patient is chair bound:	Relief of pressure by changing from lying to sitting position is insufficient if sitting is prolonged. The maximum amount of time a patient can sit before there is a need to reposition is unknown (WOCN Society, 2016).
a. Perform hand hygiene and apply clean gloves as needed. Tilt patient's chair seat to prevent sliding forward, and support arms, legs, and feet to maintain proper posture (NPUAP, EPUAP, & PPPIA, 2014).	

STEP	RATIONALE
b. Limit amount of time patient spends in a chair without pressure relief (NPUAP, EPUAP, & PPPIA, 2014).	
c. For patients who can reposition themselves while sitting, encourage pressure relief every 15 minutes using chair push-ups, forward lean, or side to side (WOCN Society, 2016).	
10. Remove gloves and discard in appropriate receptacle. Perform hand hygiene.	Reduces transmission of microorganisms.
11. Educate patient and family caregiver regarding pressure injury risk and prevention (WOCN Society, 2016).	Assists in adhering to interventions to reduce pressure injury risk.
Evaluation	
1. Observe patient's skin for areas at risk for tissue damage, noting change in color, appearance, or texture.	Enables you to evaluate success of prevention techniques.
2. Observe tolerance of patient for position change by measuring level of comfort on a pain scale.	Position changes sometimes interfere with patient's sleep and rest pattern.
3. Compare subsequent risk assessment scores and skin assessments.	Provides ongoing comparison of patient's risk level to facilitate appropriateness of plan of care.
4. Use Teach-Back: "I want you to understand why we need to assess your skin on an ongoing basis. Tell me why we will be checking your skin on a regular basis." Revise your instruction now or develop a plan for revised patient/family caregiver teaching if patient/family caregiver is not able to teach back correctly.	Determines patient's/family caregiver's level of understanding of instructional topic.

Recording and Reporting

- Record in nurses' notes in electronic health record (EHR), chart, or flow sheets any skin changes, patient's risk score, and skin assessment. Describe positions, turning intervals, pressure-redistribution devices, and other prevention measures. Note patient's response to interventions.
- Document your evaluation of patient/family caregiver understanding of need for frequent skin and pressure injury assessment.
- Report need for additional consultations for high-risk patient to health care provider.

Unexpected Outcomes and Related Interventions

- Skin becomes mottled, reddened, purplish, or bluish.
  - Refer patient to wound, ostomy, and continence nurse (WOCN); registered dietitian; clinical nurse specialist (CNS); nurse practitioner (NP), or physical therapist as necessary. Reevaluate position changes and bed surface.
- Areas under pressure develop persistent discoloration, induration, or temperature changes.
  - Refer patient to WOCN; registered dietitian; CNS; NP; or physical therapist as necessary.
  - Modify patient's positioning and turning schedule.

SKILL 17.2 Treating Pressure Injuries

Equipment

- Protective equipment: clean gloves, goggles, cover gown (if splash is a risk)
- Sterile gloves *(optional)*
- Plastic bag for dressing disposal
- Measuring device
- Sterile cotton-tipped applicators (check agency policy for use of sterile applicators)
- Topical agent (as ordered)
- Cleansing agent (as ordered)
- Sterile solution container
- Dressing of choice based on patient wound characteristics
- Hypoallergenic tape (if needed)
- Documentation records
- Scale for assessing wound healing
- Washbasin

STEP	RATIONALE
Assessment	
1. Identify the patient by using at least two identifiers (e.g., name and birthday or name and medical record number) according to agency policy.	Ensures correct patient. Complies with The Joint Commission standards and improves patient safety (TJC, 2018).

STEP	RATIONALE
2. Review accuracy of health provider's order for topical agent and/or dressing.	Ensures administration of proper medication and treatment.

Clinical decision point: Determine whether the order is consistent with established wound care guidelines and outcomes for a patient. If the order is not consistent with guidelines or varies from the identified outcome for a patient, review with health the care team.

STEP	RATIONALE
3. Determine whether the patient has allergies to topical agents.	Topical agents could contain ingredients that cause localized skin reactions.
4. Assess for factors affecting wound healing: poor perfusion, immunosuppression, or preexisting infection.	Factors will affect treatment and wound healing.
5. Assess the patient's nutrition status. Clinically significant malnutrition is present if (1) serum albumin level is less than 3.5 g/dL, (2) lymphocyte count is less than 1800/mm^3, or (3) body weight decreases more than 15% (see illustration) (WOCN Society, 2016).	Delayed wound healing occurs in patients with poor nutrition status.

Clinical decision point: When you suspect malnutrition, consider a nutrition consultation to modify the patient's diet to promote wound healing.

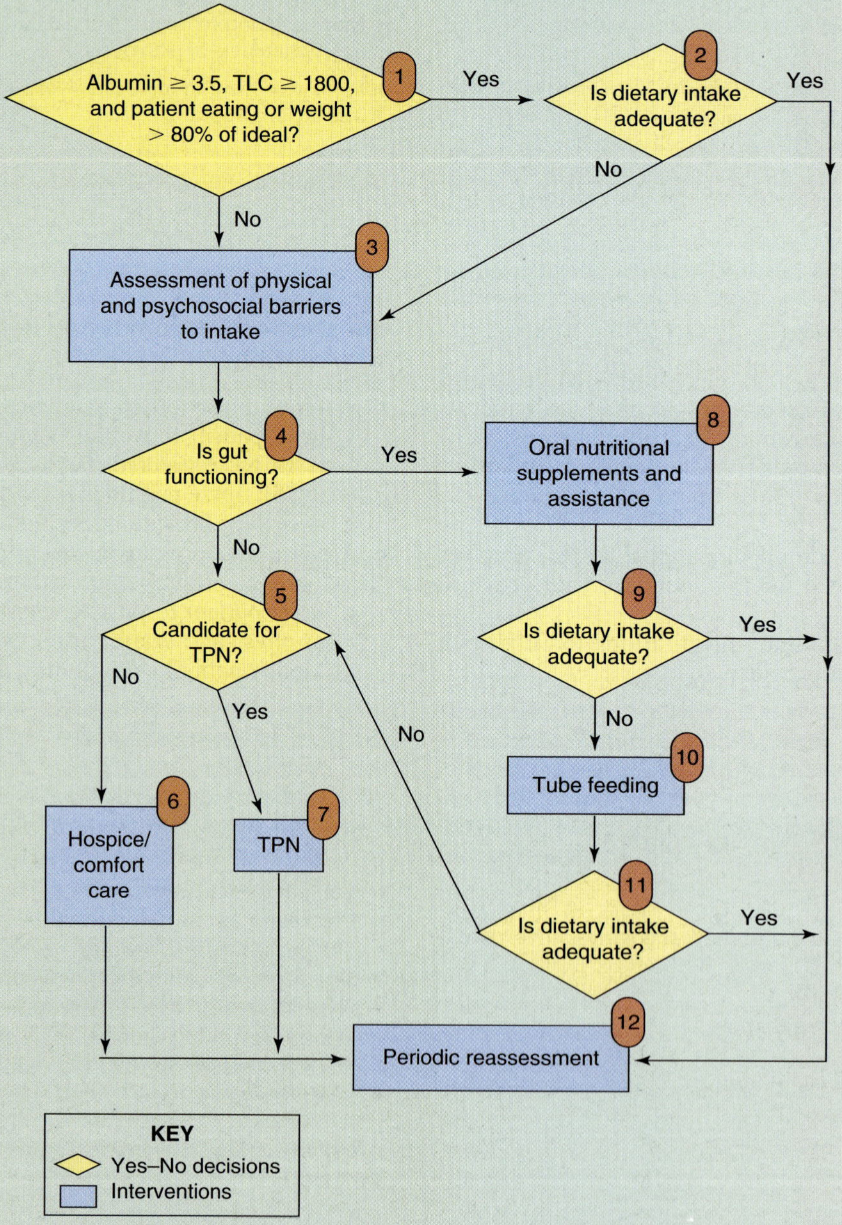

Step 5 Nutritional assessment and support. *TLC*, total lymphocyte count; *TPN*, total parenteral nutrition. (From Bergstrom N, et al: *Treatment of pressure ulcers,* AHCPR Pub. No. 95-0652, Rockville, MD, 1994, Agency for Health Care Policy and Research, Public Health Service, U.S. Department of Health and Human Services.)

STEP	RATIONALE
6. Assess the patient's level of comfort on a pain scale of 0–10. If the patient is in pain, determine whether a prn pain medication has been ordered and administer.	Dressing change should not be a traumatic event for the patient; evaluate wound pain before, during, and after wound care management (Hopf et al., 2016).
7. Close room door or bedside curtains.	Provides privacy.
8. Position the patient to allow dressing removal and position plastic bag for dressing disposal.	Provides accessible area for dressing change. Proper disposal of old dressing promotes proper handling of contaminated waste.
9. Perform hand hygiene and apply clean gloves. Remove and discard old dressing.	Reduces transmission of microorganisms and prevents accidental exposure to body fluids.
10. Assess the patient's wounds using wound parameters, and continue ongoing wound assessment per the agency policy. **Note:** This wound assessment may be performed during procedure after dressing removal.	Determines effectiveness of wound care and guides treatment plan of care (WOCN Society, 2016).
a. *Wound location:* Describe body site where the wound is located.	
b. *Stage of wound:* Describe extent of tissue destruction (see Fig. 17.3).	Staging is a way of assessing a pressure injury based on depth of tissue destruction. Wounds are documented as unstageable if the wound base is not visible (NPUAP et al., 2014).
c. *Wound size:* Length, width, and depth of wound are measured per the agency protocol. Use a disposable measuring guide for length and width. Use a cotton-tipped applicator to assess depth (see illustrations).	Injury size changes as healing progresses; therefore, the longest and widest areas of the wound change over time. Measuring width and length by measuring consistent areas provides a consistent measurement (Nix, 2016).
d. *Presence of undermining, sinus tracts, or tunnels:* Use a sterile cotton-tipped applicator to measure depth and, if needed, a gloved finger to examine wound edges.	Wound depth determines amount of tissue loss.
e. *Condition of wound bed:* Describe type and percentage of tissue in wound bed.	The approximate percentage of each type of tissue in the wound provides critical information about the progress of wound healing and choice of dressing. A wound with a high percentage of black tissue requires debridement, yellow tissue or slough tissue may indicate the presence of an infection or colonization, and granulation tissue indicates that a wound is moving toward healing.
f. *Volume of exudate:* Describe amount, characteristics, odor, and color.	Amount and type of exudate may indicate type and frequency of dressing changes (Bryant and Nix, 2016b).
g. *Condition of periwound skin:* Examine the skin for breaks; dryness; and the presence of a rash, swelling, redness, or warmth. Modify assessment based on the patient's skin color.	Impaired skin condition at the edge of an injury indicates progressive tissue damage. Maceration on periwound skin shows a need to alter the choice of wound dressing.
h. *Wound edges:* Examine edges for rolled edges, signs of moisture-associated skin damage, redness.	Provides information about epithelialization, chronicity, and etiology.
11. Assess periwound skin; check for maceration, redness, denuded tissue.	Determines whether the skin barrier is needed to protect periwound area.

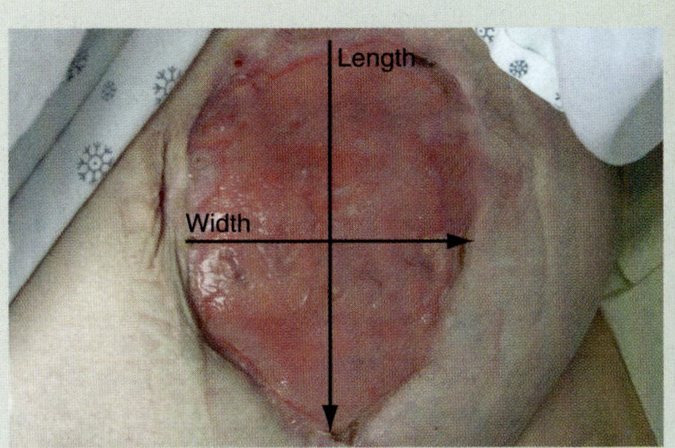

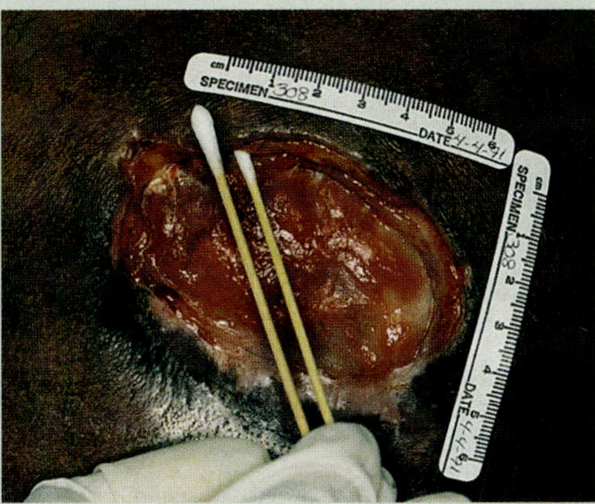

Step 10c Measuring wound width, length, and undermining of skin. (Left image from Bryant RA, Nix DP, editors: *Acute and chronic wounds: current management concepts,* ed 5, St Louis, 2016, Elsevier.)

STEP	RATIONALE
12. Remove gloves, discard appropriately, and perform hand hygiene.	Reduces transmission of microorganisms. Repeated hand hygiene is needed as you assess other pressure areas. Different organisms contaminate different wounds.
13. Assess the patient's and family caregiver's understanding of prevention, treatment, and factors contributing to recurrence of pressure injuries (WOCN Society, 2016).	The patient and caregiver need to partner with health care providers to prevent further skin breakdown.
Planning	
1. Provide privacy and prepare bedside environment for patient safety.	Providing privacy and preparing the environment before the procedure help to ensure a clean and distraction-free area for organizing procedure-related equipment.
2. Prepare and organize the following necessary equipment and supplies:	
a. Washbasin, warm water, equipment, and supplies	
b. Normal saline or other wound-cleansing agent in sterile solution container	Clean wound surface before applying topical agents and new dressing.
Clinical decision point: Use only noncytotoxic agents to clean wounds.	
c. Prescribed topical agent:	
(1) Enzyme debriding agents (follow specific manufacturer directions for frequency of application) *Or*	Enzymes debride dead tissue to clean wound surface. Enzymes are not applied to healthy tissue.
(2) Topical antibiotics	Topical antibiotics decrease bioburden of wound and should be considered for a 2-week course of treatment for nonhealing wounds (WOCN Society, 2016).
d. Prepare appropriate dressing based on stage of pressure injury, wound characteristics, principles of wound management, health care provider orders, and patient care setting (see Table 17.4). Dressing options include:	Dressing should maintain moist environment for wound while keeping surrounding skin dry (Bryant and Nix, 2016b).
(1) Gauze: Apply as a moist dressing, a dry cover dressing when using enzymes or topical antibiotics, or as a means to deliver solution to a wound.	Gauze delivers moisture to a wound and is absorptive.
(2) Transparent film dressing: Apply over superficial wounds with minimal or no exudate and skin subjected to friction.	Maintains a moist environment and offers intact skin protection.
(3) Hydrocolloid dressing	Maintains moist environment to facilitate wound healing while protecting wound base.
(4) Hydrogel—available in a sheet or in tube	Maintains moist environment to facilitate wound healing.
(5) Calcium alginate	Highly absorbent of wound exudate in heavily draining wounds.
(6) Foam dressings	Protective and prevents wound dehydration; also absorbs moderate-to-large amounts of drainage.
(7) Silver-impregnated dressings/gels	Controls bacterial burden in wound.
(8) Wound fillers	Fills shallow wounds, hydrates, and absorbs.
e. Obtain hypoallergenic tape or adhesive dressing sheet.	Used to secure nonadherent dressing. Prevents skin irritation and tearing.
3. Explain the procedure to the patient and family caregiver. Individualize teaching plan for older adults, considering normal aging changes that affect learning.	Preparatory explanations relieve anxiety, correct any misconceptions about the wound and treatment, and offer an opportunity for the patient and family education.
Implementation	
1. Perform hand hygiene and apply clean gloves. Open sterile packages and topical solution containers. Keep dressings sterile. Wear goggles, mask, and moisture-proof cover gown if potential for contamination from spray exists when cleaning wound.	Reduces transmission of microorganisms.
2. Lower side rails and position the patient.	
3. Remove bed linen and arrange the patient's gown to expose wound and surrounding skin. Keep the remaining body parts draped.	Prevents unnecessary exposure of body parts.

STEP	RATIONALE
4. Clean the wound thoroughly with normal saline or prescribed wound-cleansing agent from least contaminated to most contaminated area. For deep wounds, clean with an irrigating syringe, as ordered. Remove gloves and discard.	Cleansing wound removes wound exudate and/or dressing residue and reduces surface bacteria.
5. Perform hand hygiene and apply clean or sterile gloves.	Maintains aseptic technique during cleaning, measuring, and applying dressings. With some chronic wounds, clean versus sterile gloves are appropriate (WOCN Society, 2011). Refer to the agency policy regarding use of clean or sterile gloves.
6. Apply topical agents to wound using cotton-tipped applicators or gauze as ordered:	
a. Enzymes	Follow manufacturer directions for method and frequency of application. Be aware of which solutions inactivate enzymes and avoid their use in wound cleaning.
(1) Apply small amount of enzyme debridement ointment directly to necrotic areas in pressure wound. *Do not apply enzyme to surrounding skin.*	Thin layer absorbs and acts more effectively than a thick layer. Excess medication irritates surrounding skin (Bryant and Nix, 2016b). Proper distribution of ointment ensures effective action.
Clinical decision point: If using an enzymatic debriding agent, do not use wound-cleansing agents with metals.	
(2) Place moist gauze dressing directly over the wound and tape in place. Follow specific manufacturer recommendation for type of dressing material to use to cover a pressure injury when using enzymes. Tape dressing in place.	Protects wound and prevents removal of ointment during turning or repositioning.
b. Antibacterials (examples include bacitracin, metronidazole, and silver sulfadiazine)	Reduces bacterial growth.
7. Apply prescribed wound dressing:	
a. Hydrogel	Hydrogel dressings are designed to hydrate and donate moisture to the wound (Bryant and Nix, 2016b).
(1) Cover surface of the wound with thick layer of the amorphous hydrogel, or cut a sheet to fit wound base.	Provides moist environment to facilitate wound healing.
(2) Apply secondary dressing such as dry gauze; tape in place.	Holds hydrogel against wound surface because amorphous hydrogel (in tube) or sheet form does not adhere to wound and requires a secondary dressing to hold it in place.
(3) If using impregnated gauze, pack loosely into wound; cover with secondary gauze dressing and tape.	A loosely packed dressing delivers the gel to the wound base and allows any wound debris to be trapped in the gauze.
b. Calcium alginate	Alginate dressings absorb serous fluid or exudate forming a nonadhesive hydrophilic gel that conforms to the shape of the wound (Bryant and Nix, 2016b). Use in heavily draining wounds.
(1) Lightly pack wound with alginate using sterile cotton-tipped applicator or gloved finger.	The dressing swells and increases in size; tight packing can compromise blood flow to the tissues.
(2) Apply a secondary dressing and tape in place.	
c. Transparent film dressing, hydrocolloid, and foam dressings	
Clinical decision point: Use transparent dressings for autolytic debridement of noninfected superficial pressure injuries. Use a hydrocolloid to protect skin from friction. Some brands have custom shapes available for specific anatomical parts such as heels, elbows, and sacrum.	
8. Reposition the patient comfortably off pressure injury.	Prevents pressure to injury.
9. Remove gloves and dispose of soiled supplies. Perform hand hygiene.	Reduces transmission of microorganisms.
Evaluation	
1. Observe skin surrounding the injury for inflammation, edema, and tenderness.	Determines progress of wound healing.
2. Inspect dressings and exposed wounds observing for drainage, foul odor, and tissue necrosis. Monitor the patient for signs and symptoms of infection: fever and elevated white blood cell (WBC) count.	Wounds can become infected.
3. Compare subsequent wound measurements using one of the scales designed to measure wound healing such as Pressure Ulcer Scale for Healing (PUSH) Tool or Bates-Jensen Wound Assessment Tool (BWAT).	Use one scale consistently because this allows for comparison of serial measurements to evaluate wound healing. Use of a standard scale provides a method for consistent data collection to document wound progress or lack thereof.

STEP	RATIONALE
4. **Use teach back:** "I want to be sure that you understand why we will examine your pressure injury on an ongoing basis. Tell me why we measure your wound and examine the tissue surrounding the wound at each dressing change." Revise your instruction now or develop a plan for revised patient/family caregiver teaching if the patient/family caregiver is not able to teach back correctly.	Determines the patient's/family caregiver's level of understanding of instructional topic.

Recording and Reporting

- Record in nurses' notes in EHR or chart type of wound tissue present, wound measurements, periwound skin condition, character of drainage or exudate, type of topical agent used, and dressing applied. Note the patient's response to dressing change.
- Document your evaluation of the patient and family caregiver understanding for frequent observation and measuring of wound.
- Report any deterioration in wound appearance to the nurse in charge or health care provider.

Unexpected Outcomes

- Skin surrounding wound becomes macerated.
  - Reduce exposure of surrounding skin to topical agents and moisture.
  - Select a dressing that has increased moisture-absorbing capacity.
- Wound becomes deeper with increased drainage and/or development of necrotic tissue.
  - Review current wound care management.
  - Consult with multidisciplinary team regarding changes in wound care regimen.
  - Obtain wound cultures.
- Pressure injury extends beyond original margins.
  - Monitor for systemic signs and symptoms of poor wound healing such as abnormal laboratory results (WBC count, levels of hemoglobin/hematocrit, serum albumin, serum prealbumin, total proteins), weight loss, and fluid imbalances.
  - Assess and revise current turning schedule.
  - Consider further pressure-redistribution devices.

SKILL 17.3 Negative-Pressure Wound Therapy

Equipment

- NPWT unit (requires health care provider's order). For this skill, the vacuum-assisted closure (VAC) unit is used for illustration; several other systems are available, and their applications may differ (see manufacturer instructions).
- NPWT dressing (gauze or foam [see manufacturer recommendations], transparent dressing, adhesive drape)
- NPWT suction device
- Tubing for connection between NPWT unit and NPWT dressing
- Three pairs of gloves, clean and sterile
- Scissors, sterile
- Waterproof biohazard bag for disposal
- Skin preparation, skin barrier protectant, hydrocolloid dressing, skin barrier
- Moist washcloths
- Linen bag
- Protective equipment: gown, mask, goggles (used when splashing from wound is a risk)

STEP	RATIONALE
Assessment	
1. Identify the patient by using at least two identifiers (e.g., name and birthday or name and medical record number) according to agency policy.	Ensures correct patient. Complies with The Joint Commission standards and improves patient safety (TJC, 2018).
2. Review health care provider's orders for frequency of dressing change, amount of negative pressure, type of foam or gauze to use, and pressure cycle (intermittent or continuous).	Determines frequency of dressing change, negative pressure setting, and special instructions. Health care provider's order is also necessary for reimbursement.
3. Review electronic health record (EHR) for signs and symptoms related to condition of the patient's wound.	Provides baseline to compare your findings with previous dressing change assessments and reflects wound-healing progress.
a. Assess the patient's level of comfort on a pain scale of 0–10.	Serves as baseline to measure response to dressing therapy.
b. Administer prescribed analgesic as needed 30 min before dressing change.	A comfortable patient will be less likely to move suddenly, causing wound or supply contamination.
4. Perform hand hygiene and apply clean gloves. Assess location, appearance, and size of wound. Remove and dispose of gloves. Perform hand hygiene.	Provides information about status of wound healing, presence of complications, and proper type of supplies and assistance needed.

STEP	RATIONALE
5. Assess the patient's and family caregiver's knowledge of purpose of dressing and whether they will participate in dressing wound.	Identifies the patient's learning needs. Prepares the patient and family if dressing will need to be changed at home.
Planning	
1. Provide privacy and prepare bedside environment for patient safety.	Providing privacy and preparing the environment before the procedure helps to ensure a clean and distraction-free area for organizing procedure-related equipment.
2. Prepare and organize equipment.	Organizes procedure.
a. Verify that suction tubing is intact and suction device is working properly.	Ensures that when the nurse has prepared the wound for negative pressure, the equipment is in working order. This further increases wound care efficiency.
3. Explain procedure to the patient and family caregiver.	Relieves anxiety and promotes understanding of healing process.
Implementation	
1. Perform hand hygiene and put on clean gloves. If risk for spray exists, don protective gown, goggles, and mask.	Reduces transmission of infectious organisms from soiled dressings to nurse's hands.
2. Position the patient comfortably and drape to expose only wound site. Instruct the patient not to touch wound or sterile supplies.	Promotes the patient's cooperation and smooth completion of procedure. Prevents contamination of sterile supplies.
3. Cuff top of disposable waterproof biohazard bag and place within reach of work area.	Cuff prevents accidental contamination of top of outer bag.
4. Follow manufacturer directions for removal and replacement of wound filler and dressing.	Each NPWT unit varies slightly with wound fillers, dressing, and reattachment of suction. Knowing your agency's specific NPWT directions facilitates a smooth dressing change.
a. Turn off NPWT unit by pushing therapy on/off button.	Deactivates therapy and allows for proper drainage of fluid in drainage tubing.
b. Keeping tube connectors attached to NPWT unit, raise tubing connectors; disconnect tubes from one another, and drain fluids into drainage collector.	Prevents backflow of any drainage in tubing back into wound.
c. Before lowering, tighten clamp on canister tube, and disconnect canister and dressing tubing at connection points.	Prevents drainage from exiting tubing when removed.
5. Remove transparent film by gently stretching transparent film and slowly pull away from skin.	Prevents injury to wound tissue. Protects periwound skin breakdown from transparent adhesive.
6. Remove old dressing one layer at a time and discard in bag. Observe drainage on dressing. Use caution to avoid tension on any drains that are present.	Determines type and amount of dressings needed for replacement. Prevents accidental removal of drains.
7. Perform wound assessment. Observe surface area and tissue type, color, odor, and drainage within wound. Measure length, width, and depth of wound as ordered.	Determines condition of wound and need for replacement of dressing. Measurement of wound is necessary to assess wound healing progression and justify continuation of NPWT for third-party payers (Netsch et al., 2016).
Clinical decision point: This is a time when a wound care nurse or physician might debride the wound. Debridement of eschar or slough, if present, should be performed for removal of devitalized tissue to prepare wound bed (Netsch et al., 2016).	
8. Remove and discard gloves in waterproof bag. Avoid having the patient see old dressing because sight of wound drainage may be upsetting. Perform hand hygiene.	Reduces transmission of microorganisms. Lessens the patient anxiety during procedure.
9. Clean wound.	Irrigation removes wound debris and cleans wound bed.
a. Apply sterile or clean gloves depending on agency policy and wound status.	Cleaning periwound is essential for an airtight seal. With some chronic wounds, clean versus sterile gloves are appropriate (WOCN Society, 2011).
b. If ordered, irrigate wound with normal saline or other solution ordered by health care provider (see Skill 17.4). Gently blot periwound with gauze to dry thoroughly.	
Clinical decision point: Health care providers may order wound cultures routinely. However, when drainage looks purulent or has a foul odor or if there is a change in amount or color, obtain wound culture. This may be an indication that the wound may need to be treated for an infection and the NPWT may need to be discontinued (Netsch et al., 2016).	
10. Apply skin protectant, barrier film, solid skin barrier sheet, or hydrocolloid dressing to periwound skin.	Maintains airtight seal needed for NPWT. Protects periwound skin from moisture-associated skin damage.

STEP	RATIONALE
11. Fill any uneven skin surfaces (e.g., creases, scars, skin folds) with skin barrier product (e.g., paste, strip).	Further helps to maintain airtight seal (Netsch et al., 2016).
12. Remove and discard gloves. Perform hand hygiene.	Prevents transmission of microorganisms.
13. Depending on type of wound, apply sterile or new clean gloves (see agency policy).	Fresh sterile wounds require sterile gloves. Chronic wounds require clean technique (WOCN Society, 2011).
14. Apply NPWT.	
a. Prepare NPWT filler dressing. Consult with wound care expert for appropriate type.	Filler dressing depends on NPWT used and can include foam or gauze dressings with or without antimicrobials such as silver. The type of dressing may be adjusted based on undermining, tunneling, or sinus tracts present (Netsch et al., 2016).
(1) Measure wound and select appropriate size dressing.	Establishes baseline for wound size. Black polyurethane foam has larger pores and is most effective in stimulating granulation tissue and wound contraction. White soft foam is denser with smaller pores and is used when the growth of granulation tissue needs to be restricted (Netsch et al., 2016).
(2) Using sterile scissors, cut filler dressing foam to wound size, making sure to fit exact size and shape of wound including tunnels and undermined areas.	Proper size of foam dressing maintains negative pressure to entire wound (Netsch et al., 2016).
Clinical decision point: In some instances, an antimicrobial product such as silver-impregnated gauze or topical antibiotic is ordered. These products help reduce the bioburden of the wound.	
b. Place filler dressing in wound following manufacturer instructions. Be sure filler dressing is in contact with entire wound base, margins, and tunneled and undermined areas. Count number of filler dressings, and document in the patient's chart.	Maintains negative pressure to entire wound. Edges of foam dressing must be in direct contact with the patient's skin. Dressing count provides nurse who removes dressing with number of filler dressings that should be removed.
c. Place suction device per manufacturer instructions.	
d. Apply NPWT transparent dressing over foam wound dressing.	
(1) Trim dressing so that it will cover wound and extend onto periwound skin approximately 2.5–5 cm (1–2 inches).	Prepares dressing of appropriate size for wound.
(2) Apply transparent dressing, keeping it wrinkle-free (see illustration).	Ensures that wound is properly covered and negative-pressure seal can be achieved. Dressing should be airtight with no tunnels or gaps to ensure a good seal when suction is activated.
(3) Secure tubing to transparent film, aligning drainage holes to ensure occlusive seal. Do not apply tension.	Excessive tension may compress foam dressing and impede wound healing. It also produces pressure and/or shear force on periwound area (Netsch et al., 2016).
(4) Secure tubing several centimeters away from dressing, avoiding pressure points.	Drainage tubes over bony pressure prominences can cause medical device–related pressure injuries (Pittman et al., 2015; Netsch et al., 2016).
15. After wound is completely covered, connect tubing from dressing to tubing from canister and NPWT unit and set at ordered suction level.	Continuous therapy delivered at 125 mm Hg is most routinely used; lower levels of pressure (75–80 mm Hg) can be used to reduce pain without compromising effectiveness (Netsch et al., 2016).

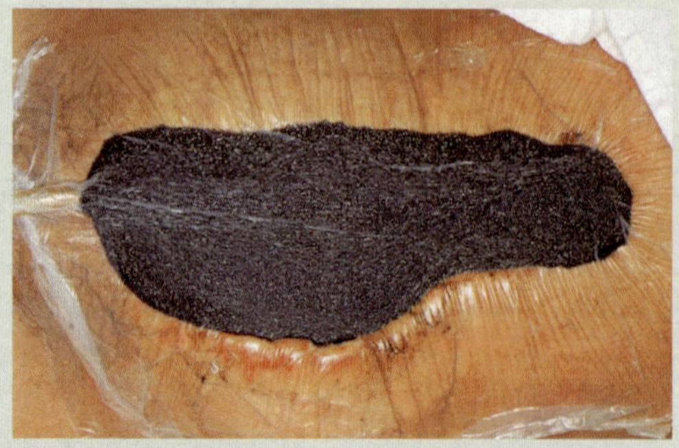

Step 14d(2) Foam wound filler, transparent dressing over existing wound. (Courtesy KCI Licensing, San Antonio, TX.)

STEP	RATIONALE
a. Remove canister from sterile packing and push unit until you hear a click. **Note:** An alarm sounds if canister is not properly engaged.	
b. Connect dressing tubing to canister tubing. Make sure that both clamps are open.	Facilitates suctioning needed for NPWT.
c. Place on level surface or hang from foot of bed. **Note:** Will deactivate therapy.	Unit alarms and deactivates therapy if it is tilted beyond 45°.
d. Press power button (commonly this is a green-lit button) and set pressure as ordered.	Activates system.
16. Inspect NPWT system.	
a. Verify that system is on. This is different for each type of NPWT unit. For example, on some units, the display screen shows "Therapy On." Check agency policy and procedure for specific information.	
b. Verify that all clamps are open and all tubing is patent.	
c. Examine the system to be sure that seal is intact and therapy is working.	Negative pressure is achieved when a tight seal is present (Netsch et al., 2016).
d. If a leak is present, use strips of transparent film to patch areas around edges of wound.	
17. Record initials and date and time on new dressing.	Provides reference for next dressing change.
18. Help the patient to comfortable position.	Enhances the patient comfort and relaxation.
Clinical decision point: Unless the patient's diagnosis contraindicates activity, patients may ambulate with NPWT. Ambulation will improve the patient's exercise tolerance and muscle strength.	
19. Discard gloves, dispose of any dressing material, and perform hand hygiene.	Prevents transmission of microorganisms.
Evaluation	
1. Inspect condition of wound on ongoing basis. Use agency wound-healing scale noting wound size, drainage, and odor.	Documents progression of wound healing.
2. Ask the patient to rate pain using scale of 0–10.	Determines the patient's level of comfort after procedure.
3. Verify airtight dressing seal and correct negative-pressure setting.	Determines effective negative pressure being applied.
4. Measure wound drainage output in canister on regular basis.	Monitors fluid balance and wound drainage.
5. **Use teach back:** "I want to be sure I explained clearly how to place the filler dressing into the wound before you are discharged. Show me how to place the filler dressings into your wound." Revise your instruction now or develop a plan for revised patient/family caregiver teaching if the patient/family caregiver is not able to teach back correctly.	Determines the patient's/family caregiver's level of understanding of instructional topic.

Unexpected Outcomes and Related Interventions

- Wound appears inflamed and tender, drainage has increased, and odor is present.
  - Notify health care provider.
  - Obtain wound culture.
  - Increase frequency of dressing changes.
- The patient reports increase in pain.
  - The patient may need more analgesia.
  - Instill normal saline to moisten foam and other filler dressings to allow them to loosen from granulation tissue.
  - If using black foam, switch to polyvinyl alcohol white soft foam.
  - Decrease pressure setting.
  - Change from intermittent to continuous cycling.
  - Change type of NPWT system.
- The patient or family caregiver is unable to perform dressing change.
  - Provide additional teaching and support.
  - Obtain services of home care agency.

Recording and Reporting

- Record in nurses' notes in EHR, chart, or flow sheets appearance of wound, characteristics of drainage, placement of NPWT (type of dressing, pressure mode and setting), and patient response to dressing change.
- Document your evaluation of the patient/family caregiver learning.
- Report brisk bright red bleeding, evidence of poor wound healing, evisceration or dehiscence, and possible wound infection to health care provider immediately.

SKILL 17.4 Applying Dressings: Dry, Damp-to-Dry, and Transparent

Equipment

- Clean gloves
- Sterile gloves *(optional)*
- Sterile dressing set (scissors, forceps) (*optional*; check agency policy)
- Sterile drape *(optional)*
- Sterile dressings: 4 × 4–inch gauze, abdominal pads
- Sterile basin *(optional)*
- Antiseptic ointment (as prescribed)
- Wound cleanser (as prescribed)
- Sterile normal saline or prescribed solution
- Debriding gel as ordered
- Tape, Montgomery ties, or hydrocolloid dressing as needed (include nonallergenic tape if necessary)
- Skin barrier (*optional* if using Montgomery ties)
- Protective waterproof underpad
- Biohazard bag
- Adhesive remover *(optional)*
- Measurement devices *(optional)*: cotton-tipped applicator, measuring guide, camera
- Personal protective equipment (PPE): gown, goggles, mask as needed
- Additional lighting if needed (e.g., flashlight, treatment light)

STEP	RATIONALE
Assessment	
1. Identify the patient by using at least two identifiers (e.g., name and birthday or name and account number) according to agency policy.	Ensures correct patient. Complies with The Joint Commission standards and improves patient safety (TJC, 2018).
2. Review accuracy of health care providers' orders for type of dressing.	Indicates dressing supplies needed.
3. Review previous nurses' notes and electronic health record (EHR).	Helps to plan for proper dressing type, securement, and supplies needed and if assistance is needed during dressing procedure.
4. Assess the patient for allergies, especially antiseptics, tape, or latex, and acquire specific orders for dressing change.	Reduces risk for localized or systemic allergic reactions to these supplies.
5. Ask the patient to rate his or her level of pain using a pain scale of 0−10 and assess character of pain. Administer prescribed analgesic as needed 30 min before dressing change.	Superficial wounds with multiple exposed nerves may be intensely painful, whereas deeper wounds with destruction of dermis should be less painful (Krasner, 2016). A comfortable patient is less likely to move suddenly, causing wound or supply contamination. Serves as baseline to measure response to dressing therapy.
6. Identify patients with risks for wound-healing problems including aging, premature infant, obesity, diabetes mellitus, circulation disorders, nutrition deficit, immunosuppression, radiation therapy, high levels of stress, and use of steroids.	Physiological changes resulting from aging, chronic illness, poor nutrition, medications that affect wound healing, and cancer treatments have potential to affect wound healing (Doughty and Sparks, 2016).
7. Assess the patient's and family caregiver's knowledge of purpose of dressing change and readiness and willingness of the patient or family caregiver to participate in dressing wound.	Determines level of support and explanation required. Identifies teaching needs to prepare the patient or family caregiver to provide dressing changes at home.
Planning	
1. Provide privacy and prepare bedside environment for patient safety.	Providing privacy and preparing the environment before the procedure helps to ensure a clean and distraction-free area for organizing procedure-related equipment.
2. Prepare and organize equipment.	
a. Place disposable biohazard bag within reach of work area (see illustration).	Ensures easy disposal of soiled dressings.
b. Prepare dressing materials.	Provides for smooth organized dressing change.
3. Explain procedure to the patient and family caregiver including type of dressing and frequency of dressing change.	Decreases the patient's and family caregiver's anxiety.
Implementation	
1. Perform hand hygiene and apply clean gloves. Apply gown, goggles, and mask if risk for splashing exists.	Reduces transmission of microorganisms.
2. Lower side rail and position the patient comfortably and drape to expose only wound site. Instruct the patient not to touch wound or sterile supplies.	Draping provides access to wound while minimizing exposure. Dressing supplies become contaminated when touched by patient's hand.
3. Gently remove tape, bandages, or ties: use nondominant hand to support dressing and with dominant hand pull tape parallel to skin and toward dressing. If dressing is over hairy area, remove in direction of hair growth. Get the patient permission to clip area (check agency policy). Remove any adhesive from skin.	Pulling tape toward dressing reduces stress on suture line or wound edges and reduces irritation and discomfort.

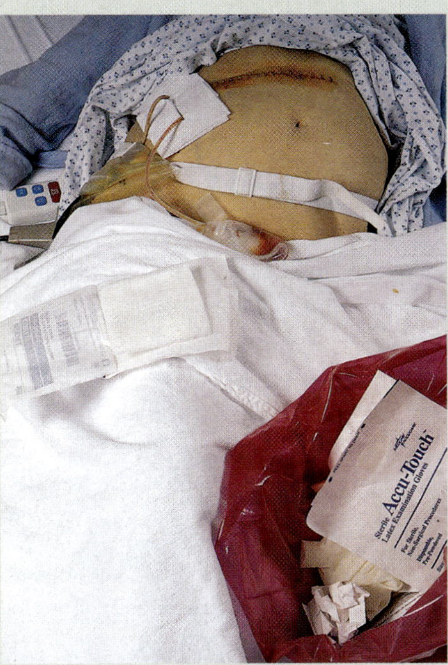

Step 2a Disposable waterproof bag placed near dressing site.

STEP	RATIONALE
4. With gloved hand or forceps remove dressing one layer at a time, observing appearance of drainage on dressing. Carefully remove outer secondary dressing first; then remove inner primary dressing that is in contact with wound bed. If drains are present, slowly and carefully remove dressings, avoiding tension on any drainage devices. Keep soiled undersurface from patient's sight.	Purpose of primary dressing is to remove necrotic tissue and exudate. Appearance of drainage may be upsetting to the patient. Avoids accidental removal of drain.
a. If dressing adheres to wound, moisten with normal saline and remove.	Prevents injury to wound surface and periwound during dressing removal.
5. Inspect wound and periwound for appearance, color, size (length, width, and depth), drainage, edema, presence and condition of drains, approximation (wound edges are together), granulation tissue, and odor. Use measuring guide or ruler to measure size of wound; see Skill 17.1, Step 10c. Gently palpate wound edges for bogginess or patient report of increased pain.	Assesses condition of wound and periwound condition. Indicates status of healing.
6. Fold dressings with drainage contained inside and remove gloves inside out. With small dressings, remove gloves inside out over dressing (see illustrations). Dispose of gloves and soiled dressing according to agency policy. Cover wound lightly with sterile gauze pad and perform hand hygiene.	Contains soiled dressings, prevents contact of nurse's hands with drainage, and reduces cross-contamination.
7. Describe appearance of wound and any indicators of wound healing to the patient.	Wounds may be unsettling and frightening to the patients. It helps the patient to know that wound appearance is as expected and whether healing is taking place.
8. Create sterile field with sterile dressing tray or individually wrapped sterile supplies on overbed table (see Chapter 9). Pour any prescribed solution into sterile basin.	Sterile dressings remain sterile while on or within sterile surface. Preparation of all supplies before dressing change prevents break in technique during dressing change.
9. Cleanse wound.	
a. Perform hand hygiene and apply clean gloves. Use gauze moistened in saline or antiseptic swab (per health care provider order) for each cleansing stroke or spray wound surface with wound cleanser.	Prevents transfer of organisms from previously cleaned area.
b. Clean from least to most contaminated area (see illustration).	Cleaning in this direction prevents introduction of organisms into wound.
c. If a drain is present, remove split gauze (see illustration A). Clean around any drain (if present) using circular strokes starting near drain and moving outward and away from insertion site (see illustration B).	Correct aseptic technique in cleaning prevents contamination.

STEP	RATIONALE

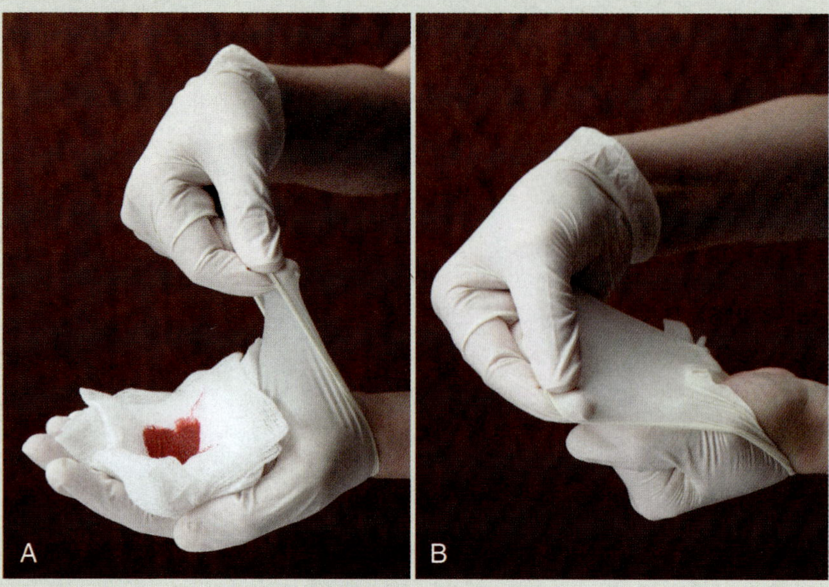

Step 6 A and **B,** Dispose of soiled dressings by placing in gloved hand and pulling glove off over dressing and then off hand.

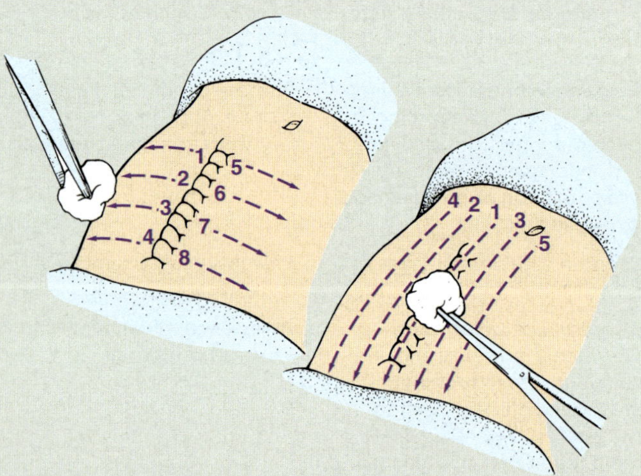

Step 9b Methods for cleansing a wound, cleansing from least to most contaminated.

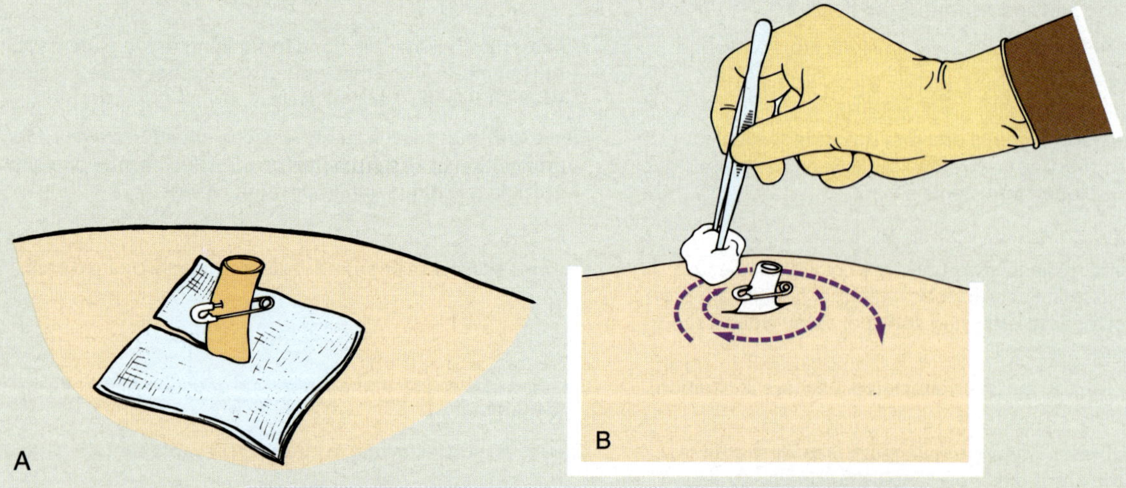

Step 9c A, Penrose drain with split gauze. **B,** Cleaning around a drain site.

STEP	RATIONALE
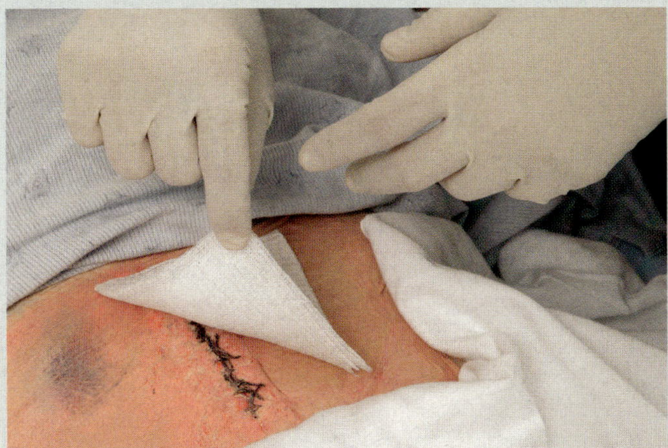 Step 12a(2) Placing dry gauze dressing over simple wound.	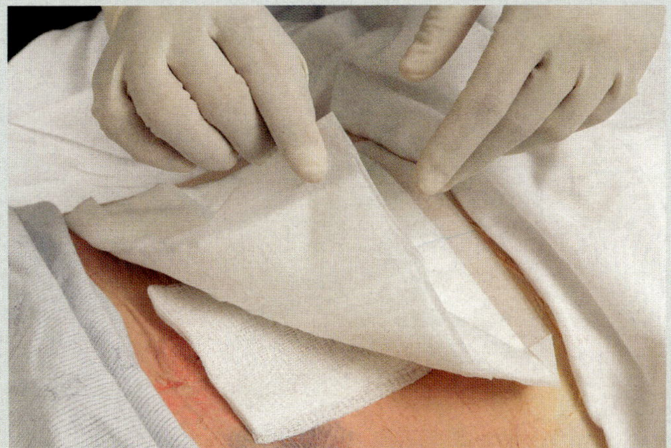 Step 12a(5) Placing abdominal pad over gauze dressing.
10. Use sterile dry gauze to blot wound bed.	Drying reduces excess moisture, which could eventually harbor microorganisms.
11. Apply antiseptic (if ordered) with sterile cotton-tipped applicator or gauze along wound edges. Dispose of gloves. Perform hand hygiene.	Helps reduce growth of microorganisms.
12. Apply dressing (see agency policy).	
a. Dry sterile dressing:	
(1) Apply clean gloves (see agency policy).	Some agencies or condition of wounds may require sterile gloves.
(2) Apply loose woven gauze as contact layer (see illustration).	Promotes proper absorption of drainage.
(3) If drain is present, apply precut, split 4 × 4–inch gauze around drain (see Step 9c).	Secures drain and promotes drainage absorption at site.
(4) Apply additional layers of gauze as needed.	Ensures proper coverage and optimal absorption.
(5) Apply thicker woven pad (e.g., Surgipad, abdominal [ABD] pad) (see illustration).	This dressing is used on postoperative wounds when there is excessive drainage.
b. Damp to dry dressing:	
(1) Apply sterile or clean gloves (see agency policy).	Reduces transmission of infection.
(2) Pour prescribed sterile solution onto 4 × 4–inch gauze. Wring out excess solution.	Moist gauze absorbs drainage and maintains a moist environment.

Clinical decision point: If using "packing strips," use sterile scissors to cut the amount of dressing that you will use to pack the wound. Do not let the packing strip touch the outside of the bottle. Pour prescribed sterile solution over packing strip. Wring out excess solution.

STEP	RATIONALE
(3) Unfold gauze and apply moist open-weave gauze as single layer directly onto wound surface. If wound is deep, gently pack gauze into wound with sterile gloved hand or forceps until all wound surfaces are in contact with moist gauze including dead spaces from sinus tracts, tunnels, and undermining (see illustrations A and B). Be sure that gauze does not touch periwound skin (see illustration C).	Inner gauze should be damp, not dripping wet, to absorb drainage and adhere to debris. When packing a wound, gauze should conform to base and side of wound (Bryant and Nix, 2016b). Wound is loosely packed to facilitate wicking of drainage into absorbent outer layer of dressing. Moisture from a dressing that is excessively wet will escape dressing and often macerates periwound area.

Clinical decision point: Be sure to count how many pieces of gauze are packed in the wound, especially deep wounds. This ensures that all gauze from previous dressing change are removed from wound.

Clinical decision point: When packing the wound, do not overpack or underpack the wound (Bryant and Nix, 2016b). Packing should fill the wound but should not be above the level of the skin.

STEP	RATIONALE
(4) Apply dry sterile 4 × 4–inch gauze over moist gauze.	Dry layer absorbs excessive moisture from wound.
(5) Cover with ABD pad, Surgipad, or gauze.	Protects wound from entrance of microorganisms.

Step 12b(3) **A** and **B,** Packing wound with fine-mesh gauze. **C,** Cross-section of deep wound packed loosely with gauze roll.

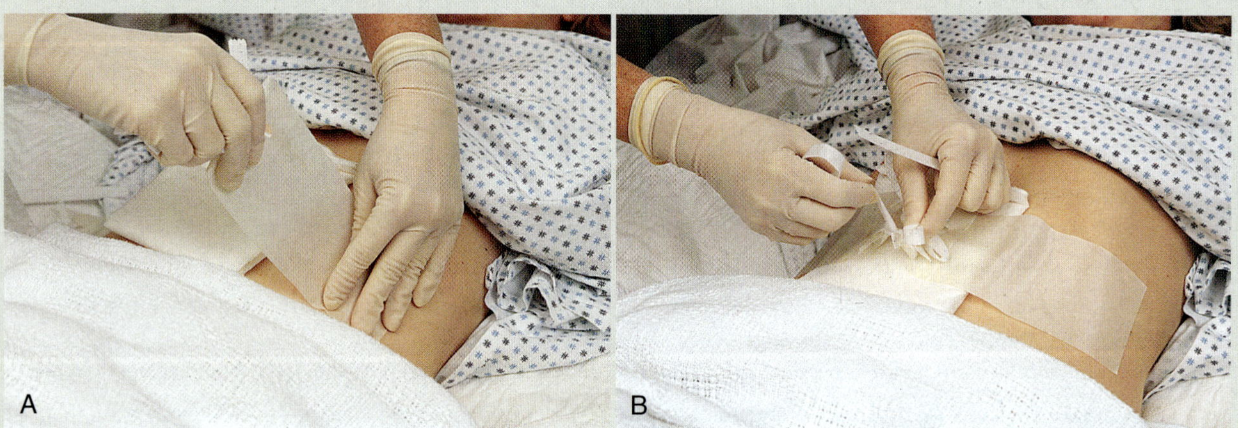

Step 13b Montgomery ties. **A,** Each tie is placed at side of gauze dressing. **B,** Securing ties encloses dressing.

STEP	RATIONALE
13. Secure dressing.	
a. Tape: Apply tape over gauze and 1–2 inches (2.5–5 cm) beyond dressing. Use nonallergenic tape when necessary.	Supports and helps dressing remain in place.
b. Montgomery ties (see illustrations):	Prevents skin irritation. Ties allow for repeated dressing changes without removal of tape.
(1) Be sure that skin is clean and dry. Application of skin barrier under adhesive tape is recommended.	
(2) Remove paper backing from adhesive surface and apply to skin 1–2 inches from the wound.	
(3) Place ties on opposite sides of dressing over skin or skin barrier.	
(4) Secure dressing by lacing ties across dressing snugly enough to hold it secure but without placing pressure on skin.	A solid skin barrier protects intact skin from stretch and tension of adhesive tape.
c. For protective window:	A protective window is an alternative to Montgomery ties for smaller wounds. There is less skin irritation by placing tape on window strips.
(1) Cut strip of hydrocolloid pad into four strips used to form a “window” around the wound.	
(2) Use skin barrier to wipe areas of skin where strips will be applied.	

STEP	RATIONALE

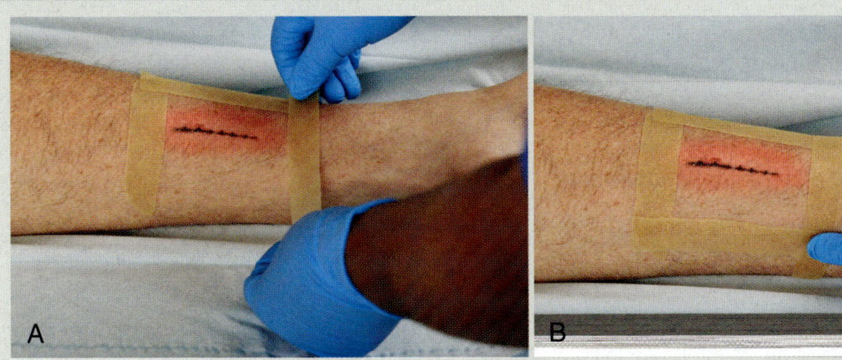
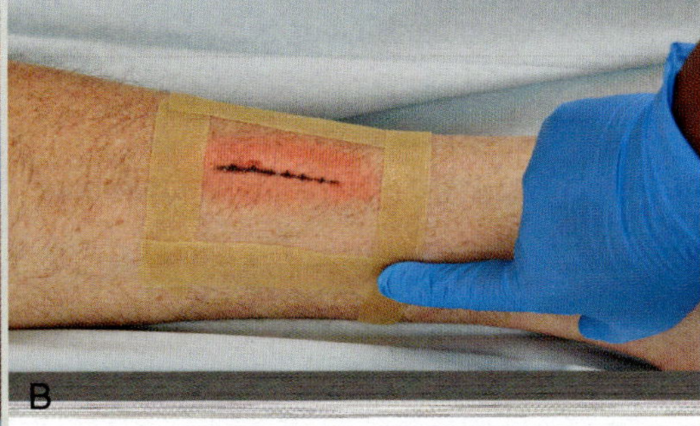

Step 13c(3) A and **B,** Apply adhesive strips to frame a "window" around the wound.

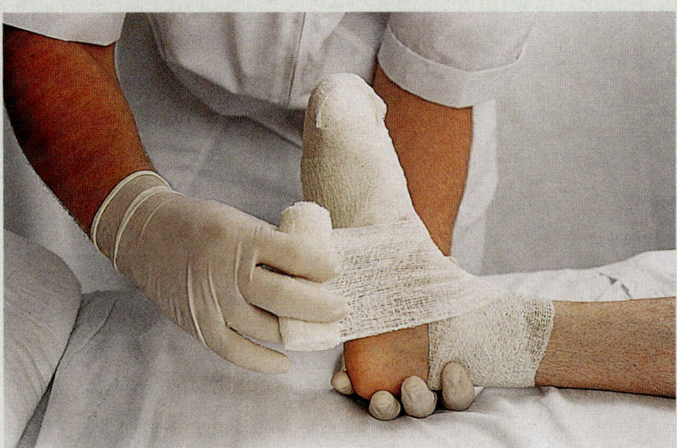

Step 13d Wrap roller gauze around extremity to secure dressing.

STEP	RATIONALE
(3) Apply adhesive strips to frame a "window" around the wound (see illustration).	
(4) Apply dressing and then secure tape ends to adhesive strips.	
d. For dressing an extremity, secure with roller gauze (see illustration) or elastic net.	Roller gauze conforms to contour of foot or hand.
14. Dispose of all dressing supplies. Remove cover gown and goggles, and remove gloves inside out; dispose of all items according to agency policy.	Reduces transmission of microorganisms. Clean environment enhances patient comfort.
15. Label tape over dressing with your initials and date dressing is changed.	Provides timeline for when next dressing change is to be scheduled.
16. Help the patient to comfortable position.	Promotes the patient's sense of well-being.
17. Perform hand hygiene.	Reduces transmission of microorganisms.
Evaluation	
1. Observe appearance of wound for healing: measure size of wound; observe amount, color, and type of drainage and periwound erythema or swelling.	Determines rate of healing.
2. Ask the patient to rate pain using a scale of 0–10.	Increased pain is often indication of wound complications such as infection or result of dressing pulling tissue.
3. Inspect condition of dressing at least every shift.	Determines status of wound drainage.
4. **Use teach back**: "I want to be sure I explained why and how often you need to continue these dressing changes in the hospital and at home. Tell me why it is important to change your dressing and how often to do so." Revise your instruction now or develop a plan for revised patient/family caregiver teaching if the patient/family caregiver is not able to teach back correctly.	Determines the patient's/family caregiver's level of understanding of instructional topic.

Recording and Reporting

- Record in nurses' notes in EHR, chart, or flow sheets relevant observations such as appearance and size of wound, characteristics of drainage, presence of necrotic tissue, type of dressing applied, patient's response to dressing change, and level of comfort.
- Document your evaluation of the patient and family caregiver learning.
- Report any unexpected appearance of wound drainage, accidental removal of drain, bright red bleeding, or evidence of wound dehiscence or evisceration.

Unexpected Outcomes and Related Interventions

- Wound appears inflamed and tender, drainage is evident, or odor is present.
  - Monitor the patient for signs of infection (e.g., fever, increased white blood cell count).
  - Notify health care provider.
  - Obtain wound cultures as ordered.
  - If there is yellow, tan, or brown necrotic tissue, notify health care provider to determine need for debridement.
- Wound bleeds during dressing change.
  - Observe color and amount of bloody drainage. If excessive, may need to apply direct dressing.
  - Inspect area along dressing and directly underneath the patient to determine amount of bleeding.
  - Obtain vital signs as needed.
  - Notify health care provider.
- Patient reports sensation that "something has given way under the dressing."
  - Observe wound for increased drainage or dehiscence (partial or total separation of wound layers) or evisceration (total separation of wound layers and protrusion of viscera through wound opening).
  - If dehiscence or evisceration occurs, protect wound. Cover with sterile moist dressing.
  - Instruct the patient to lie still.
  - Stay with the patient to monitor vital signs.
  - Notify health care provider.

SKILL 17.5 **Performing wound irrigation**

Equipment

- Irrigant/cleansing solution (volume 1.5–2 times the estimated wound volume)
- Irrigation delivery system (per order), depending on amount of pressure desired
- Sterile irrigation: It is often helpful to use a 35-mL syringe with a 19-gauge angiocatheter to facilitate optimal pressure for cleansing with minimal risk for tissue injury (Bryant and Nix, 2016b) or handheld shower.
- Protective equipment: sterile gloves, gown, and goggles if splash/spray risk exists
- Waterproof underpad if needed
- Dressing supplies
- Disposable waterproof biohazard bag
- Extra towels and padding (to use to protect bed)
- Wound assessment supplies

STEP	RATIONALE
Assessment	
1. Identify the patient by using at least two identifiers (e.g., name and birthday or name and medical record number) according to agency policy.	Ensures correct patient. Complies with The Joint Commission standards and improves patient safety (TJC, 2018).
2. Review health care provider's order for irrigation of open wound and type of solution to be used.	Open-wound irrigation requires medical order including type of solution to use.
3. Assess the patient's level of comfort using a pain scale of 0–10. If the patient is uncomfortable, offer an analgesic at least 30–45 min before the procedure.	Provides baseline to determine tolerance to procedure.
4. Review medical record for signs and symptoms related to the patient's open wound:	Provides ongoing data to indicate change in wound status (Nix, 2016).
a. Extent of impairment of skin integrity including size of wound	
b. Number of drains present	Awareness of drain position facilitates safe dressing removal and determines need for special dressings.
c. Drainage including previous amount, color, consistency, and odor	Drainage should decrease in healing wound. When drainage increases, it is often related to infection. The presence of an odor also indicates a wound infection (Doughty and Sparks, 2016).
d. Wound color	Color represents balance between necrotic tissue and new scar tissue. Proper selection of wound care products on the basis of wound color facilitates removal of necrotic tissue and promotes new tissue growth (Nix, 2016).

STEP	RATIONALE
e. Culture reports	An infected wound is colonized with bacteria. Culture reports identify type of bacteria and proper treatment. Ongoing wound cultures document resolution of infectious process (Stotts, 2016b).
f. Assessment of old dressing (e.g., dry and clean; drainage color, amount, and odor; bleeding).	Provides data of wound drainage on existing dressing.
5. Assess the patient for history of allergies to antiseptics, solutions, medications, tapes, or dressing material.	If known allergies, apply a sample of prescribed wound treatment as skin test before flushing wound with large volume of solution or select different tape or dressing material.
Planning	
1. Administer analgesic 30–45 min before starting wound irrigation procedure.	Promotes pain control and permits the patient to move more easily and be positioned to facilitate wound irrigation (Krasner, 2016).
2. Provide privacy and prepare bedside environment for patient safety.	Maintains privacy.
3. Prepare and organize appropriate supplies for wound irrigation and dressing.	
a. Cuff waterproof bag.	Cuffing helps to maintain large opening, permitting placement of contaminated dressing without touching waste bag itself.
4. Explain procedure to the patient and family members.	Promotes cooperation and reduces anxiety.
5. Perform hand hygiene, and position the patient.	Frequent hand hygiene reduces microorganisms.
6. Position the patient comfortably to permit gravitational flow of irrigating solution over wound and into collection receptacle (see illustration).	Directing solution from top to bottom of wound and from clean to contaminated area prevents further infection. Position the patient during planning stage, keeping in mind bed surfaces needed for later preparation of equipment.
a. Position the patient so that wound is vertical to collection basin. Irrigant should be at room temperature.	Room temperature solution increases comfort and reduces vascular constriction response in tissues.
b. Place padding or extra towel on bed under area where irrigation will take place.	Protects bedding from becoming wet.
c. Expose only the wound.	Prevents the patient from becoming chilled.
Implementation	
1. Perform hand hygiene.	While cleansing a wound, use meticulous hand hygiene and proper infection control procedures before and after removing soiled dressings to limit the risk for health care–acquired infection (Jaszarowski and Murphree, 2016).
2. Apply gown, mask, and goggles as indicated. Apply clean gloves and remove old dressing. Discard old dressing and gloves in biohazard bag. Perform hand hygiene.	Reduces transmission of microorganisms. Protects nurse from splashes or sprays of blood and body fluids.
3. Apply clean or sterile gloves (check agency policy). Use sterile precautions when sterile gloves are needed. Perform wound assessment and examine recent charted assessment of the patient's open wound (see Skill 17.1).	Provides ongoing wound-healing data.
4. Expose only the area near the wound.	Provides privacy and prevents chilling of the patient.
5. To irrigate wound with wide opening:	
a. Fill 35-mL syringe with irrigation solution.	Irrigating wound uses a mechanical force, which helps with separation and removal of necrotic debris and surface bacteria (Jaszarowski and Murphree, 2016). Flushing wound helps remove debris and facilitates healing by secondary intention.
b. Attach 19-gauge angiocatheter.	Catheter lumen delivers ideal pressure for cleansing and removing debris (Ramundo, 2016). Mechanical debridement may include irrigation, which can be performed through the use of a 35-mL syringe with a 19-gauge angiocatheter with irrigation pressures delivered between 4 and 15 psi (WOCN Society, 2016).
c. Hold syringe tip 2.5 cm (1 inch) above upper end of wound and over area being cleansed.	Prevents syringe contamination. Careful placement of syringe prevents unsafe pressure of flowing solution.
d. Using continuous pressure, flush wound; repeat Steps 5a–5c until solution draining into basin is clear.	Flushing wound helps to remove debris; clear solution indicates removal of all debris.

STEP	RATIONALE

Step 6 Patient position for wound irrigation.

6. Irrigate deep wound with very small opening:
   a. Attach soft catheter to filled irrigation syringe. — Catheter permits direct flow of irrigant into the wound. Expect wound to take longer to empty when opening is small.
   b. Gently insert tip of catheter into opening about 1.3 cm (0.5 inch). — Prevents tip from touching fragile inner wall of wound.

Clinical decision point: Do not force catheter into wound because this will cause tissue damage.

   c. Using slow, continuous pressure, flush the wound. — Use of slow mechanical force of stream of solution loosens particulate matter on wound surface and promotes healing (Ramundo, 2016).

Clinical decision point: Pulsatile high-pressure lavage is often the irrigation of choice for necrotic wounds. Pressure settings should be set per provider order, usually between 4 and 15 psi, and should not be used on skin grafts, exposed blood vessels, muscle, tendon, or bone. Use with caution if the patient has coagulation disorder or is taking anticoagulants (Ramundo, 2016).

   d. While keeping catheter in place, pinch it off just below the syringe. — Avoids contamination of sterile solution.
   e. Remove and refill the syringe. Reconnect to catheter and repeat until solution draining into basin is clear. Remove gloves and discard.
7. Perform hand hygiene and apply clean gloves. Cleanse wound with handheld shower.
   a. With the patient seated comfortably in shower chair or standing if condition allows, adjust spray to gentle flow; make sure that water is warm. — Useful for patients able to shower with assistance or independently. May be performed at home.
   b. Shower for 5–10 min with shower head 30 cm (12 inches) from the wound. — Ensures that the wound is thoroughly cleansed.
8. When indicated, obtain cultures after cleansing with nonbacteriostatic saline. — WOCN Society (2016) recommends using quantitative bacterial cultures (tissue biopsy or swab cultures). The most common types of wound cultures are swab technique, aspirated wound fluid, or tissue biopsy (Stotts, 2016a).

Clinical decision point: Obtain wound culture if indicated by the presence of inflammation around the wound, purulent odor or drainage, new drainage, or fever in the patient.

9. Dry wound edges with gauze; dry the patient after shower. — Prevents maceration of surrounding tissue from excess moisture.
10. Apply appropriate dressing and label with time, date, and nurse's initials. — Maintains protective barrier and healing environment for wound.
11. Remove mask, goggles, and gown. — Prevents transfer of microorganisms.
12. Dispose of equipment and soiled supplies, remove gloves, and perform hand hygiene. — Reduces transmission of microorganisms.
13. Help the patient to comfortable position.

Evaluation

1. Have the patient rate level of comfort on a scale of 0–10. — Patient's pain should not increase as a result of wound irrigation.
2. Observe type of tissue in wound bed. — Identifies wound-healing progress and determines type of wound cleansing and dressing needed.
3. Inspect dressing periodically (see agency policy). — Determines the patient's response to wound irrigation and need to modify plan of care.
4. Evaluate periwound skin integrity. — Determines whether extension of wound has occurred or signs of infection are present (warm red periwound skin).

STEP	RATIONALE
5. Observe for presence of retained irrigant.	Retained irrigant is medium for bacterial growth and subsequent infection.
6. **Use teach back**: "I want to be sure that I explained why the wound was irrigated today. Tell me why it is important to irrigate your wound." Revise your instruction now or develop a plan for revised patient/family caregiver teaching if the patient/family caregiver is not able to teach back correctly.	Determines the patient's/family caregiver's level of understanding of instructional topic.

Recording and Reporting

- Record in nurses' notes in EHR, chart, or flow sheets wound assessment before and after irrigation; amount, color, and odor of drainage on dressing removed; amount and type of solution used; irrigation device used; patient's tolerance of procedure; and type of dressing applied after irrigation.
- Document your evaluation of the patient and family caregiver learning.
- Immediately report to health care provider any evidence of fresh bleeding, sharp increase in pain, retention of irrigant, or signs of shock.

Unexpected Outcomes and Related Interventions

- Bleeding or serosanguineous drainage appears.
  - Flush wound during next irrigation using less pressure.
  - Notify health care provider of bleeding.
- Retained fluid and debris appear.
  - Increase amount of fluid during irrigation.
  - Increase amount of pressure when flushing wounds.
  - Make sure that the wound is clear of retained fluid and debris before applying new dressing.
- Suture line opening extends.
  - Notify health care provider.
  - Reevaluate amount of pressure to use for next wound irrigation.

KEY POINTS

- Wounds with partial-thickness tissue loss heal by epidermal repair, and full-thickness wounds heal by forming scar tissue.
- A clean surgical incision with little tissue loss heals by primary intention.
- When there is extensive tissue loss, a wound heals by secondary intention.
- Healing of full-thickness wounds proceeds through four overlapping phases: hemostasis, inflammation, proliferation, and remodeling.
- The chances of wound infection are greater when the wound contains dead or necrotic tissue, when foreign bodies lie on or near the wound, and when blood supply and tissue defenses are reduced.
- Physical stress from vomiting, coughing, or sudden muscular contraction can cause separation of wound edges (dehiscence).
- Wound assessment includes anatomical location, size (dimensions and depth of wound), type and percentage of wound tissue, volume and color of wound drainage, and condition of surrounding skin.
- Wound drains remove secretions within tissue layers to promote wound closure.
- Never collect a wound culture from old drainage.
- Principles of wound management include controlling or eliminating the cause, providing systemic support to reduce existing and potential cofactors, and maintaining a physiological wound environment.
- A moist environment supports wound healing.
- When cleaning wounds or drain sites, clean from the least to the most contaminated area.
- Apply a dressing or binder in a manner that does not impair circulation or irritate the skin.
- The safe use of heat or cold therapy requires an assessment of the patient's sensory function, identification of risk factors, and understanding of the physiological effects of heat and cold.
- An acute sprain, fracture, or bruise responds best to cold applications.
- Warm applications are effective for improving circulation to wound sites and promoting muscle relaxation.

REFERENCES

Ayello EA, Braden B. How and why do pressure risk assessment. Adv Skin Wound Care 2002;15(3):125.

Beitz JM. Wound healing. In: Doughty D, McNichol L, editors. Wound Ostomy and Continence Nurses Society core curriculum: wound management. Philadelphia: Wolters Kluwer; 2016.

Bergstrom N, Demuth PJ, Braden BJ. A clinical trial of the Braden Scale for predicting pressure sore risk. Nurs Clin North Am 1987a;22(2):417.

Bergstrom N, Braden BJ, Laguzza A, Holman V. The Braden Scale for predicting pressure sore risk. Nurs Res 1987b;36:205.

Bergstrom N, Braden B, Kemp M, Champagne M, Ruby E. Predicting pressure ulcer risk: a multisite study of the predictive validity of the Braden Scale. Nurs Res 1998;47(5):261.

Black J, Alves P, Brindle CT, Dealey C, Santamaria N, Call E, et al. Use of wound dressings to enhance prevention of pressure ulcers caused by medical devices. Int Wound J 2015;12(3):322.

Branson RD, Gomaa D, Rodriquez Jr D. Management of the artificial airway. Respir Care 2014;59(6):974.

Bryant RA. Types of skin damage and differential diagnosis. In: Bryant RA, Nix DP, editors. Acute and chronic wounds: current management concepts. 5th ed. St. Louis: Mosby; 2016.

Bryant RA, Nix DP. Developing and maintaining a pressure ulcer prevention program. In: Bryant RA, Nix DP, editors. Acute and chronic wounds: current management concepts. 5th ed. St. Louis: Mosby; 2016a.

Bryant RA, Nix DP. Principles of topical management. In: Bryant RA, Nix DP, editors. Acute and chronic wounds: current management concepts. 5th ed. St. Louis: Mosby; 2016b.

Burton AC, Yamada S: Relation between blood pressure and flow in the human forearm, *J ApplPhysiol* 4 (5): 329, 1951.

Doughty DB, McNichol LL. General concepts related to skin and soft tissue injury caused by mechanical factors. In: Doughty D, McNichol L, editors. Wound Ostomy and Continence Nurses Society core curriculum: wound management. Philadelphia: Wolters Kluwer; 2016.

Doughty DB, Sparks B. Wound healing physiology and factors that affect the repair process. In: Bryant RA, Nix DP, editors. Acute and chronic wounds: current management concepts. 5th ed. St. Louis: Mosby; 2016.

Edsberg LE, Black JM, Goldberg M, McNichol L, Moore L, Sieggreen M. Revised National Pressure Ulcer Advisory Panel Pressure injury staging system: revised pressure injury staging system. J Wound Ostomy Continence Nurs 2016;43(6):585.

European Pressure Ulcer Advisory Panel (EPUAP), National Pressure Ulcer Advisory Panel (NPUAP). Prevention of pressure ulcers: quick reference guide. Washington, DC: National Ulcer Advisory Panel; 2014. Available from: https://www.epuap.org/guidelines-old/.

Hopf HW, et al. Managing wound pain. In: Bryant RA, Nix DP, editors. Acute and chronic wounds: current management concepts. 5th ed. St. Louis: Mosby; 2016.

Jaszarowski KA, Murphree RW. Wound cleansing and dressing selection. In: Doughty D, McNichol L, editors. Wound Ostomy and Continence Nurses Society core curriculum: wound management. Philadelphia: Wolters Kluwer; 2016.

Krasner DL. Wound pain impact and assessment. In: Bryant RA, Nix DP, editors. Acute and chronic wounds: current management concepts. 5th ed. St. Louis: Mosby; 2016.

Maklebust J, Magnan MA. Pressure ulcer prevention. In: Doughty D, McNichol LL, editors. Wound Ostomy and Continence Nurses Society core curriculum: wound management. Philadelphia: Wolters Kluwer; 2016.

McNichol L, Watts C, Mackey D, Beitz JM, Gray M. Identifying the right surface for the right patient at the right time: generation and content validation of an algorithm for support surface selection. J Wound Ostomy Continence Nurs 2015;42(1):19.

National Pressure Ulcer Advisory Panel (NPUAP). National Pressure Ulcer Advisory Panel (NPUAP) announces a change in terminology from pressure ulcer to pressure injury and updates the stages of pressure injury. 2016. Available from: https://www.woundsource.com/blog/national-pressure-ulcer-advisory-panel-npuap-announces-change-in-terminology-pressure-ulcer#:~:text=Washington%2C%20DC%20%E2%80%93%20April%2013%2C,both%20intact%20and%20ulcerated%20skin.

National Pressure Ulcer Advisory Panel (NPUAP), European Pressure Ulcer Advisory Panel (EPUAP), Pan Pacific Pressure Ulcer Injury Alliance (PPPIA). In: Haseler E, editor. Prevention and treatment of pressure ulcers: clinical practice guideline. Osborne Park, Western Australia: Cambridge Media; 2014.

National Quality Forum (NQF). Patient Safety 2015 final report. 2016. Available from: http://www.qualityforum.org/Publications/2016/02/Patient_Safety_2015_Final_Report.aspx.

Netsch DS, Ruth Bryant and Denise Nix. Negative pressure wound therapy. In: Bryant RA, Nix DP, editors. Acute and chronic wounds: current management concepts. 5th ed. St. Louis: Mosby; 2016.

Nix DP. Skin and wound inspection and assessment. In: Bryant RA, Nix DP, editors. Acute and chronic wounds: current management concepts. 5th ed. St. Louis: Mosby; 2016.

Nix DP, Ruth Bryant and Denise Nix. Skin care needs of the neonatal and pediatric patient. In: Bryant RA, Nix DP, editors. Acute and chronic wounds: current management concepts. 5th ed. St. Louis: Mosby; 2016.

Petrofsky JS, Laymon M, Lee H. Effect of heat and cold on tendon flexibility and force to flex the human knee. Med Sci Monit 2013;19:661.

Pieper B. Pressure ulcers: impact, etiology, and classification. In: Bryant RA, Nix DP, editors. Acute and chronic wounds: current management concepts. 5th ed. St. Louis: Mosby; 2016.

Pittman J, Beeson T, Kitterman J, Lancaster S, Shelly A. Medical device-related hospital-acquired pressure ulcers: development of an evidence-based position statement. J Wound Ostomy Continence Nurs 2015; 42(2):151.

Ramundo JM. Wound debridement. In: Bryant RA, Nix DP, editors. Acute and chronic wounds: current management concepts. 5th ed. St. Louis: Mosby; 2016.

Schallom M, Cracchiolo L, Falker A, Foster J, Hager J, Morehouse T, et al. Pressure ulcer incidence in patients wearing nasal-oral versus full-face noninvasive ventilation masks. Am J Crit Care 2015;24(4):349.

Sommers MS: Color awareness: a must for patient assessment, *Am Nurs Today* 6 (1): 6, 2011.

Stotts NA. Wound infection: diagnosis and management. In: Bryant RA, Nix DP, editors. Acute and chronic wounds: current management concepts. 5th ed. St. Louis: Mosby; 2016a.

Stotts NA. Nutritional assessment and support. In: Bryant RA, Nix DP, editors. Acute and chronic wounds: current management concepts. 5th ed. St. Louis: Mosby; 2016b.

Thayer DM, Dorothy B. Doughty and Laurie L. McNichol. Top down injuries prevention and management of moisture associated skin damage, medical adhesive-related skin injury and skin tears. In: Doughty D, McNichol L, editors. Wound Ostomy and Continence Nurses Society core curriculum: wound management. Philadelphia, PA: Wolters Kluwer; 2016.

The Joint Commission (TJC). 2018 National Patient Safety Goals. Oakbrook Terrace, IL: The Joint Commission; 2018. Available from: https://www.jointcommission.org/standards_information/npsgs.aspx.

Wound, Ostomy and Continence Nurses (WOCN) Society. Clean vs. sterile dressing techniques for management of chronic wounds: a fact sheet. Mount Laurel, NJ: WOCN; 2011.

Wound, Ostomy and Continence Nurses (WOCN) Society. Guideline for prevention and management of pressure ulcers, WOCN Clinical Practice Guidelines Series. Mount Laurel, NJ: The Society; 2016.

18 Critical Thinking

OBJECTIVES

- To define critical thinking and characteristics of a professional nurse as a critical thinker.
- To explain the importance of clinical judgment in nursing practice for clinical decisions.
- To describe how reflection is helpful in clinical decision-making.
- To explain the levels of critical thinking in nursing including basic and complex thinking.
- To discuss scientific method, problem-solving, and decision-making as critical thinking competencies.
- To describe critical thinking skills used in nursing practice and utilization of nursing process as a competency.
- To explain the components of a critical thinking model for clinical decision-making.
- To discuss the critical thinking attitudes used in clinical decision-making.
- To explain influence of intellectual and professional standards in nurse's critical thinking.
- To discuss the relationship between nursing process and critical thinking for better practice.

KEY TERMS

clinical decision-making, p. 414
clinical inferences, p. 414
clinical judgment, p. 409
critical thinking, p. 410
decision-making, p. 413
diagnostic reasoning, p. 413
nursing process, p. 415
problem-solving, p. 413
reflection, p. 411
scientific method, p. 413
workarounds, p. 417

INTRODUCTION

Every day you think critically without realizing it. If your computer flashes an error warning, you think about the actions you took before the error, consider possible causes of the problem, and correct a key stroke error or reboot the computer. If you decide to walk your dogs, go to the door, and notice that it is raining, you change into your raincoat. These examples show how you use basic critical thinking skills every day.

As a professional nurse, you care for patients with unique, complicated health care problems that can change within minutes. Thus, critical thinking is embedded in your everyday routine because it involves knowing as much as possible about each patient and sorting out the information into patterns to clarify problems, recognize changes, and make appropriate decisions under pressure (Rueskin, 2015). Critical thinking is an essential process for safe, efficient, and skillful nursing intervention (Papathanasiou, 2014). Sound critical thinking enables you to face each new experience and problem involving a patient's care with open-mindedness, confidence, and continual inquiry. This skill enables you to avoid common mistakes and proceed in the most logical manner.

Critical thinking is not a simple, step-by-step, linear process. It is a thinking process that you will develop as you gain clinical nursing experience.

CLINICAL JUDGMENT IN NURSING PRACTICE

Why is the nursing role so important to health care? Nurses make the decisions and judgments that help ensure that patients receive the most appropriate, timely, and effective interventions to maintain or restore their health. A **clinical judgment** is a conclusion about a patient's needs, concerns, or health problems and/or the decisions to take or avoid action, use or modify standard approaches, or improvise new approaches based on the patient's response (Tanner, 2006). Clinical decision-making separates professional nurses from nursing assistive personnel (NAP). For example, an RN observes for changes in patients' conditions, recognizes changes and potential problems as they arise, and takes quick action when a patient's clinical condition worsens. Nurses direct technical personnel to perform basic aspects of care based on patient need; technical personnel do not have the knowledge or critical thinking skills to analyze when or why patients' clinical needs change. Good clinical decision-making requires you to investigate and analyze all aspects of a clinical situation or problem and then apply scientific and nursing knowledge to choose the best course of action.

In 2006, Dr Christine Tanner described a research-based model of clinical judgment in nursing. It included the following conclusions:

- Clinical judgments are influenced more by the nurse's experience and knowledge than by the objective data about the situation at hand. This means experience is crucial.
- Sound clinical judgment partly relies on knowing the patient and his or her typical pattern of responses as well as an engagement with the patient and his or her concerns.
- Clinical judgments are influenced by the context of clinical situations and the culture of patient care units.
- Nurses use a variety of reasoning patterns alone or in combination, including reflection.

Critical thinking and good clinical judgment enable you to creatively seek knowledge, act quickly when conditions change, and make quality decisions to protect your patient's well-being. This process requires you to be flexible and able to recognize important aspects of an undefined clinical situation, interpret their meanings, and respond appropriately (Tanner, 2006).

Critical Thinking

A critical thinker identifies the important data in each clinical situation, imagines and explores alternatives, considers ethical principles and care standards, and makes informed decisions about patient care.

Critical thinking is a continuous process characterized by open-mindedness, continual inquiry, and perseverance combined with a willingness to look at each unique patient situation and identify the assumptions that are true and relevant.

Critical thinking includes recognizing an issue (e.g., patient problem), analyzing information related to the issue (e.g., clinical and historical data about the patient), evaluating information (including assumptions and evidence), and drawing conclusions.

An effective nurse engages in critical thinking by fully assessing a patient's health condition, meaning that a nurse learns as much as possible about the patient from many sources to form a clear holistic view of a patient's problems and the approaches for resolving them. Critical thinking allows you to focus on the important issues at hand in any clinical situation and make decisions that produce desired outcomes (Raterink, 2011).

You begin to learn critical thinking early in your practice. Critical thinking is a way of thinking about a situation by asking the following:

- "Why does the patient have this condition?"
- "Are the signs and symptoms demonstrated by the patient what I would expect for the condition or situation?"
- "What do I really know about this patient's situation?"
- "What options do I have?"
- "What factors can contribute to comfort?"

Evidence-based knowledge (knowledge based on research or clinical expertise) makes nurses better informed critical thinkers.

Critical thinking requires cognitive skills, the habit of asking questions, the dedication to stay well informed, honesty in facing personal biases, the willingness to reconsider conclusions, and the ability to think clearly about issues (Facione, 1990). Table 18.1 summarizes core critical thinking skills that, when applied to nursing, show the complex nature of clinical decision-making.

Table 18.1 Core Critical Thinking Skills

Skill	Description
Interpretation	Interpretation is the process of discovering, determining, or assigning meaning. Interpretation skills can be applied to anything (e.g., written messages, charts, diagrams, maps, graphs, memes, and verbal and nonverbal exchanges). People apply their interpretive skills to behaviors, events, and social interactions when deciding what they think something means in a given context.
Analysis	Analytical skills are used to identify assumptions, reasons, themes, and the evidence used in making arguments or offering explanations. They enable us to consider all the key elements in any given situation and to determine how those elements relate to one another. People with strong analytical skills notice important patterns and details. People use analysis to gather the most relevant information from spoken language, documents, signs, charts, graphs, and diagrams.
Inference	Inference skills enable us to draw conclusions from reasons, evidence, observations, experiences, or our values and beliefs. Using inference, we can predict the most likely consequences of the options we may be considering. Inference enables us to see the logical consequences of the assumptions we may be making. Sound inferences rely on accurate information. People with strong inference skills draw logical or highly reliable conclusions using all forms of analogical, probabilistic, empirical, and mathematical reasoning.
Evaluation	Evaluative skills are used to assess the credibility of the claims people make or post, and to assess the quality of the reasoning people display when they make arguments or give explanations. We can also apply our evaluation skills to assess the quality of many other elements that are important for good thinking, such as analyses, interpretations, explanations, inferences, options, opinions, beliefs, hypotheses, proposals, and decisions. People with strong evaluation skills can judge the quality of arguments and the credibility of speakers and writers.
Explanation	Explanation is the process of justifying what we have decided to do or what we have decided to believe. People with strong explanation skills provide the evidence, methods, and considerations they actually relied on when making their judgment. Explanations can include our assumptions, reasons, values, and beliefs. Strong explanations enable others to understand and to evaluate our decisions.
Self-regulation	Self-regulation in the context of critical thinking relates to monitoring and, if necessary, correcting any mistakes that may have occurred in the process of interpreting, analyzing, inferring, evaluating, or explaining. Self-regulation occurs throughout the critical thinking process; it is not confined to the ending point only. As soon as an individual or a thinking team identifies an error as a result of the process of self-monitoring, that error can be corrected so that the overall process of critical thinking can again begin to move forward toward its culmination, which is the considered judgment about what to believe or what to do in any given context. Self-regulation can focus any of the elements in that process, including how the problem was framed, what was accepted as evidence, what methods were used, what the guiding theoretical considerations were, and what level of closure was deemed appropriate for regarding the problem as having been solved or the decision as having been made. Self-regulation is the skill that separates critical thinking from uncritical thinking.

Learning to think critically helps you care for patients by acting as their advocate and making informed choices about their care. Facione and Facione (1996) identified concepts for critical thinking (Table 18.2). These concepts are still current and essential to the use of critical thinking skills. Critical thinking is more than just problem-solving. It is an attempt to continually improve your effectiveness in facing patient care problems.

Reflection

As you care for patients, you will often review your practice experience to describe, analyze, and evaluate it (Barksby et al., 2015). You might ask yourself the following:

- How did I act?
- Why did I take such an action?
- What could I have done differently?
- What should I do in a similar situation in the future?

This is **reflection**, a part of critical thinking that involves purposefully reviewing a situation to discover its purpose or meaning. As a nurse, you will reflect on the purpose and meaning of each patient's situation as well as the purpose and meaning of your actions in that situation.

Reflection means recalling patient care situations to explore the factors that influenced your actions in handling each situation. It is like replaying a video. It is not intuitive. It means visualizing a past situation and taking time to honestly review everything you remember about the situation. This reflection allows you to gain new knowledge and raise questions about your practice, which can lead to a search for better evidence for practice (Barksby et al., 2015). Research shows that reflective reasoning improves the accuracy of making diagnostic conclusions (Mamede et al., 2012). This means that gathering information about a patient, reflecting on the meaning of your findings, and exploring the possible meaning of those findings improve your ability to identify a patient's problems (see Chapter 19). Reflection helps you to focus on learning and self-awareness and to avoid simply retelling an event (Barksby et al., 2015). Box 18.1 lists steps of a model for using reflection in your practice.

BOX 18.1 Model for Reflection

REFLECT: This model can be used individually or as a process shared with others.

R	**Recall** the events: Review the facts about a situation, and describe what happened.
E	**Examine** your responses: Think about or discuss your thoughts and actions at the time of the situation.
F	Acknowledge **feelings**: Identify any feelings you had during the situation.
L	**Learn** from the experience: Review and highlight what you learned from the situation, for example, your patient's responses and your actions.
E	**Explore** options: Think about or discuss your options for similar situations in the future.
C	**Create** a plan of action: Create a plan for action in future similar situations.
T	Set a **timescale**: Set a time by which your plan of action will be completed.

Adapted from Barksby J, et al: A new model of reflection for clinical practice, *Nurs Times* 111(34/35):21-23, 2015.

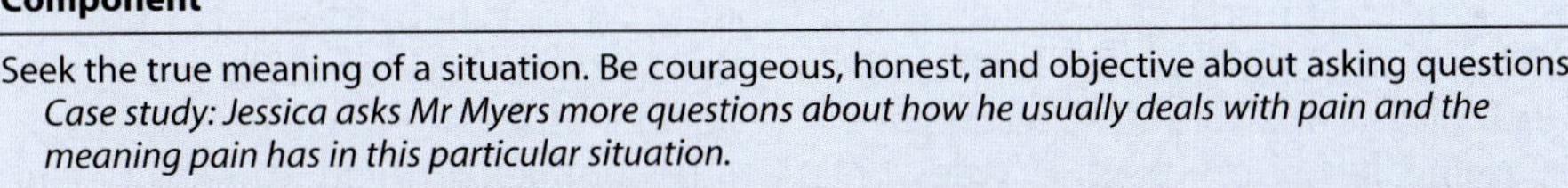

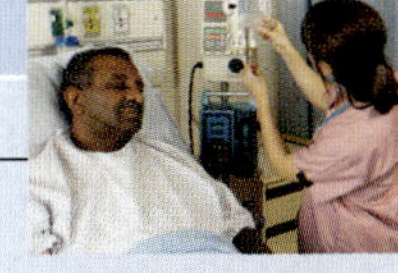

Copyright © monkey businessimages/ iStock/Thinkstock.

Table 18.2 Concepts for a Critical Thinker

Concept	Component
Truth seeking	Seek the true meaning of a situation. Be courageous, honest, and objective about asking questions. *Case study: Jessica asks Mr Myers more questions about how he usually deals with pain and the meaning pain has in this particular situation.*
Open-mindedness	Be tolerant of different views and be sure that you clearly know your patients' views. Be aware of your own biases and respect the right of others to have different opinions. *Case study: Jessica asks Mr Myers to tell her the approaches he would like to use to become mobile after surgery. Mr Myers tells Jessica that he fears walking too soon and hurting his back.*
Analyticity	Be alert to potentially problematic situations; anticipate possible results or consequences (e.g., how should a patient respond to a certain treatment?); value reason; use evidence-based knowledge. *Case study: Jessica points out to Mr Myers that he has had back pain for some time and explains that evidence shows that persistent low back pain leads to exercise intolerance and further loss of functional capacity (Atalay et al., 2012). His ability to regain mobility quickly will reduce the risk of further decline.*
Systematicity	Be organized and focused and work hard in answering your questions. Organize inquiry based on priorities of care. *Case study: Jessica focuses on pain assessment and gives Mr Myers additional analgesia after consulting with Mr Myers and his surgeon to identify the best medication considering Mr Myers' previous pain history.*
Self-confidence	Trust your own reasoning processes. *Case study: Jessica believes that by managing Mr Myers' pain well, she will build trust with him as she prepares him for the mobility protocol and use of relaxation techniques.*
Inquisitiveness	Be eager to acquire knowledge and explanations even when applications of the knowledge are not immediately obvious. Value learning for learning's sake. *Case study: Jessica decides to take some time and talk with Mr Myers' wife about her husband's experience with pain and his coping strategies.*
Maturity	Multiple solutions are acceptable. Reflect on your own judgments; develop cognitive maturity. *Case study: Jessica consults with a physical therapist who also is willing to talk with Mr Myers about the importance of early mobility. Jessica and the physical therapist will form a plan for physical therapy and nursing staff to implement an ambulation schedule during Mr Myers' waking hours.*

Modified from Facione N, Facione P: Externalizing the critical thinking in knowledge development and clinical judgment, *Nurs Outlook* 44:129, 1996.

Knowing the Patient

Clinical learning is a lifelong process. Learning to know patients results from working with many patients over time, hearing accounts of their experiences with illness, observing them, and coming to understand how they typically respond (Tanner, 2006). Knowing each patient as an individual with a unique pattern of responses enables you to individualize your responses and interventions (Tanner, 2006).

Knowing your patients occurs by engaging with them, acting responsibly, and providing excellent care. Show concern for patients and their families' well-being so that you can learn who they are, how illness has affected their lives, and how that knowledge should affect your approach to care. Make the patient and family partners in care. To make good clinical decisions, you must understand not only the pathophysiological and diagnostic aspects of a patient's clinical presentation and disease but also the effect of the illness on the patient and family and their physical, social, and emotional strengths and coping resources. Always approach your clinical work informed, and do not consider it simply a task-based, detached exercise. Reflect on your practice and knowledge to learn to think like a nurse.

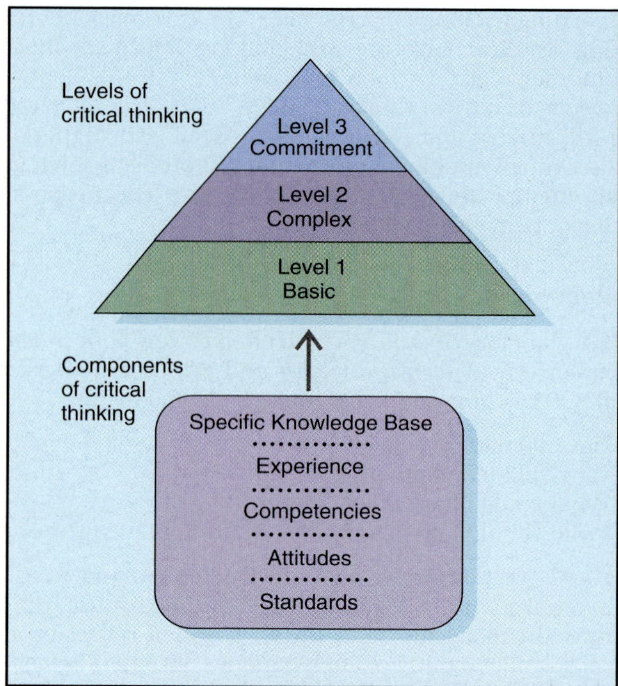

Fig. 18.1 Critical thinking model for nursing judgment. (Redrawn from Kataoka-Yahiro M, Saylor C: A critical thinking model for nursing judgment, *J Nurs Educ* 33[8]:351, 1994. Modified from Glaser E: *An experiment in the development of critical thinking,* New York, 1941, Bureau of Publications, Teachers College, Columbia University; Miller J, Malcolm N: Critical thinking in the nursing curriculum, *Nurs Health Care* 11:67, 1990; Paul R: *The art of redesigning instruction.* In Willsen J, Blinker AJA, editors: *Critical thinking: how to prepare students for a rapidly changing world,* Santa Rosa, CA, 1993, Foundation for Critical Thinking.)

LEVELS OF CRITICAL THINKING IN NURSING

Your ability to think critically grows as you gain knowledge and experience in nursing practice. Kataoka-Yahiro and Saylor (1994) developed a critical thinking model (Fig. 18.1) that includes three levels of critical thinking in nursing: basic, complex, and commitment.

Basic Critical Thinking

Beginning nursing students are very task oriented, focusing on performing skills and organizing nursing care activities correctly. At the basic level of critical thinking, a student trusts that experts have the right answers for every problem. Thinking is concrete and based on a set of rules or principles. For example, a student might rely on a hospital procedure manual or a clinical simulation guideline for inserting a nasogastric tube. The student follows the steps of the procedure without learning how to adjust his or her approach when a problem arises or a patient has a unique need (e.g., a patient has a deviated nasal septum or has difficulty swallowing). The student does not have enough experience to anticipate how to individualize or adapt the procedure when various problems arise. At this level, answers to complex problems are perceived as either right or wrong (e.g., the nasogastric tube will not advance because it is coiled in the throat), and a single solution usually resolves each problem (e.g., removing the tube and starting over). Such basic critical thinking is an early step in the development of reasoning (Kataoka-Yahiro and Saylor, 1994). A basic critical thinker learns to accept the diverse opinions and values of experts (e.g., instructors and staff nurse role models). However, inexperience, weak competencies, and inflexible attitudes can slow a nurse's ability to move to the next level of critical thinking.

Complex Critical Thinking

As a complex critical thinker, you begin to rely less on experts in daily care. You learn to analyze data and examine choices more independently. Your thinking abilities and initiative to look beyond expert opinion begin to increase. As your critical thinking skills grow, you learn that you must consider alternative and perhaps even conflicting solutions.

In complex critical thinking, you learn to synthesize knowledge. This means that you combine your experience and knowledge of patients to develop a new thought or idea. When you consider therapies for patients, you realize that each option has benefits and risks that factor into your choice. Your thinking becomes more creative and innovative. At this level, you are more willing to consider deviations from standard protocols or procedures and to provide more individualized care.

Commitment

The third level of critical thinking is commitment (Kataoka-Yahiro and Saylor, 1994). In commitment, you anticipate the need to make choices without assistance from others. You accept accountability for the decisions you make. As a nurse, you do more than just consider the complex alternatives that might resolve a problem. At the commitment level, you choose an action or belief based on the alternatives available and stand by your choice. Sometimes the choice is to avoid or delay acting.

CRITICAL THINKING COMPETENCIES

Kataoka-Yahiro and Saylor (1994) describe critical thinking competencies as the cognitive processes a nurse uses to make judgments about the clinical care of patients. The three competencies are general critical thinking, specific critical thinking in clinical situations, and specific critical thinking in nursing.

General critical thinking processes are not unique to the nursing profession. They include the **scientific method**, **problem-solving**, and **decision-making**. Specific critical thinking competencies in clinical health care situations include clinical inference, **diagnostic reasoning**, and clinical decision-making. The specific critical thinking competency in nursing is the nursing process (see Chapter 19), which involves each of the three specific critical thinking competencies.

General Critical Thinking Competencies

Scientific Method

The scientific method is a way to solve problems through reasoning. It is a systematic, ordered approach to gathering data and solving problems. Professionals use it in nursing, medicine, and a variety of other health care disciplines. This approach looks for the truth or verifies that a set of facts agrees with reality. Nurse researchers use the scientific method when testing research questions in nursing practice situations. The scientific method has five steps:

1. Identifying the problem
2. Collecting data
3. Forming a question or hypothesis
4. Testing the question or hypothesis
5. Evaluating results of the test or study

The scientific method is one formal way to approach a problem, plan a solution, test the solution, and come to a conclusion. Table 18.3 gives an example of a nursing practice issue solved by application of the scientific method in a research study.

Problem-Solving

You face problems every day. When a problem arises, you obtain information, combine it with what you already know, and develop a solution. Patients routinely present problems in practice. A traditional approach for solving problems is to clarify the problem, identify possible causes, assess and identify alternatives, choose one, implement it, and evaluate whether the problem was solved.

A systematic approach to problem-solving makes it more likely that you will find an appropriate solution. Effective problem-solving includes evaluating a solution over time to be sure that it continues to be effective. If a problem recurs, you try various options. Solving a problem in one situation adds to your clinical experience and enables you to apply the knowledge in future patient situations.

Decision-Making

When you face a problem and choose a course of action from several options, you are making a decision. Decision-making focuses on resolving a problem. Following a set of criteria helps you make a thorough and thoughtful decision. The criteria may be personal, may be based on an organizational policy, or, in the case of nursing, may be based on a professional standard.

For example, a person practices decision-making when he or she chooses a health care provider. To make a decision, the individual must recognize and define the problem (the need for a health care provider) and assess all options (e.g., consider recommended health care providers or choose one whose office is close to home). The person weighs the options against a set of personal criteria (experience, friendliness, reputation, location), tests possible options (talks directly

Table 18.3 Using the Scientific Method to Solve Nursing Practice Questions

Clinical problem: The incidence of a health care–associated infection, *Clostridium difficile* infection, has increased in a hospital general medicine patient care unit. The nursing staff on the unit practice committee, an infection control specialist, and a clinical nurse specialist in medicine have met to discuss factors that may be contributing to the problem. They note that visitors are inconsistent in the use of antiseptic hand rubs. A staff member questions whether the use of hand rubs is the best approach for this type of infection.

Step	Actions
Identify the problem.	▪ The incidence of *C. difficile* has increased among patients in a general medicine patient care unit.
Collect data.	▪ Staff members review the literature about the nature of *C. difficile* infection and the hand antiseptic techniques recommended to prevent the infection. ▪ Staff members search the literature for studies that investigated hand-hygiene practices of visitors of hospitalized patients. ▪ Staff members review performance improvement reports to monitor the occurrence of *C. difficile* in the unit. ▪ The infection control specialist is asked to discuss the trends within the hospital in the incidence of *C. difficile*.
Form a research question to study the problem.	▪ Does visitor use of antiseptic hand rub with chlorhexidine versus handwashing with soap and water reduce the incidence of *C. difficile* infection in medical patients?
Answer the question.	▪ The nurse specialist and a small team of staff members create a 4-month study approved by the hospital research board. ▪ Patients' visitors are asked to use a chlorhexidine rub on their hands before entering and leaving patient rooms. ▪ Visitors switch to handwashing with soap and water for the next 2 months. ▪ The infection control specialist tracks the incidence of *C. difficile* infection over the 4 months.
Evaluate the results of the study. Does the study answer the research question?	▪ Compare the incidence of *C. difficile* infection for the 2-month period when each hand-hygiene method was used. ▪ Results showed a decline in the number of *C. difficile* infections when visitors used chlorhexidine.

with health care providers), and makes a decision. This process leads to informed conclusions that are supported by evidence and reason. Decision-making goes hand in hand with problem-solving.

Specific Critical Thinking Competencies

Diagnostic Reasoning and Inference

Diagnostic reasoning depends on your state of readiness to apply critical thinking (Levett-Jones et al., 2010). You must be committed to doing diagnostic reasoning well. It is influenced by your attitudes, philosophical perspective, and preconceptions about nursing. For example, if you do not value a holistic approach to nursing, you will likely not complete thorough assessments of your patients. Preconceptions and inaccurate assumptions such as "most people who are poor have an alcohol use disorder" or "people who are obese are not motivated to improve their health" will negatively affect your reasoning. You must reflect on and question your assumptions and prejudices when you engage in diagnostic reasoning to become a competent thinker and to ultimately improve patient outcomes. Diagnostic reasoning involves a combination of gathering and analyzing information (Delany and Golding, 2014).

As you collect information about a patient in a clinical situation, diagnostic reasoning begins. It is the analytical process for determining a patient's health problems. You must accurately recognize a patient's health problems before you choose solutions and implement actions. Diagnostic reasoning requires you to assign meaning to the behaviors and physical signs and symptoms a patient presents. This begins when you interact with a patient, make physical or behavioral observations, and review medical history information. An expert nurse sees the context of a patient situation (e.g., a patient who has a long history of back pain is now recovering from surgery, is uniformed about postoperative care, and will require routine analgesics for reliable pain management). The nurse observes patterns and themes (e.g., symptoms that include wincing and moaning and the inability of the patient to describe what early mobility requires him or her to do). Once diagnostic reasoning is complete and problems are identified, the nurse makes clinical decisions quickly (e.g., control pain first so the patient can later attend and learn about the mobility protocol and be able to get out of bed). The information a nurse collects and analyzes leads to a diagnosis of a patient's condition and the appropriate interventions.

Nurses do not make medical diagnoses; they make nursing diagnoses (see Chapter 19). They do, however, assess and monitor patients closely and compare patients' signs and symptoms with signs and symptoms that are common to a medical diagnosis. This type of diagnostic reasoning helps health care providers pinpoint a problem and select proper therapies more quickly.

As a part of diagnostic reasoning, you make **clinical inferences**. You learn to draw conclusions from related pieces of patient data and previous experience with similar evidence. An inference is a conclusion the nurse draws from data before making a nursing diagnosis.

As a student, you confirm your judgments with more experienced nurses or your instructor. Your judgment can be wrong at times, but consulting with nurse experts gives you feedback to support future clinical judgments. Often you cannot make a precise diagnosis during your first meeting with a patient. You may sense that the patient has a problem, but you lack sufficient data to make a specific diagnosis. Some patients' physical conditions limit their ability to tell you about their symptoms. Some patients choose not to share sensitive and important information during your initial assessment. Patients' behaviors and physical responses often become observable after your initial assessment. When you are uncertain of a diagnosis, continue collecting data from all possible sources. You must critically analyze changing clinical situations on a continuous basis until you can determine a patient's unique situation. Diagnostic reasoning takes practice and must become part of your routine thinking in nursing practice.

Clinical Decision-Making

Clinical decision-making or reasoning is a problem-solving activity that involves diagnostic reasoning as well as deciding on the appropriate therapeutic actions specific to a patient's situation and wishes (Delany and Golding, 2014). When you face a clinical problem such as a patient who has an area of redness over the heel, you form a diagnostic conclusion that identifies the problem (impaired skin integrity and possible early formation of a pressure injury); then you choose the best nursing interventions (skin care, turning, and reducing heel pressure). Nurses make clinical decisions to improve a patient's health or maintain wellness. This means minimizing the severity of the problem or resolving the problem completely. **Clinical decision-making** requires problem-solving and reasoning so you can choose the options that produce the best patient outcomes based on a patient's condition and priority of the problem.

Part of developing expertise in clinical decision-making comes from knowing your patients. Expert nurses develop a level of knowing that enables them to recognize patterns of patient symptoms and responses. You begin to acquire this expertise by learning to assess patients thoroughly and by actively engaging with them. You investigate and reflect on all your clinical observations and then apply nursing and scientific knowledge to choose a course of action. For example, an expert nurse who has worked on a general surgery unit for many years knows that when a patient's blood pressure falls, it becomes necessary to further assess the patient. The nurse checks the patient's pulse and level of consciousness and quickly reviews recent laboratory tests to detect any internal hemorrhage (which could result in a fall in blood pressure, rapid pulse, a change in consciousness, or a decrease in blood count). An expert nurse can do this more quickly than a new nurse because the expert nurse has developed pattern recognition.

The expert nurse has a combination of experience, time spent in a specific clinical area, and the quality of relationships formed with patients that enables him or her to know clinical situations and quickly anticipate and select the proper course of action (Tanner, 2006). Spending more time with each patient to thoroughly observe and measure normal and abnormal findings is a way to know your patient better. In addition, consistently monitoring patients as problems develop helps you see how clinical changes evolve over time.

Select nursing interventions based on clinical knowledge and specific information that you collect from your patients, including:

- Initial assessment data about a patient's status and situation, including data collected by actively listening to a patient discuss his or her health care needs
- Knowledge of a patient's clinical variables (e.g., age, severity of the problem, preexisting disease conditions) and how the variables are linked
- Knowledge of a patient's current health risks (e.g., smoking, alcohol use, lack of immunization) related to the problem
- A judgment about the likely course and outcomes of the diagnosed problem
- Additional relevant data about a patient's needs with respect to the activities of daily living, functional capacity, and social resources
- Knowledge about the nursing intervention options available and the way in which specific interventions may affect a patient's situation

Always keep the patient your center of attention as you make clinical decisions. Making an accurate clinical decision allows you to set care priorities. Because patients bring different variables to a situation, an activity or treatment is often a higher priority in one situation than in another.

Do not assume that a particular condition is a priority. For example, you expect that a patient immediately out of surgery will experience pain, and pain treatment is often a priority of nursing care. However, if the patient is experiencing anxiety with heightened pain perception, the nurse must focus on relieving anxiety before pain-relief measures can be effective.

Clinical decision-making is challenging because nurses care for multiple patients in a fast-paced and unpredictable environment. When you work in a busy setting, use criteria such as the clinical condition of a patient, Maslow's hierarchy of needs, risks involved in treatment delays, and patients' expectations of care to decide which patients have higher priorities. Applying critical thinking to clinical decision-making enables you to attend to a high-priority patient and perhaps delegate less essential tasks to an NAP. Skillful, prioritized clinical decision-making allows you to manage the various problems associated with groups of patients.

The Nursing Process as a Competency

Nurses apply the **nursing process** as a competency when delivering patient care (Kataoka-Yahiro and Saylor, 1994). The American Nurses Association (ANA) (2010) standards set forth the framework for critical thinking in the application of the five-step nursing process (Fig. 18.2): assessment, diagnosis, planning, implementation, and evaluation (see Chapter 19). The purpose of the nursing process is to diagnose and treat human responses (e.g., patient symptoms, need for knowledge, or emotional stress) to actual or potential health problems (ANA, 2010). Using this process enables nurses to help patients meet agreed-on outcomes for better health. The nursing process requires a nurse to use the general and specific critical thinking competencies described earlier in this chapter to focus on a specific patient's unique needs. The format of the nursing process is unique to the discipline of nursing and sets a common language for nurses to "think through" patients' clinical problems (Kataoka-Yahiro and Saylor, 1994). Chapter 19 contains a detailed description of the nursing process.

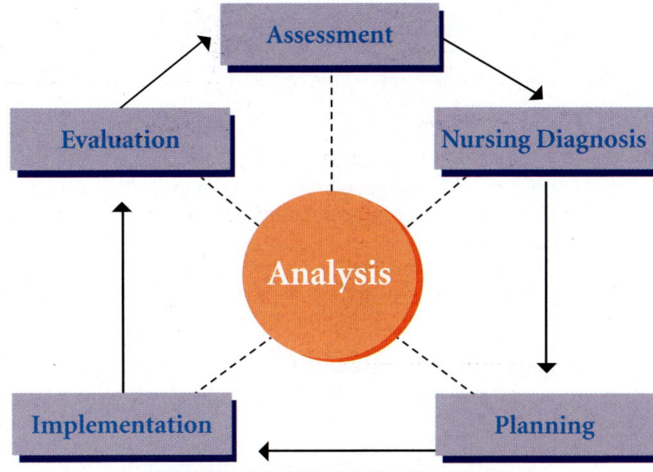

Fig. 18.2 Five-step nursing process model.

CRITICAL THINKING MODEL

Because critical thinking is complex, a model helps explain the steps in making clinical decisions and judgments about your patients. Kataoka-Yahiro and Saylor (1994) developed a model of critical thinking for nursing judgment based in part on previous works by Paul (1993), Glaser (1941), and Miller and Malcolm (1990) (see Fig. 18.1). The model defines the outcome of critical thinking: nursing judgment that is relevant to nursing problems in a variety of health care settings. The model includes five elements of critical thinking in nursing judgment: competence (e.g., problem-solving and clinical decision-making ability), knowledge, experience, attitudes, and standards (intellectual and professional). The five model elements combine to guide nurses in making clinical decisions leading to safe, effective nursing care (Box 18.2).

Competence

The first element of critical thinking is competence. Nurses perform competent critical thinking as they apply the nursing process. Throughout this text, the model shows you how to apply critical thinking as part of the nursing process.

Specific Knowledge Base

A second element of the critical thinking model is a nurse's knowledge base. A nurse's knowledge base varies according to his or her educational experience (e.g., type of basic nursing education, continuing education courses, and additional college education and degrees). In addition, a nurse builds knowledge by reading nursing literature (especially research-based literature) to maintain current knowledge of nursing science. Knowledge prepares a nurse to better anticipate and identify patient problems by understanding their origin and nature.

BOX 18.2 Components of Critical Thinking in Nursing

I. Specific knowledge base in nursing
II. Experience in nursing
III. Critical thinking competencies
  A. General critical thinking competencies
  B. Specific critical thinking competencies in clinical situations
  C. Specific critical thinking competency in nursing—the nursing process
IV. Attitudes for critical thinking
  A. Confidence
  B. Independence
  C. Fairness
  D. Responsibility
  E. Risk taking
  F. Discipline
  G. Perseverance
  H. Creativity
  I. Curiosity
  J. Integrity
  K. Humility
V. Standards for critical thinking
  A. Intellectual standards
    1. Clear: Plain and understandable (e.g., clear communication)
    2. Precise: Exact and specific (e.g., focusing on a problem and possible solution)
    3. Specific: To mention, describe, or define in detail
    4. Accurate: True and free from error; getting to the facts (objective and subjective)
    5. Relevant: Essential and crucial to a situation (e.g., a patient's situation)
    6. Plausible: Reasonable or probable
    7. Consistent: Expressing consistent beliefs or values
    8. Logical: Engaging in correct reasoning by moving from what one believes in a given instance to the conclusions that follow
    9. Deep: Containing complexities and multiple relationships
    10. Broad: Covering multiple viewpoints
    11. Complete: Thorough thinking and evaluation
    12. Significant: Focusing on what is important and not trivial
    13. Adequate (for purpose): Satisfactory in quality or amount
    14. Fair: Open-minded and impartial
  B. Professional standards
    1. Ethical criteria for nursing judgment
    2. Criteria for evaluation
    3. Professional responsibility

Modified from Kataoka-Yahiro M, Saylor C: A critical thinking model for nursing judgment, *J Nurs Educ* 33(8):351, 1994. Data from Paul R: The art of redesigning instruction. In Willsen J, Blinker AJA, editors: *Critical thinking: how to prepare students for a rapidly changing world*, Santa Rosa, CA, 1993, Foundation for Critical Thinking.

Your exposure to knowledge comes from your educational experiences and your collaboration and work at the side of knowledgeable colleagues. Your knowledge base includes information and theory from the basic sciences, humanities, behavioral sciences, science from other health care disciplines, and nursing science. This broad knowledge base gives you a holistic view of patients and their health care needs. Your depth of knowledge affects your ability to think critically about nursing problems. This is one reason why thoroughly knowing your patients is a vital part of critical thinking.

Experience

Nursing is a practice discipline. You develop the knowledge of nursing through practice—the hands-on care of patients. Experience is the body of knowledge you gain from talking and listening to patients and families, observing their courses of illness, providing interventions, and seeing the effects. You learn from these experiences by reflecting actively on your experiences alone and with faculty and fellow students. You need clinical learning to become competent at clinical decision-making.

Clinical experience is the application of nursing knowledge. Textbook approaches and simulation exercises lay an important foundation for practice, but you must adapt your practice to each setting, the unique qualities of each patient, and the experiences you gain from caring for previous patients. Benner (1984) noted that an expert nurse understands the context of a clinical situation, recognizes signs suggesting patterns, and interprets them as relevant or irrelevant. This level of competency comes with experience and a commitment to learning. Perhaps the best lesson you can learn is to value all patient experiences. Each clinical experience becomes a stepping stone to building knowledge and stimulating innovative thinking.

Attitudes for Critical Thinking

The fourth element of the critical thinking model is attitudes (see Box 18.2). There are 11 attitudes that define a critical thinker and his or her success in approaching a problem (Paul, 1993; Papathanasiou et al., 2014). To become a critical thinker, you must be motivated to develop the attitudes and dispositions of a fair-minded thinker. For example, when a patient complains of anxiety before a diagnostic procedure, a curious nurse seeks information and an explanation by asking several questions to learn what the patient does not know and the nature of the patient's concerns (Kaddoura, 2013). The nurse shows discipline in forming questions and performing a thorough assessment to learn the source of the patient's anxiety.

Assessing the reliability of information is also an important stage of critical thinking. In this step, the nurse confirms the accuracy of the information collected by checking other evidence and informants (e.g., when a patient self-reports having fallen at home, the nurse confirms the patient's story about the incident with the family caregiver and learns what factors were associated with the fall and how the patient responded).

Critical thinking attitudes give you methods for approaching a problem or making a decision. Table 18.4 summarizes the ways nurses use critical thinking attitudes in practice situations. A summary of each critical thinking attitude follows.

Table 18.4 Critical Thinking Attitudes and Applications in Nursing Practice

Critical Thinking Attitude	Application in Practice
Confidence	Learn how to introduce yourself to a patient. For example: "Mrs Tyms, I'm Chuck Lord, your nurse for this shift. I'll be responsible for your nursing care and will work with your doctor to make sure that you're comfortable." Speak with conviction when you begin a treatment or procedure. Do not let a patient think that you are not sure how to perform care safely. Always be prepared (e.g., organize equipment and provide comfort measures) before beginning a nursing activity.
Thinking independently	Read the nursing literature, especially when there are different opinions on a subject. Ask colleagues and expert staff nurses to share their ideas about nursing interventions.
Fairness	Listen to both sides in any discussion. If a patient or family member complains about a colleague, listen to the story and then speak with the colleague. Weigh all the facts.
Responsibility and accountability	Ask for help if you are not sure about how to perform a task. Report any problems immediately. Follow standards of practice in the care you give.
Risk taking	If your knowledge leads you to question a health care provider's order, speak up. Offer alternative approaches to nursing care when colleagues are having little success with patients.
Discipline	Be thorough in everything you do. Use established criteria for activities such as assessment and evaluation. Take time to be thorough.
Perseverance	Be wary of an easy answer. If colleagues give you information about a patient but some information is missing, clarify the facts or talk to the patient directly. If the same problems recur in a nursing division, bring colleagues together, look for a pattern, and find a solution.
Creativity	Seek different approaches when interventions are not working. For example, a patient may need a different positioning technique or a different instructional approach.
Curiosity	Always ask "why." A clinical sign or symptom can indicate a variety of problems. Learn more about the patient to help you make the right clinical judgments.
Integrity	Recognize when your opinions conflict with those of your patient. Review your position and work with the patient to reach agreement on how best to reach a positive outcome.
Humility	Recognize times when you need more information to make a decision. When you are new to a clinical division and unfamiliar with the patients, ask for an orientation to the area. Ask nurses regularly assigned to the area for assistance. Read professional journals regularly to keep updated on approaches to care.

Confidence

To be confident is to feel secure in your ability to accomplish a task or goal such as performing a nursing procedure or making a diagnostic decision. Confidence grows with experience as you recognize your strengths and limits. You gradually shift your focus from your own needs (e.g., remembering the steps for performing a procedure such as inserting an i.v. safely) to the patient's needs (e.g., adapting the approach to i.v. insertion to accommodate the excess swelling in the patient's arm).

When you are not confident in performing a nursing skill, you become anxious. This anxiety prevents you from attending to a patient, and this anxiety can be perceived by your patient. Always be aware of the extent and limits of your knowledge. If you have a question about a procedure, discuss it with your nursing instructor or preceptor first before performing the procedure on a patient. Patient safety is always the top priority. When an experienced nurse shows willingness to disagree with an action or expresses a doubt about an action he or she is considering, the nurse acts as a role model to colleagues and inspires them to develop their own confidence (Papathanasiou et al., 2014).

Thinking Independently

As you gain knowledge, you learn to consider a wide range of ideas and concepts before forming an opinion or making a judgment. You also are no longer limited by what you learned in school, and you become open minded in considering interventions (Papathanasiou et al., 2014). Independent thinking does not mean that you ignore other people's ideas. Instead you consider all sides of a situation. By the same token, a critical thinker does not accept another person's ideas without question. When thinking independently, you challenge the ways others think and look for rational and logical answers to problems. An independent thinker applies evidence-based practices when facing clinical decisions. You must be willing to seek answers to difficult questions as well as obvious ones.

Fairness

A critical thinker deals with situations fairly. This means that bias or prejudice does not enter into a decision. For example, regardless of what you think about illicit drug use, you do not allow your attitudes to affect the way you deliver care to patients who abuse drugs. Fairness requires that you look at each situation objectively and consider all viewpoints to understand the situation completely before making a decision. Use your imagination to help you develop an attitude of fairness. For example, imagining being in your patient's situation helps you see it through his or her eyes and appreciate its complexity.

Responsibility and Accountability

When caring for patients, you are responsible for correctly performing nursing care activities consistent with standards of practice. Standards of practice are the minimum acceptable level of performance needed to ensure high-quality care. For example, you do not take shortcuts or **workarounds** when you administer medications to a patient (e.g., failing to identify a patient or preparing medication doses for multiple patients at the same time). You are responsible for following the "six rights" of medication administration (see Chapter 26).

A professional nurse is responsible for performing nursing interventions competently. When you are competent, you make better clinical decisions about your patients. As a nurse, you are answerable, or accountable, for your decisions and the outcomes of your actions. This means that you must recognize ineffective nursing care and know the limits and scope of your practice.

Risk Taking

People often associate risk taking with danger. Using your cell phone while driving on a highway is a risk that might result in injury to you and drivers around you. However, risk taking is not always negative. Risk taking is desirable, particularly when the result can be a positive outcome. A critical thinker will take certain risks in attempting to solve problems. The willingness to take risks comes from experience with similar problems. In nursing, risk taking often produces innovations in patient care. In the past, nurses have taken risks by trying new approaches to skin care, wound care, and pain management. Some of these attempts produced interventions that are more effective than traditional approaches. When taking a risk, you must consider all options, be knowledgeable of the new intervention, identify any potential danger to a patient, and then act in a well-reasoned, logical, and thoughtful manner. In the end, the evaluation of patient outcomes is critical.

Discipline

A disciplined thinker misses few details and follows a systematic approach in collecting information, making decisions, and taking action. Being disciplined and thorough in gathering information helps you identify problems more accurately and select the most appropriate nursing interventions. Disciplined thinking does not lessen your creativity but rather ensures that your decision-making is systematic, accurate, and comprehensive.

Perseverance

A critical thinker is determined to find effective solutions to patient care problems. Perseverance is especially important when problems remain unresolved or when they recur. You must learn as much as possible about a particular problem and try various approaches to care. Perseverance also means that you continually look for additional resources until you find a successful approach. A critical thinker who perseveres is not satisfied with minimal effort but constantly tries to achieve high-quality patient care.

Creativity

Creativity arises from original thinking. This means you find solutions outside of the standard routines of care while still following standards of practice. Creativity helps you think of new options and approaches. A patient's clinical problems, living environment, and social support systems are just a few factors that can make the simplest nursing procedure more complicated. However, they also can be assets. Creativity means tailoring unique approaches to a patient's specific needs.

Curiosity

A critical thinker's favorite question is "Why?" As you care for a patient, you learn a lot of information. As you analyze this patient information, data patterns begin to emerge. Patterns may be unclear, new to you, or very unusual. Curiosity motivates you to question further, investigate the clinical situation in all possible directions, and obtain all the information needed to make a decision. For example, even if a patient who has had a recent myocardial infarction complains about chest pain, it is essential to be curious and consider other possible sources for the pain such as a pulled or strained muscle.

Integrity

Critical thinkers quickly and thoroughly question and test their own knowledge and beliefs against the knowledge and beliefs of others (Papathanasiou et al., 2014). This shows a willingness to admit and understand inconsistencies between one's own beliefs and the beliefs of other colleagues. Your integrity as a nurse builds trust in you from your coworkers. Nurses face many dilemmas in everyday clinical practice (e.g., organizing care for multiple patients, choosing the correct size of a urinary catheter for a patient, being unable to respond to a patient's nurse call system while changing a different patient's wound dressing). Everyone occasionally makes a mistake or omits care activities. A person of integrity is honest and willing to admit to any mistakes or inconsistencies in his or her performance, behavior, and beliefs. A professional always tries to follow the highest standards of nursing practice.

Humility

Always know and admit the limits in your knowledge and skill. Critical thinkers admit their knowledge gaps and try to find the knowledge they need to make proper decisions. A nurse is often an expert in one area of clinical practice (e.g., general surgery) but a novice in another area (e.g., orthopedics). You put a patient's safety and welfare at risk if you cannot admit your inability to solve a practice problem. You must rethink a situation, seek additional knowledge (e.g., literature, clinical experts), and use the information to form an opinion and draw a conclusion.

Standards for Critical Thinking

The fifth element of the critical thinking model includes intellectual and professional standards (Kataoka-Yahiro and Saylor, 1994).

Intellectual Standards

Paul (1993) identified 14 intellectual standards (see Box 18.2) universal to critical thinking. An intellectual standard is a guideline or principle for rational thought. You apply these standards when you use the nursing process competency. When you consider a patient problem, you apply intellectual standards such as precision, accuracy, and consistency to ensure that all clinical decisions are sound. A thorough use of intellectual standards in clinical practice ensures that you avoid performing critical thinking haphazardly. When you reflect on your thinking, you can begin to recognize when you are unclear, imprecise, or inaccurate.

Professional Standards

Professional standards for critical thinking include ethical criteria for nursing judgments (e.g., advocacy, patient autonomy, and beneficence), evidence-based criteria used for assessment and evaluation, and criteria for professional responsibility (Paul, 1993). Applying professional standards requires you to use critical thinking for the good of individuals or groups (Kataoka-Yahiro and Saylor, 1994). Standards of practice improve patient outcomes and thus maintain a high level of care.

Excellent nursing practice is a reflection of ethical standards (see Chapter 3). Patient care requires more than just the application of scientific knowledge and performing skills. Being able to focus on a patient's values and beliefs helps you make clinical decisions that are just, faithful to a patient's choices, and beneficial to a patient's well-being. Critical thinkers maintain a sense of self-awareness through conscious awareness of their beliefs, values, and feelings and the multiple perspectives that patients, family members, and professional peers bring to clinical situations.

Critical thinking also requires the use of evidence-based criteria for making clinical judgments. These criteria are often based on scientific research findings—practices that clinical experts developed or that institutions developed through performance improvement initiatives. For example, Dr Barbara Braden applied evidence from her research to develop the Braden Scale, which is used in many practice settings to predict pressure injury risk (see Chapter 17). Other examples are the clinical practice guidelines from the Agency for Healthcare Research and Quality (AHRQ) and the performance measures from the National Quality Forum (NQF) (e.g., asthma assessment and urinary incontinence management in older adults). The NQF performance measures are used to assess the performance of a health care institution against recognized standards. An NQF-endorsed performance measure reflects rigorous scientific and evidence-based review, input from patients and their families, and the perspectives of people throughout the health care industry (NQF, 2016).

The standards of professional responsibility that a nurse tries to achieve are the standards cited in Nurse Practice Act., institutional practice guidelines, and standards of practice of professional organizations (e.g., the ANA Scope and Standards of Practice [http://www.nursingworld.org/scopeandstandardsofpractice]). These standards raise the bar for the responsibilities and accountabilities that nurses assume in guaranteeing quality health care to the public.

Developing Critical Thinking Skills

Although you will need time to develop critical thinking skills in nursing, start now by actively engaging patients who are in your care. Apply the principles of the critical thinking model that have been presented in this chapter. Many factors in health care settings can pose barriers to critical thinking. Rising patient acuity, decreasing length of stay, and conflicts in professional relationships are just some of the factors that can challenge even experienced nurses who are adept at critical thinking. Berkow et al. (2011) argue that critical thinking is essential to nursing practice in that nurses must learn to readily see a holistic picture of their patients' conditions to recognize emerging clinical patterns.

One practice that can help you become a critical thinker is reflective journaling. Reflective journaling involves keeping a written record of your clinical experiences in your own words in a personal journal. Returning to the journal after each clinical experience gives you the chance to record the perceptions you had during patient care and develop the ability to apply theory to practice. Using a journal also improves your observational and descriptive skills. Writing skills improve as you learn to clearly describe concepts applied in practice (e.g., suffering, resilience, or hope). A journal helps you increase your experiential learning during clinical experiences (Silvia et al., 2013). Ask and answer the following questions in your daily journal entry:

- What did I learn from the experience?
- Did I respond appropriately in this situation? If not, how should I have responded?
- Were there consequences to my actions? What were they, and whom did they affect?
- Why did I react as I did? What was I thinking at that moment?
- How might I react differently in the future?
- Was I working from just instinct or from evidence-based practices?

When you begin caring for a patient with multiple health problems, you may initially have difficulty sorting out the multiple problems and how they are interrelated. With knowledge and practice, you learn to assess for problems and develop a nursing diagnosis for each one. However, you will need complex critical thinking skills to see how the problems are related and to develop a holistic view of the patient.

Concept maps help you do this. A concept map is a visual representation of meaningful relationships between concepts (e.g., patient problems or nursing diagnoses and interventions), which then form propositions. Concept maps are visual road maps that highlight the meanings of these relationships (Hunter Revell, 2012). The maps encourage students to comprehensively observe their patients and organize and process the complex information (Moattari et al., 2014). The maps come in many different designs, but the primary purpose of a concept map is to gather relevant data about a patient (e.g., assessment data, nursing diagnoses, health needs, nursing interventions, evaluation measures) and represent relationships in a visual format. Current evidence shows the value of concept maps in improving the critical thinking of nursing students (Moattari et al., 2014). You can use a concept map to organize or link information about a patient in a unique and meaningful way. You will see examples of these maps throughout this text. Chapter 19 offers examples of concept maps with details about their development.

CRITICAL THINKING SYNTHESIS

Critical thinking is a reasoning process in which you reflect on and analyze your own thoughts, actions, and knowledge and use this information to make decisions about patient care. To be a good critical thinker, you must know patients and have the dedication and desire to grow intellectually. As a beginning nurse, you must learn the steps of the nursing process and combine them with the elements of critical thinking (Fig. 18.3). These two processes go hand in hand in making clinical decisions. This text provides a model for

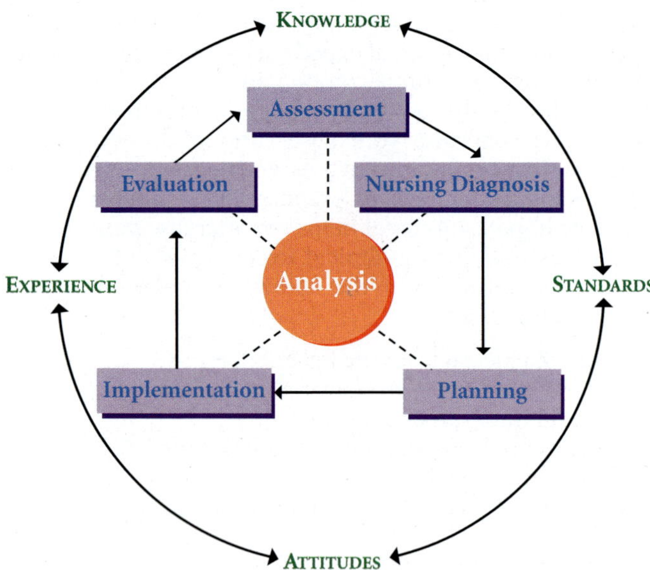

Fig. 18.3 Synthesis of critical thinking with the nursing process competency.

using critical thinking in nursing practice and emphasizes the components of critical thinking to help you better understand their relationship with the nursing process.

KEY POINTS

- Good clinical decision-making requires you to investigate and reflect on all aspects of a problem and then to apply scientific and nursing knowledge to choose the best course of action.
- Critical thinking requires recognizing that a patient has a problem, analyzing information related to the problem (e.g., clinical and historical data about a patient), evaluating information (including assumptions and evidence), and drawing conclusions.
- When you care for patients on a given day, reflection means reviewing your practice experience so that you can describe, analyze, and evaluate it.
- You learn to know patients by engaging them, caring for them over time, hearing accounts of their experiences with illness, observing them, and coming to understand how they typically respond to treatments.
- The critical thinking model includes three levels of critical thinking in nursing that you develop with time and experience: basic, complex, and commitment.
- The scientific method is a systematic and ordered approach that uses reasoning to solve problems.
- You must use the intellectual standards of clinical practice to ensure that you do not perform critical thinking haphazardly.
- To become a critical thinker, you must be motivated to develop critical thinking and clinical judgment skills, as well as the 11 attitudes of the critical thinking model.
- In complex critical thinking, you learn to analyze and examine alternatives independently and take initiative to solve problems.
- The specific critical thinking competency in nursing is the nursing process, which involves clinical inference, diagnostic reasoning, and clinical decision-making.
- Professional standards for critical thinking in nursing include ethical criteria for nursing judgments, evidence-based criteria used for assessment and evaluation, and criteria for professional responsibility.

REFERENCES

American Nurses Association (ANA). Nursing's social policy statement: the essence of the profession. Washington, DC: The Association; 2010.

Atalay A, Turhan N, Atalay B. Deconditioning in chronic low back pain: might there be a relationship between fitness and magnetic resonance imaging findings? Rheumatol Int 2012;32(1):21–5.

Barksby J, Butcher N, Whysall A. A new model of reflection for clinical practice. Nurs Times 2015;111(34/35):21–3.

Benner P. From novice to expert. Menlo Park, CA: Addison Wesley; 1984.

Berkow S, Virkstis K, Stewart J, Aronson S, Donohue M. Assessing individual frontline nurse critical thinking. J Nurs Adm 2011;41(4):168.

Delany C, Golding C. Teaching clinical reasoning by making thinking visible: an action research project with allied health clinical educators. BMC Med Educ 2014;14:20. Available from: http://bmcmededuc.biomedcentral.com/articles/10.1186/1472-6920-14-20.

Facione N, Facione P. Externalizing the critical thinking in knowledge development and clinical judgment. Nurs Outlook 1996;44:129.

Facione P. Critical thinking: a statement of expert consensus for purposes of educational assessment and instruction. The Delphi report: research findings and recommendations prepared for the American Philosophical Association. Washington, DC: ERIC; 1990. ERIC Doc No. ED 315-423.

Glaser E. An experiment in the development of critical thinking. New York: Bureau of Publications, Teachers College, Columbia University; 1941.

Hunter Revell SM. Concept maps and nursing theory: a pedagogical approach. Nurse Educ 2012;37(3):131.

Kaddoura M. New graduate nurses' perceived definition of critical thinking during their first nursing experience. Educ Res Q 2013;36(3):3.

Kataoka-Yahiro M, Saylor C. A critical thinking model for nursing judgment. J Nurs Educ 1994;33(8):351.

Kristina Ericksen. The importance of critical thinking skills in nursing. 2015. Available from: http://www.rasmussen.edu/degrees/nursing/blog/understanding-why-nurses-need-critical-thinking-skills/.

Levett-Jones, T., Sundin, D., Bagnall, M., Hague, K., Schumann, W., Taylor, C., & Wink, J. (2010). Learning to think like a nurse. HNE Handover for Nurses and Midwives, 3(1), 15–20.

Mamede S, van Gog T, Moura AS, de Faria RM, Peixoto JM, Rikers RM, et al. Reflection as a strategy to foster medical students' acquisition of diagnostic competence. Med Educ 2012;46(5):464–72.

Miller M, Malcolm N. Critical thinking in the nursing curriculum. Nurs Health Care 1990;11:67.

Moattari M, Soleimani S, Moghaddam NJ, Mehbodi F. Clinical concept mapping: does it improve discipline-based critical thinking of nursing students? Iran J Nurs Midwifery Res 2014;19(1):70–6.

National Quality Forum (NQF). Measuring performance. 2016. Available from: http://www.qualityforum.org/Measuring_Performance/Measuring_Performance.aspx.

Papathanasiou IV, Kleisiaris CF, Fradelos EC, Kakou K, Kourkouta L. Critical thinking: the development of an essential skill for nursing students. Acta Inform Med 2014;22(4):283–6.

Paul R. The art of redesigning instruction. In: Willsen J, Blinker AJA, editors. Critical thinking: how to prepare students for a rapidly changing world. Santa Rosa, CA: Foundation for Critical Thinking; 1993.

Raterink G. Critical thinking: reported enhancers and barriers by nurses in long-term care: implications for staff development. J Nurs Staff Dev 2011;27(3):136.

Silvia B, Valerio D, Lorenza G. The reflective journal: a tool for enhancing experience based learning in nursing students in clinical practice. J Nurs Educ Pract 2013;3(3). Available from: http://www.sciedu.ca/journal/index.php/jnep/article/viewFile/1388/1067.

Tanner CA. Thinking like a nurse: a research-based model of clinical judgment in nursing, J Nurs Educ 2006;45(6):204–11.

19 *Nursing Process*

OBJECTIVES

- To define nursing process and its applications.
- To explain assessment as a primary step of the nursing process.
- To describe process of data collection in nursing assessment.
- To differentiate between subjective and objective data.
- To explain different methods of data collection including patient-centered observation, observation, physical examination, and laboratory examination.
- To describe interpretation and validation of assessment data.
- To explain measures of data documentation and communication.
- To describe the relationship between critical thinking and each step of the nursing process.
- To discuss formulation of NANDA diagnosis process.
- To enlist components of nursing diagnosis and etiological factors such as PES format in detail.
- To describe cultural reference and concept mapping of nursing diagnosis.
- To explain sources of errors in diagnosis, data collection, and interpretation of data.
- To discuss the differences between a goal and an expected outcome and guidelines for writing goals and expected outcomes.
- To discuss how a nursing diagnosis guides nursing practice.
- To describe differences among health promotion, problem-focused, and risk nursing diagnoses.
- To explain the role of critical thinking in selecting nursing interventions.
- To define how consultation with other health care personnel can be done.
- To describe clinical practice guidelines and protocols for making nursing care plan.
- To explain the relationship among goals of care, expected outcomes, and evaluative measures when evaluating and revising nursing care.

KEY TERMS

activities of daily living (ADLs), p. 446
assessment, p. 422
care bundle, p. 444
clinical practice guideline, p. 443
collaborative interventions, p. 438
collaborative problem, p. 435
concept map, p. 433
consultation, p. 443
counseling, p. 447
cue, p. 423
data analysis, p. 428
data cluster, p. 427
database, p. 422
defining characteristics, p. 428
dependent nursing interventions, p. 438
direct care interventions, p. 443
etiology, p. 431
evaluation, p. 448
expected outcome, p. 436
goal, p. 436
health history, p. 422
implementation, p. 443
independent nursing interventions, p. 438
indirect care interventions, p. 443
inference, p. 423
instrumental activities of daily living (IADLs), p. 447
interdisciplinary care plans, p. 448
medical diagnosis, p. 435
NANDA International (NANDA-I), p. 428
nursing care plan, p. 439
nursing diagnosis, p. 427
nursing diagnostic process, p. 427
nursing intervention, p. 443
nursing process, p. 422
nursing-sensitive outcome, p. 436
objective data, p. 424
planning, p. 435
related factor, p. 431
scientific rationale, p. 438
standard of care, p. 450
standing order, p. 444
subjective data, p. 424
validation, p. 427

INTRODUCTION

The **nursing process** is a critical thinking process that professional nurses use to apply the best available evidence to caregiving and the promotion of human functions and responses to health and illness (American Nurses Association [ANA], 2010). It is the fundamental blueprint for patient care. Patient-centered care improves patient assessment, patient education, patient adherence to interventions, patient outcomes, and patient satisfaction (Bertakis and Azari, 2011; Burman et al., 2013). The Quality and Safety Education for Nurses (QSEN) Institute defines patient-centered care as the process of "recognizing a patient or designee as the source of control and full partner in providing compassionate and coordinated care based on respect of a patient's preferences, values, and needs" (QSEN Institute, 2014).

The nursing process is a standard of practice that, when followed correctly, protects nurses against legal problems related to nursing care. It allows you to provide timely, appropriate, and individualized care to your patients.

The five steps of the nursing process are assessment, nursing diagnosis, planning, implementation, and evaluation (Fig. 19.1). Initially you learn how to apply the process step-by-step. However, as you gain more clinical experience and care for more than one patient, you learn to move back and forth among the steps of the process. In so doing, you use critical thinking to make judgments about your patients' clinical situations, preferences, and needs. As a result, you individualize your approaches to care (Burman et al., 2013).

The nursing process is a form of scientific reasoning. Using the nursing process helps you to systematically organize and conduct your practice. You learn to make inferences from a patient's response to a health problem or generalize about a patient's functional state of health. Through the assessment process a pattern of a patient's health problems begins to form, and you gather more data to identify a patient's specific problems. Clearly defining your patient's problems provides a basis for planning and implementing relevant nursing interventions and evaluating the outcomes of care. Each time you meet a patient, you apply the nursing process, just as Rich will do throughout this chapter.

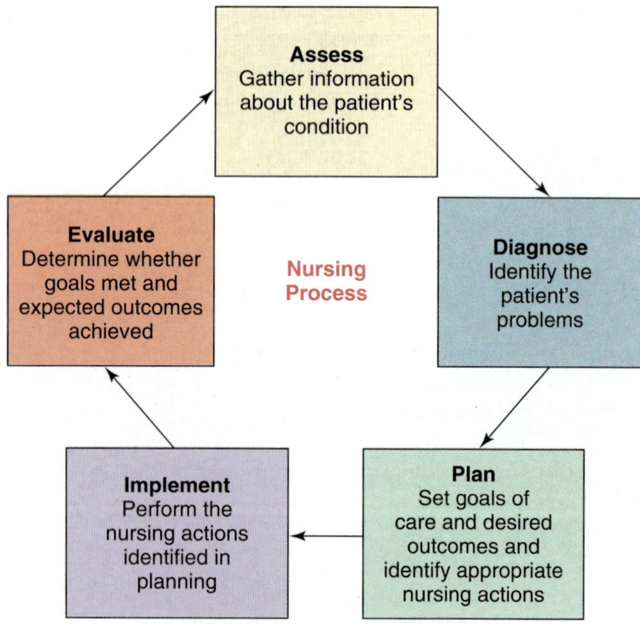

Fig. 19.1 Five-step nursing process.

ASSESSMENT

Assessment is the thorough systematic collection of patient data. The data reveal a patient's past and current health status, functional status, and past and present coping patterns (Carpenito-Moyet, 2017). Assessment requires you to apply critical thinking to have a clear picture of a patient's condition. Nursing assessment has two steps:

1. Collection and verification of data from a primary source (the patient) and secondary sources (e.g., family caregiver, friends, health professionals, medical record).
2. Interpretation and validation of data to ensure a complete database.

When you assess your patient, you collect and organize patient information into a detailed **database**. This database includes information about a patient's perceived needs, health problems, and responses to these problems. In addition, the data reveal related health issues, health practices, goals, values, and expectations about the health care delivery system.

To establish this database, you first apply knowledge that helps identify what to assess. For example, your knowledge of the physical, biological, and social sciences prepares you to ask relevant questions about a patient's health status and response to illness. You use this knowledge to collect relevant physical assessment data related to a patient's clinical condition.

Critical thinking attitudes and intellectual standards allow you to ask pertinent questions, clarify data, and gather further data for validation (see Chapter 18). Then you see the data patterns that reflect problems. Your experience allows you to recognize and anticipate what to assess. This experience leads you to ask the right questions. The answers to those questions will give you the most relevant and useful information.

An assessment database includes a patient's comprehensive **health history**. This history includes information about the patient's physical and developmental status, emotional health, social practices and resources, goals, values, lifestyle, and expectations about the health care system. The database also includes physical examination findings and a summary of results from laboratory and diagnostic testing. The knowledge you gather about a patient's medical diagnosis and treatment from the literature and medical record is also part of the database that leads you to fully understand your patient's condition and health care needs.

Critical thinking is a vital part of the assessment. As you gather data about a patient, you synthesize relevant knowledge, recall prior clinical experiences, apply critical thinking standards and attitudes, and use professional standards of practice to direct your assessment in a meaningful and purposeful way (see Chapter 18).

Data Collection

When you assess a patient, think critically about what to assess (i.e., the information you need to know to provide individualized, safe, effective care). Determine which questions or measurements are appropriate based on your clinical knowledge and experience. Once you start, select additional questions and measurements based on your patient's responses. When you meet a new patient, make a quick observational overview or screening. For example, a community health nurse assesses a patient's neighborhood and community, a surgical nurse focuses on a patient's pain control and surgical wound healing, and a home care nurse focuses on a patient's environment, health care resources, and ways to cope with illness.

You learn to differentiate important data from the total data collected. A **cue** is information that you obtain through the use of your senses. An **inference** is your judgment or interpretation of these cues (Fig. 19.2). For example, the cue of Mrs Tillman expressing a sense of feeling tired and not having energy for daily routines leads Rich to infer a problem with activity. Anything a patient says and any behaviors you observe are important cues. You can miss cues when you conduct your initial overview. Thus, you always need to be observant and interpret cues from the patient to guide your eventual assessment.

After the observational overview, you begin to focus on assessment cues and patterns of information that suggest problem areas. However, it is essential to conduct a comprehensive assessment when you can. An assessment moves from the general to the specific.

A comprehensive assessment can follow several approaches. One approach uses a structured database format, based on an agency's electronic health record (EHR). A second approach to assessment is the problem-focused approach. For example, you might focus on a patient's report of feeling tired. Then you ask the patient follow-up questions to clarify and expand. For example, Rich asks Mrs Tillman whether her lack of energy affects her ability to perform routine tasks and the extent to which it affects her physically (Table 19.1). Once he completes his initial assessment, he thoroughly analyzes the extent and nature of Mrs Tillman's sense of feeling tired. This enables him to identify her health problem correctly so that he can develop a comprehensive treatment plan.

Whichever approach you use for assessment, you begin to cluster cues, make inferences, and identify emerging patterns and potential problems. To do this well, you must always try to stay a step ahead of the assessment. For example, if you suspect that a patient has a particular health problem (e.g., fatigue), you pose questions that deal with responses typically seen with fatigue.

Remember your inferences must always have supporting cues. Inferences lead you to more questions. When you ask a question or make an observation of a patient, the information branches to an additional series of questions or observations (Fig. 19.3). Failing to anticipate assessment questions results in an incomplete assessment, or you might fail to recognize cues and dismiss relevant problems. Knowing how to probe and frame questions is a skill that grows with experience. You learn which questions are relevant to a specific sign, symptom, or situation while at the same time making sure the assessment is complete.

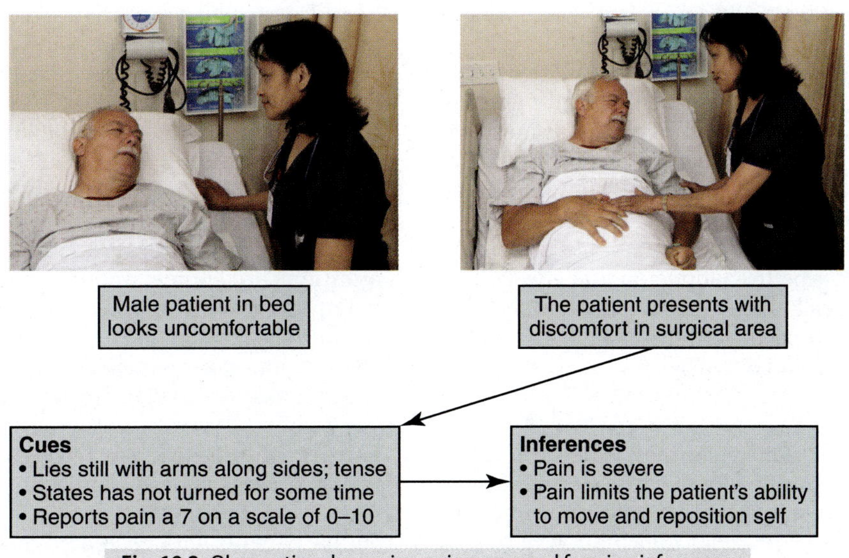

Fig. 19.2 Observational overview using cues and forming inferences.

Table 19.1 Focused Patient Assessment

Factors to Assess	Questions	Physical Assessment
Ability to perform routine tasks	Tell me how your fatigue affects your daily activities.	Observe how quickly the patient responds to questions.
	Describe what you did in a typical day before you had cancer. How has this changed?	Observe posture and body movements.
Extent to which lack of energy affects her physically	Tell me how feeling tired affects your interest in social activities. Do you have more energy after you sleep or rest?	Observe facial and other nonverbal expressions.

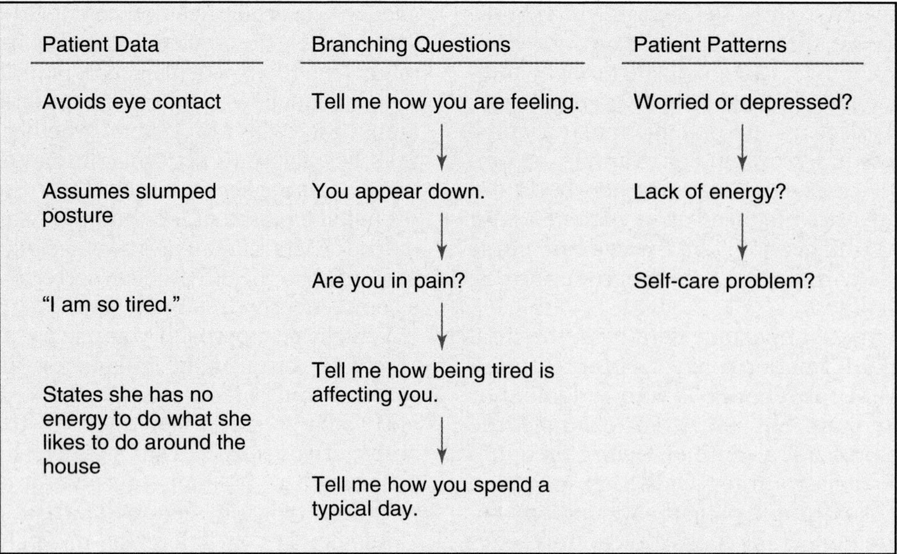

Fig. 19.3 Example of branching logic for selecting assessment questions.

Types of Data

There are two primary sources of data, subjective and objective. **Subjective data** are patients' verbal descriptions of their health problems, such as feelings of fear, anxiety, fatigue, physical discomfort, or mental stress. Patients are the only source of subjective data. For example, Mrs Tillman's comments about being worn out and dealing with a difficult experience are subjective findings. Only patients provide subjective data.

Objective data are observations or measurements of a patient's health status. Inspection of the condition of a wound or observation of a patient's posture and gait are examples of objective data. Base your measurements of objective data on an accepted standard, such as the Fahrenheit or Celsius measure on a thermometer, centimeters on a measuring tape, or known characteristics of behaviors. For example, after listening to Mrs Tillman describe her fatigue and its effects, Rich assesses her ability to walk a short distance to gather more data about how fatigue impacts her physical activity, such as change in heart rate or distance walked.

Sources of Data

You obtain data from a variety of sources. When you collect data, you apply critical thinking intellectual standards (e.g., clear, precise, and consistent) to correctly interpret your findings. Each data source provides information about the patient's level of wellness, risk factors, health practices and goals, and patterns of health and illness.

Patient

A patient is usually your best source of information. A patient who is conscious, alert, and able to answer questions appropriately provides the most accurate information about health care needs, lifestyle patterns, present and past illnesses, perception of symptoms, and changes in activities of daily living (ADLs).

Always consider the setting for your assessment. A patient experiencing acute pain in an emergency department will not offer the same depth of information as one who comes to an outpatient clinic for a routine checkup. When you communicate with your patient, always be attentive and show a caring presence with patients (see Chapter 4). Patients are more likely to fully reveal the nature of their health care problems when you show interest and focus solely on the patient and his or her concerns (Palos, 2014).

Know your patient's health literacy level. Health literacy includes specific cognitive and social skills that help determine the motivation and ability of individuals to gain access, understand, and use information in ways to promote and maintain good health (see Chapter 15). A patient with limited health literacy has difficulty obtaining, processing, and understanding basic health information (Agency for Healthcare Research and Quality [AHRQ], 2016). Because of limited health literacy, your patient may not fully understand some of your assessment questions, especially if your questions are clinical and use a lot of medical terminology. If English is not the patient's first language or the patient cannot speak English, he or she will be unable to understand you or your questions. As a result, the risk of obtaining incomplete, inaccurate assessment data increases.

Family and Significant Others

Family members and significant others are the primary sources of information for infants, children, critically ill adults, patients with decreased mental capacity, and patients who are unconscious or have reduced cognitive function. In cases of severe illness or emergencies, families are often the only available sources of information for nurses and other health care providers. The family caregiver and significant others are also good secondary sources of information for patients who are able to communicate. These additional sources confirm information that the patient provides. For example, they can tell you whether the patient regularly takes medications at home or how well he or she eats. Include the family caregiver when appropriate. The patient might not want you to question family members. However, spouses or close friends often attend the assessment and provide their views of a patient's health problems or needs. Not only do they supply information about a patient's current health status, but they can also report the timing of any changes in the patient's status. Family members who live with the patient are often well informed about the effects of health problems on the patient's ADLs. For example, Mr Tillman is an excellent resource for information about the effect of his wife's fatigue on her daily life.

Health Care Team

You frequently communicate with other health care team members when gathering information about patients. In the acute care setting, the patient hand-off is the way for nurses on one shift to communicate information to nurses or other health care providers on oncoming shifts (see Chapter 5). The hand-off is an interactive process of passing patient-specific information from one caregiver to another for the purpose of ensuring patient-centered care and safety (Boykins, 2014; Chaboyer et al., 2010). Communicating effectively during the hand-off provides an opportunity for you to collect initial information about patients assigned to your care including their health care needs and concerns and to clarify any medications or care procedures (Jahne, 2015). When nurses and other health care providers consult with one another about a patient's condition, all of them typically contribute information about the patient. This information includes the patient's adjustment to the health care environment, the patient's reactions to treatment, the results of diagnostic procedures or therapies, and the patient's responses to visitors. Every member of the health care team is a source of information about the patient.

Medical Records

The medical record is a source of a patient's medical history, laboratory and diagnostic test results, and current physical findings and a health care provider's treatment plan. The records contain baseline and ongoing information about a patient's response to illness and progress to date. The Health Insurance Portability and Accountability Act (HIPAA) of 1996, which became effective in 2003, has a privacy rule to set standards for the protection of health information. Information in a patient's record is confidential. Each health care agency has policies governing how health care providers can share information. A nurse can review a patient's medical record for assessment data but needs to know the agency policies governing how to share the information with other staff.

Other Records and the Scientific Literature

Educational, military, and employment records often contain pertinent health care information (e.g., immunizations or prior illnesses). If a patient received treatment at a community clinic or another hospital, the nurse must obtain written permission from the patient or guardian before seeing the records. HIPAA regulations dictate specifically how to obtain an information release (USDHHS, 2017). Consult agency policies.

Reviewing the most current nursing, medical, and pharmacological literature about a patient's illness provides scientific information to help refine and complete the assessment database. This review of scientific information increases your knowledge of expected signs and symptoms, recommended treatments, prognosis of the illness, and established standards of therapeutic practice.

Nurse's Experience

Another important source of data is your own experience. Your clinical experiences in caring for patients and their families help you choose the questions to ask and how and when to ask these questions. Integrating your knowledge from clinical experiences helps you understand the impact of disease on a patient and his or her family, helps you understand signs and symptoms and their patterns, and builds on your ability to know your patient. Continuity of care and experience are the elements that help you to know your patient better. When patient care is fragmented, your knowledge of the patient declines, and patient-centered care is compromised (Zolnierek, 2014).

Methods of Data Collection

As a nurse, you use the patient interview as the tool to assess a patient's health history. Once you have collected data, you proceed to a physical examination.

Patient-Centered Interview

The first step in establishing a patient-centered database is to collect subjective information by interviewing a patient (see Chapter 7). An interview is an organized conversation with a patient (see Chapter 7). The interview focuses on a patient's health history and obtaining information about the current illness (Ball et al., 2015). Obtain the patient's health history using a variety of communication techniques to promote a clear interaction (see Chapter 7) and construct a thorough database (Box 19.1).

BOX 19.1 Basic Components for a Nursing Health History

- *Biographical information:* Age, address, occupation and working status, marital status, family members, source of health care, and insurance
- *Reasons for seeking health care:* Goals of care, expectation of the services and care delivered, and expectations of the health care team and system
- *Present illness or health concern:* Onset, symptoms, nature of symptoms (e.g., sudden or gradual), duration, precipitating factors, relief measures, and weight loss or gain
- *Health history:* Prior illnesses throughout development, injuries, and hospitalizations; surgeries; blood transfusions; allergies; immunizations; habits (e.g., smoking, caffeine intake, alcohol intake, and alcohol or drug abuse); prescribed and self-prescribed medications; over-the-counter medications; work habits; relaxation activities; and sleep, exercise, and eating or nutritional patterns
- *Family history:* Health status of immediate family and living relatives; cause of death of relatives; and risk factor analyses for cancer, heart disease, diabetes mellitus, kidney disease, hypertension, and mental disorders
- *Environmental history:* Hazards, pollutants, and physical safety
- *Psychosocial and cultural history:* Primary language, cultural group, community resources, mood, attention span, and developmental stage
- *Review of systems:* Head-to-toe review of all major body systems and the patient's knowledge of and compliance with health care (e.g., frequency of breast or testicular self-examination or last visual acuity examination) (another option for an approach is to use *functional health patterns* as the method for organizing assessment data)

During the initial interview you have the opportunity to:

1. Introduce yourself to the patient, explain your role, and explain the roles of others who will provide care.
2. Establish a caring patient-centered relationship.
3. Explain how you will conduct the interview (e.g., first you will ask about the patient's current concerns and then collect other information).
4. Gain insight about the patient's concerns and worries.
5. Determine the patient's goals and expectations of the health care delivery system.
6. Obtain cues to identify topics requiring further investigation and data collection.

Later interviews allow you to further assess a patient's situation and focus on specific problem areas. The interview also helps patients explain their own interpretations and understandings of their conditions. Therefore, you and the patient are partners during the interview; you do not control it.

Always prepare for the interview. Collect all available information about the patient and create a comfortable environment for the interview (see Chapter 7).

The interview consists of three phases: orientation, working, and termination (see Chapter 7).

Observation

Observation is a powerful assessment tool. During an interview and physical examination, closely observe a patient's verbal and nonverbal behaviors. This information is important and adds depth to the objective database. Determine whether data obtained by observation match the patient's words. For example, if a patient expresses no concern about an upcoming diagnostic test but appears anxious and irritable, there is a verbal and nonverbal data conflict. Your observations lead you to persist in gathering the information needed to resolve conflicting data and form accurate conclusions about the patient's condition.

Observation also provides information about a patient's level of function—the physical, developmental, psychological, and social aspects of everyday life. Observing the patient's level of function is different from the observation you perform during the interview. At this point, you observe the patient's ability to perform tasks such as self-feeding, hygiene, or making a decision.

Physical Examination

A physical examination allows the nurse to examine the patient's body to determine his or her state of health. It involves use of the techniques of inspection, palpation, percussion, auscultation, and smell. A complete examination includes a patient's height, weight, vital signs, general appearance and behavior, and a head-to-toe examination of all body systems (see Chapter 7).

Diagnostic and Laboratory Data

Diagnostic and laboratory test results identify or confirm conditions suspected or identified during the nursing health history and physical examination. For example, during the health history, the patient reports having had a bad cold for 6 days and currently has a productive cough with dark yellow sputum and mild shortness of breath.

During a physical examination, you notice an elevated temperature, increased respirations, and decreased breath sounds in the right lower lobe. You review the results of a complete blood count (CBC) and note that the white blood cell count is elevated, indicating an infection. In addition, the radiologist's report of a chest X-ray examination shows the presence of a right lower lobe infiltrate. Such findings in combination suggest that the patient has the medical diagnosis of pneumonia and the associated nursing diagnosis of *Impaired Gas Exchange*. When a patient collects and monitors laboratory data at home such as with routine blood glucose monitoring for diabetes, ask the patient about the routine results to determine the patient's response to illness and the effects of treatment measures. Compare laboratory data with the established norms for a particular test, age group, and gender.

Cultural Considerations in Assessment

Good assessment techniques are important to patient-centered care, especially when you are caring for patients from cultural backgrounds different from your own (Box 19.2). Make a conscious effort to understand your patient's culture, including values, beliefs, lifestyle practices, language, and ways of relating to friends and family. This information will assist you in providing quality care. You must act within different value systems and with respect and understanding for the patient without imposing your own attitudes and beliefs (see Chapter 33). Culture affects the way individuals express their feelings, both verbally and nonverbally. When you learn the ways people of different cultures communicate, you will likely perform a better assessment and gather better information from these patients (Darnell

BOX 19.2 Patient-Centered Care

The nursing process is a good method for implementing patient-centered care. To be effective, it is important during the assessment phase to ask a patient and family members useful questions that explore the patient's illness or health care problem in the context of the patient's culture (Ball et al., 2015). Involvement of families encourages sharing of information and planning of care to improve the well-being of the patient (Flagg, 2015).

Implications for Practice

- When talking about a patient's illness, try to understand it "through the patient's eyes":
  - What do you think is wrong with you?
  - What do you call your problem?
  - What worries you most about your illness?
  - What types of treatments or health practices do you use?
- When talking about treatments:
  - What should we do to eliminate your problem?
  - Which types of treatments do you use?
  - What benefit do you expect from the treatment?
- When there is a cross-cultural difference between you and your patient, ask yourself the following questions (Darnell and Hickson, 2015; Suhonen et al., 2011):
  - What is unique to the patient's culture and its impact on the treatment plan?
  - Are there risk factors for cultural misunderstanding? When there is a risk, try to reduce or correct it.
  - Are there resources within the agency and community to help you to provide culturally competent care to the patient and family?

and Hickson, 2015). You show respect for your patient when you apply sensitive communication techniques. Speaking at eye level, maintaining a proper distance, and listening carefully all demonstrate respect for your patient.

Interpreting and Validating Assessment Data

Assessment requires you to use critical thinking to continuously interpret information and make accurate judgments. You want to identify any abnormal findings, recognize that further observations are needed to clarify information, and begin to identify the patient's problems. Once you have collected your data, validate the data you obtained. This helps you to more accurately analyze and interpret a patient's clinical picture. **Validation** of assessment data is the comparison of data with another source to confirm data accuracy.

You must also ask your patient to validate the information you gathered during the interview and health history. For example, when a patient describes joint pain, ask the patient to rate the pain on a scale of 0–10, ask what precipitates the pain, and ask what measures the patient uses to reduce the pain.

Validate findings from physical examination and observation of patient behavior by comparing data in the medical record and consulting with other health team members or family caregivers. Validation often leads you to gather more assessment data and occasionally to reassess previously covered areas to clarify vague or ambiguous data. The nurse continually analyzes and thinks about the patient's database to fully understand the patient's problems, measure their extent, and discover possible relationships between them.

Data Documentation and Communication

Communicating your assessment findings, either verbally or through documentation, is the last step of a complete assessment. Timely, thorough, and accurate communication of facts is vital to ensuring continuity and quality patient care. If you fail to report or record an assessment finding or problem interpretation, it is lost and unavailable to anyone else caring for the patient (see Chapter 5). If you do not report specific information, you leave another health care team member uninformed and often with only general impressions. Observing, reporting, and recording of a patient's status are legal and professional responsibilities. The Nurse Practice Act, in all states and the American Nurses Association (ANA) policy statement (2010) require accurate data collection and recording as independent functions essential to the role of a professional nurse.

NURSING DIAGNOSIS

After you review and validate the data collected in a patient assessment, the next step of the nursing process is to form diagnostic conclusions that identify a patient's problems and the level of care required. When a nurse forms an accurate diagnostic conclusion, nursing therapies will be appropriate and effective. A diagnostic conclusion takes one of two forms: a nursing diagnosis or a collaborative problem.

A **nursing diagnosis** is a clinical judgment concerning a human response to health conditions and/or life processes or vulnerability for that response by an individual, family, or community that a nurse is licensed and competent to treat (Herdman and Kamitsuru, 2014b). A nursing diagnosis provides the basis for the selection of nursing interventions to achieve outcomes for which the nurse is accountable (Herdman and Kamitsuru, 2014b).

Critical Thinking and the Nursing Diagnostic Process

The nursing diagnostic process requires you to use critical thinking. This involves logically analyzing and interpreting assessment data about a patient to form a clinical judgment, in this case a nursing diagnosis. The **nursing diagnostic process** flows from the assessment process and includes data clustering, interpreting and analyzing, identifying patient needs, and formulating the nursing diagnosis or collaborative problem (Fig. 19.4).

When you analyze assessment data accurately, you identify patients' problems and make clinical decisions about their care. You begin analysis and interpretation of assessment data by organizing all your data into meaningful and usable data clusters. A **data cluster** is a set of signs or symptoms gathered during assessment that you group together in a logical way. During clustering, a cue or an individual sign, symptom, or finding stands out more than others. Clustering also requires your knowledge of the signs

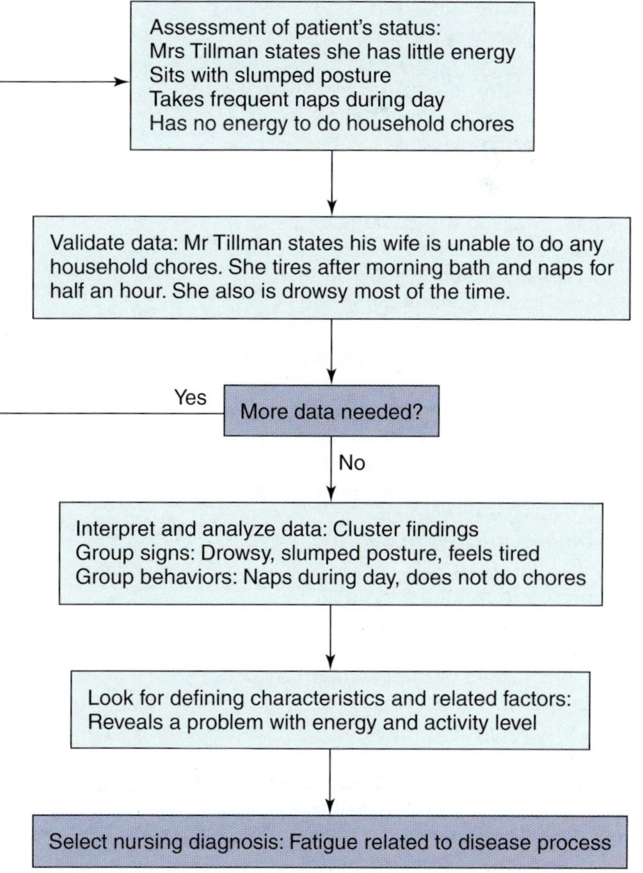

Fig. 19.4 Nursing diagnostic process for Mrs Tillman.

and symptoms and how they support the nursing diagnoses (Herdman and Kamitsuru, 2014a). For example, Mrs Tillman talks about feeling fatigued and "worn out," taking frequent naps, and being unable to perform usual activities such as preparing meals. These cues show a pattern.

Data analysis and interpretation involve recognizing patterns or trends in the clustered data, comparing them with standards, and coming to a reasoned conclusion about the patient's response to a health problem. Rich compares Mrs Tillman's signs and symptoms with normal standards for a woman her age. The typical woman might feel rested, sleeping through the night, and being able to perform daily routines. Mrs Tillman's clinical picture suggests that her cancer is producing a pattern of fatigue that affects her activity level.

You use reasoning and judgment to identify the assessment data that explains a patient's health status. Patients often present multiple cues, suggesting more than one type of health problem or need. You may need to gather additional data to clarify your interpretation.

Formulating the Nursing Diagnosis

After a nurse identifies the patterns of data that reveal a patient's health problems, the nurse must identify these problems in a way that will be clear to all health care providers. **NANDA International (NANDA-I)** has developed a model for organizing nursing diagnoses for documentation, auditing, and communication purposes. Researchers continually develop new diagnoses and add them to the NANDA-I listing (Box 19.3). The use of standard formal nursing diagnoses serves the following purposes (Gallagher-Lepak, 2014):

- Provides a precise definition that gives all members of the health care team a common language for understanding patient needs
- Allows nurses to communicate what they do among themselves, with other health care professionals, and with the public
- Distinguishes the nurse's role from that of physicians and other health care providers
- Helps nurses focus on the scope of nursing practice
- Fosters the development of knowledge and nursing science

When you finished assessing your patient, review all assessment data and compare the clusters and patterns of data with the clinical criteria that support a nursing diagnosis. **Defining characteristics** are observable cues and inferences that cluster as manifestations of a problem-focused or health promotion diagnosis or syndrome. These are the clinical criteria or assessment findings that support an actual nursing diagnosis (Gallagher-Lepak, 2014). NANDA-I-approved nursing diagnoses have identified sets

BOX 19.3 NANDA International–Approved Nursing Diagnoses, 2015–2017

Activity Intolerance
Risk for **Activity** Intolerance
Ineffective **Activity** Planning
Risk for Ineffective **Activity** Planning
Decreased Intracranial **Adaptive Capacity**
Ineffective **Airway** Clearance
Risk for **Allergy** Response
Anxiety
Risk for **Aspiration**
Risk for Impaired **Attachment**
Autonomic Dysreflexia
Risk for **Autonomic** Dysreflexia
Disorganized Infant **Behavior**
Readiness for Enhanced Organized Infant **Behavior**
Risk for Disorganized Infant **Behavior**
Risk for **Bleeding**
Risk for Unstable **Blood** Glucose Level
Disturbed **Body** Image
Risk for Imbalanced **Body** Temperature
Readiness for Enhanced **Breastfeeding**
Ineffective **Breastfeeding**
Interrupted **Breastfeeding**
Insufficient **Breast** Milk
Ineffective **Breathing** Pattern
Decreased **Cardiac** Output
Risk for Decreased **Cardiac** Output
Risk for Impaired **Cardiovascular** Function
Caregiver Role Strain
Risk for **Caregiver** Role Strain
Ineffective **Childbearing** Process
Readiness for Enhanced **Childbearing** Process
Risk for Ineffective **Childbearing** Process
Impaired **Comfort**
Readiness for Enhanced **Comfort**
Readiness for Enhanced **Communication**
Acute **Confusion**
Chronic **Confusion**
Risk for Acute **Confusion**
Constipation
Perceived **Constipation**
Risk for **Constipation**
Chronic Functional **Constipation**
Risk for Chronic Functional **Constipation**
Contamination
Risk for **Contamination**
Compromised Family **Coping**
Defensive **Coping**
Disabled Family **Coping**
Ineffective **Coping**
Ineffective Community **Coping**
Readiness for Enhanced **Coping**
Readiness for Enhanced Community **Coping**
Readiness for Enhanced Family **Coping**
Death Anxiety
Readiness for Enhanced **Decision-Making**
Decisional Conflict
Ineffective **Denial**
Impaired **Dentition**
Risk for Delayed **Development**
Diarrhea
Risk for **Disuse** Syndrome
Deficient **Diversional** Activity
Risk for **Dry** Eye
Risk for **Electrolyte** Imbalance
Impaired **Emancipated** Decision-Making
Readiness for Enhanced **Emancipated** Decision-Making
Risk for Impaired **Emancipated** Decision-Making
Labile **Emotional** Control
Risk for **Falls**
Dysfunctional **Family** Processes

BOX 19.3 **NANDA International–Approved Nursing Diagnoses, 2015–2017—cont'd**

Interrupted **Family** Processes
Readiness for Enhanced **Family** Processes
Fatigue
Fear
Ineffective Infant **Feeding** Pattern
Readiness for Enhanced **Fluid** Balance
Deficient **Fluid** Volume
Excess **Fluid** Volume
Risk for Deficient **Fluid** Volume
Risk for Imbalanced **Fluid** Volume
Frail Elderly Syndrome
Risk for **Frail** Elderly Syndrome
Impaired **Gas** Exchange
Dysfunctional **Gastrointestinal** Motility
Risk for Dysfunctional **Gastrointestinal** Motility
Risk for Ineffective **Gastrointestinal** Perfusion
Grieving
Complicated **Grieving**
Risk for Complicated **Grieving**
Risk for Disproportionate **Growth**
Deficient Community **Health**
Risk-Prone **Health** Behavior
Ineffective **Health** Maintenance
Ineffective **Health** Management
Readiness for Enhanced **Health** Management
Ineffective Family **Health** Management
Impaired **Home** Maintenance
Readiness for Enhanced **Hope**
Hopelessness
Risk for Compromised **Human** Dignity
Hyperthermia
Hypothermia
Risk for **Hypothermia**
Risk for Perioperative **Hypothermia**
Ineffective **Impulse** Control
Functional Urinary **Incontinence**
Overflow Urinary **Incontinence**
Reflex Urinary **Incontinence**
Stress Urinary **Incontinence**
Urge Urinary **Incontinence**
Risk for Urge Urinary **Incontinence**
Bowel **Incontinence**
Risk for Sudden **Infant** Death Syndrome
Risk for **Infection**
Risk for **Injury**
Risk for Corneal **Injury**
Risk for Perioperative-Positioning **Injury**
Risk for Thermal **Injury**
Risk for Urinary Tract **Injury**
Insomnia
Neonatal **Jaundice**
Risk for Neonatal **Jaundice**
Deficient **Knowledge**
Readiness for Enhanced **Knowledge**
Latex Allergy Response
Risk for **Latex** Allergy Response
Sedentary **Lifestyle**
Risk for Impaired **Liver** Function
Risk for **Loneliness**
Risk for Disturbed **Maternal/Fetal Dyad**
Impaired **Memory**
Impaired Bed **Mobility**
Impaired Physical **Mobility**
Impaired Wheelchair **Mobility**
Impaired **Mood** Regulation
Moral Distress
Nausea
Unilateral **Neglect**
Noncompliance
Imbalanced **Nutrition:** Less Than Body Requirements
Readiness for Enhanced **Nutrition**
Obesity
Impaired **Oral** Mucous Membrane
Risk for Impaired **Oral** Mucous Membrane
Overweight
Risk for **Overweight**
Acute **Pain**
Chronic **Pain**
Labor **Pain**
Chronic **Pain** Syndrome
Impaired **Parenting**
Readiness for Enhanced **Parenting**
Risk for Impaired **Parenting**
Risk for **Peripheral** Neurovascular Dysfunction
Disturbed **Personal** Identity
Risk for Disturbed **Personal** Identity
Risk for **Poisoning**
Post-trauma Syndrome
Risk for **Post-trauma** Syndrome
Readiness for Enhanced **Power**
Powerlessness
Risk for **Powerlessness**
Risk for **Pressure** Injury
Ineffective **Protection**
Rape-Trauma Syndrome
Risk for **Reaction** to Iodinated Contrast Media
Ineffective **Relationship**
Risk for Ineffective **Relationship**
Readiness for Enhanced **Relationship**
Impaired **Religiosity**
Readiness for Enhanced **Religiosity**
Risk for Impaired **Religiosity**
Relocation Stress Syndrome
Risk for **Relocation** Stress Syndrome
Risk for Ineffective **Renal** Perfusion
Impaired **Resilience**
Readiness for Enhanced **Resilience**
Risk for Impaired **Resilience**
Parental **Role** Conflict
Ineffective **Role** Performance
Readiness for Enhanced **Self-Care**
Bathing **Self-Care** Deficit
Dressing **Self-Care** Deficit
Feeding **Self-Care** Deficit
Toileting **Self-Care** Deficit
Readiness for Enhanced **Self-Concept**
Chronic Low **Self-Esteem**
Risk for Chronic Low **Self-Esteem**
Situational Low **Self-Esteem**
Risk for Situational Low **Self-Esteem**
Self-Mutilation
Risk for **Self-Mutilation**
Self-Neglect
Sexual Dysfunction
Ineffective **Sexuality** Pattern
Risk for **Shock**
Impaired **Sitting**
Impaired **Skin** Integrity
Risk for Impaired **Skin** Integrity
Sleep Deprivation
Readiness for Enhanced **Sleep**
Disturbed **Sleep** Pattern

Continued

BOX 19.3 NANDA International–Approved Nursing Diagnoses, 2015–2017—cont'd

Impaired **Social** Interaction
Social Isolation
Chronic **Sorrow**
Spiritual Distress
Risk for **Spiritual** Distress
Readiness for Enhanced **Spiritual** Well-Being
Impaired **Standing**
Stress Overload
Risk for **Suffocation**
Risk for **Suicide**
Delayed **Surgical** Recovery
Risk for Delayed **Surgical** Recovery
Impaired **Swallowing**
Ineffective **Thermoregulation**
Impaired **Tissue** Integrity
Risk for Impaired **Tissue** Integrity
Ineffective Peripheral **Tissue** Perfusion
Risk for Ineffective Peripheral **Tissue** Perfusion
Risk for Decreased Cardiac **Tissue** Perfusion
Risk for Ineffective Cerebral **Tissue** Perfusion
Impaired **Transfer** Ability
Risk for **Trauma**
Risk for Vascular **Trauma**
Impaired **Urinary** Elimination
Readiness for Enhanced **Urinary** Elimination
Urinary Retention
Risk for Self-Directed **Violence**
Risk for Other-Directed **Violence**
Impaired Spontaneous **Ventilation**
Dysfunctional **Ventilatory** Weaning Response
Impaired **Verbal** Communication
Impaired **Walking**
Wandering

From Herdman TH, Kamitsuru S, editors: *Nursing diagnoses—definitions and classification 2015–2017.* Copyright © 2014, 1994–2014 NANDA International. Used by arrangement with John Wiley & Sons, Inc. To make safe and effective judgments using NANDA-I nursing diagnoses, it is essential that nurses refer to the definitions and defining characteristics of the diagnoses listed in this work.

of defining characteristics that support identification of each nursing diagnosis (Herdman and Kamitsuru, 2014b). As you gain clinical experience, you become familiar with the defining characteristics for the more common nursing diagnoses in your practice. This helps you identify nursing diagnoses. Box 19.4 shows an example of an approved nursing diagnosis and its associated defining characteristics and related factors. As you analyze clusters of data, you begin to consider possible nursing diagnoses that may apply to your patient. *For example, a nurse reviews findings pertaining to a patient, who reported feeling fatigue. The defining characteristics of tiredness and fatigue apply to the nursing diagnoses of* Fatigue *and* Activity Intolerance. *However, the nurse's assessment probed further and revealed the particular patient's inability to maintain the usual levels of activity or routines, pointing him toward the nursing diagnosis of* Fatigue. The absence of certain defining characteristics suggests that you must reject a nursing diagnosis under consideration. Carefully review all defining characteristics that support or eliminate a nursing diagnosis.

While focusing on patterns of defining characteristics, you also compare a patient's pattern of data with data that are consistent with normal, healthful patterns. Use accepted norms as the basis for comparison and judgment. These norms include laboratory and diagnostic test values, professional standards, and normal anatomical or physiological limits. When you compare patterns, determine whether the patient's grouped signs and symptoms are normal for the patient and within the range of healthful responses.

As you isolate the defining characteristics that are not within healthy norms, you identify a patient's need or problem. Let's try to understand through a case scenario; *for example, a nurse assessed a patient's verbal report of feeling tired and lacking energy. These symptoms are not necessarily common for an elderly and indicate a basic problem involving the patient's ability to participate in normal activity.*

The nurse also learned that the patient sometimes has difficulty completing routine chores and requires frequent naps during the day. The nurse recognized that the patient had a problem, but he reviewed the NANDA-I classifications to define her problem more specifically. He looked first at the domain of activity/rest. NANDA-I has a variety of nursing diagnoses that can apply to activity/rest (e.g., Activity Intolerance, Risk for Activity Intolerance, Fatigue, *and* Impaired Walking).

After carefully reviewing the patient's presenting symptoms, the nurse selected Fatigue. *The key to the nurse's diagnosis was his assessment showing that the patient's lack of energy affected her daily activities.* It is critical to identify the correct diagnostic label for a patient's need. A nurse usually moves from

BOX 19.4 Example of a NANDA International–Approved Nursing Diagnosis With Defining Characteristics and Related Factors

Diagnosis: Fatigue

DEFINING CHARACTERISTICS	RELATED FACTORS (EXAMPLES)
Impaired ability to maintain usual physical activity	Psychological: Anxiety, stress, depression
Impaired ability to maintain usual routines	Physiological: Physical deconditioning, malnutrition
Insufficient energy	Environmental: Humidity, lights, noise
Lethargy	Situational: Negative life events, occupation
Increase in rest requirements	

Used with permission from Herdman TH, Kamitsuru S, editors: *NANDA International nursing diagnoses: definitions & classification 2015–2017*, Oxford, 2014, Wiley Blackwell.

general to specific. It helps to think of the problem identification phase as the identification of a general health care problem and the formulation of the nursing diagnosis as the identification of a specific health problem. When you begin to identify a problem, review the NANDA-I domains to help you focus on nursing diagnoses pertinent to a particular domain.

Types of Nursing Diagnoses

NANDA-I identifies three types of nursing diagnoses: problem-focused diagnoses, risk diagnoses, and health promotion diagnoses. A problem-focused diagnosis is a clinical judgment concerning an undesirable human response to a health condition and/or life process that exists in an individual, family, group, or community (Gallagher-Lepak, 2014). Selecting a problem-focused diagnosis means that there are sufficient assessment data to support the nursing diagnosis. In Mrs Tillman's case, *Fatigue* and *Death Anxiety* are problem-focused nursing diagnoses.

A risk nursing diagnosis is a clinical judgment concerning the vulnerability of an individual, family, group, or community for developing an undesirable human response to health conditions and/or life processes (Gallagher-Lepak, 2014). These diagnoses do not have related factors or defining characteristics because they have not yet occurred. Instead, a risk diagnosis has risk factors. Risk factors are the environmental, physiological, psychosocial, genetic, and chemical elements that place a person at risk for a health problem. *Risk for Falls* is an example of a risk diagnosis.

A health promotion nursing diagnosis is a clinical judgment concerning motivation and desire to increase well-being and actualize human health potential. These responses are expressed by a readiness to enhance specific health behaviors and can be used in any health state. Health promotion responses may apply to an individual, family, group, or community (Gallagher-Lepak, 2014). This readiness is supported by defining characteristics (Herdman and Kamitsuru, 2014a). *Readiness for Enhanced Comfort* is an example of a health promotion diagnosis.

Components of a Nursing Diagnosis

The identification of a nursing diagnosis flows from the assessment and diagnostic processes. Throughout this text, nursing diagnoses are worded in a two-part format: the diagnostic label followed by a statement of a related factor (Table 19.2). This two-part format provides a diagnosis that is relevant for a specific patient.

Table 19.2 NANDA International Nursing Diagnosis Format

Diagnostic Label	Related Factors (Examples Listed)
Fatigue	▪ Psychological: Anxiety, depression, stressors ▪ Physiological: Malnutrition, physical deconditioning ▪ Environmental: Humidity, lights, ambient noise ▪ Situational: Negative life events, occupational demands
Death Anxiety	▪ Perceived imminence of death ▪ Anticipation of pain ▪ Anticipation of suffering ▪ Discussions on topic of death ▪ Uncertainty of prognosis

Diagnostic Label

The diagnostic label is the name of the nursing diagnosis as approved by NANDA-I, and it describes the essence of a patient's response to a health condition in as few words as possible (see Box 19.3). Each NANDA-I-approved diagnosis also has a definition. The definition describes the characteristics of the particular human response. Use these definitions to help you identify a patient's correct diagnoses. The definitions are especially helpful when selecting between two diagnoses with similar defining characteristics. The diagnostic labels include descriptors that further support the nursing diagnosis. For example, the diagnosis *Impaired Physical Mobility* includes the descriptor *impaired*. The term *impaired* describes the nature of or change in mobility that best describes the patient's response. Examples of other descriptors are *compromised, decreased, delayed,* or *ineffective*.

Related Factor

The **related factor** is an integral component of all problem-focused nursing diagnoses. The related factor is associated with a patient's actual or potential response to the health problem and can change by using specific nursing interventions (Herdman and Kamitsuru, 2014b). The related factor comes from the patient's assessment data. Thus, the assessment data must be accurate. A related factor provides context for the defining characteristics (see Box 19.4). It is a condition associated with or contributing to the diagnosis. For example, a nursing diagnostic statement applicable to Mrs Tillman includes the diagnostic label (e.g., *Fatigue*) and the related factor (e.g., *chronic disease process*).

Related factors include four categories: pathophysiological (biological or psychological), treatment-related, situational (environmental or personal), and maturational (Carpenito-Moyet, 2017). The "related to" phrase does not always imply a cause-and-effect relationship. It indicates that the etiology contributes to or is associated with the problem (Fig. 19.5). The "related to" phrase requires you to use critical thinking skills to individualize the nursing diagnosis and select appropriate nursing interventions.

Related factors are not listed for risk diagnoses (e.g., *Risk for Infection, Risk for Falls,* and *Risk for Injury*). The diagnosis is supported by various risk factors. For example, Mrs Tillman has sleeplessness, metastatic disease, and lack of strength. These risk factors all contribute to her increased vulnerability for a *Risk for Falls* nursing diagnosis.

The **etiology** is always within the domain of nursing practice and a condition that responds to nursing interventions. Nurses sometimes record medical diagnoses as the etiologies of nursing diagnoses. This is incorrect. Nursing interventions cannot change a medical diagnosis. For example, in Mrs Tillman's case, nursing interventions cannot change cancer. Thus, the diagnosis of *Fatigue related to cancer* is incorrect. Instead, you direct nursing interventions toward behavior or conditions that you can treat or manage. For example, the nursing diagnosis *Fatigue related to chronic disease process* is correct. Rich, Mrs Tillman's nurse, can develop interventions that are known to help manage fatigue related to the chronic and progressive nature of cancer.

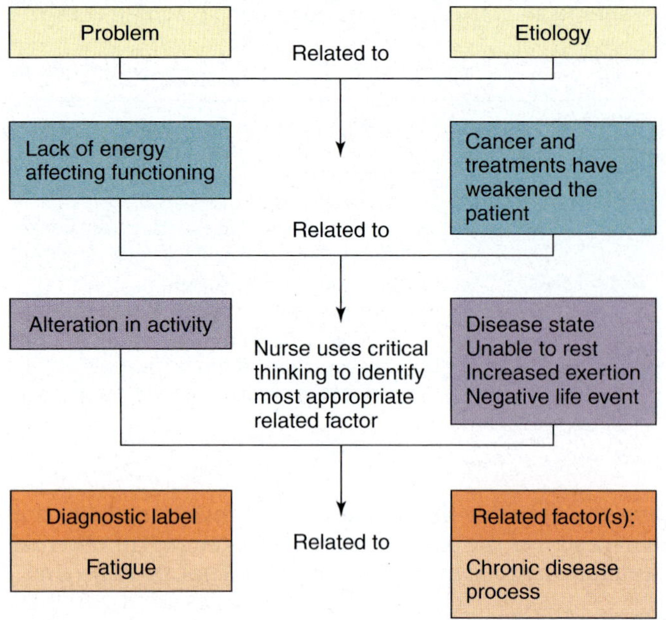

Fig. 19.5 Relation between diagnostic label and etiology (related factor). (Redrawn from Hickey P: *Nursing process handbook*, St Louis, 1990, Mosby.)

Table 19.3 demonstrates the association between a nurse's assessment of a patient, the clustering of defining characteristics, and the formulation of two different nursing diagnoses. The diagnostic process results in the formation of a total diagnostic statement that enables a nurse to develop an appropriate, patient-centered plan of care. The defining characteristics and relevant etiologies are from NANDA-I (Herdman and Kamitsuru, 2014b).

Definition

NANDA-I approves a definition for each diagnosis following clinical use and testing. The definition describes the characteristics of the human response identified. For example, the definition of the diagnostic label *Fatigue* is an "overwhelming sustained sense of exhaustion and decreased capacity for physical and mental work at usual level" (Herdman and Kamitsuru, 2014b). Always refer to a definition to help you further identify a patient's diagnosis.

PES Format

Some health care agencies prefer a three-part nursing diagnostic label. In this case, the diagnostic label consists of the NANDA-I label, the related factor, and the defining characteristics (Ackley and Ladwig, 2016). A problem-focused nursing diagnosis, including a diagnostic label and the related factor exhibited by defining characteristics, is the best practice (Herdman and Kamitsuru, 2014b). This approach makes a diagnosis even more specific to the patient. The acronym *PES* stands for *p*roblem, *e*tiology, and symptoms. Following is an example using the nursing diagnosis in Mrs Tillman's care plan:

P (Problem) NANDA-I label: *Death Anxiety*
E (Etiology or related factors): Anticipation of suffering
S (Symptoms or defining characteristics): Increased expression of worries, difficulty breathing (examples)
PES diagnostic statement: *Death Anxiety* related to anticipation of suffering, evidenced by increased expression of worries, difficulty breathing

Cultural Relevance of Nursing Diagnoses

When you select nursing diagnoses, always consider your patient's culture, which in its broadest sense reflects the whole of human behavior, including ideas, beliefs, values, ways of relating to one another, language and manners of speaking, and work and lifestyle practices (Ball et al., 2015; Flagg, 2015) (see Chapter 33). Consideration of the patient's culture is more than just knowing the cultural differences; it is assessing how those cultural differences affect patient-centered care (Ball et al., 2015; Flagg, 2015). Lai et al. (2013) noted that certain NANDA-I nursing diagnoses were difficult for nurses to apply considering the cultural beliefs of a Chinese health care setting, which emphasizes holistic harmony and balance. The patient's culture influences health care preferences and a patient's desire to resolve health care problems (Burman et al., 2013; Nielsen et al., 2015).

A patient's culture influences the type of health care problems that he or she experiences as well as the importance of those problems (Nielsen et al., 2015). When you make a nursing diagnosis, consider the effect of culture on the related factor in the diagnostic statement. For example, *Impaired Verbal Communication related to cultural differences*

Table 19.3 Formulation of Nursing Diagnoses

Assessment Activities	Defining Characteristics (Clustering Cues)	Nursing Diagnosis	Etiologies ("Related to")
Ask the patient to describe usual daily physical activities.	Impaired ability to maintain usual level of physical activity	Fatigue	Chronic disease process
Observe the patient during care activities.	Lethargy Drowsiness		
Question the patient about frequency of rest periods.	Increase in rest requirements		
Ask the patient to talk about any concerns or worries related to diagnosis of cancer.	Fear of suffering related to dying	Death Anxiety	Anticipation of suffering
Have the patient describe her emotions.	Reports deep sadness		
Ask the patient to discuss how she thinks her illness will affect her relationship with her husband.	Reports worry about impact of her own death on significant others		

reflects a diagnostic conclusion that considers a patient's unique cultural needs. *Deficient Knowledge* is a common nursing diagnosis and may be related to a patient's culture. When a nurse is aware of the effects of culture on a patient's health care practices, the nurse can improve the cultural effectiveness of the nursing diagnoses by asking some of the following questions:

- How has this health problem affected you and your family?
- What worries you most about this problem?
- What do you believe will help or fix the problem?
- What health care practices do you use to keep yourself and family well?

Using a patient-centered approach when asking these questions helps you see the patient's problems through his or her eyes (Cope, 2015). This leads you to culturally relevant nursing diagnoses and interventions (Lai et al., 2013; Nielsen et al., 2015).

Concept Mapping Nursing Diagnoses

Your patients usually will have multiple nursing diagnoses. When you care for multiple patients, prioritizing and focusing on all patients' multiple diagnoses becomes challenging. Developing a **concept map** helps you critically think about your patients' nursing diagnoses, their relationship with one another, and their effect on the nursing care plan (Lhussier et al., 2015; Pilcher, 2011). Concept mapping helps you logically organize and link data about a patient's multiple diagnoses. The concept map graphically represents the connections between concepts (e.g., a nursing diagnosis) that relate to a central subject (e.g., a patient's health problems). As you apply each step of the nursing process, your concept map includes more detail about planned interventions (see the section Planning).

For example, Mrs Tillman's *Death Anxiety* makes it more difficult for her to sleep, and this results in *Fatigue*. Fatigue in turn is a risk factor that increases the *Risk for Falls*. Finally, the diagnoses of *Deficient Knowledge* and *Death Anxiety* also are related. Having a poor understanding of her conditions heightens Mrs Tillman's anxiety. Being anxious can make it hard for her to sleep. This concept map will show you how the diagnoses relate to one another.

Sources of Diagnostic Errors

Errors can occur in the diagnostic process during data collection, data interpretation, clustering, and statement of the nursing diagnosis. Apply methodical critical thinking to make an accurate nursing diagnosis.

Errors in Data Collection

To avoid errors in data collection, be knowledgeable of, and skillful in, all assessment techniques. Ensure that data are complete and accurate, and collect data in an organized way. The following practice tips are essential in avoiding data collection errors:

- Review your level of comfort and competence with interview and physical assessment skills before you begin the data collection step.
- Approach assessment in steps. Focus on completing the patient history and interview before starting the examination. Consider focusing on a single body system to learn how to perform an examination. Then move to a more complex head-to-toe examination.
- Review your assessments in clinical or classroom settings to gain feedback and learn to revise an assessment or gather more information.
- Organize the examination. Prepare the patient and environment for the examination (see Chapter 7).

Errors in Interpretation and Analysis of Data

After you complete the data collection step, review your database to determine whether it is accurate and complete. Review your data to validate that measurable, objective physical findings support the subjective data. For example, when a patient reports "difficulty breathing," you auscultate lung sounds and assess respiratory rate and rhythm.

When data are not validated, the result is a mismatch between clinical cues and the nursing diagnosis. Consider any conflicting cues and determine whether you have sufficient cues to form a diagnosis.

Consider the patient's cultural background or developmental stage when you interpret the meaning of cues. For example, male and female patients might express pain very differently. Misinterpreting the patient's expression of pain could easily lead to an inaccurate diagnosis.

Errors in Data Clustering

Errors result when you cluster data prematurely, incorrectly, or not at all. When you make the nursing diagnosis before grouping all data, you are clustering data prematurely. For example, a patient has urinary incontinence and states that he has urgency and nocturia. You cluster the available data and identify *Impaired Urinary Elimination* as a probable nursing diagnosis. Incorrect clustering occurs when you try to make the nursing diagnosis fit the signs and symptoms obtained. In this example, further assessment reveals that the patient also has bladder distention and dribbling; thus, the correct diagnosis is *Urinary Retention*. The nursing diagnosis comes from the data, not the other way around. An incorrect nursing diagnosis affects the quality of nursing care.

Errors in the Diagnostic Statement

A correct diagnostic statement, supported by relevant assessment data, is more likely to result in the appropriate selection of appropriate nursing interventions and outcomes (Herdman and Kamitsuru, 2014b). To reduce errors, phrase the diagnostic statement in appropriate, concise, and precise language. Use correct terminology reflecting a patient's response to the illness or condition. Use standardized nursing language from NANDA-I to ensure accuracy. Follow these guidelines:

1. Identify the patient's response, not the medical diagnosis (Carpenito-Moyet, 2017). Because a medical diagnosis requires medical interventions, it is legally inadvisable to include it in the nursing diagnosis. Change the diagnosis *Fatigue related to cancer* to *Fatigue related to chronic disease process*.
2. Identify a NANDA-I diagnostic statement, not a symptom. Identify nursing diagnoses from a cluster of defining

characteristics that apply to a patient. A single symptom is insufficient for identifying a problem. For example, shortness of breath alone does not identify a diagnosis. In contrast, shortness of breath, pain on inspiration, and productive cough in a postoperative patient form the cluster for *Ineffective Breathing Pattern related to increased airway secretions*.

3. Identify a treatable related factor or risk factor, rather than a clinical sign or chronic problem that is not treatable through nursing intervention. Identifying a related factor allows you to select nursing interventions for resolving the etiology of the problem or minimizing the patient's risk. A diagnostic test or chronic dysfunction is not an etiology that a nursing intervention can treat. A patient with cancer often develops anemia, reflected in low red blood cell counts. The diagnosis *Fatigue related to low red blood cell counts* is an incorrect diagnostic statement. *Fatigue related to chronic disease process* is appropriate because it allows you to focus interventions on the physical responses common in chronic progressive disease.
4. Identify the problem caused by the treatment or diagnostic study rather than the treatment or study itself. Patients can respond to diagnostic tests and medical treatments in many ways. These responses are the area of nursing concern. The patient who has severe chest pain and is scheduled for a cardiac catheterization may have a nursing diagnosis of *Anxiety related to lack of knowledge about cardiac catheterization*.
5. Identify the patient response to the equipment rather than the equipment itself. Change the diagnosis *Anxiety related to cardiac monitor* to *Deficient Knowledge regarding the need for cardiac monitoring*.
6. Identify the patient's problems rather than your problems with nursing care. Nursing diagnoses are always patient-centered and form the basis for goal-directed care. The statement "potential for electrolyte complications related to severe gastroenteritis" directs the nurse to focus on the patient's need for i.v. therapy and observing and controlling the patient's symptoms related to gastroenteritis. The diagnosis *Deficient Fluid Volume related to severe vomiting and diarrhea* centers attention on the patient's signs and symptoms.
7. Identify the patient's problem rather than the nursing intervention. You plan nursing interventions later when you plan care to alleviate the patient's problems. The statement "Offer bedpan frequently because of altered elimination patterns" changes to the diagnosis *Diarrhea related to food intolerance*. This corrects the misstatement and allows proper implementation of the nursing process.
8. Identify the patient's problem rather than the goal. You set goals during the planning step of the nursing process. Goals serve as a basis for determining whether you have resolved a health problem, not as a tool for identifying the problem. Change the statement "Patient needs high-protein diet related to potential alteration in nutrition" to *Imbalanced Nutrition: Less Than Body Requirements related to inadequate protein intake*. This diagnosis identifies the correct etiology and enables you to then plan a proper treatment.
9. Make professional rather than prejudicial judgments. Base nursing diagnoses on subjective and objective patient data rather than on your personal beliefs and values. Remove your judgment from *Impaired Skin Integrity related to poor hygiene habits* by changing the nursing diagnosis to *Impaired Skin Integrity related to lack of knowledge about perineal care*.
10. Avoid legally inadvisable statements that imply blame, negligence, or malpractice (Carpenito-Moyet, 2017). The diagnosis *Chronic Pain related to insufficient pain medication* implies that the health care provider prescribed inadequate analgesia prescription. The correct way to identify the problem is to write *Chronic Pain related to incorrect adherence of analgesic schedule*.
11. Identify the problem and etiology to avoid a circular statement. Circular statements are vague and give no direction to nursing care. Change the diagnosis *Acute Pain related to alteration in comfort* to the specific patient problem and cause: *Acute Pain related to incisional trauma*.
12. Identify only one patient problem in a diagnostic statement. Problems have different expected outcomes. Including multiple problems in a nursing diagnosis causes confusion during the planning step. However, it is permissible to include multiple etiologies contributing to one patient problem. For example, you might restate *Pain and Anxiety related to difficulty in ambulating* as two nursing diagnoses. These could be *Impaired Physical Mobility related to pain in right knee* and *Anxiety related to fear of falling*.

Documentation and Informatics

After identifying a patient's nursing diagnoses, enter them on his or her written plan of care or in the EHR of the health care agency. Start-of-the art EHRs contain the following:

- NANDA-I-approved nursing diagnoses, interventions, and outcomes
- Related or risk factors
- Defining characteristics (Herdman and Kamitsuru, 2014b)

With this type of EHR, the nurse enters assessment data, and the computer organizes the data into clusters. This feature improves the nurse's ability to select accurate nursing diagnoses. Once the diagnoses are identified, the computer system will direct the nurse to possible outcomes and interventions to select for the patient. This helps to make the patient care plan more theoretically based. When agencies use EHR systems that do not use NANDA-I, entry of nursing diagnoses is more tedious.

List nursing diagnoses chronologically as you identify them. When you initiate a care plan, always list the diagnoses in order from highest priority to lowest. The highest priority diagnosis depends on a patient's condition and the nature of the nursing diagnosis. (For example, an acute physical health problem ranks above a long-term, chronic health problem.)

Add nursing diagnoses to the list and date each nursing diagnosis. When caring for a patient, always review the list of nursing diagnoses and identify the diagnoses with the highest priority, regardless of chronological order.

DIFFERENCE BETWEEN MEDICAL AND NURSING DIAGNOSIS

Never confuse a medical diagnosis with a nursing diagnosis. A **medical diagnosis** is the identification of a disease condition based on an evaluation of physical signs, symptoms, history, and diagnostic tests and procedures. A medical diagnosis stays constant as long as the disease condition remains. Health care providers are licensed to treat diseases or pathological processes described in medical diagnostic statements. An advanced practice nurse can also treat medical diagnoses but does not perform surgery.

In contrast, a patient's responses to cancer such as symptoms of pain and nausea and insufficient knowledge about treatment are nursing diagnoses that nurses manage. What makes a nursing diagnostic process unique is having patients involved in the process when possible.

A **collaborative problem** is an actual or potential physiological complication that nurses monitor to detect the onset of changes in a patient's status (Carpenito-Moyet, 2017). When collaborative problems develop, nurses intervene in cooperation with social workers, dietitians, or personnel from other health care disciplines.

The Canadian Interprofessional Health Collaborative (2010) defines interprofessional collaboration as a partnership between a team of health care providers (e.g., nurses, health care providers, therapists, and dietitians) and a patient in a participatory collaborative and coordinated approach for shared decision-making about the patient's health care issues. Nurses manage collaborative problems such as hemorrhage or infection using both physician-prescribed and nursing-prescribed interventions. For example, a patient who has a surgical wound is at risk for developing an infection. Thus, a physician or advanced practice nurse prescribes antibiotics. The nurse monitors the patient for signs of infection, provides meticulous wound care, and administers the prescribed antibiotics.

PLANNING

After you identify a patient's nursing diagnoses and collaborative problems, you begin the planning step of the nursing process. **Planning** involves setting priorities, identifying patient-centered goals and expected outcomes, and prescribing nursing interventions. The most important principle in planning is the individualization of a plan of care for each patient's unique needs. The nursing diagnoses you select direct your selection of nursing interventions and goals and outcomes you hope to achieve. The individualized nursing diagnoses and problems that you identify direct your selection of individualized nursing interventions and the goals and outcomes you hope to achieve (Flagg, 2015; Nielsen et al., 2015).

Establishing Priorities

A single patient often has multiple diagnoses and collaborative problems. Eventually you will care for multiple patients at one time. You must be able to set priorities for these patients carefully and wisely to ensure timely, safe, and effective care.

Priority setting is the ordering of nursing diagnoses or patients' problems considering their urgency and importance to establish an order for nursing actions. In other words, you must provide some types of care before others. By ranking nursing diagnoses in the order of importance, you attend to your patient's most important needs and better prioritize your care activities.

A priority list helps you anticipate and sequence nursing interventions when a patient has multiple problems. Together with your patients, you select mutually agreed-on priorities based on the urgency of the problem, the patient's safety and desires, and the nature of the treatment indicated. Establishing priorities is not just a matter of numbering the nursing diagnoses based on severity or physiological importance.

Classify priorities as high, intermediate, or low. Nursing diagnoses that, if left untreated, result in harm to the patient or others have the highest priority. One way to prioritize diagnoses is to consider Maslow's hierarchy of needs. For example, you want to attend to a patient's oxygen, fluid, and nutrition needs before you focus on shelter or sexual needs. However, it is always important to consider each patient's unique case. High priorities are sometimes both psychological and physiological. Avoid classifying only physiological nursing diagnoses as high priority.

Consider Mrs Tillman's case. The nursing diagnosis of *Death Anxiety* is a high-priority diagnosis because it has the potential to impair Mrs Tillman's ability to participate in her own care and maintain a healthy relationship with her husband. Intermediate-priority nursing diagnoses involve the nonemergent, non-life-threatening needs of a patient. In Mrs Tillman's case, *Fatigue* is an intermediate diagnosis. Mrs Tillman's activity problem is linked to the progressive nature of her cancer. Her fatigue will be an ongoing challenge, but not a life-threatening issue. Energy conservation and management therapies are important but not critical.

Low-priority nursing diagnoses are patient needs that are usually directly related to a specific illness or prognosis but also affect a patient's future well-being. Rich, Mrs Tillman's nurse, knows that she will have more health care needs as her disease progresses. Her husband, the family caregiver, may assume even more responsibility for in-home care. *Deficient Knowledge regarding palliative care related to inexperience* is a relevant diagnosis but currently of lower priority than the other diagnoses. In future clinic visits, Rich will plan a discussion about palliative care with the Tillman family.

Priorities change as the patient's condition changes. Each time you begin a sequence of care such as the beginning of a nursing care shift or during a clinic visit, you must reorder priorities. Continually assess the patient to determine the status of a patient's nursing diagnoses. Following the order of priorities helps to ensure that you meet your patients' needs in a timely and effective way.

Priority setting includes prioritizing specific interventions that you plan to use with the patient. For example, as Rich considers the high-priority diagnosis of *Death Anxiety*, he decides whether to counsel Mrs Tillman first or conduct a care conference with the patient, her husband, and the clinic nurse practitioner. Rich must prioritize interventions to be most effective in meeting the desired goals and outcomes. It is always important to involve the patient in priority setting. In some situations, you and the patient assign different priority rankings to nursing diagnoses and collaborative problems. Resolve these differences through open communication. When a patient's physiological and emotional needs are at stake, you must assume primary responsibility for setting priorities.

Ethical care must factor into priority setting. When ethical issues cloud priorities, you must maintain an open dialogue with the patient, family, and other health care providers. For example, when caring for patients with cancer and other disabling illnesses, discuss the situation with the patient and understand his or her expectations. Understand your professional responsibility in providing care, and work with the health care team, patient, and family caregivers when developing a patient-centered care plan.

Critical Thinking in Setting Goals and Expected Outcomes

After you identify a nursing diagnosis for your patient, ask yourself the following questions:

- What is the best approach to address and resolve the problem?
- What does my patient need to achieve? What are the goals and expected outcomes?
- How will I know when my patient has achieved them?

Goals and expected outcomes are specific statements of patient behavior or physiological responses that you select to resolve a nursing diagnosis or collaborative problem. They serve two purposes: to set a clear direction for the selection and use of nursing interventions and to set specific measures for evaluating the effectiveness of the interventions.

Goals of Care

A patient-centered **goal** is a broad statement that describes a desired change in a patient's condition or behavior. For Mrs Tillman, who has a diagnosis of *Fatigue related to chronic disease process*, a goal of care would be "Patient will achieve improved energy level within 2 weeks." A goal is realistic and based on patient needs and resources. A patient goal is a predicted resolution of a problem, evidence of progress toward problem resolution, progress toward improved health status, or continued maintenance of good health or function (Carpenito-Moyet, 2017).

Each goal is time limited so the health care team has a common time frame for problem resolution. The time frame depends on the nature of the problem, etiology, overall condition of the patient, and treatment setting. A *short-term goal* is an objective behavior or response that you expect the patient to achieve in a short time, usually less than a week. In an acute care setting, you may set goals to be achieved within just a few hours; for example, "Patient will maintain a balanced fluid status within the next 12 hours." A *long-term goal* is an objective behavior or response that you expect the patient to achieve over a longer period, usually several days, weeks, or months. Goal setting establishes the framework for the nursing care plan. Table 19.4 shows the progression from nursing diagnoses to goals and expected outcomes, which you individualize to meet patient needs.

Goals are often based on standards of care or clinical guidelines established for minimal safe practice. For example, the Infusion Nurses Society (INS) has standards of care to prevent the i.v. complication of phlebitis. When a nurse cares for a patient with a peripheral i.v. catheter, the goal "The i.v. site will remain free of phlebitis" is established based on sound nursing practice standards.

Role of the Patient in Goal Setting

Always collaborate with your patients when setting goals. Mutual goal setting involves the patient and family caregiver (when appropriate) in prioritizing the goals of care and developing a plan of action to achieve those goals. Unless goals are mutually set and include a clear plan of action, patients or family caregivers will not participate. Patients need to understand and see the value of nursing therapies even though they are often totally dependent on you as the nurse. When developing goals, you act as an advocate or supporter for the patient when developing nursing interventions to promote the patient's return to health or prevent further deterioration when possible.

Expected Outcomes

For Rich to determine whether Mrs Tillman has shown progress and achieved the goal of an improved energy level within 2 weeks, expected outcomes are necessary. An **expected outcome** is the measurable change in the patient that must be achieved to reach a goal. Expected outcomes provide a focus or direction for nursing care because they are the desired physical, psychological, behavioral, social, emotional, developmental, or spiritual responses that show resolution of a patient's health problems. Expected outcomes must also be singular.

For example, in Mrs Tillman's case, measurable outcomes for the goal of improved energy level include "Patient's self-report of fatigue is 3 or less on a scale of 0–10" and "Patient is able to complete bathing without taking rest periods." These outcomes help Rich determine the success of selected interventions that effectively lessen Mrs Tillman's fatigue. An outcome includes measurable criteria (e.g., 3 or less on a scale of 0–10, completes bathing without taking rest) to evaluate goal achievement (Table 19.5). Achieving outcomes means that a goal has been met.

Typically, all health care providers contribute to achievement of patient outcomes. A **nursing-sensitive outcome** is a measurable patient or family state, behavior, or perception largely influenced by and sensitive to nursing interventions

Table 19.4 Examples of Goal Setting With Expected Outcomes for Mrs Tillman

Nursing Diagnoses	Goals	Expected Outcomes
Fatigue related to chronic disease process	Mrs Tillman will achieve an improved energy level within 2 weeks.	The patient's self-report of fatigue is 3 or less on a scale of 0–10 in 2 weeks. The patient is able to increase some daily activities in 1 week.
Death Anxiety related to anticipation of suffering	Mrs Tillman will express belief that she will gain a stable level of comfort in 3 weeks.	The patient seeks information about palliative care treatment in 1 week. The patient reports acceptable comfort level in 2 weeks. The patient participates in health care decisions in 1 week.

Table 19.5 Examples of NANDA International Nursing Diagnoses and Suggested NOC Linkages

Nursing Diagnosis	Suggested NOC Outcomes (Examples)	Outcome Indicators (Examples)
Fatigue	Activity tolerance	Walking pace Ease of performing ADLs Pulse rate with activity Ease of breathing with activity
	Energy conservation	Balances activity and rest Uses naps to restore energy Adapts lifestyle to energy level
Deficient Knowledge regarding palliative care	Knowledge of treatment regimen	Rationale for treatment Self-care responsibilities for ongoing treatment Expected effects of treatment

ADLs, activities of daily living; *NOC*, Nursing Outcomes Classification.

(Moorhead et al., 2013). Examples of nursing-sensitive outcomes include reduction in pain severity, incidence of pressure injuries, and incidence of falls. In comparison, outcomes largely influenced by medical interventions include patient mortality and hospital readmission.

Outcomes are measurable, reliable, valid, suited to the patient, and sensitive to change (Moorhead et al., 2013). Consider the example of Mrs Tillman's problem of fatigue. One outcome measure is a self-report fatigue scale. The scale provides an objective measure of the patient's level of fatigue. Current evidence shows that self-report scales are reliable (consistently measure an outcome) and valid (accurately measure an outcome). A self-report scale is easy for a patient to complete without causing anxiety or physical distress as in the case of an exercise test for fatigue. The patient's perceptions of fatigue change over time and are reflected by differences in the fatigue scale.

You normally develop several expected outcomes for each nursing diagnosis and goal. The reason for multiple outcomes is that sometimes one nursing action is not enough to resolve a patient problem. The listing of step-by-step expected outcomes guides you in planning interventions. Always write expected outcomes sequentially with time frames. Time frames give you progressive steps in which to move a patient toward recovery. They also give an order for when to perform nursing interventions. In addition, time frames set limits for problem resolution.

Nursing Outcomes Classification

Health care agencies are very interested in measuring nursing-sensitive outcomes because of the effect they have on patient outcomes, quality of care, and health care costs. The *Nursing Outcomes Classification (NOC)*, published by the Iowa Intervention Project, classifies, identifies, labels, and validates nursing-sensitive outcomes (Moorhead et al., 2013). NOC links evidence-based outcomes to every NANDA-I nursing diagnosis (Moorhead et al., 2013). NOC-suggested outcomes describe the focus of nursing care and provide ways to measure the success of nursing interventions (see Table 19.5). NOC helps you select appropriate nursing interventions to improve the quality of care for individuals, families, and communities in all health care settings (Moorhead et al., 2013). Using a common language allows nurses to plan effective patient care and provides a standardized way to measure the success of nursing interventions. In addition, the use of NOC facilitates the evaluation of the effects of nursing interventions over time and across a variety of health care settings.

Guidelines for Writing Goals and Expected Outcomes

Goals and expected outcomes direct your nursing care. After you set a patient-centered goal for a nursing diagnosis, the expected outcomes set the desired physiological, psychological, behavioral, social, developmental, or spiritual responses that measure the resolution of the patient's health problem.

Use the *SMART* acronym (*s*pecific, *m*easureable, *a*ttainable, *r*ealistic, *t*imed) as an approach for writing goals and expected outcomes:

1. *Specific:* Outcomes and goals reflect a specific patient behavior or response that you expect as a result of nursing interventions. A proper goal statement is "Patient will ambulate independently in 3 days." A proper outcome statement is "Patient ambulates in the hall three times a day by 4/22." A common error is to write an outcome as an intervention, such as "Ambulate patient in the hall three times a day."
   In addition, the outcome must address only one behavior or response. For example, an outcome might read "Patient's lungs are clear to auscultation, and respiratory rate is 24 breaths/min by 8/22." How would you evaluate the outcome when you determine that the lungs are clear but the respiratory rate is 28 breaths/min? You would be unable to determine whether the expected outcome has been achieved.
   By splitting the statement into two parts, "Lungs are clear to auscultation by 8/22" and "Respiratory rate is 24 breaths/min by 8/22," you can determine whether the patient achieves each outcome separately. This focus on a single outcome enables you to determine whether you need to modify the plan of care.
2. *Measurable:* You must be able to measure or observe whether a change takes place in a patient's status. Examples such as "Body temperature remains 98.6°F" and "Apical pulse remains between 60 and 100 beats/min" allow you to objectively measure changes in a patient's status. Do not use vague qualifiers such as "normal," "acceptable," "stable," or "sufficient" in the expected outcome statement. Vague terms make it difficult to determine a patient's response to care. Terms describing quality, quantity, frequency, length, or weight allow you to accurately evaluate whether outcomes are met.
3. *Attainable:* A goal and an outcome are more attainable when mutually set with the patient. This ensures that the patient and the nurse agree on the direction and time limits of care. Mutual goal setting increases a patient's motivation and cooperation. As a patient advocate, you apply standards of practice, patient safety, and basic human needs when helping patients set goals.
4. *Realistic:* Set goals and expected outcomes that a patient can achieve. Achieving a goal gives a patient a sense of accomplishment. This sense of accomplishment further increases the patient's motivation and cooperation. When you establish realistic goals, consider the resources of the health care agency, family, and patient.

For example, do the patient's cultural beliefs affect the goals you set? Does the patient have the necessary resources in the home to successfully meet the goals?

5. *Timed:* A time limit is set for each goal and outcome so the health care team has a common time frame for problem resolution, for example, "Patient will be able to ambulate the hospital corridor in 2 days." Time frames help you and your patient determine whether progress is being made at a reasonable rate. If not, revision of the plan of care is necessary.

Critical Thinking in Planning Nursing Care

During planning, you make clinical decisions by choosing the nursing interventions most appropriate to your patient's nursing diagnoses and collaborative problems. The actual implementation of these interventions occurs during the implementation phase of the nursing process. Choosing suitable nursing interventions involves critical thinking applied in decision-making. To select interventions, you need to be competent in three areas: (1) knowing the **scientific rationale**, or reason, for the interventions; (2) possessing the necessary psychomotor and interpersonal skills to perform the interventions; and (3) being able to function within a particular setting to use the available health care resources effectively (Bulechek et al., 2013).

Types of Nursing Interventions

Nursing interventions include three categories: nurse-initiated, health care provider–initiated, and collaborative interventions.

Nurse-initiated interventions are **independent nursing interventions** or actions that nurses initiate. These do not require direction or an order from another health care professional. Nurse-initiated interventions (independent nursing interventions) are autonomous actions based on scientific rationales. Examples include elevating an edematous extremity, offering counseling on coping, and instructing patients about medication side effects. These interventions benefit patients in a predicted way related to nursing diagnoses and patient goals (Bulechek et al., 2013). They require no supervision or direction from others.

Health care provider–initiated interventions are **dependent nursing interventions** or actions that require an order from a health care professional. Such interventions are based on a health care provider's response to treat or manage a medical diagnosis. Advanced practice nurses who have collaborative agreements with physicians or who are licensed independently by state Nurse Practice Acts also write dependent interventions. As a nurse, you intervene by carrying out the independent provider's written and/or verbal orders. Administering a medication, implementing an invasive procedure, and preparing a patient for diagnostic tests are examples of dependent nursing interventions.

Collaborative interventions, or interdependent nursing interventions, are therapies that require the combined knowledge, skill, and expertise of multiple health care professionals. When you plan care for a patient, you review the necessary interventions and determine whether the collaboration of other health care professionals is necessary.

Selection of Interventions

Never select interventions for a patient randomly. For example, patients with the diagnosis of *Anxiety* do not always need care in the same way with the same interventions. You treat *Anxiety related to the uncertainty of results from a diagnostic test* differently from *Anxiety related to a threat of loss of a loved one.* When choosing interventions, consider the following six factors: (1) desired patient outcomes, (2) characteristics of the nursing diagnosis, (3) evidence base (research or clinical practice guidelines) for the intervention, (4) feasibility of implementing the intervention, (5) acceptability to the patient, and (6) your own competency (Box 19.5) (Bulechek et al., 2013).

BOX 19.5 Selecting Nursing Interventions

Characteristics of the Nursing Diagnosis

- Interventions should alter the etiological (related to) factor associated with the diagnostic label.
- When an etiological factor cannot change, direct interventions toward treating the signs and symptoms (e.g., NANDA-I defining characteristics).
- For potential or high-risk diagnoses, direct interventions at altering or eliminating risk factors for the nursing diagnoses.

Expected Outcomes

- Specify expected outcomes before choosing interventions.
- Identify for each patient the outcomes that can be reasonably expected and attained as the result of nursing care.
- Use the Nursing Outcomes Classification to specify outcomes.

Evidence Base

- Know the research base for an intervention.
- Research will indicate the effectiveness of using an intervention with certain types of patients.
- When research is not available, use scientific principles (e.g., safety) or consult experts.

Feasibility of the Intervention

- A specific intervention has the potential for interacting with other interventions.
- Consider cost: Is the intervention clinically effective and cost-efficient?
- Consider time: Are time and personnel resources available?

Acceptability to the Patient

- An intervention must be acceptable to the patient and family caregiver and match a patient's goals, beliefs, health care values, and culture.
- Promote informed choice; help a patient know how he or she is expected to participate.

Capability

- Be prepared to carry out the intervention.
- Be competent in knowing the scientific rationale for the intervention, possessing necessary psychomotor and interpersonal skills, and being able to function in the particular setting.

Modified from Bulechek GM, et al: *Nursing interventions classification (NIC)*, ed 6, St Louis, 2013, Mosby.

When choosing interventions, review resources such as evidence in the literature, standard protocols or guidelines, the Nursing Interventions Classification (NIC), critical pathways, and current textbooks. Collaborating with other health care professionals is also useful, especially when a patient moves from one setting to another, such as hospital to home or hospital to a rehabilitation agency (Lemetti et al., 2015). Review your patient's needs, values, priorities, and previous experiences to select the nursing interventions that have the best potential for achieving the expected outcomes.

Nursing Interventions Classification

Just as with the standardized NOC, the Iowa Intervention Project developed a set of nursing interventions that provides a level of standardization to enhance communication of nursing care across all health care settings and to compare outcomes (Bulechek et al., 2013). The NIC model includes three levels for ease of use: domains, classes, and interventions. The seven domains (level 1) are the highest level of the model, using broad terms (e.g., *physiological, safety*) to organize the more specific classes and interventions (Table 19.6). The second level of the model includes 30 classes, which offer useful clinical categories to refer to when selecting interventions. The third level includes interventions, defined as any treatment based on clinical judgment and knowledge that a nurse performs to enhance patient outcomes (Bulechek et al., 2013). Each intervention has a variety of nursing activities from which to choose (Box 19.6). The NIC interventions link with NANDA-I nursing diagnoses. For example, Mrs Tillman has the problem of *Fatigue*, which falls under the domain of Physiological: Basic and the class of Activity and Exercise Management. Under the class of Activity and Exercise Management, there are a variety of interventions to choose from (e.g., Energy Management, Exercise Therapy: Ambulation). When you refer to an intervention within NIC such as energy management, there are numerous nursing activities or interventions to choose from (see Mrs Tillman's Care Plan [see Fig. 19.6]). NIC is a valuable resource for selecting interventions for your unique patients.

BOX 19.6 Examples of Level 3 Interventions and Activities for Activity and Exercise Management

Activity and Exercise Management

Interventions to organize or assist with physical activity and energy conservation and expenditure

Level 3 Interventions

- Body Mechanics Promotion
  Examples of Nursing Activities for Body Mechanics Promotion: Instruct to use a firm mattress; assist to demonstrate appropriate sleeping positions; assist to avoid sitting in same position for prolonged periods.
- Energy Management
- Exercise Promotion
- Exercise Therapy: Ambulation
- Teaching Prescribed Activity/Exercise

Examples of Linked Nursing Diagnoses

- Activity Intolerance
- Fatigue
- Impaired Physical Mobility

From Bulechek GM, et al: *Nursing interventions classification (NIC)*, ed 6, St Louis, 2013, Mosby.

Systems for Planning Nursing Care

In every health care setting, the nurse is responsible for developing a plan of nursing care for each patient. The plan of care can take one of several forms (e.g., standardized care plan, computerized plan). EHRs typically include a documentation system for nursing care plans. These programs use standardized nursing language, including NANDA, NOC, and NIC taxonomies. This enables nurses and other health care providers to quickly identify a patient's needs and situation. Although EHR plans often follow a standard format, you customize each plan to the needs of the unique patient. Patients also benefit from standardized language because it promotes continuity of care and standardizes communications.

A **nursing care plan** includes nursing diagnoses, goals and/or expected outcomes, and individualized nursing interventions. This plan promotes continuity of care because it allows all health care providers to identify a patient's needs and interventions and reduces the risk for incomplete, incorrect, or inaccurate care. The plan is a guideline for coordinating nursing care, promoting continuity of care, and listing outcome criteria for the evaluation of care.

Besides addressing a patient's short-term problems, the care plan also addresses the patient's long-term needs. You incorporate the goals of the care plan into discharge planning. All patients benefit from this level of continuity of care, especially those who need long-term rehabilitation in the community and those who require home care. Same-day surgeries and earlier discharges from hospitals also require you as the nurse to begin planning discharge needs from the moment a patient enters a health care agency. The adaptation of the care plan enhances the continuity of nursing care between nurses working in hospital settings and nurses working in community agencies (Nielsen et al., 2015). Fig. 19.6 provides an example of the care plan format used throughout this text.

Hand-Off Reporting

Part of planning is transferring essential information from one nurse to another. This is often called hand-off reporting, which offers a health care provider accepting the care of a patient the opportunity to ask questions to clarify and confirm important details about the patient's plan of care, patient progress, and continuing needs during the transfer of information. A correctly formulated nursing care plan facilitates a hand-off report as one nurse communicates to another nurse (see Chapter 5). You learn to focus your reports on the nursing care, treatments, and expected outcomes documented in your care plans. During end-of-shift hand-off or when transferring a patient, you can discuss the care plan and the patient's overall progress with the next caregiver. Thus, all nurses are able to discuss current and relevant information about the patient's plan of care.

Table 19.6 Nursing Interventions Classification (NIC) Taxonomy

Domain 1	Domain 2	Domain 3	Domain 4	Domain 5	Domain 6	Domain 7
LEVEL 1 DOMAINS						
1. **Physiological: Basic** Care that supports physical functioning	2. **Physiological: Complex** Care that supports homeostatic regulation	3. **Behavioral** Care that supports psychosocial functioning and facilitates lifestyle changes	4. **Safety** Care that supports protection against harm	5. **Family** Care that supports the family unit	6. **Health system** Care that supports effective use of the health care delivery system	7. **Community** Care that supports the health of the community
LEVEL 2 CLASSES						
A *Activity and Exercise Management:* Interventions to organize or assist with physical activity and energy conservation and expenditure B *Elimination Management:* Interventions to establish and maintain regular bowel and urinary elimination patterns and manage complications caused by altered patterns C *Immobility Management:* Interventions to manage restricted body movement and the sequelae D *Nutrition Support:* Interventions to modify or maintain nutritional status E *Physical Comfort Promotion:* Interventions to promote comfort using physical techniques F *Self-Care Facilitation:* Interventions to provide or assist with routine activities of daily living G *Electrolyte and Acid–Base Management:* Interventions to regulate electrolyte/acid–base balance and prevent complications	H *Drug Management:* Interventions to facilitate desired effects of pharmacological agents I *Neurological Management:* Interventions to optimize neurological functions J *Perioperative Care:* Interventions to provide care before, during, and immediately after surgery K *Respiratory Management:* Interventions to promote airway patency and gas exchange L *Skin/Wound Management:* Interventions to maintain or restore tissue integrity M *Thermoregulation:* Interventions to maintain body temperature within a normal range N *Tissue Perfusion Management:* Interventions to optimize circulation of blood and fluids to the tissue	O *Behavior Therapy:* Interventions to reinforce or promote desirable behaviors or alter undesirable behaviors P *Cognitive Therapy:* Interventions to reinforce or promote desirable cognitive functioning or alter undesirable cognitive functioning Q *Communication Enhancement:* Interventions to facilitate delivering and receiving verbal and nonverbal messages R *Coping Assistance:* Interventions to assist another to build on own strengths, adapt to a change in function, or achieve a higher level of function S *Patient Education:* Interventions to facilitate learning T *Psychological Comfort Promotion:* Interventions to promote comfort using psychological techniques	U *Crisis Management:* Interventions to provide immediate short-term help in both psychological and physiological crises V *Risk Management:* Interventions to initiate risk reduction activities and continue monitoring risks over time	W *Childbearing Care:* Interventions to assist in understanding and coping with the psychological and physiological changes during the childbearing period X *Childrearing Care:* Interventions to assist in rearing children Z *Life Span Care:* Interventions to facilitate family unit functioning and promote the health and welfare of family members throughout the life span	Y *Health System Mediation:* Interventions to facilitate the interface between patient/family and the health care system a *Health System Management:* Interventions to provide and enhance support services for the delivery of care b *Information Management:* Interventions to facilitate communication among health care providers	c *Community Health Promotion:* Interventions that promote the health of the whole community d *Community Risk Management:* Interventions that assist in detecting or preventing health risks to the whole community

From Bulechek GM, et al: *Nursing interventions classification (NIC)*, ed 6, St Louis, 2013, Mosby.

CARE PLAN Death Anxiety

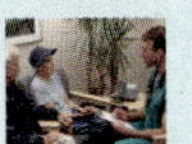

Assessment

Rich learns in his initial discussions with Mrs Tillman that she feels a sense of dread and uncertainty about the course of cancer. Mrs Tillman shares her emotions through crying and sadness in the way she looks down and has difficulty talking about her condition. She admitted to Rich that her greatest fear is not knowing whether she might suffer from her disease. Rich knows from his review of pathophysiology the probable course of the patient's disease and the type of palliative care treatments her physician will recommend. He decides to assess further the extent of her death anxiety.

Assessment Activities	Findings[a]
Ask Mrs Tillman to discuss her concerns about the effect her illness will have on her husband.	The patient is **concerned about strain on her husband** and that he will begin to have more physical problems.
Have Mrs Tillman explain what she fears most about having a terminal illness.	The patient states that she **fears loss of her mental thought processes and Pain.**
Question Mrs Tillman about her desire to be able to make decisions regarding palliative care.	The patient expresses fear of ***powerlessness*** and having little control over what will happen.

[a]**Defining characteristics/risk factors** are shown in **bold** type.

Nursing Diagnosis: Death Anxiety related to anticipation of suffering

Planning

Goal	Expected Outcomes (NOC)[b]
	Anxiety Level
Mrs. Tillman will state, within 3 weeks, that she believes she will have a comfortable death.	The patient will verbalize feeling less anxious about the course of her disease in 1 week.
	The patient uses relaxation techniques when anxiety heightens by 2 weeks.
	Participation in Health Care Decisions
	The patient is able to specify her priorities in palliative care plan in 2 weeks.
	The patient and husband establish end-of-life care plan in 3 weeks.

[b]Outcomes classification labels from Moorhead S, et al, editors: *Nursing outcomes classification (NOC)*, ed 5, St Louis, 2013, Mosby.

Interventions (NIC)[c]	Rationale
Anxiety Reduction	
Plan a palliative care conference with the patient, husband, and health care team and provide factual information about treatment options and availability of respite care for husband.	Information that helps patients understand their condition, disease course, and the benefits and burdens of treatment options reduces anxiety (Suhonen et al., 2011). Interventions designed to meet individualized needs preserve autonomy and lessen uncertainty (Suhonen et al., 2011).
Instruct the patient in guided imagery and passive relaxation exercises.	Patients with advanced disease such as cancer require a moderate expenditure of energy to perform active progressive relaxation exercise. This can increase a person's existing fatigue. Passive relaxation and guided imagery are more appropriate options (Koithan, 2017).
Explore community resources for a short-term education group for Carl that teaches self-care tools to reduce stress.	Education groups help caregivers develop self-care tools to reduce stress, charge negative self-talk, communicate more effectively, and make difficult decisions (Cope, 2015; Flagg, 2015).

Fig. 19.6 Nursing care plan.

Continued

CARE PLAN Death Anxiety—cont'd

Interventions (NIC)[c]	Rationale
Explain specifically how palliative care measures will reduce symptoms the patient is most anxious about.	You can lessen anxiety in terminally ill patients by explaining and managing underlying causes of anxiety (Matzo and Sherman, 2015). For example, improving a patient's breathing and oxygenation helps to decrease anxiety (McClurg, 2017).
Decision-Making Support	
Provide information requested by patient, and help to identify advantages and disadvantages of all alternatives.	Respect for a patient's autonomy involves a commitment to support a patient's ability to make decisions in a well-informed way.
Facilitate a discussion between the patient and husband about end-of-life treatment preferences regarding life-extending treatment.	Difficult end-of-life decisions complicate the survivor's grief and create family divisions. When these decisions are handled well and patient's symptoms are controlled, families experience a meaningful conclusion to the loved one's death (McClurg, 2017).

[c]Intervention classification labels from Bulechek GM et al, editors: *Nursing interventions classification (NIC)*, ed 6, St Louis, 2013, Mosby.

Evaluation

Nursing Actions	Patient Response/Finding	Achievement of Outcome
Question Mrs Tillman about level of anxiety she feels.	The patient states she feels less worried about suffering. "I know what I'm facing, and I know what they can give me when I have trouble breathing."	The patient obtaining control over anxiety; accepting course of her disease.
Ask Mr Tillman whether Mrs Tillman practices guided imagery at home.	Husband reports that the patient uses guided imagery each afternoon for a period of 20 min.	The patient is applying anxiety control technique effectively in the home.
Have Mrs Tillman discuss her feelings about an end-of-life care plan.	The patient is planning to discuss feelings with husband; has not finalized plan yet; wants to know more about respite care for husband.	Further discussion and support necessary to help the patient and husband finalize an end-of-life care plan.

Fig. 19.6, cont'd

Student Care Plans

Student care plans help you learn the problem-solving technique, the nursing process, skills of written communication, and organizational skills needed for nursing care. Most important, the student care plan enables you to apply knowledge gained from the nursing and medical literature and the classroom to a practice situation.

Students typically write care plans for each nursing diagnosis, using a columnar format with columns for assessment findings, goals, expected outcomes, nursing interventions with supporting rationales, and evaluative outcome criteria. The student care plan is more detailed than a care plan in a hospital or community health care agency because its purpose is to teach the process of planning care. Each nursing school uses a different format for its student care plans.

Concept Mapping

In the section Nursing Diagnosis, you were introduced to a concept map for Mrs Tillman that displayed relevant assessment data and four interrelated nursing diagnoses. To complete Mrs Tillman's concept map, you add individualized nursing interventions (Fig. 19.8). As you further develop the concept map, you must think critically, organize information, understand complex relationships among nursing diagnoses and nursing interventions, and integrate theoretical knowledge into practice (Daley and Torre, 2010; Lhussier et al., 2015).

Using a concept map will help you make better clinical decisions, develop better clinical judgment, and provide better patient-centered care (Gerdeman et al., 2013). It forms a picture of each patient's diagnoses and the interconnections between the assessment data and nursing interventions associated with the patient problems.

Concept mapping also helps you develop reflective thinking skills. These skills will help you understand that patient care, patient information, nursing diagnoses, interdisciplinary interventions, and patient outcomes all are interrelated and prioritized to produce a plan of care.

As Mrs Tillman's nurse, Rich's next step is to plan interventions for each of her nursing diagnoses. At the same time, he must recognize that each intervention can apply to more than one diagnosis (see Fig. 19.8).

Use the following tips to help you develop a complete concept map:

1. Begin by reviewing the patient's clinical assessment data. Verify that this information is current.
2. Review all information about the patient's health problems, treatments, and medications in course textbooks, scientific literature, and other related resources.
3. Review any standardized nursing care plans, clinical pathways, protocols, or patient education materials developed for patients on the nursing unit.
4. Prepare the concept map by first developing a skeleton diagram of the patient's health problems. Write the patient's primary health problems and key assessment priorities in the middle of the map. Next add boxes for the patient's nursing care needs like spokes on a wheel.
5. In each box identify and group clinical assessment data that seem to form patterns. Do not worry if you have difficulty labeling nursing diagnoses at first. It is important to first recognize the major nursing care focus for the patient. Remember that sometimes symptoms apply to more than one nursing diagnosis. Repeat symptoms under different categories when appropriate.
6. Analyze relationships among the nursing diagnoses. Draw lines between nursing diagnoses to show relationships. The links must be accurate, meaningful, and complete. You must be able to explain how the nursing diagnoses are related. For example, Mrs Tillman's nursing diagnoses of *Death Anxiety* and *Deficient Knowledge* are interrelated. In addition, her *Fatigue* nursing diagnosis influences her *Risk for Falls* nursing diagnosis.
7. List on the map the nursing interventions that you select to attain the outcomes for each nursing diagnosis.
8. While caring for your patient, write down the patient's responses to each nursing activity. Also write your clinical impressions and inferences about the patient's progress toward expected outcomes and the effectiveness of interventions. Use the concept map as a working tool and revise as needed.

Consulting Other Health Care Professionals

Planning requires consultation with other members of the health care team. Consultation can occur at any step in the nursing process, but you consult most often during planning and implementation. During these steps, you are more likely to identify a problem requiring additional knowledge, skills, or community or agency resources.

Consultation is a process in which you seek the expertise of a specialist to help you identify methods of handling problems in patient care or implementation of therapies. For example, you might consult a clinical nurse specialist. Consultation is based on the problem-solving approach, and the consultant is the stimulus for change. An experienced nurse often is a valuable consultant when you face an unfamiliar patient care situation. Through consultation and collaboration, you use the best available resources to individualize nursing actions to produce expected outcomes.

IMPLEMENTATION

Implementation, the fourth step of the nursing process, begins after you develop the care plan. It involves providing care to patients. **Implementation** is the performance of nursing interventions necessary for achieving the goals and expected outcomes of nursing care. A **nursing intervention** is any treatment based on clinical judgment and knowledge that a nurse performs to enhance patient outcomes (Bulechek et al., 2013). Ideally the nurse uses evidence-based nursing interventions. Interventions include both direct and indirect care measures provided to individuals, families, and the community.

Direct care interventions are treatments performed through interactions with patients. Examples are medication administration, insertion of an i.v. catheter, and counseling during a time of grief. **Indirect care interventions** are treatments performed away from but on behalf of the patient or group of patients (Bulechek et al., 2013). Examples are actions aimed at managing the patient's environment (safety and infection control), documentation, and interdisciplinary collaboration.

Both direct and indirect care interventions fall under the categories discussed earlier: independent nursing (nurse-initiated), dependent nursing (health care provider–initiated), and collaborative interventions. For example, the direct care intervention of patient education is an independent nursing intervention. The indirect intervention of consultation is a collaborative intervention.

Standard Nursing Interventions

Health care settings offer opportunities for nurses to create and individualize patient care plans. Although it is critical for each patient to have his or her own unique set of interventions, many health care systems have mechanisms for standardizing the more common types of interventions or approaches to care. Many patients have common health problems. Thus, standardized interventions assist nurses to intervene more efficiently. Standard interventions are set at a level of excellence for practice. Nurse-initiated and health care provider–initiated standardized interventions include clinical practice guidelines, protocols, standing orders, and NIC. The ANA defines standards of professional nursing practice, which include standards for the implementation step of the nursing process (ANA, 2010).

Clinical Practice Guidelines and Protocols

A **clinical practice guideline** or protocol is a systematically developed set of statements. Guidelines are based on an authoritative examination of current scientific evidence. The guideline helps nurses and other health care providers choose appropriate interventions for specific clinical circumstances. Guidelines are key tools for improving the quality of patient care.

The AHRQ National Guideline Clearinghouse (NGC) is a resource for evidence-based clinical practice guidelines (NGC, n.d.). This site is continually updated and provides nurses and other health care providers easy access to current guidelines on many topics such as low back pain, dizziness, or deep vein thrombosis.

Clinicians within a health care agency review the scientific literature and their own standard of practice to create a clinical practice guideline. Some guidelines are already developed by national health groups such as the National Institutes of Health, INS, and NGC. These clinical guidelines are available to any clinician or agency that wishes to adopt evidence-based guidelines in patient care.

Ongoing review of scientific literature and best practices leads to the development of care bundles for a variety of conditions. A **care bundle** is a group of interventions related to a disease process or condition. These interventions, when executed together, result in better patient outcomes than when implemented individually. The aim for the care bundle is to ensure that patients receive quality care and achieve positive outcomes while preventing the most common complications associated with their diagnoses (Goodstone et al., 2015). Examples of care bundles include, but are not limited to, sepsis management, prevention of central line–associated bloodstream infection (CLABSI), and prevention of ventilator-associated pneumonia (VAP). As you move through clinical practice, you will study specific bundles in later chapters of this text.

In acute care settings, it is common to find clinical protocols that outline independent nursing interventions for specific conditions. Examples are protocols for admission and discharge, pressure injury care, and fall prevention. Protocols are also used in interdisciplinary settings for diagnostic testing and physical, occupational, and speech therapies.

A **standing order** is a preprinted document containing orders for conducting routine therapies, monitoring guidelines, or diagnostic procedures for specific patients with identified clinical problems. A standing order directs the specific interventions to be used in specific clinical settings. Licensed, prescribing health care providers in charge of care at the time of implementation approve and sign standing orders. These orders are common in critical care settings and other specialized practice settings in which patients' needs can change rapidly and require immediate attention. For example, a standing order might specify certain medications such as diltiazem or propranolol for an irregular heart rhythm. After assessing a patient and identifying the irregular rhythm, the critical care nurse gives the specified medication without first notifying the health care provider because his or her initial standing order covers the nurse's action. After completing a standing order, the nurse notifies the health care provider. Standing orders are also common in the community health setting, where nurses face situations that do not permit immediate contact with a physician or health care provider. Standing orders give you the legal protection to intervene appropriately in the patient's best interest.

Nursing Intervention Classification Interventions

The NIC system developed by the University of Iowa differentiates nursing practice from practice of other health care professionals by offering a language that nurses can use to describe sets of actions in delivering nursing care (see Table 19.6). The NIC interventions offer a level of standardization to improve communication of nursing care across settings and compare outcomes.

Critical Thinking in Implementation

Selecting nursing interventions for your patient is part of clinical decision-making. Strong clinical reasoning and decision-making skills help you accurately identify appropriate nursing interventions for a patient's specific nursing diagnoses and achieve appropriate patient outcomes. The critical thinking model discussed in Chapter 18 provides a framework for decision-making when implementing nursing care. Your knowledge about your patient's health problems leads you to select appropriate therapies.

Apply prior clinical experiences in performing specific interventions. Consider which interventions have worked before and which have not worked in previous clinical situations. Be aware of both professional and agency standards of practice. Standards of practice offer guidelines for selection of interventions, their frequency, and the determination of whether the procedures may be delegated. In Mrs Tillman's case, the NGC has a guideline for cancer pain management that would be very helpful (NGC, n.d.). As you perform any nursing intervention, apply intellectual standards. For example, when teaching patients a self-care procedure, your language should be relevant, clear, and logical to promote patient learning (see Chapter 15). All critical thinking attitudes such as confidence, creativity, and discipline apply to implementation. A beginning student needs supervision from an instructor or experienced nurse to guide the decision-making process for implementation.

Implementation Process

Preparation for implementation ensures efficient, safe, and effective nursing care. Perform the following five preparatory activities: reassess the patient, review and revise the existing nursing care plan, organize resources and care delivery, anticipate and prevent complications, and implement nursing interventions.

Reassessing the Patient

Patient assessment is a continuous process that occurs each time you interact with a patient. When you gather new data and identify a new nursing diagnosis, you might need to reestablish priorities and modify the care plan. Creating a concept map helps you understand the relationship between nursing diagnoses and interventions. You also modify a plan when you resolve a patient's health care need. Just before implementing a nursing activity, reassess your patient. This is a partial assessment and sometimes focuses on one dimension such as level of comfort or on one system such as the cardiovascular system. The reassessment helps you decide whether the proposed nursing activity is still appropriate for the patient's level of wellness. For example, you plan to assist a patient with ambulation after lunch. However, a reassessment reveals shortness of breath and increased fatigue. The occurrence of these signs and symptoms requires you to help the patient back to bed.

Reviewing and Revising the Care Plan

Reassessment allows you to validate the patient's nursing diagnoses, review the care plan, and determine whether the nursing interventions are still appropriate. If the patient's status has changed and the nursing diagnosis and related interventions are no longer appropriate, modify the nursing care plan. An out-of-date or incorrect care plan puts the quality of nursing care at risk. Reviewing and modifying the care plan enables you to provide timely nursing interventions to best meet a patient's current needs.

There are four steps to modifying the written care plan:

1. Revise data in the assessment section to reflect a patient's current status. Date any new data to inform other health team members of the time that the change occurred.
2. Revise nursing diagnoses. Delete diagnoses that are no longer relevant and add and date any new diagnoses. Revise related factors and the patient's goals, outcomes, and priorities as needed.
3. Revise specific interventions that correspond to the new nursing diagnoses and goals. This revision should reflect the patient's present status.
4. Choose the method of evaluation for determining whether the patient achieved his or her outcomes.

Organizing Resources and Delivering Care

Organize time, equipment, and personnel to prepare for implementing nursing actions. Organizing equipment and personnel makes timely, efficient, and skilled patient care possible. Preparing for care delivery also includes preparing the environment and patient for nursing interventions.

Time Management

Providing patient-centered care is the focus of your nursing practice. You will practice within work environments that are part of the sociocultural context of a health care organization. These are busy environments, and you will assume dual roles: a patient care provider and an organizational employee. In this dual role, you need to be aware of efficiency and cost control of the organization. You need to provide timely, safe, competent, and efficient care. This conveys caring and concern to your patient. Poor patient care results when you are hurried, experience interruptions, or are disorganized.

Equipment

Most nursing procedures require some equipment or supplies. Decide which supplies are necessary and determine their availability before you start implementation. Equipment should be in safe working order. Place supplies in a convenient, uncluttered location for easy access during the procedure. Be sure extra supplies are available in case of errors or accidents, but do not take them into a patient's room or open them unless they are needed. Unused equipment left in rooms must be thrown away as a loss to an agency. Wise use of supplies controls health care costs. After a procedure, return any unopened supplies.

Personnel

Nursing care delivery models determine how nursing personnel deliver patient care. For example, the accountabilities of an RN in a team nursing model differ from the accountabilities of an RN in a primary nursing model. A team nurse is accountable for the specific shift in which he or she works. A primary nurse is accountable for the nursing care that a patient receives during his or her length of stay or course of visits. You are responsible for determining whether to perform an intervention or delegate it to another member of the nursing team. Your ongoing assessment of a patient directs the decision about delegation and not the intervention alone. For example, you know nursing assistive personnel (NAP) can competently ambulate patients. However, you learn that a patient experienced an increased pulse rate after walking during the previous shift; thus, you decide to personally assist the patient with ambulation and evaluate his or her cardiac status.

Patient care staff work together as patients' needs demand it. If a patient makes a request such as for use of a bedpan, position the patient on the pan if you have time rather than trying to find NAP. When interventions are complex or physically difficult, you may need assistance from colleagues. For example, you are more effective in performing procedures when NAP help you position a patient and hand you supplies during the procedure.

Environment

A patient care environment needs to be safe and conducive for implementing therapies. Patient safety is your first concern. When the patient has sensory deficits, physical disabilities, or an alteration in level of consciousness, arrange the environment to prevent injury (e.g., provide assistive devices such as walkers or eyeglasses, rearrange furniture and equipment, and make rooms free of clutter). Make sure that lighting is adequate to perform procedures correctly.

Patient

Before you deliver interventions, be sure your patients are as physically and psychologically comfortable as possible. For example, symptoms such as nausea or pain interfere with a patient's full concentration and cooperation. Offer comfort measures before initiating interventions to help the patient participate more fully. If you need a patient to be alert, give a dose of pain medication to relieve discomfort but not impair mental faculties (e.g., ability to follow instruction, reasoning, and communication). If a patient is fatigued, delay ambulation until after he or she has had a chance to rest. Be aware of the patient's level of endurance and plan the amount of activity that the patient can tolerate comfortably. Even if symptoms are not a factor, make the patient physically comfortable during interventions. Start any intervention by controlling environmental factors, positioning, and taking care of other physical needs (e.g., elimination).

Knowing a patient's psychosocial needs enables you to create a supportive emotional climate. Some patients feel reassured by having a significant other present for encouragement and moral support. Other strategies include planning sufficient time or multiple opportunities for patients to work through and vent feelings and anxieties. Adequate preparation allows a patient to obtain maximal benefit from each intervention.

Anticipating and Preventing Complications

Risks to patients come from both illness and treatment. Observe for and recognize these risks, adapt your choice of interventions to each situation, evaluate the relative benefit of the treatment versus the risk, and take risk prevention measures. Many conditions place patients at risk for complications. For example, a patient who had a stroke has limited mobility and is at risk for developing pressure injury.

Nurses are often the first ones to detect changes in patients' conditions. Your knowledge of pathophysiology and previous patient care experiences help identify or anticipate possible complications. A thorough assessment reveals the level of a patient's current risk. Scientific rationales for the effectiveness of certain interventions (e.g., turning and use of pressure relief devices) to prevent or minimize complications help you select the most useful preventive measures. Some nursing procedures pose risks for patients. Be aware of potential complications and take precautions. For example, the patient with a urinary catheter is at risk for infection. In this situation, implementing catheter-associated urinary tract infection (CAUTI) guidelines for urinary tract infection prevention reduces infection risk (see Chapter 21).

Identifying Areas of Assistance

Certain patient care situations require you to obtain assistance by seeking additional personnel, knowledge, or nursing skills. Before beginning care, review the plan to determine the need for assistance and the type required. Sometimes you need help performing a procedure, providing comfort measures, or preparing a patient for a procedure. For example, when you care for a patient who is overweight and immobilized, you require safe patient handling equipment and additional personnel to safely turn and position the patient. Be sure to determine in advance the number of additional personnel and when you need them. Discuss your need for assistance with potential resources such as other nurses or NAP.

You require additional knowledge and skills in situations in which you are less familiar or experienced. For example, seek additional knowledge when you give a new medication or implement a new procedure. You find such information in a hospital formulary or procedure book. If you are still uncertain about the new medication or procedure, ask other members of the health care team for help.

Because of the continual growth in health care technology, you may lack the skills needed to perform a new procedure. When this occurs, first locate information about the procedure in the literature and in the agency's policies and procedures. The agency's policies and procedures are usually available online or in print. Second, collect all equipment necessary for the procedure. Last, ask another nurse who is experienced in performing the procedure to provide assistance and guidance. The assistance can come from another staff nurse, supervisor, educator, or nurse specialist. Requests for assistance are common, are part of the learning process, and continue during education and into professional development.

Implementation Skills

Nursing practice requires cognitive, interpersonal, and psychomotor (technical) skills. You need each of these skills to implement direct and indirect nursing interventions. You are responsible for knowing when one type of implementation skill is preferred over another and for having the necessary knowledge and skill to perform each.

Cognitive Skills

Cognitive skills involve the application of critical thinking in the nursing process. Always use good judgment and sound clinical decision-making when performing any intervention. This ensures that no nursing action is automatic. Always think and anticipate so that you individualize patient care appropriately. Know the rationale for therapeutic interventions and understand normal and abnormal physiological and psychological responses. Know the evidence to ensure that you deliver the most current and relevant nursing interventions.

Interpersonal Skills

Interpersonal skills are essential to effective nursing action. Develop a trusting relationship, express caring, and communicate clearly with the patient and family caregiver (see Chapter 7). Effective communication is critical for keeping patients informed, for teaching, and for supporting patients who have challenging emotional needs. Your interpersonal skills should enable you to perceive a patient's verbal and nonverbal communications accurately. As a member of the health care team, you must communicate patient problems and needs clearly, intelligently, and promptly.

Psychomotor Skills

Psychomotor skills require the integration of cognitive and motor activities. For example, when you take a pulse, you must understand anatomy and physiology (cognitive) and assume the proper positioning and use of touch to detect the pulse correctly (motor). With time and practice, you learn to perform skills correctly, smoothly, and confidently. This is critical in establishing patient trust. You are responsible for acquiring necessary psychomotor skills. In the case of a new skill, assess your level of competency and obtain the necessary resources to ensure that the patient receives safe treatment.

Direct Care

Nurses provide a wide variety of direct care measures (i.e., activities that nurses perform with patient interaction). Remain sensitive to a patient's clinical condition, values and beliefs, expectations, and cultural views. All direct care measures require competent, safe practice. Show a caring approach when you provide direct care.

Activities of Daily Living

Activities of daily living (ADLs) are activities usually performed during a normal day and include ambulation, eating, dressing, bathing, and grooming. A patient's need for assistance with ADLs may be temporary or permanent. A patient with impaired mobility because of bilateral arm casts has a temporary need for assistance. After the casts are removed, the patient gradually regains the strength and range of motion needed to perform ADLs. A patient with an irreversible injury to the cervical spinal cord is paralyzed and thus has a permanent need for assistance. It is unrealistic to plan a rehabilitation goal for this patient to be independent with ADLs. Instead, through restorative care, the patient learns new ways to perform ADLs to be less dependent on others.

When an assessment reveals that a patient is experiencing fatigue, a limitation in mobility, confusion, or pain, assistance with ADLs is likely needed. This assistance ranges from partial to complete care. Always consider a patient's preferences when assisting with ADLs. Consulting with a physical or occupational therapist may be helpful. Involving the patient in planning the timing and types of interventions can also increase the patient's self-esteem and willingness to become more independent.

Instrumental Activities of Daily Living

Illness or disability sometimes alters a patient's ability to be independent in society. **Instrumental activities of daily living (IADLs)** include skills such as shopping, preparing meals, handling finances (e.g., writing checks), and taking medications. Nurses in home care and community nursing often help patients find new ways to perform IADLs. Family caregivers and friends can be excellent resources for assisting patients. In acute care, you must anticipate the effect of patients' illnesses on their ability to perform IADLs so that you can make appropriate referrals.

Physical Care Techniques

You routinely perform a variety of physical care techniques in patient care. Physical care techniques involve the safe and competent administration of nursing procedures (e.g., inserting a urinary catheter, performing range-of-motion exercises). The specific knowledge and skills needed to perform these procedures are in subsequent clinical chapters of this text. Common methods for administering physical care techniques appropriately include protecting you and the patient from injury, using proper infection control practices, staying organized, and positioning patients correctly. When you apply physical care during a procedure, know the clinical practice guidelines and how to perform the procedure, the standard frequency, and the expected outcomes.

Lifesaving Measures

A lifesaving measure is a physical care technique that you use when a patient's physiological or psychological state is threatened. The purpose of lifesaving measures is to restore physiological and psychological balance. Such measures include administering emergency medications, performing cardiopulmonary resuscitation, and protecting a violent patient. When an inexperienced nurse encounters a situation requiring emergency measures, it is critical to obtain the assistance of an experienced professional.

Counseling

Counseling helps patients use a problem-solving process to recognize and manage stress and facilitate interpersonal relationships. As a nurse, you counsel patients to accept actual or impending changes resulting from stress. Counseling includes emotional, intellectual, spiritual, and psychological support (see Chapters 28 and 31). Examples of counseling strategies are behavior modification, bereavement counseling, biofeedback, and crisis intervention. A patient and family caregiver who need nursing counseling may have normal adjustment difficulties and are upset or frustrated, but they are not necessarily psychologically disabled. A good example is the case of Mr Tillman, who faces normal grief and the uncertainty of how cancer will affect his wife and his relationship with her.

Nurse counseling encourages patients to examine available alternatives and make useful and appropriate choices. When patients can examine alternatives, they develop a sense of control and can better manage stress. Patients with severe depression, schizophrenia, or other psychiatric diagnoses require specialized therapy provided by mental health care nurses, social workers, psychologists, or psychiatrists.

Teaching

Teaching is an important nursing responsibility. The teaching-learning process is an active interaction between the teacher and the learner in which you, the teacher, address specific learning objectives.

The focus of teaching is intellectual growth or the acquisition of new knowledge or psychomotor skills. You teach correct principles, procedures, and techniques of health care to inform patients about their health status and prepare them for self-care (see Chapter 15). When patients are unable to assume self-care, nurses focus teaching efforts on family caregivers. Teaching takes place in all health care settings. As a nurse, you are responsible for assessing the learning needs and readiness of patients and family caregivers, and you are accountable for the quality of education you deliver. Know your patients; be aware of the cultural and social factors that influence their willingness and ability to learn. Know your patient's health literacy level. Can he or she read directions or make calculations that are necessary for self-care skills?

Controlling for Adverse Reactions

An adverse reaction is a harmful or unintended effect of a medication, diagnostic test, or therapeutic intervention. Adverse reactions can follow any nursing intervention. Learn to anticipate them and know which adverse reactions to expect. Nursing actions that control for adverse reactions reduce or counteract the reaction. For example, when applying a moist heat compress, you want to prevent burns to the patient's skin. First, assess the area requiring the compress. After applying the compress, check the area every 5 minutes for any adverse reaction such as excessive reddening of the skin from the heat. When administering a medication, understand the known and potential side effects of the drug. After administration of the medication, evaluate the patient's response for adverse effects. Remember that certain drugs are available to counteract side effects. Although adverse reactions are uncommon, they do occur. You must recognize the signs and symptoms of an adverse reaction and intervene promptly.

Preventive Measures

Preventive nursing actions promote health and prevent illness. Prevention includes promoting a patient's health potential, applying prescribed measures (e.g., immunizations), health teaching, and identifying risks for illness and/or trauma. Consider Mrs Tillman's situation. Rich worries that, with her fatigue and the progressive nature of her cancer, she is likely to become weaker and less mobile and have an increased risk for falling. He recommends preventive measures to make the Tillman's home setting safer. He assesses their home environment and chooses the interventions (e.g., installing grab bars in the bath and rearranging furniture) that will improve Mrs Tillman's safety and ability to move about in her home. All patients need nursing interventions aimed at promoting health and preventing illness. As changes in the health care system continue, there is and will be greater emphasis on health promotion and illness prevention.

Indirect Care

Indirect care measures are actions that support the effectiveness of direct care measures (Bulechek et al., 2013). Many measures are managerial in nature such as emergency cart maintenance and supply management. Much of a nurse's time is spent in indirect care activities such as consultation and preparing a hand-off report. These activities promote communication of patient information. Accurate communication ensures that direct care activities are planned and coordinated with proper resources. Delegation of care to NAP is another indirect care activity. Proper delegation ensures that the right care providers perform the right tasks so that RNs and NAP work most efficiently for their patients.

Communicating Nursing Interventions

Communicate all patient interventions in an electronic, written, or oral format (see Chapter 5). EHRs or written charts have sections for individualized interventions, which are part of a patient's nursing care plan and permanent medical record. All entries usually have a brief description of pertinent patient assessment findings, the specific interventions, and the patient's response. A patient's medical record validates that a procedure or intervention was performed, and provides valuable information to subsequent caregivers. Some institutions have **interdisciplinary care plans**, which represent the contributions of all disciplines caring for a patient. Enter your nursing interventions into the plan, documenting the treatment and patient's response (see Chapter 5). Effective communication and teamwork among all health care professionals reduce medical errors and prevent adverse events. Miscommunication is often the root cause for most reported or sentinel events that occur in health care organizations (ECRI, 2017).

Delegating, Supervising, and Evaluating Work of Other Staff Members

The nurse who develops the care plan frequently does not perform all the nursing interventions. Nurses delegate some activities to other members of the health care team. Remember that an RN delegates components of care but not the nursing process itself (ANA and National Council of State Boards of Nursing [NCBSN], 2012). You can assign noninvasive and repetitive interventions to certified nurse assistants and other NAP. These activities include skin care, ambulation, grooming, and hygiene measures. Licensed practical nurses (LPNs) perform these measures in addition to medication administration and many invasive tasks. For example, LPNs may perform dressing care and catheterization.

The nursing tasks or activities that members of the nursing team perform under the direction of an RN are identified according to legal parameters defined by each state in its Nurse Practice Act and by the scope of practice and standards established by professional nursing organizations (ANA, 2010). When you delegate aspects of care to another staff member, you are responsible for assigning the task and ensuring that the staff member completes the task according to the standard of care. You are also responsible for delegating direct care interventions to personnel competent to provide the care.

EVALUATION

Evaluation is the crucial step of determining whether a patient's condition or well-being improved after an intervention was delivered (see Fig. 19.6). During evaluation, you examine the patient's condition or situation and then decide whether change has occurred.

The evaluation determines whether the nursing care was effective. Apply all that you know about a patient and the patient's condition together with experience with previous patients. You conduct this evaluation to determine whether expected outcomes are met, not whether nursing interventions were completed. *For example, in Rich's plan of care for Mrs Tillman, he established the outcome of "The patient will verbalize feeling less anxious about the course of her disease within 1 week." Rich implements educational interventions to improve Mrs Tammana's knowledge and anxiety reduction exercises.* Evaluation *does* involve questioning Mrs Tammana about her feelings toward her disease. Evaluation *does not* involve observation of her performing anxiety reduction exercises. Expected outcomes are the standards against which you judge whether goals have been met and care is successful.

Critical Thinking and Evaluation

Critical thinking is key to evaluation. Evaluation is an ongoing process that you conduct while caring for a patient. After you complete an intervention, use evaluative measures to gather subjective and objective data from the patient, family, and health care team members. This includes reviewing knowledge about a patient's current condition, treatment, and resources available for recovery. By referring to previous experiences caring for similar patients, you are in a better position to know how to evaluate outcomes of care. Then apply critical thinking attitudes and standards to determine whether outcomes of care are achieved. If outcomes are met, the overall goals for the patient are also met.

The evaluation process includes a before-and-after comparison. Compare patient behavior and responses assessed before delivering nursing interventions with behavior and responses that occur after administering nursing care.

During evaluation, you make clinical decisions and continually redirect nursing care. For example, when evaluating a patient for a change in pain severity, you apply knowledge of disease processes, physiological responses to interventions, and the correct procedure for measuring pain severity to interpret whether a change has occurred and whether it is desirable. If a patient continues to report pain at a higher level on the pain scale than expected, you consult with the health care provider to increase an analgesic dose or try different noninvasive approaches to help the patient relax and concentrate less on the pain. You continue to evaluate until the patient achieves pain relief.

When expected outcomes are met, you conclude that the nursing interventions effectively met the patient's goals. Negative evaluations or undesired results indicate that the interventions were not effective in meeting the outcomes of care (e.g., resolving the actual problem or avoiding a potential problem). Sometimes new data reveal that a patient's condition altered the patient's ability to meet the expected outcome. As a result, change the care plan and try different therapies or a different approach in administering existing therapies.

This sequence of critically evaluating and revising therapies continues until you and the patient appropriately resolve the problems. Outcomes must be realistic and adjusted based on the patient's prognosis and nursing diagnoses. Evaluation is dynamic and ever changing, depending on a patient's nursing diagnoses and condition. A patient whose health status continuously changes requires more frequent evaluation. In addition, priority diagnoses are usually evaluated first. For example, you evaluate a patient's *Acute Pain* before evaluating the status of *Deficient Knowledge*.

Evaluation Process

The evaluation process includes five elements: (1) comparing achieved effect with goals and outcomes, (2) collecting data to determine whether your patient met the criteria or standards, (3) interpreting and summarizing findings, (4) recognizing errors or unmet outcomes, and (5) revising the care plan as needed.

Comparing Achieved Effect With Goals and Outcomes

Evaluation is most effective when you know what to observe or measure. During evaluation, you compare your findings with the goals and expected outcomes set for your patient. Critical thinking directs you to analyze evaluation data. Did the patient reach a level of wellness or recovery that was reflected in the goals of care? Are there factors that prevent achievement of goals? Has the patient's condition changed?

Collecting Data

Evaluate a patient's response to nursing care using evaluative measures, which are simply assessment skills and techniques (e.g., auscultation of lung sounds, observation of a patient's skill performance, or discussion of the patient's feelings). In fact, evaluative measures are the same as assessment measures, but you perform them after the nursing intervention at the point of care when you prepare to make decisions about a patient's status and progress. The intent of the original assessment is to identify what, if any, problem exists. The purpose of the evaluation is to determine whether the identified problems have remained the same, improved, worsened, or otherwise changed.

In many clinical situations, you need to collect evaluative measures over a period of time to determine whether a pattern of improvement or change exists. For example, observing a pressure injury one time will not sufficiently determine whether the area of impaired skin integrity is healing. You want to see consistency in change. For example, over a period of 2 days, is the pressure injury decreasing in size? Is the amount of drainage declining? Recognizing a pattern of improvement or decline allows you to reason and decide whether the patient's problems are resolved.

The primary source of data for evaluation is the patient. However, you also use input from the family and other caregivers. For example, you ask a family caregiver to report on the amount of food a patient eats during a meal or how well the patient is able to sleep during the night. You sometimes consult with colleagues about how patients responded to therapies (e.g., pain control measures) during a previous shift. In addition to outcomes, it is important to evaluate whether you met a patient's expectations of care. You evaluate patients about their perceptions of care such as, "Did you receive the type of pain relief you expected? Were you able to feel comfortable?" This level of evaluation is important to determine the patient's satisfaction with care and strengthen partnering between you and the patient.

Interpreting and Summarizing Findings

An expert nurse recognizes relevant evidence, even if it does not match clinical expectations, and makes judgments about the patient's condition. To develop clinical judgment, you learn to match the results of evaluative measures with expected outcomes to determine whether or not a patient's status is improving. When interpreting findings, you compare the patient's behavioral responses and the physiological signs and symptoms you expect to see with those you actually see during evaluation. To objectively evaluate the degree of success in achieving outcomes of care, use the following steps:

1. Examine the outcome criteria to identify the exact desired patient behavior or response.
2. Measure the patient's actual behavior or response.
3. Compare the established outcome criteria with the actual behavior or response.
4. Judge the degree of agreement between outcome criteria and the actual behavior or response.
5. If there is no agreement (or only partial agreement) between outcome criteria and patient response, why did they not agree? What barriers prevented achievement of outcomes?

Evaluation is easier to perform after you have cared for a patient over a period of time. You can then make subtle comparisons of patient responses and behaviors. When you have not had the chance to care for a patient over an extended time, you can improve your evaluation by referring to previous experiences and asking colleagues familiar with the patient to confirm evaluation findings.

Remember to evaluate each expected outcome and its place in the sequence of care. If you do not, you will have trouble identifying the unmet outcomes. This prevents you from revising and redirecting the plan of care when necessary.

Recognizing Errors or Unmet Outcomes

During evaluation, recognizing errors or unmet outcomes requires you to have an open mind, to actively pursue truth, to be patient and confident, and to engage in self-reflections (Chao et al., 2013). You cannot assume that all your interventions will be successful. Applying your observational skills, critical thinking intellectual standards, and knowledge help you recognize the actual results of nursing interventions. You reflect on your patient care and identify possible reasons for unmet outcomes. Was the intervention specific for the patient's health care need? Did the patient's status change? Did the patient have an adverse reaction? During reflection, use problem-solving techniques to analyze and explain unmet outcomes and to identify new interventions to achieve a desired outcome.

Revising the Care Plan

The result of the evaluation helps you decide whether to discontinue or revise the plan of care. If your patient meets a goal successfully, discontinue that part of the care plan. Unmet and partially met goals require you to continue intervention. During the evaluation process, you often modify or add nursing diagnoses with appropriate goals and expected outcomes and then establish interventions. You must also redefine priorities. This is an important step in critical thinking (i.e., knowing how the patient is progressing and how problems either resolve or worsen).

Documentation

Discontinuing a Care Plan

After you determine that expected outcomes and goals were met, you confirm this evaluation with the patient whenever possible. If you and the patient agree, you discontinue that part of the care plan. Documentation of a discontinued plan ensures that other nurses will not unnecessarily continue interventions for that portion of the plan of care. Continuity of care assumes that care provided to patients is relevant and timely. You waste time when you do not communicate achieved goals.

Modifying a Care Plan

When goals are not met, you must identify the factors that interfered with achieving them. A change in a patient's condition, needs, or abilities makes modifications to the care plan necessary.

A failure to achieve a goal can also result from an error in nursing judgment or a failure to follow each step of the nursing process. Patients often have multiple problems. Always remember the possibility of overlooking or misjudging something. When a goal is not achieved, no matter what the reason, repeat the entire nursing process sequence for that nursing diagnosis to discover changes the plan needs. Reassess the patient, determine accuracy of the nursing diagnosis, establish new goals and expected outcomes, and select new interventions.

When you modify a plan, you must completely reassess all patient factors relating to the nursing diagnosis and etiology. Apply critical thinking as you compare new data about the patient's condition with previous data. Knowledge from previous experiences helps you direct the reassessment process. Caring for patients who have had similar health problems gives you a strong background of knowledge to use for anticipating patient needs and knowing what to assess. Reassessment ensures that the database is accurate and relevant (standards for critical thinking). It also reveals any missing link or piece of information that was overlooked and perhaps responsible for preventing goal achievement.

After reassessment, determine which nursing diagnoses are accurate for the situation. Ask yourself whether you selected the correct diagnosis and whether the diagnosis and the etiological factors are current. Revise the problem list to reflect the patient's changed status. You may make a new diagnosis. You base nursing care on an accurate list of nursing diagnoses. Accuracy is more important than the number of diagnoses selected. As the patient's condition changes, the diagnoses do as well.

When you modify a care plan, also review the goals and expected outcomes for needed changes. Examine the goals for unchanged nursing diagnoses. Are they still appropriate? A change in one diagnosis may affect others. For example, if Mrs Tillman now has *Impaired Gas Exchange*, it likely will require Rich to alter goals and outcomes with respect to her diagnosis of *Fatigue*. It is also important to determine that each goal and expected outcome is realistic for the problem, etiology, and time frame. Unrealistic expected outcomes and time frames make goal achievement difficult.

Clearly document goals and expected outcomes for new or revised nursing diagnoses so that all team members are aware of the revised care plan. When the goal is still appropriate but has not yet been met, you may change the evaluation date to allow more time. You may also decide at this time to change interventions. For example, when a patient's wound does not heal with a transparent dressing, you choose a different dressing material such as a colloid dressing. All goals and expected outcomes are patient centered, with realistic expectations for patient achievement.

The evaluation of interventions examines two factors: the appropriateness of the interventions selected and the correct application of the intervention. The appropriateness of an intervention is based on the standard of care for a patient's health problem. A **standard of care** is the minimum level of care accepted to ensure high quality of care to patients. Standards of care define the types of therapies typically administered to patients with specific problems or needs. For example, if a patient who is receiving chemotherapy for leukemia has the nursing diagnosis *Nausea related to pharyngeal irritation*, the standard of care established by a nursing department for this problem includes pain control measures, mouth care guidelines, and diet therapy. The nurse reviews the standard of care to determine whether the right interventions have been chosen or whether additional ones are needed.

You may need to increase or decrease the frequency of interventions when you revise a care plan. Use clinical judgment based on previous experience and a patient's actual response to therapy. For example, if a patient continues to have congested lung sounds, you increase the frequency of coughing and deep-breathing exercises to remove secretions.

During evaluation, you may find that some planned interventions deliver an inappropriate level of nursing care. If you need to change the level of care, substitute a different action verb, such as *assist* in place of *provide*, or *demonstrate* in place of *describe*. For example, assisting a patient with walking requires a nurse to be at the patient's side during ambulation, whereas providing an assistive device suggests that the patient is more independent. Sometimes the level of care is appropriate, but the interventions are unsuitable because of a change in the expected outcome. In this case, discontinue the interventions and plan new ones.

Make any changes in the plan of care based on the nature of the patient's unfavorable response. Consulting with other health care providers often yields suggestions for improving the approach to care delivery. Practicing nurses are usually excellent resources because of their experience.

Simply changing the care plan is not enough. Implement the new plan and reevaluate the patient's response to the nursing actions. Remember, *evaluation is continuous*.

KEY POINTS

- The nursing process has five steps: assessment, nursing diagnosis, planning, implementation, and evaluation.
- Using critical thinking skills with each step of the nursing process helps to develop and refine clinical decision-making.
- When you first meet a patient, you conduct an initial assessment screening and then focus on cues and patterns of information to complete a more comprehensive assessment.
- Subjective data are obtained from the patient's perception of a sign or symptom (e.g., level of pain or shortness of breath).
- Objective data are obtained for specific validated measures (e.g., body temperature, blood pressure).
- Data analysis involves recognizing patterns or trends, comparing data with standards, and forming a reasoned conclusion about the meaning of the data.
- Data clustering organizes assessment data into meaningful clusters of defining characteristics or sets of signs and symptoms.
- The diagnostic process includes analysis and interpretation of data, identification of patient and family needs, and formulation of nursing diagnoses and collaborative problems.
- Nursing diagnoses provide the basis for selection of nursing interventions to achieve outcomes for which a nurse is accountable.
- The absence of certain defining characteristics following a patient assessment suggests that you reject a nursing diagnosis under consideration.
- Nursing diagnostic errors may lead to inappropriate and/or inadequate nursing care.
- During the planning component, you determine patient goals, establish priorities, develop expected outcomes of nursing care, and write a nursing care plan.
- The NOC has labels for describing the focus of nursing care and includes indicators for use in measuring success with interventions.
- A nurse begins a care plan by first addressing the nursing diagnoses that have the highest priority.
- The care plan is a guideline for patient care so that all members of the health care team can quickly understand the care given.
- A concept map organizes and links data about a patient's multiple diagnoses in a logical way.
- There are three types of nursing interventions: nurse-initiated, physician initiated, and collaborative.
- The NIC is a comprehensive standardized classification of the interventions that nurses use in the care of patients.
- You evaluate by comparing the patient's response to nursing actions with expected outcomes established during planning.
- When goals of care are not met, you identify factors that interfere with goal achievement, reassess the patient's condition, revise existing or develop new nursing diagnoses, and select appropriate interventions.

REFERENCES

Ackley BJ, Ladwig GB. Nursing diagnosis handbook. 11th ed. St. Louis: Mosby; 2016.

Agency for Healthcare Research and Quality (AHRQ). Health literacy measurement tools (revised). 2016. Available from: http://www.ahrq.gov/professionals/quality-patient-safety/quality-resources/tools/literacy/index.html.

American Nurses Association (ANA). Nursing's social policy statement: the essence of the profession. 3rd ed. Washington, DC: The Association; 2010.

American Nurses Association (ANA) and the National Council of State Boards of Nursing (NCBSN). Joint statement on delegation. 2012. Available from: https://www.ncsbn.org/Delegation_joint_statement_NCSBN-ANA.pdf.

Ball JW, Dains J, Flynn J, Solomon B, Stewart R. Seidel's guide to physical examination. 8th ed. St. Louis: Mosby; 2015.

Bertakis KD, Azari R. Determinants and outcomes of patient-centered care. Patient Educ Couns 2011;85(10):46.

Boykins A. Core communication competencies in patient-centered care. ABNF J 2014;25(2):40.

Bulechek GM, Butcher H, Dochterman JM, Wagner C. Nursing interventions classification (NIC). 6th ed. St. Louis: Mosby; 2013.

Burman ME, Robinson B, Hart AM. Linking evidence-based nursing practice and patient-centered care through patient preferences. Nurs Adm Q 2013;37(3):231.

Canadian Interprofessional Health Collaborative (2010). A National Interprofessional Competency Framework, University of British Columbia. https://www.mcgill.ca/ipeoffice/ipe-curriculum/cihc-framework.

Carpenito-Moyet LJ. Nursing diagnosis: application to clinical practice. 15th ed. Philadelphia: Lippincott Williams & Wilkins; 2017.

Chaboyer W, McMurray A, Wallis M. Bedside nursing handover: a case study. Int J Nurs Pract 2010;16(1):27.

Chao SY, Liu HY, Wu MC, Clark MJ, Tan JY. Identifying critical thinking indicators and critical thinker attributes in nursing practice. J Nurs Res 2013;21(3):204.

Cope DG. Cultural competency in nursing research. Oncol Nurs Forum 2015;42(3):305.

Daley BJ, Torre DM. Concept maps in medical education: an analytical literature review. Med Educ 2010;44:440.

Darnell LK, Hickson SV. Culturally competent patient-centered nursing care. Nurs Clin North Am 2015;50(1):99.

ECRI Institute. Top 10 patient safety concerns for healthcare organizations. 2017. Available from: https://www.ecri.org/EmailResources/PSRQ/Top10/2017_PSTop10_ExecutiveBrief.pdf.

Flagg AJ. The role of patient-centered care in nursing. Nurs Clin North Am 2015;50(1):75.

Gallagher-Lepak S. Nursing diagnosis basics. In: Herdman TH, Kamitsuru S, editors. NANDA International nursing diagnoses: definitions & classification 2015-2017. Oxford: Wiley-Blackwell; 2014.

Gerdeman JL, Lux K, Jacko J. Using concept mapping to build clinical judgment skills. Nurse Educ Pract 2013;13(1):11.

Goodstone L, Cherkis F, Glaser C, Nikolaidou M, Maggio N. Bundle up: introducing care bundles to increase knowledge and confidence of senior nursing students, Teach Learn Nurs 2015;10(3):143.

Herdman TH, Kamitsuru S. From assessment to diagnosis. In: Herdman TH, Kamitsuru S, editors. Nursing diagnoses: definitions & classification 2015-2017. Oxford: Wiley-Blackwell; 2014a.

Herdman TH, Kamitsuru S, editors. Nursing diagnoses: definitions & classification 2015-2017. Oxford: Wiley-Blackwell; 2014b.

Jahne J. Palliative care: patient-centered assessment and communication to improve quality of life. N M Nurse 2015;60(4):4.

Lai WS, Chao CS, Yang WP, Liu HC, Chen CH. "Does one size fit all?" Exploring the cultural applicability of NANDA nursing diagnoses to Chinese nursing practice. J Transcult Nurs. 2013 Jan;24(1):43–50.

Lemetti T, Stolt M, Rickard N, Suhonen R. Collaboration between hospital and primary care nurses: a literature review. Int Nurs Rev 2015;62:248.

Lhussier M, Eaton S, Forster N, Thomas M, Roberts S, Carr SM. Care planning for long-term conditions – a concept mapping. Health Expect 2015;18:605.

Moorhead S, Johnson M, Maas M, Swanson E. Nursing outcomes classification (NOC). 5th ed. St. Louis: Mosby; 2013.

National Guideline Clearinghouse (NGC). Guidelines, Agency for Healthcare Research and Quality. n.d. Available from: http://www.guideline.gov.

Nielsen LS, Angus JE, Howell D, Husain A, Gastaldo D. Patient-centered care or cultural competence: negotiating palliative care at home for Chinese Canadian immigrants. Am J Hosp Palliat Care 2015;32(4):372.

Palos GR. Care, compassion, and communication in professional nursing: art, science, or both. Clin J Oncol Nurs 2014;18(2):247.

Pilcher J. Teaching and learning with concept maps. Neonatal Netw 2011;30(5):336.

QSEN Institute. Pre-licensure KSAS. 2014. Available from: http://qsen.org/competencies/pre-licensure-ksas/.

Suhonen R, Papastavrou E, Efstathiou G, Lemonidou C, Kalafati M, da Luz MD, et al. Nurses' perceptions of individualized care: an international comparison. J Adv Nurs 2011;67(9):1895.

U.S. Department of Health and Human Services (USDHHS). Summary of the health information privacy rule. 2017. Available from: http://www.hhs.gov/hipaa/for-professionals/privacy/laws-regulations/index.html.

Zolnierek CD. An integrative review of knowing the patient. J Nurs Scholarsh 2014;46(1):3.

20 Nutritional Needs

OBJECTIVES

After reading this chapter, the student should be able to:

- Understand the significance and principles of essential nutrients in human nutrition.
- Enlist the different types of nutrients required for development of body.
- Explain environmental and developmental factors influencing nutritional needs.
- Describe the alternative food pattern and their use in planning meals for balanced nutrition.
- Explain the importance of dietary guidelines and dietary reference intakes.
- Discuss the major areas of nutrition assessment including assessment and screening.
- Identify patients at risk for nutritional problems.
- Conduct physical examination, anthropometric assessment, laboratory values, and dysphagia assessment.
- Prepare a plan of care that meets the nutritional needs of a patient.
- Identify methods for feeding patients who require oral intake assistance.
- Make nursing diagnosis and care plan based on priority needs of clients with nutritional problems.
- Describe the importance of parenteral nutrition.
- Demonstrate the procedure for initiating and maintaining parenteral nutrition.
- Explain medical nutrition therapy and its requirement for patients with gastrointestinal diseases, diabetes, cardiovascular diseases, cancer, and so on.

KEY TERMS

amino acids, p. 454
anthropometry, p. 462
carbohydrates, p. 454
dysphagia, p. 465
jejunostomy tube, p. 469
lipids, p. 454
medical nutrition therapy (MNT), p. 463
minerals, p. 455
monounsaturated fatty acids, p. 454
nitrogen balance, p. 454
nutrient, p. 453
omega-3 fatty acid, p. 454
omega-6 fatty acid, p. 454
parenteral nutrition (PN), p. 470
polyunsaturated fatty acids, p. 454
saturated fatty acids, p. 454
unsaturated fatty acids, p. 454
vitamins, p. 454
xerostomia, p. 461

INTRODUCTION

Nutrition is a key component of health and is essential for normal growth and development, tissue maintenance and repair, cellular metabolism, and organ function. The human body needs an adequate supply of all nutrients for essential functions of cells.

Scientific principles regarding nutrition and the role of various nutrients in metabolism and health form a basis for the nutrition plan of care that you and the dietitian develop with your patients. Age, gender, activity level, medications, and disease processes all affect the use of nutrients and nutritional requirements.

PRINCIPLES OF NUTRITION

The body requires food to provide nutrients for growth and development, cellular metabolism, synthesis and repair of tissues, organ function, movement, and maintenance of body temperature. The gastrointestinal (GI) system allows for the nourishment of the body following food ingestion. Each organ or structure in the GI tract has a specific function aimed toward preparing food for the digestion and absorption of its nutrients.

NUTRIENTS

A **nutrient** is a chemical substance that provides nourishment and affects metabolic and nutritive processes. The essential nutrients include carbohydrates, proteins, lipids, vitamins, minerals, and water. Only carbohydrates, proteins, and lipids provide energy and are thus known as the energy-yielding nutrients. Although not a *nutrient*, alcohol also provides energy. Vitamins and minerals serve as catalysts or coenzymes necessary for the use of nutrients for energy. Minerals and water regulate many body processes.

Carbohydrates

Carbohydrates are composed of carbon, hydrogen, and oxygen. They are starches and sugars obtained mainly from plant foods, with the exception of lactose, which is found only in milk of animal origin (e.g., cow's milk, goat milk). Carbohydrates provide 4 kcal/g.

Fiber, a type of carbohydrate, is the structural part of plants and is sometimes called *nonstarch polysaccharides*. It also includes some nonpolysaccharides such as lignins and tannins. Human digestive enzymes cannot break down fiber. Therefore, it does not contribute calorically to the diet. However, it does provide several benefits. Fiber is categorized as either soluble or insoluble. Soluble fiber becomes a gel in water and delays GI transit time; because of this, soluble fiber helps prevent diarrhea in patients receiving tube feedings. Insoluble fiber does not change in water and accelerates intestinal transit; this helps to prevent or relieve constipation.

Proteins

Amino acids are the building blocks of proteins and are made of hydrogen, oxygen, carbon, and nitrogen. They are vital for the synthesis of body tissue in growth, maintenance, and repair. The body synthesizes some amino acids. These are known as dispensable amino acids, meaning that they are *dispensable in the diet*. Amino acids that the body cannot synthesize are referred to as indispensable amino acids (formerly referred to as essential amino acids). Indispensable amino acids must be obtained from food sources. Protein can be used as a source of energy when carbohydrates and fatty acids are not available. It provides 4 kcal/g.

The required daily intake of protein (per kilogram of body weight) varies according to age and growth rates. For example, rapidly growing infants younger than 6 months require 2.2 g/kg daily. Adolescents require 1 g/kg daily. Most healthy adults require only about 0.8 g/kg of ideal body weight (IBW) per day. Women who are pregnant or lactating need 25 g more than the usual daily need (Food and Nutrition Board [FNB] and Institute of Medicine [IOM], 2002). Other factors that influence the body's need for protein include tissue repair, dietary quality of the protein consumed, and illness or disease state. For example, in patients with major burns, protein requirements often double or triple.

Protein is composed of 16% nitrogen. The body uses nitrogen for building, repairing, and replacement of body tissues. **Nitrogen balance** is achieved when nitrogen intake equals nitrogen output. When nitrogen intake is greater than output, the patient is in positive nitrogen balance. The body needs a positive nitrogen balance for growth (including pregnancy and muscle building) and wound healing. Negative nitrogen balance occurs when the output of nitrogen is greater than the intake. It occurs in states of infection, sepsis, fever, burns, starvation, and trauma. Protein provides energy; however, because of the essential roles of protein, a balanced diet provides adequate kilocalories from nonprotein sources, thus sparing protein from being used for energy. When there are insufficient carbohydrates in the diet to meet the energy needs of the body, protein stores are broken down and used for energy.

Fats

Fats (**lipids**) are insoluble in water but soluble in organic solvents such as ethanol and acetone. Fatty acids are the building blocks of fat. Lipids are a source of energy, providing 9 kcal/g.

Triglycerides are made up of three fatty acids attached to glycerol. Most lipids in foods and the human body are triglycerides. High blood levels of triglycerides in the blood are a risk factor for cardiovascular diseases.

Saturated fatty acids are saturated with as much hydrogen as they can hold. **Monounsaturated fatty acids** have a single double bond, and **polyunsaturated fatty acids** have two or more double bonds. Most animal fats have a high proportion of saturated fatty acids, whereas most vegetable fats have higher amounts of **unsaturated fatty acids**. For example, olive oil contains 14% saturated fatty acids, 77% monounsaturated fatty acids, and 9% polyunsaturated fatty acids. Trans fatty acids are created when vegetable oils are hydrogenated during food processing. Diets high in *trans* fats are associated with cardiovascular disease and mortality (de Souza et al., 2015).

The two essential fatty acids (EFAs) in human nutrition are linoleic acid (an **omega-6 fatty acid**) and linolenic acid (an **omega-3 fatty acid**). EFAs have many roles in the body, including producing cell membranes and hormones and regulating blood pressure, blood clot formation, and immune response. Studies indicate that there is a reduction in cardiovascular disease risk when people replace dietary sources of saturated fats with polyunsaturated fats (Sanders, 2014).

Vitamins

Vitamins are organic substances present in small amounts in food and are essential for life. They generally serve as coenzymes or catalysts in cellular enzyme reactions. The body is unable to synthesize vitamins in adequate amounts and depends on regular dietary intake. The exception to this is vitamin K. A significant portion of the body's vitamin K needs is supplied by the bacteria found in the intestines; the rest is supplied by consuming dark, leafy green vegetables. Food processing, storage, and preparation all affect the bioavailability of vitamins. The bioavailability is usually highest in foods that are fresh and used quickly after minimal exposure to heat, air, or water. Vitamins A, C, and E are also important antioxidants. They neutralize *free radicals*, which produce oxidative damage to body cells and tissues.

Vitamins are categorized as either water-soluble or fat-soluble. Water-soluble vitamins (C and B-complex vitamins) are stored in limited amounts for short periods of time in the body, requiring daily consumption. Water-soluble vitamins are absorbed easily from the GI tract.

Fat-soluble vitamins (A, D, E, and K) are stored in the body for longer periods; however, dietary intake is still necessary. In addition, the body produces some needed vitamin D through a series of steps beginning with sunlight exposure to the skin. Because the body has a high storage capacity for fat-soluble vitamins, toxicity is possible, particularly from excess supplementation. For this reason, always ask patients whether they are taking supplements and in what quantities.

Minerals

Minerals are inorganic elements that catalyze biochemical reactions. They are classified as macrominerals when the daily requirement is 100 mg or more and microminerals or trace elements when the body needs less than 100 mg daily. Minerals have many functions and are required for most of the body's metabolic processes. Interactions occur among some minerals. For example, zinc absorption is inhibited with large doses of iron supplements.

Vitamins and minerals are best obtained from a healthy diet of varied food choices. When deficiencies exist, these nutrients can also be provided through supplementation. However, dietary supplements should not contain more than 100% of the recommended dietary allowance (RDA) for any nutrient unless specifically prescribed by a health care provider. Excessively high doses may be toxic.

Water

Normal cell function depends on an aqueous environment. Water is an essential nutrient with many functions in the body including transporting nutrients and waste products; providing a structure to large molecules (protein, glycogen); promoting metabolic reactions; serving as solvent, lubricant, and cushion; regulating body temperature; and maintaining blood volume.

Water makes up 60%–70% of the total body weight. Infants have the greatest percentage of total body weight as water, and older adults have the least percentage of total body weight as water. Subsequently, infants and older adults are the most vulnerable to water deprivation and water loss. Muscle tissue is about 75% water, whereas fat tissue is only about 10% water. Thus, a lean person contains a higher percentage of water in the body than an obese person does.

The human body requires approximately 1–1.5 mL of water for every kilocalorie of energy used (FNB and IOM, 2004). Ingesting liquids and solid foods such as fresh fruits and vegetables helps meet fluid needs. The body also produces water when food is oxidized during digestion.

Thirst is a protective mechanism that alerts an oriented person to the need for fluids. It is less reliable in infants and patients who are confused because they are unable to communicate that they are thirsty.

FACTORS INFLUENCING NUTRITION

Nutritional requirements depend on many factors. Individual caloric and nutrient requirements vary by stage of development, body composition, activity levels, conditions such as pregnancy and lactation, and the presence of disease. Registered dietitian nutritionists (RDNs) may use predictive equations that consider each of these factors as a starting point for estimating a patient's nutritional requirements.

Environmental Factors

Environmental factors beyond the control of individuals contribute to the development of obesity. Obesity is an epidemic in the developed countries. Proposed contributing factors for obesity are sedentary lifestyle, work schedules, and poor meal choices often related to the increasing frequency of eating away from home and eating fast food (Wang et al., 2013). Environmental factors can limit a person's likelihood of healthy eating and participation in exercise or other activities of healthy living. Lack of access to full-service grocery stores, high cost of healthy food, widespread availability of less healthy foods in fast food restaurants, widespread advertising of less healthy food, and lack of access to safe places to play and exercise are environmental factors that contribute to obesity (Hedwig et al., 2013).

Developmental Needs

Infants to School Age

Infancy is marked by rapid growth requiring high protein, vitamin, mineral, and energy availability. Infants need an energy intake of approximately 108 kcal/kg of body weight in the first half of infancy and 98 kcal/kg in the second half (FNB and IOM, 2002). Infants from birth to 12 months of age need approximately 700–800 mL/day of fluid because a large portion of total body weight is water (FNB and IOM, 2004).

Breastfeeding

The Indian Academy of Pediatrics (IAP), World Health Organization (WHO), and Institute of Medicine (IOM) recommend exclusive breastfeeding for approximately 6 months, with the continuation of breastfeeding for at least 1 year or as long as mutually desired by mother and infant. The benefits include an enhanced immune system, reduced food allergies and intolerances, reduced infant morbidity and mortality, and easier digestion. In addition, breast milk is convenient, fresh, always the correct temperature, and economical. Breastfeeding provides increased time for mother and infant bonding.

Breast Milk Substitutes

Commercially available infant formulas contain the approximate nutrient composition of human milk and are an acceptable alternative. Infants should not have regular cow's milk during the first year of life. Cow's milk does not meet infants' nutrient needs and has excessive sodium, potassium, and protein. Such high solute loads are dangerous to an infant's GI tract and renal system.

Introduction to Solid Food

Breast milk, or breast milk substitute, remains the major source of nutrition throughout the entire first year of life. However, the nutrient needs and physiological development of the infant warrant the introduction of solid foods to the basic diet of breast milk beginning around 6 months of age. Iron-fortified cereals are usually the first semisolid food introduced and are an important nonmilk source of protein and iron. Ideally, new foods are introduced one at a time, approximately 4–7 days apart, to identify and remove any allergens from the diet. Teach your patients to introduce new foods immediately before giving milk to increase acceptance and avoid satiety. Honey and corn syrup are potential sources of botulism toxin and should not be used in an infant's diet before the age of 1 year.

The growth rate slows during toddler years, requiring fewer kilocalories per kilogram of body weight. Toddlers are naturally intuitive eaters, and their appetite reflects these changing energy needs. Toddlers often exhibit strong food preferences and may become picky eaters. They are not able to consume enough volume of food to meet their nutrient needs in only three meals per day. Snacks are an important part of the overall diet for toddlers and should consist of high–nutrient density foods to help improve the quality of the diet. Data from *What We Eat in America* indicate that snacks provide 30% of total energy, 22% of protein intake, and about 25% of all vitamins and minerals in the diets of children 2–5 years of age.

Toddlers (older than 1 year) should drink full-fat milk or a milk substitute until the age of 2 years to ensure adequate intake of fatty acids necessary for brain and neurological development. Certain foods such as hot dogs, hard candy, nuts, grapes, chopped raw vegetables, and popcorn increase the risk for choking and should be avoided or consumed only with supervision. Preschoolers' (3–5 years of age) dietary requirements are similar to those of toddlers. They consume slightly more volume than toddlers, and nutrient density continues to be a very important aspect of their diet.

School-age children (6–12 years of age) grow at a slower and steadier rate, with a gradual decline in energy requirements per unit of body weight. Despite the better appetites and more diverse food intake of school-age children, you still need to assess their diets carefully for balance and variety. There is no room for excess intake of empty calories at this age. The intake of sugar-sweetened beverages prevents the intake of nutrient-dense foods and beverages. Although there are many contributing factors to obesity, diet and lifestyle are two readily modifiable factors. Researchers continue to find that the key to childhood obesity prevention is to increase current levels of physical activity and ensure a well-balanced diet for children (Kumar and Kelly, 2017; Wang et al., 2015).

Adolescents

Throughout the adolescent years, energy and protein requirements increase to meet greater metabolic demands of growth. Calcium is essential for rapid bone growth, and girls need a continuous source of iron to replace menstrual losses. Boys also need adequate iron for muscle development. B-complex vitamins are necessary to support heightened metabolic activity. Figure-conscious adolescents are susceptible to dieting, meal skipping, and subsequent nutrient deficiencies during the period of puberty and body changes. In extreme circumstances, eating disorders can develop. Snacks continue to be an important source of nutrient intake for teenagers, providing approximately 25% of their total dietary intake. Fast food is commonly eaten during this stage of life and adds excess salt, fat, and often "empty" kilocalories.

Young and Middle-Age Adults

Adults need nutrients for energy, maintenance, and tissue repair. Energy needs usually decline over the years along with the metabolic rate. Adults who do not adjust their energy intake in response to a slowing metabolism will likely gain weight. Obesity is one of the most significant health care problems in the United States with 69.5% of adults (older than 20 years) currently overweight or obese (as defined by a body mass index [BMI] 25 kg/m^2 or higher).

Pregnancy

Poor nutrition and inadequate maternal weight gain during pregnancy contribute to low birth weight in infants, preterm birth, and poor pregnancy outcomes (Han et al., 2011). The nutrition status of a mother at the time of conception is critically important to the developing embryo. Energy requirements during pregnancy are related to the mother's body weight, activity level, and stage of pregnancy. On average, a pregnant woman needs 15%–20% more kilocalories than she needs when not pregnant. This is equal to approximately 340 kcal/day extra beginning in the second trimester and 450 kcal/day extra during the third trimester (FNB and IOM, 2002). Protein requirements throughout pregnancy increase by 25 g over nonpregnancy needs (FNB and IOM, 2002). Iron needs increase dramatically during pregnancy to provide for increased maternal blood volume, fetal blood storage, and blood loss during delivery. Most women benefit from taking supplemental iron.

The active form of folate, tetrahydrofolic acid, is particularly important for DNA synthesis and cell division. Inadequate intake is associated with increased risk of neural tube defects such as spina bifida and anencephaly (Copp and Greene, 2013). It is recommended that all women of childbearing age consume 400 mcg of folic acid daily, increasing to 600 mcg daily during pregnancy (FNB and IOM, 1998).

Lactation

A woman needs an additional 330–400 kcal/day and 25 g of protein above her usual requirements to meet the nutrient demands of milk production (FNB and IOM, 2002). The increase in food consumption usually meets the increased needs for most vitamins and minerals. Women who are breastfeeding should drink about 3 L of fluid daily while limiting caffeine and avoiding alcohol and drugs because they are excreted in the breast milk. Remind women to talk with their health care provider about prescription drugs that may be excreted in breast milk.

Older Adults

Adults 65 years of age and older have similar needs for vitamins and minerals as younger adults but a decreased need for calories because of a slowing metabolic rate. This makes it even more important that older adults have well-balanced diets and ingest foods with high nutritional value. Numerous physiological and socioeconomic factors influence the nutrition status of older adults. For example, living on a fixed income may limit funds available to purchase food. Older adults are more likely to have a chronic disease that requires a therapeutic diet and medications and increases the risk for drug–nutrient interactions. They may have difficulty eating because of physical symptoms, lack of teeth, or dentures. Changes in cognition may limit an older adult's ability to select nutritious foods and to prepare meals. Some older adults need a vitamin and mineral supplement (Box 20.1).

Alternative Food Patterns

Individuals' patterns of food intake are based on religion, cultural background, ethics, health beliefs, concern about the environment, or any number of other reasons. A

BOX 20.1 Care of an Older Adult

Dietary Teaching

- Eat a balanced diet that contains a variety of foods. Avoid too much fat, cholesterol, sugar, and sodium.
- Eat foods that have adequate amounts of starch and fiber such as fruits and vegetables and whole-grain cereals and breads.
- Consult with a pharmacist about the potential for medication and food–nutrient interactions.
- Drink adequate fluids because the thirst sensation diminishes with age. Water requirements do not decrease with age.
- If unable to eat meat because of cost or difficulty chewing, find alternative sources of protein.
  - Cream soups and meat-based vegetable soups are nutrient-dense sources of protein.
  - Cheese, eggs, and peanut butter are also useful high-protein alternatives.
- Drink milk or fortified milk-substitute products for calcium and vitamin D to protect against osteoporosis. Provide calcium supplements if lactose intolerance is present or the patient declines to consume fortified milk-substitute products (e.g., soy milk, rice milk, almond milk).
- Take vitamin and nutrient supplements as recommended.

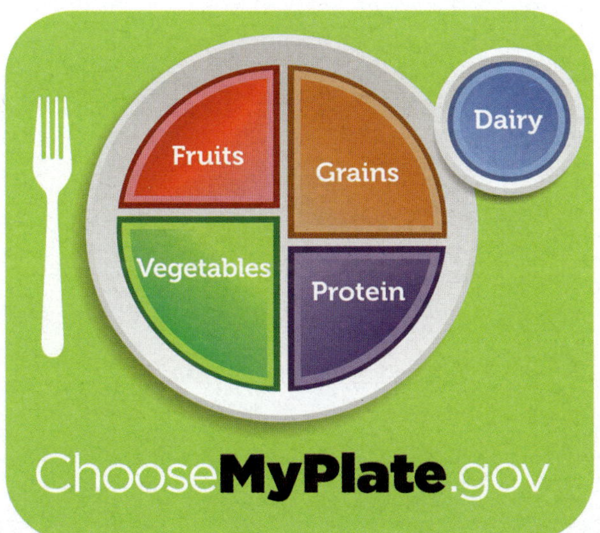

Fig. 20.1 ChooseMyPlate. (From U.S. Department of Agriculture: ChooseMyPlate, 2011.)

patient's food preferences and choices may not meet nutrition recommendations based on ChooseMyPlate or the Dietary Guidelines for Americans (Fig. 20.1). Optimal nutrition intake depends on balanced consumption of all required nutrients. The vegetarian diet is an example of a dietary pattern that is commonly consumed because of religious beliefs or personal preferences. There are several types of vegetarian diets, which are primarily plant based and eliminate many animal-based foods. Ovolactovegetarians avoid meat, fish, and poultry but eat eggs and milk products. Lactovegetarians consume milk and milk products but avoid eggs and other animal-based foods. Ovovegetarians consume egg products but avoid all other animal-based foods. Vegans eat only foods of plant origin. Individuals consuming a vegan diet are more susceptible to vitamin B_{12} deficiency because this vitamin is found only in animal products. However, with the abundance of fortified and enriched plant-based foods (e.g., B_{12}- and calcium-fortified plant-based milk), it is not a limitation to this diet. Vegans consuming a comprehensive vegan diet score higher on the Healthy Eating Index compared with those who eat vegetarian diets (Clarys et al., 2014).

DIETARY GUIDELINES

Several agencies and organizations in the United States regularly publish and update dietary guidelines based on current scientific evidence. The guidelines change as nutrition researchers discover new knowledge.

Dietary Reference Intakes

Dietary intake requirements are country specific, which are determined by various sociocultural, economic, environmental, personal, and dietary factors. The National Institute of Nutrition, Indian Council of Medical Research, Hyderabad, published the first edition of "*Dietary Guidelines for Indians*" in the year 1998, which is revised at several times and latest guidelines published in 2020. The latest edition of *Dietary Guidelines for Indians* was published in 2020, which highlighted the EARs for adults, infants, children, and adolescents (Table 20.1) and the number of proportion for balanced diet for moderate active man (Table 20.2), sedentary man (Table 20.3), moderate active woman (Table 20.4), sedentary woman (Table 20.5), and pregnant woman (Table 20.6). The RDA is the average needs of 97.5% of the population, not the exact needs of an individual. To plan healthy diets, however, it is important to match the dietary guidelines with the food preferences of a specific individual and his or her cultural, socioeconomic, and personal inclinations. Indian RDA recommendations are based on single value, which need to be revised based on strong scientific evidence base.

NUTRITIONAL ASSESSMENT

Screening

Nutrition screening is part of your initial assessment of a patient. Standardized nutrition screening tools are a quick method of identifying malnutrition. Nutrition screening tools commonly include objective measures such as age, BMI, weight change, and the presence of acute disease. A single objective measure alone does not predict a person's nutritional risk.

Several standardized nutrition screening tools are available to use in the inpatient and outpatient settings. One example is the Malnutrition Universal Screening Tool (MUST), a validated clinical method that uses current BMI, unintentional weight loss, and the presence of compromised nutrient intake for more than 5 days because of acute disease. The MUST is a simple, inexpensive tool that highly correlates with the medical diagnostic criteria for malnutrition (Poulia et al., 2017).

Table 20.1 ICMR-NIN Recommended Dietary Allowances (RDA) and Estimated Average Requirement (EAR) of nutrients for Indians-2020

		Body Wt	Energy (**)	Protein	Cal cium	Magnes ium	Iron	Zinc	Iodine	Thiamine	Ribo flavin	Niacin	Vit B6	Folate	Vit B12	Vit C	Vit A	Vit D
Age Group	**Category of work**	**(kg)**	**(Kcal/d)**	**(g/d)**	**(mg/d)**	**(mg/d)**	**(mg/d)**	**(mg/d)**	**(µg/ day)**	**(mg/d)**	**(mg/d)**	**(mg/d)**	**(mg/d)**	**(µg/d)**	**(µg/d)**	**(mg/d)**	**(µg/d)**	**(IU/d)**
	Sedentary		2110							1.2	1.6	12	1.6					
Men	Moderate	65	2710	43.0	800	370	11	14.1	95	1.5	2.1	15	2.1	250	2	65	460	400
	Heavy		3470							1.9	2.7	19	2.6					
	Sedentary		1660							1.1	1.6	9	1.6					
	Moderate	55	2130	36.0	800	310	15	11.0	95	1.4	2.0	12	1.6	180	2	55	390	400
	Heavy		2720							1.8	2.6	15	2.1					
Women	Pregnant woman	55 + 10	+350	+7.6 (2nd trimester) +17.6 (3rd trimester)	800	370	21	12.0	160	1.6	2.3	+2	1.9	480	+0.2	+10	406	400
	Lactation		+600	+13.6							2.5		+0.22					
	0–6m	–			1000	335	16	11.8	200	1.7		+4		280	+0.8	+40	720	400
	7–12m		+520	+10.6							2.4		+0.16					
Infants	0–6 m*	5.8	530	7.0	–	–	–	–	–	–	–	–	–	–	–	–	–	–
	6–12m	8.5	680	9.0	–	–	2	2.1	–	–	–	–	0.5	71	1	–	170	–
	1–3y	12.9	1110	10.0	400	73	6	2.8	65	0.6	0.8	6	0.8	97	1	24	180	
Children	4–6y	18.3	1360	13.0	450	104	8	3.7	65	0.8	1.1	8	1.0	111	2	27	240	400
	7–9 y	25.3	1700	19.0	500	144	10	4.9	65	1.0	1.3	10	1.3	142	2	36	290	
Boys	10–12y	34.9	2220	27.0	650	199	12	7.0	70	1.3	1.7	12	1.7	180	2	45	360	400
Girls	10–12y	36.4	2060	27.0	650	207	16	7.1	70	1.2	1.6	12	1.6	186	2	44	370	400
Boys	13–15y	50.5	2860	36.0	800	287	15	11.9	100	1.6	2.2	16	2.2	238	2	60	430	400
Girls	13–15y	49.6	2400	35.0	800	282	17	10.7	100	1.3	1.9	13	1.8	204	2	55	420	400
Boys	16–18y	64.4	3320	45.0	850	367	18	14.7	100	1.9	2.5	19	2.5	286	2	70	480	400
Girls	16–18y	55.7	2500	37.0	850	317	18	11.8	100	1.4	1.9	14	1.9	223	2	57	400	400

* Adequate Intake (AI)

** There is no RDA for energy, the EAR for energy is equivalent to the Estimated Energy Requirement (EER)

Note: For adequate intake of Biotin and Pantothenic acid, refer to the text on summary of recommendations.

Source: "ICMR-NIN Expert Group on Nutrient Requirement for Indians, Recommended Dietary Allowances (RDA) and Estimated Average Requirements (EAR) - 2020".

Table 20.2 Balanced Diet for Moderate Active Man with Nutrient Content Values

Food Composition	Amount (g/Day)	Nutrient	Vegetarian Diet	Non-vegetarian Diet	EAR	RDA
Cereals & Millets	360	Energy (kcal)	2690	2650	2710	-
		Protein (g)	87.5	81.7	43	54
Pulses (Legumes)/ flesh foods	120	Visible fat (g)	35	35	30	30
Green leafy vegetables	100	Calcium (mg)	1084	1054	800	1000
Other vegetables	200	Iron (mg)	33.3	31.1	11	19
Roots & Tubers (excluding Potatoes)	100	Zinc (mg)	16.3	15.9	14.1	17
Fruits	150	Magnesium (mg)	968	891	370	440
Milk	300	Vitamin A (μg)*	1802	1796	460	1000
Fats & Oils	30	β Carotene	9842	9779	2760	6000
Oil seeds & Nuts (gingely seeds & Pea nuts)	30	Thiamine (mg)	2	1.9	1.5	1.8
		Riboflavin (mg)	1.9	1.9	2.1	2.5
		Niacin (mg)	19	20	15	18
		Vitamin B_6 (mg)	2.4	2.4	2.1	2.4
		Vitamin C (mg)	209	209	65	80
		Total Folates (μg)	559	491	250	300
		Vitamin B_{12} (μg)	1.5	2.4	2	2.2

Note: Total protein from the above diet = 88g, Digestible protein = 71g, PDCAAS = 84%
[1]Pulses can be replaced with animal foods (egg, meat, fish and chicken) for non-vegetarians.
*Retinol derived from β carotene from diet was also added to the total Vitamin A.
For cereals and millets, it is recommended to consume 50% as whole grains.
Source: "ICMR-NIN Expert Group on Nutrient Requirement for Indians, Recommended Dietary Allowances (RDA) and Estimated Average Requirements (EAR) – 2020".

Table 20.3 Balanced Diet for Sedentary Man with Nutrient Content Values

Food Composition	Amount (g/Day)	Nutrient	Vegetarian Diet	Non-vegetarian Diet	EAR	RDA
Cereals & Millets	275	Energy (kcal)	2130	2084	2110	–
		Protein (g)	67.2	69.1	43	54
Pulses (Legumes)/ flesh foods	80	Visible fat (g)	25	25	25	25
Green leafy vegetables	100	Calcium (mg)	968	958	800	1000
Other vegetables	200	Iron (mg)	27.4	26.3	11.0	19.0
Roots & Tubers (excluding Potatoes)	100	Zinc (mg)	13.5	13.2	14.1	17.0
Fruits	150	Magnesium (mg)	798	762	370	440
Milk	300	Vitamin A (μg)*	1768	1765	460	1000
Fats & Oils	25	β-Carotene (μg)	9638	9605	2760	6000
Oil seeds & Nuts (gingely seeds & Pea nuts)	30	Thiamine (mg)	1.7	1.6	1.2	1.4
		Riboflavin (mg)	1.6	1.6	1.6	2.0
Spices	10	Niacin (mg)	15.6	16.0	12	14
		Vitamin B_6 (mg)	2.0	2.0	1.6	1.9
		Vitamin C (mg)			65	80
		Total Folates (μg)	483	450	250	300
		Vitamin B_{12} (μg)	1.5	2.0	2.0	2.2

Note: Total protein from the above diet = 71g, Digestible protein = 58g, PDCAAS = 85%
[1]Pulses can be replaced with animal foods (egg, meat, fish and chicken) for non-vegetarians.
*Retinol derived from β carotene from diet was also added to the total Vitamin A.
For cereals and millets, it is recommended to consume 50% as whole grains.
Source: "ICMR-NIN Expert Group on Nutrient Requirement for Indians, Recommended Dietary Allowances (RDA) and Estimated Average Requirements (EAR) – 2020".

Nutrition Assessment

Refer patients at risk for nutritional problems to an RDN for a more in-depth nutrition assessment. Nutrition assessment is different from nutrition screening. The RDN completes a nutrition assessment, which includes an in-depth exploration of medical history, dietary history, physical examination, anthropometric measurements, and laboratory data (Table 20.7). Nutrition assessment determines nutrient and energy needs. In an acute care setting, the RDN is available to make these calculations. In an outpatient setting, make a referral if an RDN is not available on-site.

Table 20.4 Balanced Diet for Moderate Active Woman with Nutrient Content Values

Food Composition	Amount (g/Day)	Nutrient	Vegetarian Diet	Non-vegetarian Diet	EAR	RDA
Cereals & Millets	300	Energy (kcal)	2135	2084	2130	–
		Protein (g)	74.2	73.3	36.0	46.0
Pulses (Legumes)[1]	90	Visible fat (g)	20	20	25	20
Green leafy vegetables	100	Calcium (mg)	999	989	800	1000
Other vegetables	200	Iron (mg)	29.0	27.9	15.0	29.0
Roots & Tubers (excluding Potatoes)	100	Zinc (mg)	14.0	13.6	11.0	13.2
Fruits	150	Magnesium (mg)	841	806	310	370
Milk	300	Vitamin A (μg)*	1804	1741	390	840
Fats & Oils	20	β-carotene (μg)	9489	9457	–	–
Oil seeds & Nuts (gingely seeds & Pea nuts)	30	Thiamine (mg)	1.75	1.70	1.4	1.7
		Riboflavin (mg)	1.65	1.64	2.0	2.4
Spices	10	Niacin (mg)	16.3	16.8	12	14
		Vitamin B_6 (mg)	1.96	1.97	1.6	1.9
		Vitamin C (mg)	187	187	55	65
		Total Folates (μg)	191	459	180	220
		Vitamin B_{12} (μg)	1.5	2.0	2	2.2

Note: Total protein from the above diet = 76g, Digestible protein = 62g, PDCAAS = 85%
[1]Pulses can be replaced with animal foods (egg, meat, fish and chicken) for non-vegetarians.
*Retinol derived from β carotene from diet was also added to the total Vitamin A.
For cereals and millets, it is recommended to consume 50% as whole grains.
Source: "ICMR-NIN Expert Group on Nutrient Requirement for Indians, Recommended Dietary Allowances (RDA) and Estimated Average Requirements (EAR) – 2020".

Table 20.5 Balanced Diet for Sedentary Woman with Nutrient Content Values

Food Composition	Amount (g/Day)	Nutrient	Vegetarian Diet	Non-vegetarian Diet	EAR	RDA
Cereals & Millets	200	Energy (kcal)	1690	1650	1660	–
		Protein (g)	58.2	57.4	36.0	46.0
Pulses (Legumes)[1]	60	Visible fat (g)	15	15	20	20
Green leafy vegetables	100	Calcium (mg)	905	895	800	1000
Other vegetables	200	Iron (mg)	23.8	22.8	15.0	29.0
Roots & Tubers (excluding Potatoes)	100	Zinc (mg)	11.0	10.5	11.0	13.2
Fruits	150	Magnesium (mg)	684	649	310	370
Milk	300	Vitamin A (μg)*	1730	1727	390	840
Fats & Oils	15	β-carotene (μg)	9412	9380	–	–
Oil seeds & Nuts (gingely seeds & Pea nuts)	30	Thiamine (mg)	1.36	1.30	1.1	1.4
		Riboflavin (mg)	1.5	1.48	1.6	1.9
Spices	10	Niacin (mg)	13.0	13.5	9.0	11
		Vitamin B_6 (mg)	1.7	1.7	1.6	1.9
		Vitamin C (mg)	187	187	55	65
		Total Folates (μg)	426	395	180	220
		Vitamin B_{12} (μg)	1.5	2.0	2	2.2

Note: Total protein from the above diet = 60g, Digestible protein = 50g, PDCAAS = 87%
[1]Pulses can be replaced with animal foods (egg, meat, fish and chicken) for non-vegetarians.
*Retinol derived from β carotene from diet was also added to the total Vitamin A.
For cereals and millets, it is recommended to consume 50% as whole grains.
Source: "ICMR-NIN Expert Group on Nutrient Requirement for Indians, Recommended Dietary Allowances (RDA) and Estimated Average Requirements (EAR) – 2020".

Diet History

A diet history focuses on usual intake of food and liquids along with information about preferences, allergies, and digestive problems (Box 20.2). Open-ended questions encourage a patient to provide more information on food intake during the interview. For example, ask a patient who reports avoiding dairy products, "Tell me what led you to avoid dairy products?" The patient's answer to this question leads to physiological, psychological, sociological, religious, cultural, or food preference factors that you can further explore.

When indicated, the RDN will ask the patient to keep a detailed record of food intake over 3 days, including one weekend

Table 20.6 Balanced Diet for Pregnant Woman with Nutrient Content Values

Food Composition	Amount (g/Day)	Nutrient	Vegetarian Diet	Non-vegetarian Diet	EAR	RDA
Cereals & Millets	325	Energy (kcal)	2060	2040	2480	–
		Protein (g)	71.7	71.6	54	68
Pulses (Legumes)[1]	90	Visible fat (g)	15	15	30	30
Green leafy vegetables	100	Calcium (mg)	980	970	800	1000
Other vegetables	200	Iron (mg)	27.2	26	21	27
Roots & Tubers (excluding Potatoes)	100	Zinc (mg)	13.1	12.8	12	14.5
Fruits	150	Magnesium (mg)	786	747	370	440
Milk	400	Vitamin A (μg)*	1821	1818	406	900
Fats & Oils	25	β-carotene (μg)	9634	9597	–	–
Oil seeds & Nuts (gingely seeds & Pea nuts)	40	Thiamine (mg)	1.64	1.6	1.6	2
		Riboflavin (mg)	1.8	1.84	2.3	2.7
Spices	10	Niacin (mg)	16	16.7	14	16
		Vitamin B_6 (mg)	2	2	1.9	2.3
		Vitamin C (mg)	210	210	65	80
		Total Folates (μg)	484	447	480	570
		Vitamin B_{12} (μg)	2	2.4	2.2	2.5

Note: Total protein from the above diet = 78.8g, Digestible protein = 70g, PDCAAS = 88%
[1]Pulses can be replaced with animal foods (egg, meat, fish and chicken) for non-vegetarians.
*Retinol derived from β carotene from diet was also added to the total Vitamin A.
For cereals and millets, it is recommended to consume 50% as whole grains.
Source: "ICMR-NIN Expert Group on Nutrient Requirement for Indians, Recommended Dietary Allowances (RDA) and Estimated Average Requirements (EAR) – 2020".

Table 20.7 Focused Patient Assessment

Factors to Assess	Questions	Physical Assessment
Food and nutrient intake	How many meals and snacks a day do you eat? What times do you normally eat meals and snacks? What portion sizes do you eat at each meal? Are you on a special diet because of a health problem? Who purchases and prepares the food?	Observe percentage of food consumed from meal tray. Inspect condition of skin, hair, and nails. Inspect oral cavity for signs of malnutrition such as cheilosis, stomatitis, and dry lesions at corners of mouth.
Patterns and dietary history	Which types of food do you like? Are you allergic to any foods? What type of problems do you have with these foods? Have you noticed any changes in taste? Do you have any problems with chewing or swallowing?	Observe patient swallowing. Inspect oral cavity for physical barriers to eating (e.g., tooth decay, poor-fitting dentures).
Changes in weight	Has your appetite changed? What is your normal weight? Have you noticed a change in your weight? Was this change anticipated (e.g., were you on a weight-reduction diet)? Over what period of time did your weight change?	Weigh the patient and analyze for changes. Observe the patient's muscle tone.
Skin	Have you noticed any changes in your skin such as scaliness, dryness, rashes, or bruising? Do you use skin moisturizers regularly?	Observe skin for color, moisture, changes in pigment, or bruising. Assess skin turgor.

day, to determine a typical eating pattern and whether routine intake meets nutrient dietary reference intakes (DRIs).

Medication History

Prescribed and over-the-counter medications have the potential for drug–nutrient interactions. Consultation with a pharmacist determines the specific risks for nutrient–drug interactions for your patients.

Older Adult Considerations

Multiple age-related factors may affect nutrition status in older adults. The presence of chronic illness, anorexia, slowed digestion and peristalsis, decreased physical and cognitive function, ability to feed self, medication side effects, loss of dentition, and **xerostomia** all may contribute to development of malnutrition.

The Mini Nutritional Assessment (MNA) is a nutrition screening tool developed specifically for adults older than 65 years. It is a more sensitive tool than other universal tools such as the MUST in the geriatric population for early identification of malnutrition or risk for malnutrition (Donini et al., 2016).

Patients at Risk for Nutritional Problems

Assess patients for conditions that may interfere with the ability to ingest, digest, or absorb adequate nutrients. Use a

BOX 20.2 Diet History

A trained nutrition professional interviews the patient about the number and timing of meals and snacks eaten per day, the patient's appetite and food dislikes, the presence or absence of gastrointestinal distress, the use of dietary supplements (vitamins, minerals, and herbal products), and other lifestyle choices. A trained interviewer can assess usual nutrient intake, seasonal changes in food choices, and data about all nutrients consumed.

Other information contained in a diet history includes the following:

- Specific foods consumed for breakfast, lunch, dinner, and snacks
- Food preferences, allergies, and aversions
- Use of enteral or parenteral nutrition
- Dietary restrictions or medically prescribed and/or modified-consistency diets
- Use of weight-reduction, vegetarian, macrobiotic, vegan, fad, or other diets
- Foods that cause indigestion, diarrhea, or gas
- Impact of any functional disabilities or limitations (e.g., food shopping, preparation, self-feeding, socioeconomic limitations)
- Potential drug–nutrient interactions including drug dose and treatment duration
- Chewing or swallowing difficulties (e.g., use of dentures, dysphagia, xerostomia, mucositis, mouth sores, tooth decay)
- Usual bowel movements; presence and duration of constipation or diarrhea
- Symptoms of malabsorption such as clay-colored or frequent fatty stools
- Weight history including percentage of weight lost over period of time lost

standardized tool to assess nutritional risks when possible. Congenital anomalies and surgical revisions of the GI tract interfere with normal function. Patients receiving only i.v. infusions of 5%–10% dextrose are at risk for nutrient deficiencies. Older adults, infants, and patients who are malnourished are at the greatest risk.

Physical Examination

Examine a patient for signs of actual or potential nutrition complications (Table 20.8). You can conduct a portion of the examination while performing or assisting the patient with hygiene. The skin and hair are primary areas that reflect nutrient and hydration deficiencies. Be alert for rashes; dry, scaly skin; poor skin turgor; skin lesions; hair loss; easily pluckable hair; hair without luster; and excessively dry or scaly scalp.

Anthropometry

Anthropometry is a systematic measurement of the size and makeup of the body using height and weight as the principal measures. Height and weight measurements typically are obtained during a patient's admission to any health care setting. If a patient is unable to stand, estimate height by measuring the patient's length with a tape measure while the patient lies supine. Assess weight with bed scales, and then compare height and weight with usual measurements, called *usual body weight (UBW)*, and standard norms for normal height–weight relationships, called **IBW**. Serial measures of weight over time provide more useful information than one measurement. When collecting serial measurements of weight, weigh a patient at about the same time each day, on the same scale, and with the same amount of clothing. Unintentional changes in body weight indicate a risk factor for malnutrition. Refer patients who have lost 5% or more of their body weight in 1 month or 10% or more of their body weight over any amount of time for unknown reasons to an RDN for a nutrition evaluation.

Laboratory Values

No single laboratory or biochemical test is diagnostic for malnutrition. Factors that frequently alter test results include fluid balance, liver function, kidney function, and the presence of disease. Laboratory values useful in nutrition assessment include complete blood count, albumin, prealbumin, electrolytes, blood urea nitrogen (BUN), 24-hour urine urea nitrogen (UUN), creatinine, glucose, cholesterol, and triglycerides. Individual laboratory measures alone are not specific enough to indicate nutritional risk; therefore, they are combined with multiple objective measures to determine malnutrition risk. A low red blood cell count and low hemoglobin value indicate anemia. Hemoglobin, hematocrit, electrolyte, and BUN values also help to reflect the state of hydration. Serum proteins such as prealbumin and albumin levels are affected by acute inflammation, injury, and illness and are not sensitive to protein or energy deprivation until the point of overt starvation (e.g., BMI less than 12 kg/m^2) in an otherwise healthy individual (Lee et al., 2015). Thus, albumin and prealbumin levels should not be used alone as indicators of nutrition status. Nitrogen balance, which is measured through laboratory analysis of 24-hour UUN, is important to establish adequacy of protein and calorie intake.

Dysphagia Screening

Dysphagia screening quickly identifies problems with swallowing so that you can refer at-risk patients for a more in-depth assessment (see Skill 20.1). It includes medical record review and observation of a patient at a meal for change in voice quality, posture, and head control; percentage of meal consumed; eating time; drooling of liquids and solids; cough during and/or after a swallow; facial or tongue weakness; difficulty with secretions; pocketing; and presence of voluntary and dry cough. Bedside screening tools are designed for multidisciplinary use by RNs, RDNs, physicians, or speech-language pathologists (SLPs). However, the gold standard for diagnosis is videofluoroscopy because current bedside assessment protocols are not sufficiently sensitive (O'Horo et al., 2015). Refer at-risk patients to the SLP. The SLP administers trials of several consistencies of foods and fluids to obtain a comprehensive assessment of a patient's phases of swallowing to determine the degree of dysfunction and aspiration risk.

Therapeutic Diets

It is common for oral intake to decrease during periods of stress and acute illness. This occurs because of the anorexic effects of stress-induced hormones. It is important to monitor a patient's nutrient intake, identify influences that

Table 20.8 Physical Signs of Nutrition Status

Body Area	Indicators of Malnutrition
General appearance	Easily fatigued, no energy, falls asleep easily, looks tired, apathetic, cachectic
Weight	Overweight, obese, or underweight (special concern for underweight); unplanned weight loss over period of time
Posture	Poor posture, sagging shoulders, sunken chest, humped back
Muscles	Flaccid, weak, poor tone, tender; "wasted" appearance; impaired mobility
Mental status	Inattentive, irritable, confused
Neurological function	Burning and tingling of hands and feet (paresthesia), loss of position and vibratory sense, decrease or loss of ankle and knee reflexes
Gastrointestinal function	Anorexia, indigestion, constipation or diarrhea, symptoms of malabsorption, liver or spleen enlargement, abdominal distention
Cardiovascular function	Tachycardia, abnormal rhythm, elevated blood pressure
Hair	Stringy, dull, brittle, dry, thin and sparse, depigmented
Skin (general)	Rough, dry, scaly, pale, pigmented, irritated; bruises; petechiae
Face and neck	Swollen; skin dark over cheeks and under eyes
Lips	Dry, scaly, swollen; redness and swelling at corners of mouth (cheilosis); angular lesions at corners of mouth; fissures or scars (stomatitis)
Mouth, oral mucous membranes	Swollen, deep red oral mucous membranes; oral lesions
Gums	Spongy, bleed easily, inflamed, receding
Tongue	Swollen, scarlet and raw, magenta color, beefy (glossitis)
Teeth	Missing teeth, broken teeth
Eyes	Eye membranes pale (pale conjunctivae), redness of membrane (conjunctival injection), dryness or infection
Nails	Spoon-shaped (koilonychia), brittle, ridged
Legs and feet	Edema, tender calf, tingling, weakness, lesions
Skeleton	Bowlegs, knock-knees, chest deformity at diaphragm, beaded ribs, prominent scapulae

Data from Jelliffe DB: The assessment of the nutritional status of the community, *WHO Monograph No. 53*, Geneva, 1966; Clinical Assessment of Nutritional Status. Am J Public Health. 1973 Nov;63(11 Suppl):18–27; and Williams SR: Nutritional assessment and guidance in prenatal care. In Worthington-Roberts BS, Williams SR: *Nutrition in pregnancy and lactation*, ed 5, New York, 1993, McGraw-Hill.

reduce appetite, and plan interventions to manage stress and support nutrient needs.

Some patients have decreased intake in acute care settings because of diagnostic testing. Some blood and radiographic studies require a patient to receive nothing by mouth (NPO) until testing is completed. This disrupts mealtimes, and sometimes patients must wait for extended periods of time to eat or experience discomfort related to the test. Continue to assess a patient's nutrition status. Nutritional support is recommended when patients are NPO and receive only standard i.v. fluids for more than 5–7 days.

Emotional stress also influences food intake. Patients who are worried about their families, finances, employment, or illness are not always able to eat or eat well enough to compensate for the effect of stress on metabolism.

Medications may also affect dietary intake and in some cases the body's use of nutrients. Some medications cause reduced appetite, slowed motility and constipation, anorexia, or malabsorption. For example, opioids (e.g., morphine sulfate, codeine) used for pain relief usually cause constipation. Medication-induced and condition-related nausea, vomiting, and diarrhea have a significant impact on nutrient intake. This is common with chemotherapy for cancer treatment. Taste changes often occur with chemotherapy, diuretics, and mineral preparations such as zinc. Work with an RDN to help a patient select foods that are tolerated and do not worsen the nausea or other symptoms. Sometimes medications need to be provided to decrease nausea or pain, and other medications can be changed or their administration dose or timing altered.

Symptoms associated with illness often have a major effect on appetite. Pain, nausea, and shortness of breath make it difficult for patients to chew, swallow, and tolerate stomach filling. Patients may refuse to eat to avoid discomfort. Patients who are ill, have had surgery, or have been NPO for a long period of time often have specialized dietary needs. The lack of taste in low-sodium or low-fat diets may lead to reduced dietary intake or reduced compliance. In this situation, you need to consider the benefits associated with the **therapeutic diet** against the detrimental effects of weight loss and malnutrition. Table 20.9 describes commonly prescribed diets for patients in health care settings.

Food presentation also affects appetite. Hot foods that are cold or cold foods that are warm are not appetizing. Overcooked or undercooked foods are generally unappealing. A meal tray balanced on a crowded, soiled overbed table does not support an appetite. Removing the tray lid outside of a patient's room helps to decrease distress in patients who are sensitive to odors (e.g., patients with nausea). Support your patient's appetite through environmental adaptations, meal scheduling, attention to food preferences and patient symptoms, consultation with an RDN, and patient and family counseling.

Medical Nutrition Therapy

Optimal nutrition is important. Optimal nutrition is patient-centered and individualized. **Medical nutrition therapy (MNT)** is the diagnosis, therapy, and counseling services provided by an RDN for disease management. Patients with specific diseases often need to modify their diet to achieve balanced nutrition. These include GI diseases such as irritable bowel syndrome and malabsorption syndromes, metabolic

Table 20.9 Therapeutic Diets

Diet	Description
Clear liquid	Broth, bouillon, coffee, tea, carbonated beverages, clear fruit juices, gelatin, popsicles
Full liquid	As for clear liquid with addition of smooth-textured dairy products (e.g., ice cream, yogurt drinks, milk), custards, very thin refined cooked cereals, vegetable juice, pureed vegetables, all fruit juices
Mechanical soft	As for full liquid with addition of ground or finely diced meats, flaked fish, cottage cheese, cheese, rice, potatoes, pancakes, light breads, cooked vegetables, cooked or canned fruits, bananas, soups, peanut butter
Fiber-restricted	Addition of easily digested foods such as pastas, casseroles, tender well-cooked meats (without added fat), and canned or cooked fruits and vegetables (without skin); desserts, cakes, cookies without nuts or coconut
High fiber	Addition of fresh uncooked fruits, steamed vegetables, bran, oatmeal, dried fruits
Low sodium	4-g, 2-g, 1-g, or 500-mg sodium diets; vary from no added salt (4-g sodium diet) to severe sodium restriction (500-mg sodium diet) that requires selective food purchases
Low cholesterol	300 mg/day or less cholesterol, in keeping with American Heart Association guidelines for serum lipid reduction
Diabetic	Nutrition recommendations by American Diabetes Association: focus on total energy and balanced intake of carbohydrates from fruits, vegetables, whole grains, legumes, and low-fat milk; fats; and proteins; caloric recommendations vary to accommodate the patients' metabolic demands
Gluten-free	Eliminates wheat, barley, rye, and their derivatives
Dysphagia diet	*National Dysphagia Diet* has three stages depending on the patient's swallowing capacity; foods included vary according to stage
Regular	No restrictions unless specified

disorders such as diabetes mellitus (DM) and hypoglycemia, cardiovascular disease, renal disease, liver disease, and cancer. Diet modifications need to correspond with the body's ability to metabolize certain nutrients, correct nutritional deficiencies, and eliminate harmful foods from the diet. Always work with the health care provider and RDN when planning and implementing modified diets. MNT includes the four steps of the nutrition care process: nutrition assessment, nutrition diagnosis, nutrition intervention, and nutrition monitoring and evaluation (AND, 2016).

Diet in Gastrointestinal Diseases

Control peptic ulcers with regular meals and medications such as histamine receptor antagonists that block secretion of HCl or proton pump inhibitors. Marshall and Warren first identified *Helicobacter pylori* in 1984. *H. pylori*, a bacterium that causes up to 85% of peptic ulcers, is confirmed by laboratory tests or a biopsy during endoscopy (Nix, 2012). Antibiotics treat and control the bacterial infection. Stress and overproduction of gastric HCl also irritate a preexisting ulcer. Encourage patients to avoid foods that increase stomach acidity and pain such as caffeine, decaffeinated coffee, frequent milk intake, citric acid juices, and certain seasonings (hot chili peppers, chili powder, black pepper). Discourage smoking, alcohol, aspirin, and nonsteroidal anti-inflammatory drugs (NSAIDs). Teach patients to eat a well-balanced, healthy diet; avoid eating large meals; and eat three regular meals (or several small meals) without snacks, especially at bedtime (Nix, 2012). Family members of the patient with *H. pylori* infection also need to be tested and, if indicated, treated.

Inflammatory bowel disease includes Crohn disease and idiopathic ulcerative colitis. Treatment of acute inflammatory bowel disease includes elemental diets (formula with the nutrients in their simplest form ready for absorption) or parenteral nutrition (PN) when symptoms such as diarrhea and weight loss are prevalent. In the chronic stage of the disease, a regular highly nourishing diet is appropriate. Vitamins and iron supplements are often required to correct or prevent anemia. Patients manage irritable bowel syndrome by increasing fiber, reducing fat, avoiding large meals, and avoiding lactose- or sorbitol-containing foods for susceptible individuals.

The treatment of **malabsorption** syndromes such as celiac disease includes a gluten-free diet. Gluten is present in wheat, rye, barley, and oats. Short bowel syndrome results from extensive resection of bowel, after which patients suffer from malabsorption caused by lack of intestinal surface area. These patients require lifetime feeding with either elemental enteral formulas or PN.

Diverticulitis is a condition that results from an inflammation of diverticula, which are abnormal but common pouchlike herniations that occur in the bowel lining. Nutritional treatment for diverticulitis includes a moderate- or low-residue diet until the infection subsides. Afterward, prescribing a high-fiber diet for chronic diverticula problems ensues.

Diet in Diabetes Mellitus

Type 1 DM requires both insulin and dietary restrictions for optimal control, with treatment beginning at diagnosis (ADA, 2012). By contrast, patients often control type 2 DM initially with exercise and diet therapy. If these measures prove ineffective, it is common to add oral medications. Insulin injections often follow if type 2 DM worsens or fails to respond to these initial interventions.

Individualize the diet according to a patient's age, build, weight, and activity level. Maintaining a prescribed carbohydrate intake is the key in diabetes management. The ADA recommends a diet that includes carbohydrates from fruits, vegetables, whole grains, legumes, and low-fat milk (American Dietetic Association, 2010). Monitoring carbohydrate consumption is a key strategy in achieving glycemic control (ADA, 2012). Limit saturated fat to less than 7% of the total calories and cholesterol intake to less than 200 mg/day. In addition, varieties of foods containing fiber are recommended. Patients are able to substitute sucrose-containing foods for carbohydrates but need to make sure to avoid excess energy intake. Patients with diabetes can eat sugar alcohols and nonnutritive sweeteners as long as they follow the recommended daily intake level (ADA, 2012). Patients with diabetes and normal renal function should continue to consume usual amounts of protein (15%–20% of energy) (ADA, 2012).

The goal of MNT treatment is to have glycemic levels that are normal or as close to normal as safely possible; lipid and lipoprotein profiles that decrease the risk of microvascular (e.g., renal and eye disease), cardiovascular, neurological, and peripheral vascular complications; and blood pressure in the normal or near-normal range (ADA, 2012). Be aware of signs and symptoms of hypoglycemia and hyperglycemia.

Diet in Cardiovascular Diseases

The goal of the American Heart Association (AHA) dietary guidelines (AHA, 2010) is to reduce risk factors for the development of hypertension and coronary artery disease. Diet therapy for reducing the risk of cardiovascular disease includes balancing calorie intake with exercise to maintain a healthy body weight; eating a diet high in fruits, vegetables, and whole-grain high-fiber foods; eating fish at least two times per week; and limiting food and beverages that are high in added sugar and salt. The AHA guidelines also recommend limiting saturated fat to less than 7%, trans fats to less than 1%, and cholesterol to less than 300 mg/day. To accomplish this goal, patients choose lean meats and vegetables, use fat-free dairy products, and limit intake of fats and sodium (Nix, 2012).

Diet in Cancer and Cancer Treatment

Malignant cells compete with normal cells for nutrients, increasing a patient's metabolic needs. Most cancer treatments cause nutritional problems. Patients with cancer often experience anorexia, nausea, vomiting, and taste distortions. The goal of nutrition therapy is to meet the increased metabolic needs of a patient (Nix, 2012). Malnutrition in cancer is associated with increased morbidity and mortality. Enhanced nutritional status often improves a patient's quality of life.

Radiation therapy destroys rapidly dividing malignant cells; however, normal rapidly dividing cells such as the epithelial lining of the GI tract are often affected. Radiation therapy causes anorexia, stomatitis, severe diarrhea, strictures of the intestine, and pain. Radiation treatment of the head and neck region causes taste and smell disturbances, decreased salivation, and dysphagia. Nutrition management of a patient with cancer focuses on maximizing intake of nutrients and fluids. Individualize diet choices to a patient's needs, symptoms, and situation (Nix, 2012). Use creative approaches to manage alterations in taste and smell. For example, patients with altered taste often prefer chilled foods or foods that are spicy. Encourage patients to eat small, frequent meals and snacks that are nutritious and easy to digest.

Diet in Human Immunodeficiency Virus/Acquired Immunodeficiency Syndrome

Patients with HIV/AIDS typically experience body wasting and severe weight loss related to anorexia, stomatitis, oral thrush infection, nausea, or recurrent vomiting, all resulting in inadequate intake. Factors associated with weight loss and malnutrition include severe diarrhea, GI malabsorption, and altered metabolism of nutrients. Systemic infection results in hypermetabolism from cytokine elevation. The medications that treat HIV infection often cause side effects that alter patients' nutritional status.

Restorative care of malnutrition resulting from AIDS focuses on maximizing kilocalories and nutrients. Diagnose and address each cause of nutritional depletion in the care plan. The progression of individually tailored nutrition support begins with administering oral, to enteral, and finally to parenteral. Good hand hygiene and food safety are essential because of a patient's reduced resistance to infection. For example, minimization of exposure to *Cryptosporidium* in drinking water, lakes, or swimming pools is important. Small, frequent, nutrient-dense meals that limit fatty and overly sweet foods are easier to tolerate. Patients benefit from eating cold foods and drier or saltier foods with fluid in between (Nix, 2012).

CARING PATIENT WITH DYSPHAGIA

Dysphagia refers to difficulty with swallowing. It occurs because of damage to muscles and nerves or physical obstruction (Box 20.3). Physiological consequences of dysphagia include dehydration, malnutrition, and pneumonia; other consequences include increased length of hospital stay, health care cost, morbidity, and mortality (Sura et al., 2012).

Signs of dysphagia include coughing during or after a swallow, difficulty or painful chewing or swallowing, change in voice, unintentional weight loss, frequent clearing of throat, and recurrent chest infections (i.e., pneumonia) (Malhi, 2016). Other signs are abnormal gag, delayed swallowing, incomplete oral clearance or pocketing, regurgitation,

BOX 20.3 Causes of Dysphagia[a]

Myogenic (Muscle)

- Aging-related changes
- Muscular dystrophy
- Myasthenia gravis
- Myopathy
- Polymyositis

Neurogenic (Nerve)

- Amyotrophic lateral sclerosis (Lou Gehrig disease)
- Cerebral palsy
- Diabetic neuropathy
- Guillain–Barré syndrome
- Huntington disease
- Multiple sclerosis
- Parkinson disease
- Stroke
- Traumatic brain injury

Obstructive

- Anterior mediastinal masses
- Benign peptic stricture
- Candidiasis
- Cervical spondylosis
- Head and neck cancer
- Inflammatory masses
- Lower esophageal ring
- Trauma/surgical resection

Others

- Connective tissue disorders
- Gastrointestinal or esophageal resection
- Rheumatological disorders
- Vagotomy

[a]This is not an exhaustive list. Other disorders may lead to dysphagia.

pharyngeal pooling, drooling, delayed or absent trigger of swallow, and inability to speak consistently. Patients with dysphagia do not always exhibit overt signs such as coughing when food enters the airway. *Silent aspiration*, or aspiration that occurs without a cough, is a common cause of complications.

Dysphagia often results in decreased food intake, which may then lead to malnutrition caused by inability to consume an adequate volume of food. Malnutrition resulting from inadequate protein, calorie, and micronutrient intake significantly slows down recovery. Early nurse-initiated screening with a dysphagia screening protocol improves patient outcome by reducing the risk for inpatient deaths and respiratory infections (Hines et al., 2016).

Dysphagia Diet Management

In October 2002, the American Dietetic Association (now known as the Academy of Nutrition and Dietetics) published the National Dysphagia Diet Task Force (NDDTF) *National Dysphagia Diet* (NDDTF, 2002). The *National Dysphagia Diet* provides guidelines and standard terminology for food and texture modifications. There are three levels of solid foods: dysphagia pureed, dysphagia mechanically altered, and dysphagia advanced. The four levels of liquid are thin liquids (low viscosity), nectar-like liquids (medium viscosity), honey-like liquids (viscosity of honey), and spoon-thick liquids (viscosity of pudding) (AND, 2016; NDDTF, 2002).

Thickened liquids are commonly prescribed to prevent aspiration pneumonia. However, thickening agents alter the flavor and texture qualities of food. The period of adjustment to new dietary restrictions and the rehabilitation period may reduce intake for long periods of time, subsequently reducing quality of life and further increasing the risk for malnutrition and dehydration, particularly in the elderly (Cichero, 2013; Swan et al., 2015; Takeuchi et al., 2014).

The specified thickness of a liquid depends on a patient's swallowing deficit. Always use foods and fluids with the appropriate viscosity as determined by the SLP. Thin fluids (e.g., water) are generally the most difficult to swallow properly. Read the label directions carefully when modifying liquids to prepare the desired thickness correctly. Instructions are not universal for all thickening agents. Excessive thickness also has consequences. The risk of postswallow residue in the pharynx will increase with high-viscosity liquids (Steele et al., 2015).

Before each meal, position the patient in a chair or raise the head of the bed to an upright, seated position (Malhi, 2016). Have the patient slightly flex the head to a chin-down position to help prevent aspiration. If a patient has unilateral weakness, teach the patient and caregiver to place food in the stronger side of the mouth. Feed a patient with dysphagia slowly, provide small bites, and allow the patient to chew thoroughly and swallow the bite before taking another. Frequently assess the patient's chewing and swallowing throughout the meal. Allow the patient time to empty the mouth after each spoonful, matching the speed of feeding to the patient's readiness. If the patient begins to cough or choke, remove the food immediately.

MEETING NUTRITIONAL NEEDS

Evidence-based guidelines help the RDN set goals and plan care for the patient who is unable to maintain adequate nutrition by the oral route. These guidelines focus on enhancing oral nutrition as a priority. To improve intake, modify food choices to increase the nutrient value of food ingested, manage symptoms, administer medication to relieve nausea or pain if it interferes with oral intake, adjust mealtimes, or help with the process of eating. When these interventions fail to improve voluntary oral intake or when oral intake is not deemed safe, enteral nutrition (EN) is considered to maintain adequate nutrition. PN is considered only when nutrition support via the GI tract is not physiologically possible, when the bowel must be rested, or when nutrient needs cannot otherwise be met. EN is preferred to PN because it maintains the structure and function of the gut and the gut-associated lymphoid tissue, prevents bacteria translocation, decreases the risk for infection, and is less expensive (AND, 2016; McClave et al., 2016). Work with the patient, family caregiver, and other health care team members to maintain adequate nutrition in the safest, most physiological, and most cost-effective manner possible.

Assisting Patients With Oral Feeding

Some patients are unable to feed themselves adequately because of the severity of their illness, fatigue, or debilitation of their condition. Improve patient feeding by carefully protecting their dignity and actively involving them in the eating process. Encourage the patient to eat a small amount of food at a comfortable pace when helping with feeding. Provide independence using adaptive devices (Fig. 20.2) or finger foods. Position the patient in a chair or high Fowler's position to improve swallowing and digestion. Allow the patient time to empty the mouth after every spoonful, attempting to match the speed of feeding to the patient's readiness. Encourage patients to direct the order in which they wish to eat food items. Mealtime is a good time to instruct patients and their families about a balanced diet and the selection of appropriate foods.

Patients with visual deficits also need special assistance. Patients with decreased vision are often able to feed themselves independently when they are given adequate information. Identify the food location on the plate as if it were a clock (e.g., meat at 9 o'clock and vegetable at 3 o'clock). Tell the patient where the beverages are located in relation to the plate. Be sure that other care providers set the meal tray and plate in the same manner. Patients with impaired vision may be more

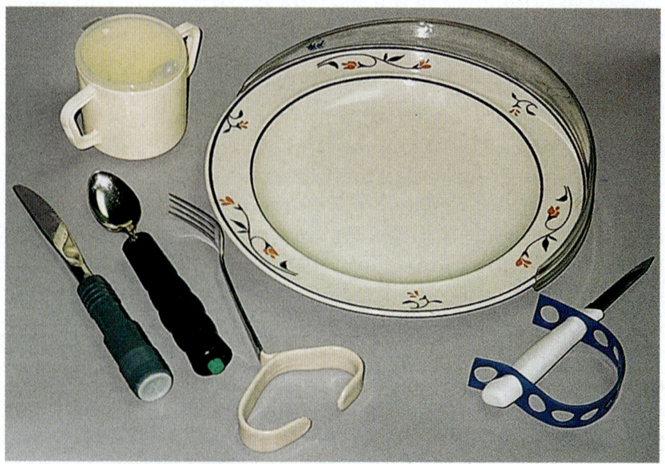

Fig. 20.2 Assistive devices for self-feeding.

independent during mealtimes with the use of large-handled adaptive utensils, which are easier to grip and manipulate.

Enteral Tube Feedings

EN refers to the use of the GI tract for the intake of nutrition. According to this definition, oral intake is also a form of EN. However, in a clinical setting, EN refers only to when nutrients and fluids are administered into the stomach or GI tract via a feeding tube. Nasogastric (NG) feedings are delivered through a feeding tube introduced through the nose and into the stomach. Nasointestinal feedings are delivered through a feeding tube inserted through the nose and passed through the stomach to the small intestine (duodenum or jejunum). When patients have nasopharyngeal obstructions or are not candidates for nasally placed tubes or when the need for EN is anticipated to be longer than 4–6 weeks, feeding tubes may be inserted directly into the stomach (gastrostomy) or jejunum (jejunostomy) (Table 20.10). A variety of enteral feeding formulas are available including products either with or without fiber. Special enteral formulas are designed to meet the nutrient needs of certain diseases (e.g., diabetes, kidney disease, hepatic failure). However, there is little evidence that supports the use of such formulas. The American Society for Parenteral and Enteral Nutrition (ASPEN) guidelines are to use standard polymetric formulas when initiating EN (McClave et al., 2016). When provided in amounts to meet a patient's protein and calorie needs, products will usually also meet the patient's DRIs for micronutrients. As a rule, enteral formulas do not meet most patients' needs for fluid. After accounting for water provided through tube flushes, additional water must be provided to meet hydration needs. Consult with an RDN to ensure that a patient's nutrient and fluid needs are met. The skills presented in this chapter focus on the administration of nutrition feedings directly into the GI tract with the goal of restoring and maintaining the patient's nutrition status.

Skill 20.2 describes insertion of a small-bore feeding tube. Feeding tubes are usually referred to as being nasally placed because that is the route most frequently used. The nose provides natural stability for tubes and it is the least invasive route. However, feeding tubes are sometimes placed orally if there has been trauma to the nose or if a patient already has an endotracheal tube placed in the mouth. Use the smallest gauge tube that is appropriate for a patient for comfort and to avoid irritation to the nasopharyngeal and esophageal mucosa. Occasionally, the large-bore tube, initially inserted for gastric decompression, is used to initiate enteral feeding because it is already in place. If feeding continues for more than a few days, consult with the health care provider about placing a softer small-bore feeding tube (Miller et al., 2014). For an adult, most of these tubes are 8–12 Fr and 43–55 inches long. A stylet is often used during insertion of a small-bore tube to stiffen it for placement purposes and then removed when the correct position of the tube is confirmed.

Initiating Tube Feedings

When making the decision regarding enteral access, the health care provider considers the patient's rate of gastric emptying, GI anatomy and functionality, risk for gastric reflux and aspiration, anticipated duration of requirement for enteral access, and disease state. The prolonged use of NG tubes is associated with inconvenience, discomfort, psychological stress, and displacement requiring reinsertion (Gomes et al., 2015). It is not recommended to use them for long-term enteral access (AND, 2016). Feeding tubes that end in the stomach are used for gravity bolus or continuous infusion feedings. The small intestine does not have the storage capability of the stomach, and therefore a tube feeding administered into the small intestine is delivered more slowly and continuously with an infusion pump.

Aspiration into the lung can occur from secretions or other material in the oral pharyngeal area, or it may occur as a result of reflux of gastric contents including tube feeding formula. Aspiration irritates the bronchial mucosa and provides growth material for pneumonia or other infections. Specific factors that increase a patient's risk for aspiration include neuromuscular or structural interference with swallowing (e.g., dysphagia, intubation), nasoenteric tubes (especially large-bore tubes), incorrectly placed feeding tube, inadequate nursing staff, delayed gastric emptying, vomiting, prolonged supine position, sedation, and advanced age (Elke et al., 2015). To reduce the risk of aspiration, keep the head of the bed elevated to a minimum of 30° and monitor tolerance to EN daily by physical

Table 20.10 Comparison of Enteral Feeding Tubes

Tube	Features	Nursing Considerations
Gastrostomy	Placed surgically (laparoscopic or open) with endoscope or fluoroscopy Held in place internally with balloon or semisolid "bolster"- or "bumper"-type end Uses external disc to prevent tube from migrating internally Uses low-profile tubes for patients who are conscientious of their body image or may be prone to pull at tube	Monitor external tube length as guide for placement. Internal migration can block pylorus, leading to gastric retention, patient discomfort, and emesis or large residual volumes. Check for tube tightness if the person gains weight or is bloated or distended. If external disc is too tight, circulation is restricted, and skin breakdown often occurs. Use small gauze dressing under external disc. It may be used for stomach decompression. Usual gastric returns are expected. If tube is placed high in stomach, repositioning the patient may help obtain returns. Use adapter for administration through low-profile tubes.
Jejunostomy	Placed surgically with endoscope or fluoroscopy Held in place by sutures, Dacron cuff, or small-volume balloon	Ability to use for gravity bolus feeding (meal-like feedings) is limited because jejunum lacks storage capacity of stomach. Monitor external tube length to watch for internal or external migration. High gastric-like residual volumes are not expected.
Gastrojejunostomy	Has gastric and small bowel ports Low-profile gastrojejunostomy tubes that have small bowel access may be used	Label port to be used for feeding and medications. Gastric port typically is used for decompression. Jejunal port is used for feeding. Monitor gastric returns. Gastric returns may indicate that jejunal port has flipped into stomach and is no longer appropriate for jejunal feeding.

examination, radiological evaluation, presence of abdominal distention, and patient-reported pain or discomfort (McClave et al., 2016). Most health care providers order measurement of gastric residual volume (GRV) every 4–6 hours in patients receiving continuous feedings and immediately before a feeding in patients receiving intermittent feedings. However, the amount of GRV in a patient's stomach is not a sensitive indicator of aspiration risk (McClave et al., 2016).

The Society for Critical Care Medicine and ASPEN made the following recommendations regarding GRV: (1) do not use GRV as part of routine care to monitor patients in the intensive care unit (ICU) receiving EN; (2) in cases where GRV is still used, evaluate the patient for aspiration, and use nursing measures to reduce the risk for aspiration if GRV is between 200 and 500 mL; and (3) do not withhold feedings when GRV is less than 500 mL and there are no other signs of EN intolerance (McClave et al., 2016). Inadequate nutrient delivery through EN is a significant problem, particularly in patients in the ICU, when feedings are stopped without proper evidence of intolerance.

Ensure that enteral feedings are correctly connected to an enteral feeding tube. The bedside method of testing feeding tube placement by injecting air into the tube while listening over the stomach with a stethoscope is ineffective and no longer used. The gold standard for determining tube location is X-ray confirmation. Monitor the tube location every 4 hours by assessing the color and pH of the gastric aspirate (Box 20.4), observe changes in the length of the tube that is external from the nose or abdomen, and review any available chest or abdominal X-ray reports for information about tube placement (American Association of Critical Care Nurses [AACN], 2016b).

Gastrostomy/Jejunostomy Tube Placement

When patients cannot tolerate nasally or orally placed tubes or when EN will be needed for more than several weeks, tubes may be placed into the GI tract through the abdomen. A surgeon inserts a gastrostomy tube through a small incision in the left upper quadrant of the stomach

BOX 20.4 Procedural Guidelines

Verifying Enteral Tube Placement by Obtaining Gastrointestinal Aspirate for pH Measurement via Large-Bore and Small-Bore Feeding Tubes: Intermittent and Continuous Feeding

Equipment

Sixty-milliliter ENfit syringe, stethoscope, clean gloves, pH indicator strip (scale of 1.0–11.0), small medication cup, water (tap water or sterile [see agency policy]) in a dated and initialed container at the patient's bedside

Steps

1. Identify the patient by using at least two identifiers (e.g., name and birthday or name and medical record number) according to agency policy.
2. Review agency policy and procedures for frequency and method of checking tube placement. *Do not insufflate air into tube to check placement.*
3. Observe for signs and symptoms of respiratory distress such as coughing, choking, or reduced oxygen saturation during feeding.
4. Identify conditions that increase risk for spontaneous tube migration or dislocation (e.g., altered level of consciousness or agitation, retching or vomiting, nasotracheal suction).
5. Observe external portion of tube for movement of ink or tape mark away from mouth or naris.
6. Review the patient's medication record for orders for continuous feeding or a gastric acid inhibitor (e.g., cimetidine [Tagamet], ranitidine [Zantac], famotidine [Pepcid AC], nizatidine [Axid]) or a proton pump inhibitor (e.g., omeprazole [Prilosec]).
7. Review the patient's medical record for history of prior tube displacement.
8. Explain procedure to the patient and/or family caregivers.
9. Prepare equipment at the patient's bedside, perform hand hygiene, and apply clean gloves.
10. Verify tube placement at the following times:
    a. For intermittently tube-fed patients, test placement immediately before each feeding (usually a period of at least 4 h will have elapsed since previous feeding) and before medications (AACN, 2016b).
    b. Follow agency policy regarding when to test pH for patients receiving continuous tube feeding. Tube feedings should never be stopped exclusively for the purpose of pH testing (AACN, 2016b). If feedings have been interrupted for more than a few hours, testing of the pH at this time may be useful in distinguishing placement (Bourgault et al., 2015).
    c. Wait to verify placement at least 1 h after medication administration by tube or mouth.
11. *Continuous feeding:* Turn off or place feeding on hold. Clamp or kink feeding tube and disconnect from nasogastric (NG) or nasointestinal (NI) tube. *Intermittent feedings:* Remove plug at end of tube. Draw up 30 mL of air into a 60-mL ENFit syringe. Place tip of syringe into end of NG or NI tube. Flush NG or NI tube with 30 mL of air before attempting to aspirate fluid. Repositioning the patient from side to side is helpful. In some cases, more than one bolus of air is necessary.
12. Draw back on syringe slowly and obtain 5–10 mL of gastric aspirate. Observe appearance of aspirate (see illustration). Aspirates from NG tubes of continuously tube-fed patients often look like curdled enteral formula. During fasting, gastric aspirates from tube-fed patients are typically grassy green or clear. Small bowel fluid is often bile stained. If gastric aspirates are bile stained, it may indicate that intestinal fluid has refluxed into the stomach (AACN, 2016b).
13. Gently mix aspirate in syringe. Expel a few drops into clean medicine cup. Measure pH of aspirated gastrointestinal contents by dipping pH strip into fluid or by applying a few drops of fluid to strip. Compare color of strip with color on chart (see illustration) provided by manufacturer.
    a. Gastric fluid from a patient who has fasted for at least 4 h usually has pH range of 5.0 or less.
    b. Fluid from tube in small intestine of a fasting patient usually has pH greater than 6.0.
14. Consider the use of radiographic confirmation of tube if the bedside techniques used raise doubt about the location of the tube (AACN, 2016b).
15. Irrigate tube.
16. Remove and dispose of gloves and supplies in appropriate receptacle. Perform hand hygiene.
17. Observe the patient for signs of respiratory distress including persistent gagging, paroxysms of coughing, drop in oxygen saturation, and respiratory patterns (e.g., rate and depth) that are inconsistent with baseline measures.
18. Verify that external length of tube, pH, and appearance of aspirate are consistent with initial tube placement.

BOX 20.4 Procedural Guidelines—cont'd

19. Use the principles of teach-back to evaluate patient/family caregiver learning. To determine that the patient and family understand about tube placement confirmation, state, "I want to make sure you understand what I explained earlier. Tell me why it is important for me to test gastric pH and the color of the gastric secretions before feedings."

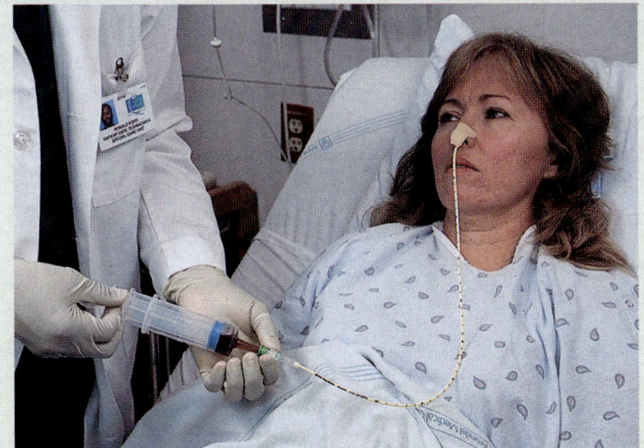

Step 12 Obtain gastric aspirate.

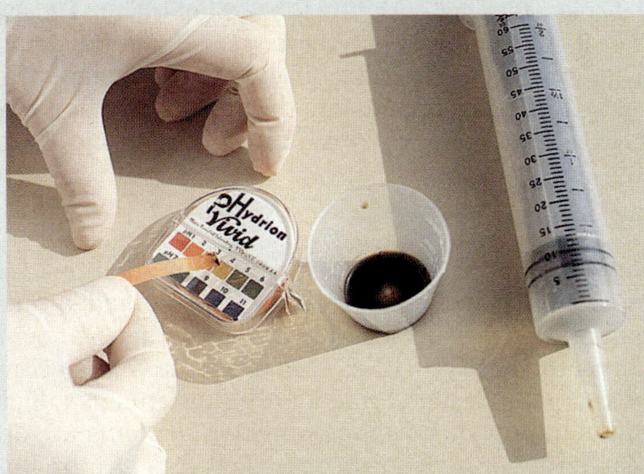

Step 13 Compare color on test strip with color on pH chart.

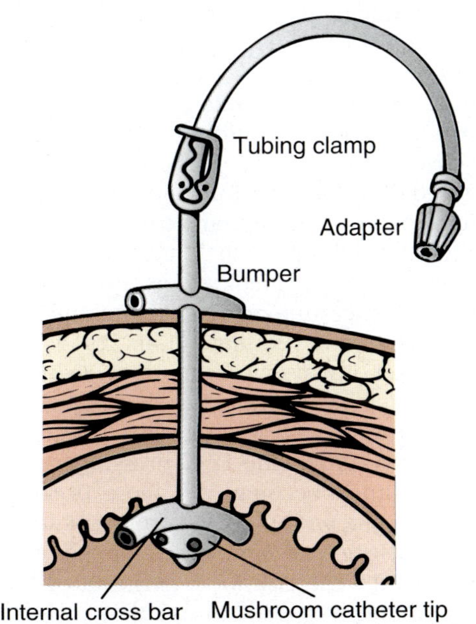

Fig. 20.3 Percutaneous endoscopic gastrostomy tube.

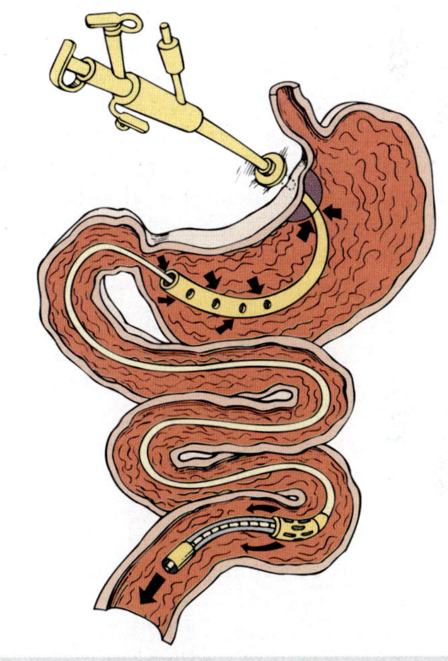

Fig. 20.4 Endoscopic insertion of jejunostomy tube.

either laparoscopically or with an open surgical technique. The tube is held in place internally by a balloon, pigtail design, or other design. A *percutaneous endoscopic gastrostomy (PEG) tube* is placed with an endoscope. The design of the PEG tube holds it in place (Fig. 20.3). You administer feedings into the stomach via a gastrostomy tube using gravity bolus in small volumes or continuously by a slow infusion. Because gastrostomy tubes provide more options for feeding delivery and thus more freedom and flexibility for patients, they are used for longer term feeding instead of jejunal tubes when possible (AND, 2016; Boullata et al., 2017).

When patients have delayed gastric emptying or gastric resection or other surgery in the upper GI tract such as a pancreatectomy, a **jejunostomy tube** may be inserted to deliver nutrition (see Skill 20.3). Feedings delivered via a jejunostomy tube are usually delivered even more slowly (e.g., over a period of hours overnight) because the jejunum lacks the storage and regulated emptying capacity of the stomach. Jejunostomy tubes are inserted either directly into the small intestine through a percutaneous incision or through a gastrostomy opening into the small intestine. Gastrojejunostomy tubes provide access to both the stomach and the small intestine. The gastric port may be used for decompression of accumulated stomach content while feeding is delivered into the jejunal port (Fig. 20.4). You need to know which port is gastric and which port is jejunal.

It is important to prevent and monitor for feeding tube displacement. Gastrostomy tubes that migrate internally sometimes block the pylorus or exit from the stomach to the small intestine. This results in increased GRV, discomfort, emesis, or leaking around the tube. An external disk helps prevent migration of a gastrostomy tube. Tubes that are too tight impair circulation between the external disc and the insertion site and quickly lead to breakdown of the site. Perform site care and assess the insertion site daily. Daily cleaning and evaluation of the site detects problems. Prevent displacement of a feeding tube by taping it to the abdomen or tucking it into clothing for security as indicated or applying an abdominal binder if necessary. Displaced tubes can lead to infusion of fluid into the peritoneal space, which leads to serious complications (check agency policy).

Parenteral Nutrition

Parenteral nutrition (PN) administers a solution of glucose, amino acids, minerals, electrolytes, and vitamins through a peripherally inserted venous catheter or central venous catheter (CVC). PN is used when the GI tract cannot be used or cannot digest and absorb nutrients in sufficient amounts to provide adequate nutrition. Patients are at an increased risk for infection because PN requires intravascular access and because of the high concentration of glucose in PN solutions. Patients on PN do not experience the many physiological benefits from being fed from the GI tract. PN is also significantly more costly than EN. The health care team evaluates the need for PN on a daily basis. The goal is to discontinue PN as soon as the patient can tolerate greater than 60% of energy needs enterally (McClave et al., 2016).

PN solutions that contain 10% or greater dextrose are hyperosmolar (i.e., highly concentrated) and irritate small peripheral veins. As a result, PN at this concentration is administered through CVCs where the blood flow is very rapid. This is called *central PN*. PN solutions with osmolality less than 900 mOsm may be administered through peripheral veins. Peripheral PN is usually used only for a short period (10–14 days or less) because it is still irritating to the blood vessels. In addition, it is challenging to meet a patient's nutritional needs with less concentrated solutions. A PN solution meets a patient's specific nutritional needs and is adjusted based on a patient's laboratory values and metabolic and nutrition status. Some PN solutions contain fat emulsions (lipids) with concentrations ranging from 10% to 30%. They are mostly composed of omega-6 fatty acids.

Fat emulsions can be combined with the other nutrients in a PN prescription to make a total nutrient admixture (TNA), or they can be provided in a separate bag via i.v. piggyback. Do not administer TNA if you observe oil droplets or an oily or creamy layer on the surface of the solution. Administer lipid emulsions peripherally or via a larger blood vessel (centrally).

Initiating Parenteral Nutrition

PN therapy requires a CVC inserted into the superior vena cava via the subclavian vein or, less ideally, the jugular vein. PN can also be administered via a peripherally inserted central catheter (PICC). Nurses assist physicians during CVC insertion. Specially trained nurses insert PICCs (see agency policy and Chapter 25) (DiMaria-Ghalili et al., 2016). A chest X-ray confirms the location of the CVC after initial placement and when misplacement is suspected. Some patients needing long-term PN have a central venous access device (CVAD) such as a tunneled catheter or an implanted port. When administering PN, be sure that the formula ordered is being delivered into a catheter or CVAD that terminates in the appropriate position. Thus, you need to assess for catheter displacement.

Before beginning an infusion, inspect the solution and check the contents carefully to make sure that it is formulated according to the health care provider order. Administer the solution at the prescribed rate using an infusion pump. PN is usually started at a lower rate (e.g., 40–60 mL/h) and advanced to meet the patient's goal rate as tolerance is demonstrated (generally within 72–96 hours of PN initiation). Reactions to lipid infusion include dyspnea, cyanosis, vomiting, headache, and chest pain. If a reaction occurs, stop the infusion and notify the health care provider immediately.

Caring for the Patient Receiving Parenteral Nutrition

Nursing care for the patient receiving PN focuses on seven major nursing goals: (1) preventing infection; (2) maintaining the PN system; (3) preventing metabolic, electrolyte, or fluid balance complications; (4) ensuring that the patient's nutrient and fluid needs are being met; (5) evaluating the continued need for PN or if oral intake or EN may be initiated; (6) planning for home PN if this is indicated; and (7) supporting the patient and family during major lifestyle changes.

Infection prevention includes strict aseptic management of the catheter hub, proper care of the CVC and dressing, maintaining policy recommendations for frequency of tubing and filter changes, and minimizing manipulation of the catheter (Ayers et al., 2014). Make sure that PN solutions do not exceed their 24-hour infusion limit. If you are using a CVC that has multiple lumens, use a port that is exclusively dedicated for the PN. Label the port for PN, and do not infuse other solutions or medications through the port, unless clinical evidence supports the compatibility and stability of the combination (Boullata et al., 2014). During CVC dressing changes, always wear a mask to reduce the risk of introducing airborne contaminants. Assess the insertion site for signs of infection. Wear sterile gloves if you need to touch the site. Change the CVC dressing per institution policy and anytime it becomes wet, loose, or contaminated. Chlorhexidine gluconate (CHG)–impregnated dressings and cleaning solutions are preferred for skin antisepsis because they reduce the risk for CVAD-related bloodstream infections (Ullman et al., 2016). Scrub the catheter hub or port with 70% alcohol solution, tincture of iodine, or CHG using friction every time the system is entered. An in-line 0.22-mcg filter is typically used to remove air and particulate matter such as bacteria. Because fat molecules are large, you need to bypass the filter or use a larger filter (0.5 mcg) if a patient is receiving a fat emulsion.

Closely assess patients receiving PN for tolerance, the need for adjustments to the solution, and efficacy of the nutrition provided. Analyze laboratory findings for metabolic or electrolyte abnormalities and assess fluid balance, weight trends, and the ability to heal during administration. Laboratory monitoring includes frequent blood glucose testing because the high dextrose (glucose) content of the solution easily leads to hyperglycemia. Some patients need supplemental insulin (Ayers et al., 2014). Stopping the high-dextrose solution suddenly often leads to hypoglycemia. To reduce the risk of hypoglycemia, taper the solution before it is discontinued, especially if the patient is not currently receiving another source of carbohydrate. Be alert for changes in vital signs, changes in fluid balance, and laboratory results that indicate osmotic diuresis and dehydration, infection (e.g., an increased temperature or white blood cell count), electrolyte imbalance or hyperglycemia, and clinical symptoms of high or low blood glucose. Report any unusual symptoms to the health care provider.

SAFETY GUIDELINES FOR NURSING SKILLS

Ensuring patient safety is an essential role of the nurse. To ensure patient safety, communicate clearly with members of the health care team, assess and incorporate the patient's priorities of care and preferences, and use the best evidence when making decisions about your patient's care. When performing the skills in this chapter, remember the following points to ensure safe, individualized care:

- Verify tube position and connector type (current or ENFit) at the beginning of each initial nursing assessment and before administration of feedings or medications and as needed (prn) (Boullata et al., 2017). The ENFit device will not be compatible with a Luer-Lock connection or any other type of small-bore medical connector, thus preventing misadministration of an enteral feeding (Institute for Safe Medication Practices [ISMP], 2015).
- Label enteral equipment with patient information, formula type, enteral access delivery site/access, administration method, individuals responsible for preparing and hanging the formula, and time and date formula is prepared and hung (Boullata et al., 2017).
- Ensure "right patient, right formula, right tube" by matching formula and rate to feeding order and verifying that enteral tubing set connects formula to feeding tube (see the ASPEN *Be ALERT* safety campaign for enteral feeding at www.nutritioncare.org).
- Elevate the head of the bed a minimum of 30–45° for patients receiving enteral feedings unless medically contraindicated (AACN, 2016a; McClave et al., 2016).
- Trace all lines and tubing back to the patient to ensure that you have only enteral-to-enteral connections and that they are secure (Boullata et al., 2017).
- Monitoring tube placement is essential in early detection of tube misplacement. Auscultation is not a reliable method for verification of NG or nasointestinal tube placement because a tube inadvertently placed in the lungs, pharynx, or esophagus transmits a sound similar to that of air entering the stomach (AACN, 2016b).
- Food safety is especially important in providing EN. Feeding products and equipment used to deliver them are good growth media for bacteria. Clean, dry, and store syringes as two pieces to prevent moisture accumulation. Keep other equipment clean and dry, and change according to agency protocol.
- Refer to manufacturer guidelines to determine hang time for enteral feedings. Maximum hang time for formula is 8 hours in an open system and 24 hours in a closed, ready-to-hang system (if it remains closed) (Boullata et al., 2017). There is increased risk for bacterial growth in feedings that exceed the recommended hang time.
- To prevent tube clogging, flush tube with at least 30 mL of water (for adults without volume restriction) following enteral feedings. Use freshly obtained tap water as the flush and fluid administration solution unless normal saline is ordered or agency protocol is to use sterile water for patients who are immunocompromised (Boullata et al., 2017).
- Use liquid medications whenever possible or crush and adequately dilute medications administered via the feeding tube. Do not mix medications. Flush tube with at least 15 mL of water before, between, and after each medication administration in adult patients without volume restriction (Boullata et al., 2017).
- Administer continuous EN and PN with an infusion pump.

SKILL 20.1 Aspiration Precautions

Equipment

- Chair or bed that allows the patient to sit upright
- Thickening agents as designated by speech-language pathologist (SLP)—rice, cereal, yogurt, gelatin, and commercial thickener
- Tongue blade
- Penlight
- Oral hygiene supplies
- Suction equipment
- Clean gloves

STEP	RATIONALE
Assessment	
1. Identify the patient by using at least two identifiers (e.g., name and birthday or name and medical record number) according to agency policy.	Ensures correct patient. Complies with The Joint Commission standards and improves patient safety (TJC, 2018).
2. Review results of nutrition screening in medical record.	Reveals risk patterns (e.g., patients with dysphagia may alter their eating patterns or choose foods that are easy to swallow but do not provide adequate nutrition).
3. Ask the patient or family caregiver whether the patient has difficulties with chewing or swallowing various food textures.	Patients are likely to aspirate certain foods more than others.
4. Assess for conditions that cause dysphagia and thus present risk for aspiration (see Box 20.3). Also assess signs and symptoms of dysphagia (e.g., coughing, voice change, food pocketing). Use dysphagia screening tool if available.	Patients with neurological or neuromuscular disease and patients with trauma to or surgery of the oral cavity or throat are at increased risk.

STEP	RATIONALE
5. Assess mental status including alertness, orientation, and ability to follow simple commands (e.g., open your mouth; stick out your tongue).	Dementia and cognitive impairment increase risk for dysphagia and aspiration (Rösler et al., 2015).
6. Assess the patient's oral cavity, level of dental hygiene, missing teeth, or poorly fitting dentures (apply clean gloves if needed).	Poor oral hygiene can result in decayed teeth, plaque, and periodontal disease; these increase the risk for aspiration and pneumonia in patients with dysphagia (Sørensen et al., 2013).
7. Observe the patient during mealtime for signs of dysphagia such as coughing, voice change, or fatigue. Observe the patient attempt to feed self; note type of food consistencies and liquids the patient is able to swallow.	Detects a change in eating habits or abnormal eating patterns that indicate a risk for dysphagia (AND, 2016; Hines et al., 2016; Malhi, 2016).
8. Indicate on the patient's electronic medical record (EMR), chart, or Kardex that dysphagia/aspiration risk is present. *Option:* Some agencies use different-colored meal trays to signify patients at risk for aspiration.	Identifying a patient as having dysphagia reduces the risk that the patient will receive improperly prepared oral nutrition without supervision.
9. Assess the patient and family caregiver knowledge of aspiration precautions.	Encourages cooperation, minimizes risks and anxiety, and identifies teaching needs.
Planning	
1. Provide the patient rest time before meals.	Some practitioners recommend rest time before meals (Metheny, 2012). Muscle weakness and fatigue may increase risk of aspiration.
2. Explain to the patient why you are observing him or her while eating.	Signs or symptoms associated with aspiration indicate need for further swallowing evaluation such as fluoroscopic examination.
3. Explain to the patient and family caregiver about the aspiration precautions you are implementing.	Increases patient cooperation and prepares family caregiver for being able to assist.
Implementation	
1. Perform hand hygiene and have the patient or family caregiver (if going to assist with feeding) perform hand hygiene.	Prevents transmission of microorganisms. Educates the patient and family caregiver about need to maintain infection control practices.
2. Apply clean gloves. Provide thorough oral hygiene including brushing of tongue before meal.	Intensified oral hygiene reduces risk for aspiration pneumonia (Sørensen et al., 2013).
3. Position the patient in chair or raise head of the bed to upright, seated position (45–90° angle or highest position allowed by medical condition during meal).	Upright position aids safe swallowing and helps prevent aspiration (AACN, 2016a; Malhi, 2016).
4. Using penlight and tongue blade, gently inspect mouth for pockets of food.	Pockets of food found inside the cheeks may indicate that a patient has difficulty moving food from mouth into the pharynx to swallow. Food pocketing because of impaired swallowing increases risk for aspiration (Jeng et al., 2001).
5. Add thickener to thin liquids to create desired consistency per SLP assessment.	For patients unable to safely control swallowing of thin liquids, thickening agents slow the process of swallowing and increase safety by helping to prevent aspiration (Newman et al., 2016).
6. Objectively measure viscosity of liquids to ensure consistency with recommendation by SLP.	Different thickening agents yield variable consistencies. Subjective measurements of viscosity are unreliable. Only thickening agents with reliable viscosity data should be used (Popa Nita et al., 2013).
7. Have the patient assume chin-tuck position. Remind the patient to not tilt head backward when eating or while drinking.	Hyperextension of neck makes it easier for food to enter airway. Chin-tuck or chin-down position reduces aspiration in some patients. Patients need a minimum of 17.5° of neck flexion to achieve a beneficial effect (Ra et al., 2014).
8. Provide tactile and temperature stimulation techniques if recommended by the SLP. Examples include increasing pressure on the tongue by a spoon during feeding and using cold utensils to stimulate oral cavity.	Provides tactile cue to food being eaten and may promote effective swallowing (Wirth et al., 2016).
9. Provide verbal coaching. Remind the patient to chew and think about swallowing: ■ "Open your mouth." ■ "Feel the food in your mouth." ■ "Chew and taste the food." ■ "Raise your tongue to the roof of your mouth." ■ "Think about swallowing." ■ "Close your mouth and swallow." ■ "Swallow again." ■ "Cough to clear your airway."	Verbal cueing and positive reinforcement help patients focus on steps of normal swallowing. Instructing patients to repeat-swallow or practice effortful swallowing may help clear remaining food from the airway (Park et al., 2016).

STEP	RATIONALE
10. Monitor swallowing and observe for throat clearing, coughing, choking, change in voice, and drooling of food; suction airway as needed.	Detects abnormal eating patterns that indicate a risk for aspiration from dysphagia (Hines et al., 2016; Malhi, 2016).
11. Minimize distractions and do not rush the patient through a meal. Allow time for adequate chewing and swallowing. Provide rest period as needed during meal.	Environmental distractions and conversations during mealtime may increase the risk for aspiration.
12. Ask the patient to remain sitting upright for at least 30–60 min after meal.	Allows additional time for food particles in pharynx to clear.
13. Provide thorough oral hygiene after meal.	Oral hygiene reduces plaque and secretions containing bacteria that can cause pneumonia (Sørensen et al., 2013).
14. Remove gloves if worn. Return the patient's tray to appropriate place and perform hand hygiene.	Reduces spread of microorganisms.
Evaluation	
1. Throughout meal, observe the patient's ability to swallow food and fluids of various textures and thickness without choking.	Indicates whether there is ease with swallowing and absence of signs related to aspiration. The ability to swallow safely may improve or deteriorate over time and within a single meal.
2. Monitor the patient's intake and output (I&O), calorie count, and food intake.	Aids in detection of malnutrition and dehydration resulting from dysphagia.
3. Weigh the patient daily or weekly.	Determines whether weight is stable and reflects nutrition status.
4. Observe the patient's oral cavity after meal.	Determines presence of food pockets after meal.
5. **Use teach back:** "We talked about why your loved one is at risk to aspirate food. Tell me the things to watch for that indicate trouble swallowing. What should you do if these things happen?" Revise your instruction now or develop a plan for revised patient/family caregiver teaching if the patient/family caregiver is not able to teach back correctly.	Determines the patient's/family caregiver's level of understanding of instructional topic.

Recording and Reporting

- Document in the patient's electronic health record (EHR) or chart assessment findings the patient's tolerance of liquids and food textures, amount of assistance required, position during meal, absence or presence of any symptoms of dysphagia during feeding or fluid intake, and total amount eaten.
- Document your evaluation of patient/family caregiver learning.
- Report any coughing, choking, voice changes, or other swallowing difficulties to health care provider.
- Communicate with other health care staff that the patient has dysphagia during hand-off communication.

Unexpected Outcomes and Related Interventions

- The patient coughs, gags, complains of food "stuck in throat," and has wet quality to voice when eating.
  - Stop feeding immediately and place the patient on NPO. Notify health care provider, and suction as needed.
  - Schedule consultation with SLP for swallowing exercises and techniques to improve swallowing.
- The patient experiences weight loss over next several days/weeks.
  - Discuss findings with health care provider and registered dietitian nutritionist (RDN). Determine whether increasing frequency or quality of foods is needed.
  - Nutritional supplements may be needed.

SKILL 20.2 Inserting a Nasogastric or Nasointestinal Feeding Tube

Equipment

Insertion

- Small-bore nasogastric (NG) or nasoenteric tube with or without stylet (select the smallest diameter possible to enhance patient comfort)
- Sixty-milliliter ENFit syringe
- Stethoscope, pulse oximeter, and capnography *(optional)*
- Hypoallergenic tape, semipermeable (transparent) dressing, or tube fixation device
- Tincture of benzoin or other skin barrier protectant
- pH indicator strip (scale 1.0–11.0)
- Cup of water and straw or ice chips (for patients able to swallow)
- Water-soluble lubricant
- Emesis basin
- Towel or disposable pad
- Facial tissues
- Clean gloves
- Suction equipment in case of aspiration
- Penlight to check placement in nasopharynx
- Tongue blade

Removal

- Disposable pad
- Tissues
- Clean gloves
- Disposable plastic bag
- Towel

STEP	RATIONALE
Assessment	
1. Identify the patient by using at least two identifiers (e.g., name and birthday or name and medical record number) according to agency policy.	Ensures correct patient. Complies with The Joint Commission standards and improves patient safety (TJC, 2018).
2. Verify health care provider's order for type of tube and enteric feeding schedule. Also check order to determine whether health care provider wants a prokinetic agent (e.g., metoclopramide) given before tube placement.	Health care provider's order is needed to insert a feeding tube. Prokinetic agent given before tube placement may help advance the tube into intestine.
3. Assess the patient's knowledge of procedure.	Encourages cooperation, reduces anxiety, and minimizes risks. Identifies teaching needs.
4. Perform hand hygiene.	Reduces transmission of microorganisms.
5. Have the patient close each nostril alternately and breathe. Examine each naris for patency and skin breakdown (apply clean gloves if drainage present).	Sometimes nares are obstructed or irritated, or a septal defect or facial fractures are present. Place tube in the most patent nostril.
6. Review the patient's medical history (e.g., for basilar skull fracture, nasal problems, nosebleeds, facial trauma, nasal-facial surgery, head or neck cancer, deviated septum, anticoagulant therapy, coagulopathy).	History of these problems may require you to consult with the health care provider to change route of nutrition support. Passage of tube intracranially can cause morbid complications (Miller et al., 2014).
Clinical decision point: If a patient is at risk of intracranial passage of the tube, avoid the nasal route. Oral placement or placement under medical supervision using fluoroscopic direct visualization is preferable. Insertion of a gastrostomy or jejunostomy tube is another alternative.	
7. Assess the patient's height, weight, hydration status, electrolyte balance, caloric needs, and I&O.	Provides baseline information to measure nutrition improvement and metabolic parameters after enteral feedings are instituted (Boullata et al., 2017).
8. Assess the patient's level of consciousness, presence of cough and gag reflex, ability to sit upright, obstructive or restrictive lung disease, and presence of mechanical ventilation.	These are risk factors for inadvertent tube placement into tracheobronchial tree (Sparks et al., 2011).
Clinical decision point: Recognize situations in which blind placement of a feeding tube poses an unacceptable risk for placement. Devices designed to detect pulmonary intubation such as carbon dioxide (CO_2) sensors or obtaining a radiograph enhances patient safety. To avoid insertion complications from blind placement in high-risk situations, clinicians trained in the use of radiographic confirmation should place tubes (AACN, 2016b).	
9. Perform physical assessment of abdomen. Perform hand hygiene, and remove and dispose of gloves (if worn).	Abdominal pain, tenderness, or distention may indicate medical problem that contraindicates feedings.
10. Assess the patient's and family caregiver's knowledge of procedure for NG feeding tube insertion.	Encourages cooperation, minimizes risks and anxiety, and identifies teaching needs.
Planning	
1. Provide privacy and prepare bedside environment for patient safety.	Preparing the environment helps the nurse think about the steps in the procedure; removing clutter from overbed or bedside table removes barriers to insertion.
2. Prepare and organize equipment needed for insertion of NG feeding tube.	Ensures an organized approach for insertion of NG feeding tube.
3. Explain procedure to the patient including sensations (e.g., discomfort or burning sensation in nasal passages) that will be felt during insertion.	Increases the patient's cooperation with tube insertion procedure and helps lessen anxiety.
4. Explain to the patient how to communicate during intubation by raising index finger to indicate gagging or discomfort.	The patient must have a way of communicating to alleviate stress and enhance cooperation.
Implementation	
1. Perform hand hygiene. Prepare supplies at bedside.	Reduces transmission of microorganisms. Ensures organized procedure.
2. Stand on same side of bed as naris chosen for insertion and position the patient upright in high Fowler's position (unless contraindicated). If the patient is unresponsive, raise head of bed as tolerated in semi-Fowler's position with head tipped forward, using a pillow chin to chest. If necessary, have an NAP help with positioning of confused or unresponsive patients. If the patient is forced to lie supine, place in reverse Trendelenburg position.	Allows for easier manipulation of tube. An upright position aids safe swallowing and helps prevent aspiration (AACN, 2016a; Malhi, 2016). Forward head position assists with closure of airway and passage of tube into esophagus.

STEP	RATIONALE
3. Apply pulse oximeter/capnograph and measure vital signs.	Provides baseline for objective assessment of respiratory status during tube insertion.
a. If the patient has an increase in end-tidal CO_2 or decrease in oxygen saturation, do not insert tube until you determine the patient's stability.	CO_2 detectors are helpful in detecting when the tube is placed in the tracheobronchial tree. However, X-ray confirmation of placement is necessary (AACN, 2016b).
4. Place bath towel over the patient's chest. Keep facial tissues within reach.	Prevents soiling of gown. Insertion of tube frequently produces tearing.
5. Determine length of tube to be inserted and mark location with tape or indelible ink.	
a. Measure distance from tip of nose to earlobe to xyphoid process of sternum (see illustration). Mark this distance on tube with tape.	Length approximates distance from nose to stomach. Tip of NG tube must reach stomach to avoid risk for pulmonary aspiration, which increases when tubes terminate in the esophagus (AACN, 2016a).
b. Measure distance from tip of nose to earlobe to midumbilicus for a pediatric patient.	
c. Add additional 20–30 cm (8–12 inches) for nasojejunal tubes.	Length approximates distance from nose to jejunum.
6. Prepare NG or nasojejunal tube for intubation. **Note:** Do not ice tubes.	Iced tube becomes stiff and inflexible, causing trauma to nasal mucosa.
a. Obtain order for stylet tube and check agency policy for trained clinician to insert tube.	
b. If tube has a guidewire or stylet, inject 10 mL of water from ENFit syringe into tube.	Activates lubrication of tube for easier passage and ensures that tube is patent. Aids in guidewire or stylet removal. ENFit devices are not compatible with any other type of small-bore medical connector, thus preventing inappropriate connections and misadministration of an enteral feeding (ISMP, 2015).
c. If using stylet, make certain that it is positioned securely within tube.	Promotes smooth passage of tube into gastrointestinal (GI) tract. Improperly positioned stylet can cause tube to kink or injure the patient. Once tube insertion is confirmed, have trained clinician remove stylet.
7. Prepare tube fixation materials. Cut hypoallergenic tape 10 cm (4 inches) long or prepare membrane dressing or other tube fixation device.	Used to secure tubing after insertion. Fixation devices allow tube to float free of the nares, thus reducing pressure on the nares and preventing medical device–related pressure injury.
8. Apply clean gloves.	Reduces transmission of microorganisms.
9. *Option:* Dip tube with surface lubricant into glass of room-temperature water or apply water-soluble lubricant (see manufacturer directions).	Activates lubricant to facilitate passage of tube into naris and GI tract.
10. Hand an alert patient a cup of water with straw (if able to swallow).	The patient is asked to swallow water to facilitate tube passage.
11. Explain the next steps and gently insert tube through nostril to back of throat (posterior nasopharynx). This may cause the patient to gag. Aim back and down toward ear (see illustration).	Natural contours facilitate passage of tube into GI tract.

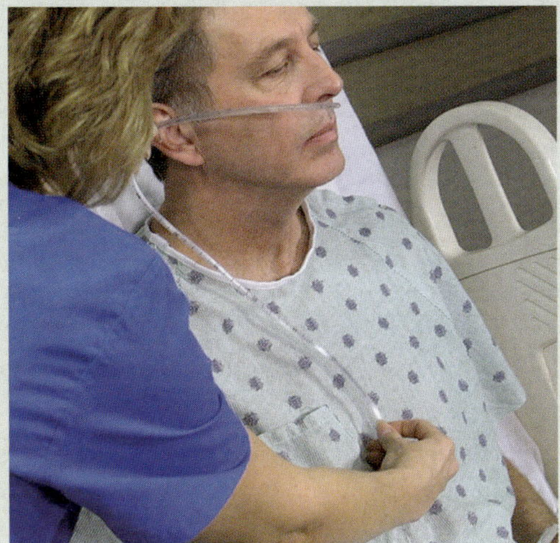

Step 5a Measure to determine length of tube to insert.

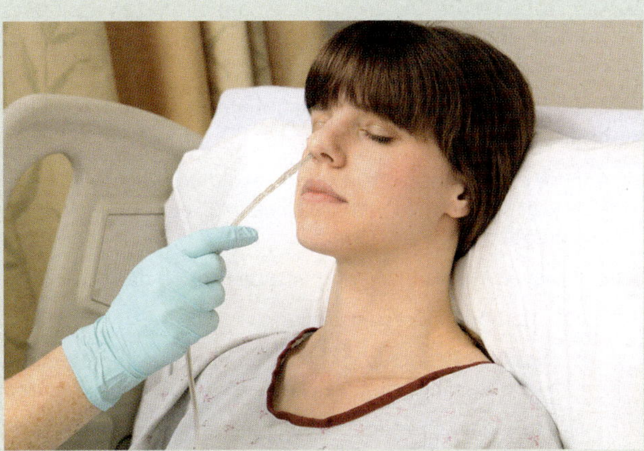

Step 11 Insert tube through nostril to back of throat.

STEP	RATIONALE

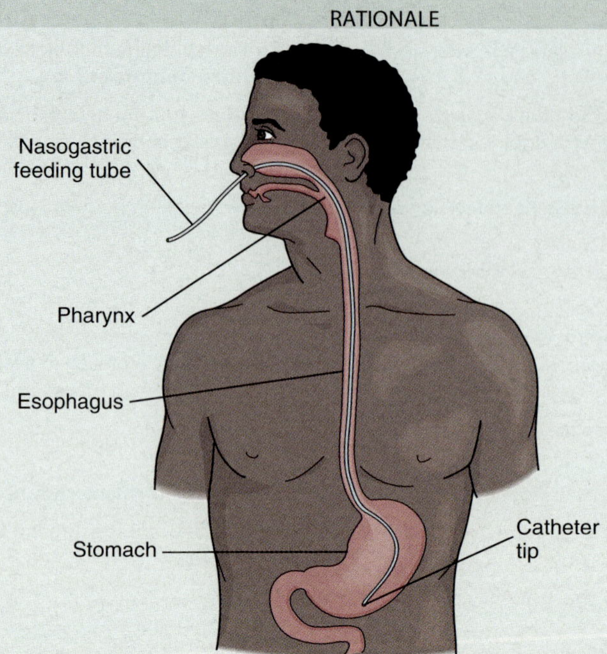

Step 16 Nasogastric tube inserted through nasopharynx and esophagus into stomach.

STEP	RATIONALE
12. Have the patient take a deep breath and relax and flex head toward chest after tube has passed through nasopharynx.	Closes off glottis and reduces risk for tube entering trachea.
13. Encourage the patient to swallow small sips of water. Advance tube as the patient swallows. Rotate tube gently 180° while inserting.	Swallowing facilitates passage of tube past oropharynx. Distinct tug may be felt as the patient swallows, indicating that tube is following expected path.
14. Emphasize need to breathe through mouth and swallow during insertion.	Helps facilitate passage of tube and decreases the patient's anxiety reaction during procedure.
15. Do not advance tube during inspiration or coughing because it is more likely to enter the respiratory tract. Monitor oximetry and capnography.	Can cause tube to inadvertently enter the patient's airway, which will be reflected in changes in oxygen saturation and/or capnography.
16. Advance tube each time the patient swallows until desired length has been reached (see illustration).	Reduces discomfort and trauma to the patient. Helps facilitate tube passage.

Clinical decision point: Do not force the tube or push against resistance. If the patient starts to cough, experiences a drop in oxygen saturation, or shows other signs of respiratory distress, withdraw the tube into posterior nasopharynx until normal breathing resumes.

STEP	RATIONALE
17. Check for position of tube in back of throat using penlight and tongue blade.	Tube may be coiled, kinked, or entering trachea.
18. Temporarily anchor tube to nose with small piece of tape.	Movement of tube stimulates gagging. Allows assessment of general position before anchoring tube more securely.
19. Keep tube secure and check placement of tube by aspirating stomach contents to measure gastric pH. Also, assess amount, color and quality of return.	Proper tube position is essential before initiating feeding. (Confirm by radiograph before feeding is initiated.)

Clinical decision point: Insufflation of air into tube while auscultating abdomen is not a reliable means to determine position of feeding tube tip (AACN, 2016b).

STEP	RATIONALE
20. Anchor tube to the patient's nose, avoiding pressure on nares. Mark exit site on tube with indelible ink. Select one of the following options for anchoring:	Marking tube can alert nurses to possible displacement of tube (AACN, 2016b; Boullata et al., 2017). Properly secured tube allows the patient more mobility and prevents trauma to nasal mucosa.
a. Apply membrane dressing or tube fixation device.	Permits longer securement without need to change dressing.
(1) Membrane dressing:	
(a) Apply tincture of benzoin or other skin protectant to the patient's cheek and area of tube to be secured.	Allows membrane to adhere to skin and protects skin.
(b) Place tube against the patient's cheek and secure tube with membrane dressing, out of the patient's line of vision.	Eliminates application of tape around naris. Decreases risk for inadvertent extubation.

STEP	RATIONALE

Step 20a(2)(a) Applying tube fixation device to bridge of nose.

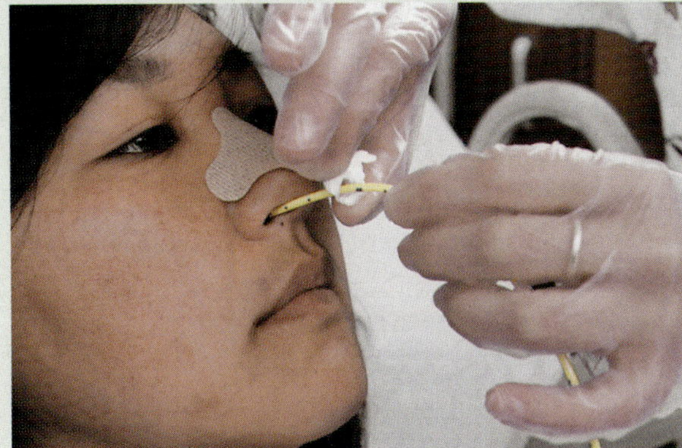

Step 20a(2)(b) Slip connector around feeding tube.

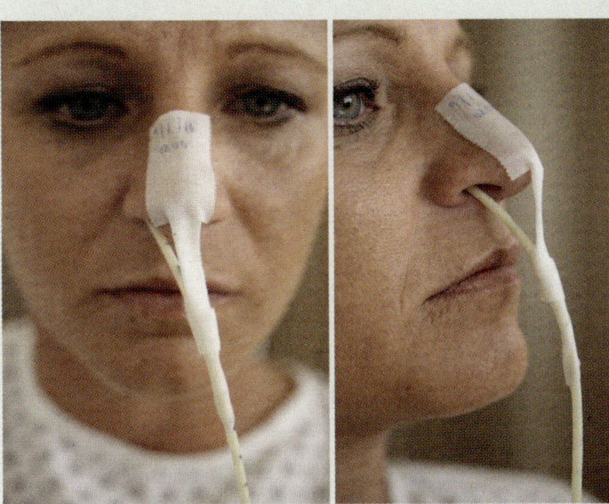

Step 20b(4) Securing tape to nose.

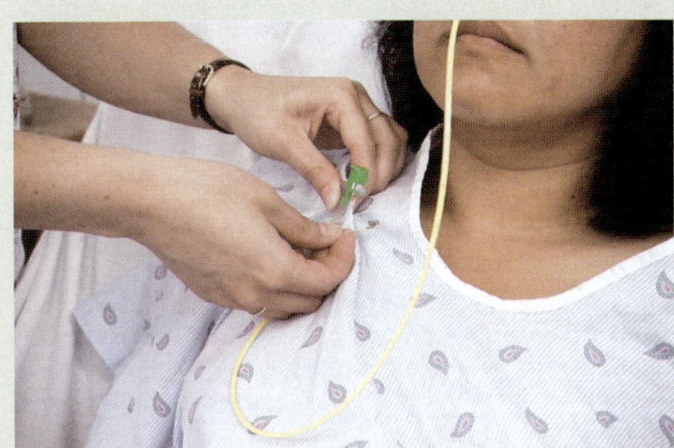

Step 21 Fastening feeding tube to patient's gown.

STEP	RATIONALE
(2) Tube fixation device:	Secures tube and reduces friction on naris.
(a) Apply wide end of patch to bridge of nose (see illustration).	
(b) Slip connector around feeding tube as it exits nose (see illustration).	
b. Apply tape:	Prevents pulling of tube. May require frequent change if tape becomes soiled.
(1) Apply tincture of benzoin or other skin adhesive on tip of the patient's nose and allow it to become "tacky."	Helps tape adhere better. Protects skin.
(2) Remove gloves and tear two horizontal slits on each side of tape at one-third and two-third length. Do not split tape. Fold middle sections forward.	Creates gap in tape that will allow tube to float and exert less pressure on naris.
(3) Tear vertical strip at bottom of tape. Print date and time on nasal portion of the tape.	Secures tube firmly. Documents when tube and tape were applied.
(4) Place intact end of tape over bridge of the patient's nose. Wrap each strip around tube as it exits (see illustration).	Tube is free floating in the naris with this taping method, resulting in movement of tube in the pharynx. Securing tape to naris in this way reduces pressure on naris and reduces risk for medical device–related pressure injury (Markowitz et al., 2013).
21. Fasten end of tube to the patient's gown using clip (see illustration) or piece of tape. Do not use safety pins to secure tube to gown.	Reduces traction on naris if tube moves, which can cause medical device–related pressure injury. Safety pins become unfastened and cause injury to patients.
22. Assist the patient to comfortable position, but keep head of bed elevated at least 30° (preferably 45°) unless contraindicated. For intestinal tube placement, place the patient on right side when possible until correct placement is confirmed by radiograph.	Promotes patient comfort and lowers risk of aspiration should the patient receive tube feeding (AACN, 2016a; Metheny and Frantz, 2013). Placing the patient on right side promotes passage of tube into small intestine.

STEP	RATIONALE
23. Remove gloves and perform hand hygiene.	Reduces transmission of microorganisms.
Clinical decision point: Leave stylet in place until correct position is verified by X-ray film. Never try to reinsert a partially or fully removed stylet while feeding tube is in place. This can cause perforation of tube and injure the patient.	
24. Contact radiology to obtain X-ray film of chest/abdomen.	Radiographic examination is the most accurate method to determine feeding tube placement (AACN, 2016b; Boullata et al., 2017).
25. Perform hand hygiene. Apply clean gloves and administer oral hygiene. Clean tubing at nostril with washcloth dampened in mild soap and water.	Reduces transmission of microorganisms. Promotes patient comfort and integrity of oral mucous membranes.
26. Remove gloves, dispose of equipment, and perform hand hygiene.	Reduces transmission of microorganisms.
Tube Removal	
1. Verify health care provider's order for tube removal.	Health care provider's order is needed to remove feeding tube.
2. Gather equipment.	Ensures organized procedure.
3. Explain procedure to the patient.	Encourages cooperation, reduces anxiety, and minimizes risks. Identifies teaching needs.
4. Perform hand hygiene. Apply clean gloves.	Reduces transmission of microorganisms.
5. Position the patient in high Fowler's position unless contraindicated.	Reduces risk for pulmonary aspiration in the event the patient vomits.
6. Place disposable pad or towel over the patient's chest.	Prevents mucous and gastric secretions from soiling the patient's clothing.
7. Disconnect tube from feeding administration set (if present) and clamp or cap end.	Prevents formula from spilling from tube as it is removed.
8. Remove tape or tube fixation device from the patient's nose. Unclip tube from the patient's gown.	Allows tube to be removed easily.
9. Instruct the patient to take a deep breath and hold it. Then as you kink end of tube securely (folding it over on itself), completely withdraw tube by pulling it out steadily and smoothly onto towel or disposable bag. Dispose of it into appropriate receptacle.	Prevents inadvertent aspiration of gastric contents while tube is removed. Kinking prevents leakage of fluid from tube. Promotes patient comfort. Reduces transmission of microorganisms.
10. Offer tissues to the patient to blow nose.	Clears nasal passages of remaining secretions.
11. Offer mouth care.	Promotes patient's comfort.
12. Remove gloves; perform hand hygiene.	Reduces transmission of microorganisms.
Evaluation	
1. Observe the patient's response to tube placement. Assess lung sounds; have the patient speak; check vital signs; note any coughing, dyspnea, cyanosis, or decrease in oxygen saturation or capnography.	Symptoms may indicate placement in respiratory tract. Auscultation of crackles or wheezes, dyspnea, or fever may be delayed response to aspiration. Capnography indicates change in CO_2 concentration.
2. Confirm X-ray results with health care provider.	Verifies position of tube before initiating enteral feeding.
3. Remove stylet after radiographic verification of correct placement.	If placement needs adjustment, stylet is still in place.
4. Routinely check condition of nares, location of external exit site marking on tube, and color and pH of fluid aspirated from tube.	Routine evaluation ensures no formation of medical device–related pressure injury and correct placement of tube.
5. After removal, assess the patient's level of comfort.	Provides for continued comfort of patient.
6. **Use teach back:** "I want to be sure that I explained to you what you can do during insertion of the nasogastric tube so that you can communicate with me. Tell me what you are going to do to communicate with me during tube insertion." Revise your instruction now or develop a plan for revised patient/family caregiver teaching if the patient/family caregiver is not able to teach back correctly.	Determines the patient's/family caregiver's level of understanding of instructional topic.

Recording and Reporting

- Record type and size of tube placed, location of distal tip of tube, patient's tolerance of procedure, condition of naris, and confirmation of tube position by X-ray.
- Document your evaluation of patient/family caregiver learning.
- Record removal of tube, condition of naris, and patient's tolerance.
- Report any type of unexpected outcome and the interventions performed.

Unexpected Outcomes and Related Interventions

- Aspiration of stomach contents into respiratory tract (delayed response or small-volume aspiration) occurs,

evidenced by auscultation of crackles or wheezes, dyspnea, or fever.
- Report change in the patient's condition to health care provider; if a chest X-ray film has not been recently obtained, suggest ordering one.
- Position the patient on side to protect airway.
- Suction nasotracheally and orotracheally.
- Prepare for possible initiation of antibiotics.

- Displacement of feeding tube to another site (e.g., from duodenum to stomach) possibly occurs when the patient coughs or vomits.
  - Aspirate GI contents and measure pH.
  - Remove displaced tube, and insert and verify placement of new tube.
  - If there is a question of aspiration, obtain chest X-ray film.

SKILL 20.3 Administering Enteral Nutrition Via Nasoenteric, Gastrostomy, or Jejunostomy Tubes

Equipment

- Disposable feeding bag, tubing, or ready-to-hang system
- ENFit syringe 60 mL or larger
- Stethoscope, pulse oximeter, and capnography *(optional)*
- Enteral infusion pump for continuous feedings
- pH indicator strip (scale 1.0–11.0)
- Prescribed enteral formula
- Clean gloves
- ENFit connector

STEP	RATIONALE
Assessment	
1. Identify the patient by using at least two identifiers (e.g., name and birthday or name and medical record number) according to agency policy.	Ensures correct patient. Complies with The Joint Commission standards and improves patient safety (TJC, 2018).
2. Assess the patient's clinical status to determine potential need for tube feedings: decreased level of consciousness, nutrition deficits, head or neck surgery, facial trauma, or impaired swallowing. Consult with nutrition support team and health care provider.	Identify candidates for enteral nutrition (EN) before they become nutritionally depleted. Health care provider order is necessary for feedings.
3. Assess the patient for food allergies.	Prevents the patient from developing localized or systemic allergic responses to feeding.
4. Perform physical assessment of abdomen. Objective measures for assessing tolerance include changes in bowel sounds, expanding girth, tenderness and firmness on palpation, increasing nasogastric tube output, and vomiting.	These symptoms may indicate intolerance for feeding (McCarthy and Martindale, 2015). Report findings to health care provider to determine whether tube feeding can proceed safely (Boullata et al., 2017).
5. Obtain baseline weight. Assess the patient for fluid volume excess or deficit, electrolyte abnormalities, and metabolic abnormalities (e.g., hyperglycemia).	Enteral feedings should restore or maintain the patient's nutrition status. Measures provide objective data and baseline to determine selection of formula and measure effectiveness of feedings.
6. Verify health care provider's order for type of formula, rate, route, and frequency.	Ensures that correct formula will be administered in appropriate volume. Enteral formulas are not interchangeable.
7. Assess the patient's and family caregiver's knowledge of the rationale for and the administration of enteral feedings.	Encourages cooperation, minimizes risks and anxiety, and identifies teaching needs.
Planning	
1. Provide privacy and prepare bedside environment for patient safety.	Preparing the environment helps the nurse think about the steps needed; removing clutter from overbed or bedside table removes barriers to administration of feeding.
2. Prepare and organize equipment for enteral feeding administration.	Ensures organized approach for administration of feedings.
3. Explain enteral feeding administration procedure to the patient and/or caregiver.	Decreases patient anxiety. Promotes patient cooperation and increases compliance.
Implementation	
1. Perform hand hygiene. Apply clean gloves.	Reduces transmission of microorganisms and potential contamination of enteral formula.
2. Obtain formula to administer.	
a. Verify correct formula and check expiration date; note condition of container.	Ensures that correct therapy is to be administered and checks integrity of formula.
b. Provide formula at room temperature.	Cold formula may cause gastric cramping and discomfort because liquid is not warmed by mouth and esophagus.
3. Prepare formula for administration, following manufacturer's guidelines.	
a. Use aseptic technique when manipulating components of feeding system (e.g., formula, administration set, connections).	Bag, connections, and tubing must be free of contamination to prevent bacterial growth (Boullata et al., 2017).

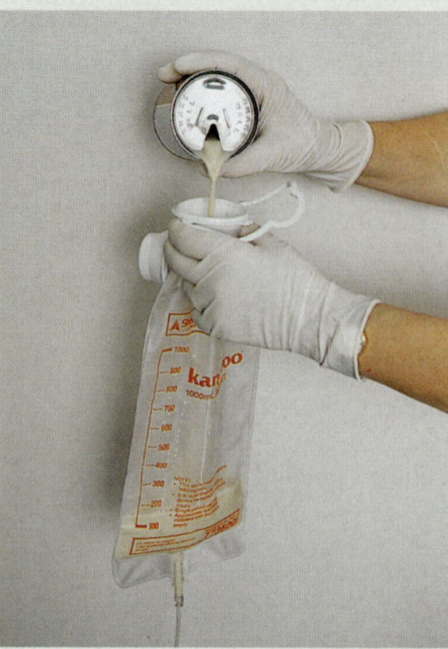

Step 3c Pour formula into open feeding container.

STEP	RATIONALE
b. Shake formula container well. Clean top of canned formula with alcohol swab before opening it.	Ensures integrity of formula; prevents transmission of microorganisms (Boullata et al., 2017).
c. For closed systems, connect administration tubing to container. If using open system, pour formula from brick pack or can into administration bag (see illustration).	Formulas are available in closed-system containers that hold a 24- to 48-h supply of formula or in an open system, in which formula must be transferred from brick packs or cans to a bag before administration.
4. Open roller clamp and allow administration tubing to fill. Clamp off tubing with roller clamp. Hang container on i.v. pole.	Prevents introduction of air into stomach once feeding begins.
5. Place the patient in high Fowler's position or elevate head of bed at least 30° (preferably 45°). For a patient forced to remain supine, place in reverse Trendelenburg position, which raises head.	Elevated head helps prevent pulmonary aspiration (AACN, 2016a).
6. Verify tube has remained in correct place. Observe appearance of aspirate and measure pH.	Verifies whether tip of tube is in stomach or intestine based on pH value (AACN, 2016b). pH testing is not always a reliable indicator (e.g., continuous feedings or medications can alter pH) (Simons and Abdallah, 2012). See agency procedure guidelines regarding other verification methods.
a. *Nasoenteric tube:* Attach ENFit syringe and aspirate gastric contents. Observe appearance of aspirate, and note pH.	Gastric fluid for a patient who has fasted for at least 4 h usually has a pH of 1.0–4.0 (especially when the patient is not receiving gastric acid inhibitor).
b. *Gastrostomy tube:* Attach ENFit syringe and aspirate gastric contents. Observe appearance of aspirate, and note pH.	Continuous administration of tube feeding elevates pH (Metheny and Stewart, 2002; Simons and Abdallah, 2012).
c. *Jejunostomy tube:* Attach ENFit syringe and aspirate intestinal secretions. Observe appearance and whether significant amounts are returned or resemble gastric secretions, and note pH.	Presence of intestinal fluid indicates that end of tube is in small intestine. If fluid tests acidic on pH test or looks like gastric fluid, tube may be displaced into stomach (AACN, 2016b).
7. Check gastric residual volume (GRV) before each feeding for bolus and intermittent feedings and every 4–6 h for continuous feedings per agency policy. Do not use GRV as part of routine assessment for EN tolerance in patients in the intensive care unit (ICU).	GRV may indicate whether gastric emptying is compromised in patients who are not critically ill. Intestinal residual is usually very small. If there is a substantial increase in GRV, displacement of tube into stomach may have occurred (AACN, 2016b). Measuring GRV in critically ill patients is not validated as a means of measuring tolerance. Instead, use physical examinations, review of abdominal X-ray films, and evaluation of clinical risk factors for aspiration to monitor EN feedings in patients in the ICU (McClave et al., 2016).
a. Draw 10–30 mL of air into ENFit syringe and connect to end of feeding tube. Inject air slowly into tube. Pull back slowly and aspirate total amount of gastric contents you can aspirate.	GRV may not be easy to obtain from a small-bore feeding tube. A large-volume syringe (e.g., 60 mL) may prevent gastric tube collapse.
b. Return aspirated contents to stomach unless volume exceeds maximum GRV (see agency policy for maximum GRV).	Prevents loss of nutrients and electrolytes in discarded fluid. There is insufficient evidence to define an exact amount or the safety of returning aspirated contents to the patient. More research is needed.

STEP	RATIONALE
c. GRV of 200–500 mL should raise concern and lead to implementation of measures reducing the risk of aspiration. Automatic cessation of feeding should not occur for GRV less than 500 mL in absence of other signs of intolerance.	Raising the cutoff value for GRV from a lower number to a higher number does not increase risk for regurgitation, aspiration, or pneumonia. However, you should take measures to reduce the risk for aspiration when GRV is high (McClave et al., 2016).
d. Flush feeding tube with 30 mL of water.	Prevents clogging of tubing.
8. Use ENFit devices when administering enteral feedings.	These devices are not compatible with a Luer-Lock connection. Use of ENFit prevents misadministration of an enteral feeding or medication by the wrong route such as i.v. tubing (ISMP, 2015).
9. Intermittent feeding (administered at certain times during the day):	
a. Pinch proximal end of feeding tube and remove cap. Connect distal end of administration set tubing to ENFit device on feeding tube and release tubing.	Prevents excessive air from entering the patient's stomach and leakage of gastric contents. Ensures feeding will be administered into correct tubing (ISMP, 2015).
b. Set rate by adjusting roller clamp on tubing or attach tubing to feeding pump. Allow bag to empty gradually over 30–45 min (the length of time of a comfortable meal). Label bag with tube-feeding type, strength, and amount. Include date, time, and initials.	Gradual emptying of tube feeding reduces risk for abdominal discomfort, vomiting, or diarrhea induced by bolus or too-rapid infusion of tube feedings. Labeling provides means to determine when to change administration set and confirms that the right patient is receiving feeding.

Clinical decision point: Use pumps designated for tube feeding, not i.v. fluids.

STEP	RATIONALE
c. Immediately follow feeding with water (per health care provider's orders or agency policy). Cover end of feeding tube with cap when not in use. Keep bag as clean as possible. Change administration set every 24 h.	Prevents tube from clogging. Prevents air from entering stomach between feedings, and limits microbial contamination of system.
10. Continuous infusion method:	Method delivers prescribed hourly rate of feeding and reduces risk for abdominal discomfort.
a. Remove cap on tubing and connect distal end of administration set tubing to feeding tube using ENFit connector as in Step 9a.	Prevents excess air from entering the patient's stomach and leakage of gastric contents. Ensures feeding will be administered into correct tubing (ISMP, 2015).
b. Thread tubing through feeding pump; set rate on pump and turn on (see illustration).	Delivers continuous feeding at steady rate and pressure. Feeding pump sounds alarm for increased resistance.
c. Advance rate of tube feeding (and concentration of feeding) gradually, as ordered.	Tube feeding can usually begin with full-strength formula. In the absence of critical illness (including metabolic or systemic complications), enteral feedings can advance to goal rate within 24–48 h (McClave et al., 2016). Conservative initiation and advancement of EN depend on the patient's age, medical condition, nutrition status, and expected patient tolerance (Kozeniecki and Fritzshall, 2015).

Clinical decision point: Maximum hang time for formula is 8 h in an open system and 24–48 h in a closed, ready-to-hang system (if it remains closed). The risk for contamination increases in formulas hanging more than 24 h (Boullata et al., 2017). Refer to manufacturer guidelines.

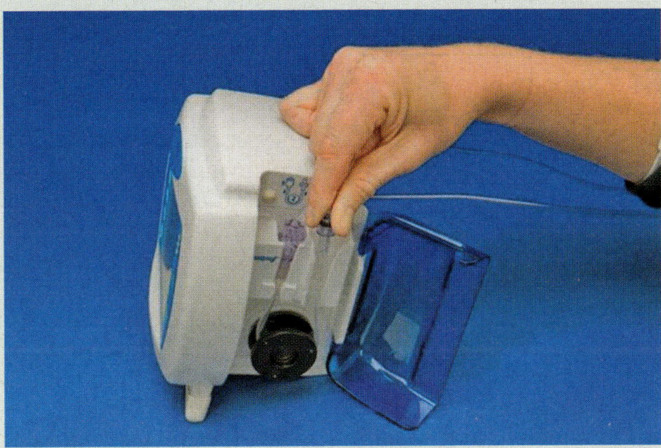

Step 10b Connect tubing through infusion pump. (Image used with the permission of Covidien. All rights reserved.)

STEP	RATIONALE
11. Flush tubing with 30 mL of water every 4 h during continuous feeding (see agency policy) and before and after an intermittent feeding. Have registered dietitian recommend total free water requirement per day and obtain health care provider's order.	Provides the patient with source of water to help maintain fluid and electrolyte balance. Clears tubing of formula.
12. Rinse bag and tubing with warm water whenever feedings are interrupted. Use new administration set every 24 h.	Rinsing bag and tubing with warm water clears old tube feedings and reduces bacterial growth.
13. Dispose of supplies and perform hand hygiene.	Reduces transmission of microorganisms.
Evaluation	
1. Measure GRV per agency policy, usually every 4–6 h, and ask whether nausea or abdominal cramping is present.	Gastrointestinal tolerance of tube feedings must be closely monitored to avoid complications.
2. Monitor intake and output at least every 8 h (or as ordered), and calculate daily totals every 24 h.	Intake and output are indications of fluid balance—fluid volume excess or deficit.
3. Weigh patient daily until maximum administration rate is reached and maintained for 24 h; then weigh patient three times per week.	Slow weight gain is an indicator of improved nutrition status; however, sudden gain of more than 2 lb (0.9 kg) in 24 h usually indicates fluid retention.
4. Monitor laboratory values as ordered by health care provider.	Determines correct administration of formula rate and strength.
5. Observe the patient's respiratory status.	Change in respiratory status may indicate aspiration of tube feeding into respiratory tract. Symptoms may include coughing, dyspnea, tachypnea, change in oxygen saturation, crackles, and hoarseness.
6. Examine abdomen and auscultate bowel sounds.	Estimates status of gastric emptying and peristalsis.
7. For gastrostomy tubes, inspect site for signs of impaired skin integrity, symptoms of infection, injury, or tightness of tube.	Enteral tubes often cause pressure and excoriation at insertion site.
8. Observe nasoenteral tube insertion site at least daily (see agency policy). Note skin integrity and look for edema under device, excoriation, or presence of pressure injury.	Allows for early detection of excoriation that can progress to medical device–related pressure injury.
9. **Use teach back:** "I want to be sure that I explained to you what you need to look out for that may tell us you are not tolerating your tube feeding. Tell me two things that may tell us that you are not tolerating your tube feedings." Revise your instruction now or develop a plan for revised patient/family caregiver teaching if the patient/family caregiver is not able to teach back correctly.	Determines the patient's/family caregiver's level of understanding of instructional topic.

Recording and Reporting

- Record amount and type of feeding, infusion rate, method of infusion, and the patient's response to tube feeding (e.g., GRV, cramping, bowel sounds, patency of tube, condition of skin at tube site).
- Document your evaluation of patient/family caregiver learning.
- Record volume of formula and any additional water on intake and output form.
- Report type of feeding, status of feeding tube, patient's tolerance, and adverse outcomes.

Unexpected Outcomes and Related Interventions

- Feeding tube becomes clogged.
  - Attempt to flush tube with water.
  - Special products are available for unclogging feeding tubes; do not use carbonated beverages or juice.
  - Hold feeding and notify health care provider.
  - Maintain the patient in semi-Fowler's position.
  - Contact pharmacist to change medications to liquid form and flush before and after intermittent feedings and medications (Kozeniecki and Fritzshall, 2015).
- The patient develops large amount of diarrhea (more than three loose stools in 24 hours).
  - Notify health care provider.
  - Consult dietitian about need to change formula to prevent malabsorption.
  - Identify and treat underlying medical/surgical issues and infections (Kozeniecki and Fritzshall, 2015).
  - Provide perianal skin care after each stool.
  - Determine other causes of diarrhea such as *Clostridium difficile* infection, contaminated tube feeding, or medication containing sorbitol.
- The patient develops nausea and vomiting.
  - Administer antiemetic as ordered.
  - Administer medications (ordered by health care provider) to increase gastric motility (e.g., prokinetic agents) and evaluate need for medications that slow gastric emptying (Kozeniecki and Fritzshall, 2015).
  - Ensure that formula and water flushes are administered at room temperature (Kozeniecki and Fritzshall, 2015).
  - Temporarily reduce infusion rate or withhold tube feeding and notify health care provider.
  - Be sure that tube is patent; aspirate for residual.

KEY POINTS

- Digestion is the mechanical and chemical process by which food is broken down into its simplest form for absorption. Digestion and absorption occur mainly in the small intestine.
- Eating a balanced diet including carbohydrates, protein, lipids, vitamins, minerals, and water provides the essential nutrients to carry out the normal physiological functioning of the body.
- IBW is maintained when energy intake in food or fluids equals energy output.
- DRIs for macronutrients and micronutrients were formulated for population groups, not individuals.
- Guidelines for dietary change advocate (1) for a limitation of added sugars, saturated fats, and sodium intake; (2) for people to focus on variety, nutrient density, and amount; and (3) for a shift to healthier food and beverage choices.
- Age, developmental stages, and clinical conditions affect the requirements for essential nutrients. Periods of rapid growth increase the need for protein, vitamins, and minerals.
- Because improper nutrition affects all body systems, nutrition assessment includes a review of total physical assessment findings.
- Special hospital diets alter the composition, texture, digestibility, and residue of foods to meet a patient's needs.
- Enteral nutrition (EN) is for patients who are unable to ingest food safely or adequately but are able to digest and absorb nutrition via the gastrointestinal (GI) tract.
- EN preserves intestinal structure and function and maintains immunity.
- Parenteral nutrition (PN) supplies essential nutrients through a concentrated nutrient solution administered into the superior vena cava and is used when nutrition via the GI tract is not possible or cannot effectively meet patient needs.
- Medical nutrition therapy is a recognized treatment modality for both acute and chronic disease states.

REFERENCES

American Diabetes Association (ADA): Management of hyperglycemia in type 2 diabetes: a patient centered approach, *Diabetes Care* 2012;35(6):1364.

American Dietetic Association: Position of the American Dietetic Association, American Society for Nutrition, and Society for Nutrition Education: Food and nutrition programs for community-residing older adults, *J Am Diet Assoc* 2010;110(3):463.

American Heart Association (AHA): Diet and lifestyle recommendations revision, 2010, http://www.heart.org/HEARTORG/GettingHealthy/Diet-and-Lifestyle-Recommendations_UCM_305855_Article.jsp. Accessed November 2019.

Academy of Nutrition and Dietetics (AND). Nutrition care manual. 2016. Available from: http://www.nutritioncaremanual.org.

American Association of Critical Care Nurses (AACN). AACN Practice Alerts: prevention of aspiration in adults. Crit Care Nurse 2016a;36(1):e20.

American Association of Critical Care Nurses (AACN). AACN Practice Alerts: initial and ongoing verification of feeding tube placement in adults. Crit Care Nurse 2016b;36(2):e8.

Ayers P, Adams S, Boullata J, Gervasio J, Holcombe B, Kraft MD, et al. A.S.P.E.N. parenteral nutrition safety consensus recommendations. JPEN J Parenter Enteral Nutr 2014;38(3):296.

Boullata JI, Gilbert K, Sacks G, Labossiere RJ, Crill C, Goday P, et al. A.S.P.E.N. clinical guidelines: parenteral nutrition ordering, order review, compounding, labeling, and dispensing. JPEN J Parenter Enteral Nutr 2014;38(3):334.

Boullata JI, Carrera AL, Harvey L, Escuro AA, Hudson L, Mays A, et al. ASPEN safe practices for enteral nutrition therapy. JPEN J Parenter Enteral Nutr 2017;41(1):15.

Bourgault AM, Heath J, Hooper V, Sole ML, Nesmith EG. Methods used by critical care nurses to verify feeding tube placement in clinical practice. Crit Care Nurse 2015;35:e1.

Cichero JA. Thickening agents used for dysphagia management: effect on bioavailability of water, medication and feelings of satiety. Nutr J 2013; 12:54.

Clarys P, Deliens T, Huybrechts I, Deriemaeker P, Vanaelst B, De Keyzer W, et al. Comparison of nutritional quality of the vegan, vegetarian, semi-vegetarian, pesco-vegetarian and omnivorous diet. Nutrients 2014; 6:1318.

Copp AJ, Greene ND. Neural tube defects—disorders of neurulation and related embryonic processes. Wiley Interdiscip Rev Dev Biol 2013; 2(2):213.

de Souza RJ, Mente A, Maroleanu A, Cozma AI, Ha V, Kishibe T, et al. Intake of saturated and trans unsaturated fatty acids and risk of all cause mortality, cardiovascular disease, and type 2 diabetes: systematic review and meta-analysis of observational studies. BMJ 2015; 351:h3978.

DiMaria-Ghalili RA, Gilbert K, Lord L, Neal T, Richardson D, Tyler R, et al. Standards of nutrition care practice and professional performance for nutrition support and generalist nurses. Nutr Clin Pract 2016;31(4):527.

Donini LM, oggiogalle E, Molfino A, Rosano A, Lenzi A, Rossi Fanelli F, et al. Mini-nutritional assessment, malnutrition universal screening tool, and nutrition risk screening tool for the nutritional evaluation of older nursing home residents. J Am Med Dir Assoc 2016;17(10):959.e11.

Elke G, Felbinger TW, Heyland DK. Gastric residual volume in critically ill patients: a dead marker or still alive? Nutr Clin Pract 2015;30(1):59.

Food and Nutrition Board (FNB), Institute of Medicine (IOM). Dietary reference intakes for thiamin, riboflavin, niacin, vitamin B6, folate, vitamin B12, pantothenic acid, biotin, and choline. Washington, DC: National Academies Press; 1998.

Food and Nutrition Board (FNB), Institute of Medicine (IOM). Dietary reference intakes for energy, carbohydrate, fiber, fat, fatty acids, cholesterol, protein, and amino acids. Washington, DC: National Academies Press; 2002.

Food and Nutrition Board (FNB), Institute of Medicine (IOM). Dietary reference intakes for water, potassium, sodium, chloride, and sulfate. Washington, DC: National Academies Press; 2004.

Gomes Jr CA, Andriolo RB, Bennett C, Lustosa SA, Matos D, Waisberg DR, et al. Percutaneous endoscopic gastrostomy versus nasogastric tube feeding for adults with swallowing disturbances. Cochrane Database Syst Rev 2015;(5):CD008096.

Han Z, Lutsiv O, Mulla S, Rosen A, Beyene J, McDonald SD et al. Low gestational weight gain and the risk of preterm birth and low birthweight: a systematic review and meta-analyses. Acta Obstet Gynecol Scand 2011;90(9):935.

Hedwig L, et al: Multiple levels of social disadvantage and links to obesity in adolescence and young adults, J School Health 2013;83:139.

Hines S, Kynoch K, Munday J. Nursing interventions for identifying and managing acute dysphagia are effective for improving patient outcomes: a systematic review update. J Neurosci Nurs 2016;48(4):215.

Institute for Safe Medication Practices (ISMP). Safety Alert: ENFit enteral devices are on their way...Important safety considerations for hospitals. 2015. Available from: http://www.ismp.org/newsletters/acutecare/showarticle.aspx?id=105.

Jeng C, Sheu PY, Chen CM, Chen SR, Tseng IG. Clinical validation of the related factors and defining characteristics of impaired swallowing for patients with stroke. J Nurs Res 2001;9(4):105.

Kozeniecki M, Fritzshall R. Enteral nutrition for adults in the hospital setting. Nutr Clin Pract 2015;30(5):634.

Kumar S, Kelly AS. Review of childhood obesity: from epidemiology, etiology, and comorbidities to clinical assessment and treatment. Mayo Clin Proc 2017;92(2):251.

Lee JL, Oh ES, Lee RW, Finucane TE. Serum albumin and prealbumin in calorically restricted, nondiseased individuals: a systematic review. Am J Med 2015;128(9):1023.e1.

Malhi H. Dysphagia: warning signs and management. Br J Nurs 2016; 25(10):546.

Markowitz J, Spurgeon H, Rupp E. Device-related pressure ulcers. American Association of Critical-Care Nurses (AACN) Clinical Scene Investigator Academy; 2013. Available from: http://www.aacn.org/wd/csi/

docs/FinalProjects/IU%20Methodist%20ACC%20-%20Power%20Point%20Presentation.pdf.
McCarthy MS, Martindale RG. What's on the menu? Delivering evidence-based nutritional therapy. Nursing 2015;45(8):36.
McClave SA, Taylor BE, Martindale RG, Warren MM, Johnson DR, Braunschweig C, et al. Guidelines for the provision and assessment of nutrition support therapy in the adult critically ill patient: Society of Critical Care Medicine (SCCM) and American Society for Parenteral and Enteral Nutrition (A.S.P.E.N.). JPEN J Parenter Enteral Nutr 2016;40(2):159.
Metheny NA, Frantz RA. Head-of-bed elevation in critically ill patients: a review. Crit Care Nurse 2013;33(3):53.
Metheny NA, Stewart BJ. Testing feeding tube placement during continuous tube feedings. Appl Nurs Res 2002;15(4):254.
Miller KR, McClave SA, Kiraly LN, Martindale RG, Benns M. A tutorial on enteral access in adult patients in the hospitalized setting. JPEN J Parenter Enteral Nutr 2014;38(3):282.
National Dysphagia Diet Task Force (NDDTF). National Dysphagia Diet: standardization for optimal care, Chicago: American Dietetic Association; 2002.
Newman R, Vilardell N, Clavé P, Speyer R. Effect of bolus viscosity on the safety and efficacy of swallowing and the kinematics of the swallow response in patients with oropharyngeal dysphagia: White Paper by the European Society for Swallowing Disorders (ESSD). Dysphagia 2016;31(2):232.
Nix S: Williams' basic nutrition and diet therapy, 14th ed., St Louis: Mosby; 2012.
O'Horo JC, Rogus-Pulia N, Garcia-Arguello L, Robbins J, Safdar N. Bedside diagnosis of dysphagia: a systematic review. J Hosp Med 2015;10(4):256.
Park JS, Oh DH, Hwang NK, Lee JH. Effects of neuromuscular electrical stimulation combined with effortful swallowing on post-stroke oropharyngeal dysphagia: a randomised controlled trial. J Oral Rehabil 2016;43(6):426.
Popa Nita S, Murith M, Chisholm H, Engmann J. Matching the rheological properties of videofluoroscopic contrast agents and thickened liquid prescriptions. Dysphagia 2013;28(2):245.
Poulia KA, Klek S, Doundoulakis I, Bouras E, Karayiannis D, Baschali A, et al. The two most popular malnutrition screening tools in the light of the new ESPEN consensus definition of the diagnostic criteria for malnutrition. Clin Nutr 2017;36(4):1130.
Ra JY, Hyun JK, Ko KR, Lee SJ. Chin tuck for prevention of aspiration: effectiveness and appropriate posture. Dysphagia 2014;29(5):603.
Rösler A, Pfeil S, Lessmann H, Höder J, Befahr A, von Renteln-Kruse W. Dysphagia in dementia: influence of dementia severity and food texture on the prevalence of aspiration and latency to swallow in hospitalized geriatric patients. J Am Med Dir Assoc 2015;16(8):697.
Sanders TA. Protective effects of dietary PUFA against chronic disease: evidence from epidemiological studies and intervention trials. Proc Nutr Soc 2014;73(1):73–9.
Simons SR, Abdallah LM. Bedside assessment of enteral tube placement: aligning practice with evidence. Am J Nurs 2012;112(2):40.
Sørensen RT, Rasmussen RS, Overgaard K, Lerche A, Johansen AM, Lindhardt T. Dysphagia screening and intensified oral hygiene reduce pneumonia after stroke. J Neurosci Nurs 2013;45(3):139.
Sparks DA, Chase DM, Coughlin LM, Perry E. Pulmonary complications of 9931 narrow-bore nasoenteric tubes during blind placement: a critical review. JPEN J Parenter Enteral Nutr 2011;35(5):625.
Steele CM, Alsanei WA, Ayanikalath S, Barbon CE, Chen J, Cichero JA, et al. The influence of food texture and liquid consistency modification on swallowing physiology and function: a systematic review. Dysphagia 2015;30(1):2.
Sura L, Madhavan A, Carnaby G, Crary MA. Dysphagia in the elderly: management and nutritional considerations. Clin Interv Aging 2012;7:287.
Swan K, Speyer R, Heijnen BJ, Wagg B, Cordier R. Living with oropharyngeal dysphagia: effects of bolus modification on health-related quality of life—a systematic review. Qual Life Res 2015;24:2447.
Takeuchi K, Aida J, Ito K, Furuta M, Yamashita Y, Osaka K. Nutritional status and dysphagia risk among community-dwelling frail older adults. J Nutr Health Aging 2014;18(4):352.
The Joint Commission (TJC). 2018 National Patient Safety Goals. Oakbrook Terrace, IL: The Joint Commission; 2018. Available from: https://www.jointcommission.org/standards_information/npsgs.aspx.
Ullman AJ, Cooke ML, Mitchell M, Lin F, New K, Long DA, et al. Dressing and securement for central venous access devices (CVADs): a Cochrane systematic review. Int J Nurs Stud 2016;59:177.
Wang J, et al: Factors associated with health-related quality of life among overweight or obese adults, J ClinNurs 2013;22:2172.
Wang Y, Cai L, Wu Y, Wilson RF, Weston C, Fawole O, et al. What childhood obesity prevention programmes work? A systematic review and meta-analysis. Obes Rev 2015;16(7):547.
Wirth R, Dziewas R, Beck AM, Clavé P, Hamdy S, Heppner HJ, et al. Oropharyngeal dysphagia in older persons—from pathophysiology to adequate intervention: a review and summary of an international expert meeting. Clin Interv Aging 2016;11:189.

21 *Urinary Elimination*

OBJECTIVES

- To define the process of urine elimination.
- To explain anatomy and physiology of the urinary system.
- To enlist factors influencing urination.
- To discuss the characteristics of urine including color, clarity, and odor.
- To describe the common urinary elimination problems including urinary retention, urinary tract infections, urinary incontinence, and urinary diversions.
- To understand to perform physical assessment, assessment of urine, and intake and output that focuses on urinary elimination.
- To discuss about different types of urinalysis including timed urine test, clean-catch midstream specimen, and urine for culture and sensitivity.
- To explain nursing responsibilities associated with common diagnostic tests of the urinalysis.
- To prioritize nursing diagnoses and care plan associated with alterations in urinary elimination.
- To understand the importance of patient education and promoting normal micturition for health promotion.
- To describe how to maintain elimination habits and fluid intake, promote bladder emptying, and prevent infections among patients.
- To implement nursing measures required in acute care including catheter changes and catheter care to reduce urinary tract infections.
- To describe how to apply a condom catheter, insert an indwelling urinary catheter, and measure postvoid residual using a bladder scan.
- To perform catheter irrigations and instillations to maintain the patency of indwelling urinary catheter.
- To understand the need of restorative and continuing care to improve bladder emptying and restore urinary continence.

KEY TERMS

bacteremia, p. 488
bacteriuria, p. 488
catheter-associated urinary tract infection (CAUTI), p. 497
catheterization, p. 497
condom catheter, p. 500
cystitis, p. 488
dysuria, p. 488
graduated measuring container, p. 493
hematuria, p. 486
micturition, p. 486
postvoid residual, p. 497
proteinuria, p. 486
pyelonephritis, p. 488
residual urine, p. 497
stoma, p. 488
suprapubic catheter, p. 500
ureterostomy, p. 490
urinal, p. 494
urinalysis, p. 494
urinary diversion, p. 488
urinary incontinence (UI), p. 488
urinary reflux, p. 486
urinary retention, p. 488
urinary tract infections (UTIs), p. 488
urine hat, p. 493
urometer, p. 493
urosepsis, p. 488
voiding, p. 486

INTRODUCTION

Providing effective nursing care requires you to support patients as they respond to alterations in their physical, psychological, spiritual, and emotional health. A basic human function is urinary elimination, which can be affected by a wide variety of illnesses and conditions. Many factors influence urine production, such as fluid intake, physical activity, and body temperature. Nurses support patients' urinary elimination needs by supporting normal micturition. Sometimes, you will insert and maintain urinary catheters for close monitoring of urine output or to facilitate bladder emptying when bladder function is impaired. Some patients require long-term urethral or suprapubic indwelling catheters when the bladder fails to empty effectively. You will consistently implement measures to minimize the risk for urinary tract infection (UTI) during the administration of nursing care. Nurses in all health care settings play a key role in teaching patients about bladder health.

URINE ELIMINATION

Urinary elimination is the last step in the removal and elimination of excess water and the by-products of body metabolism. Adequate elimination depends on the coordinated function of the ureters, bladder, and urethra (Fig. 21.1). The kidneys filter waste products of metabolism from the blood. The ureters transport urine from the kidneys to the bladder. The bladder holds urine until the volume in the bladder triggers a sensation of urge, sending impulses to the sacral level of the spinal cord indicating the need to pass urine. When the brain allows the bladder to empty, the bladder contracts, the urinary sphincter relaxes, and urine leaves the body through the urethra (Huether and McCance, 2016).

Anatomy and Physiology of the Urinary Tract

Kidneys

The kidneys lie on either side of the vertebral column behind the abdominal peritoneum and against the deep muscles of the back level with the 12th thoracic and 3rd lumbar vertebrae. Normally the left kidney is higher than the right because of the anatomical position of the liver. Nephrons, the functional unit of the kidneys, remove waste products from the blood and play a major role in the regulation of fluid and electrolyte balance. Each nephron contains a cluster of capillaries called the *glomerulus*. The glomerulus filters water, glucose, amino acids, urea, uric acid, creatinine, and major electrolytes. Large proteins and blood cells do not normally filter through the glomerulus. Suspect glomerular injury when protein **(proteinuria)** or blood **(hematuria)** is found in the urine.

Not all glomerular filtrate is excreted as urine. Approximately 99% is resorbed into the plasma by the proximal convoluted tubule of the nephron, the loop of Henle, and the distal tubule. The remaining 1% is excreted as urine.

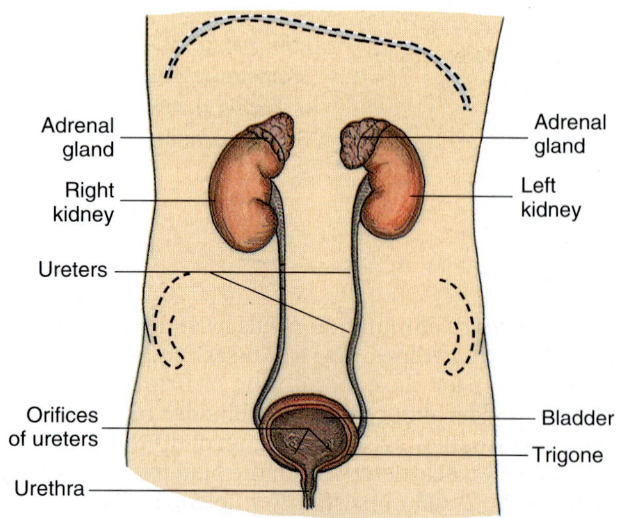

Fig. 21.1 Organs of the urinary system.

The delicate balance of fluid and electrolytes is maintained during the resorption process (Huether and McCance, 2016). The kidneys normally produce 1–2 L of urine daily (Huether and McCance, 2016).

Ureters

A ureter is attached to each kidney pelvis and carries urinary wastes to the bladder. Urine draining from the ureters to the bladder is sterile. Peristaltic waves cause the urine to enter the bladder in spurts rather than steadily. Contractions of the bladder during micturition compress the lower portion of the ureters to prevent urine from backflowing into them (Huether and McCance, 2016). Obstruction of urine flow through the ureters such as by a kidney stone can cause a backflow of urine **(urinary reflux)** into the ureters and pelvis of the kidney, causing distention (hydroureter/hydronephrosis), infection from stasis, and in some cases permanent damage to sensitive kidney structures and function.

Bladder

The urinary bladder is a hollow, distensible, muscular organ that holds urine. When empty, the bladder lies in the pelvic cavity behind the symphysis pubis. The bladder rests against the rectum in males and rests against the anterior wall of the uterus and vagina in females. It expands as it fills with urine. Normally the pressure in the bladder during filling remains low; this prevents the dangerous backward flow of urine into the ureters and kidneys. In a pregnant woman, the developing fetus pushes against the bladder, reducing capacity and causing a feeling of fullness.

Urethra

Urine travels from the bladder to the urethra and passes to the outside of the body through the urethral meatus. The urethra passes through a thick layer of skeletal muscles called the *pelvic floor muscles*. These muscles stabilize the urethra and contribute to urinary continence. The external urethral sphincter, composed of striated muscles, contributes to voluntary control over the flow of urine (Huether and McCance, 2016). The female urethra is approximately 3–4 cm (1.18–1.5 inches) long, and the male urethra is approximately 18–20 cm (7–7.8 inches) long (Huether and McCance, 2016). The shorter length of the female urethra increases the risk for UTI because of close access to the bacteria-contaminated perineal area.

Act of Urination

Urination, **micturition**, and **voiding** all are terms that describe the process of bladder emptying. Micturition is a complex interaction between the bladder, urinary sphincter, and central nervous system. Several areas in the brain are involved in bladder control including the cerebral cortex, thalamus, hypothalamus, and brain stem. There are two micturition centers in the spinal cord; one coordinates inhibition of bladder contraction, and the other coordinates bladder contractility. As the bladder fills and stretches, bladder contractions are inhibited by sympathetic stimulation from the thoracic micturition center. Normal bladder capacity in adults is approximately 300–600 mL. With a strong sensation of urge and when in the appropriate place to void, the central nervous system sends a message to the micturition centers stopping sympathetic stimulation and starting parasympathetic stimulation from the sacral micturition center. The urinary sphincter relaxes, and the bladder contracts. When the time and place are inappropriate, the brain sends messages to the micturition centers to contract the urinary sphincter and relax the bladder muscle.

COMPOSITION AND CHARACTERISTICS OF URINE

Inspect urine for color, clarity, and odor. Monitor and document any changes.

Color

Normal urine ranges in color from pale yellow (like straw) to amber depending on its concentration. Urine is usually more concentrated in the morning or in the presence of fluid volume deficits. As a patient drinks more fluids, urine becomes less concentrated, and the color lightens. Patients taking diuretics commonly void dilute urine while the medication is active.

Hematuria, or blood in the urine, is never a normal finding. Bleeding from the kidneys or ureters usually causes urine to become dark red; bleeding from the bladder or urethra usually causes bright red urine. Hematuria and blood clots commonly cause urinary catheter blockage. Report these findings immediately to the patient's health care provider.

Various medications and foods can change the color of urine. Patients taking phenazopyridine, a urinary analgesic, void urine that is bright orange. Eating beets, rhubarb, and blackberries sometimes causes red urine. The kidneys excrete special dyes used in i.v. diagnostic studies, which discolor the urine. Patients with liver disease who have high concentrations of bilirubin (urobilinogen) often have dark amber urine. Report unexpected color changes to the health care provider.

Clarity

Normal urine appears transparent at the time of voiding. Urine that stands several minutes in a container becomes cloudy. Sometimes, a patient's first voided urine of the day is cloudy because the urine is stored in the bladder overnight; urine normally clears on the next voiding. Patients with bacteria and white blood cells in their urine usually have thick and cloudy urine. In patients with renal disease, freshly voided urine often appears cloudy because of protein concentration.

Odor

Urine has a characteristic ammonia odor. The more concentrated the urine, the stronger the odor. As urine remains standing (e.g., in a collection device), more ammonia breakdown occurs, and the odor becomes stronger. A foul odor often indicates a UTI. Some foods such as asparagus and garlic can change the odor of urine.

FACTORS INFLUENCING URINATION

Physiological factors, psychosocial conditions, and diagnostic or treatment-induced factors sometimes affect normal urinary elimination (Box 21.1). Understanding these factors helps you anticipate possible elimination problems and intervene when or before they develop.

BOX 21.1 Factors Influencing Urinary Elimination

Growth and Development

- Children cannot voluntarily control voiding until 18–24 months of age when myelination is complete.
- Readiness for toilet training includes the ability to recognize the feeling of bladder fullness, hold urine for 1–2 h, and communicate the sense of urgency.
- Some older adults experience a decrease in bladder capacity, increased bladder irritability, and increased frequency of bladder contractions during bladder filling.
- In older adults, the ability to hold urine between the initial desire to void and an urgent need to void decreases.
- Older adults are at increased risk for urinary incontinence as a result of chronic illnesses and factors that interfere with mobility, cognition, and manual dexterity.

Sociocultural Factors

- Cultural and gender norms vary. North Americans expect toilet facilities to be private, whereas some cultures accept communal toilet facilities; gender-neutral bathrooms are becoming more common in the United States.
- Religious or cultural norms may dictate who is acceptable to assist in elimination practices.
- Social expectations (e.g., school recesses, work breaks) can interfere with timely voiding.

Psychological Factors

- Anxiety and stress sometimes affect a sense of urgency and increase frequency of voiding.
- Anxiety can impact bladder emptying because of inadequate relaxation of the pelvic floor muscles and urinary sphincter.
- Depression can decrease the desire for urinary continence.

Personal Habits

- The need for privacy and adequate time to void often influences the ability to adequately empty the bladder.

Fluid Intake

- If fluids, electrolytes, and solutes are balanced, increased fluid intake increases urine production.
- Alcohol decreases the release of antidiuretic hormones, thus increasing urine production.
- Fluids containing caffeine and other bladder irritants can prompt unsolicited bladder contractions, resulting in frequency, urgency, and incontinence.

Pathological Conditions

- Diabetes mellitus, multiple sclerosis, and stroke can alter bladder contractility and the ability to sense bladder filling. Patients experience either bladder overactivity or deficient bladder emptying.

Continued

BOX 21.1 Factors Influencing Urinary Elimination—cont'd

- Arthritis, Parkinson disease, dementia, and chronic pain can interfere with timely access to a toilet.
- Spinal cord injury or intervertebral disk disease (above S1) can cause the loss of urine control because of bladder overactivity and impaired coordination between the contracting bladder and the urinary sphincter.
- Prostatic enlargement (e.g., benign prostatic hyperplasia) can cause obstruction of the bladder outlet, which results in urinary retention.

Surgical Procedures

- Local trauma during lower abdominal and pelvic surgery sometimes obstructs urine flow, requiring temporary use of an indwelling urinary catheter.
- Anesthetic agents and other agents given during surgery decrease bladder contractility and/or sensation of bladder fullness, often causing urinary retention (Woodward, 2015a).

Medications

- Diuretics increase urinary output by preventing resorption of water and certain electrolytes.
- Some drugs change the color of urine (e.g., phenazopyridine—orange; riboflavin—intense yellow).
- Anticholinergics (e.g., atropine, overactive bladder agents) increase the risk for urinary retention by inhibiting bladder contractility (Rantell, 2014).
- Hypnotics and sedatives (e.g., analgesics, antianxiety agents) may reduce the ability to recognize and act on the urge to void.

Diagnostic Examinations

- Cystoscopy may cause localized trauma of the urethra, resulting in transient (1–2 days) dysuria and hematuria.
- Whenever the sterile urinary tract is catheterized, there is a risk for infection.

COMMON URINARY ELIMINATION PROBLEMS

The most common urinary elimination problems involve the inability to store urine or to fully empty urine from the bladder. Problems can result from infection; irritable or overactive bladder; obstruction of urine flow; impaired bladder contractility; or issues that impair innervation to the bladder, resulting in sensory or motor dysfunction.

Urinary Retention

Urinary retention is the inability to partially or completely empty the bladder. Acute or rapid-onset urinary retention stretches the bladder, causing feelings of pressure, discomfort and/or pain, and tenderness over the symphysis pubis; restlessness; and sometimes diaphoresis. Patients often have no urine output over several hours and in some cases experience frequency, urgency, small-volume voiding, or incontinence of small volumes of urine. Chronic urinary retention has a slow, gradual onset during which patients may report decreased voiding volumes, straining to void, frequency, urgency, incontinence, and sensations of incomplete emptying. Complete urinary retention occurs when there is no voiding; during partial retention, the bladder never empties completely. Incontinence caused by urinary retention is called *overflow incontinence*. The pressure in the bladder exceeds the ability of the sphincter to prevent the passage of urine, and the patient dribbles urine (Table 21.1).

Urinary Tract Infections

Urinary tract infection (UTI) are the most common health care–associated infections (HAI) (Galiczewski, 2016). The Centers for Disease Control and Prevention (CDC, 2017) reports that 75% of these infections result from the use of an indwelling urinary catheter. *Escherichia coli*, a bacterium commonly found in the colon, is the most common causative pathogen (Nicolle, 2014). Risk for a UTI increases when a patient has an indwelling catheter, urinary retention, urinary and fecal incontinence, or poor perineal hygiene practices.

Bacteriuria (bacteria in the urine) can lead to serious upper UTI (pyelonephritis) and life-threatening bloodstream infection (**bacteremia** or **urosepsis**). Symptoms of a lower UTI (bladder) include burning or pain with urination **(dysuria)** or irritation of the bladder **(cystitis)** characterized by urgency, frequency, incontinence, suprapubic tenderness, and foul-smelling, cloudy urine. In some cases, there is obvious blood in the urine (hematuria). If infection spreads to the upper urinary tract **(pyelonephritis)**, patients frequently experience fever (39°C [102.2°F]), chills, diaphoresis, flank pain, and lower back pain (Casey, 2014). Older adults with a UTI often experience *delirium* (a change in mental status), new or increased incontinence, agitation or absence of normal behavior, decreased appetite, and deteriorating mobility resulting in increased falls.

Urinary Incontinence

Urinary incontinence (UI) is defined by the International Continence Society as "any involuntary loss of urine" (Wilson, 2016). The highest incidence of UI occurs in older adults—17% of men older than 60 years and 30%–50% of women older than 60 years (Testa, 2015). The most common forms of UI are urge or urgency UI and stress UI. Mixed UI occurs when both stress and urgency symptoms are present. Table 21.1 summarizes the most common types, characteristics, and selected nursing interventions for UI.

Urinary Diversions

Patients who have their bladder removed (cystectomy) because of cancer or significant bladder dysfunction (e.g., related to radiation injury or neurogenic dysfunction with frequent UTI) require surgical procedures that divert urine to the outside of the body through an opening in the abdominal wall called a **stoma**. A **urinary diversion** is constructed from a section of intestine to create a storage reservoir or conduit for urine.

Table 21.1 Types of Urinary Incontinence

Definition	Characteristics	Selected Nursing Interventions
TRANSIENT INCONTINENCE		
Incontinence caused by medical conditions that in many cases are treatable and reversible	Common reversible causes include: ▪ Delirium and/or acute confusion ▪ Inflammation (e.g., UTI, urethritis) ▪ Medications (diuretics) (Kehinde, 2016) ▪ Excessive urine output (e.g., hyperglycemia, heart failure) ▪ Mobility impairment ▪ Fecal impaction ▪ Depression ▪ Acute urinary retention ▪ Conditions that increase blood pressure or blood osmolality (e.g., dehydration) (Testa, 2015)	Look for reversible causes with new-onset or increased incontinence. Notify health care provider of any suspected reversible causes.
FUNCTIONAL INCONTINENCE		
Loss of continence from causes outside the urinary tract; usually related to functional deficits such as altered mobility and manual dexterity, cognitive impairment, or environmental barriers impairing ability to reach or use toilet (Bardsley, 2016)	Toilet access restricted by: ▪ Sensory impairments (e.g., vision) ▪ Cognitive impairments cause poor motivation for or inability to attend to continence (e.g., delirium, dementia, severe retardation) ▪ Altered mobility (e.g., hip fracture, arthritis, chronic pain, spastic paralysis associated with multiple sclerosis; slow movements associated with Parkinson disease, hemiparesis) ▪ Altered manual dexterity (e.g., arthritis, upper extremity fracture) ▪ Environmental barriers (e.g., caregiver unavailable to help with transfers, pathway to bathroom not maneuverable with walker, tight clothing that is difficult to remove, incontinence briefs)	Ensure adequate lighting in bathroom. Provide individualized toileting program designed for degree of cognitive impairment: habit training program, scheduled toileting program, and prompted voiding program. Provide mobility aids (e.g., raised toilet seats, toilet grab bars). Clear toilet area to allow access for walker or wheelchair. Suggest use of elastic waist pants without buttons or zippers. Stress that call bell always be within reach. Use incontinence containment product that the patient can easily remove such as pull-up type pant or pad that can be moved aside easily for voiding.
OVERFLOW URINARY INCONTINENCE		
Involuntary loss of urine caused by overdistended bladder; often related to bladder outlet obstruction or poor bladder emptying caused by weak or absent bladder contractions	Distended bladder on palpation High postvoid residual Frequency Involuntary leakage of small volumes of urine Nocturia Common causes include neurological impairment, pelvic surgery, constipation, fecal impaction, pregnancy, prolapse, medication, and benign prostatic hyperplasia (Bardsley, 2016)	Interventions are individualized related to severity of urinary retention, ability of bladder to contract, and kidney damage. **Mild retention with some bladder function:** ▪ Timed voiding ▪ Double voiding ▪ Monitor postvoid residual per health care provider's direction ▪ Intermittent catheterization **Severe retention, no bladder function:** ▪ Intermittent catheterization ▪ Indwelling catheterization
STRESS URINARY INCONTINENCE		
Involuntary leakage of small volumes of urine associated with increased intra-abdominal pressure and urethral hypermobility or weakness of or injury to urinary sphincter (e.g., weak pelvic floor muscles, trauma after childbirth, radical prostatectomy)	Small volume loss of urine with coughing, sneezing, laughing, exercise, walking, bending, lifting, or getting up from a chair Usually does not leak urine at night when sleeping	As directed by health care provider, instruct the patient in pelvic muscle (Kegel) exercises (Box 21.5): eight contractions performed three times a day (Bardsley, 2016).
URGE URINARY INCONTINENCE		
Involuntary passage of urine often associated with strong sense of urgency related to overactive bladder (involuntary bladder contractions) caused by neurological problems, bladder inflammation, or bladder outlet obstruction	May experience one or all of the following symptoms: ▪ Urgency ▪ Frequency ▪ Nocturia ▪ Difficulty or unable to hold urine once urge to void occurs ▪ Leaks on way to bathroom ▪ Leaks larger volumes of urine, sometimes enough to wet outer clothing ▪ Dribbling small amounts on way to bathroom ▪ Strong urge/leaks when hears water running, washes hands, drinks fluids	Ask the patient about symptoms of UTI. Avoid bladder irritants (e.g., caffeine, smoking tobacco, alcohol). Instruct the patient in pelvic muscle (Kegel) exercises, urge inhibition exercises, or bladder training. If ordered by health care provider, monitor the patient's symptoms and for presence of side effects of antimuscarinic medications.

Continued

Table 21.1 Types of Urinary Incontinence—cont'd

Definition	Characteristics	Selected Nursing Interventions
REFLEX URINARY INCONTINENCE		
Involuntary loss of urine occurring at predictable intervals when the patient reaches specific bladder volume related to spinal cord damage from C1 to S2	Diminished or absent awareness of bladder filling and urge to void Leakage of urine without awareness May not completely empty bladder because of dyssynergia of urinary sphincter (i.e., inappropriate contraction of sphincter when bladder contracts, causing obstruction to urine flow) **Caution:** Patients with reflex incontinence are at risk for developing autonomic dysreflexia, a life-threatening condition that causes severe elevation of blood pressure and pulse rate and diaphoresis	Follow prescribed schedule for emptying bladder either through voiding or by intermittent catheterization. Use urine containment products: condom catheter, undergarments, pads, and briefs. Monitor for signs and symptoms of urinary retention and UTI. Monitor for autonomic dysreflexia; this is a medical emergency requiring immediate intervention. Notify health care provider immediately.

UTI, urinary tract infection.

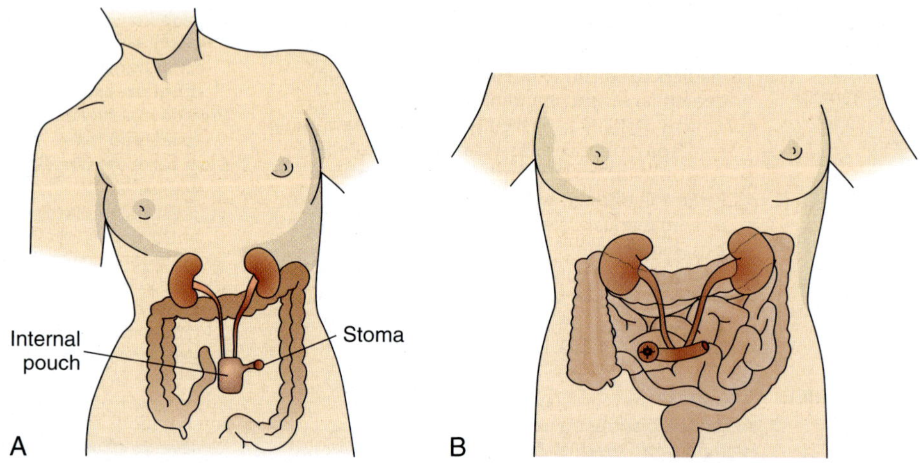

Fig. 21.2 Types of incontinent and continent urinary diversions. **A,** Continent urinary reservoir. **B,** Urostomy (ileal conduit).

There are two types of continent urinary diversions. The continent urinary reservoir (Fig. 21.2A) is created from a distal portion of the ileum and proximal portion of the colon. The ureters are embedded in the reservoir, which is placed under the abdominal wall. A narrow segment of the ileum is brought out through the abdominal wall to form a small stoma. The ileocecal valve creates a one-way valve in the pouch. A catheter is inserted through the stoma to empty urine from the pouch. Patients catheterize the pouch four to six times a day for the rest of their lives.

The other type of continent urinary diversion, an orthotopic neobladder, uses an ileal pouch to replace the bladder. Anatomically the pouch is in the same position as the bladder was before removal, allowing a patient to void through the urethra using the Valsalva technique.

An ileal conduit or **ureterostomy** is a permanent incontinent urinary diversion created by transplanting the ureters into a closed-off portion of the intestinal ileum. The other end of the ureters come out onto the abdominal wall, forming a stoma (Fig. 21.2B). Patients have no sensation or control over the continuous flow of urine through the ileal conduit, requiring the effluent (drainage) to be collected in a pouch.

Nephrostomy tubes are small tubes tunneled through the skin into the renal pelvis to drain the renal pelvis when the ureter is obstructed. Patients go home with these tubes and need careful teaching about site care and signs of infection.

FACILITATING URINE ELIMINATION

Assessment

To identify urinary elimination problems and ensure patient-centered diagnosis and care, use your scientific and nursing knowledge, conduct a thorough nursing history of a patient's problem, perform a physical examination, assess a patient's urine, and review information from diagnostic tests and examinations.

Nursing History

The nursing history includes a review of a patient's elimination patterns, symptoms of urinary alterations, and assessment of factors affecting normal urination. Because urination is often considered a private matter, some patients find it difficult to talk about their voiding habits. Approach patients in a professional manner, and assure them that you will maintain their confidentiality.

Pattern of Urination

Information about a patient's normal pattern of urination establishes a baseline for comparison. Ask a patient about daily voiding patterns including frequency and times of day, normal volume at each voiding, and history of recent changes. Frequency of voiding varies among individuals depending on fluid intake, medications such as diuretics, and the intake of alcohol and caffeine. Be sure to ask whether a patient is awakened from sleep with an urge to void and how many times this occurs. It is normal for hospitalized patients to experience an urge to void when they awaken at night because of noise, pain, or required treatments (e.g., nebulizer treatment).

Symptoms of Urinary Alterations

During assessment, ask about the presence of symptoms listed in Table 21.2. Also determine whether a patient is aware of conditions or factors that precipitate or aggravate the symptoms.

Table 21.2 Common Symptoms of Urinary Alterations

Description	Common Causes
URGENCY	
Immediate and strong desire to void that is not easily deferred	Full bladder UTI Inflammation or irritation of bladder Overactive bladder
DYSURIA	
Pain or discomfort associated with voiding	UTI Inflammation of prostate Urethritis Trauma to lower urinary tract Urinary tract tumors
FREQUENCY	
Voiding more than eight times during waking hours and/or at decreased intervals such as less than every 2 h	High volumes of fluid intake Alcohol intake Bladder irritants (e.g., caffeine) UTI Increased pressure on bladder (e.g., pregnancy) Bladder outlet obstruction (e.g., prostate enlargement, pelvic organ prolapse) Overactive bladder Uncontrolled diabetes mellitus or diabetes insipidus
HESITANCY	
Delay in start of urinary stream when voiding	Anxiety (e.g., voiding in public restroom or in front of others) Bladder outlet obstruction (e.g., prostate enlargement, urethral stricture)
POLYURIA	
Voiding excessive amounts of urine	High volumes of fluid intake Uncontrolled diabetes mellitus Diabetes insipidus Diuretic therapy
OLIGURIA	
Diminished urinary output in relation to fluid intake	Fluid and electrolyte imbalance (e.g., dehydration) Kidney dysfunction or failure Increased secretion of ADH Urinary tract obstruction
NOCTURIA	
Awakened from sleep by urge to void	Excessive intake of fluids (especially coffee or alcohol before bedtime) Bladder outlet obstruction (e.g., prostate enlargement) Overactive bladder Medications (e.g., diuretic taken in the evening) Cardiovascular disease (e.g., hypertension) UTI
DRIBBLING	
Leakage of small amounts of urine despite voluntary control of micturition	Bladder outlet obstruction (e.g., prostatic enlargement) Incomplete bladder emptying Stress incontinence
HEMATURIA	
Presence of blood in urine Gross hematuria—blood easily seen in urine Microscopic hematuria—blood not visualized but detected on urinalysis	Tumors (e.g., kidney, bladder) Infection (e.g., glomerular nephritis, cystitis) Urinary tract calculi Trauma to urinary tract
RETENTION	
Acute retention: Suddenly unable to void when bladder is adequately full or overfull Chronic retention: Bladder does not empty completely during voiding, and urine retained in bladder	Bladder outlet obstruction (e.g., prostatic enlargement, urethral obstruction) Absent or weak bladder contractility (e.g., neurological dysfunction such as caused by diabetes, multiple sclerosis, lower spinal cord injury) Side effects of certain medications (e.g., anesthesia, anticholinergics, antispasmodics, antidepressants)

ADH, antidiuretic hormone; *UTI*, urinary tract infection.

Factors Affecting Voiding

Focused assessment enables you to gather data relevant to your patient's elimination pattern and identify factors that impact the ability to void normally (Table 21.3).

Older Adult Considerations

Normal aging causes changes in the urinary system and the rest of the body that increase the risk for bladder dysfunction (Box 21.2; see also Box 21.1). Aging and long-term neurological conditions such as multiple sclerosis, stroke, and dementia can also affect the urinary system and create elimination changes (Jones, 2015). These changes usually include decreased bladder capacity, decreased ability to delay voiding, loss of bladder contractility, and increased incidence of overactive bladder.

Physical Assessment

Assessment of the urinary system helps you identify signs and severity of urinary problems and monitor responses to medical and nursing interventions. The primary areas

Table 21.3 Focused Patient Assessment

Factors to Assess	Questions	Physical Assessment
Fluid intake	Do you have any fluid restrictions? How much do you normally drink in 24 h? Describe the types of fluids you drink. Are you decreasing your fluid intake because you need to use the toilet too often? How often do you drink beverages that contain caffeine or alcohol (e.g., coffee, tea, soft drinks, beer)?	Observe skin and mucous membranes for adequate hydration. Obtain intake and output over 24 h.
Urinary symptoms (see Table 21.2)	Are you experiencing a sudden urge to urinate, burning or painful urination, frequent urination, difficulty urinating, excessive urination, the need to urinate at night, dribbling or blood in the urine, straining when you urinate, leaking urine on the way to the bathroom, or leaking urine when you cough or sneeze? Do you feel like you have completely emptied your bladder after you have urinated? When did you last urinate? How many times did you urinate in the last 24 h?	Observe urine for: ▪ Red color ▪ Cloudiness ▪ Foul odor ▪ Amount with each voiding Assess vital signs for fever and tachycardia. Assess 24-h intake and output. Start a bladder diary to record frequency and episodes of incontinence. Inspect the abdomen for distention. Inspect the perineal skin for evidence of incontinence-associated dermatitis. Palpate bladder for tenderness or distention. Determine postvoid residual by bladder scan if available.
Medication usage	Which medications including prescription, over-the-counter, and herbal supplements do you take, and how often do you take them?	Assess for signs of fluid and electrolyte disturbances (see Chapter 25).
	Do you take blood pressure medicine or a diuretic?	Inspect urine for pale color and dilute concentration. Start a bladder diary to record frequency and episodes of incontinence.
	Are you taking pain medicine?	Assess output for decreased frequency and amount. Palpate bladder for distention. Assess bowel pattern for constipation.
Functional ability	Do you have trouble getting to the bathroom or toilet on time?	Observe the patient's ability to get up or out of bed and walk safely to bathroom.
	What type of help do you need when using the bathroom?	Observe the patient's ability to safely get on and off toilet.
	Do you have trouble removing your clothing to use the toilet?	Observe the patient's ability to remove clothing for toileting and perform hygiene.
	Do you have difficulty cleaning yourself after urinating? Do you use a product to contain urine leakage (e.g., brief or incontinence pad)?	Assess the patient's ability to understand instructions related to toileting (cognition, language, culture).
Environment	Does anything prevent you from getting to the bathroom on time? Do you use assistive devices in the bathroom (e.g., elevated toilet seat, handrails)?	Assess for adequate lighting in bathroom and need for assistive devices to facilitate safe toileting; easy access to nurse call system; clear path to bathroom, especially if a walker is used; and prompt response of nursing assistive personnel to patient requests for toileting.
Medical history that possibly affects urinary system	Do you have a history of a UTI, urinary incontinence, urinary retention, kidney stones, prostate disease, pregnancy, neurological disease, pelvic organ prolapse, or diabetes mellitus? Do you have any difficulty feeling the need to urinate?	Start a bladder diary to record frequency, amount, and episodes of incontinence.
Recent surgery and critical illness (some anesthesia affects sensory and motor function of the bladder)	Do you feel the urge to urinate? Have you urinated since your surgery? Did you have a catheter before or after surgery?	Assess intake and output record for adequate frequency and amounts of voiding. Using a bladder scan, assess for urinary retention.

UTI, urinary tract infection.

BOX 21.2 Care of an Older Adult

Bladder Dysfunction

- The prevalence of overactive bladder (OAB) (urgency, urge incontinence, frequency, and nocturia in the absence of UTI) increases with age (Rantell, 2014).
- The risk for urinary incontinence increases in patients as a result of aging, cognitive impairment, and chronic disease (Jones, 2015; Nazarko, 2015).
- Assess all possible causes of new-onset incontinence, which includes taking a comprehensive history for urinary incontinence (onset, duration, aggravating factors, characteristics, medical history, associated symptoms, attempted treatments, and severity) and performing a focused physical assessment of physical indicators within each body system (coughing, sensory impairment, skin breakdown) (Testa, 2015).
- Carefully assess older adults taking an antimuscarinic medication to treat urgency, urge incontinence, and OAB for mental status changes. Side effects of these medications include cognitive impairment, sedation, and inability to concentrate (Bardsley, 2016).
- Implement plans to maximize self-care and continence (e.g., toileting program, mobility aides, assistance with hygiene) when caring for older adults with impaired mobility and incontinence.
- Teach older women with stress incontinence about pelvic muscle (Kegel) exercises. There is no age limit on their effectiveness.
- The sensation of thirst decreases with aging. Remind older adults to drink adequate amounts of water.

to assess include the kidneys, bladder, external genitalia, urethral meatus, and perineal skin (see Chapter 7).

Assessment of Urine

To assess a patient's urine, measure a patient's fluid intake and urinary output (I&O), and observe the characteristics of the urine.

Intake and Output

You assess I&O to evaluate bladder emptying, renal function, and fluid and electrolyte balance. Although often written as part of a health care provider's order, placing a patient on I&O is also nursing judgment. Obtaining accurate I&O measurement often requires cooperation and assistance from a patient and family. Include all oral liquids and semiliquids, enteral feedings, and any parenteral fluids as intake (see Chapter 20). Include urine and any other fluid that leaves the body that can be measured, such as vomitus, gastric drainage in tubes, and wound drainage that is collected as output.

Urinary output is more than a key indicator of kidney and bladder function. A change in urine volume is significant, often indicating fluid imbalance, kidney dysfunction, or decreased blood volume. If a patient has an indwelling catheter after surgery, assess urinary output hourly to indirectly measure circulating blood volume. Continually assess your patient for signs of blood loss, and notify the health care provider if the urinary output falls below 30 mL/h for more than 2 consecutive hours or if the patient has excessive urine output (called polyuria). Evaluate patients who have not voided for longer than 3–6 hours and have had fluid intake recorded for urinary retention. Assess for extreme increases or decreases in urine volume. Sometimes, just helping a patient to a normal position to void prompts urinary elimination.

Measure urine volume with containers that have volume measurement markings. Use a **graduated measuring container** after a patient voids in a bedside commode, bedpan, or urinal or after emptying urine from a catheter drainage bag. Each patient needs to have a graduated container for individual use to prevent potential cross-contamination. Label each container with the patient's name. Rinse the container after each use to minimize odor and bacterial growth. A **urine hat** (Fig. 21.3) collects urine in a toilet, allowing for patient privacy in the bathroom. Some catheters have a specialized drainage bag with a **urometer** attached between the drainage tubing and the drainage bag that allows for accurate hourly urine measurement (Fig. 21.4). Empty drainage bags every 8 hours or as needed and record the output. When emptying catheter drainage bags, make sure that the drainage tube is reclamped and secured.

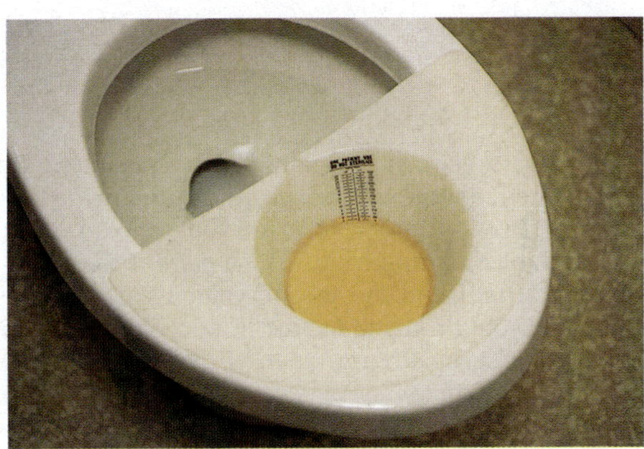

Fig. 21.3 Urine hat.

Characteristics of Urine

Inspect urine for color, clarity, and odor. Monitor and document any changes.

Laboratory and Diagnostic Testing

You are responsible for collecting urine specimens for laboratory testing. The type of test determines the method of collection. Label all specimens at the bedside with the patient's name, date, time, and type of collection. Complete laboratory requisition forms with specific information required by the testing laboratory. Most urine specimens need to reach the laboratory within 2 hours of collection or be preserved according to the laboratory protocol (Pagana et al., 2017). Urine that stands in a container at room temperature without the required preservative grows bacteria and experiences changes that affect the accuracy of the test. Follow agency infection control policies and standard precautions when handling urine specimens (see Chapter 9). Urine specimens commonly collected include

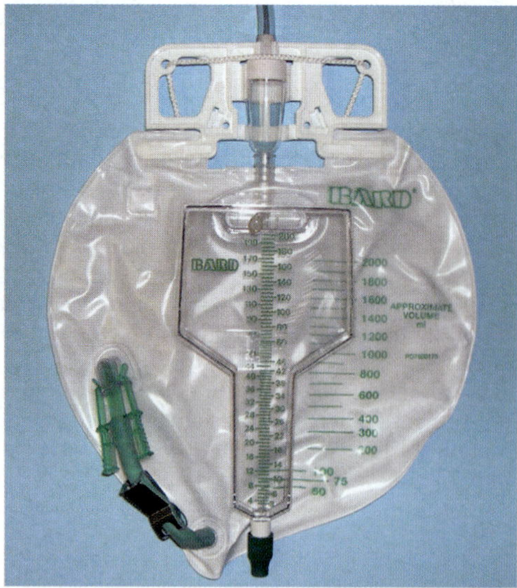

Fig. 21.4 Urometer. (Courtesy Michael Gallager, RN, BSN, MSN, OSF, Saint Francis Medical Center, Peoria, IL.)

first morning specimen, random urine specimen, timed urine specimen, double-voided specimen, and urine for culture and sensitivity. To obtain urine that is freshly voided, ask the patient to double void. Ask a patient to empty the bladder, and then send the second voided specimen to the laboratory. To obtain urine as free of bacterial contamination as possible, a midstream, clean-catch urine specimen is sometimes required.

Urinalysis

When a routine urinalysis is ordered, collect a random or first morning specimen. A routine urinalysis requires no special preparation and is collected either by the patient voiding into an appropriate clean container or by urethral catheterization. You can obtain specimens from an indwelling catheter as long as you use the specimen port and not the drainage bag. **Urinalysis** includes a number of tests that are used for diagnostic screening for fluid and electrolyte disturbances, UTI, presence of blood, and other metabolic problems (Table 21.4). In some health care settings, you test urine using reagent strips. Follow manufacturer instructions when performing the test and reading the strips. Dip the reagent strip into fresh urine, and observe for color changes on the strip. Compare the colors on the strip with a color chart on the reagent strip container. Be sure to examine each color at the exact time indicated on the container.

Timed Urine Tests

Timed testing requires urine collection and testing either at a specific time of day or urine collected over a specific time period. These tests measure substances that may be excreted at higher levels at specific times of the day such as glucose 2 hours after a meal or substances that are to be measured over a specific time period such as sodium, potassium, and chloride as indicators of fluid and electrolyte disturbance (Pagana et al., 2017). For most 24-hour specimen collections, discard the first voided specimen and start collecting all urine with the next void for a 24-hour period in a special container that has a preservative added. Depending on the

Table 21.4 Routine Urinalysis Values

Measurement (Normal Value)	Interpretation
pH (4.6–8.0)	Indicates acid–base balance (average 6.0). Acid pH helps protect against bacterial growth. Urine that stands for several hours becomes alkaline from bacterial growth.
Protein (up to 8 mg/100 mL)	Protein is normally not present in urine. Presence of protein is a very sensitive indicator of kidney disease. Damage to glomerular membrane (such as in glomerulonephritis) allows for filtration of larger molecules such as protein to seep through.
Glucose (not normally present)	Patients with poorly controlled diabetes have glucose in the urine because of inability of tubules to resorb high serum glucose concentrations (greater than 180 mg/100 mL). Ingestion of high concentrations of glucose causes some glucose to appear in urine of healthy individuals.
Ketones (not normally present)	With poor control of type 1 diabetes, patients experience breakdown of fatty acids. End products of fatty acid metabolism are ketones. Patients with dehydration, starvation, high-protein diets, alcoholism, or excessive aspirin ingestion also have ketonuria.
Blood	A positive test for occult blood occurs when intact erythrocytes, hemoglobin, or myoglobin is present. Damage to glomerulus or tubules causes blood cells to enter urine. Trauma or disease of lower urinary tract also causes hematuria.
Specific gravity (1.005–1.030)	Measures concentration of particles in urine. High specific gravity reflects concentrated urine, and low specific gravity reflects diluted urine. Dehydration, reduced renal blood flow, and increase in ADH secretion elevate specific gravity. Overhydration, early renal disease, and inadequate ADH secretion reduce specific gravity.
Microscopic examination	
RBCs (up to 2)	Damage to glomeruli or tubules allows RBCs to enter the urine. Trauma, disease, presence of urethral catheters, or surgery of the lower urinary tract also causes RBCs to be present.
WBCs (0–4 per low-power field)	Elevated numbers indicate inflammation or infection.
Bacteria (not normally present)	Usually indicates infection or colonization (presence of bacteria and the patient shows no symptoms of infection).
Casts (not normally present)	Casts are microscopic cylindrical bodies that look like objects within the renal tubule. There are two main categories of casts: acellular and cellular. Acellular casts include hyaline, granular, waxy, and fatty; cellular casts include WBC, RBC, bacterial, and epithelial cell casts. Their presence often indicates renal disease.
Crystals (not normally present)	Crystals indicate increased risk for development of renal calculi (stone). Some patients with high uric acid levels (gout) develop uric acid crystals. Patients with parathyroid abnormalities or malabsorption often develop phosphate and calcium oxalate crystals.

ADH, antidiuretic hormone; *RBC*, red blood cell; *WBC*, white blood cell.
Data from Pagana TJ, et al: *Mosby's diagnostic and laboratory test reference*, ed 13, St Louis, 2017, Mosby.

test, you need to keep the urine container cool by placing it in a container of ice. Provide patient education including an explanation of the test, an emphasis on the need to collect all urine voided during the prescribed time period, and how to avoid contaminating the specimen with stool or toilet paper. Carefully document the start and stop time of the test, as requested by the laboratory, to improve testing accuracy.

Clean-Catch Midstream Specimen

Collect a clean-catch midstream specimen when you want to obtain a specimen relatively free of contaminating microorganisms. A clean-catch urine specimen kit includes a sterile cup and disinfectant wipes. Illustrated instructions are often included. Teach the patient how to cleanse the urinary meatus effectively two to three times with a separate clean wipe each time, and remind female patients to clean the meatus by wiping front to back. Instruct male patients to retract their foreskin if not circumcised and to cleanse the meatus in a circular motion, moving from the center of the meatus to the outside. After cleansing, the patient opens the sterile urine cup. Caution your patient not to touch the inside of the cup. To collect the specimen, instruct the patient to start voiding in the toilet or other receptacle, stop the stream, position the sterile cup to collect urine, and then continue voiding into the cup. When finished, you or your patient puts the lid on the cup, and you send the specimen to the laboratory for testing.

Urine for Culture and Sensitivity

Urine specimens collected for culture and sensitivity determine the presence of bacteria and identify the appropriate antibiotic needed. Collect the specimen using clean-catheter midstream urine or by sterile catheterization (see Skill 21.1). Catheterize the stoma of a patient with a urinary diversion to obtain an accurate specimen. Sometimes, a preliminary report is available in 24 hours, but usually 48–72 hours are needed for bacterial growth and sensitivity testing (Pagana et al., 2017).

Diagnostic Examinations

The urinary system is one of the few organ systems accessible to accurate diagnostic study by radiographic techniques. Studies are either simple and noninvasive or complex and invasive (Table 21.5). Before testing, nursing responsibilities include ensuring that a signed consent is completed (check agency policy). Assess whether the patient has allergies or

Table 21.5 Common Diagnostic Testing

Procedure	Description	Special Nursing Considerations
NONINVASIVE PROCEDURES		
Abdominal radiograph (plain film; KUB or flat plate)	X-ray film of abdomen to determine size, shape, symmetry, and location of structures of lower urinary tract. Common uses: Detects and measures size of urinary calculi.	**Preparation:** ▪ No special preparation. ▪ Previous GI barium contrast study could alter results. ▪ Contraindicated in pregnant patients.
CT scan	Noninvasive, detailed, three-dimensional, real-time display imaging of abdominal structures provided by computerized reconstruction of cross-sectional images. Common uses: Identifies anatomical abnormalities, renal tumors, cysts, calculi, and obstruction of ureters.	**Preparation:** ▪ Follow bowel cleansing protocol. ▪ Assess for allergy to shellfish (iodine) or previous reaction to contrast media (if contrast agent is ordered). ▪ Restrict food and fluid up to 4 h before test (see agency protocol). **After procedure:** ▪ Encourage fluids to promote excretion of dye. ▪ Assess for delayed hypersensitivity reaction to contrast media. **Patient teaching:** ▪ Explain that the patient will be placed on a special bed that will move through a tunnel-like imaging chamber. The patient needs to lie still when instructed by the technician. Some patients feel claustrophobic and may need an order for a mild sedative.
IVP	Imaging of urinary tract that views collecting ducts and renal pelvis and outlines ureters, bladder, and urethra; after i.v. injection of contrast media (iodine-based that converts to a dye), a series of X-ray films are taken to observe passage of urine from renal pelvis to bladder. Common uses: Detects and measures urinary calculi, tumors, hematuria, and obstruction of urinary tract.	**Preparation:** ▪ Assess for allergies and dehydration. ▪ Follow bowel cleansing protocol. ▪ Restrict food and fluid up to 4 h before test (see agency protocol). **After procedure:** ▪ Assess for delayed hypersensitivity to contrast media. ▪ Encourage fluids after test to dilute and flush dye from the patient. ▪ Assess urine output; less than 30 mL/h increases risk for contrast-induced nephropathy. **Patient teaching:** ▪ Facial flushing and salty taste in the mouth is a normal response during dye injection. Patients also often feel dizzy, warm, or nauseated.
Ultrasound renal bladder	Imaging of kidneys, ureters, and bladder using sound waves. Identifies gross structural abnormalities and estimates volume of urine in bladder. Common uses: Detects masses, cysts, obstruction, presence of hydronephrosis or hydroureter, abnormalities of bladder wall, and renal and pelvic calculi; measures postvoid residual.	**Preparation:** ▪ Patients need to come to study with full bladder. ▪ Fasting is not required. **Patient teaching:** ▪ Test is completed in about 1 h. ▪ The patient will experience little or no discomfort during procedure.

Continued

Table 21.5 Common Diagnostic Testing—cont'd

Procedure	Description	Special Nursing Considerations
INVASIVE PROCEDURES		
Endoscopy—cystoscopy	Introduction of cystoscope through urethra into bladder to provide direct visualization, specimen collection, or treatment of bladder and urethra. Procedure is performed using local anesthesia in most cases, but under certain circumstances, general anesthesia or conscious sedation may be used. Common uses: Microscopic hematuria; detects bladder tumors and obstruction of bladder outlet and urethra.	**Preparation:** ▪ Encourage the patient to drink fluids several hours before procedure to ensure steady flow of urine and prevent infection. ▪ When applicable, follow agency protocol for preoperative preparation (see Chapter 23). **During procedure:** ▪ Instruct the patient to lie still. ▪ The patient may feel need to void as cystoscope passes bladder neck. **Patient teaching:** ▪ Urine is sometimes tinged pink after test. Assess for signs and symptoms of UTI. Antibiotics are often ordered before and after procedure to reduce risk of UTI.

CT, computed tomography; *GI*, gastrointestinal; *IVP*, intravenous pyelogram; *KUB*, kidney, ureter, bladder; *UTI*, urinary tract infection.
Data from Pagana TJ, et al: *Mosby's diagnostic and laboratory test reference*, ed 13, St Louis, 2017, Mosby.

has experienced a previous reaction to a contrast agent (Pagana et al., 2017). Administer bowel cleansing agents as ordered; check agency policy. Ensure that the patient adheres to the appropriate pretest diet, which may be clear liquids or nothing by mouth (NPO). Nursing responsibilities after testing include assessing I&O and voiding and urine (color, clarity, presence of blood, dysuria, problems emptying). Also encourage fluid intake, especially if using radiopaque dye.

Promoting Normal Micturition

Maintaining normal urinary elimination prevents many problems. Instruct the patient to void at regular intervals, usually every 3–4 hours, depending on fluid intake. Teach patients to report to their health care provider any changes in bladder habits, frequency, urgency, pain when voiding, or blood in the urine. Many measures that promote normal voiding are independent nursing interventions.

Maintaining Elimination Habits

When in a hospital or long-term care facility, institutional routines often conflict with a patient's normal voiding routine. Create as much privacy as possible such as closing the door and bedside curtains; asking visitors to leave a room when a bedside commode, bedpan, or urinal is used; and masking the sounds of voiding with running water. Respond to requests for assistance with toileting as quickly as possible. Embarrassing accidents are easily avoided when help comes in time. Avoid the use of incontinence containment products unless needed for uncontrolled urine leakage. Some containment products are difficult to remove, increase the incidence of skin breakdown when not removed quickly, and interfere with prompt toilet access. Patients should avoid straining when voiding or moving the bowels. Encourage them to take enough time to empty the bladder completely, up to 5–10 minutes for some patients. Instruct patients to keep the bowels regular. A rectum full of stool irritates the bladder, causing urgency and frequency.

Maintaining Adequate Fluid Intake

A simple method to promote normal micturition is maintaining optimal fluid intake. A patient with normal renal function and no health problems requiring fluid restriction (e.g., heart failure) needs up to 2300 mL of fluid in a 24-hour period. Adequate fluid intake helps flush out solutes or particles that collect in the urinary system and decreases bladder irritability. Help patients increase their fluid intake by teaching the importance of adequate hydration, setting a schedule for drinking extra fluids, identifying fluid preferences, increasing high-fluid foods such as fruits, and encouraging frequent fluid intake in small volumes. Avoid or limit drinking beverages that contain caffeine (coffee, tea, chocolate drinks, soft drinks). Instruct patients to not limit fluids if experiencing incontinence. Concentrated urine often irritates the bladder and increases bladder symptoms. To prevent nocturia, suggest that a patient avoid drinking fluids 2 hours before bedtime.

Promoting Complete Bladder Emptying

It is normal for a small volume of urine to remain in the bladder after micturition. When the bladder does not empty completely, and **residual urine** volumes are high, there is risk for incontinence and dangerous urinary retention. Excessive accumulation of urine in the bladder is painful for the patient; increases the risk for UTI; and can cause backward flow of urine into the ureters to the kidneys, causing kidney damage. Adequate bladder emptying depends on feeling an urge to urinate, contracting the bladder, and relaxing the urethral sphincter. Help patients into the normal position for voiding to promote relaxation and stimulate bladder contractions. Squatting is the normal anatomical position for female voiding. Women empty the bladder better when sitting on the toilet or bedside commode with the feet on the floor. If a female patient cannot use a toilet, position her on a bedpan (see Chapter 16). After bedpan use, help the patient perform perineal hygiene (see Chapter 16). A man voids more easily while standing. If the patient is unable to reach a toilet, have him stand at the bedside and void into a **urinal** (a plastic or metal receptacle for urine) (Fig. 21.5A). Always assess mobility status to determine whether a male patient can stand safely, and implement safety measures such as having someone assist him if needed. If a patient is unable to stand at the bedside, help him use the urinal in bed. Some patients need help positioning the penis completely within the urinal and holding the urinal in place. Once the patient finishes voiding, carefully remove the urinal and perform perineal hygiene (see Chapter 16). Most urinals are used by men, but some are

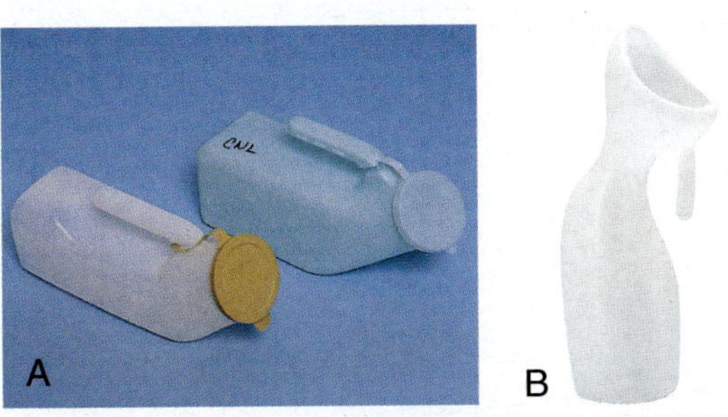

Fig. 21.5 Types of male urinals **(A)** and female urinals **(B)**. (**B,** Courtesy Medegen Medical Products.)

specially designed for women (Fig. 21.5B). A female urinal has a larger opening at the top with a defined rim that helps position the urinal closely against the genitalia.

Educate your patients about ways to enhance their urinary health and improve bladder emptying. To promote relaxation and stimulate bladder contractions, use sensory stimuli (e.g., turning on running water, putting a patient's hand in a pan of warm water, or stroking the female patient's inner thigh) and provide privacy. To improve bladder emptying, encourage patients to wait until the urine flow completely stops when voiding, and encourage them to attempt a second void (double voiding). Also encourage patients to attempt voiding according to the clock, not according to urge; this is called *timed voiding*. Do not implement the Credé method or manual compression of the bladder (i.e., placing the hands over the bladder and compressing it to assist in emptying) unless ordered by the health care provider. In the presence of a high **postvoid residual** or a complete inability of the bladder to empty, either intermittent or indwelling urinary catheterization is often required.

Preventing Infection

UTIs are one of the most common infections encountered in a primary care practice, accounting for 15% of antibiotic prescriptions that are ordered (Haddock, 2015). As a nurse, you play a key role in implementing evidenced-based practices to avoid this common and potentially dangerous infection. Some key interventions include promoting adequate fluid intake, perineal hygiene, and voiding at regular intervals. Encourage female patients to wipe from front to back after voiding and defecation; to avoid perfumed perineal washes and sprays, bubble baths, and tight clothing; to void before and after sexual intercourse; and to wear cotton underwear. If a patient has a problem with urine leakage, stress the importance of hygiene. Patients who use containment products need to use products that are designed for urine and wick wetness away from the body. Teach patients to avoid prolonged periods of urine wetness to prevent skin breakdown.

CATHETERIZATION

Urinary **catheterization** is the placement of a tube through the urethra into the bladder to drain urine. Because of the risk of **catheter-associated urinary tract infections (CAUTIs)**, the ANA developed an evidenced-based tool, the *ANA CAUTI Prevention Tool*, to guide the health care team with decision making regarding indwelling catheter insertion and care, maintenance of sterile technique, and best practices for timely catheter removal (Panchisin, 2016). Skill 36.1 lists steps for performing female and male urethral catheterization.

Patients can have urinary catheterization for short-term (up to 7 days), medium-term (up to 28 days), or long-term (up to a maximum of 12 weeks) periods (Yates, 2016). Conditions that require urinary catheter insertion include the need for accurate monitoring of urine output during some surgical procedures, critical illness, acute urinary retention, bladder outlet obstruction, and prolonged immobilization from spinal or multiple traumatic injuries. Catheterization should not be used routinely in surgical patients or in patients in nursing homes with incontinence (Gould et al., 2017). Indwelling catheters are also used for promotion of wound healing in sacral or perineal wounds and as a comfort measure in end-of-life care (Panchisin, 2016). Intermittent catheterization is used to measure postvoid residual when a bladder scanner is not available or as a way to manage chronic urinary retention.

Types of Catheters

Urinary catheters differ based on the number of catheter lumens. Some have balloons to keep the indwelling catheter in place, and some have a closed drainage system. Urinary catheters are made with one to three lumens (Fig. 21.6). You use single-lumen catheters (see Fig. 21.6A) for intermittent/straight catheterization (i.e., insertion of a catheter for one-time bladder emptying). Double-lumen catheters, designed for indwelling catheters, provide one lumen for urinary drainage and a second lumen that is used to inflate a balloon that keeps the catheter in place (see Fig. 21.6B). Use triple-lumen catheters (see Fig. 21.6C) for continuous bladder irrigation (CBI) or when it is necessary to instill medications into a patient's bladder. One lumen drains the bladder, a second lumen inflates the balloon, and a third lumen delivers irrigation fluid into the bladder.

A health care provider chooses a catheter on the basis of factors such as latex allergy, history of catheter encrustation, and susceptibility to infection. Indwelling catheters are made of latex or silicone. Latex catheters with a special coating such as polytetrafluoroethylene reduce urethral irritation (Yates, 2016). All silicone catheters have a larger internal diameter and are often helpful for patients who require frequent catheter changes because of encrustation. Antimicrobial catheters are coated with silver or an antibiotic. Current evidence shows that silver-coated catheters may reduce the incidence of CAUTI for short-term use (Yates, 2016). Intermittent/straight catheters are made of rubber (softer and more flexible) or polyvinyl chloride. Patients who self-catheterize have a large selection of catheters, some with special coatings that do not require lubrication and others that are self-contained systems consisting of a prelubricated catheter and packaged with a preconnected drainage bag.

Catheter Sizes

The size of a urinary catheter is based on the French (Fr) scale, which reflects the internal diameter of the catheter. Use the smallest indwelling catheter size possible, 10–12 Fr for women and 12–14 Fr for men, to minimize trauma and

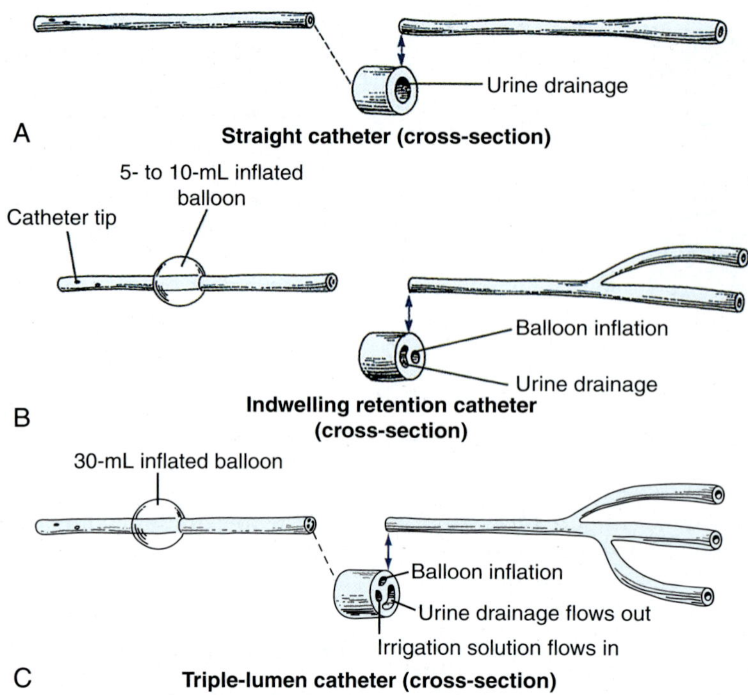

Fig. 21.6 **A,** Straight catheter (cross-section). **B,** Indwelling retention catheter (cross-section). **C,** Triple-lumen catheter (cross-section).

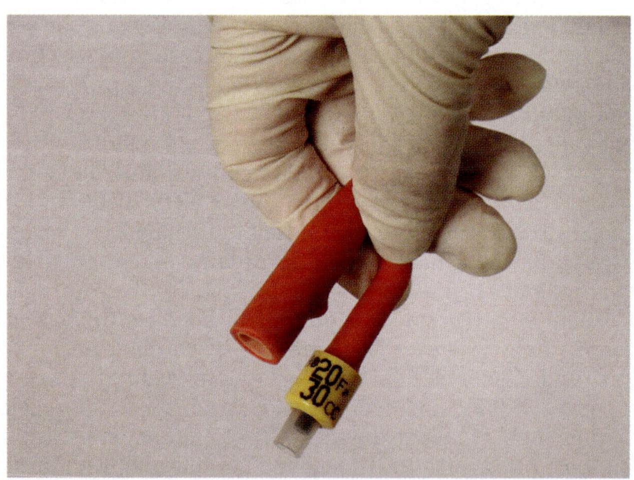

Fig. 21.7 Size of catheter and balloon printed on catheter.

risk for infection (Bardsley, 2015). Use of larger catheter diameters increases the risk for urethral trauma and bypassing, when the urine leaks between the urethral mucosa and the shaft of the catheter (Yates, 2016). Larger sizes may be used under special circumstances such as following urological surgery or in the presence of gross hematuria. Use smaller sizes for children: 5–6 Fr for infants, 8–10 Fr for children, and 10–12 Fr for adolescent girls.

Indwelling catheters come in balloon sizes ranging from 3 mL (for a child) to 30 mL for CBI. The size of the balloon is usually printed on the catheter port (Fig. 21.7). The recommended balloon size for an adult is a 10-mL balloon (the balloon is 5 mL and requires 10 mL to fill completely) (Yates, 2016). Long-term use of larger balloons (30 mL) is associated with increased patient discomfort, irritation and trauma, increased risk of catheter expulsion, and incomplete emptying of the bladder because of urine that pools below the level of the catheter drainage eyes.

Catheter Changes

Use clinical indicators such as obstruction, prior treatment of a symptomatic infection, malfunction of the catheter, or compromise of the closed system to determine when to change long-term indwelling catheters and drainage bags (Gesmundo, 2016). In many cases, you need to change catheters every 4–6 weeks. Change long-term catheters if they leak or become blocked and before obtaining a sterile specimen for urine culture. Avoid use of long-term catheterization because of the increased risk of CAUTI. Make every attempt to remove catheters as soon as a patient can void. See Box 21.3 for evidence-based nursing interventions to prevent CAUTI.

Closed Drainage Systems

An indwelling catheter is attached to a closed-system drainage bag to collect the continuous flow of urine. Do not separate the drainage system unless absolutely necessary to avoid introducing pathogens (Fig. 21.8). Always hang the bag below the level of the bladder on the bedframe or a chair so that urine drains down, out of the bladder. Do *not* let the bag touch the floor or secure it on a side rail. When a patient ambulates, carry the bag below the level of the patient's bladder. The only exception to this rule is when a patient has a catheter that is attached to a specially designed drainage bag (belly bag) worn across the abdomen. This system has a one-way valve to prevent the backflow of urine into the bladder. To keep the drainage system patent, check for kinks or bends in the tubing, avoid

BOX 21.3 Preventing Catheter-Associated Urinary Tract Infections

- Use aseptic technique with sterile equipment when inserting urinary catheters into patients in an acute care setting.
- Secure indwelling catheters to prevent movement and pulling on the catheter.
- Maintain a closed urinary drainage system.
- Maintain an unobstructed flow of urine through the catheter, drainage tubing, and drainage bag.
- Keep the urinary drainage bag below the level of the bladder at all times.
- Avoid dependent loops in urinary drainage tubing.
- Prevent the urinary drainage bag from touching or dragging on the floor.
- When emptying the urinary drainage bag, use a separate measuring receptacle for each patient. Do not let the drainage spigot touch the receptacle.
- Before transfers or activity, drain all urine from tubing into bag and empty drainage bag.
- Empty the drainage bag when half full.
- Perform routine perineal hygiene daily and after soiling.
- Obtain urine samples using the sampling port. Cleanse the port with disinfectant. Use a sterile syringe/cannula.
- Ensure quality improvement programs alert providers when a patient has a catheter and include regular educational programming about catheter care.

Data from Centers for Disease Control and Prevention: *Guideline for prevention of catheter-associated urinary tract infections*, 2009, http://www.cdc.gov/hicpac/pdf/CAUTI/CAUTIguideline2009final.pdf.

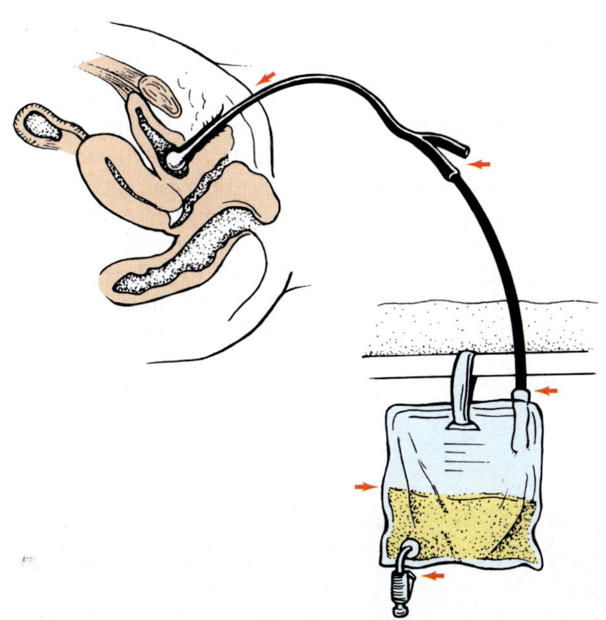

Fig. 21.8 Potential sites *(arrows)* for introduction of infection.

positioning the patient on the drainage tubing, prevent tubing from becoming dependent, and observe for clots or sediment that can cause blockage.

Routine Catheter Care

Patients with indwelling catheters require regular perineal hygiene (see Chapter 16), especially after bowel movements,

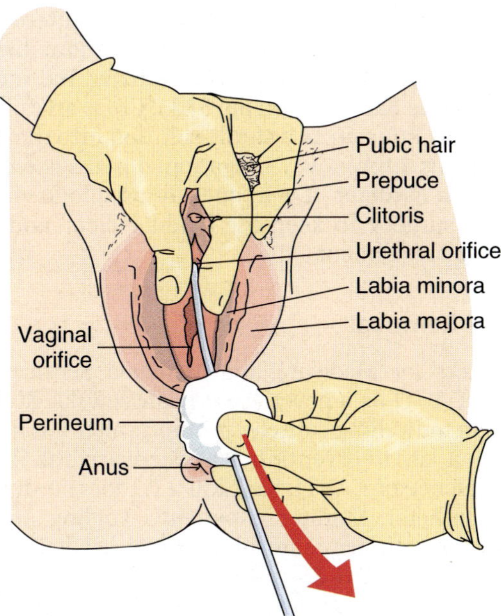

Fig. 21.9 Cleansing the catheter during catheter care. (From Sorrentino SA, Remmert LA: *Mosby's textbook for nursing assistants*, ed 8, St Louis, 2012, Mosby.)

to reduce the risk for CAUTI (Yates, 2016). In many institutions, patients receive catheter care every 8–12 hours as the minimal standard of care. Provide catheter care during perineal hygiene. You cleanse the catheter with the labia of a female patient separated or the foreskin of a male patient retracted so you can visualize the urethral meatus. Note any discharge, odor, or inflammation. Grasp the catheter with two fingers to prevent unnecessary traction. Using a clean washcloth, soap, and water, or a CHG bathing cloth, start cleansing the catheter close to the urinary meatus and move outward approximately 10 cm (4 inches) in a circular motion to remove any secretions that adhere to the catheter (Fig. 21.9). Remove all traces of soap and replace the foreskin if pulled back. Replace the catheter securement device as necessary (see Skill 21.1). Empty the drainage bag when it is three-quarters full, and record output. An overfull drainage bag creates tension and pulls on the catheter, resulting in trauma to the urethra and/or urinary meatus (Yates, 2016) (see Box 21.3).

Catheter Irrigations and Instillations

To maintain the patency of indwelling urinary catheters, it is sometimes necessary to irrigate or flush a catheter with sterile solution. However, irrigation poses the risk for causing a UTI and thus must be done maintaining a closed urinary drainage system. Generally, if a catheter becomes occluded, it is best to change it rather than risk flushing debris into the bladder. In some instances, the health care provider will determine that irrigations are needed to keep a catheter patent such as after genitourinary surgery when there is high risk for catheter occlusion from blood clots. Bladder instillations are used to instill medication into the bladder. Refer to specific instructions for these medications in terms of how long the medication needs to stay in the bladder.

Closed catheter irrigation provides intermittent or continuous irrigation of a urinary catheter without disrupting the sterile connection between the catheter and the drainage system (see Skill 21.2 on pp. 511). CBI is an example of a continuous infusion of a sterile solution into the bladder, usually using a three-way irrigation closed system with a triple-lumen catheter. It is frequently used following genitourinary surgery to keep the bladder clear and free of blood clots or sediment.

Catheter Removal

The Centers for Medicare and Medicaid Services (CMS) identified CAUTI as a never event (Galiczewski, 2016). Removing an indwelling catheter promptly after it is no longer needed is a key intervention that decreases the incidence and prevalence of CAUTI. See Skill 21.1 for the steps to remove a catheter. Monitor a patient's voiding and urine output after catheter removal by using a voiding record, bladder diary, or I&O documentation. A bladder diary records the time and amount of each voiding including any incontinence. Use a bladder scan when needed to monitor bladder functioning and measure postvoid residual. Abdominal pain and distention, a sensation of incomplete emptying, incontinence, constant dribbling of urine, and voiding in very small amounts indicate possible inadequate bladder emptying, which requires intervention.

The risk of UTI increases with the use of an indwelling catheter (Carter et al., 2014). Symptoms of infection can develop 2 or 3 or more days after catheter removal. Patients need to be informed of the risk for infection, prevention measures, and signs and symptoms that need to be reported to a nurse and health care provider.

The patient care unit is evaluating a quality improvement (QI) project focused on reducing CAUTIs (a never event). UTIs are common HAIs. A high percentage of HAI UTIs are caused by urinary catheterization, resulting in longer hospital stays, increased costs, and increased mortality.

- Which nursing care interventions would Carly, the nursing student, expect to find on the QI tool, and which data would indicate that the QI project was successful?

Suprapubic Catheters

A **suprapubic catheter** is a urinary drainage tube inserted surgically into the bladder through the abdominal wall above the symphysis pubis (Fig. 21.10). The catheter is sutured to the skin, secured with an adhesive material, or retained in the bladder with a fluid-filled balloon similar to an indwelling catheter.

Suprapubic catheters are placed when there is blockage of the urethra (e.g., enlarged prostate, urethral stricture, after urological surgery) and in situations when a long-term urethral catheter causes irritation or discomfort or interferes with sexual functioning. Because of the abdominal pressure on the catheter, the suprapubic catheter is usually size 16 Fr or larger (Yates, 2016).

Care of a suprapubic catheter involves daily cleansing of the insertion site and catheter. The same care for the tubing and drainage bag of a urethral catheter applies for a suprapubic catheter. Assess the insertion site for signs of inflammation and growth of overgranulation tissue. If insertion is new, expect slight inflammation as part of normal wound healing; however, monitor the site carefully because inflammation also indicates infection. Overgranulation tissue can develop at the insertion site as a reaction to the catheter. In some instances, intervention is needed. Site care follows principles of applying a dry dressing (see Chapter 17), and institutional policy indicates whether aseptic or sterile technique is required.

Condom Catheters

An external catheter, also called a **condom catheter**, *penile sheath*, or *Texas catheter*, is a soft, pliable, condom-like sheath that fits over the penis, providing a safe and noninvasive way to contain urine. Most external catheters are made of soft silicone that aids in reducing friction. They are clear to allow for easy visualization of skin under the catheter. Latex catheters are used by some patients. Verify that a patient does not have a latex allergy before applying this type of catheter. Condom-type external catheters are held in place by an adhesive coating of the internal lining of the sheath, a double-sided self-adhesive strip, brush-on adhesive applied to the

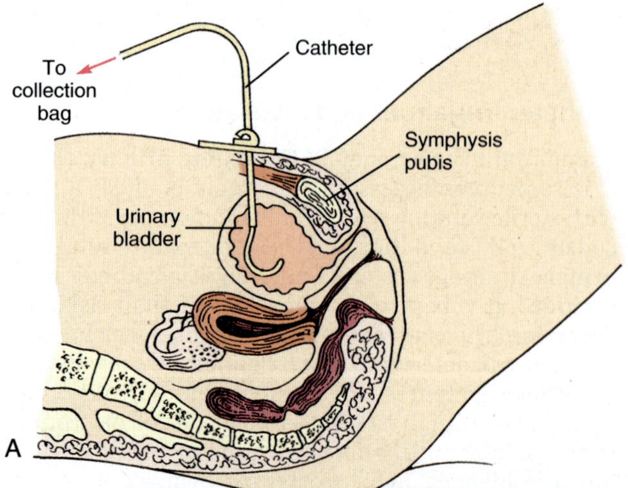

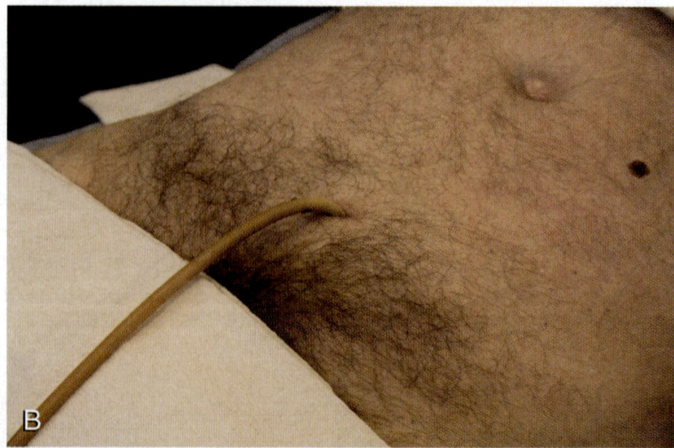

Fig. 21.10 A, Placement of suprapubic catheter above the symphysis pubis. **B,** Suprapubic catheter without a dressing.

penile shaft, or (in rare cases) an external strap. They may be attached to a small-volume (leg) drainage bag or a large-volume (bedside) urinary drainage bag, both of which need to be kept lower than the level of the bladder. A condom-type external catheter is suitable for patients who are incontinent and have complete and spontaneous bladder emptying. Condom catheters come in a variety of styles and sizes. Refer to manufacturer guidelines to ensure the best fit and correct application. See Box 21.4 for the steps in applying a condom catheter. Condom catheters are associated with less risk for UTI than indwelling catheters; thus, they are an excellent option for a male patient with UI (Smart, 2014). Other externally applied catheters are available for men who cannot be fitted for a condom catheter. One type attaches to the glans

BOX 21.4 Procedural Guidelines

Applying a Condom Catheter

Equipment

Condom catheter kit (condom sheath of appropriate size, securement device [internal adhesive or strap], skin preparation solution [per manufacturer directions]); urinary collection bag with drainage tubing or leg bag and straps; basin with warm water and soap; towels and washcloths; bath blanket; clean gloves; scissors, hair guard, or paper towel

Steps

1. Identify the patient by using at least two identifiers (e.g., name and birthday or name and medical record number) according to agency policy.
2. Review medical record and assess urinary pattern, ability to empty bladder effectively, and presence of urinary continence.
3. Assess the patient's mental status, knowledge of purpose of using condom-type catheter, and ability to apply device. Include family caregivers as appropriate.
4. Review medical record for history of allergy to rubber or latex. Check the patient's allergy wristband.
5. Perform hand hygiene. Provide privacy by closing room door and bedside curtain.
6. Raise bed to appropriate working height. Lower side rail on working side.
7. Apply gloves. Verify the patient's size and type of condom catheter, or use manufacturer measuring guide. Prepare condom catheter, urinary drainage collection bag, and tubing (large-volume drainage bag or leg bag). Clamp off drainage bag port. Place nearby ready to attach to condom after applied.
8. Help the patient into supine position or sitting position. Place bath blanket over upper torso. Fold sheets so that only penis is exposed.
9. Provide perineal care. Dry thoroughly before applying device. In an uncircumcised patient, ensure that foreskin has been replaced to normal position before applying condom catheter. Do not apply barrier cream.
10. Assess skin of penis for rashes, erythema, or open areas. (This may be deferred until just before catheter application.)
11. Clip hair at base of penis if necessary before application of condom sheath. If hair guard is available, place over penis before applying device. Remove hair guard after applying catheter. An alternative to a hair guard is to tear a hole in a paper towel, place it over penis, and remove after application of device (Woodward, 2015b).
12. Apply condom catheter. With nondominant hand, grasp penis along shaft. With dominant hand, hold rolled condom sheath at tip of penis with head of penis in the cone. Smoothly roll sheath onto penis. Allow 2.5–5 cm (1–2 inches) of space between tip of glans penis and end of condom catheter (see illustration).
13. Apply appropriate securement device as indicated in manufacturer guidelines.
    a. Self-adhesive condom catheters: After application, apply gentle pressure on penile shaft for 10–15 s to secure catheter.
    b. Outer securing strip–type condom catheters: Spiral wrap penile shaft with strip of supplied elastic adhesive. Strip should not overlap itself. Elastic strip should be snug, not tight (see illustration). **Caution:** Never use tape.
14. Remove hair guard if used. Connect drainage tubing to end of condom catheter. Be sure that condom is not twisted. If using large drainage bag, place excess tubing on bed and secure to bottom sheet.
15. Help the patient to safe, comfortable position. Lower bed and place side rails accordingly.
16. Dispose of contaminated supplies, and remove and dispose of gloves. Perform hand hygiene.
17. Remove and reapply daily unless an extended-wear device is used. To remove condom, wash penis with warm, soapy water and gently roll sheath and adhesive off penile shaft.
18. **Use teach back:** "We talked about what you need to do to prevent the drainage tube from blocking urine flow. Please tell me what you need to do."

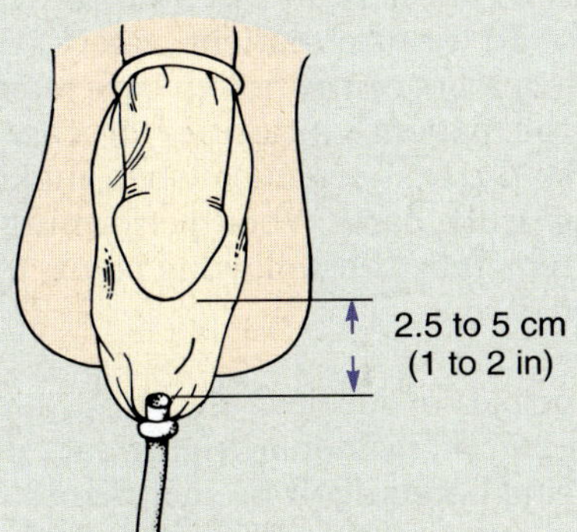

Step 12 Condom catheter.

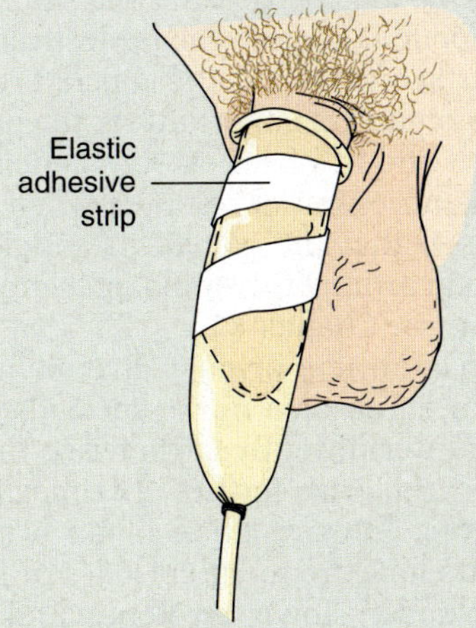

Step 13b Spiral application of adhesive strip.

BOX 21.5 Patient Teaching

Pelvic Muscle (Kegel) Exercises

Outcome

At the end of the teaching session, the patient will describe and demonstrate how to perform pelvic muscle (Kegel) exercises.

Teaching Strategies

- Use pictures to teach the patient pelvic anatomy and the location of the pelvic muscles.
- Teach the patient to identify and contract the correct muscle.
  - Women: Instruct the patient to squeeze the anus as if to hold in gas or to insert a finger into the vagina and feel the muscle squeeze around her finger.
  - Men: Instruct the patient to stand in front of a mirror, squeeze the anus as if to hold in gas, and watch to see if the penis moves up and down as he contracts the pelvic floor muscles.
  - Tell the patient to avoid contracting the abdomen, buttocks, or thighs when contracting the pelvic muscles.
- Teach pelvic muscle contraction exercises.
  - Quick flicks: Squeeze the muscle for 2–3 s and relax.
  - Sustained contractions: Squeeze the muscle for 5–10 s and relax after each contraction for 10 s.
- Teach the patient to maintain a daily exercise schedule.
  - Perform 3–5 quick flicks followed by 5–10 sustained contractions.
  - Repeat these exercises three to four times a day.

Evaluation Strategies

- Use the principles of teach-back to evaluate patient/family caregiver learning:
  - "Tell me how you will perform pelvic muscle exercises."
  - "Describe your plan for exercise for the next week."

penis using hydrocolloid strips that stay in place for multiple days and allows intermittent/straight catheterization (Woodward, 2015b). Another option available is a reusable condom-like device that is held in place by specially designed underwear.

Urinary Diversions

Immediately after surgery, a patient with an incontinent urinary diversion wears a pouch to collect the urine (drainage). The pouch keeps the patient clean and dry, protects the skin from damage, and provides a barrier against odor. Urinary pouches with an antireflux flap are opaque or clear, drainable one-piece or two-piece pouches with cut-to-fit or precut wafers. Change the pouch every 5–7 days (National Institute of Diabetes and Digestive and Kidney Diseases [NIDDK], 2013). You can connect pouches to a bedside drainage bag for use at night.

When changing a pouch, gently cleanse the skin surrounding the stoma with warm tap water using a clean washcloth and pat dry (Schreiber, 2016). Observe the appearance of the stoma and surrounding skin. The stoma is normally red and moist and is located in the right lower quadrant of the abdomen. Measure the stoma and cut the opening in the pouch. Remove the protective backing from the adhesive surface, and apply the pouch. Press firmly into place over the stoma. It is important for the patient to have the correct type and fit of an ostomy pouch. A specialty ostomy nurse is an essential resource when selecting the right appliance so that the pouch fits snugly against the surface of the skin around the stoma, preventing damaging leakage of urine (see Chapter 17).

Patients with continent urinary diversions do not wear external pouches. You or a nurse specialist will teach a patient how to intermittently catheterize the stoma. Patients need to catheterize four to six times a day for the rest of their lives. After creation of an orthotopic neobladder, patients have frequent episodes of incontinence until the neobladder slowly stretches and the urinary sphincter is strong enough to contain the urine (Leaver, 2016). The postoperative care of patients with continent urinary diversions varies widely with the surgical techniques used. Learn the surgeon's preferred routine and health care agency procedures before caring for these patients.

Intermittent Catheterization

Some patients experience chronic inability to completely empty the bladder because of neuromuscular damage related to multiple sclerosis, diabetes, spinal cord injury, and urinary retention. To minimize the risk of UTI, teach patients or family caregivers to catheterize the bladder using clean technique. In institutions where there is increased risk for exposure to multiple pathogens, intermittent catheterization follows the principles of sterile asepsis as discussed earlier in the chapter. Teach patients and family caregivers the importance of adequate fluid intake and signs of infection, and about their individualized catheterization schedule. The goal for intermittent catheterization is drainage of 400 mL of urine every 2–3 hours while awake. Individualize the schedule to meet this goal.

SAFETY GUIDELINES FOR NURSING SKILLS

Ensuring patient safety is an essential role of the professional nurse. To ensure patient safety, communicate clearly with members of the health care team, assess and incorporate the patient's priorities of care and preferences, and use the best evidence when making decisions about your patient's care. When performing the skills in this chapter, remember the following points to ensure safe, individualized care:

- Follow principles of medical and surgical asepsis when performing catheterizations, helping patients with toileting needs, and handling urine specimens.
- Identify patients at risk for latex allergies.
- Identify patients with allergies to povidone-iodine (Betadine). Provide alternatives such as chlorhexidine.

SKILL 21.1 Inserting and Removing Straight/Intermittent or Indwelling Catheters

Equipment

- Catheter kit containing sterile items (**Note:** Catheter kits vary):
  - Straight catheterization kit: Single-lumen catheter, drapes (one fenestrated—has an opening in the center), sterile gloves, lubricant, cleansing solution incorporated in an applicator or to be added to cotton balls, and specimen container
  - Indwelling catheterization kit: Drapes (one fenestrated—has an opening in the center), sterile gloves, lubricant, antiseptic cleansing solution incorporated in an applicator or to be added to cotton balls, specimen container, and prefilled syringe with sterile water (to inflate balloon); some kits contain a catheter with attached drainage bag; others contain only a catheter; others have no catheter
- Sterile drainage tubing and bag (if not included in indwelling catheter insertion kit)
- Device to secure catheter (catheter strap or other device)
- Extra sterile and clean gloves and catheter *(optional)*
- Basin with warm water, washcloth, towel, and soap for perineal care
- Flashlight or other additional light source
- Bath blanket and waterproof absorbent pad
- Measuring container for urine

STEP	RATIONALE
Assessment	
1. Identify the patient by using at least two identifiers (e.g., name and birthday or name and medical record number) according to agency policy.	Ensures correct patient. Complies with The Joint Commission standards and improves patient safety (TJC, 2018).
2. Review the patient's medical record including health care provider's order and nurses' notes. Note previous catheterization including catheter size, response of the patient, and time of catheterization.	Identifies purpose of inserting catheter (e.g., for measurement of postvoid residual, preparation for surgery, or specimen collection) and potential difficulty with catheter insertion.
3. Review medical record for any pathological condition that may impair passage of catheter (e.g., enlarged prostate gland in men, urethral strictures).	Obstruction of urethra may prevent passage of catheter into bladder.
4. Ask the patient and check health record for allergies.	Identifies allergy to antiseptic, tape, latex, and lubricant.
5. Assess the patient's weight, level of consciousness, developmental level, ability to cooperate, and mobility.	Determines positioning for catheterization; indicates how much assistance is needed to properly position the patient, ability of the patient to cooperate during procedure, and level of explanation needed.
6. Assess the patient's gender and age.	Determines catheter size.
7. Perform hand hygiene and apply clean gloves. Assess for pain and bladder fullness. Palpate bladder over symphysis pubis or use bladder scanner (if available).	Palpation of full bladder causes pain and/or urge to void, indicating full or overfull bladder.
8. Inspect perineal region, observing for perineal anatomical landmarks, erythema, drainage or discharge, and odor. Remove gloves and perform hand hygiene.	Assessment of female perineal landmarks improves accuracy and speed of catheter insertion.
9. Assess the patient's knowledge, health literacy, prior experience with catheterization, and feelings about procedure.	Reveals need for patient instruction and/or support.
Planning	
1. Provide privacy by closing room door and bedside curtain.	Promotes comfort and protects patient confidentiality.
2. Check the patient's plan of care for size and type of catheter (if this is a reinsertion). Use smallest size catheter possible. Collect all required equipment.	Ensures that the patient receives correct size and type of catheter. Larger catheter diameters increase risk for urethral trauma (Yates, 2016). Small catheter allows for adequate drainage of periurethral glands.
3. Explain procedure to the patient or family caregiver and arrange for extra personnel to help as necessary.	Promotes cooperation and informs the patient about what to expect. Some patients are unable to assume positioning independently for procedure.
Implementation	
1. Perform hand hygiene.	Reduces transmission of microorganisms.
2. Raise bed to appropriate working height. If side rails in use, raise side rail on opposite side of bed and lower side rail on working side.	Promotes good body mechanics. Use of side rails in this manner promotes patient safety.
3. Place waterproof pad under the patient.	Prevents soiling of bed linen.

Clinical decision point: Obtain assistance to position and support patients who are weak, frail, obese, or confused.

STEP	RATIONALE
4. Position the patient:	
a. **Female patient:**	
(1) Help to dorsal recumbent position (on back with knees flexed). Ask the patient to relax thighs so you can rotate hips.	Exposes perineum and allows hip joints to be externally rotated.
(2) Alternative female position: Position side-lying (Sims') position with upper leg flexed at knee and hip. Support the patient with pillows if necessary to maintain position.	Alternative position is more comfortable if the patient cannot abduct leg at hip joint (e.g., the patient has arthritic joints or contractures).
b. **Male patient:**	
(1) Position supine with legs extended and thighs slightly abducted.	Comfortable position for the patient aids in visualization of penis.
5. Drape patient: a. **Female patient:**	Protects patient dignity by avoiding unnecessary exposure of body parts.
(1) Drape with bath blanket. Place blanket diamond fashion over the patient, with one corner at the patient's midsection, side corners over each thigh and abdomen, and last corner over perineum (see illustration).	Protects patient dignity by avoiding unnecessary exposure of body parts.
b. **Male patient:**	
(1) Drape the patient by covering upper part of body with small sheet or towel; drape with separate sheet or bath blanket so that only perineum is exposed (see illustration).	Protects patient dignity by avoiding unnecessary exposure of body parts.
6. Apply clean gloves. Cleanse perineal area with soap and water, rinse, and dry. Use gloves to re-examine the patient and identify urinary meatus. Remove and discard gloves. Perform hand hygiene.	Perineal hygiene removes secretions, urine, and feces that could contaminate sterile field and increase risk for catheter-associated urinary tract infection (CAUTI) (Yates, 2016).
7. Position light to illuminate genitals or have assistant available to hold light source to visualize urinary meatus.	Adequate visualization of urinary meatus helps with speed and accuracy of catheter insertion.
8. Open outer wrapping of catheterization kit. Place inner wrapped catheter kit tray on clean, accessible surface such as bedside table or, if possible, between the patient's open legs. Patient size and positioning dictate exact placement.	Provides easy access to supplies during catheter insertion.
9. Open inner sterile wrap covering tray containing catheterization supplies using sterile technique. Fold back each flap of sterile covering one at a time, with last flap opened toward the patient.	Sterile wrap serves as sterile field.

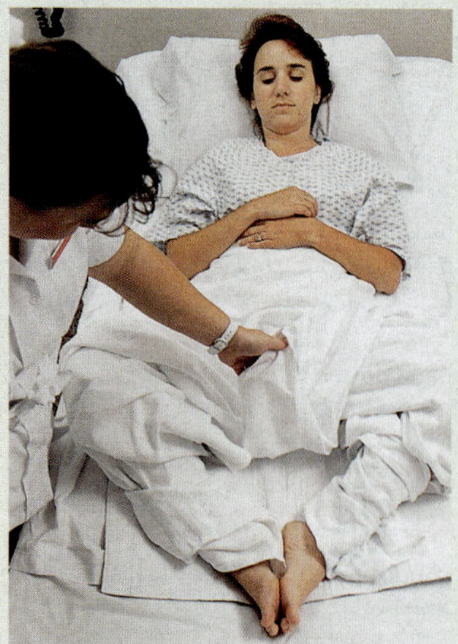

Step 5a(1) Female patient draped and in dorsal recumbent position.

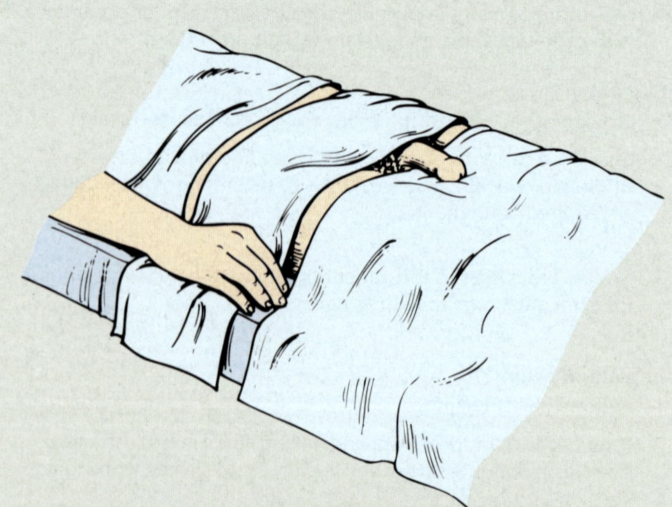

Step 5b(1) Draping male patient with blankets.

STEP	RATIONALE
a. Indwelling catheterization open system: Open separate package containing drainage bag, check to make sure that clamp on drainage port is closed, and place drainage bag and tubing in easily accessible location. Open outer package of sterile catheter, maintaining sterility of inner wrapper.	Open drainage bag systems have separate sterile packaging for sterile catheter, drainage bag and tubing, and insertion kit.
b. Indwelling catheterization closed system: All supplies are in sterile tray and are arranged in sequence of use.	Closed drainage bag systems have catheter preattached to drainage tubing and bag.
c. Straight catheterization: All needed supplies are in sterile tray that contains supplies and can be used for urine collection.	
10. Put on sterile gloves. (*Option:* Apply sterile drape with ungloved hands when drape is packed as first item. Touch only edges of drape. Then apply sterile gloves.)	Maintains surgical asepsis.
11. Drape perineum, keeping gloves and working surface of field sterile.	Sterile drapes provide sterile field over which you will work during catheterization.
a. **Drape female patient:**	
(1) Pick up square sterile drape touching only edges (2.5 cm [1 inch]).	When creating the cuff over sterile gloved hands, sterility of gloves and workspace is maintained.
(2) Allow drape to unfold without touching unsterile surfaces. Allow top edge of drape (2.5–5 cm [1–2 inches]) to form cuff over both hands.	
(3) Place drape with shiny side down on bed between the patient's thighs. Slip cuffed edge just under buttocks as you ask the patient to lift hips. Take care not to touch contaminated surfaces with sterile gloves.	
(4) Pick up fenestrated sterile drape out of tray. Allow drape to unfold without touching unsterile surfaces. Allow top edge of drape to form cuff over both hands. Apply drape over perineum, exposing labia (see illustration).	Opening in drape creates sterile field around labia.
b. **Drape male patient:**	
(1) Use of square drape is optional; you may apply fenestrated drape instead.	
(2) Pick up edges of square drape and allow to unfold without touching unsterile surfaces. Place over thighs, with shiny side down, just below penis.	
(3) Place fenestrated drape with opening centered over penis (see illustration).	
12. Move tray closer to the patient. Arrange remaining supplies on sterile field, maintaining sterility of gloves. Place sterile tray with cleaning medium (premoistened swab sticks or cotton balls, forceps, and solution), lubricant, catheter, and prefilled syringe for inflating balloon (indwelling catheterization only) on sterile drape.	Provides easy access to supplies during catheter insertion and helps to maintain aseptic technique. Appropriate placement is determined by size of the patient and position during catheterization.

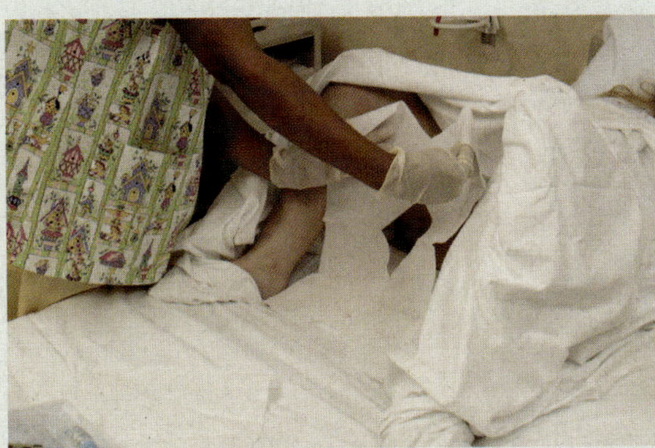

Step 11a(4) Place sterile fenestrated drape (with opening in center) over perineum of female patient.

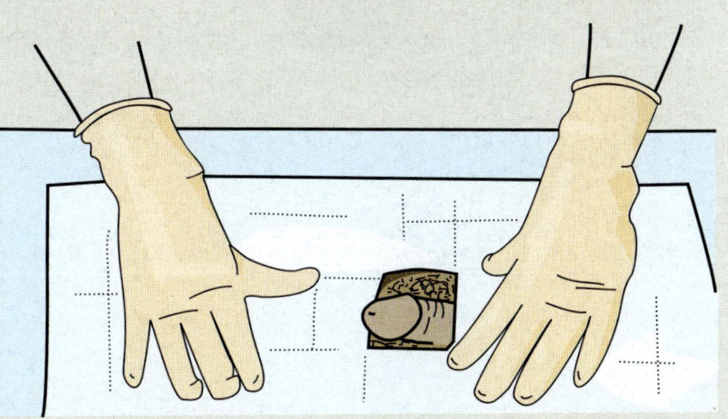

Step 11b(3) Draping male patient with fenestrated drape.

STEP	RATIONALE
a. If kit contains sterile cotton balls, open package of sterile antiseptic solution and pour over cotton balls. Some kits contain a package of premoistened swab sticks. Open end of package for easy access (see illustration).	Use of sterile supplies and antiseptic solution reduces risk of CAUTI (Galiczewski, 2016).
b. Open sterile specimen container if specimen is to be obtained.	Makes container accessible to receive urine from catheter if specimen is needed.
c. For indwelling catheterization, open sterile wrapper of catheter and leave catheter on sterile field. If part of a closed system kit, remove tray with catheter and preattached drainage bag and place on sterile drape. Make sure that clamp on drainage port of bag is closed. If needed and if part of sterile tray, attach catheter to drainage tubing.	Indwelling catheterization trays vary. Some have preattached catheters; others need to be attached but are part of the sterile tray; others do not have catheter or drainage system as part of tray.
d. Open packet of lubricant and squeeze out on sterile field. Lubricate catheter tip by dipping it into water-soluble gel 2.5–5 cm (1–2 inches) for women and 12.5–17.5 cm (5–7 inches) for men (see illustration).	Lubrication minimizes trauma to urethra and discomfort during catheter insertion. Male catheter needs enough lubricant to cover length of catheter inserted.
Clinical decision point: Pretesting a balloon on an indwelling catheter by injecting fluid from the prefilled sterile water syringe into the balloon port is no longer recommended. Testing the balloon may distort and stretch it and lead to damage, causing increased trauma on insertion.	
13. Clean urethral meatus:	
a. **Female patient:**	
(1) Separate labia with fingers of nondominant hand (now contaminated) to fully expose urethral meatus.	Optimal visualization of urethral meatus is possible.
(2) Maintain position of nondominant hand throughout procedure.	Closure of labia during cleaning means that area is contaminated and requires cleaning procedure to be repeated.
(3) Holding forceps in dominant hand, pick up one moistened cotton ball or pick up one swab stick at a time. Clean labia and urinary meatus from clitoris toward anus. Use new cotton ball or swab for each area that you clean. Clean by wiping far from labial fold, near labial fold, and directly over center of urethral meatus (see illustration).	Front-to-back cleaning moves from area of least contamination toward highly contaminated area. Follows principles of medical asepsis. Dominant gloved hand remains sterile.
b. **Male patient:**	
(1) With nondominant hand (now contaminated), retract foreskin (if uncircumcised) and gently grasp penis at shaft just below glans. Hold shaft of penis at right angle to body. Nondominant hand remains in this position for remainder of procedure.	When grasping shaft of penis, avoid pressure on dorsal surface to prevent compression of urethra. Losing grasp during cleaning means that area is contaminated and requires cleaning procedure to be repeated.
(2) Using uncontaminated dominant hand, clean meatus with cotton balls or swab sticks, using circular strokes, beginning at the meatus and working outward in a spiral motion.	Circular cleaning pattern follows principles of medical asepsis.
(3) Repeat cleansing three times using clean cotton ball or swab stick each time (see illustration).	

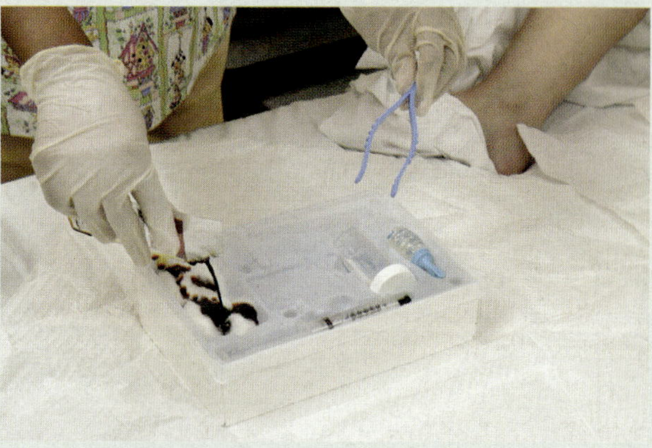

Step 12a Sterile kit includes antiseptic swabs.

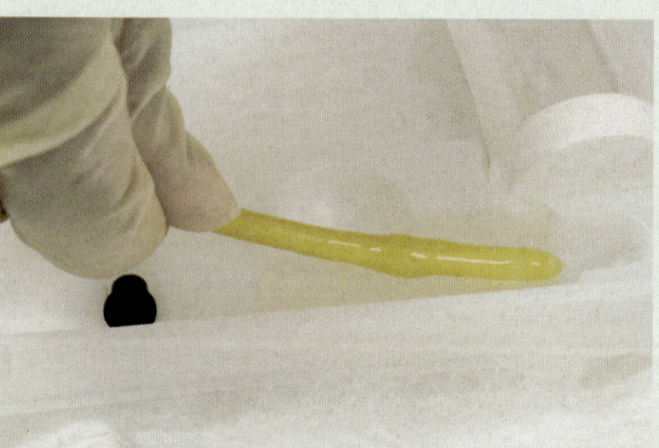

Step 12d Lubricating catheter.

STEP	RATIONALE

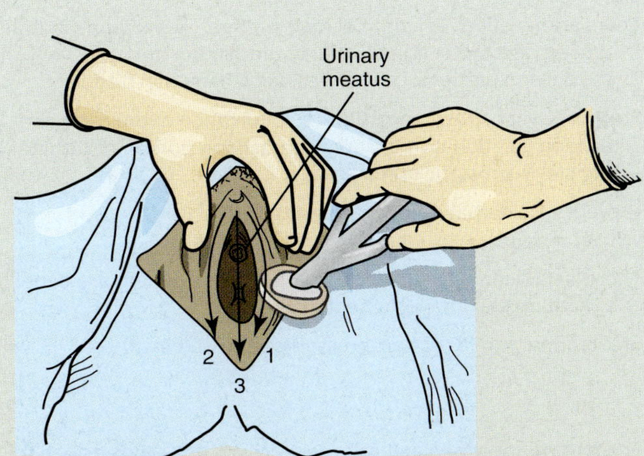

Step 13a(3) Cleaning perineum of female patient.

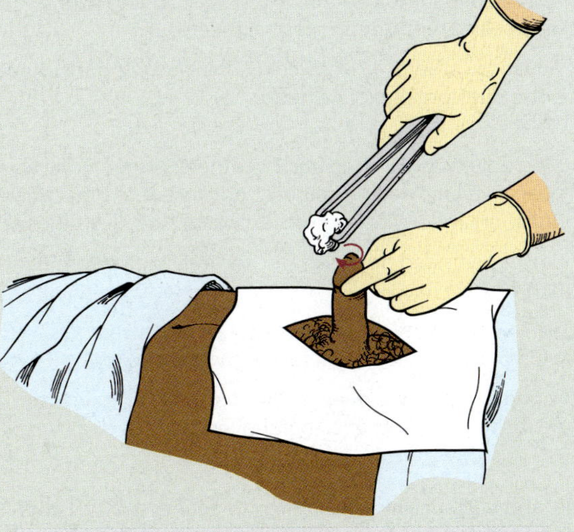
Step 13b(3) Cleaning urinary meatus of male patient.

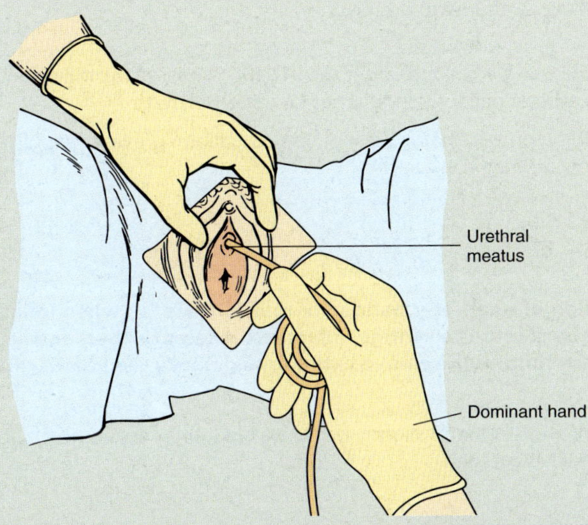

Step 15a(1) Inserting catheter into urinary meatus of female patient.

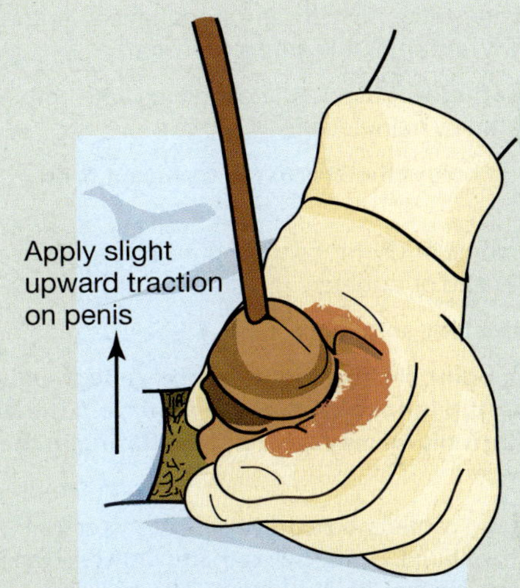

Step 15b(1) Inserting catheter into urinary meatus of male patient.

STEP	RATIONALE
14. Pick up and hold catheter 7.5–10 cm (3–4 inches) from catheter tip with catheter loosely coiled in palm of hand. If catheter is not attached to drainage bag, make sure to position urine tray so that end of catheter can be placed there once insertion begins.	Holding catheter near tip allows for its easier manipulation during insertion. Coiling catheter in palm prevents distal end from striking nonsterile surface.
15. Insert catheter. Explain to the patient that a feeling of burning, pinching, or pressure may be experienced as the catheter is inserted into the urethra. This sensation is normal and will go away quickly.	Information on what to expect during procedure helps reduce patient anxiety.
a. **Female patient:**	
(1) Ask the patient to bear down gently, and slowly insert catheter through urethral meatus (see illustration).	Bearing down may help visualize urinary meatus and promotes relaxation of external urinary sphincter, aiding in catheter insertion.
(2) Advance catheter 5–7.5 cm (2–3 inches) or until urine flows out of catheter. When urine appears, advance catheter another 2.5–5 cm (1–2 inches). Do not use force to insert catheter.	Urine flow indicates that catheter tip is in bladder or lower urethra.
(3) Release labia and hold catheter securely with nondominant hand.	Prevents accidental dislodgment of catheter.
b. **Male patient:**	
(1) Lift penis to a position perpendicular (90°) to the patient's body and apply gentle upward traction (see illustration).	Straightens urethra to ease catheter insertion.

STEP	RATIONALE
(2) Ask the patient to bear down as if to void and slowly insert catheter through urethral meatus.	Relaxation of external sphincter aids in insertion of catheter.
(3) Advance catheter 17–22.5 cm (7–9 inches) or until urine flows out from end of catheter.	There are variations in length of male urethra. Flow of urine indicates that tip of catheter is in bladder or urethra but not necessarily that the balloon portion of an indwelling catheter is in bladder.
(4) Stop advancing with a straight catheter. When urine appears in an indwelling catheter, advance it to bifurcation (inflation and deflation ports exposed) (see illustration).	Further advancement of catheter to bifurcation of drainage and balloon inflation port ensures that balloon portion of catheter is not still in prostatic urethra.
(5) Lower penis and hold catheter securely in nondominant hand.	Prevents accidental dislodgment of catheter.
16. Allow bladder to empty fully unless agency policy restricts maximum volume of urine drained (see agency policy).	There is no definitive evidence regarding whether there is benefit in limiting maximal volume drained.
17. Collect urine specimen as needed. Fill specimen container to 20–30 mL by holding end of catheter over cup.	Sterile specimen for culture analysis can be obtained.
a. Label and bag specimen according to agency policy. Label specimen in front of the patient. Send to laboratory as soon as possible.	Fresh urine specimen ensures more accurate findings. Labeling ensures that diagnostic results will be connected to the correct patient.
18. Straight catheterization: When urine stops flowing, withdraw catheter slowly and smoothly until removed.	Minimizes trauma to urethra.
19. **Indwelling catheter:** Inflate catheter balloon with amount of fluid designated by manufacturer.	Avoid using a balloon larger than 10 mL (Yates, 2016). Indwelling catheter balloons should not be underinflated.
a. Continue to hold catheter with nondominant hand.	Holding onto catheter before inflating balloon prevents expulsion of catheter from urethra.
b. With free dominant hand, connect prefilled syringe to injection port at end of catheter.	
c. Slowly inject total amount of solution (see illustration).	

Clinical decision point: If the patient reports sudden pain during inflation of a catheter balloon or resistance is felt when inflating the balloon, stop inflation, allow the fluid from the balloon to flow back into the syringe, advance catheter further, and reinflate balloon. The balloon may have been inflating in the urethra. If pain continues, remove catheter and notify the health care provider.

STEP	RATIONALE
d. After inflating catheter balloon, release catheter from nondominant hand. *Gently* pull catheter until resistance is felt. Then advance catheter slightly.	By moving catheter slightly back into bladder, pressure on bladder neck is avoided.
e. Connect drainage tubing to catheter if it is not already preconnected.	

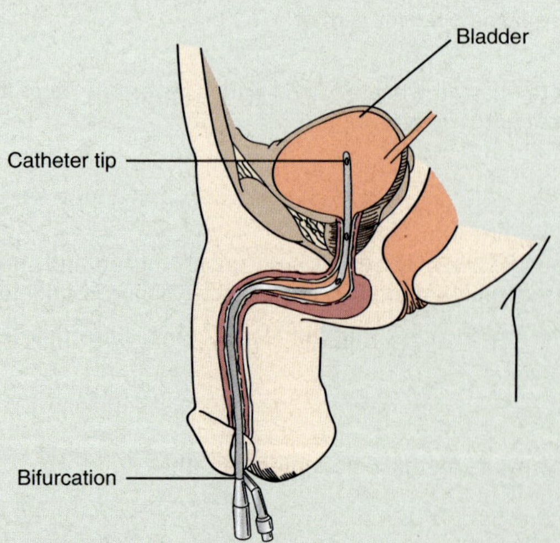

Step 15b(4) Male anatomy with correct catheter insertion to bifurcation.

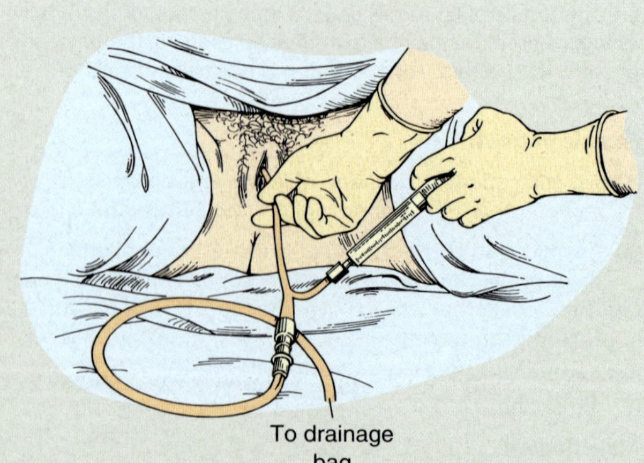

Step 19c Inflating balloon (indwelling catheter).

STEP	RATIONALE
20. Secure indwelling catheter with catheter strap or other securement device. Leave enough slack to allow leg movement. Attach securement device at tubing just above catheter bifurcation.	Securing the catheter prevents traction on the catheter and ensures the balloon is not pulled into the neck of the bladder (Yates, 2016). Attachment of securement device at catheter bifurcation prevents occlusion of catheter.
a. **Female patient:**	
(1) Secure catheter tubing to inner thigh, allowing enough slack to prevent tension (see illustration).	
b. **Male patient:**	
(1) Secure catheter tubing to upper thigh (see illustration) or lower abdomen (with penis directed toward chest). Allow slack in catheter so that movement does not create tension on catheter.	Anchoring catheter reduces pulling and unnecessary pressure on the bladder neck, urethral–penile–scrotal junction, and urinary meatus (Ansell, 2016).
(2) If retracted, replace foreskin over glans penis.	Leaving foreskin retracted can cause discomfort and dangerous edema.
21. Clip drainage tubing to edge of mattress. Position drainage bag lower than bladder by attaching to bed frame. Do not attach to side rails of bed (see illustration) or place on the floor.	Drainage bags that are below level of bladder ensure free flow of urine to prevent reflux and contamination, decreasing risk for CAUTI (Gould, 2017; Yates, 2016). Bags attached to movable objects such as a side rail increase risk for urethral trauma because of pulling or accidental dislodgment.
22. Check to ensure that there is no obstruction to urine flow. Coil excess tubing on bed and fasten to bottom sheet with clip or other securement device.	Obstruction to flow of urine increases risk for CAUTI (Gould et al., 2017; Nicolle, 2014).

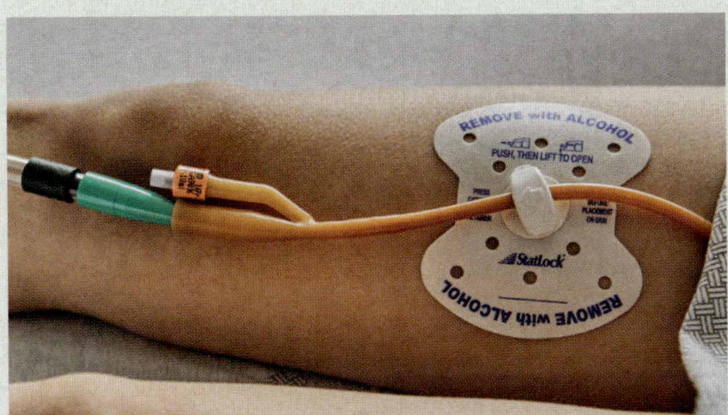

Step 20a(1) Securing indwelling catheter on female patient with adhesive securement device.

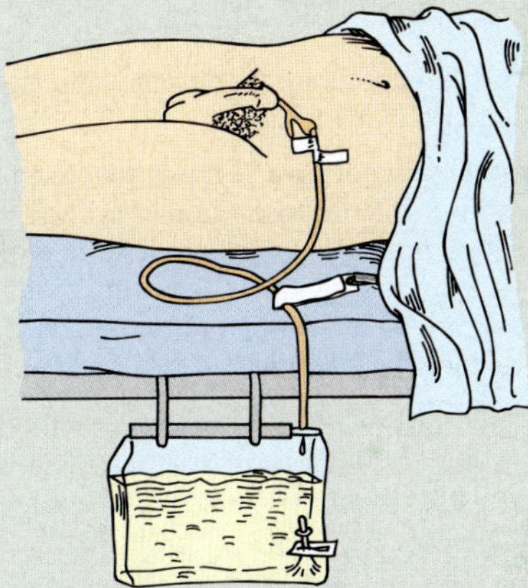

Step 20b(1) Securing indwelling catheter on male patient with tape.

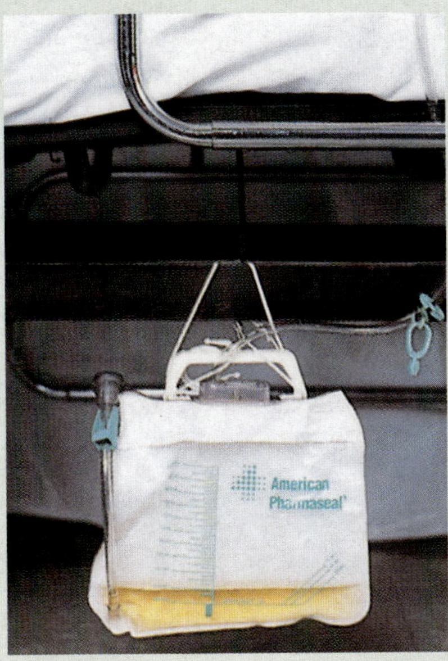

Step 21 Drainage bag below level of bladder.

STEP	RATIONALE
23. Provide hygiene as needed. Help the patient to comfortable position.	
24. Dispose of supplies in appropriate receptacles.	Reduces transmission of microorganisms.
25. Measure urine and record. If specimen is collected, label container for culture, place in biohazard container, and send to laboratory.	Provides baseline for urine output and ensures prompt diagnostic analysis of urine.
26. Remove and dispose of gloves. Perform hand hygiene.	Reduces transmission of microorganisms.
27. **Removal of indwelling Foley catheter:**	
a. Close room door and bedside curtain.	Provides patient privacy.
b. Perform hand hygiene.	Reduces transmission of microorganisms.
c. Raise bed to appropriate working height. If side rails are raised, lower side rail on working side.	Promotes use of proper body mechanics.
d. Organize equipment for perineal care and/or removal of catheter.	Increases efficiency of procedure.
e. Position the patient with waterproof pad under buttocks and cover with bath blanket, exposing only genital area and catheter.	Shows respect for patient dignity by exposing only genital area and catheter.
(1) Female patient in dorsal recumbent position	
(2) Male patient in supine position	
f. Apply clean gloves.	Reduces transmission of microorganisms.
g. Remove catheter securement device while maintaining connection with drainage tubing.	Provides ability to easily clean around catheter or to remove it.
h. Move syringe plunger up and down to loosen and then pull back plunger to 0.5 mL. Insert hub of syringe into inflation valve (balloon port). Allow balloon fluid to drain into syringe by gravity. Syringe should fill. Make sure that entire amount of fluid is removed by comparing removed amount with volume needed for inflation.	Partially inflated balloon can traumatize urethral wall during removal. Passive drainage of catheter balloon prevents formation of ridges in balloon. These ridges can cause discomfort or trauma during removal.
i. Pull catheter out smoothly and slowly. Examine it to ensure that it is whole. Catheter should slide out easily. Do not use force. If you note any resistance, repeat Step 27h to remove remaining water.	Nonwhole catheter means that pieces of catheter may still be in bladder. Notify health care provider immediately.
j. Wrap contaminated catheter in waterproof pad. Unhook collection bag and drainage tubing from bed.	Prevents transmission of microorganisms.
k. Reposition the patient and provide hygiene as needed. Lower level of bed and position side rails accordingly.	Promotes patient comfort and safety.
l. Empty, measure, and record urine present in drainage bag.	Documents urinary output.
m. Encourage the patient to maintain or increase fluid intake (unless contraindicated).	Maintains normal urine output.
28. Initiate voiding record or bladder diary. Instruct the patient to tell you when need to empty bladder occurs and that all urine needs to be measured. Make sure that the patient understands how to use collection container.	Evaluates bladder function.
29. Explain that many patients experience mild burning, discomfort, or small-volume voiding with first voiding, which soon subsides.	Burning results from urethral irritation.
30. Inform the patient to report any signs of UTI.	
31. Ensure easy access to toilet, commode, bedpan, or urinal. Place urine hat on toilet seat if the patient is using toilet. Place call bell within easy reach.	Reduces incidence of falls during toileting. Urine hat collects first voided urine.
32. Dispose of all contaminated supplies in appropriate receptacle, remove gloves, and perform hand hygiene.	Reduces transmission of microorganisms.
Evaluation	
1. Palpate bladder for distention or use bladder scan.	Determines whether distention is relieved.
2. Ask the patient to describe level of comfort.	Determines whether the patient's sensation of discomfort or fullness has been relieved.

STEP	RATIONALE
3. Indwelling catheter: Observe character and amount of urine in drainage system.	Determines whether urine is flowing adequately.
4. Indwelling catheter: Ensure that there is no urine leaking from catheter or tubing connections.	Prevents injury to the patient's skin and ensures closed sterile system.
5. Observe time and measure amount of first voiding after catheter removal.	Indicates return of bladder function after catheter removal.
6. Evaluate the patient for signs and symptoms of UTI.	Any patient who has recently had catheter removed is at risk for UTI.
7. Use principles of teach back to evaluate patient/family caregiver learning. State, "I want to be sure I explained information about your urinary catheter. What can you do to ensure the urine flows out of the catheter?" Revise your instruction or develop plan for revised patient teaching if the patient is unable to teach back correctly.	Determines the patient and family caregiver level of understanding of instructional topic.

Recording and Reporting

- Record and report the reason for catheterization, type and size of catheter inserted, amount of fluid used to inflate balloon, specimen collection (if applicable), characteristics and amount of urine, patient's response to procedure, and education provided in nurses' notes in the electronic health record (EHR) or chart.
- Record amount of urine on intake and output (intake and output) flow sheet record in EHR or chart.
- Report persistent catheter-related pain, inadequate urine output, and discomfort to health care provider.
- Record time for catheter care and appearance of urine; describe condition of meatus and catheter in EHR or chart.
- Record and report time of catheter removal, amount of water removed from balloon, and condition of urethral meatus and catheter as well as time, amount, and characteristics of first voided urine in EHR or chart.
- Record teaching and patient response related to catheter care, catheter removal, and fluid intake in EHR or chart.
- Report hematuria, dysuria, inability or difficulty voiding, and any new incontinence after catheter is removed.

Unexpected Outcomes and Related Interventions

- Catheter goes into vagina.
  - Leave catheter in vagina.
  - Clean urinary meatus again. Using another catheter kit, reinsert sterile catheter into meatus (check agency policy). **Note:** If gloves become contaminated, start procedure over.
  - Remove catheter in vagina after successful insertion of second catheter.
- The patient has fever, chills, burning, flank pain, back pain, hematuria, painful urination, urgency, frequency, lower abdominal pain, change in mental status, and lethargy (Haddock, 2015).
  - Assess for bladder distention and tenderness.
  - Monitor vital signs and urine output.
  - Report findings to health care provider; signs and symptoms may indicate UTI.
- The patient is unable to void after catheter removal, has sensation of not emptying, strains to void, or experiences small voiding amounts with increasing frequency.
  - Assess for bladder distention.
  - Help to normal position for voiding and provide privacy.
  - Perform bladder ultrasound to assess for excessive urine volume in bladder.
  - If the patient is unable to void within 6–8 hours of catheter removal and/or experiences abdominal pain, notify health care provider.

SKILL 21.2 Closed Catheter Irrigation

Equipment

Closed intermittent irrigation

- Antiseptic swabs
- Sterile irrigation solution at room temperature as prescribed
- Sterile container
- Syringe to access system: Luer-Lok syringe without needle for needleless access port (per manufacturer directions)
- Screw clamp or rubber band (used to temporarily occlude catheter as irrigant is instilled)

Closed continuous irrigation

- Antiseptic swabs
- Sterile irrigation solution at room temperature (as prescribed)
- Irrigation tubing with clamp to regulate irrigation flow rate
- Y connector (optional) to connect irrigation tubing to double-lumen catheter
- Intravenous (i.v.) pole (closed continuous or intermittent)

STEP	RATIONALE
Assessment	
1. Review the patient's record to determine:	
a. Purpose of bladder irrigation. Confer with health care provider as needed.	Allows you to anticipate observations to make (e.g., blood or mucus in urine).
Clinical decision point: It is recommended to avoid catheter irrigation in these situations: Do not perform continuous irrigation of the bladder with antimicrobials as a routine infection prevention measure. If continuous irrigation is being used to prevent obstruction, maintain a closed system (Lo et al., 2014).	
b. Prescriber's order for method (continuous or intermittent), type, and amount of irrigant (e.g., saline, medicated solutions).	Health care provider's order is required to initiate therapy. Frequency and volume of solution used for irrigation may be in the order or standardized as part of agency policy. Each type of irrigation requires different equipment. Procedure (frequency, dosage, and duration of time dwelling in bladder) for instilling medications into bladder are specific to medication.
c. Type of catheter used.	Triple-lumen catheters are used for both intermittent and continuous closed irrigation. Double-lumen catheters can be used only for intermittent irrigation.
2. Identify the patient by using two identifiers (e.g., name and birthday or name and medical record number) according to agency policy.	Ensures correct patient. Complies with The Joint Commission standards and improves patient safety (TJC, 2016).
3. Assess the patient:	
a. Perform hand hygiene and apply gloves.	Reduces transmission of microorganisms.
b. Inspect urine for color, amount, and clarity and presence of mucus, blood clots, or sediment.	Indicates whether the patient is bleeding or sloughing tissue, which would require increased irrigation rate or frequency of catheter irrigation.
c. Palpate bladder for distention and tenderness.	Bladder distention and tenderness may indicate that urine is not draining freely from bladder. Make sure that there is free flow of urine through catheter drainage tubing (e.g., tubing kinked, occlusion with mucus or blood clots).
d. Observe the patient for abdominal pain, spasms, sensation of bladder fullness, or catheter bypassing (leaking).	May indicate overdistention of bladder caused by blockage of catheter. Offers baseline to determine whether therapy is successful.
4. Review input and I&O record.	If continuous bladder irrigation (CBI) is being used, amount of fluid draining from bladder should exceed amount of fluid infused into bladder. If output does not exceed irrigant infused, catheter obstruction (i.e., blood clots, kinked tubing) should be suspected, irrigation stopped, and prescriber notified.
5. Remove gloves and perform hand hygiene.	Reduces transmission of microorganisms.
6. Assess the patient's knowledge and experience regarding purpose of performing catheter irrigations.	Reveals extent of patient instruction needed.
Planning	
1. Gather supplies needed for catheter irrigation.	Type of irrigation indicates supplies needed to take into the patient's room.
2. Explain procedure to the patient.	Reduces anxiety and promotes cooperation.
Implementation	
1. Perform hand hygiene and apply clean gloves.	Reduces transmission of microorganisms.
2. Provide privacy by closing room door and bed curtains.	Protects patient confidentiality.
3. Raise bed to appropriate working height. If side rails are raised, lower side rail on working side.	Promotes use of good body mechanics and patient safety.
4. Position the patient in dorsal recumbent or supine position and expose catheter junctions (catheter and drainage tubing).	Position provides access to catheter and promotes patient dignity as much as possible.
5. Remove catheter securement device.	Eases access to catheter irrigation ports.
6. Organize supplies according to type of irrigation prescribed.	Ensures easy access to supplies during procedure.
7. Closed intermittent irrigation or instillation with double-lumen catheter:	
Clinical decision point: Closed intermittent irrigation should be done only in cases in which catheter is occluded and health care provider deems that removal of catheter can injure the patient.	

STEP	RATIONALE
a. Draw up in syringe the prescribed amount of medication or sterile solution. Place sterile cap on tip of needleless syringe.	Ensures that irrigation or instillation fluid remains sterile.
b. Clamp indwelling retention catheter just below specimen port.	Occlusion of catheter ensures that irrigation solution goes into bladder, not down into drainage tubing.
Clinical decision point: Avoid irrigating with or instilling cold solution because it results in bladder spasm and discomfort.	
c. Using circular motion, thoroughly clean injection port with antiseptic swab (same port used for specimen collection). Allow to dry.	Reduces transmission of infection. Drying achieves full antimicrobial properties.
d. Insert tip of needleless syringe with twisting motion into irrigation port (see manufacturer instructions for possible variation).	Ensures that hub enters lumen of catheter and flow is directed into bladder.
e. Slowly and evenly inject fluid into catheter and bladder.	Slow injection minimizes potential trauma to bladder mucosa.
Clinical decision point: If catheter does not irrigate easily, stop the irrigation. The catheter may be totally occluded, or the end of the catheter may have been displaced into the urethra. Contact the prescriber; the catheter may need to be removed and replaced.	
f. Withdraw syringe, cleanse port with antiseptic swab, remove clamp, and allow solution to drain into drainage bag. Some medicated irrigants may need to dwell in bladder for a prescribed period of time, requiring catheter to be clamped temporarily.	Allows drainage by gravity. Some irrigation solutions require time in catheter and bladder to exert therapeutic effect. Clamped catheters should not be left unattended.
8. Closed continuous irrigation (see illustration):	
a. Close clamp on tubing and hang bag of solution on intravenous (i.v.) pole. Insert (spike) tip of sterile irrigation tubing into designated port of irrigation solution bag using aseptic technique.	Closing clamp on tubing allows tubing drip chamber to fill after tip of tubing is inserted into port of irrigation solution bag.
b. Fill drip chamber half full by squeezing chamber; then open clamp and allow solution to flow (prime) through tubing, keeping end of tubing sterile. Once fluid has completely filled tubing, close clamp and recap end of tubing.	Priming tubing with fluid prevents introduction of air into bladder.
c. Use aseptic technique to wipe off irrigation port of triple-lumen catheter and attach to irrigation tubing.	Third lumen provides means for irrigation solution to enter bladder.
d. Be sure that drainage bag and tubing are securely connected to drainage port of triple-lumen catheter.	Ensures that urine and irrigation solution drain from bladder without leaking.
e. Calculate drip rate and adjust rate at roller clamp. If urine is bright red or has clots, increase irrigation rate until drainage appears pink (according to ordered rate or agency protocol).	Continuous drainage is expected. It helps with prevention of clotting in the presence of active bleeding in bladder and flushes blood clots out of bladder.
f. Observe for outflow of fluid into drainage bag. Empty catheter drainage bag as needed.	Discomfort, bladder distention, and possibly injury can occur from overdistention of bladder when bladder irrigant cannot adequately flow from bladder. Bag will fill rapidly and may need to be emptied every 1–2 h.
g. Compare urine output with infusion of irrigation solution every hour.	Determines urinary output and ensures that irrigant is draining freely.
9. When procedure is completed, dispose of contaminated supplies in appropriate receptacle, replace catheter securement device if removed, remove gloves, help the patient to safe and comfortable position with bed in low position, and perform hand hygiene.	Promotes patient comfort and safety and reduces transmission of microorganisms.
Evaluation	
1. Measure actual urine output by subtracting total amount of irrigation fluid infused from total volume drained.	Determines accurate urinary output.
2. Review I&O flow sheet to verify that hourly output into drainage bag is in appropriate proportion to irrigating solution entering bladder. Expect more output than fluid instilled because of urine production.	Determines urinary output in relation to irrigation.
3. Observe for catheter patency, inspect urine for blood clots and sediment, and ensure that tubing is not kinked or occluded.	Decrease in blood clots means that therapy is successful in maintaining catheter patency. Ensures that bladder is emptying freely.
4. Assess patient comfort.	An indicator of catheter patency by absence of symptoms of bladder distention.
5. Assess for signs and symptoms of infection.	Evaluates for presence of infection.

STEP	RATIONALE

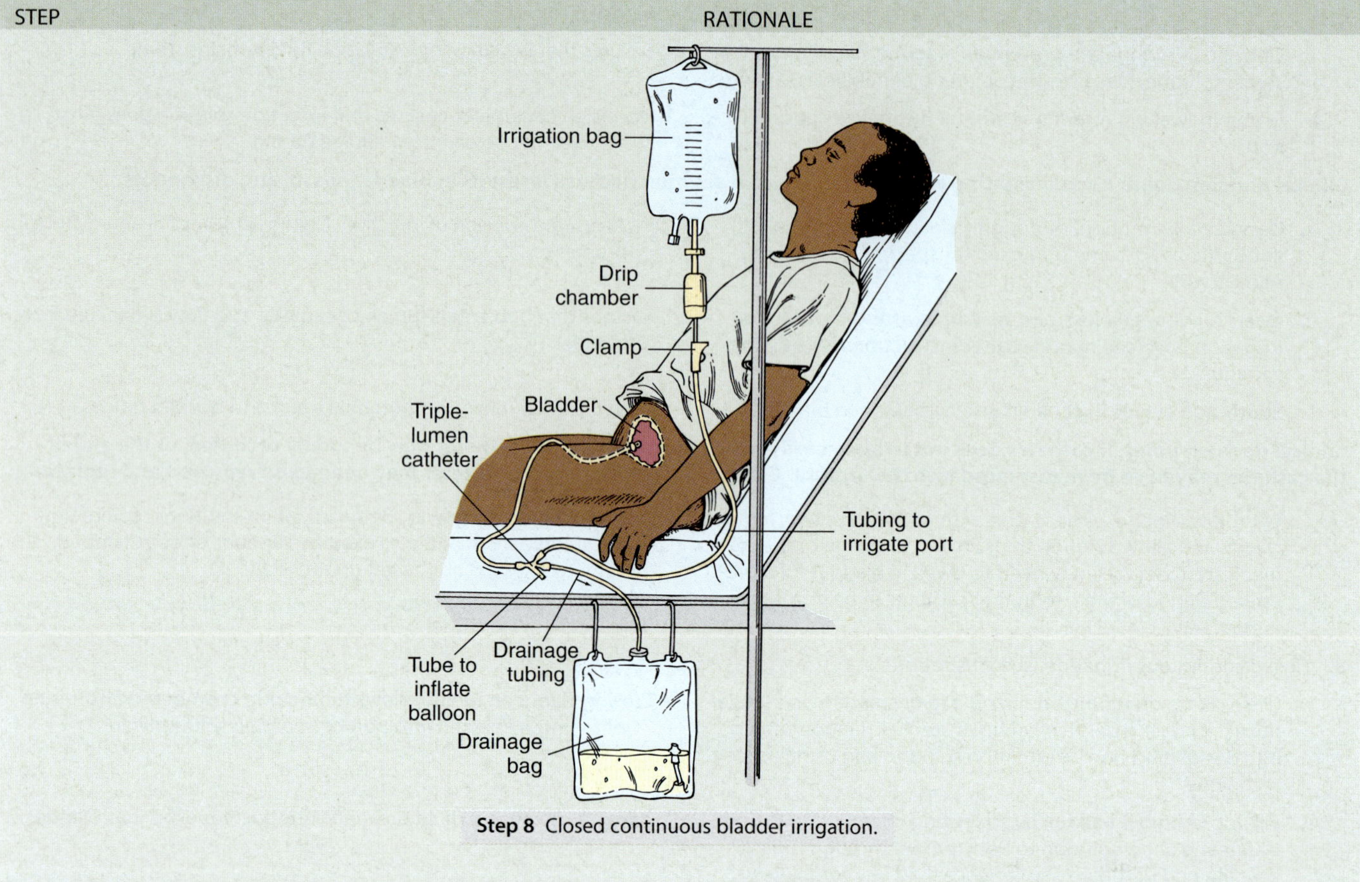

Step 8 Closed continuous bladder irrigation.

STEP	RATIONALE
6. Use ***teach back*** to determine the patient's understanding about irrigation. State, "I want to go over the reason we discussed about why we are irrigating your urinary catheter. Can you tell me the reason we need to irrigate it?" Revise your instruction now or develop plan for revised patient teaching if the patient is not able to teach back correctly.	Evaluates what the patient is able to explain or demonstrate.

Unexpected Outcomes and Related Interventions

1. Irrigating solution does not return (intermittent irrigation); drainage is less than amount of irrigation solution infused or is not flowing at prescribed rate (CBI).
   - Examine tubing for clots, sediment, and kinks.
   - Inspect urine for presence of or increase in blood clots and sediment.
   - Evaluate the patient for pain and distended bladder.
   - Notify health care provider if irrigant does not flow freely from the bladder, the patient complains of pain, or bladder distention occurs.
2. Bright red bleeding with irrigation (CBI) drip is wide open.
   - Assess for hypovolemic shock (vital signs, skin color and moisture, anxiety level).
   - Leave irrigation drip wide open and notify health care provider.
3. The patient experiences pain with irrigation.
   - Examine drainage tubing for clots, sediment, or kinks.
   - Evaluate urine for presence of or increase in blood clots and sediment.
   - Evaluate for distended bladder.
   - Notify health care provider.

Recording and Reporting

- Record irrigation method, amount of and type of irrigation solution, amount returned as drainage, characteristics of output, and urine output.
- Report catheter occlusion, sudden bleeding, infection, or increased pain.
- Record I&O.
- Document your evaluation of patient learning.

Home Care Considerations

- Patients and/or family caregivers can be taught to perform catheter irrigations with adequate support, demonstration/return demonstration, and written instructions.
- Teach patients and/or family caregivers to observe urine color, clarity, odor, and amount.

- Arrange for home delivery and storage of catheter/irrigation supplies.
- Teach patients and/or family caregivers signs of catheter obstruction or urinary tract infection.

KEY POINTS

- Voiding is a complex interaction that takes place among the bladder, urinary sphincter, and central nervous system.
- Many factors affect voiding such as growth and development, sociocultural implications, personal habits, fluid intake, pathological conditions, surgical procedures, medications, and diagnostic examinations.
- When completing a nursing history, collect data from a patient about patterns of urination, symptoms of urinary alterations, and factors affecting voiding.
- Normal urine is pale yellow to amber, is free of hematuria, appears transparent at time of voiding, and is free from odor. Medications and certain foods can alter normal urine characteristics.
- Nursing interventions to promote normal urination and control incontinence include educating patients to have adequate hydration, develop good voiding habits, maintain regular bowel movements, reduce or eliminate smoking, and report changes in bladder function to health care providers.
- Use the smallest catheter size with a 10-mL balloon to minimize trauma and risk for infection when inserting an indwelling Foley catheter. Any patient with an indwelling catheter or who has recently had a catheter is at risk for a catheter-associated urinary tract infection (CAUTI).
- Use of a bladder scanner to measure postvoid residual avoids unnecessary catheterization and decreases the risk for developing a urinary tract infection (UTI).
- Monitoring a patient's intake and output is a common health care provider order or can be initiated per nursing judgment to evaluate bladder emptying, renal function, and fluid balance.

REFERENCES

Ansell T. Indwselling urinary catheters: should we secure them? Br J Nurs 2016;25(18):S22.

Bardsley A. Safe and effective catheterisation for patients in the community. Br J Community Nurs 2015;20(4):166.

Bardsley A. An overview of urinary incontinence. Br J Nurs 2016;25(18):S14.

Carter N, Reitneier L, Goodloe LR. An evidence-based approach to the prevention of catheter-associated urinary tract infections. Urol Nurs 2014;34(5):238.

Casey G. Understanding urinary tract infections. Nurs N Z 2014;20(5):20.

Centers for Disease Control and Prevention (CDC). Urinary tract infection (catheter-associated urinary tract infection [CAUTI] and non-catheter-associated urinary tract infection [UTI]) and other urinary system infection [USI]) events. 2017. Available from: https://www.cdc.gov/nhsn/PDFs/pscManual/7pscCAUTIcurrent.pdf.

Galiczewski JM. Interventions for the prevention of catheter associated urinary tract infections in intensive care units: an integrative review. Intensive Crit Care Nurs 2016;32:1.

Gesmundo M. Managing indwelling urinary catheters. Nurs N Z 2016; 22(6):14.

Gould CV, Umscheid CA, Agarwal RK, Kuntz G, Pegues DA, and the Healthcare Infection Control Practices Advisory Committee (HICPAC). Guideline for prevention of catheter-associated urinary tract infections. 2009. February 15, 2017. Available from: https://www.cdc.gov/infectioncontrol/pdf/guidelines/cauti-guidelines.pdf.

Haddock G. Improving the management of urinary tract infection. Nurs Resid Care 2015;17(1):22.

Huether SE, McCance KL. Understanding pathophysiology. 6th ed. St. Louis: Mosby; 2016.

Jones ML. Elimination of urine and incontinence of urine. Br J Healthc Assist 2015;9(8):375.

Kehinde O. Common incontinence problems seen by community nurses. J Community Nurs 2016;30(4):46.

Leaver R. Managing the aftercare of patients with a Mitrofanoff pouch. J Community Nurs 2016;30(1):40.

Lo E, et al: Strategies to prevent catheter-associated urinary tract infections in acute care hospitals, *Infect Control HospEpidemiol* 35(5):464, 2014.

National Institute of Diabetes and Digestive and Kidney Diseases (NIDDK). Urinary diversion. 2013. Available from: https://www.niddk.nih.gov/health-information/urologic-diseases/urinary-diversion.

Nazarko L. Person-centered care of women with urinary incontinence. Nurse Prescr 2015;13(6):288.

Nicolle L. Catheter-related urinary tract infection: practical management in the elderly. Drugs Aging 2014;31:1.

Pagana TJ, Pagana KD, Pagana TN. Mosby's diagnostic and laboratory test reference. 13th ed. St. Louis: Mosby; 2017.

Panchisin T. Improving outcomes with the ANA CAUTI Prevention Tool. Nursing 2016;46(3):55.

Rantell A. Pharmacological management of overactive bladder in women. Nurse Prescr 2014;12(5):232.

Schreiber M. Ostomies: nursing care and management. Medsurg Nurs 2016;25(2):127.

Smart C. Male incontinence: using the urinary sheath. Nurs Resid Care 2014;16(10):568.

Testa A. Understanding urinary incontinence in adults. Urol Nurs 2015;35(2):82.

The Joint Commission (TJC): 2016 *National Patient Safety Goals*, Oakbrook Terrace, IL, 2016, The Commission, Available at http://www.jointcommission.org/standards_information/npsgs.aspx. Accessed November 2019.

The Joint Commission (TJC). 2018 National Patient Safety Goals, Oakbrook Terrace, IL: The Joint Commission; 2018. Available from: http://www.jointcommission.org/standards_information/npsgs.aspx.

Wilson M. Urinary incontinence: considering the physical and psychological implications. Br J Community Nurs 2016;21(5):222.

Woodward S. Intermittent catheterization for postoperative urinary retention. Br J Nurs 2015a;24(14):732.

Woodward S. Selecting and fitting a penile sheath. Br J Nurs 2015b;24(5):290.

Yates A. Indwelling urinary catheterization: what is best practice? Br J Nurs 2016;25(9):84.

22 Bowel Elimination

OBJECTIVES

- To explain the physiology of digestion, absorption, and bowel elimination.
- To understand anatomy and physiology of GI tract.
- To describe characteristics of feces and factors that influence bowel elimination.
- To explain common physiological alterations in bowel elimination, which include constipation, impaction, diarrhea, fecal incontinence, flatulence, hemorrhoids, and intestinal diversion ostomies.
- To discuss nursing process for patients with problems in bowel elimination.
- To describe lab and diagnostic examination including colonoscopy for diagnosing bowel problems.
- To assess the patient's need and able to prioritize nursing diagnosis based on that.
- To describe the steps used in the nursing interventions that promote normal elimination and defecation.
- To evaluate outcomes of bowel elimination interventions.
- To explain the need of laxatives and nasogastric tube for gastric decompression as a part of acute care for bowel elimination.
- To understand different types of enemas and its importance in treating bowel problems.
- To describe the management of patients with fecal incontinence and restorative care including bowel training and ostomy care.
- To understand guidelines for nursing skills required for treating patients with bowel problems.

KEY TERMS

cathartics, p. 526	fecal impaction, p. 519	laxatives, p. 526
colon, p. 517	fecal incontinence, p. 520	melena, p. 518
constipation, p. 519	feces, p. 517	ostomy, p. 521
defecation, p. 518	flatus, p. 517	peristalsis, p. 517
diarrhea, p. 520	hemorrhoids, p. 521	stoma, p. 521
enema, p. 527	ileus, p. 526	

INTRODUCTION

Regular bowel elimination is essential to maintain a healthy body. Alterations in bowel elimination are often early signs or symptoms of problems within either the gastrointestinal (GI) or other body systems. Bowel function depends on the balance of several factors such as age, diet, fluid intake, activity level, and medications. Elimination patterns and habits vary among individuals.

Individuals of any age are at risk for changes in intestinal activity. These changes are the result of illness, medications, diagnostic testing, or surgical intervention. Aging when accompanied by chronic illness, cognitive decline, decreased mobility, and a decrease in food and fluid intake changes digestive system function; however, aging alone does not necessarily alter the digestive process. Alterations in intestinal elimination respond to both preventive and therapeutic interventions.

ANATOMY AND PHYSIOLOGY OF THE GASTROINTESTINAL TRACT

The GI tract is a series of hollow mucous membrane–lined muscular organs that begin at the mouth and end at the anal orifice. The functions of the GI tract are to break down ingested food for use as energy by body cells and promote the absorption of fluid and nutrients. It is a complex system, and changes in any one part can alter the function of other parts (Fig. 22.1).

Mouth

The mouth mechanically and chemically breaks down nutrients into usable size and form. The teeth chew food, breaking it down into a size suitable for swallowing. Saliva, produced by the salivary glands in the mouth, dilutes

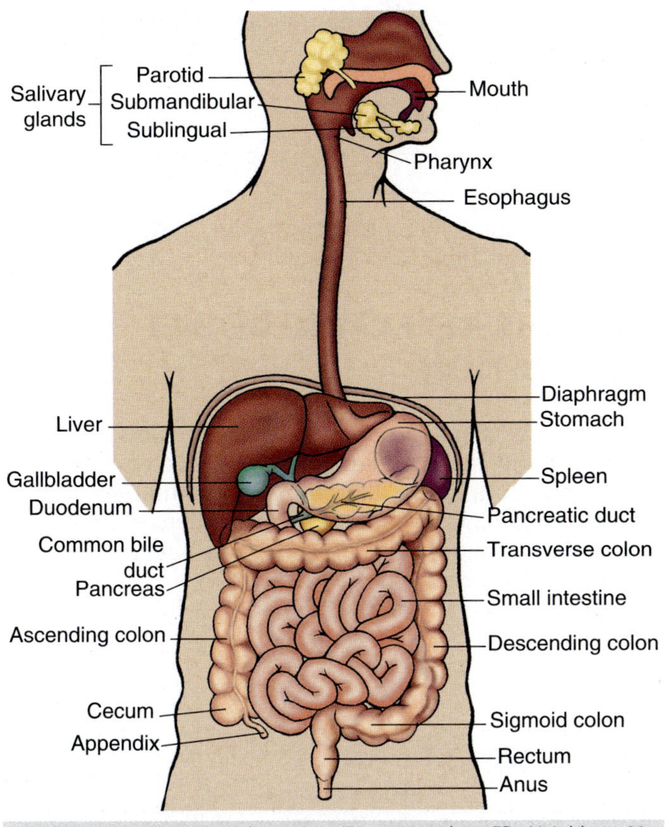

Fig. 22.1 **Gastrointestinal system.** (From Monahan FD, Neighbors M: *Medical-surgical nursing*, ed 2, Philadelphia, 1998, Saunders.)

and softens the food in the mouth for easier swallowing. Enzymes in saliva begin the breakdown of food.

Esophagus

As food enters the upper esophagus, it passes through the upper esophageal sphincter, a circular muscle that prevents air from entering the esophagus and food from refluxing into the throat. The bolus of food travels down the esophagus with the aid of **peristalsis**, which is a contraction that propels food through the length of the GI tract. The food moves down the esophagus and reaches the cardiac sphincter, which lies between the esophagus and the upper end of the stomach. The sphincter prevents reflux of stomach contents back into the esophagus.

Stomach

The stomach performs three tasks: storing swallowed food and liquid, mixing food with digestive juices, and regulating emptying of its contents into the small intestine. The stomach produces and secretes hydrochloric acid (HCl), mucus, the enzyme pepsin, and intrinsic factor. Pepsin and HCl facilitate the digestion of protein. Mucus protects the stomach mucosa from acidity and enzyme activity. Intrinsic factor is essential in preparing vitamin B_{12} for absorption in the ileum.

Small Intestine

Movement within the small intestine, occurring by peristalsis, facilitates both digestion and absorption. Food comes into the small intestine as a semifluid material and mixes with digestive juices. Resorption in the small intestine is so efficient that by the time the fluid reaches the end of the small intestine, it is semisolid in consistency. The small intestine is divided into three sections: the duodenum, the jejunum, and the ileum.

The duodenum is approximately 8–11 inches long and continues to process the fluid from the stomach. The second section, the jejunum, is approximately 8 feet long and absorbs carbohydrates and proteins. The ileum is approximately 12 feet long and absorbs water, fats, and bile salts. The duodenum and jejunum absorb most nutrients and electrolytes in the small intestine. The ileum absorbs certain vitamins, iron, and bile salts. Digestive enzymes and bile enter the small intestine from the pancreas and liver to further break down nutrients into a form usable by the body.

When small intestine function is impaired, it greatly alters the digestive process. Conditions such as inflammation, infection, surgical resection, or obstruction disrupt peristalsis, reduce absorption, or block the passage of the fluid. Electrolyte and nutrient deficiencies then develop.

Large Intestine

The lower GI tract is called the *large intestine* because it is larger in diameter than the small intestine. However, its length (1.5–1.8 m [5–6 feet]) is much shorter. The large intestine is divided into the cecum, ascending colon, transverse colon, descending colon, sigmoid colon, and rectum (see Fig. 22.1). It is the primary organ of bowel elimination.

The digestive fluid enters the large intestine by waves of peristalsis through the ileocecal valve, a circular muscle layer that prevents regurgitation back into the small intestine. The muscular tissue of the colon allows it to accommodate and eliminate large quantities of waste and gas **(flatus)**. The **colon** has three functions: absorption, secretion, and elimination. It resorbs a large volume of water (up to 1.5 L) and significant amounts of sodium and chloride daily. The amount of water absorbed depends on the speed at which colonic contents move. Normally, the fecal matter becomes a soft, formed solid or semisolid mass. If peristalsis is abnormally fast, there is less time for water to be absorbed, and the stool is watery. If peristaltic contractions slow, water continues to be absorbed, and a hard mass of stool forms, resulting in constipation.

Peristaltic contractions move contents through the colon. Intestinal content is the main stimulus for contraction. Mass peristalsis pushes undigested food toward the rectum. These mass movements occur only three or four times daily, with the strongest during the hour after mealtime.

The rectum, located at the end of the large intestine, is normally empty of waste products **(feces)** until just before defecation. It contains vertical and transverse folds of tissue that help to control expulsion of fecal contents during defecation. Each fold contains veins that can become distended from pressure during straining. This distention results in hemorrhoid formation.

Anus

The body expels feces and flatus from the rectum through the anus. Contraction and relaxation of the internal and external sphincters, which are innervated by sympathetic and parasympathetic nerves, aid in the control of defecation. The anal canal contains a rich supply of sensory nerves that allow people to sense when there is solid, liquid, or gas that needs to be expelled and aids in maintaining continence.

Defecation

The physiological factors essential to bowel function and **defecation** include normal GI tract function, sensory awareness of rectal distention and rectal contents, voluntary sphincter control, and adequate rectal capacity and compliance (Steele et al., 2016). Normal defecation begins with movement in the left colon, moving stool toward the anus. When stool reaches the rectum, the distention causes relaxation of the internal sphincter and an awareness of the need to defecate. At the time of defecation, the external sphincter relaxes, and abdominal muscles contract, increasing intrarectal pressure and forcing the stool out. Normally, defecation is painless, resulting in passage of soft, formed stool. Straining while having a bowel movement indicates that the patient may need changes in diet or fluid intake or that there is an underlying disorder in GI function.

COMPOSITION AND CHARACTERISTICS OF FECES

Inspect feces for color, consistency, odor, and several other characteristics (Table 22.1).

FACTORS AFFECTING BOWEL ELIMINATION

To manage your patient's elimination problems, you need to understand normal elimination and factors that promote, impede, or cause alterations in elimination such as constipation, diarrhea, and fecal incontinence (Box 22.1). Supportive nursing care respects each patient's privacy and emotional needs and includes interventions designed to promote normal bowel elimination while minimizing discomfort.

Table 22.1 Fecal Characteristics

Characteristic	Normal	Abnormal	Abnormal Cause
Color	Infant: Yellow Adult: Brown	White or clay	Absence of bile
		Black or tarry (**melena**)	Iron ingestion or GI bleeding
		Red	GI bleeding, hemorrhoids, ingestion of beets
		Pale and oily	Malabsorption of fat
Odor	Malodorous; may be affected by certain foods	Noxious change	Blood in feces or infection
Consistency	Soft, formed	Liquid	Diarrhea, reduced absorption
		Hard	Constipation
Frequency	Varies: Infant: Four to six times daily (breastfed) or one to three times daily (bottle-fed) Adult: Twice daily to three times a week	Infant: more than six times daily or less than once every 1–2 days Adult: More than three times a day or less than once a week	Hypermotility or hypomotility
Shape	Resembles diameter of rectum	Narrow, pencil shaped	Obstruction, increased peristalsis
Constituents	Undigested food, dead bacteria, fat, bile pigment, cells lining intestinal mucosa, water	Blood, pus, foreign bodies, mucus, worms	Internal bleeding, infection, swallowed objects, irritation, inflammation, infestation of parasites
		Oily stool	Malabsorption syndrome, enteritis, pancreatic disease, surgical resection of intestine
		Mucus	Intestinal irritation, inflammation, infection, or injury

GI, gastrointestinal.

BOX 22.1 **Factors Influencing Bowel Elimination**

Age

- Infants have a smaller stomach capacity, less secretion of digestive enzymes, and more rapid intestinal peristalsis. The ability to control defecation does not occur until 2–3 years.
- Adolescents experience rapid growth of the large intestine and increased secretion of gastric acids to dissolve food fibers and act as a bactericide against swallowed organisms.
- Older adults may have decreased chewing ability. Partially chewed food is not digested as easily. Peristalsis declines, and esophageal emptying slows. This impairs absorption by the intestinal mucosa. Muscle tone in the perineal floor and anal sphincter weakens, causing difficulty in controlling defecation (National Institute of Diabetes, Digestive and Kidney Diseases [NIDDK], 2016).

Diet

- Regular daily food intake promotes peristalsis.
- High-fiber foods (e.g., fruits, greens, and other vegetables) and whole grains (cereals and breads) promote peristalsis and defecation by creating bulk.

BOX 22.1 Factors Influencing Bowel Elimination—cont'd

- Low-fiber foods (e.g., pasta, white rice, white bread, cheese) slow peristalsis.
- Gas-producing foods (e.g., broccoli, cauliflower, onions, dried beans) stimulate peristalsis.
- People with lactose intolerance lack the enzyme lactase, which is needed to digest the simple sugars in milk. Lactose intolerance leads to diarrhea and cramping.
- People with gluten intolerance experience pain, bloating, diarrhea, or constipation.

Position During Defecation

- A sitting position allows a person to lean forward, exert intra-abdominal pressure, and contract thigh muscles for normal defecation.
- Older adults and patients with chronic pain or immobility may have difficulty sitting down on or rising from a toilet seat. An elevated toilet seat and chairs with arms on the sides of the toilet help to promote defecation.
- Patients required to use a bedpan while lying down cannot contract muscles to defecate.

Pregnancy

- As pregnancy advances and a fetus enlarges, pressure is exerted on the rectum. Constipation commonly occurs.

Diagnostic Tests

- Examinations involving visualization of GI structures require the emptying of bowel contents. Patients receive nothing by mouth (NPO) or only clear liquids, bowel evacuants, and enema administration to cleanse the bowel before the test. This is called *bowel prep* and temporarily interferes with normal elimination.
- Barium examinations require ingestion of barium, a mixture that can cause constipation unless the barium is eliminated soon after a test.

Fluid Intake

- When there is adequate fluid intake (1.5–2 L/day), the body absorbs fluid into the fecal mass and increases bulk for easier passage.
- Warm beverages and fruit juices soften stool and increase peristalsis.
- Caffeinated drinks in moderation may stimulate peristalsis.

Activity

- Immobilization depresses colon motility, whereas regular physical exercise promotes peristalsis.

Psychological Factors

- Stress, anxiety, or fear initiates parasympathetic impulses, causing the acceleration of digestion and peristalsis. Diarrhea and gaseous distention result.
- Emotional depression decreases peristalsis and leads to constipation.

Personal Habits

- Failing to respond to the need to defecate and lack of privacy interfere with normal elimination patterns and lead to constipation.
- Hospitalized patients often share toilet facilities or use bedpans or bedside commodes. The resulting embarrassment causes them to ignore the urge to defecate.

Pain

- Hemorrhoids, rectal surgery, and abdominal surgery cause a patient to suppress defecation because of pain; constipation develops.

Medications

- Laxatives and cathartics soften stool and promote peristalsis.
- Antidiarrheal agents inhibit peristalsis.
- Opiates and anticholinergic drugs depress peristalsis and cause constipation.
- Antibiotics alter normal bowel flora and often produce diarrhea.
- Drugs that contain iron sometimes turn the stool black. Antacids cause a white discoloration. Anticoagulants can cause frank or occult blood in the stool.

Surgery and Anesthesia

- General anesthetics slow or halt peristalsis.
- Surgery involving bowel manipulation may temporarily stop peristalsis, creating a condition called *paralytic ileus*, which lasts for hours or days and resolves spontaneously.

BOWEL ELIMINATION PROBLEMS

Alterations in bowel elimination are caused by a variety of factors.

Constipation

Constipation is defined as having fewer than three bowel movements per week, but based on the American Society of Gastroenterologists recommendations, health care providers now also define constipation as one or more of the following:

- Hard or dry stools
- Decreased frequency of stooling
- Sensation of incomplete evacuation following a bowel movement
- Pain or straining associated with stool elimination (Steele et al., 2016)

Constipation is commonly caused by changes in diet, medications, mobility, inflammation, environmental factors (e.g., unavailability of toilet facilities or lack of privacy), and lack of knowledge about regular bowel habits. It is not a physiological response to aging, but changes in mobility and comorbidities that occur with aging make this condition more prevalent in older adults (Steele et al., 2016). Regardless of cause, intestinal motility slows, causing prolonged exposure of the feces to the intestinal wall. Liquid from the feces continues to be absorbed, leaving the stool hard and dry (Box 22.2).

Constipation has significant health implications. Straining during defecation causes problems for patients with recent abdominal, gynecological, or rectal surgery. An effort to pass a stool can cause stress and pain in the surgical site. Patients with cardiovascular disease, diseases causing elevated intraocular pressure (glaucoma), and increased intracranial pressure need to prevent constipation and avoid straining to have a bowel movement. The constipation can be prevented by help of bowel hygiene practices (Box 22.3).

Impaction

Fecal impaction results from unrelieved constipation. A patient is unable to expel the hardened feces retained in the

BOX 22.2 Common Causes of Constipation

- Irregular bowel habits and ignoring the urge to defecate
- Chronic illnesses (e.g., Parkinson disease, multiple sclerosis, rheumatoid arthritis, chronic bowel diseases, depression, eating disorders)
- Low-fiber diet high in animal fats (e.g., meats and carbohydrates); low fluid intake
- Stress (e.g., illness of a family member, death of a loved one, divorce)
- Physical inactivity
- Medications and overuse of laxatives
- Changes in life or routine such as pregnancy, aging, and travel
- Neurological conditions that block nerve impulses to the colon (e.g., stroke, spinal cord injury, tumor)
- Chronic bowel dysfunction (e.g., colonic inertia, irritable bowel)

Data from National Institute of Diabetes, Digestive and Kidney Diseases (NIDDK): *Health information*, 2016, https://www.niddk.nih.gov/health-information.

BOX 22.3 Bowel Hygiene for Prevention of Constipation

Helping patients and their families in healthy food selection and preparation practices reduces the risks of gastrointestinal (GI) disorders. There is increasing evidence that weight control with a body mass index of 25 or below; a diet rich in fruits, vegetables, and whole grains and low in fat and red meat; and daily exercise reduce risk for colorectal cancers, digestive diseases, and other cancers (ACS, 2017). Consider whether a patient is able to afford the foods recommended. In addition to solid foods, a patient with elimination problems needs to drink 1.5–2 L of fluids daily if not contraindicated by other medical conditions.

Application to Nursing Practice

- Recommend fluid intake of at least 1.5 L/day.
- Teach patients to limit alcohol because of its diuretic properties and not to count any alcoholic beverage as part of their daily intake of fluids.
- Suggest a high-fiber diet (25–30 g/day) to reduce constipation; as fiber passes through the colon, it retains fluid. As a result, bulkier and softer stools develop. In addition, the waste moves through the colon more easily and results in more regular bowel movements.
- Teach patients to use a combination of insoluble and soluble fiber (e.g., bran, fruits, and vegetables) to prevent constipation.
- Assess the patient's ability to afford foods.
- Encourage physical activity in combination with adequate fluid intake and high-fiber diet to manage constipation. Walking once or twice a day for 30 min is sufficient.
- Explain need to use laxatives with caution. A stepwise progression of laxatives is recommended: first bulk-forming laxatives, followed by stool softeners and osmotic stimulants. Use suppositories and/or enemas if diet, fluid, and laxative regimen are not successful.

rectum. In severe impaction, the hardened fecal mass extends up into the sigmoid colon. Patients at greatest risk for impaction include those who are confused, weak, unconscious, or unaware of the need to defecate and patients who have an interruption in nerve supply to the bowel. An obvious sign of impaction is the inability to pass a stool for several days, despite a repeated urge to defecate. Continuous oozing of liquid stool after several days with no fecal output may indicate an impaction. Loss of appetite, abdominal distention and cramping, nausea and/or vomiting, and rectal pain can also occur.

Diarrhea

Diarrhea is an increase in the number of stools and the passage of liquid, unformed stools (Table 22.2).

- It is associated with disorders affecting digestion, absorption, and secretion in the GI tract.
- Intestinal contents pass too quickly through the small intestine and colon to allow for the usual absorption of fluid and nutrients.
- Dehydration leading to fluid and electrolyte and acid–base imbalances can result. Older adults and very young children are at the greatest risk for dehydration (Box 22.4).
- Persistent diarrhea may cause skin breakdown in the perianal region.

A common cause of diarrhea in health care facilities is *Clostridium difficile*; symptoms of *C. difficile* infection range from mild to severe diarrhea. This infection is acquired by use of antibiotics that depress natural intestinal flora, allowing an overgrowth of *C. difficile*, and by contact with the *C. difficile* organism. The best ways to prevent the occurrence and spread of *C. difficile* is cautious use of antibiotics and rigorous hand hygiene with soap and water (Mayo Clinic, 2016). Communicable foodborne pathogens also cause diarrhea. Thorough handwashing after using the bathroom and before and after meal preparation and careful cleansing and storing of fresh produce and meats help to reduce foodborne illnesses.

Fecal Incontinence

Fecal incontinence is the temporary or permanent inability to control the passage of feces and gas from the anus. It is underreported because of shame or a sense that nothing can be done about it, yet it affects up to 20% of community-living adults and nearly 50% of nursing home residents (Callan and Wilson, 2016). It is embarrassing and may cause social isolation and loss of intimacy. It is often assumed that a loss of cognitive function is the primary reason that an older person is unable to remain continent; however, a person may be mentally alert but physically unable to avoid uncontrolled defecation. Impairment of anal sphincter function or control may cause incontinence. Conditions that create frequent, large-volume, watery stools predispose to fecal urgency and incontinence. Similar to diarrhea, incontinence predisposes a patient to skin breakdown. Management of fecal incontinence requires a complete understanding of the causes.

Flatulence

Flatulence (accumulated gas) is one of the most common GI disorders. It is a sensation of bloating and abdominal distention accompanied by excess gas. As gas accumulates in the lumen of the intestines, the bowel wall stretches and distends. Normally, intestinal gas escapes through the mouth (belching) or the anus. However, when intestinal motility is reduced as a result of medications, general

Table 22.2 Conditions That Cause Diarrhea

Condition	Physiological Effects
Intestinal infection (streptococcal or staphylococcal enteritis)	Inflammation of intestinal mucosa, increased mucus secretion
Food allergies	Abnormal digestion of food elements, increased mucus secretion
Food intolerance (lactose, gluten, high fat, coffee, alcohol, spicy foods)	Abnormal digestion of food elements, increased mucus secretion
Tube feedings	Hyperosmolarity of some enteral solutions results in diarrhea because hyperosmolar fluids draw fluids into the GI tract
Medications	
Iron supplements	Irritation of intestinal mucosa
Antibiotics	Loss of normal flora, susceptibility to opportunistic infection
Laxatives (short term)	Increased intestinal motility and irritability
Inflammatory bowel disease (colitis, Crohn disease)	Inflammation and ulceration of intestinal walls, reduced absorption of fluids, increased intestinal motility
Surgical alterations	
Gastrectomy	Loss of reservoir function of stomach, improper absorption because food moves into duodenum too quickly
Intestinal resection	Reduced length of intestine, reduced amount of absorptive surface
Emotional stress (anxiety)	Increased intestinal motility

GI, gastrointestinal.

BOX 22.4 **Signs of Dehydration**

Signs of dehydration in adults include the following:

- Thirst
- Less frequent urination than usual
- Dark-colored urine
- Dry skin
- Fatigue
- Dizziness
- Light-headedness

Signs of dehydration in infants and young children include the following:

- Dry mouth and tongue
- No tears when crying
- No wet diapers for 3 h or more
- Sunken eyes, cheeks, or soft spot in the skull
- High fever
- Listlessness or irritability

anesthetics, abdominal surgery, or immobilization, flatulence may become severe, causing abdominal distention and sharp pain.

Hemorrhoids

Hemorrhoids are dilated, engorged veins in the lining of the rectum. Increased venous pressure resulting from straining at defecation, pregnancy, and chronic illnesses such as congestive heart failure and chronic liver disease are causative factors. A hemorrhoid forms either within the anal canal (internal) or through the opening of the anus (external). Passage of hard stool causes hemorrhoid tissue to stretch and bleed. Hemorrhoid tissue becomes inflamed and tender, and patients may report itching and burning. Because pain worsens during defecation, the patient sometimes ignores the urge to defecate, resulting in constipation.

Intestinal Diversions/Ostomies

Certain diseases or surgical alterations make the normal passage of intestinal contents throughout the small and large intestines difficult or inadvisable. When these conditions are present, a temporary or permanent opening **(stoma)** is surgically created by bringing a portion of the intestine out through the abdominal wall. These surgical openings are called an *ileostomy* or *colostomy*, depending on which part of the intestinal tract is used to create the stoma (Figs 22.2 and 22.3). Newer surgical techniques allow more patients to have portions of their small and large intestines removed and the remaining portions to be reconnected so that they can continue to defecate through the anal canal.

The location of an **ostomy** determines stool consistency. The more intestine remaining, the more formed and normal the stool. For example, an ileostomy bypasses the entire large intestine, creating frequent, liquid stools. A person with a sigmoid colostomy has a more formed stool.

Loop ostomies are performed on an emergency basis and are reversible stomas that may be constructed in the ileum or the colon. The surgeon pulls a loop of intestine onto the abdomen and places a plastic rod, bridge, or rubber catheter temporarily under the bowel loop to keep it from slipping back. The surgeon then opens the bowel and sutures it to the skin of the abdomen. The loop ostomy has two openings through the stoma. The proximal end drains fecal effluent, and the distal portion drains mucus.

An end colostomy consists of a stoma formed by bringing a piece of intestine out through a surgically created opening in the abdominal wall, turning it down like a turtleneck and suturing it to the abdominal wall (see Fig. 22.2). The intestine distal to the stoma is either removed or sewn closed (called *Hartmann pouch*) and left in the abdominal cavity. End ostomies may be permanent or reversible. The rectum may be left intact or removed.

Managing a stoma that produces frequent passage of liquid stool (e.g., an ileostomy) can be challenging. Skin protection is important because of the liquid and caustic nature of the output, which may cause irritant dermatitis. The more

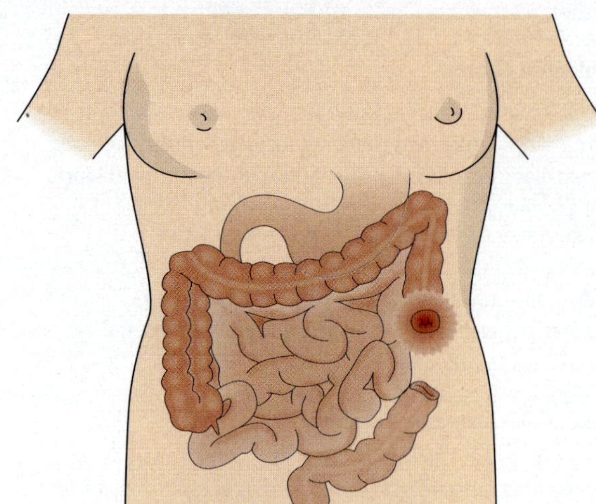
Fig. 22.2 Sigmoid colostomy.

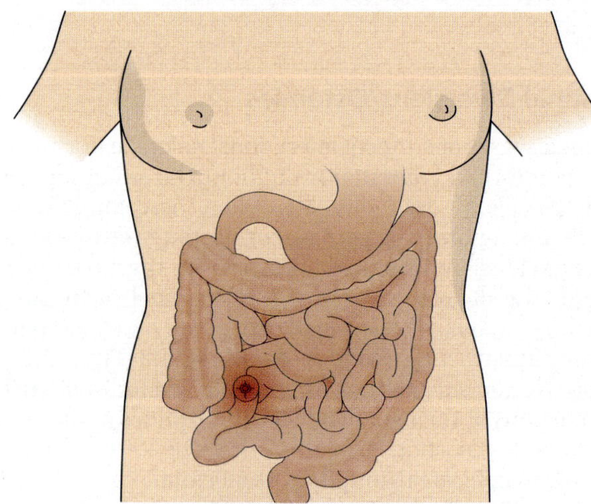
Fig. 22.3 Ileostomy.

common peristomal skin problems are contact dermatitis, fungal infections, or folliculitis (Salvadalena, 2016). An ostomy is managed with an odor-proof pouch with a skin barrier surrounding the stoma. Empty the pouch when it is one-third to one-half full. If the pouch becomes full of gas, open the pouch and expel the air. Change the pouching system approximately every 3–7 days, depending on the patient's individual needs.

Other Diversion Procedures

The ileoanal pouch anastomosis is a surgical procedure that is an option for some patients who need to undergo a colectomy (removal of the colon) for treatment of ulcerative colitis or familial polyposis. In this procedure, the colon is removed, a pouch is created from the end of the small intestine, and the pouch is attached to the anus (Fig. 22.4). The ileoanal pouch provides for collection of waste material in a fashion similar to that of the rectum. The patient is continent of stool because stool evacuates via the anus. When surgeons create the ileal pouch, they also make a temporary ileostomy to allow the pouch anastomosis to heal.

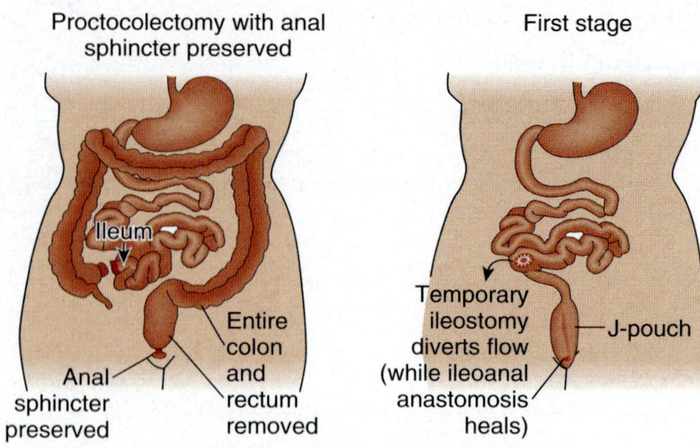

Fig. 22.4 Ileal pouch anal anastomosis.

A continent ileostomy involves creating a pouch from the small intestine. This procedure is rarely done now; however, some patients may have had this procedure in the past. The pouch has a continent stoma on the abdomen created with a valve that can be drained only when the patient places a large catheter into the stoma. The patient empties the pouch several times a day.

PROMOTION OF NORMAL DEFECATION

Assess for the consistency of the stool using Bristol Stool Form Scale (Fig. 22.5). To help patients evacuate contents normally and without discomfort, recommend interventions that stimulate the defecation reflex or increase peristalsis. Helping a patient into an upright sitting position increases pressure on the rectum and facilitates the use of intra-abdominal muscles. Patients who have had surgery or have muscular weakness or mobility limitations benefit from the use of elevated toilet seats. Regular toilets may be too low for patients to lower themselves to a sitting position because of pain or altered mobility. With an elevated seat, the patient exerts less effort to sit and stand.

Providing Bedpan

A patient restricted to the use of a bedpan for defecation usually needs help. Sitting on a bedpan is uncomfortable and awkward. Help position a patient comfortably. Two types of bedpans are available (Fig. 22.6). The regular bedpan, made of hard plastic, has a curved smooth upper end and a sharper-edged lower end and is about 5 cm (2 inches) deep. A fracture pan is used for patients with low-extremity fractures or any patient for whom raising the hips to get on a bedpan is too painful. It has a shallow upper end about 2.5 cm (1 inch) deep. The shallow end of the pan fits under the buttocks toward the sacrum, and the deeper end goes just under the upper thighs. The pan needs to be high enough so that the stool can enter the pan.

When positioning or assisting patients on bedpans, focus on preventing muscle strain and discomfort (Box 22.6). Never place a patient on a bedpan and then leave the bed flat unless activity restrictions demand it. This forces the patient to hyperextend the back to lift the hips onto the pan

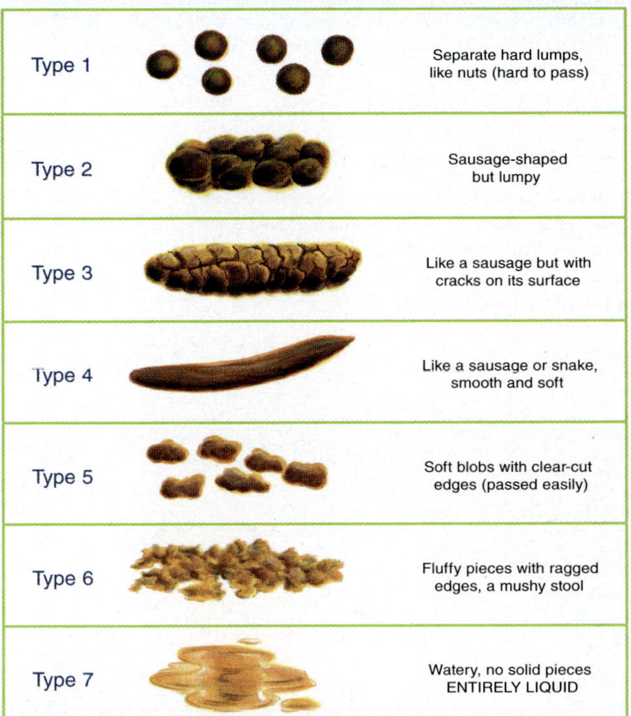

Fig. 22.5 Bristol Stool Form Scale. (Distributed with the kind permission of Dr K. W. Heaton; formerly reader in Medicine at the University of Bristol. Reproduced as a service to the medical profession by Norgine Ltd. ©2017 Norgine group of companies.)

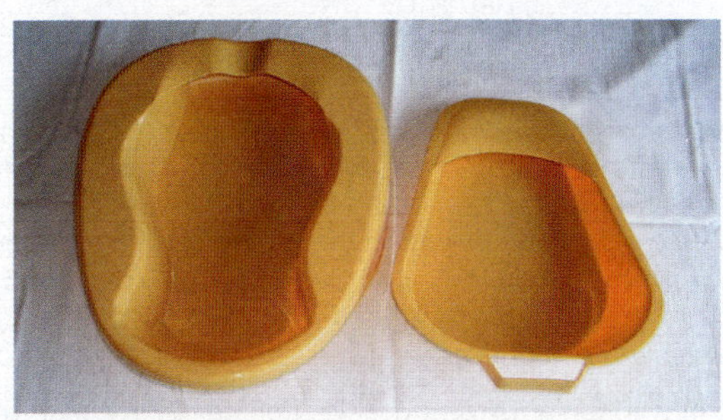

Fig. 22.6 Types of bedpans. *From left:* Regular bedpan and fracture pan.

(Fig. 22.7A). It is often necessary to have the bed flat when placing a patient on a bedpan. Rolling the patient onto the bedpan is the most comfortable way to position a patient with impaired mobility. After it is positioned under the patient, raise the head of the bed 30–45° (Fig. 22.7B). Patients who have overhead trapeze frames are able to lift themselves by grasping the trapeze bar. Always be sure to come back to the patient frequently to see whether he or she is ready to get off. The patient who is sedated or cognitively impaired could fall asleep on the bedpan and develop serious pressure injury to the buttocks if left on it for a prolonged period of time.

For the more mobile patient, a bedside commode is a safe, effective alternative to a bedpan. Its use is less exhausting and allows the patient to assume a more normal or familiar position for defecation.

BOX 22.5 Procedural Guidelines

Measuring Fecal Occult Blood

Equipment

Soap, water, washcloth, and towel; paper towel; clean gloves; wooden applicators; guaiac fecal occult blood test (gFOBT) kit or immunochemical fecal occult blood test (iFOBT, or FIT) kit

Steps

1. If nurse is performing test: Identify the patient by using at least two identifiers (e.g., name and birthday or name and medical record number) according to agency policy.
2. Assess the patient's or family member's understanding of need for stool test.
3. Explain procedure to the patient and/or family member. Discuss reason for specimen collection and how the patient can help or perform. Explain that feces must be free of urine and toilet tissue.
4. Perform hand hygiene and apply clean gloves.
5. Use tip of wooden applicator to obtain small portion of feces. Obtain uncontaminated stool specimen and place in clean, dry container not contaminated with urine, water, or toilet tissue.
6. Measure for occult blood.
   a. **To perform gFOBT test:**
      (1) Open flap of test slide. Apply thin smear of stool on paper in the first box.
      (2) Obtain second fecal specimen from different portion of stool and apply thinly to the second box of slide (see illustration).
      (3) Close slide cover and turn slide over to reverse side. Open cardboard flap and apply two drops of developing solution on each box of guaiac paper (see illustration).
      (4) Read results of test after 30–60 s. Note color changes.
      (5) Dispose of test slide in proper receptacle.
   b. **To perform iFOBT or FIT:**
      (1) Read manufacturer's directions.
      (2) Use special spoon or other device provided in kit to collect a sample of stool.
      (3) Place in collection container that comes with the test kit.
7. If the patient performs gFOBT or FIT test at home:
   a. Have the patient flush the toilet before having a bowel movement.
   b. After passing stool, have the patient put the used toilet paper in the waste bag provided. DO NOT put it into the toilet bowl.
      (1) gFOBT test: Have the patient collect a stool sample from each of two or three bowel movements in a clean container, usually on consecutive days. Use the applicator stick to apply a smear of stool to a specific area of the test card. After the samples are dry, have the patient return them to their doctor (directly or by mail).
      (2) FIT test: Have the patient use the brush from the kit to brush the surface of the stool, and then dip the brush into the toilet water. Touch the brush on the space indicated on the test card. Add the brush to the waste bag and throw it away. Have the patient return test card to doctor (directly or by mail).

Continued

BOX 22.5 Procedural Guidelines—cont'd

Clinical decision point: Instruct the patient to not perform test if the patient has bleeding hemorrhoids; there is blood in the urine; it is during or within 3 days of menstrual period; there is any bleeding cuts or wounds on the patient's hands; the test card has passed its expiration date; the test kit is damaged, dirty, or appears to have been tampered with in any way; or toilet water is saltwater or rusty.

8. Wrap wooden applicator or collection device in paper towel, grasp in nondominant hand, and remove gloves over wrapped applicator. Discard in proper receptacle. Perform hand hygiene.
9. Record the results of the test; note color changes in guaiac paper. Note character of stool specimen.
10. **Use teach back:** "You will need to check your stool two more times for blood when you go home. I want to be sure I explained the procedure correctly. Please repeat the steps back to me." Revise your instruction now or develop a plan for revised patient/family caregiver teaching if the patient/family caregiver is not able to teach back correctly.

Clinical decision point: A single positive test result does not confirm bleeding or indicate colorectal cancer. To confirm positive results, test must be repeated while the patient is on meat-free, high-residue diet with more in-depth diagnosis (Van Leeuwen et al., 2015).

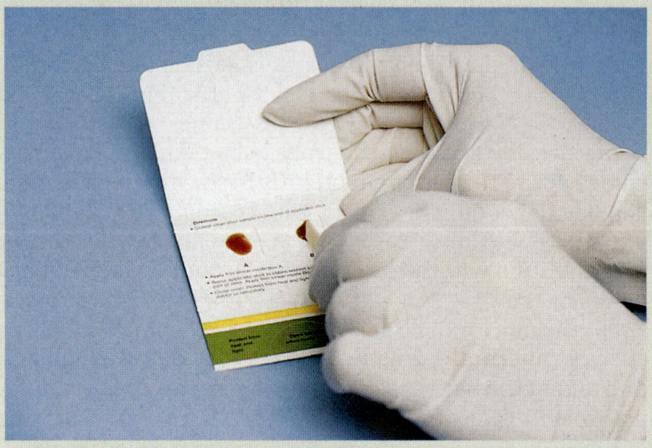

Step 6a(2) Application of stool specimen to both spots on Hemoccult slide.

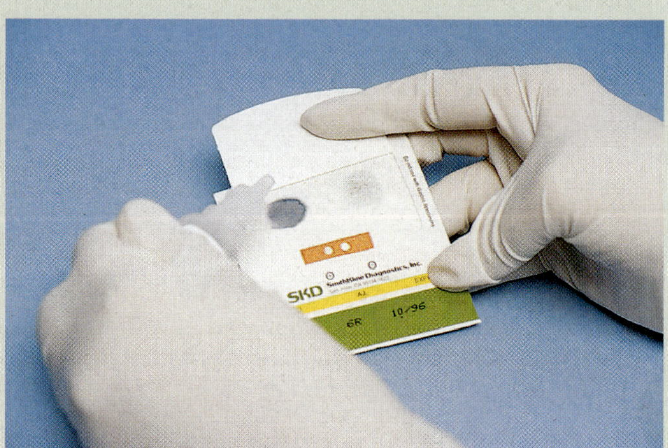

Step 6a(3) Application of developing solution.

BOX 22.6 Procedural Guidelines

Assisting Patient on and off a Bedpan

Equipment

Clean gloves; bedpan (regular or fracture) (see Fig. 22.6); bedpan cover; toilet tissue; specimen container (if necessary); plastic bag clearly labeled with date, patient's name, and identification number; basin, washcloths, towels, and soap; waterproof, absorbent pads (if necessary); clean draw-sheet (if necessary)

Steps

1. Perform hand hygiene. Assess the patient's level of mobility, strength, ability to help, and presence of any condition (e.g., orthopedic) that interferes with the use of bedpan.
2. Review medical record to determine the need for stool specimen.
3. Explain procedure that you will use in turning and positioning, and include patient self-help tips (e.g., how to use a trapeze, how to move hips).
4. Obtain assistance from additional nursing personnel as warranted.
5. Apply clean gloves.

Clinical decision point: Use a fracture pan if the patient has had a total hip replacement. An abduction pillow must be placed between the legs when turning to prevent dislocation of new joint.

6. Provide privacy by closing door of room or curtains around bed.
7. Lower side rail on side of bed where you are standing. Raise bed horizontally according to your height. Position the patient high in bed with head of the patient's bed raised 30–45° (as tolerated) (see Chapter 14).

Clinical decision point: Observe for the presence of drains, dressings, i.v. fluids, and traction. These devices make it difficult for a patient to assist with positioning, and you will likely need more personnel to help place the patient on a bedpan.

8. Fold back top linen to the patient's knees, but do not expose the patient. Place bedpan on bed.
9. **Positioning a patient who can help on a bedpan:**
   a. Raise side rail and instruct the patient to grasp both side rails
   b. Have the patient flex knees and lift hips upward.
   c. Place your hand closest to the patient's head palm up under the patient's sacrum to help lift. Ask the patient to bend knees and raise hips. As the patient raises hips, use other hand to slip bedpan under him or her (see illustration and Fig. 22.7). Be sure that open rim of bedpan is facing toward foot of bed. Do not force pan under the patient's hips. (*Optional:* Have the patient use overhead trapeze frame to raise hips.)
   d. *Optional:* If using fracture pan, slip it under the patient as hips are raised (see illustration). Be sure that deep, open, lower end of bedpan is facing toward foot of bed.
10. **Positioning a patient who is immobile or has mobility restrictions on a bedpan:**
   a. Lower head of bed flat or raise head slightly (if tolerated by medical condition).
   b. Help the patient roll onto side with back toward you. Place bedpan firmly against the patient's buttocks and down into

BOX 22.6 **Procedural Guidelines—cont'd**

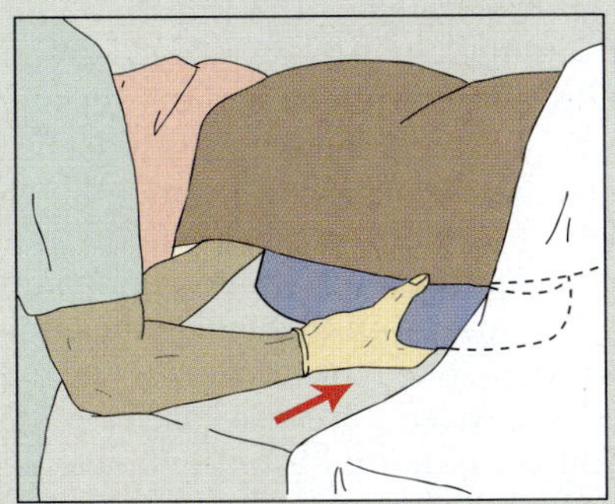

Step 9c Placing bedpan under patient's hips.

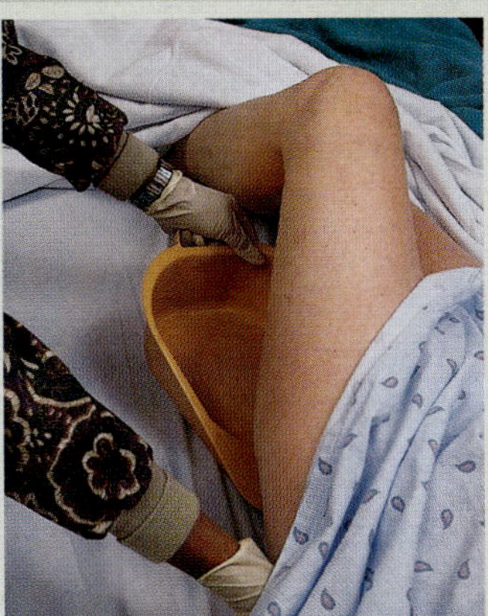

Step 9d Patient lifts hips as fracture pan is positioned.

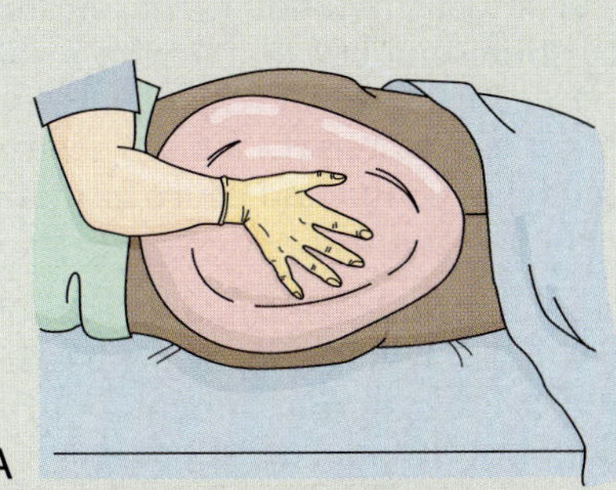

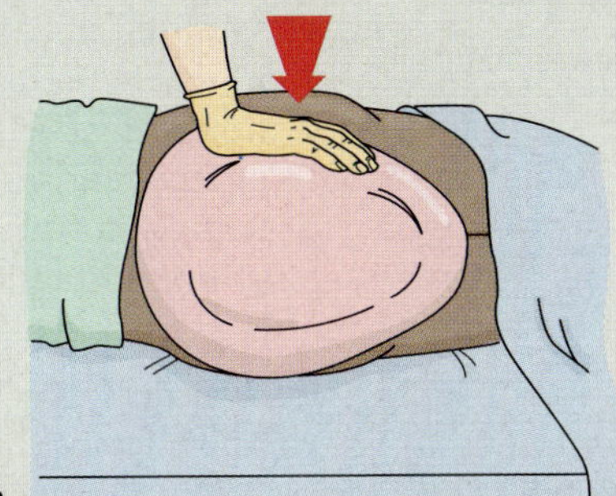

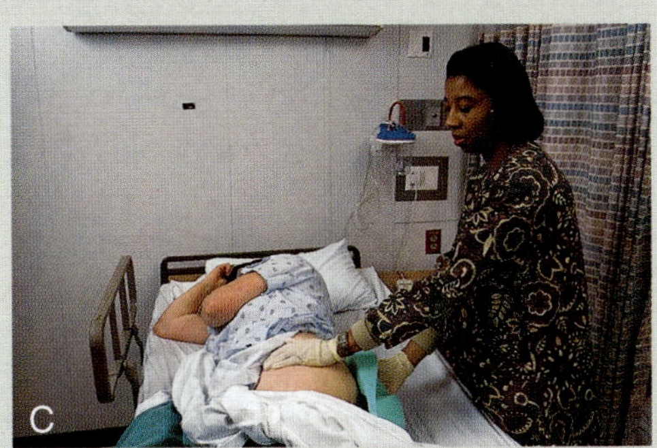

Step 10b A, Position patient on one side and place bedpan firmly against buttocks. **B,** Push down on bedpan and toward patient. **C,** Nurse places bedpan in position. (**A** and **B** from Sorrentino SA, Remmert LN: *Mosby's textbook for nursing assistants*, ed 9, St Louis, 2017, Elsevier.)

mattress. Be sure that open rim of bedpan is facing toward foot of bed (see illustrations).

Clinical decision point: If the patient has had a total hip replacement, use a fracture pan. Make sure that abduction pillow remains between the patient's legs while the patient is transferring to and from and using the fracture pan.

c. Keep one hand against bedpan; place other around far hip of the patient. Ask the patient to roll back onto bedpan, flat in bed. Do not force pan under the patient.
d. Raise the patient's head 30° or to a comfortable level (unless contraindicated).
e. Have the patient bend knees (unless contraindicated).

11. Maintain the patient's comfort, privacy, and safety. Cover the patient for warmth. Place small pillow or rolled towel under lumbar curve of back.
12. Have call bell and toilet tissue within reach for the patient. Give the patient time to defecate.
13. Ensure that bed is in lowest position and raise side rails.
14. Remove and discard gloves and perform hand hygiene.
15. Remove bedpan.
    a. Perform hand hygiene and apply clean gloves
    b. Place the patient's bedside chair close to working side of bed. Place towel on chair seat.
    c. Maintain privacy; determine whether the patient is able to wipe own perineal area. If you clean perineal area, use several layers of toilet tissue or disposable washcloths. For female patients, clean from mons pubis toward rectal area. Deposit contaminated tissue in bedpan if no specimen or intake and output (I&O) is needed.
    d. Remove gloves and perform hand hygiene. Reapply gloves.
    e. **For mobile patients:** Ask the patient to flex knees, placing body weight on lower legs, feet, and upper torso; lift buttocks up from bedpan. At the same time, place hand farther from the patient on side of bedpan to support it (prevent spillage) and place other hand (closer to the patient) under sacrum to help lift. Have the patient lift and remove bedpan. Place bedpan on draped bedside chair and cover.
    f. **For immobile patients:** Lower head of bed. Help the patient roll onto side away from you and off bedpan. Hold bedpan flat and steady while the patient is rolling off; otherwise, spillage will occur. Place bedpan on draped bedside chair and cover.
16. Assist the patient to comfortable position. Allow the patient to perform hand hygiene. Change soiled linens; remove and dispose of gloves.
17. Place bed in its lowest position. Ensure that call bell, phone, drinking water, and desired personal items (e.g., books) are within easy access.
18. *Optional:* Obtain stool specimen as ordered (see Box 22.6). Wear gloves when emptying contents of bedpan into toilet or in special receptacle in utility room. Use spray faucet attached to most institution toilets to rinse bedpan thoroughly. Use disinfectant if required by agency, and then store pan. Remove gloves.
19. Perform hand hygiene.
20. Assess characteristics of stool. Note color, odor, consistency, frequency, amount, shape (see Fig. 22.5), and constituents. Assess characteristics of urine if the patient voided in bedpan. Document findings.
21. **Use teach back:** "Since your leg is immobilized, I want to make sure you are comfortable getting off and on the bedpan by using the trapeze to pull your torso off the bed. Show me how you will position your arms on the trapeze." Revise your instruction now or develop a plan for revised patient/family caregiver teaching if the patient/family caregiver is not able to teach back correctly.

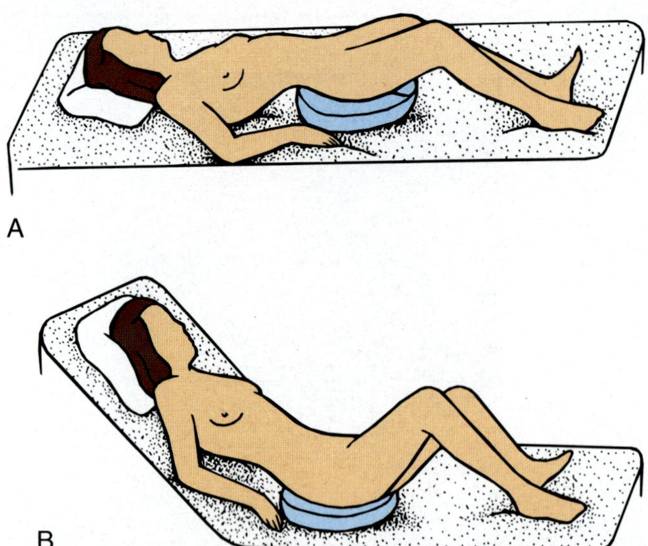

Fig. 22.7 Positions on bedpan. **A,** Improper positioning of patient. **B,** Proper position reduces patient's back strain.

FACILITATING BOWEL ELIMINATION

When patients become acutely ill, the GI system is often affected. Simple changes in activity levels, sleeping patterns, diet, and medications directly affect regular bowel habits. Surgical intervention creates additional elimination problems for the patient in acute care (e.g., discomfort from an abdominal incision, absent or decreased GI peristalsis, or increased accumulation of intestinal gas following surgery). Whenever possible, help the patient to the toilet or bedside commode and allow for privacy for a bowel movement. This facilitates the return of normal bowel habits.

Laxatives and Cathartics

Medications that initiate and facilitate stool passage include **laxatives** and **cathartics**, which have the short-term action of emptying the bowel. These agents are also used to cleanse the bowel for patients undergoing GI tests and abdominal surgery. Although the terms *laxative* and *cathartic* are often used interchangeably, cathartics generally have a stronger and more rapid effect on the intestines.

Although patients usually take medications orally, laxatives prepared as **suppositories** may act more quickly because of their stimulant effect on the rectal mucosa. Suppositories such as bisacodyl act within 30 minutes. Give the suppository shortly before a patient's usual time to defecate or immediately after a meal. Teach patients about the potential harmful effects of overuse of laxatives such as impaired bowel motility and decreased response to sensory stimulus. Make sure that a patient understands that laxatives are not to be used long term for maintenance of bowel function.

Before administering a laxative, assess for signs of a fecal impaction. The impaction must be removed before laxative therapy is initiated.

Laxatives and cathartics are classified by the method by which the agent promotes defecation. They are listed as follows in the order in which they should be used with patients:

- Bulk-forming agents, also known as *fiber supplements*, are considered the safest and least irritating to the intestine. They absorb water in the intestine and make the stool softer and bulkier. The fecal bulk stretches the intestinal walls, stimulating peristalsis. Passage of stool occurs in 12–24 hours. These agents must be taken with water and should be used with patients who have an adequate food and fluid intake. Patients may note increased gas formation and flatus when they first start taking these laxatives, but this will abate after 4–5 days.
- Emollient laxatives soften the fecal mass and make it easier to evacuate. These agents are also called *stool softeners*.
- Osmotic laxatives pull fluid into the bowel to soften the stool and distend the bowel to stimulate peristalsis. Some are saline based; others contain lactulose, sorbitol, and polyethylene glycol.
- Stimulant laxatives cause local irritation to the intestinal mucosa, increase intestinal motility, and inhibit resorption of water in the large intestine. The rapid movement of feces causes retention of water in the stool. The drugs usually contain bisacodyl or senna and cause formation of a soft to fluid stool in 6–8 hours.

There are newer drugs for chronic constipation or motility disorders. It is too soon to tell whether these medications will be effective and safe for long-term treatment, but they are not used for the relief of occasional constipation.

The most commonly used antidiarrheal agents are loperamide or diphenoxylate with atropine. Antidiarrheal agents decrease intestinal muscle tone to slow the passage of feces. As a result, the body absorbs more water through the intestinal walls. However, the cause of diarrhea must be determined before effective treatment can be ordered by the health care provider. For example, if an infection is the causative factor, an antibiotic may be used for treatment; if inflammation is the cause, steroids may be given.

Nasogastric Tube for Gastric Decompression

At times following abdominal or pelvic surgery, an **ileus** or temporary cessation of peristalsis occurs. A patient cannot eat or drink fluids without causing abdominal distention, nausea, and vomiting. The insertion of a nasogastric (NG) tube into the stomach serves to decompress the stomach, keeping it empty until normal peristalsis returns. An NG tube is a pliable tube that is inserted through the patient's nose, through the nasopharynx, and into the stomach. The tube has a hollow lumen that allows the removal of gastric secretions and the introduction of solutions into the stomach. The Levin and Salem sump tubes are most commonly used for stomach decompression. The Levin tube is a single-lumen tube with holes near the tip. You connect the tube to a drainage bag or an intermittent suction device to drain stomach secretions. The Salem sump tube is preferable for stomach decompression. The tube has two lumens: one for removal of gastric contents and one to provide an air vent. A blue "pigtail" is the air vent that connects with the second lumen. When you connect the main lumen of the sump tube to suction, the air vent permits free, continuous drainage of secretions. *Never clamp the air vent if the tube is connected to suction, and never use for irrigation.*

NG tube insertion is done using clean technique. The procedure is uncomfortable; patients experience a burning sensation as the tube passes through the sensitive nasal mucosa. One of the greatest nursing care challenges is keeping the patient comfortable because the tube is a constant irritation to mucosa and can cause a pressure injury. Routinely assess the condition of the nares and mucosa for inflammation and excoriation. Supportive care includes changing soiled tape or fixation devices daily when they become soiled, keeping the nares lubricated and clean, and providing frequent mouth care to minimize dehydration from mouth breathing.

Enemas

An **enema** is an instillation of a solution into the rectum and sigmoid colon to primarily promote defecation by stimulating peristalsis. The volume of fluid instilled breaks up the fecal mass, stretches the rectal wall, and begins the defecation reflex. Enemas are also used to administer drugs that exert a local effect on rectal mucosa. For example, sodium polystyrene sulfonate (Kayexalate) is used to treat patients with dangerously high serum potassium levels.

The most common use for an enema is temporary relief of constipation. Other indications include removing impacted feces, emptying the bowel before diagnostic tests and some surgical procedures, and beginning a program of bowel training. Discourage patients from relying on enemas at home to maintain bowel regularity. Enemas do not treat the cause of constipation. As with overuse of laxatives, frequent use may affect normal defecation reflexes.

- **Cleansing enemas:** Cleansing enemas promote complete evacuation of feces from the colon.
  - They act by stimulating peristalsis through the infusion of a large volume of solution or through local irritation of the mucosa of the colon.
  - Cleansing enemas include tap water, normal saline, low-volume hypertonic saline, and soapsuds solution.
  - Each solution exerts a different osmotic effect, causing the movement of fluids between the colon and interstitial spaces beyond the intestinal wall.
  - Infants and children should be given only normal saline enemas because they are at greater risk for fluid imbalance (Hockenberry and Wilson, 2014).
- **Tap water:** Tap water is hypotonic and exerts a lower osmotic pressure than fluid in interstitial spaces.
  - After infusion into the colon, tap water escapes from the bowel lumen into interstitial spaces.
  - The net movement of water is low; the infused volume stimulates defecation before large amounts of water leave the bowel.
  - Do not repeat tap-water enemas because water toxicity or circulatory overload develops if the body absorbs large amounts of water.
- **Normal saline:** Physiologically normal saline is the safest solution to use because it exerts the same osmotic pressure as fluids in interstitial spaces around the bowel.
  - The volume of infused saline stimulates peristalsis. Giving normal saline enemas does not create the danger of excess fluid absorption.
  - At times a soap solution is ordered to be added to tap water or saline to create the additional effect of intestinal irritation.
  - Only pure castile soap is safe because harsh soaps or detergents cause bowel inflammation.
- **Hypertonic solutions:** Hypertonic solutions infused into the bowel exert osmotic pressure that pulls fluids into the colon.
  - The colon fills with fluid, and the resultant distention promotes defecation. Patients unable to tolerate large volumes of fluid benefit most from this type of enema. A hypertonic solution of 120–180 mL (4–6 oz) is usually effective.
  - A health care provider sometimes orders a high or low cleansing enema. The terms *high* and *low* refer to the height and pressure with which you deliver the fluid. You give high enemas to clean the entire colon. A low enema cleans only the rectum and sigmoid colon.
  - After you infuse the enema, ask the patient to turn from the left lateral to the dorsal recumbent and over to the right lateral position. The position changes help fluid reach the large intestine.
- **Oil-retention enemas:** Oil-retention enemas lubricate the rectum and colon.
  - The feces absorb the oil and become softer and easier to pass.
  - To enhance action of the oil, the patient retains the enema for several hours if possible. Skill 22.1 outlines the steps for enema administration.

Other Types of Enemas

Carminative enemas provide relief from gaseous distention. They improve the ability to pass flatus. An example of a carminative enema is MGW solution, which contains 30 mL of magnesium, 60 mL of glycerin, and 90 mL of water.

Medicated enemas contain drugs. An example is sodium polystyrene sulfonate (Kayexalate), used to treat patients with dangerously high serum potassium levels. This drug contains a resin that exchanges sodium ions for potassium ions in the large intestine. Another medicated enema is neomycin solution, an antibiotic used to reduce bacteria in the colon before bowel surgery. An enema containing steroid medication may be used for acute inflammation in the lower colon.

Digital Removal of Stool

For patients with an impaction, the fecal mass is sometimes too large to pass voluntarily. If enemas fail, the mass needs to be broken up digitally. Patients with an impaction frequently have a continuous oozing of liquid stool because liquid passes around the impacted feces. Disimpaction is done only when all other measures have failed (Box 22.7).

The procedure is uncomfortable for the patient. Excess rectal manipulation irritates the mucosa and can cause bleeding. There is also risk of stimulation of the vagus nerve, which can result in a reflex slowing of the heart rate. Disimpaction in patients with spinal cord injury can cause autonomic dysreflexia (University of Michigan, 2013). Because of the potential complications of the procedure, some institutions restrict nurses from removing impactions digitally. Before you perform the procedure, check your agency policy regarding a health care provider's order.

Management of Patients With Fecal Incontinence or Diarrhea

You may apply a fecal collector around a patient's anal opening if the skin is intact. The devices are difficult to apply when there is a deep fold between the buttocks and there

BOX 22.7 Procedural Guidelines

Digital Removal of Stool/Fecal Impaction

Equipment

Clean gloves; water-soluble local anesthetic lubricant (**Note:** Some agencies require use of water-soluble lubricant without anesthetic when nurse performs procedure); waterproof, absorbent pads; bedpan; bedpan cover *(optional)*; bath blanket; basin, washcloths, towels, and soap; sphygmomanometer *(optional)*

Steps

1. Identify the patient by using at least two identifiers (e.g., name and birthday or name and medical record number) according to agency policy.

Clinical decision point. Because of the potential to stimulate the sacral branch of the vagus nerve, patients with a history of dysrhythmias or heart disease have a greater risk for changes in heart rhythm. Monitor the patient's pulse before and during procedure. This procedure is often contraindicated in cardiac patients; if in doubt, verify with the health care provider.

2. Perform hand hygiene. Pull curtains around bed, obtain the patient's baseline vital signs, assess level of comfort, and palpate for abdominal distention before procedure.
3. Explain procedure to the patient, including positioning and expected discomfort. Have the patient demonstrate ability to take slow, deep breaths to relax.
4. Obtain assistance to help change the patient's position if necessary. Raise bed horizontally to comfortable working height.
5. Lower side rail on the patient's right side. Keeping far side rail raised, help the patient to left side-lying position with knees flexed and back.
6. Drape the patient's trunk and lower extremities with bath blanket and place waterproof pad under the patient's buttocks.
7. Perform hand hygiene and apply clean gloves and place bedpan next to the patient.
8. Lubricate gloved index finger and middle finger of dominant hand with anesthetic lubricant.
9. Instruct the patient to take slow deep breaths during procedure. Gradually and gently insert gloved index finger and feel anus relax around finger. Insert middle finger. Gradually advance fingers slowly along rectal wall toward umbilicus.
10. Gently loosen fecal mass by moving fingers in scissors motion to fragment the fecal mass. Work fingers into hardened mass. Work stool downward toward end of rectum. Remove small sections of feces and discard into bedpan.
11. Observe the patient's response and periodically assess heart rate and look for signs of fatigue.

Clinical decision point: Stop procedure if heart rate drops or rhythm changes from the patient's baseline or if the patient has dyspnea or reports palpitations.

Clinical decision point: Patients who have a spinal cord injury and are unable to sense the need to defecate are at risk for autonomic dysreflexia from a full bowel. Rectal stimulation may aggravate this risk. Stop procedure if the patient develops pounding headache, flushing of face, increased muscle spasms, blurred vision, and a blood pressure increase of 20–40 mm Hg. This is a medical emergency.

12. Continue to clear rectum of feces allowing the patient to rest at intervals.
13. After removal of impaction, perform perineal hygiene.
14. Remove bedpan and inspect feces for color and consistency. Dispose of feces in toilet.
15. If needed, help the patient to toilet or clean and store the bedpan. (Procedure may be followed by enema or cathartic.)
16. Remove gloves by turning them inside out and discarding in proper receptacle. Perform hand hygiene.
17. Record results of procedure by describing fecal characteristics and amount.
18. Reassess vital signs and compare with baseline values. Continue to monitor the patient for 1 h for bradycardia. Monitor blood pressure in patients with spinal cord injury.
19. **Use teach back:** "I want to make sure you include high-fiber foods and fluids in your diet to help increase the passage of stool. Tell me what foods you will add to your diet." Revise your instruction now or develop a plan for revised patient/family caregiver teaching if the patient/family caregiver is not able to teach back correctly.

is hair in the area. There are fecal management systems available for short-term use with high-volume diarrhea. The devices have an intra-anal soft silicone catheter with a retention balloon, much like a Foley catheter for insertion into the rectal vault. The catheter connects to a drainage bag for collection of fecal effluent.

CONTINUING AND RESTORATIVE CARE

Before a patient is able to return home or is transferred to an extended care facility, you need to help establish regular elimination patterns.

Bowel Training

A bowel training program helps patients who still have some neuromuscular control to achieve normal defecation. The training program involves setting up a daily routine. By attempting to defecate at the same time each day and using measures that promote defecation, the patient gains control of bowel reflexes. The program requires time, patience, and consistency. A patient with cognitive impairment needs to have a caregiver available to devote time to the training program. A health care provider determines the patient's physical readiness and ability to benefit from bowel training.

Ostomy Care

Immediately after a surgical diversion, it is necessary to place a pouch over the newly created stoma because in some ostomies output of effluent begins soon after surgery. The pouch collects all effluent and protects the skin from irritating dermatitis. A proper pouch fits comfortably, with its skin barrier covering the skin surface around the stoma and creating a good seal. The postoperative pouch is transparent to allow visibility of the stoma.

For up to 6 weeks, the new stoma may be edematous. The stoma itself often has a series of small stitches around its perimeter. Apply a pouch and skin barrier that fits right around the stoma and protects the surrounding skin. Take care to avoid disrupting the suture line. It may be several days after surgery before bowel function returns. In the case of an ileostomy, the patient has frequent liquid stools when peristalsis returns. With a colostomy, the fecal output may be loose in the first few days after surgery, but a more formed stool would be expected after the patient is eating again.

Many types of pouches and skin barriers are available (Colwell, 2016). Some pouches have skin barriers attached and are one-piece pouching systems (Fig. 22.8). Some of these one-piece pouches already are precut to size by the manufacturer, whereas others are custom cut to size for the patient's stoma measurement. Other systems have two separate pieces (Fig. 22.9). Attach the pouch to the skin barrier by attaching it to the flange (a plastic ring) on the barrier. Often you have to custom cut the skin barrier to the patient's specific stoma size. For two-piece systems, use the skin barrier with flange corresponding to the size of the ring on the pouch, making sure that both pieces are from the same manufacturer. Understand how to use each of these different pouching systems before attempting to teach ostomy care to the patient. If possible, change the pouch when the stoma is less active, usually before meals.

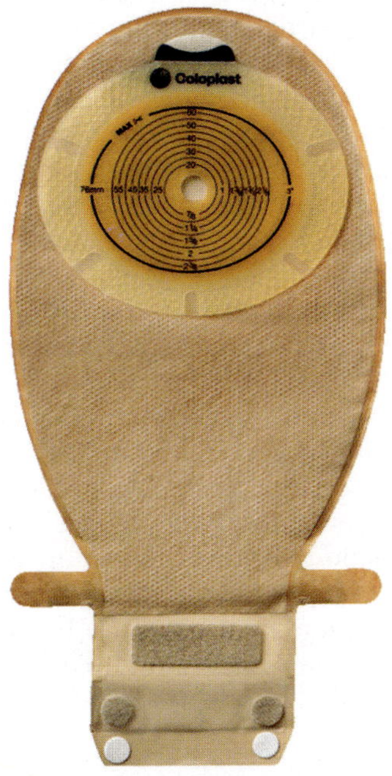

Fig. 22.8 One-piece pouch with Velcro closure. (Courtesy: Coloplast, Minneapolis, MN.)

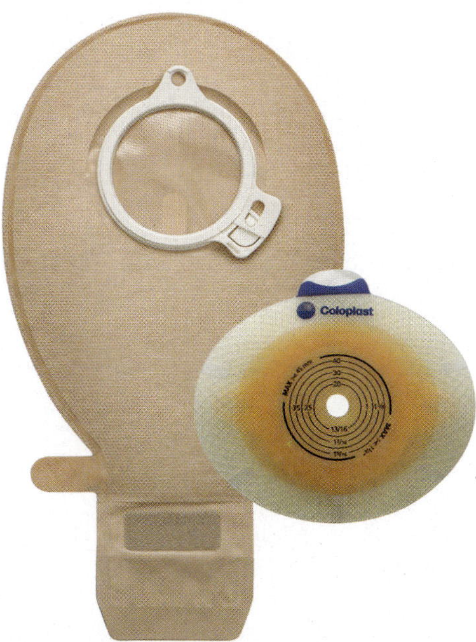

Fig. 22.9 Two-piece pouch system with separate skin barrier and attachable pouch. (Courtesy: Coloplast, Minneapolis, MN.)

Have patients participate in pouching because they need to learn to recognize the normal appearance of a stoma. It should be red and moist. By 6 weeks after surgery, the size should not change. If there are noticeable changes in the size of the stoma, either smaller or larger than normal, it should be reported to the health care provider. Skill 22.2 describes the steps for pouching an ostomy.

A patient with an ostomy experiences a change in body image. The appearance of the stoma and accompanying effluent and odor can cause psychological stress. For the patient with a new ostomy, it is important for you to encourage self-care and acceptance of the ostomy. Early involvement in self-care promotes confidence. Even simple tasks such as holding pieces of equipment during stoma pouching and learning to open and close the pouch help the patient begin to adjust to bodily changes. Whenever possible, have an ostomy nurse provide care and teaching for the patient with a new stoma (Box 22.8). In addition, patients may benefit from information and encouragement from an ostomy support group.

BOX 22.8 Patient Teaching

The Patient With an Ostomy

Outcome

The patient/caregiver can demonstrate changing an ostomy pouch.

Teaching Strategies

- Provide a comprehensive list of products needed to care for the ostomy.
- Provide the patient/family caregiver with supplies to last 1–2 weeks and the contact number of the closest medical supply store.
- Demonstrate how to empty pouch and have the patient/family caregiver begin emptying it while still in the hospital.
- Show the patient/family caregiver the step-by-step approach for changing an ostomy pouch; provide at least one opportunity to change the ostomy pouch while the patient is in hospital.
- Set up visits with an ostomy nurse or home care nurse and provide contact numbers.
- Provide detailed discharge instructions for skin care, driving, lifting, resuming exercise, and when to contact the health care provider.

Evaluation

- Use the principles of teach back to evaluate patient/family caregiver learning:
  - "Show me how you empty and change your ostomy pouch."
  - "Tell me the signs of peristomal skin irritation and how you would relieve it."
  - "Tell me about the type and amount of output that you should get from the stoma and when you need to call the health care provider."

Irrigating a Colostomy

Although this practice is not as common because of improved odor-proof pouches, some patients irrigate their sigmoid colostomies to regulate colon emptying. This process takes about an hour a day to complete but usually means that a patient wears only a mini-pouch afterward to absorb mucus from the stoma and contain gas. Specific equipment designed for ostomies is used. The equipment has a silicone cone attached by plastic tubing to a bag that will hold the irrigation fluid, which is usually warm water. Follow the routine that the patient has established for this care. Occasionally a patient with a colostomy who has constipation will have an irrigation or enema ordered. Use equipment that is designed specifically for the irrigation rather than an enema administration set used by patients without a stoma.

Maintenance of Skin Integrity

The patient with diarrhea or fecal incontinence is at risk for skin breakdown when fecal contents remain on the skin (see Chapter 17). The same problem exists for the patient with an ostomy that drains liquid stool. Liquid stool is usually acidic and contains digestive enzymes. Irritation from repeated wiping with toilet tissue causes skin breakdown. To prevent skin irritation, cleanse and dry the skin immediately after soiling occurs.

Instruct a patient or family caregiver about cleansing the perineal area with a no-rinse perineal cleanser and warm water or a prepackaged perineal wipe after each passage of stool. When caring for a patient who is debilitated, incontinent, and unable to ask for assistance, check frequently for defecation and cleanse the skin. Protect the skin around the anal area with barrier ointments. Baby powder or cornstarch is contraindicated because it does not provide a barrier to protect the skin. Check the skin for rashes that could indicate a yeast infection. Patients with incontinence who are taking antibiotics are particularly susceptible to yeast infections. This type of rash is raised and deep red with satellite lesions, and usually the patient will report itching. This rash should be reported promptly so that topical treatment can be started.

SAFETY GUIDELINES FOR NURSING SKILLS

Ensuring patient safety is an essential role of the professional nurse. To ensure patient safety, communicate clearly with the members of the health care team, assess and incorporate the patient's priorities of care and preferences, and use the best evidence when making decisions about your patient's care. When performing the skills in this chapter, remember the following points to ensure safe, individualized patient care:

- If a patient has cardiac disease or is taking cardiac or hypertensive medication, obtain a pulse rate before an enema because manipulation of rectal tissue stimulates the vagus nerve and can cause a sudden decline in pulse rate, which can increase the patient's risk for fainting while on the bedpan, commode, or toilet.
- Instruct patients who self-administer enemas to use the side-lying position. Administering an enema with the patient sitting on the toilet is unsafe because it is impossible to safely guide the tubing into the rectum.
- Keep the patient in a sitting high Fowler's position during NG intubation to prevent aspiration (Shlamovitz and Shah, 2016).

SKILL 22.1 Administering a Cleansing Enema

Equipment

- Clean gloves
- Water-soluble lubricant
- Waterproof, absorbent pads
- Toilet tissue
- Bedpan, bedside commode, or access to toilet
- Bath blanket
- Basin, washcloths, towel, and soap
- Stethoscope

Enema Bag Administration

- Enema container with tubing and clamp
- I.v. pole
- Appropriate-size rectal tube (adult: 22–30 Fr; child: 12–18 Fr)
- Correct volume of warmed (tepid) solution (adult: 750–1000 mL; adolescent: 500–700 mL); for pediatric patients, the child's weight usually determines the volume for the enema, usually 5–10 mL/kg (Nurko and Zimmerman, 2014)

Prepackaged Enema

- Prepackaged enema container with lubricated rectal tip (Fig. 22.10)

STEP	RATIONALE
Assessment	
1. Identify the patient by using at least two identifiers (e.g., name and birthday or name and medical record number) according to agency policy.	Ensures correct patient. Complies with The Joint Commission Standards and improves patient safety (TJC, 2018).
2. Review health care provider's order for enema and clarify reason for administration.	Health care provider's order is usually required for a hospitalized patient. The order states which type of enema the patient will receive.

STEP	RATIONALE

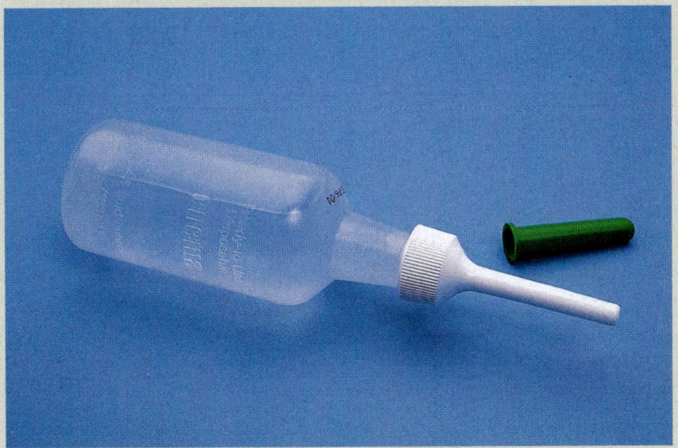

Fig. 22.10 Prepackaged enema container with rectal tip.

STEP	RATIONALE
3. Perform hand hygiene. Assess last bowel movement, normal versus most recent bowel pattern, presence of hemorrhoids, mobility, and presence of abdominal pain or cramping.	Determines need for enema and type of enema used. Also establishes baseline for bowel function. Hemorrhoids may obscure rectal opening and cause discomfort or bleeding during evacuation.
4. Inspect abdomen for presence of distention and auscultate for bowel sounds.	Establishes baseline for determining effectiveness of enema.
5. Assess the patient's mobility and ability to turn and position on side. Perform hand hygiene.	Determines whether assistance is needed for positioning the patient.
6. Assess the patient for allergy to any active ingredients of Fleet enema.	Reduces risk for allergic reaction.
7. Assess the patient's level of understanding of purpose of enema.	Allows for planning appropriate teaching measures.

Clinical decision point: "Enemas until clear" order means that you repeat enemas until the patient passes fluid that is clear of fecal matter. The fluid the patient passes may be tinted and have small flecks of fecal matter. Check agency policy, but usually the patient should receive only three consecutive enemas to avoid disruption of fluid and electrolyte balance. It is essential to observe contents of solution passed.

Planning

STEP	RATIONALE
1. Provide privacy by closing curtains around bed or closing door and prepare bedside environment for patient safety.	Preparing the environment early helps the nurse think about the steps needed; removing clutter from overbed table removes barriers to completing procedure. Reduces embarrassment for the patient.
2. Prepare and organize equipment for enema at bedside.	Ensures organized approach for enema administration.
3. Explain to the patient the steps of enema procedure.	Promotes patient cooperation and increases compliance.

Implementation

STEP	RATIONALE
1. If enema is medicated, the skill may or may not be delegated to NAP (see agency policy). Check accuracy and completeness of each medication administration record (MAR) with health care provider's written order. Check the patient's name, type of enema, and time for administration. Compare MAR with label of enema solution.	The order is the most reliable source and only legal record of drugs or procedure that the patient is to receive. Ensures that the patient receives correct enema.
2. Place bedpan or bedside commode in easily accessible position. If the patient will be expelling contents in toilet, ensure that toilet is available, and place the patient's nonskid slippers and bathrobe in easily accessible position.	Bedpan is used if the patient is unable to get out of bed. Nonskid slippers help prevent falling of a patient who may be rushing to the bathroom. Extra gown provides modesty for the patient.
3. Perform hand hygiene.	Reduces transmission of microorganisms.
4. With side rail raised on the patient's right side and bed raised to appropriate working height, help the patient turn onto left side-lying (Sims') position with right knee flexed. Encourage the patient to remain in position until procedure is complete. Children are placed in dorsal recumbent position.	Allows enema solution to flow downward by gravity along natural curve of sigmoid colon and rectum, improving retention of solution.

Clinical decision point: Patients with poor sphincter control require placement of a bedpan under the buttocks. Administering enema with the patient sitting on toilet is unsafe because curved rectal tubing can abrade rectal wall.

STEP	RATIONALE
5. Apply clean gloves and place waterproof pad, absorbent side up, under hips and buttocks. Cover the patient with bath blanket, exposing only rectal area, clearly visualizing anus.	Pad prevents soiling of linen. Blanket provides warmth, reduces exposure of body parts, and allows the patient to feel more relaxed and comfortable.
6. Separate buttocks and examine perianal region for abnormalities including hemorrhoids, anal fissure, and rectal prolapse (protrusion of rectal tissue outside anus).	Findings influence approach for inserting enema tip. Prolapse contraindicates enema.
7. Administer enema.	
a. Administer prepackaged disposable enema.	
(1) Remove plastic cap from tip of container. Tip may already be lubricated. Apply more water-soluble lubricant as needed.	Lubrication provides for smooth insertion of rectal tube without causing rectal irritation or trauma. Extra lubricant provides added comfort in presence of hemorrhoids.
(2) Gently separate buttocks and locate anus. Instruct the patient to relax by breathing out slowly through mouth.	Breathing out promotes relaxation of external rectal sphincter.
(3) Expel any air from enema container.	Introducing air into colon causes further distention and discomfort.
(4) Insert lubricated tip of container gently into anal canal toward umbilicus (see illustration). *Adult:* 7.5–10 cm (3–4 inches) *Adolescent:* 7.5–10 cm (3–4 inches) *Child:* 5–7.5 cm (2–3 inches) *Infant:* 2.5–3.75 cm (1–1½ inches)	Gentle insertion prevents trauma to rectal mucosa.

Clinical decision point: If pain occurs or you feel resistance at any time during procedure, stop and discuss with health care provider. Do not force insertion.

STEP	RATIONALE
(5) Roll plastic bottle from bottom to tip until all of solution has entered rectum and colon. Instruct the patient to retain solution until urge to defecate occurs, usually 2–5 min.	Prevents instillation of air into colon and ensures that all solution enters rectum. Hypertonic solutions require only small volumes to stimulate defecation.
b. Administer enema in standard enema bag.	
(1) Add warmed prescribed type of solution and amount to enema bag: Warm tap water as it flows from faucet, place saline container in basin of warm water before adding saline to enema bag, and check temperature of solution by pouring small amount of solution over inner wrist.	Hot water burns intestinal mucosa. Cold water causes abdominal cramping and is difficult to retain.
(2) If soapsuds enema (SSE) is ordered, add castile soap after water.	Reduces suds in enema bag.
(3) Raise container, release clamp, and allow solution to flow long enough to fill tubing.	Removes air from tubing.

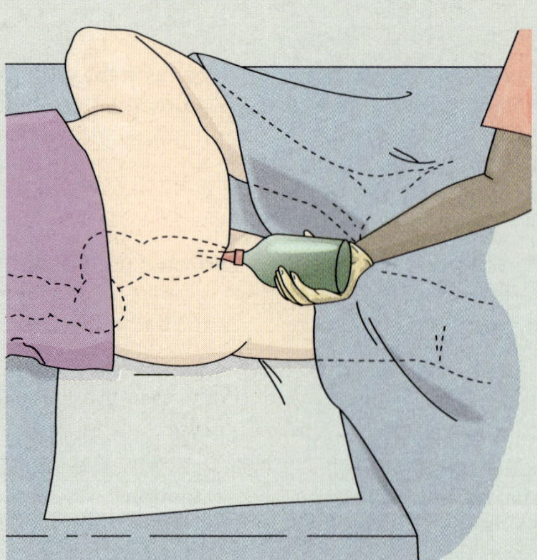

Step 7a(4) With patient in left lateral Sims' position, insert tip of commercial enema into rectum. (From Sorrentino SA, Remmert LN: *Mosby's textbook for nursing assistants*, ed 9, St Louis, 2017, Elsevier.)

STEP	RATIONALE
(4) Reclamp tubing.	Prevents further loss of solution.
(5) Lubricate 6–8 cm (2½–3 inches) of tip of rectal tube with lubricant.	Allows smooth insertion of rectal tube without risk for irritation or trauma to mucosa.
(6) Gently separate buttocks and locate anus. Instruct the patient to relax by breathing out slowly through mouth. Touch the patient's skin next to anus with tip of rectal tube.	Breathing out and touching skin with tube promotes relaxation of external anal sphincter.
(7) Insert tip of rectal tube slowly by pointing it in the direction of the patient's umbilicus. Length of insertion varies.	Careful insertion prevents trauma to rectal mucosa from accidental lodging of tube against rectal wall. Insertion beyond proper limit can cause bowel perforation.

Clinical decision point: If tube does not pass easily, do not force. Consider allowing a small amount of fluid to infuse and then try to reinsert tube slowly. The instillation of fluid relaxes the sphincter and provides additional lubrication. If impaction is present, remove it before administering enema.

STEP	RATIONALE
(8) Hold tubing in rectum constantly until end of fluid instillation.	Prevents expulsion of rectal tube during bowel contractions.
(9) Open regulating clamp and allow solution to enter slowly with container at the patient's hip level.	Rapid infusion may stimulate evacuation of tubing and can cause cramping.
(10) Raise height of enema container slowly to appropriate level above anus: 30–45 cm (12–18 inches) for high enema, 30 cm (12 inches) for regular enema (see illustration), and 7.5 cm (3 inches) for low enema. Instillation time varies with volume of solution administered (e.g., 1 L may take 10 min). You may use an i.v. pole to hold enema bag once you get a slow flow of fluid established.	Allows for continuous, slow instillation of solution. Raising container too high causes rapid instillation and possible painful distention of colon. High pressure causes rupture of bowel in an infant.

Clinical decision point: Temporary cessation of infusion minimizes cramping and promotes ability to retain solution. Lower container or clamp tubing if the patient complains of cramping or if fluid escapes around rectal tube.

STEP	RATIONALE
(11) Instill all solution and clamp tubing. Tell the patient that procedure is completed and that you will be removing tubing.	Prevents entrance of air into rectum. Patients may misinterpret sensation of removing tube as loss of control.
8. Place layers of toilet tissue around tube at anus and gently withdraw rectal tube and tip.	Provides for the patient's comfort and cleanliness.
9. Explain to the patient that some distention and abdominal cramping is normal. Ask the patient to retain solution as long as possible until urge to defecate occurs. This usually takes a few minutes. Stay at bedside. Have the patient lie quietly in bed if possible. (For an infant or young child, gently hold buttocks together for few minutes.)	Solution distends bowel. Length of retention varies with type of enema and the patient's ability to contract rectal sphincter. Longer retention promotes stimulation of peristalsis and defecation.

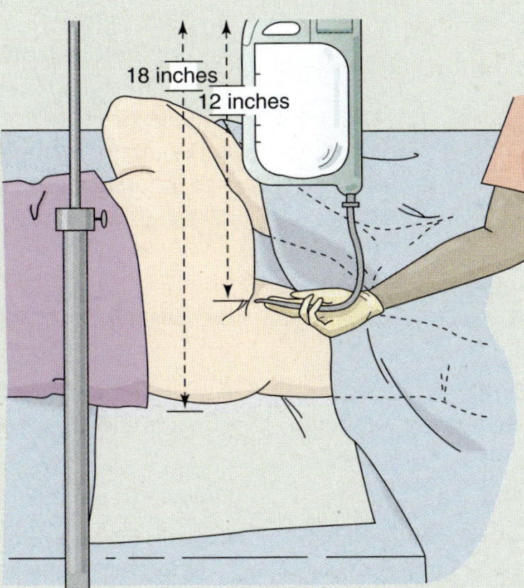

Step 7b(10) I.v. pole is positioned so that the bottom of the enema bag is 18 inches above the anus.

STEP	RATIONALE
10. Discard enema container or disposable bag and tubing in proper receptacle. Remove gloves and perform hand hygiene.	Reduces transmission and growth of microorganisms.
11. Help the patient to bathroom or commode if possible. If using bedpan, help to as near normal position for evacuation as possible (wearing gloves).	Normal squatting position promotes defecation.
12. Observe character of stool and solution (caution the patient against flushing toilet before inspection).	Determines whether enema was effective.
13. Help the patient as needed to wash anal area with warm soap and water (if nurse administers perineal care, use gloves).	Fecal contents irritate skin. Hygiene promotes patient comfort.
14. Remove and discard gloves and perform hand hygiene.	Reduces transmission of microorganisms.
Evaluation	
1. Inspect color, consistency, and amount of stool; odor; and fluid passed.	Determines whether stool is evacuated or fluid is retained. Note abnormalities such as presence of blood or mucus.
2. Assess for abdominal distention.	Determines whether distention is relieved.
3. **Use teach back:** "I want to be sure I explained how to administer a Fleet enema to yourself. I want to be sure you understand the correct position for lying down to administer the enema. Please show me how you would lie down." Revise your instruction now or develop a plan for revised patient/family caregiver teaching if the patient/family caregiver is not able to teach back correctly.	Determines the patient's/family caregiver's level of understanding of instructional topic.

Recording and Reporting

- Record the type and volume of enema given, time of administration, characteristics of results, and the patient's tolerance of the procedure on flow sheet or nurses' notes in electronic health record (EHR) or chart.
- Record the patient's understanding through teach back for self-administration of Fleet enema.
- Report failure of the patient to defecate and any unexpected outcomes to health care provider or nurse.

Unexpected Outcomes and Related Interventions

- Severe abdominal cramping, bleeding, or sudden abdominal pain develops and is unrelieved by temporarily stopping or slowing flow of solution.
  - Stop enema.
  - Notify health care provider.
  - Obtain vital signs.
- The patient is unable to hold enema solution.
  - If this occurs during instillation, slow rate of infusion.

SKILL 22.2 Pouching an Ostomy

Equipment

- Skin barrier/pouch—clear, drainable one-piece or two-piece, cut-to-fit or precut size
- Pouch closure device such as a clip if needed
- Ostomy measuring guide
- Adhesive remover *(optional)*
- Clean gloves
- Washcloth, towel, or disposable waterproof barrier
- Basin with warm tap water
- Scissors
- Waterproof bag for disposal of pouch
- *Optional:* Gown or goggles if there is any risk of splashing when emptying pouch

STEP	RATIONALE
Assessment	
1. Identify the patient by using at least two identifiers (e.g., name and birthday or name and medical record number) according to agency policy.	Ensures patient safety. Complies with The Joint Commission Standards and improves patient safety (TJC, 2018).
2. Perform hand hygiene and apply clean gloves.	Reduces transmission of microorganisms.
3. Observe existing skin barrier and pouch for leakage and length of time in place. Pouch should be changed every 3–7 days, not daily (Colwell, 2016). If an opaque pouch is being used, remove it to fully observe stoma (dispose of pouch in proper receptacle).	Assesses effectiveness of pouching system and detects potential for problems. To minimize skin irritation, avoid unnecessary changing of entire pouching system. When pouch leaks, skin damage from effluent causes more skin trauma than early removal of wafer.

STEP	RATIONALE
Clinical decision point: Repeated leaking may indicate need for different type of pouch or addition of products such as stoma putty. If pouch is leaking, change it. Taping or patching pouch to contain effluent leaves skin exposed to chemical or enzymatic irritation.	
4. Observe amount of effluent in pouch and empty it if it is more than one-third to one-half full by opening pouch and draining it into a container for measurement of output. Note consistency of effluent and record intake and output.	Weight of pouch may disrupt seal of adhesive on skin. Monitors fluid balance and bowel function after surgery. Normal colostomy effluent is soft or formed stool, whereas normal ileostomy effluent is liquid.
5. Observe stoma for type, location, color, swelling, presence of sutures, trauma, and healing or irritation of peristomal skin. Determine if it is budded, flush with skin level, or retracted below skin level (see illustrations).	Stoma characteristics influence selection of appropriate pouching system. Convexity in skin barrier is often necessary with flush or retracted stoma.
6. Observe placement of stoma in relation to abdominal contours or presence of scars or incisions. Remove and dispose of gloves, and perform hand hygiene.	Determines whether current pouching system is effective or whether new selection is needed. Abdominal contours, scars, or incisions affect type of system and adhesion to skin surface. Reduces transmission of microorganisms.
7. Explore the patient's attitudes, perceptions, knowledge, and acceptance of stoma; discuss interest in learning self-care. Identify family caregiver who will be helping the patient after leaving hospital.	Determines the patient's willingness to learn. Facilitates teaching plan and timing of care to coincide with availability of family caregivers.
Planning	
1. Provide privacy by closing curtains around bed or closing door and prepare bedside environment for patient safety.	Preparing the environment early helps the nurse think about the steps needed; removing clutter from overbed table removes barriers completing procedure. Reduces embarrassment for the patient.
2. Assemble equipment needed to change ostomy pouch.	Ensures organized approach for changing ostomy pouch.
3. Explain procedure to the patient; encourage patient's interaction and questions.	Lessens patient's anxiety and promotes patient's participation.
Implementation	
1. Have the patient assume semi-reclining or supine position (same position assumed during assessment and pouching). (**Note:** Some patients with established ostomies prefer to stand.) If possible, provide the patient with mirror for observation.	When the patient is in semi-reclining position, there are fewer skin folds, which allows for ease of application of pouching system.
2. Perform hand hygiene and apply clean gloves.	Reduces transmission of microorganisms.
3. Place towel or disposable waterproof barrier under the patient and across the patient's lower abdomen.	Protects bed linen; maintains patient's dignity.
4. If not done during assessment, remove used pouch and skin barrier gently by pushing skin away from barrier. Use an adhesive remover to facilitate removal of skin barrier. Empty pouch and dispose of it in appropriate receptacle. Measure output if needed. **Note:** There may be no output at time of first pouch change.	Reduces skin trauma. Improper removal of pouch and barrier can cause peristomal skin irritation or breakdown.

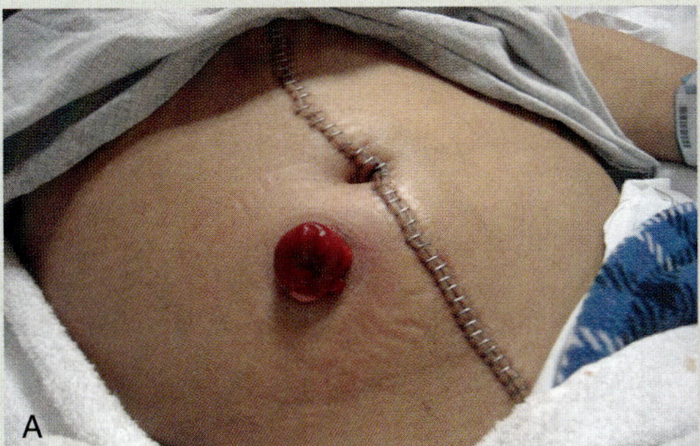

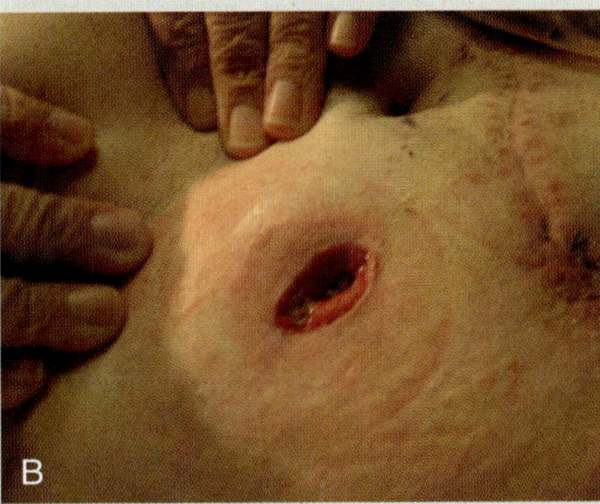

Step 5 A, Budded stoma. **B,** Retracted stoma. (Courtesy Jane Fellows.)

STEP	RATIONALE
5. Clean peristomal skin gently with warm tap water using washcloth; do not scrub skin. If you touch stoma, minor bleeding is normal. Pat skin dry. Have washcloth handy for additional cleansing if there is output from stoma while preparing pouch. Remove and dispose of gloves. Perform hand hygiene.	Soap leaves residue on skin, which may irritate skin. Pouch does not adhere to wet skin. Do not use products containing moisturizers, such as cleansers and baby wipes, because the pouch will not adhere well. Ileostomies have frequent output, especially after eating.
6. Measure stoma (see illustration). Expect size of stoma to change for the first 4–6 weeks after surgery.	Allows for proper fit of pouch that will protect peristomal skin.
7. Trace pattern of stoma measurement on pouch backing or skin barrier (see illustration).	Prepares for cutting opening in pouch.
8. Cut opening on backing or skin barrier wafer (see illustration). If using a moldable or shape-to-fit barrier, use fingers to mold the shape to fit the stoma.	Customizes pouch to provide appropriate fit over stoma.
9. Remove protective backing from adhesive backing or wafer (see illustration).	Prepares skin barrier for placement.
10. Apply gloves. Apply pouch over stoma (see illustration). Press firmly into place around stoma and outside edges. Have the patient hold hand over pouch to apply heat to secure seal.	Pouch adhesives are heat and pressure sensitive and hold more securely at body temperature.
11. Close end of pouch with clip or integrated closure. Remove drape from the patient. Assist the patient to assume comfortable position.	Ensures pouch is secure. Contains effluent.
12. Remove and dispose of gloves and other disposables. Perform hand hygiene.	Reduces transmission of microorganisms.

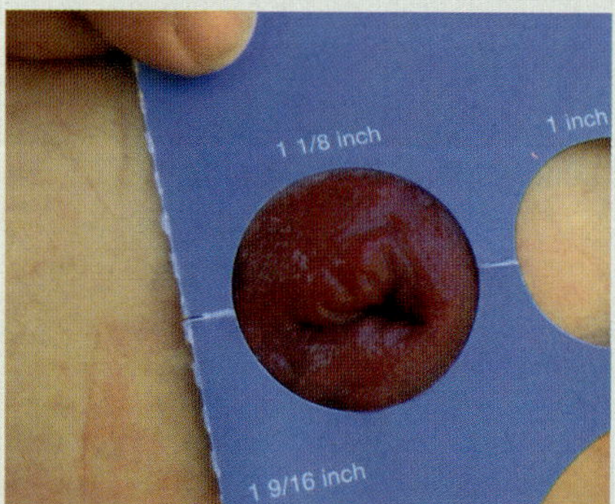

Step 6 Measure stoma. (Courtesy Coloplast, Minneapolis, MN.)

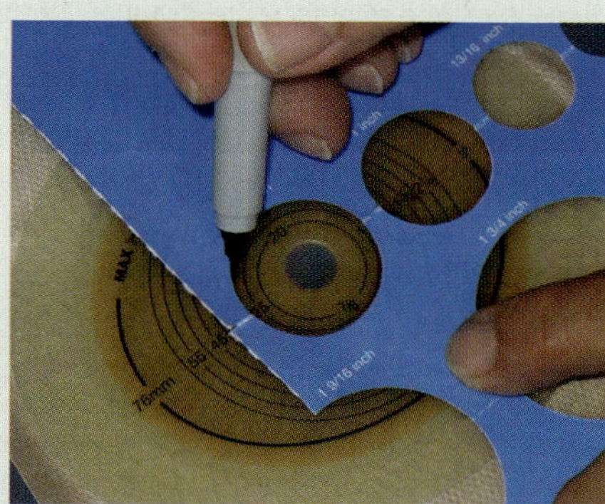

Step 7 Trace measurement on skin barrier. (Courtesy Coloplast, Minneapolis, MN.)

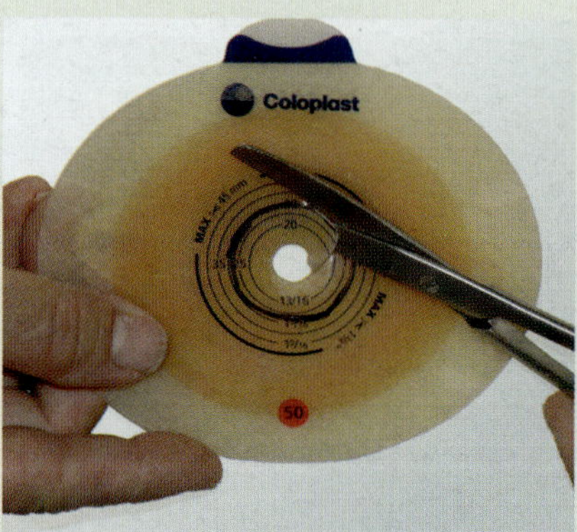

Step 8 Cut opening in wafer. (Courtesy Coloplast, Minneapolis, MN.)

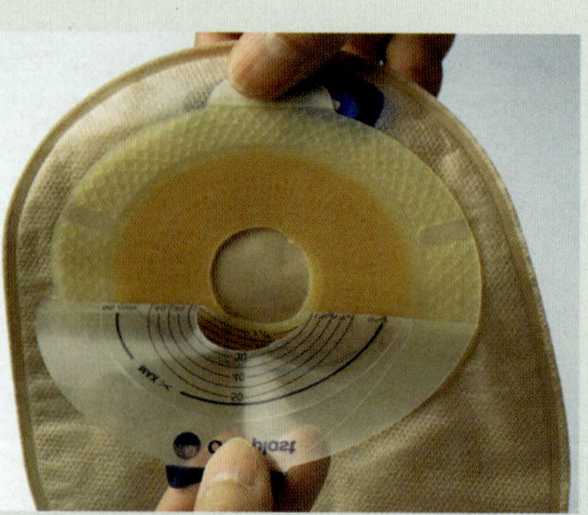

Step 9 Remove protective backing. (Courtesy Coloplast, Minneapolis, MN.)

STEP	RATIONALE

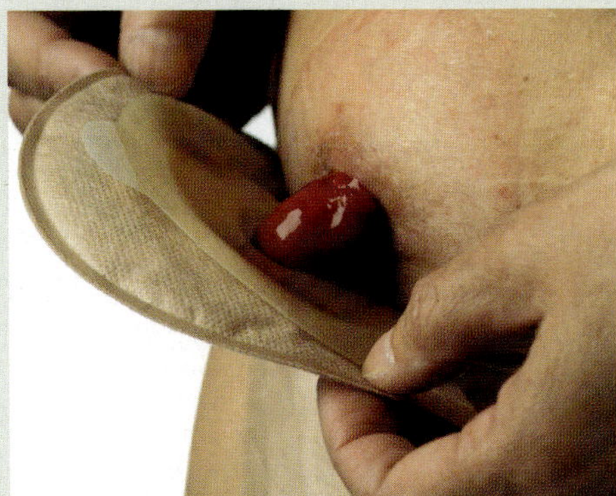

Step 10 Apply pouch over stoma. (Courtesy Coloplast, Minneapolis, MN.)

Evaluation

STEP	RATIONALE
1. Observe condition of skin barrier and adherence of pouch to abdominal surface.	Determines presence of leaks.
2. Observe appearance of stoma, peristomal skin, abdominal contours, suture line, and presence of any flatus during pouch change.	Determines condition of stoma and peristomal skin and progress of wound healing.
3. Note whether there is presence of any flatus during pouch change.	Determines whether peristalsis is returning.
4. Observe the patient's and family caregiver's willingness to view stoma and ask questions about procedure.	Determines level of adjustment and understanding of stoma care and pouch application. Allows planning for future education needs and progress toward acceptance of altered body image.
5. **Use teach back:** "I want to be sure you understand what is involved in changing your ostomy pouch. Tell me what you should do to prevent your skin from becoming irritated and how often you should empty your pouch." Revise your instruction now or develop a plan for revised patient/family caregiver teaching if the patient/family caregiver is not able to teach back correctly.	Determines the patient's/family caregiver's level of understanding of instructional topic.

Recording and Reporting

- Record type of pouch and skin barrier applied; time of procedure; amount and appearance of effluent in pouch; location, size, and appearance of stoma; and condition of peristomal skin in nurses' notes in EHR or chart.
- Document your evaluation of patient/family caregiver learning.
- Report to nurse and/or health care provider: abnormal appearance of stoma, suture line, peristomal skin, or character of output.

Unexpected Outcomes and Related Interventions

- Skin around stoma is irritated, blistered, or bleeding, or a rash is noted; may be caused by undermining of pouch seal by fecal contents causing irritant dermatitis, adhesive removal causing skin stripping, or fungal or other skin eruption.
  - Remove pouch more carefully.
  - Change pouch more frequently or use different type of pouching system.
  - Consult ostomy care nurse.
  - Avoid use of acetone-based products.
- Necrotic stoma may be bluish, purple, or black in color; dry instead of moist in texture; fail to bleed when washed gently; or show signs of tissue sloughing.
  - Report to nurse in charge or health care provider.
  - Document appearance.
- The patient refuses to view stoma or participate in care.
  - Obtain referral for ostomy care nurse.
  - Allow the patient to express feelings.
  - Encourage family support.

KEY POINTS

- Mechanical breakdown of food elements, gastrointestinal (GI) motility, and selective absorption and secretion of substances by the large intestine influence the character of feces.
- Food high in fiber content and increased fluid intake keep feces soft.
- Daily exercise is important for maintenance of normal bowel function.
- The greatest dangers from diarrhea are dehydration and fluid and electrolyte imbalance.

- A patient with a fecal diversion (colostomy or ileostomy) requires teaching in the care of the stoma and support in adjusting to the change in body image and function.
- The location of an ostomy influences the consistency of stool.
- A fecal occult blood test (FOBT) or fecal immunochemical test (FIT) determines whether blood is present in a stool sample See Box 22.5. Both are screening tools for colon cancer for patients older than 50 years.
- Consider frequency of defecation, fecal characteristics, effect of foods on GI function, and patient's food preferences when selecting a diet promoting normal elimination.
- Proper enema administration requires the slow instillation of the correct volume of a solution.
- Dangers during digital removal of stool include traumatizing the rectal mucosa and promoting vagal stimulation.
- Skin breakdown occurs after repeated exposure to liquid stool; prevention of this is an important nursing responsibility.

REFERENCES

Anne M. Van Leeuwen and Mickey L. Bladh. Davis's comprehensive handbook of laboratory and diagnostic tests with nursing implications. 6th ed. Philadelphia: Davis; 2015.

American Cancer Society (ACS). American Cancer Society recommendations for colorectal cancer early detection. 2017. Available from: https://nccrt.org/resource/american-cancer-society-recommendations-colorectal-cancer-early-detection/.

Callan L, Wilson M. Fecal incontinence: pathology, assessment and management. In: Doughty D, Moore K, editors. Wound Ostomy Continence Nursing Society core curriculum: continence management. Philadelphia: Wolters Kluwer; 2016.

Colwell J. Selection of a pouching system. In: Carmel J, et al., editors. Wound, Ostomy and Continence Nurses Society®. core curriculum: ostomy management. Philadelphia: Wolters Kluwer; 2016.

Hockenberry MJ, Wilson D. Wong's nursing care of infants and children. 10th ed. St. Louis: Mosby; 2014.

Mayo Clinic. *C. difficile* infection. 2016. Available from: http://www.mayoclinic.org/diseases-conditions/c-difficile/home/ovc-20202264.

National Institute of Diabetes, Digestive and Kidney Diseases (NIDDK). Health information. 2016. Available from: https://www.niddk.nih.gov/health-information.

Nurko S, Zimmerman LA. Evaluation and treatment of constipation in children and adolescents. Am Fam Physician 2014;90(2):82.

Salvadalena G. Peristomal skin conditions. In: Carmel J, et al., editors. Wound Ostomy Continence Nursing Society®. core curriculum: ostomy management. Philadelphia: Wolters Kluwer; 2016.

Shlamovitz G, Shah N. Nasogastric intubation. 2016. Available from: http://emedicine.medscape.com/article/80925-overview.

Steele S, et al. Motility disorders. In: Carmel J, et al., editors. Wound Ostomy Continence Nursing Society®. core curriculum continence management. Philadelphia: Wolters Kluwer; 2016.

The Joint Commission (TJC). 2018 National Patient Safety Goals. Oakbrook Terrace, IL: The Joint Commission; 2018. Available from: http://www.jointcommission.org/standards_information/npsgs.aspx.

University of Michigan. Troubleshooting autonomic dysreflexia. 2013. Available from: http://www.med.umich.edu/1libr/SpinalCordInjuryProgram/AutomonicDysreflexia.pdf.

23 Diagnostic Testing

OBJECTIVES

After reading this chapter, the student should be able to:

- Enumerate various diagnostic tests that can be performed to detect certain disorders.
- Describe the phases of diagnostic testing and the nurse's role in these phases.
- Illustrate about various blood laboratory tests and electrolyte levels in the blood.
- Demonstrate the blood glucose monitoring.
- Describe the method to collect the specimen and analyze various types of urine specimens.
- Explain about the collection and testing of the specimens for culture and sensitivity.
- Illustrate about sputum culture and throat culture.
- Describe about various radiological and endoscopic investigations.
- Explain about the role of nurse in laboratory diagnostic tests procedures.

KEY TERMS

albuminuria, p. 546
angiography, p. 548
anoscopy, p. 548
bronchoscopy, p. 549
colonoscopy, p. 548
complete blood count, p. 540
cystoscopy, p. 548
echocardiogram, p. 549
guaiac test, p. 544
hemoccult, p. 545
hemoglobin A1C (HbA1C), p. 543
intravenous pyelography, p. 548
laryngoscopy, p. 549
liver function test (LFT), p. 541
lung scan, p. 549
magnetic resonance imaging (MRI), p. 549
occult blood, p. 544
positron emission tomography (PET), p. 549
proctoscopy, p. 548
proctosigmoidoscopy, p. 548
retrograde pyelography, p. 548
serum glucose, p. 541
specific gravity, p. 546
steatorrhea, p. 544
stress electrocardiography, p. 548
urine culture, p. 546

INTRODUCTION

Diagnostic testing is the basic tool to determine or identify the cause of any disease or disorder. There are various types of diagnostic tests that are done in regard to the type of test required to rule out the cause. Testing helps us to be aware about the current health status of the patient and to implement necessary interventions as soon as the cause is identified. The most vital part in this is the communication with the patient undergoing these tests and the necessary information needs to be provided to the patient therapeutically. Nurses need to be thorough about these tests and are required to be the essential part of the process to provide care to the patient on the basis of the results of the tests.

PHASES OF DIAGNOSTIC TESTING

Diagnostic testing is done in various settings in health care and the sites may be hospitals and clinics; nowadays diagnostic testing also includes testing at homes, shopping malls, workplaces, and mobile units. The testing is done following a specific set of guidelines and standards for accurate results of a test. Advancements in technology are in progress that are making the testing an easy way of providing effective and quick results. The team in the entire process is responsible to create a safe and protective environment.

There are three phases of diagnostic testing: pretest, intratest, and post-test.

Pretest

Pretest phase may also be referred to as preanalytical phase. This phase involves preparing the patient and educating the family about the testing. It focuses on thorough assessment; data collection including physical, biological, sociological, cultural, and spiritual aspects; and what needs to be known, that is, indications, contraindications, and identification of high-risk patients. An informed consent is required to be taken before the tests. The nurse needs to confirm about the use of any dye or agent before the test and any previous allergy related to the dye or injection. Complete information about the test is necessary to avoid any error or mistake related to the procedure.

Intratest

This phase is called analytical phase in which procedural care is provided and the specific specimen is collected. Standard and universal precautions are maintained per the diagnostic test and sterility has to be maintained following the institutional policies or protocols. A patient needs emotional and physical support during the procedure and the essential parameters need to be assessed, that is, vital signs, pulse oximetry, and ECG. The specimen should be collected appropriately following the guidelines and labeling, storage, and transportation should be done to promote accuracy in results and avoid delay in the diagnosis.

Post-test

This phase is the postanalytical phase and is focused on aftercare of the patient. The test results are interpreted and nursing care is provided based on the diagnosis of the patient. The nurse should monitor the patient for the posteffect of the test or any complications related to the procedure. The results should be reported to the other team members involved in the care of the patient and an appropriate care plan needs to be formulated for the client.

COMPLETE BLOOD COUNT

Complete blood count is done to obtain information about certain components in blood such as hemoglobin, hematocrit values, erythrocyte count, leukocyte count, red blood cell count, differential count, and platelet count. The basic findings associated with these indices are presented in Table 23.1.

Table 23.1 Complete Blood Count

Component	Normal Value	Increased	Decreased
Red blood cell (RBC) count (cells/mm^3)	Male (adult): 4.7–6.1 Female (adult): 4.2–5.4 Children: 4.0–5.5	Erythrocytosis Polycythemia vera Major burns Lung disease (chronic)	Anemia Infection Hemorrhage Deficiency of vitamin B_6, vitamin B_{12}, folic acid Renal diseases Bone marrow suppression Thalassemia
Hemoglobin (g/dL)	Male: 13.5–18 Female: 12–15	Polycythemia vera Major burns Cardiovascular disease Chronic lung disease Congenital heart defect	Hemolytic anemia Bone marrow suppression Sickle cell anemia Chronic infection Hemorrhage Deficiency of vitamin B_6, vitamin B_{12}, folic acid Renal disease
Hematocrit (%)	Male: 42–52 Female: 37–47	Polycythemia vera Dehydration Major burns Cardiovascular disease Chronic lung disease Congenital heart defect	Anemia Hypervolemia Bone marrow suppression Chronic infection Hemorrhage Deficiency of vitamin B_6, vitamin B_{12}, folic acid Renal disease
Red blood cell indices			
MCV (cells/mm^3)	Male: 80–98 Female: 78–102	Pernicious anemia Folic acid deficiency Alcoholism Chronic liver disease	Iron-deficiency anemia Lead poisoning Thalassemia minor and major
Mean corpuscular hemoglobin (pg/cell)	25–35	Alcohol abuse Chronic liver disease Folic acid deficiency Hypothyroidism	Iron-deficiency anemia Lead poisoning Rheumatoid arthritis Sickle cell anemia
Mean corpuscular hemoglobin concentration (g/dL)	32–36	Normal in infancy	Iron-deficiency anemia Lead poisoning
White blood cell (WBC) (cells/mm^3)	4600–11,000	Leukocytosis Infection	Leukopenia Autoimmune disease
Differential WBC count			
Neutrophils (cells/mm^3)	50%–70%	In stress conditions Acute infection Injuries	Viral diseases Drugs (chemotherapy, antibiotics such as nafcillin, penicillin, and cephalosporins)
Lymphocytes	20%–40%	Infections such as viral or bacterial tuberculosis Lymphocytic leukemia Mononucleosis	Immunosuppressive agents Diseases that are autoimmune Malnutrition
Monocytes	2%–8%	Inflammatory diseases Chronic tuberculosis Infections: Protozoal	Drugs: Prednisone

Table 23.1 Complete Blood Count—cont'd

Component	Normal Value	Increased	Decreased
Eosinophils	1%–3%	Allergic reactions Hypersensitivity Parasitic infestations	Corticosteroids
Basophils	0.5%–1.0%	Blood or bone marrow cancer	Allergic reaction Acute use of corticosteroids Infections: Acute
Platelet count (mm^3)	150,000–350,000	Polycythemia vera Tumors that are malignant	Thrombocytopenic purpura Aplastic anemia Folate deficiency Iron deficiency Viral infections Systemic lupus erythematosus Chemotherapy, radiation, and chemical toxicity

SERUM ELECTROLYTES

Testing for serum electrolytes is done to rule out electrolyte and acid–base imbalances in the body. The electrolytes such as sodium, potassium, chloride, carbon dioxide, glucose, blood urea nitrogen, and serum creatinine values are assessed. The normal values and the increase and decrease in values are seen in various conditions that are shown in Table 23.2.

LIVER FUNCTION TEST

Liver function test (LFT) is performed to monitor the functioning of the liver and to rule out liver disease and damage. There are certain enzymes that are tested and their values are monitored for any abnormality in association with the liver disease. This test is done to assess the four liver enzymes, that is, alanine aminotransferase (ALT), alkaline phosphatase (ALP), aspartate aminotransferase (AST), and gamma-glutamyl transferase (GGT). Other indices such as albumin, prealbumin, bilirubin, and ammonia values are also monitored. The parameters that are tested are presented in Table 23.3.

LIPID PROFILE

Lipid profile is a measure of concentration of lipoproteins and is a tool to estimate the level of lipid in blood (hyperlipidemia) and to assess the effectiveness of treatment. It includes estimating total cholesterol, high-density lipoprotein (HDL) cholesterol, low-density lipoprotein (LDL) cholesterol, and triglycerides.

Cholesterol

It is a sterol synthesized in the liver and is found in the cell plasma membrane. Cholesterol is needed for hormones, and is a precursor for vitamin D and sex hormones. The desirable level of cholesterol is less than 200 mg/dL. The values are estimated as a screening for heart disease. High levels of total cholesterol are seen in patients with atherosclerosis, biliary cirrhosis, diet containing high amount of fats and cholesterol, cardiovascular disease, nephritic syndrome, chronic renal failure, uncontrolled diabetes mellitus, and alcoholism. Certain conditions in which total cholesterol decreases are AIDS, malnutrition, malabsorption, stress, sepsis, chronic anemia, severe burns, and severe hepatocellular disease.

High-Density Lipoprotein Cholesterol

HDL is known as "good cholesterol." It is produced and secreted by the liver and small intestine. Its value ranges from 40 to 60 mg/dL. Its excess levels are seen in chronic liver disease, vigorous or long-term aerobic exercise, and alcoholism. A fall in its level can be seen in hypolipoproteinemia, hypertriglyceridemia, uncontrolled diabetes mellitus, end-stage liver disease, obesity, smoking, stress, and renal failure.

Low-Density Lipoprotein Cholesterol

LDL cholesterol is known as "bad cholesterol" and comprises 70% of the total serum cholesterol. It carries cholesterol from the liver to various parts of the body. The level of LDL must be less than 130 mg/dL and its rise is seen in conditions such as diabetes mellitus, chronic renal failure, diet high in cholesterol, hyperlipidemia, nephrotic syndrome, multiple myeloma, and chronic renal failure. LDL is low in conditions such as cancer, malabsorption, malnutrition, chronic anemia, hyperthyroidism, and severe hepatocellular disease.

Triglycerides

Triglyceride is formed from three fatty acids and is an ester that is derived from glycerol. The triglycerides are stored in the adipose tissues and muscles. The desirable level of triglycerides is less than 150 mg/dL. Their rise is seen in malnutrition, alcohol abuse, cirrhosis of the liver, diabetes mellitus, diet low in protein and high in carbohydrate, hypertension, hyperlipoproteinemia, gout, and nephrotic syndrome. Triglycerides are seen to be low in conditions such as COPD, low-fat diet, malabsorption, and malnutrition.

SERUM GLUCOSE

Serum glucose is blood sugar that is carried to all cells and provides energy. Serum blood glucose testing is done to monitor the level of blood glucose. Carbohydrates

Table 23.2 Serum Electrolytes—Normal and Altered Values

Component	Normal Value	Increased	Decreased
Sodium (mEq/L)	135–145	Excessive sodium intake Less water intake Increased insensible water loss Infusion of hypertonic solutions Diarrhea	Hypovolemic hyponatremia Excessive use of diuretics Excessive diaphoresis Water intoxication Hypotonic solution infusion SIADH
Potassium (mEq/L)	3.5–5.1	Excess intake of potassium Impaired renal excretion Addison disease Potassium-sparing diuretic use Hemolysis Burns Diabetic ketoacidosis	Inadequate intake of potassium Vomiting Gastric suctioning Diarrhea Excessive use of loop diuretics
Chloride (mEq/L)	98–106	Prolonged vomiting Diarrhea Dehydration Hypernatremia Renal failure Metabolic acidosis Hyperventilation	Vomiting or gastric suctioning Addison disease Overhydration Burns Metabolic alkalosis SIADH Heart failure
Calcium (mg/dL)	8.6–11	Hyperparathyroidism Use of thiazide diuretics Prolonged immobilization Lung cancer and breast cancer	Hypoparathyroidism Deficiency of vitamin D Pancreatitis Renal failure Rhabdomyolysis
Magnesium (mEq/L)	1.5–2.5	Addison disease Lithium therapy Hypothyroidism Excessive use of magnesium containing drugs Renal failure Milk alkali syndrome	Impaired GI absorption Diarrhea Inadequate intake of magnesium
Blood urea nitrogen (mg/dL)	10–20	Acute glomerulonephritis Congestive heart failure Urinary tract obstruction High intake of protein Renal disease Dehydration Diabetes mellitus Infections	Alcohol abuse Hepatitis Liver failure Malnutrition Low intake of protein
Serum creatinine (mg/dL)	0.6–1.3	Chronic kidney disease Dehydration High protein intake Excessive exercise Use of medications or certain antibiotics such as trimethoprim	Low muscle mass (aging and muscular dystrophy) Excessive weight loss Pregnancy
Carbon dioxide (mEq/L)	23–30	Hypoventilation Severe vomiting Metabolic alkalosis COPD Emphysema Sleep apnea	Renal failure Salicylate toxicity Diabetic ketoacidosis Metabolic acidosis Lung disease
Glucose (mg/dL)	70–120	Diabetes mellitus Pancreatitis Obesity Liver disease Corticosteroid therapy Increased stress	Excessive alcohol consumption Overuse of diabetic medications Overproduction of insulin Excessive exercise Malabsorption

when taken break down in small parts, which include sugar or glucose, in the small intestine. Glucose gets absorbed in the bloodstream from the small intestine. It provides energy to all the body tissues and organs. For the transport of glucose, insulin is required, which is produced by the pancreas. Alterations in the level of glucose need to be monitored to rule out hyperglycemia or hypoglycemia.

These values can be a tool to diagnose pancreas-related issues such as hyperglycemia that occurs when insulin is not produced by the pancreas such as in pancreatitis. Serum glucose level can be assessed after fasting of 7–10 hours,

Table 23.3 Liver Function Tests

Test	Normal Findings	Significance	Increased	Decreased
Alanine aminotransferase (ALT) or serum pyretic transaminase (SGPT)	Male: 10–55 U/L Female: 7–30 U/L	Specific marker for injury to liver.	Hepatitis Liver cirrhosis Acute pancreatitis Myocardial infarction Cardiac failure Liver tumors	Insignificant
Aspartate aminotransferase (AST) or serum glutamic oxaloacetic transaminase (SGOT)	Male: 10–40 U/L Female: 9–25 U/L	Present mostly in heart and liver, and in skeletal muscles to a lesser extent. Marker for liver injury.	Hepatitis Alcoholism Skeletal muscle disease Myocardial infarction Acute anemia	Renal dialysis; chronic renal failure Deficiency of vitamin B_6
Alkaline phosphatase (ALP)	25–100 U/L	Found mostly in bone and liver.	Diseases of bone and liver Myocardial infarction Chronic renal failure Heart failure hyperparathyroidism	Pernicious anemia Malnutrition or protein deficiency Hypothyroidism
Gamma-glutamyl transferase (GGT)	Male: 1–94 U/L Female: 1–70 U/L	Present mostly in liver, kidney, spleen, and prostate.	Liver disease Alcoholism Damage in bile ducts	Not significant
Albumin	3.5–5.1 g/dL	Plasma protein synthesized by liver, helps in fluid balance and maintains oncotic pressure.	Acute infections Rise is not significant in liver disease	Malnutrition Liver disease or dysfunction Infections Severe burns
Bilirubin	Total: 0.3–1.0 mg/dL Direct: 0.0–0.2 mg/dL Indirect: 0.1–1.0 mg/dL	Component of bile; synthesized in liver, spleen and bone marrow; result of breakdown of hemoglobin.	**Total:** Hepatitis, common bile duct obstruction, pernicious anemia, sickle cell anemia **Direct:** Cancer of head of pancreas, bile duct stones **Indirect:** Hemolytic anemia, reactions related to blood transfusion	Insignificant
Ammonia	15–45 mcg/dL	Produced after protein breakdown or metabolism. Liver converts ammonia into urea and is excreted by the kidneys.	Cirrhosis of liver Reye syndrome Bleeding in stomach, intestine, or esophagus Alcoholism or drug use	Liver failure

which is referred to as fasting blood sugar or fasting blood serum (FBS) value. It is referred to as postprandial serum glucose or postprandial blood glucose (PPBS) when the test is performed after 2 hours of meal. When the test is performed by giving a standardized amount of glucose to the patient orally, it is referred to as oral glucose tolerance test (OGTT).

Fasting Blood Sugar

The test is performed to evaluate the level of sugar in blood after fasting overnight. The level must be less than 100 mg/dL. The client is considered to be prediabetic if the blood sugar values fall between 100 and 125 mg/dL and client is diabetic if the value is 126 mg/dL or exceeds this value. The client is instructed to fast overnight or 7–8 hours before blood test.

Postprandial Blood Glucose

For a PPBS test, the blood is withdrawn 2 hours after the meal. The levels are monitored for alterations, if any, for example, PPBS is elevated in diabetics and is normal in healthy clients. Patients with diabetes may need to monitor PPBS regularly to monitor their blood sugar levels to keep an eye on the alteration in the values.

Hemoglobin A1C (HbA1C)

Hemoglobin A1C (HbA1C) is a term that is referred to as glycated hemoglobin. Red blood cells contain a protein called hemoglobin that carries oxygen throughout the body and combines with glucose present in blood and becomes glycated. This means that the hemoglobin now contains an added molecule, that is, sugar, after undergoing the process of glycation. Therefore, it is called HbA1C or A1C. This test measures accurate glycemic levels and helps to rule out complications related to diabetes. The value of HbA1C ranges between 4% and 6%. A level between 6.0% and 6.4% reflects prediabetes and a level of 6.5% or more depicts diabetes.

CAPILLARY BLOOD GLUCOSE

Capillary blood glucose testing is done by piercing the skin of a finger and withdrawing blood. This is done when regular testing of blood glucose is required; this test can be performed by self and is less painful as compared with a venipuncture. This technique is used to measure the blood glucose in clients with diabetes.

There has been advancement in technology and nowadays there are several types of glucose monitors such as voice-activated glucose meters and meters that have a large visual display. There are meters that can perform testing automatically; such meters can rest on the forearm but the accuracy is less than that of fingertip testing. Testing from the forearm can be done before or after taking a meal, after physical activity or exercise, or when an insulin dose is administered. The client's teaching about the use of a particular device is important. Self-management of blood glucose is essential and the patient develops confidence in using the device and feels empowered.

Purposes

- To obtain the blood glucose sample and monitor the values to know the risk of hyperglycemia or hypoglycemia
- To teach the client about the use of glucose testing device effectively
- To promote regulation of blood glucose by the client after knowing the values obtained by testing

Equipment

- Glucometer
- Blood glucose reagent strip
- Sterile swabs
- Clean gloves
- Lancet (sterile)
- Lancet pen or injector to hold lancet

The basic care during capillary blood glucose monitoring is illustrated in Box 23.1 and instructions for care to be taken by people at home during capillary blood glucose monitoring are depicted in Box 23.2. The skill of capillary blood glucose testing is described in Skill 23.1.

BOX 23.1 General Care During Capillary Blood Glucose Testing

Infants

- For neonates and infants, the outer aspect of heel is the site for blood glucose monitoring. A warm cloth is placed over the infant's heel that increases the blood flow to the site.

Children

- Side of the fingertip for a child older than 2 years is the site for blood glucose monitoring, unless contraindicated.
- The child may be allowed to choose the site for the puncture if possible and is encouraged for cooperation.

Older Adults

- Because of joint changes in older adults such as in arthritis, poor vision, and hand tremors, assistance is needed for the use of glucometer.
- Financial issues may be present to obtain diabetic supplies.
- Warming the hands before the procedure is necessary because older adults have poor circulation. A warm cloth is wrapped around the hand for 3–5 min; placing the hand in a dependent position also promotes circulation.

BOX 23.2 Home Care During Capillary Blood Glucose Testing

- Willingness to perform the procedure at home must be evaluated.
- Proper instructions must be conveyed about the use of a lancet and guidelines or manual provided for the same.
- A return demonstration is important and the client may require several visits to obtain skills to perform the procedure completely.
- The client must be encouraged about obtaining the supplies needed for the procedure.
- Keeping the record of the values is essential information that must be conveyed to a client and he or she is instructed to notify the health care provider in case abnormal results are found.
- Children must be taught about the safe practices to be followed while performing a puncture on the site and also appropriate measures to keep the equipment safe in home or school settings.

Evaluation

- Evaluate and compare the patient's blood glucose level with the normal values of the blood glucose and note the difference. Encourage the patient about self-testing of blood glucose and teach the technique to the patient.
- Physician should be notified in case abnormal results are found and immediate care is needed or a venipuncture is required if policy recommends.
- Follow up the client to explain what the results mean and demonstrate to him/her about the test that is scheduled next.

STOOL ROUTINE EXAMINATION

A stool specimen provides information concerning the client's health position or functioning of the gastrointestinal (GI) system. Most commonly, **occult blood** testing is performed to determine the presence of occult (hidden) blood in the stool. It indicates the presence of bleeding in the GI tract and it also detects the presence of ova and parasites that are responsible for causing parasitic infections.

Purpose of Collecting Stool Specimen

- It helps to determine the presence of occult blood. This is also known as **guaiac test** that shows presence of occult blood. In this test, guaiac is used to coat the fecal occult blood test (FOBT) cards.
- Digestive secretions and dietary products such as fat in stool (**steatorrhea**) are analyzed, which indicate faulty absorption of fat from the small bowel. To determine these specific types of tests, a whole quantity of stool that is expelled is tested at once instead of a small sample.

- To see the existence of parasitic infections, the sample needs to be transported promptly when it is warm and the test needs three specimens that are evaluated for the presence of specific organisms.
- The test helps to detect bacteria and viruses in the specimen and the same is cultured. It is done by following certain guidelines and protocols for the culture test.

Collection of Specimen

Collection of specimen requires some guidelines to be followed by a nurse who determines the reason for the collection of stool specimen. This may require a single specimen or timed specimens may also be ordered. The quantity of the specimen needs to be noted and the correct method of collection and handling the specimen is an important aspect. The nurse needs to know whether preservative should be added to the stool or whether the specimen should be sent immediately to the laboratory.

The specimen may be obtained by the Unlicensed assistive personnel (UAP) if it is a random stool specimen. In case a specimen is required for culture and needs sterile swab in a test tube, it must be performed by the nurse. The UAP can also perform occult blood testing by obtaining the specimen. Caution is required to maintain the sterility if culture is required so that accurate results can be obtained. The UAP has to inform the nurse in case presence of blood is noted or detected and the test results are positive or negative.

Special Instructions

- The nurse must instruct the client to void before the procedure to avoid contamination of the specimen and also avoid contamination with menstrual discharge.
- A clean bedpan or bedside commode is required for the test.
- Once the sample is collected, avoid placing tissue paper over the bedpan following defecation.
- Following sample collection, it needs to be notified to the nurse so that the specimen can be sent to the laboratory immediately.
- Medical asepsis is required while shifting the stool sample to a specimen container as well as while disposing the content of the bedpan.
- Contamination is prevented by using clean gloves and avoiding direct contact with the specimen.
- If tongue blades are used to shift the specimen to the container, discard the tongue blades after wrapping in a paper towel.
- For a formed stool, about 2.5 cm and 15–30 mL of stool if liquid is considered adequate for the specimen.
- If there is visible pus, blood, or mucus, it should be included in the sample specimens.
- Sterility needs to be maintained carefully while collecting the specimen for the stool culture.
- Labeling the sample with accurate information per the requisition form is necessary to avoid errors related to identification and risk of wrong diagnosis.
- Stool specimen left at room temperature has chances of bacterial contamination or changes, so the sample may need to be refrigerated but do not place it along with the food or medication.
- Documentation is an important aspect that needs to be maintained after the collection of the specimen and the results need to be noted specifying the date and time of collection and considering the color, odor, consistency, and quantity of feces.
- Consider findings that are abnormal and discomfort during or after defecation. Note for the presence of fresh blood after defecation or any irritation caused following defecation.

Fecal Occult Blood Testing

FOBT is performed to detect the presence of blood in the stool. Presence of blood indicates GI bleeding. There are two types of tests to perform FOBT, that is, the traditional guaiac smear (Hemoccult) and flushable reagent pads (EZ-Detect or ColoCARE).

Hemoccult Test

Hemoccult test requires a chemical reagent that detects a specific substance such as enzyme peroxidase in the molecule of hemoglobin. A tongue blade is usually used to take a small amount of stool or feces and place it over a slide or card and the card is then closed. Then the drop of reagent is added over each smear on the back of the card and the nurse notes change in the color. The test is positive if a blue color appears. No change in color or any other color except blue color is considered to be negative, which means that there is no presence of blood in stool. The following are the considerations that need to be maintained while following this method of testing:

- Test results may be inaccurate because of certain foods, medications, or vitamin C.
- Red meat (beef, lamb, liver, or processed meats) and raw vegetables or fruits including radishes, turnips, horseradish, and melons may cause false-positive results. Use of medications that irritate the gastric mucosa causing bleeding, aspirin, nonsteroidal anti-inflammatory drugs, iron preparations, and anticoagulants is also responsible for causing false-positive results.
- Consumption of more than 250 mg of vitamin C per day by the patient either in diet or supplementary for 3 days before the test—even if bleeding persists—can cause false-negative results.

Flushable Reagent Pads (EZ-Detect or ColoCARE)

Flushable reagent pads are used to detect presymptomatic occult bleeding that may be the result of GI diseases.

A test pad is placed in the toilet after a motion and is watched for a change in the color. If blood is present, the hemoglobin will react with the chromogen and the reaction will show blue or green color. The pad is flushed after noting the reaction and is biodegradable. The results can appear within 2 minutes.

URINE TESTING

Collecting urine specimens provides significant information about disorders, helps in monitoring client recovery or deterioration, helps in assessment of functioning of kidneys and liver, and detects the presence of legal or illegal drugs, pregnancy, or disease-causing microorganisms. There are a number of tests that are performed such as testing of urine to check the presence of albumin in urine, to know the pH of urine to determine whether it is acidic and alkaline, and to find out the specific gravity of urine. Culture may be required as a routine examination or timed urine specimens are also ordered. A clean void urine specimen examination is done to perform routine urinalysis, a clean-catch or midstream urine specimen is obtained for the culture of urine, and timed urine specimen is obtained for performing various other tests.

Testing for Albumin

Albumin is a protein naturally made by the liver and is present in blood. Its presence in urine is called **albuminuria**, which may be indicative of a kidney disease that allows the albumin to pass from the blood into the urine. It may be a result of kidney damage because of diabetes, high blood pressure, heart failure, cirrhosis of the liver, or lupus. If a large amount of albumin is present in the urine, it can eventually lead to chronic kidney disease. Albumin test can be done randomly, over a 24-hour period or over a specific period of time or overnight.

There are two types of test that we can perform to detect the presence of albumin in the urine: cold test and hot test.

Cold Test

Pour a small quantity or 0.5 inch of nitric acid or sulfosalicylic acid 2% in a clean test tube. Then about 2 inches from the sides of the test tube, allow equal quantity of urine to trickle down the sides of the test tube. If albumin is present, a white precipitate or white opaque ring will appear at the junction of urine and nitric acid. After noting the findings, discard the urine and clean the test tube.

Hot Test

Fill three-fourth of the test tube with filtered urine. Hold the test tube from the bottom and over the flame of the spirit lamp; heat up the upper part of urine in the tube. The test tube is rotated during the process to avoid break in the tube. Note that if a cloudy layer appears in the hot urine, it indicates the presence of proteins and phosphates. By using a dropper, acetic acid is added to urine. If cloud disappears, phosphates are present in the urine; and if cloud still remains, albumin is present in the urine.

Testing for Acetone

Acetone is a by-product of metabolism of fat and fatty acids providing energy for the cells. It is the simplest and smallest ketone that enters the bloodstream and is completely metabolized in the liver. If the presence of acetone in the blood is higher than normal or if acetone shows higher levels, it can be excreted in the urine. Acetone test is used to differentiate between diabetic coma and insulin shock, and to monitor the glucose control in patients who are diabetic, for screening, in pregnancy, and in patients who suffer from ketoacidosis. Increased levels are seen in ethanol hangover or after consumption of a large amount of alcohol.

Rothera Test

This test requires a clean urine container and acetone testing strips.

- An amount of 5 mL of urine is taken in a test tube and ammonium sulfate is added for saturation.
- A small crystal of sodium nitroprusside is added and is mixed well in it.
- Formation of purple-colored ring of permanganate at the junction indicates a positive test result.

Testing for pH

The pH of urine is tested to determine the acidity or alkalinity of the urine sample. A simple dipstick method is used to know the acidic or alkaline nature of the urine. Urine specimen is collected by instructing the client about the procedure and after the collection of urine (15–20 mL), testing strip is dipped in the urine by holding it horizontally for 15 seconds. The color of the ketone patch on the strip of the color chart is compared on the container of acetone testing strips. The color ranging from orange to yellow is considered acidic with a pH of 3–6 and blue color indicates alkalinity.

Specific Gravity

Specific gravity of the urine compares the density of urine with the density of water, which is 1.000. The specific gravity may alter by the presence of blood, protein, or casts in the urine. The urine specific gravity ranges from 1.010 to 1.030. There are various methods to determine the specific gravity of urine such as multiple-test dipstick or by using a urinometer in which urine is placed in a small cylinder and the urinometer is allowed to float in the urine. The reading of the specific gravity is measured at the level of the meniscus.

The specific gravity alters with the amount of fluid present in the body. Usually, it decreases if the fluid intake is high and increases when the fluid intake is low. A decrease in the specific gravity of urine is also noted in certain conditions such as diabetes insipidus, glomerulonephritis, renal failure, excessive fluid intake, acute tubular necrosis, and pyelonephritis. The specific gravity of urine increases in diabetes mellitus, nephritis, dehydration, renal artery stenosis, and decreased blood flow to the kidneys.

URINE CULTURE

A **urine culture** is a noninvasive method that can find microorganisms (bacteria) in the urine. Urine culture test is performed to discover the bacteria and germs that are responsible for urinary tract infection. A clean-catch or a midstream urine specimen is obtained for urine culture. It is important to avoid contamination of the specimen and the specimen must be free from microorganisms. A specimen container (sterile disposable clean catch kits) is required to collect the specimen for culture. The method to obtain the urine specimen for culture by clean-catch or midstream approach is described in Skill 23.2.

Purpose

- To identify the presence and type of microorganisms that are responsible for causing the disease
- To determine the antibiotics to which certain microorganisms are sensitive

Equipment

- Clean gloves
- Sterile specimen container
- Antiseptic swabs or wipes
- Identification label for specimen

Routine Urinalysis

A clean voided specimen is collected as a part of routine examination of urine. The client is provided the instructions to collect the urine for a routine examination. The male patients are instructed to void directly into the specimen container, whereas the female patients have to sit over the toilet seat to void into the container. It is usually performed in the morning because the urine has a higher and uniform concentration and a more acidic pH in the morning. An amount of 10 mL of urine is usually adequate for a routine analysis. Assistance is provided for the clients who are dependent or physically incapacitated or disoriented or who require a bedpan or urinal to void.

Special Considerations

- A clean specimen is collected free of contamination such as fecal contamination.
- Avoid keeping any tissue paper on the bedpan because it may alter the results and make it difficult to analyze.
- Avoid touching the outer surface of the container to avoid contamination and a disinfectant is used to clean the same if touched accidently.
- Labeling the specimen accurately avoids errors in diagnosis and therapy for the patient.

TIMED URINE SPECIMEN

Urine examination can also be performed by collecting the urine specimen in a particular time that ranges from 1–2 to 24 hours. These specimens may require refrigeration or may contain preservative to prevent bacterial growth. Because hormones, proteins, and electrolytes are excreted in small amounts in urine, the specimen is collected over an extended period so as to produce quantities of diagnostic value.

Purposes

- To monitor or assess kidneys' ability to concentrate and dilute urine
- To detect disorders related to glucose metabolism such as diabetes mellitus
- To detect presence of specific constituents such as albumin, amylase, creatinine, and urobilinogen in the urine

Steps of Urine Collection

- Identify the patient and the procedure is explained to the patient to enlist cooperation.
- A specimen container with preservative is obtained and labeling is done to avoid errors in diagnosis. The interval of collection needs to be noted.
- Provide a bedpan, commode, or collection container or urinal to the client.
- Instruct the client to save all obtained urine during the period of collection of urine and to notify the nurse after each voiding and avoid touching the specimen with tissue paper and also prevent contamination with feces.
- The obtained specimen during the period of timed collection is saved, refrigerated, or placed on ice as indicated.
- The entire amount is taken to the laboratory for investigation following filling of the laboratory requisition form.
- The time the collection of specimen is started and completed is recorded.

SPUTUM CULTURE

Sputum is secreted by the mucous membranes lining the bronchioles, bronchi, and trachea. It is helpful in protecting the respiratory tract from infection and it is a mixture of saliva, nasal, sinus secretions, dead cells, and normal oral bacteria in the respiratory tract. Various types of pathogens are detected in culture of the sputum. Sputum specimens are usually collected in the morning. Specimens can be obtained by expectoration that may need nebulization, chest percussion, and hydration or by performing postural drainage. If expectoration is not possible, pharyngeal suctioning can be done. It is usually indicated in conditions such as pneumonia, bronchiectasis, bronchitis, pulmonary abscess, productive cough, fever, hemoptysis, and pulmonary infections

Purposes

- To identify the causative microorganism and antibiotic resistance
- To determine the cell pathology
- To identify any cancerous cell type
- To detect acid-fast bacillus by obtaining serial collection of sputum for 3 consecutive days
- To diagnose nosocomial pneumonia and community-acquired pneumonia

Expectoration Method

- Identify the patient and explain about the procedure to the patient. (Instruct the patient priorly that the specimen will be collected in the morning because overnight wait will promote accumulation of secretions.)
- Position the patient on a chair or at the side of the bed or in high Fowler's position if unable to sit to promote chest expansion, prevent aspiration, and promote better expectoration of sputum.
- Provide water to perform mouth care. Wear gloves and PPE to avoid contact with the sputum. Special

precautions need to be followed if the client is suspected to have tuberculosis and obtain specimen in a room with special airflow system or outdoors.

- Instruct the patient to cough deeply and expectorate into the specimen container. Tell him or her to produce 15–30 mL of sputum. Clean the container with disinfectant if sputum is spilled and has contaminated the container.
- Offer mouth care to the patient after the procedure.
- Remove gloves and discard them following biomedical waste management protocol and wash hands thoroughly. Label the container containing specimen including the patient's name, bed number, IP number, and date and time of the procedure.
- Document the procedure on the patient's chart. Note the quantity, color, odor, consistency (thick, clinging, watery), presence of blood, or any discomfort caused to the client after the procedure.

Tracheal Suctioning Method

This method is preferred if the patient is not able to expectorate the required amount of sputum. If this fails too, bronchoscopy may be done to collect the sputum.

The following steps are followed to obtain the specimen:

- Explain the procedure to the patient to promote cooperation and clarification, and reduce anxiety in the patient.
- Ensure that suction machine is functioning. Position the patient in high Fowler's or semi-Fowler's position and promote oxygenation.
- Perform hand hygiene and wear PPE. Sterility needs to be maintained while obtaining the specimen.
- Connect the suction tubing to the male adapter of the suction trap because the suctioned amount will be trapped inside the container directly.
- Lubricate the catheter with normal saline solution and insert it through the nostril without applying suction to ensure smooth entry of the catheter from the nostril and prevent injury to mucosa.
- Instruct the patient to take a deep breath while inserting to promote ease in insertion and advance the catheter to the trachea from the larynx.
- Apply suction for 5–10 seconds but no longer than 15 seconds to avoid hypoxia. Discontinue the suction, withdraw the catheter, and provide oxygen to the patient.
- Detach catheter from the in-line trap and close the trap tightly after collection to send the container to the laboratory. Offer mouth care to the patient after the procedure.
- Note the consistency of the sputum to differentiate between saliva and sputum and send it to the laboratory following labeling and filling up of laboratory requisition form if applicable.

RADIOLOGICAL DIAGNOSTIC TESTS

Radiological diagnostic tests involve direct visualization of the organ or site with the help of various techniques. Radiological investigations include X-ray, computed tomography (CT) scan, and magnetic resonance imaging (MRI). There are various tests done for visualization that depend on the system of the body that is to be monitored.

Gastrointestinal System

A number of tests are performed such as **colonoscopy** (visualizes the large intestine), **proctoscopy** (visualizes the rectum), **proctosigmoidoscopy** (visualizes the rectum and sigmoid), and **anoscopy** (visualizes the anal canal) to identify the alterations in the GI system. X-rays can be performed to identify any abnormalities such as strictures, obstructions, tumors, ulcers, and inflammation. A radiopaque substance is introduced through the GI tract and the obstructions may be seen here. The client is asked to swallow barium sulfate and as it travels down the GI tract, the examination is done for the upper GI tract. For the visualization of the lower GI tract, barium enema is administered. These tests are performed with the fluoroscopic examination that shows the flow of barium in the tract and detects any obstruction in the tract.

Urinary System

To identify the problems related to the genitourinary system, X-ray of kidneys, ureters, or bladder may be performed. **Pyelography (intravenous and retrograde)** is also performed to rule out problems in the urinary tract.

Intravenous pyelography involves using a contrast medium that is injected intravenously, whereas while performing **retrograde pyelography**, the contrast medium is instilled directly into the pelvis of the kidney via the urethra, bladder, and ureters. X-ray is then performed to visualize the tract. Another technique used to visualize the kidneys and note abnormalities is ultrasonography, which involves reflection of sound waves.

Cystoscopy is performed by inserting a cystoscope into the tract to visualize the bladder, urethral orifices, and urethra.

Cardiovascular System

Electrocardiography is performed to record the graphics of the electrical activity of the heart. Various electrodes are placed over specific sites to produce electrical impulses to a graphic recorder. The waveforms are recorded and are read to note any abnormality found in ECG such as dysrhythmias, changes in the ST segment in myocardial infarction, and T-wave abnormalities in ischemia; in addition, changes related to potassium imbalance (hyperkalemia or hypokalemia) may also be seen in the ECG waveform.

Stress electrocardiography is a method that monitors the heart's electrical rhythms and measures response of the client when cardiac workload is increased. The blood pressure as well as chest discomfort caused to the client during exercise is monitored, which may rule out coronary artery disease.

Angiography is a type of imaging test and an invasive procedure to visualize the blood vessels of the heart and detect blockage in the vessels. It is done under fluoroscopic guidance and X-ray is taken to see the flow in the vessels. It detects the blockage and enlargement of arteries or veins by injecting a radiopaque dye in the radial or femoral artery to visualize the path.

Echocardiogram is a noninvasive procedure that involves the use of ultrasound to see the structures of the heart (muscles or valves) to note abnormalities related to the anatomy and functioning of the chambers of the heart. It is done to determine left ventricular function through images formed by an ultrasound scan. Abnormalities in the functioning of valves can also be detected and images are saved. The client is allowed to be in the supine position; a pillow can be placed under the right side of the patient unless contraindicated. The client must be instructed to refrain from talking during the procedure and lie still or breathe normally.

Lung scan is a type of nuclear imaging test performed to diagnose lung problems. It is also known as ventilation/perfusion (V/Q) scan. It involves the use of a radioactive material to determine the flow of air (ventilation) and blood (perfusion) in the lungs. To detect the abnormalities related to perfusion, the radioisotope is injected intravenously to see the flow of blood and blockage is noted if present. The radioisotope is inhaled by the client through a gas mask and exhaled into room air if ventilation scan is performed.

Laryngoscopy is a sterile procedure performed to visualize the larynx, vocal folds, or glottis.

Computed Tomography

A CT scan is a noninvasive technique that distinguishes minor differences in the density of the tissues. A narrow beam of X-rays is directed at the patient and is rotated around the whole body to produce electrical signals. These signals are then processed by the machine and cross-sectional images are formed on a computer.

Magnetic Resonance Imaging

An **magnetic resonance imaging (MRI)** technique is a noninvasive procedure in which images of the anatomy and physiological processes of the body are taken by placing the client in a magnetic field. The clients with a pacemaker and hip prosthesis are not able to undergo this procedure because a strong magnetic field is produced during the procedure. The client is instructed to remove all metallic items such as jewelry, cell phones, watches, or other metal items before the procedure. Instructions must be given to the client to lie still during the procedure. The client is asked whether he/she has a tattoo over the body because recent reports have suggested that tattoos may hinder the quality of an MRI and in some cases, it has been seen to cause burns or edema over the area of the tattoo. Inform the client that he/she may experience claustrophobia while he/she is in the scanner. MRI is performed to visualize the brain, spine, heart, blood vessels, extremities, joints, abdomen, and pelvis.

Nuclear Imaging Studies

Radioactive isotopes (radiopharmaceuticals) are used in this procedure and are targeted to specific organs. It allows the radiotracer to travel through the area which is being examined and it releases energy in the form of gamma rays that are detected by the camera and the images are formed on the computer. It is a method that tells about the disease in an early stage. Dark images are formed if an organ is hyperfunctioning and are referred to as "hot" spots. Hypofunctioning forms lighter images that are called "cold" spots.

Positron emission tomography (PET) is also a noninvasive procedure in which images are created following injection or inhalation of a radioisotope. It reveals the functioning of the tissues and organs.

ENDOSCOPIC DIAGNOSTIC TESTS

Endoscopy is a general term to describe the visual examination and inspection of body organs or cavities by using an endoscope. An endoscope is an instrument with a light source and a lens. It may be rigid or flexible; rigid endoscopes are used in arthroscopy and flexible endoscopes are used to visualize pulmonary or GI tracts. Endoscopes vary in size and length and can accommodate special instruments that can be inserted through an endoscope to perform certain procedures such as obtaining specimens, removing objects, and cauterizing bleeding.

It requires an informed consent from the patient or parents in case of a minor child. There are different types of endoscopes that are named according to the areas that are examined such as an arthroscope (visualizes the joints), bronchoscope (visualizes the lungs), cystoscope (visualizes the urinary bladder), and laparoscope (visualizes the ovaries, abdominal organs). **Bronchoscopy** is the visualization of the respiratory tract such as the larynx, trachea, and smaller airways of the lungs. For both procedures, a local anesthetic (spray) is given before the procedure is performed to prevent gag reflex.

Before the Procedure

- Patients undergoing pulmonary and GI endoscopy are prepared by explaining the procedure to them and informed consent is obtained.
- The client must be instructed to keep on nil per oral (NPO) status or nothing by mouth for 8–12 hours before the procedure to reduce the chances of vomiting and aspiration.
- The nurse must assure that dentures are removed if present and see for loose teeth and the same must be recorded before the procedure. The bowel must be cleansed before colonoscopy.
- History about specific allergy or bleeding tendencies must be obtained before the procedure.

During the Procedure

- The endoscopy is usually performed in well-equipped endoscopy rooms or it may be performed at bedside in case of emergency.
- Resuscitation equipment must be available for potential complications that may arise during the procedure. For better visualization of the bowel lumen, room air is instilled into the bowel.

After the Procedure

- Complications such as perforation and bleeding after endoscopy need to be assessed immediately after the procedure.

- The patient is kept NPO for 2 hours following the procedure and is not allowed to swallow anything until gag reflex returns.
- The patient is monitored for any discomfort after the procedure. Perforation of an organ or cavity may occur, which can be assessed by observing abdominal tenderness, pain, and distension.
- Bleeding from a biopsy site can be assessed by monitoring vitals, for example, hypotension and tachycardia denote hemorrhage.
- The patient must be monitored or assessed for respiratory function because sedation may cause respiratory depression, so care must be taken to avoid breathing-related complications.
- Observe the patient for signs of infection that may occur as a result of use of cystoscope.
- Instruct the patient to drink more fluids to prevent accumulation of bacteria.

SKILL 23.1 Capillary Blood Glucose Monitoring

S. NO.	STEPS	RATIONALE
1.	Identify the patient and explain the procedure to the patient about the use of the monitor to measure blood glucose.	To obtain consent and gain confidence of the patient.
2.	Assemble the articles needed at the bedside.	To avoid delay in procedure.
3.	Perform hand hygiene and wear gloves.	To prevent cross-infection.
4.	Get the equipment ready by inserting the reagent strip into the meter.	The device turns on when the strip is inserted.
5.	Prepare the site for puncture, preferably the side of the finger of an adult, avoiding the prick next to bone.	Vascular site is preferred.
6.	Hold the finger in a dependent position or below heart level.	To increase blood flow to the area and accuracy of results is assured.
7.	Clean the site using sterile swab and let it dry.	Wet site affects the accuracy and it stings when punctured.
8.	Place the pen or injector against the site to prick and release the needle so that skin may be pierced.	The injector must fully touch the skin of the finger and must be hold perpendicularly to allow it to puncture at specific depth.
9.	Squeeze the site, avoiding touching the site, and form a blood drop (0.3 mL) to be taken up by lancet.	Touching the site will wipe away the blood drop and another sample will be required.
10.	Hold the reagent strip with glucometer lower than puncture site and allow the drop of blood to cover the square on the strip.	Covering the whole square will prevent errors in results and ensure accuracy.
11.	Apply sterile swab over the punctured site and apply pressure.	To promote hemostasis.
12.	Wait for some time for the results to appear on the glucometer.	Do not remove the testing strip until it gives result after reading the blood testing strip.
13.	Measure the blood glucose when it displays on the screen and note the timings.	Correct value and time prevents further errors.
14.	Turn the meter off, remove the testing strip from glucometer, and discard it following biomedical waste protocol.	Device safety is also important by keeping its functioning proper.
15.	Remove the gloves and discard.	To avoid cross-contamination after the procedure.
16.	Document the readings in the patient's record file or in a flow sheet if applicable, noting the results of testing and the amount, type, route, and time of insulin administration.	Diabetic flow sheet provides the whole information about the patient's progress and deterioration.

SKILL 23.2 Urine Culture Specimen Collection

S. NO.	STEPS	RATIONALE
1.	Identify the patient, introduce self, and explain that the urine specimen will be collected and describe the method to collect the urine.	Identification is needed to avoid errors in wrong patient procedure and explaining the details of procedure reduces anxiety and promotes cooperation from the patient.
2.	Gather needed articles for the collection of urine.	To save time and prepare the patient.
3.	Perform hand hygiene and wear PPE as required.	To avoid cross-contamination.
4.	Maintain the client's privacy.	Privacy reduces anxiety and promotes confidence in the patient.
5.	If the client can ambulate, provide directions to obtain the specimen. Assist the patient to washroom and ask to wash the perineal area using soap and water or antiseptic towelettes.	Reduces the chances of infection with bacteria and prevents contamination of the specimen. Using antiseptic agents reduces chances of contamination of specimen.
6.	Instruct the client to avoid any antiseptic if he/she is sensitive to that agent.	Prevents irritation to the perineal area.

S. NO.	STEPS	RATIONALE
7.	Female clients: Using one stroke with one swab, clean from front to back. Discard the swab after each use.	Cleaning from least contaminated area to more contaminated area reduces spread of infection.
8.	Male clients: Retract the foreskin slightly to clean the area if uncircumcised. By using the circular motion, wipe the meatus from proximal to distal part of penis using one swab for one stroke.	Cleaning from least contaminated area to more contaminated area reduces spread of infection.
9.	Dependent clients: Wear clean gloves and wash the perineal area using soap and water or else use the antiseptic swab and follow the steps discussed above.	To prevent contamination to the specimen.
10.	Assist the client over a bedpan as required and position the client upright or as tolerated.	To facilitate urine by forming normal anatomical position.
11.	Collect urine in a clean catch kit and make sure to avoid contamination of the inner side of the specimen container.	Sterility is needed to prevent specimen to get contaminated.
12.	Discard the gloves after use and apply new gloves to clean the perineal area again after collection.	Cleaning the area in the same way as discussed earlier prevents further contamination.
13.	Nonambulatory clients: Instruct the client to start voiding and hold the container into the midstream of urine and avoid touching container to perineal area as well as avoid spilling of urine.	Promoting this practice will prevent contamination of the specimen.
14.	Clean the outer side of the container using a disinfectant if required.	Prevents further transfer of microorganisms.
15.	Label the specimen and send to laboratory per protocol and fill necessary information on the specimen.	To avoid any error in identification and diagnosis.
16.	Document the findings after collection and the method of collection that is used to collect the urine. Note the color, amount, consistency, and discomfort faced by the client during the procedure.	To provide correct information about the procedure and prevent errors on communication.

KEY POINTS

- Diagnostic testing is a tool to determine the cause of a particular disease and helps promote better patient care and improves the quality of care.
- The nurse plays a major role in providing information to the client about the tests that are ordered by the physician and provides support to the client during the phases of diagnostic testing.
- Repeated diagnostic procedures for clients with chronic illness lead to fear and anxiety. The nurse has to provide psychological support in this situation and encourage patient participation in these tests.
- Essential information regarding any allergic reactions must be ruled out before the procedure to avoid giving rise to any complication because some diagnostic tests require injection of dye to visualize certain areas.
- To help prevent any complications related to the procedure, thorough assessment and need of the test must be identified by the nurse.
- The client must be monitored for any discomfort caused during or after the procedure and the nurse must be aware about the treatment to be provided.
- Pretest education or instructions reduces anxiety in patients, promotes confidence, and establishes patient trust.
- Special consideration must be taken for older patients while performing any test such as venipuncture in which one should assess the site carefully because the veins may not be accessible easily. These patients may require assistance in some procedures, so care must be considered to prevent any injury to them.
- Care must be taken while performing any procedure on infants and young children because they are not stable and the nurse needs to pacify them sometimes to avoid any injury to them and to create a sense of trust.
- Confidentiality related to procedures is also an important aspect in diagnostic testing.

REFERENCES

Aggarwal I, Bharat A, Bharat S, Aggarwal SK. AIIMS Medeasy. 2nd ed. CBS Publishers & Distributors Pvt. Ltd; 2018. Available from: https://books.google.co.in/books?id=U4lfDwAAQBAJ&pg. Accessed March 24, 2020.

Audrey JB, Shirlee S.. Kozier & Erb's fundamentals of nursing: concepts, process, and practice. 9th ed. Noida (UP): Dorling Kindersley (India) Pvt. Ltd;.2014.

Button BM, Button B. Structure and function of the mucus clearance system of the lung. Cold Spring Harb Perspect Med. 2013 Aug 1;3(8):a009720. doi: 10.1101/cshperspect.a009720. PMID: 23751214; PMCID: PMC3721269.

Chernecky CC, Berger BJ. Laboratory tests and diagnostic procedures. 6th ed. USA: Elsevier Health Sciences; 2012. Available from: https://books.google.co.in/books?id=dWHYcOJK-cgC&pg. Accessed March 20, 2020.

Daniels R. Manual of laboratory and diagnostic tests. 2nd ed. USA: Cengage Learning; 2009. Available from: https://books.google.co.in/books?id=DRgEAAAAQBAJ&printsec. Accessed March 10, 2020.

ENA. Sheehy's manual of emergency care. 7th ed. Elsevier Health Sciences; 2012. Available from: https://books.google.co.in/books?id=mAwCmKpnFsOC&printsec. Accessed March 11, 2020.

Fischbach FT, Dunning MB. A manual of laboratory and diagnostic tests. 8th ed. Philadelphia: Williams & Wilkins; 2009. Available from: https://books.google.co.in/books?id=CQuBkXDspBkC&source=gbs_navlinks_s. Accessed March 25, 2020.

Grant LR. Hammitt LL, Murdoch DR, O'Brien KL, Scott JA. Procedures for collection of induced sputum specimens from children. Clin Infect Dis 2012;54(Suppl. 2):S140–5. doi:10.1093/cid/cir1069.

Jacob A, Rekha R, Jadhav TS. CLINICAL NURSING PROCEDURES. 3rd ed. New Delhi (India): JAYPEE Brothers MEDICAL P45; 2019.

Jewkes FE, McMaster DJ, Napier WA, Houston IB, Postlethwaite RJ. Home collection of urine specimens—boric acid bottles or Dipslides? Arch Dis Child. 1990;65(3):286–9. doi:10.1136/adc.65.3.286.

Leeuwen AMV, Bladh ML. Textbook of laboratory and diagnostic testing. Philadelphia: 2016. Available from: https://books.google.co.in/books?id=DEq8CwAAQBAJ&printsec. Accessed March 12, 2020.

Meers PD, Chow CK. Bacteriostatic and bactericidal actions of boric acid against bacteria and fungi commonly found in urine. J Clin Pathol 1990;43(6):484–7. doi:10.1136/jcp.43.6.484.

Murdoch DR, Morpeth SC. The diagnostic utility of induced sputum microscopy and culture in childhood pneumonia. Clin Infect Dis 2017; 64(Suppl. 3):S280–8. doi:10.1093/cid/cix090.

Pagana KD, Pagana TJ, Pike-MacDonald SA. Mosby's Canadian manual of diagnostic and laboratory tests. Canada: Elsevier Health Sciences; 2012. Available from: https://books.google.co.in/books?id=Qxmj3nE8-fUC&pg. Accessed March 16, 2020.

Pernille H, Lars B, Marjukka M, Volkert S, Anne H. Sampling of urine for diagnosing urinary tract infection in general practice - First-void or mid-stream urine? Scand J Prim Health Care 2019;37(1):113–9. doi:10.1080/02813432.2019.1568708.

Rosdahl CB, Kowalski MT. Textbook of basic nursing. 9th ed. Lippincott Williams & Wilkins; 2008. Available from: https://books.google.co.in/books?id=tB1YiYj_kdkC&pg. Accessed March 10, 2020.

Suzanne CS, Brenda GB, Janice LH, Kerry HC. Brunner & Suddharth's textbook of medical surgical nursing. 12th ed. America: Wolter Kluwers; 2010.

Wilson W, Grande C, Hoyt D. Critical care. 1st ed. New York: Informa Healthcare; 2007.

Yoost BL, Crawford LR. Fundamentals of nursing: active learning for collaborative practice. 2nd ed. Canada: Elsevier Health Sciences; 2019. Available from: https://books.google.co.in/books?id=jP2EDwAAQBAJ&pg. Accessed March 22, 2020.

24 Oxygenation Needs

OBJECTIVES

- To define oxygen as a basic human need and its importance.
- To explain the structure and function of the cardiopulmonary physiology.
- To identify the physiological processes of ventilation, perfusion, cardiac output, and respiratory gas exchange.
- To describe the alterations of pulmonary system including factors affecting ventilation and oxygen transport.
- To understand the structure and function of circulatory system that explains regulatory blood flow and conduction system.
- To explain different types of alterations that results because of problems in the circulatory system such as disturbances in conduction, altered cardiac output, impaired valvular function, myocardial ischemia, and impaired tissue perfusion.
- To discuss nursing process and perform assessment along with diagnostic test.
- To plan nursing diagnosis and patient care based on priority needs of the client.
- To describe the effects of a patient's health status, age, lifestyle, and environment on tissue oxygenation.
- To explain maintenance or promotion of lung expansion and perform restoration of cardiopulmonary functioning (CPR).
- To identify nursing interventions for promotion, maintenance, and restoration of cardiopulmonary function in all health care settings.
- To describe clinical outcomes for hyperventilation, hypoventilation, and hypoxemia.

KEY TERMS

afterload, p. 557
atelectasis, p. 559
cardiac index (CI), p. 557
cardiac output (CO), p. 557
cardiopulmonary rehabilitation, p. 577
cardiopulmonary resuscitation (CPR), p. 577
chest percussion, p. 574
chest physiotherapy (CPT), p. 573
chest tube, p. 575
compliance, p. 554
cough, p. 563
depolarization, p. 558
diaphragmatic breathing, p. 578
diastolic heart failure, p. 558
diffusion, p. 554
dyspnea, p. 563
dysrhythmia, p. 558
hemoptysis, p. 563
hemothorax, p. 575
high-frequency chest wall compression (HFCWC), p. 575
humidification, p. 572
hypercapnia, p. 556
hyperventilation, p. 556
hypoventilation, p. 556
hypovolemia, p. 558
hypoxemia, p. 555
hypoxia, p. 555
myocardial contractility, p. 557
myocardial infarction, p. 558
myocardial ischemia, p. 558
nebulization, p. 572
normal sinus rhythm (NSR), p. 558
orthopnea, p. 558
oxygen therapy, p. 569
perfusion, p. 554
pleural effusion, p. 575
pneumothorax, p. 575
postural drainage, p. 573
preload, p. 557
productive cough, p. 563
pursed-lip breathing, p. 578
repolarization, p. 558
respiration, p. 554
stress, p. 561
stroke volume (SV), p. 557
surfactant, p. 554
systolic heart failure, p. 558
tension pneumothorax, p. 575
ventilation, p. 554
vibration, p. 574
wheezing, p. 563

INTRODUCTION

Oxygen is a basic human need. The heart and lungs supply the body with oxygen necessary for carrying out the respiratory and metabolic processes needed to sustain life. You will frequently care for patients who are unable to meet their oxygenation needs. This often results from ineffective gas exchange (lungs) or an ineffective pump (heart). Any condition that affects cardiopulmonary functioning directly affects the ability of the body to meet oxygen demands.

CARDIOPULMONARY PHYSIOLOGY

Respiration is the act of breathing with the exchange of oxygen and carbon dioxide (CO_2) during cellular metabolism. The airways of the lung transfer oxygen from the atmosphere to the alveoli, where the oxygen is exchanged for CO_2. Through the alveolar capillary membrane, oxygen transfers to the blood, and CO_2 transfers from the blood to the alveoli. This occurs through the three steps of oxygenation: ventilation, diffusion, and perfusion. **Ventilation** is the movement of air in and out of the lungs, and **diffusion** is the movement of gases between the alveoli and the bloodstream. The heart supports **perfusion**, the transport of oxygenated blood to the cells and tissues (Giddens, 2017; Lewis et al., 2017).

Structure and Function of the Pulmonary System

The pulmonary system consists of two lungs, their numerous airways, the respiratory muscles and chest walls, pleural space, and the blood vessels that support them (Fig. 24.1). The right lung is composed of three lobes: the upper, middle, and lower lobes. The left lung has two lobes: the upper and lower lobes. The trachea enters the thorax and bifurcates, or branches out, into the right and left mainstem bronchus. The bronchi branch into smaller and smaller bronchioles, similar to a tree. The last branch of the airways ends at the alveoli, the exchanging unit of the lung. The blood flows through capillaries around the alveoli, allowing for diffusion of oxygen and CO_2 across the alveolar capillary membrane. The alveoli are lined with a phospholipid, **surfactant**, which decreases the pressure needed to open the alveoli and prevents them from collapsing. Surfactant is essential for normal lung function. Without adequate amounts of surfactant, the alveoli would collapse on expiration, leading to impaired gas exchange.

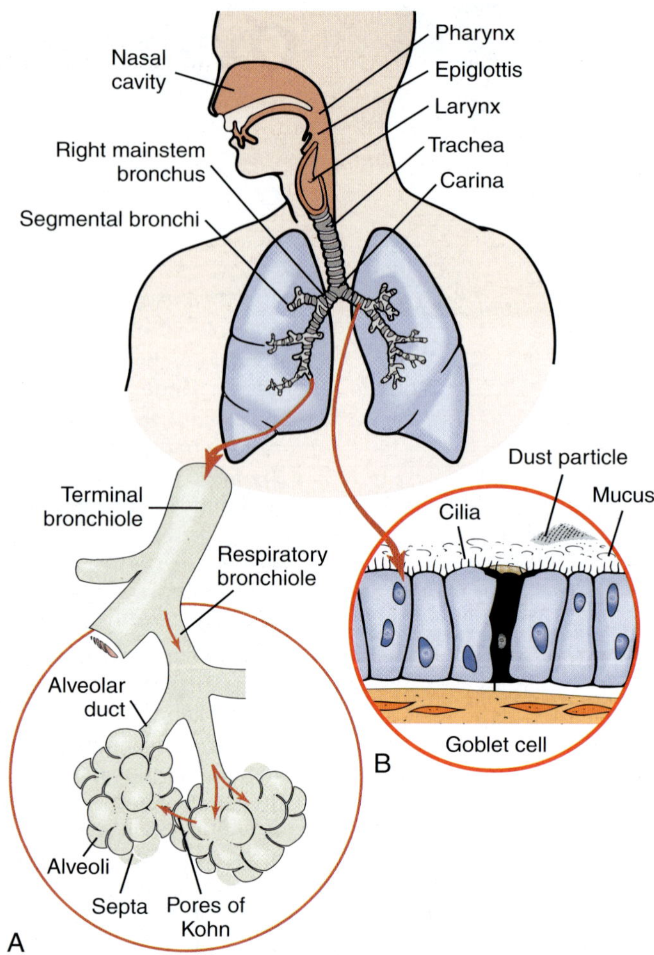

Fig. 24.1 Structures of the respiratory tract. **A,** Pulmonary functional unit. **B,** Ciliated mucous membrane. (From Lewis SM, et al: Medical surgical nursing: assessment and management of clinical problems, ed 10, St Louis, 2017, Mosby.)

Ventilation

Ventilation is the process of moving gases into and out of the lungs. It requires coordination of the muscular and elastic properties of the lungs and thorax. Gases move into and out of the lungs through pressure changes. Intrapleural pressure is negative, or less than atmospheric pressure (760 mm Hg at sea level). For air to flow into the lungs, intrapleural pressure becomes more negative, setting up a pressure gradient between the atmosphere and the alveoli. The diaphragm and external intercostal muscles contract to create a negative pleural pressure and increase the size of the thorax for inspiration. Relaxation of the diaphragm and contraction of the internal intercostal muscles allow air to escape from the lungs.

Successful ventilation depends on neuroreceptors and chemoreceptors in the lungs and central nervous system (CNS), muscles that support inspiration and exhalation, and **compliance**. Compliance is the ability of the lungs to distend or expand in response to increased intra-alveolar pressure. It depends on the elasticity of the lungs and reflects how easily the lungs can expand. Appropriately controlled ventilation provides for adequate oxygen to meet a person's metabolic demands such as exercise, infection, or pregnancy. Ventilation promotes exhalation of metabolically produced CO_2, which is a determinant of acid–base status (see Chapter 25).

Neural and chemical regulators control ventilation. The CNS sends signals to maintain the rhythm and depth of ventilation, respiratory rate, and the balance between inspiration and expiration. Voluntary control of respiration delivers impulses to respiratory motor neurons by way of the spinal cord for control of respiration during speaking, eating, and swimming. Chemical regulation involves the activity of chemoreceptors located in the medulla, aortic bodies, and carotid bodies. Changes in blood concentration of oxygen (O_2), CO_2, and hydrogen ions (H^+) stimulate the chemoreceptors, which stimulate neural regulators to adjust the rate and depth of ventilation to maintain normal arterial blood gas levels. Chemical regulation occurs during physical exercise and emotional distress.

Lung volumes are determined by a person's age, gender, and height. Tidal volume is the amount of air exhaled after a normal inspiration. Residual volume is the amount of air left in the alveoli after a full expiration. Forced vital capacity is the maximum amount of air that can be removed from the lungs during forced expiration (McCance and Huether, 2014).

Oxygen Transport

The delivery of oxygen to the cells and tissues depends on the amount of oxygen entering the lungs (oxygenation) from the atmosphere, the person's ability to exchange gases in the alveoli, and the ability of the heart to pump oxygenated blood to the cells and tissues (MacIntyre, 2014). Ventilation allows for movement of oxygen and CO_2 into and out of the lungs. Once oxygen has reached the alveoli, diffusion occurs. The thickness of the alveolar capillary membrane affects the rate of diffusion. Increased thickness of the membrane impedes diffusion because gas takes longer to transfer across the membrane. Patients with pulmonary edema or effusion have slow diffusion. Normally oxygen crosses the alveolar–capillary membrane and dissolves into the plasma (Fig. 24.2). It then moves into the red blood cells (RBCs) and binds with hemoglobin (Hgb) molecules. Hgb transports most oxygen and serves as a carrier for both oxygen and CO_2. The Hgb molecule combines with oxygen to form oxyhemoglobin. The formation of oxyhemoglobin is easily reversible, allowing Hgb and oxygen to dissociate, which frees oxygen to enter tissues. The amount of dissolved oxygen in the plasma, the amount of Hgb, and the tendency of Hgb to bind with oxygen all influence the capacity of the blood to carry oxygen. Perfusion of oxygenated blood occurs in the capillary beds of the organs and tissues.

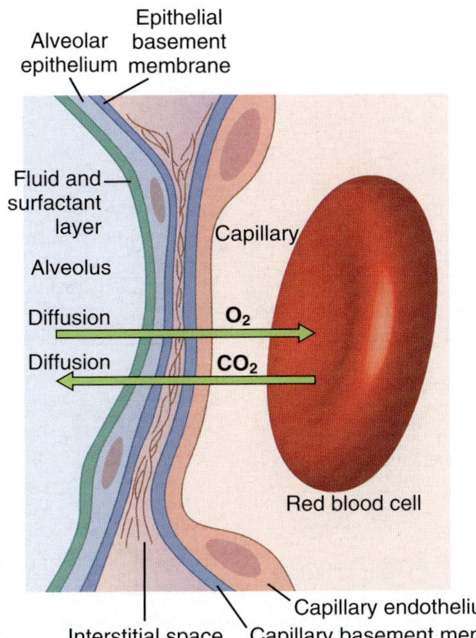

Fig. 24.2 Diffusion: gas-exchange membrane. (From Hall JE: *Guyton and Hall textbook of medical physiology*, ed 13, Philadelphia, 2016, Elsevier.)

Carbon Dioxide Transport

CO_2 is a product of cellular metabolism. The blood carries CO_2 in three ways: (1) dissolved in plasma, (2) as carbamino compounds, and (3) as bicarbonate. At the capillary level, most CO_2 diffuses from the cells into the plasma, and the remaining CO_2 is dissolved in the plasma (PCO_2). The rest of the CO_2 rapidly moves into the RBCs and forms carbonic acid (H_2CO_3). The carbonic acid dissociates (separates) into hydrogen (H^+) and bicarbonate (HCO_3^-) ions. The H^+ ion binds to Hgb, which has released its oxygen, to form HHb and deoxyhemoglobin ($HbCO_2$); 23% of CO_2 is transported as $HbCO_2$. The HCO_3^- ion moves out of the RBCs and back into the plasma (see Chapter 25). To help maintain acid–base balance, 70% of CO_2 is carried as HCO_3^-. Once the CO_2 is transported by the venous blood to the lungs, diffusion occurs again, and CO_2 quickly crosses the permeable gas membrane into the alveoli. Through ventilation, the CO_2 is then exhaled.

ALTERATIONS OF THE PULMONARY SYSTEM: FACTORS AFFECTING VENTILATION AND OXYGEN TRANSPORT

Illnesses and conditions that affect ventilation or oxygen transport alter respiratory functioning. The primary alterations are hypoxia, hypoxemia, hypoventilation, and hyperventilation.

Hypoxia

Hypoxia is a state of inadequate tissue oxygenation. Mild hypoxia stimulates peripheral chemoreceptors to increase heart and respiration rates. The central mechanisms that regulate breathing fail in severe hypoxia, leading to irregular respiration, Cheyne–Stokes respiration, apnea, and respiratory and cardiac failure. The tissues most sensitive to hypoxia are the brain, heart, and liver. Causes of hypoxia typically include the following:

- **Hypoxemia**, or low arterial concentrations of oxygen in the blood
- Inability of the tissues to extract oxygen from the blood, such as in septic shock and cyanide poisoning
- Impaired delivery of oxygen to the tissues, which can be seen in cases of low cardiac output (CO), sepsis, thyroid storm, or exercise (MacIntyre, 2014)
- Obstructive or restrictive pulmonary diseases
- Impaired ventilation from multiple rib fractures, spinal cord injury, neuromuscular diseases, or CNS depression resulting from medications or overdose

Signs and symptoms of hypoxia include tachycardia, tachypnea and dyspnea, peripheral vasoconstriction, dizziness, and mental confusion. Treatment aims to correct the cause and may include oxygen therapy, cardiac and respiratory stimulant drugs, and mechanical ventilation.

Hypoxemia

Hypoxemia is an abnormal deficiency in the concentration of oxygen in arterial blood. Partial pressure of oxygen

(PaO_2) less than 60 mm Hg is typically considered to be hypoxemic. Chronic hypoxemia stimulates RBC production by the bone marrow, leading to secondary polycythemia. Causes of hypoxemia include the following:

- Decreased diffusion of oxygen from the lung (alveoli) into the blood, as in pneumonia, asthma exacerbation, or atelectasis
- High altitudes
- Shunting of blood from the right side of the heart to the left side without exchange of gases in the lungs, as seen in some congenital heart defects

Symptoms of acute hypoxemia are similar to symptoms of hypoxia and include tachypnea, dyspnea, hypertension, hypotension, pallor, cyanosis, mental status changes (e.g., headache, anxiety, impaired judgment, confusion, euphoria, lethargy), and motor function changes (e.g., loss of coordination, weakness, tremors, restlessness, stupor, coma, death). Hypoxemia may also cause dysrhythmias, diaphoresis, blurred or tunnel vision, and nausea and vomiting. Treatment for hypoxemia includes administration of oxygen and correction of the underlying cause.

Hypoventilation

Hypoventilation occurs when ventilation is inadequate to meet the oxygen demands of the body or to have it eliminate CO_2. It can result from a decreased respiratory rate or a breathing pattern that is too shallow. This results in hypoxia or **hypercapnia** (arterial carbon dioxide [$PaCO_2$] level greater than 45 mm Hg) and respiratory acidosis. Causes of hypoventilation include the following:

- Impaired ventilation related to trauma, pain, infection, obstructive diseases (emphysema or sleep apnea), or fluid volume overload
- Alterations in neurological regulation of breathing, such as occurs with head or spinal cord injuries
- Alterations in chemical regulation of breathing

As ventilation decreases, $PaCO_2$ is elevated. Clinical signs and symptoms of hypoventilation include dizziness, occipital headache on awakening, lethargy, disorientation, decreased ability to follow instructions, dysrhythmias, hypertension, seizures, and possible coma or cardiac arrest.

When caring for patients with chronic obstructive pulmonary disease (COPD) and hypercapnia (high CO_2 levels), remember that administering excessive oxygen *may* result in hypoventilation and subsequent decrease in oxygenation. These patients have adapted to the higher CO_2 level, and the CO_2-sensitive chemoreceptors are no longer sensitive to increased CO_2 as a stimulus to breathe. Theoretically, their stimulus to breathe is a decreased PaO_2, or hypoxemia. Administering excessive oxygen to patients with COPD and hypercapnia satisfies the oxygen requirement of the body and *may* negate the stimulus to breathe. However, other factors are associated with the hypoxic drive to breathe, such as ventilation and perfusion. It should also be noted that not every patient with COPD retains CO_2 and has hypercapnia (Lewis et al., 2017).

Any patient with hypoventilation may retain CO_2, which leads to respiratory acidosis and ultimately respiratory arrest. If untreated, a patient's status rapidly declines, and death is possible. Treatment for hypoventilation involves treating the underlying cause, improving tissue oxygenation, restoring ventilation, and achieving acid–base balance.

Hyperventilation

Hyperventilation is an increase in respiratory rate, resulting in excess amounts of CO_2 elimination. This causes a decrease in $PaCO_2$, or hypocapnia, and respiratory alkalosis. Causes of hyperventilation include severe anxiety, infection, head injury, medications (e.g., stimulants), and acid–base imbalance. Acute anxiety and the subsequent increased respiratory rate may cause loss of consciousness from excess CO_2 exhalation. An increase of 1°F in body temperature causes a 7% increase in metabolic rate, thereby increasing CO_2 production. The clinical response is increased rate and depth of respiration. Hypoxia associated with pulmonary embolus or shock also results in hyperventilation.

Hyperventilation produces signs and symptoms of tachycardia, shortness of breath, chest pain, dizziness, lightheadedness, decreased concentration, paresthesia, circumoral and/or extremity numbness, tinnitus, blurred vision, and disorientation. Treatment involves treating the underlying cause, improving tissue oxygenation, restoring ventilation, reducing respiratory rate, and achieving acid–base balance.

STRUCTURE AND FUNCTION OF THE CIRCULATORY SYSTEM

The circulatory system delivers oxygen, nutrients, and other substances to bodily tissues to support cellular life. During cellular metabolism, waste products accumulate. The system then removes waste products such as CO_2 and delivers them to the lungs and/or kidneys, where the wastes are eliminated. The pumping action of the heart supports the circulatory system. The four heart valves (tricuspid, pulmonic, mitral, and aortic) ensure the one-way flow of blood through the heart (Fig. 24.3).

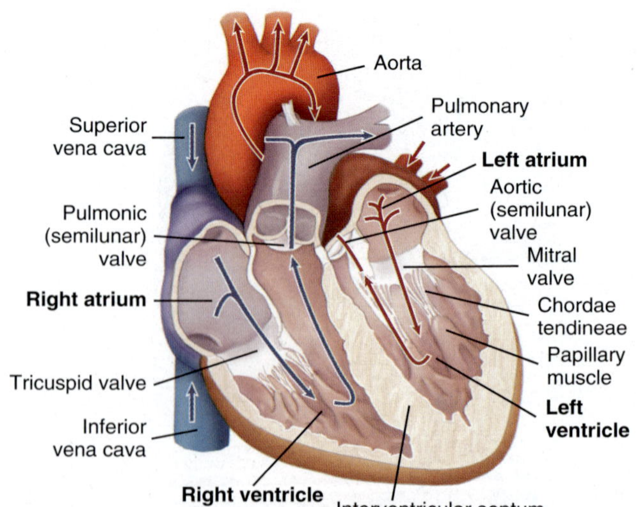

Fig. 24.3 Schematic representation of blood flow through the heart. Arrows indicate direction of flow. (Modified from Lewis SM, et al: *Medical surgical nursing: assessment and management of clinical problems*, ed 10, St Louis, 2017, Mosby.)

Regulation of Blood Flow

There are multiple regulators of blood flow (Table 24.1). The heart muscle (myocardium) relaxes and contracts to support the regulation of blood flow. A cardiac cycle consists of two phases, contraction and relaxation. The contraction phase, also called systole, occurs when blood is ejected from the ventricles into the systemic circulation. The relaxation phase is called diastole, in which blood fills the ventricles.

The amount of blood ejected from the left ventricle each minute is termed **cardiac output (CO)**. A normal CO for a healthy adult is 4–8 L/min. The CO is calculated as follows:

$$\text{CO} = \text{Stroke volume (SV)} \times \text{Heart rate (HR)}$$

Table 24.1 Regulation of Blood Flow

Regulator	Definition
Cardiac output (CO)	Amount of blood ejected from the ventricles per minute Normal range (adult): 4–8 L/min
Cardiac index (CI)	Measure of adequacy of CO: CI equals CO divided by the patient's body surface area Normal range (adult): 2.5–4 L/min/m^3
Stroke volume	Amount of blood ejected from the ventricle with each contraction Normal range (adult): 50–75 mL per contraction
Preload	Amount of blood remaining in the ventricles at end of diastole, before the next contraction
Afterload	Resistance of the ejection of blood from the left ventricle
Myocardial contractility	Ability of the heart to contract and eject blood from the ventricles and prepare for the next contraction

Stroke volume (SV) is the amount of blood ejected from the ventricle with each contraction. The normal range for a healthy adult is 50–75 mL per contraction. SV is determined by preload, afterload, and myocardial contractility. **Preload** is the amount of blood at the end of ventricular diastole, before the next contraction. **Afterload** is the resistance to the ejection of blood from the left ventricle. The left ventricular pressure must be greater than the peripheral pressure to eject blood from the heart. **Myocardial contractility** is the ability of the heart to squeeze blood from the ventricles and prepare for the next contraction. Contractility is difficult to accurately measure because preload, afterload, and HR must remain constant. The HR, or beats per minute, is regulated by the sympathetic and parasympathetic systems. Normal limits for HR are between 60 and 100 beats/min. **Cardiac index** (CI) is a measure of adequacy of the CO. This calculation gives health care providers a more accurate calculation of cardiac function because it is more patient specific.

Conduction System

The heart's conduction system generates impulses that initiate the electrical/mechanical chain of events for a normal heartbeat. The rhythmic relaxation and contraction of the atria and ventricles depend on continuous, organized transmission of electrical impulses to the muscle. The conduction system generates, controls, and transmits these impulses (Fig. 24.4). The autonomic nervous system influences the rate of impulse generation, the transmission speed through the conductive pathway, and the strength of contractions through sympathetic and parasympathetic nerve fibers in the atria and ventricles. The vagus nerve (parasympathetic) also innervates sinoatrial (SA) and atrioventricular (AV) nodes and is able to reduce the rate of impulse generation.

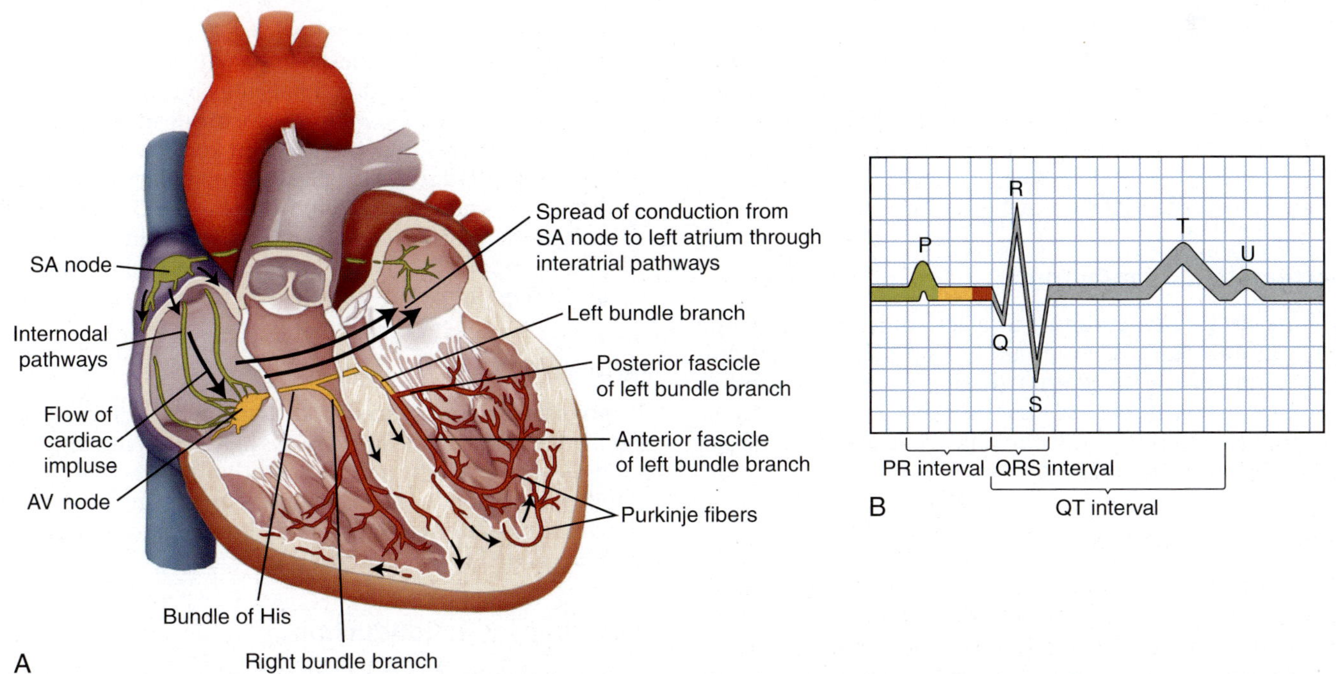

Fig. 24.4 Conduction system of the heart. *AV*, atrioventricular; *LA*, left atrium; *LV*, left ventricle; *RA*, right atrium; *RV*, right ventricle; *SA*, sinoatrial. (From Lewis SM, et al: *Medical surgical nursing: assessment and management of clinical problems*, ed 10, St Louis, 2017, Mosby.)

The conduction system originates with the **SA node**, the "pacemaker" of the heart. The SA node is in the right atrium next to the entrance of the superior vena cava. Impulses begin at the SA node at an intrinsic rate of 60–100 beats/min. Electrical impulses travel along interatrial and internodal pathways to the **AV node**. The AV node mediates impulse transmission between the atria and the ventricles. Delaying the impulse at the AV node before transmitting it through the bundle of His and ventricular Purkinje network assists atrial emptying.

An electrocardiogram (ECG) records the electrical activity of the conduction system as waves and complexes. It monitors the rate, regularity, and path of the electrical impulse through the conduction system; however, it does not reflect the muscular work of the heart. The normal sequence of electrical impulses on the ECG is called **normal sinus rhythm (NSR)** (see Fig. 24.4). A normal ECG waveform consists of a P wave (atrial **depolarization**), QRS complex (ventricular depolarization), and T wave (ventricular **repolarization**). Depolarization is the electrical event occurring just before contraction of the cardiac chambers, whereas repolarization reflects the period of time when the heart is resting and the chambers are filling. Health care providers interpret the size, appearance, and sequence of waves to identify dysrhythmias and recognize the area of the heart affected.

ALTERATIONS OF THE CIRCULATORY SYSTEM

Conditions that affect cardiac rate, rhythm, strength of contraction, blood flow through the chambers, myocardial blood flow, and peripheral circulation alter cardiac functioning. Controllable risk factors for heart disease include smoking, hypertension, physical inactivity, obesity, diabetes, alcohol intake, high-fat/high-sodium diets, and high low-density lipoprotein (LDL or "bad cholesterol") levels and low high-density lipoprotein (HDL or "good cholesterol") levels. Uncontrollable risk factors include male gender, family history of heart disease, and ethnicity (Centers for Disease Control and Prevention [CDC], 2015a). Black people, Caucasians, and Hispanics are at the greatest risk (Mozaffarian et al., 2015). Several genetic disorders lead to an increased risk of early heart attacks.

Decreased Cardiac Output

Failure of the myocardium to eject sufficient CO to the systemic and pulmonary circulations results in heart failure. Failure of the myocardial pump results from primary coronary artery disease (CAD), valvular disorders, cardiomyopathic conditions, congenital heart defects, conduction disorders, and pulmonary disease.

Myocardial Ischemia

Myocardial ischemia occurs when the coronary artery does not supply sufficient blood to the heart muscle (myocardium). This condition results in chest pain, especially with activity. Angina pectoris is the result of decreased blood flow to the myocardium, often as a result of coronary artery spasms or other temporary constriction of the coronary arteries. When decreased myocardial blood perfusion is extensive or perfusion is completely blocked, the tissue becomes necrotic, and **myocardial infarction** occurs. Symptoms of myocardial infarction include severe or crushing chest pain, jaw pain, left arm pain, shortness of breath, and diaphoresis. Some people, particularly women, present with nonspecific symptoms of discomfort, weakness, and fatigue.

Impaired Valvular Function

Valvular heart disease is an acquired or congenital disorder of a cardiac valve characterized by stenosis, which obstructs blood flow, or valvular degeneration and regurgitation, which result in backflow of blood. When stenosis occurs in the aortic and pulmonic valves, the adjacent ventricles work harder to move the ventricular volume beyond the stenotic valve. When regurgitation occurs, there is a backflow of blood into an adjacent chamber, which causes either pulmonary or systemic congestion.

Left-Sided Heart Failure

Left-sided heart failure is characterized by impaired functioning of the left ventricle. It can be further classified as either systolic or diastolic failure. **Systolic heart failure** is an inability of the ventricle to adequately eject blood. **Diastolic heart failure** is the inability of the ventricle to relax and fill with blood during diastole. Left-sided heart failure is typically because of hypertension or CAD. In this type of heart failure, blood eventually backs up into the pulmonary veins, causing patients to present with pulmonary symptoms such as crackles on auscultation and complaints of fatigue, dyspnea, and **orthopnea** (difficulty breathing while lying down) (Lewis et al., 2017).

Right-Sided Heart Failure

Right-sided heart failure results from impaired functioning of the right ventricle, which is typically caused by pulmonary disease or pulmonary hypertension. An increase in pressure in the pulmonary system causes increased resistance in the right ventricle. The right ventricle fails as a result of this pressure. The patient then develops venous congestion in the systemic circulation, and on assessment you often identify distended jugular veins and peripheral edema. Right-sided heart failure may also result from untreated or end-stage left-sided heart failure.

Hypovolemia

Hypovolemia is a reduced circulating blood volume resulting from extracellular fluid losses that occurs in conditions such as shock and severe dehydration. If the fluid loss is significant, the body tries to adapt by increasing the HR and constricting peripheral vessels to increase the volume of blood returned to the heart and the CO.

Disturbances in Conduction

A **dysrhythmia** is a disturbance in the formation or conduction of the heart's electrical impulse. Any rhythm not generated at the SA node is classified as a dysrhythmia.

Dysrhythmias are primary conduction disturbances that occur as a response to ischemia, valvular abnormalities, anxiety, and drug toxicity (e.g., digoxin toxicity). They also occur as a result of excess caffeine, alcohol, or tobacco use; following cardiothoracic surgery; or as a complication of acid–base or electrolyte imbalance, such as altered serum potassium levels (see Chapter 25).

Dysrhythmias are classified by their site of origin and cardiac response. The cardiac response can be an increase in HR such as tachycardia (greater than 100 beats/min), a decrease in HR such as bradycardia (less than 60 beats/min), premature (early beat) atrial or ventricular beats, or blocked (delayed or absent beat) atrial or ventricular beats. Dysrhythmias often affect the pumping mechanism of the heart.

FACTORS AFFECTING OXYGENATION

Alterations in oxygenation result from a decrease in oxygen-carrying capacity of blood, decreased inspired oxygen concentration, an increase in the metabolic demands of the body, and any alteration that affects a patient's chest wall movement.

Decreased Oxygen-Carrying Capacity

The Hgb molecule carries 97% of oxygen. Any process that decreases or alters Hgb, such as anemia or inhalation of toxic substances, decreases the oxygen-carrying capacity of blood. Anemia is the reduction in the number of RBCs or a decrease in Hgb, the oxygen-carrying protein of RBCs. Acute blood loss or certain chronic diseases can result in anemia.

Carbon monoxide, a colorless and odorless gas, is a common toxic inhalant that decreases the oxygen-carrying capacity of blood. It has a 230–300 times greater affinity for Hgb than oxygen, which can create a functional hypoxemia (Huether and McCance, 2017). Because of the strength of the bond, it is not easy for carbon monoxide to dissociate (break away) from Hgb, making it unavailable for oxygen transport.

Decreased Inspired Oxygen Concentration

When the concentration of inspired oxygen declines, the oxygen-carrying capacity of the blood decreases. An upper or lower airway obstruction limiting delivery of inspired oxygen to alveoli decreases the fraction of inspired oxygen concentration (FiO_2). Decreased environmental oxygen (the effect at high altitudes) or decreased delivery of inspired oxygen (e.g., incorrect oxygen concentration setting on respiratory therapy equipment) results in decreased FiO_2.

Increased Metabolic Rate

Increases in metabolism increase oxygen demand. Oxygen levels fall when the body is unable to meet an increased oxygen demand. An increased metabolism is a normal response of the body to pregnancy, infection, fever, wound healing, and exercise. Most people are able to meet increased oxygen demands and do not display signs of oxygen deprivation.

In patients with increased metabolic rates, CO_2 production also increases. If the condition, such as a fever, lasts for a period of time and the metabolic rate remains high, the body begins to break down protein stores resulting in muscle wasting and decreased muscle mass. Respiratory muscles such as the diaphragm and intercostals are also wasted. The body attempts to adapt to the increased CO_2 (hypercapnia) levels by increasing the rate and depth of respiration to eliminate the excess CO_2. The patient's work of breathing increases, and the patient eventually displays signs and symptoms of hypoxemia, such as anxiety and restlessness.

As the hypoxemia worsens, some patients develop cardiac dysrhythmias, develop cyanosis, and/or lose consciousness. Patients with pulmonary diseases are at greater risk for hypoxemia and hypercapnia (elevated $PaCO_2$ level). Patient assessments often show an increased rate and depth of respiration along with pursed-lip breathing and use of accessory muscles for respiration.

Conditions Affecting Chest Wall Movement

Any condition that reduces chest wall movement decreases ventilation. If the diaphragm is unable to fully descend with breathing, the volume of inspired air decreases, delivering less oxygen to the alveoli and subsequently to tissues.

Musculoskeletal Abnormalities

Thoracic abnormalities such as abnormal structural shapes and muscle disease contribute to decreased oxygenation and ventilation. Structural abnormalities impairing oxygenation include conditions that affect the rib cage such as pectus excavatum and those that affect the spinal column such as kyphosis or scoliosis. The angle of curvature in kyphosis or scoliosis can progress with time, resulting in severe hypoventilation and eventual hypoxemia. Muscle diseases such as muscular dystrophy decrease diaphragmatic movement (i.e., the patient's ability to expand and contract the chest). This impairs ventilation and often causes **atelectasis** (collapsed alveoli), hypercapnia, and hypoxemia.

Nervous System Diseases

Myasthenia gravis and Guillain–Barré syndrome are examples of nervous system diseases that result in hypoventilation. These diseases impair nervous and muscular control, causing reduced ventilation (hypoventilation).

Disease or trauma involving the brain stem and spinal cord can impair respiration. When the brain stem is affected, neural regulation of respiration is damaged, and abnormal breathing patterns develop. Damage to the spinal cord affects respiration in two ways. If the phrenic nerve is damaged, the diaphragm does not descend, reducing inspiratory lung volumes and causing hypoxemia. Cervical trauma at C3–C5 levels can paralyze the phrenic nerve. Spinal cord trauma below the fifth cervical vertebra usually leaves the phrenic nerve intact but damages nerves that innervate the intercostal muscles, preventing anteroposterior chest expansion.

Trauma

Trauma to the chest wall also impairs inspiration. The patient with multiple rib fractures sometimes develops a flail chest, a life-threatening condition in which fractures cause instability in part of the chest wall. This causes paradoxical breathing in which the lung underlying the injured area contracts on inspiration and expands on expiration, making ventilation ineffective. Chest wall or upper abdominal incisions also decrease chest wall movement because incisional pain causes patients to inhale shallowly, which decreases chest wall movement.

Developmental Factors

The age and developmental level of a patient as well as the normal aging process can affect tissue oxygenation. Thus, you need to identify developmental risk factors in your patients.

Premature Infants

Premature infants are at risk for respiratory distress syndrome, which is caused by surfactant deficiency and immature lung development. Surfactant is a chemical in the lung that maintains the integrity of the alveoli, preventing alveolar collapse. When surfactant is inadequate, infants are unable to keep their alveoli open, which impedes the exchange of respiratory gases. The surfactant-synthesizing ability of the lung develops at about 24 weeks of gestation, but surfactant-producing cells are not fully mature until 36 weeks of gestation. Premature infants are at risk for developing long-term lung issues such as chronic lung disease (bronchopulmonary dysplasia), particularly if they need mechanical ventilation or supplemental oxygen therapy. Premature infants and children younger than 1 year are at increased risk for contracting respiratory illnesses such as respiratory syncytial virus (Hockenberry et al., 2017).

Infants and Toddlers

Healthy full-term infants younger than 3 months are presumed to have a lower infection rate because of the protective function of maternal antibodies. The infection rate increases in infants from 3 to 6 months of age. Infants and toddlers are at risk for upper respiratory tract infections, especially when they are exposed to secondhand smoke or other children. Upper respiratory tract infections are usually not dangerous, and infants and toddlers recover with little difficulty. Infants and toddlers are also at risk for airway obstruction because of their anatomically smaller airways and their tendency to place foreign objects in the mouth (Hockenberry et al., 2017).

School-Age Children and Adolescents

School-age children and adolescents are exposed to respiratory infections and respiratory risk factors such as secondhand smoke and are at risk to experiment with cigarette smoking and other recreational inhalants. A healthy child usually does not have adverse pulmonary effects from respiratory infections. However, a person who starts smoking in adolescence and continues to smoke into middle age has an increased risk for cardiopulmonary disease and lung cancer. School-age children and adolescents possess other cardiopulmonary disease risk factors such as obesity, inactive lifestyles, unhealthy diets, and excessive use of caffeinated or other energy drinks (Hockenberry et al., 2017).

Young and Middle-Age Adults

Young and middle-age adults are exposed to many cardiopulmonary risk factors including an unhealthy diet, lack of exercise, stress, excessive use of highly caffeinated energy drinks, and cigarette smoking. Reducing these modifiable factors sometimes decreases a patient's risk for cardiac or pulmonary diseases. Pregnancy causes changes in ventilation. As the fetus grows during pregnancy, the enlarged uterus pushes abdominal contents up against the diaphragm. During the last trimester of pregnancy, the inspiratory capacity declines, resulting in dyspnea on exertion and increased fatigue.

Older Adults

The cardiac and pulmonary systems change throughout the aging process (Table 24.2). Normal changes of aging place an older adult at risk for complications in oxygenation, particularly when hospitalized. Older adults are at increased risk for the development of influenza and community-acquired pneumonia, which sometimes results in death. Because of these risks, this age group should have the pneumonia vaccine and an annual flu vaccine (CDC, 2016b, 2016c).

Lifestyle Factors

Patients are exposed to numerous lifestyle factors that, either alone or in combination, affect cardiopulmonary function. Knowledge of these factors enables a nurse to consider the health promotion needs of patients.

Nutrition

Good nutrition affects cardiopulmonary function by supporting normal metabolic functions. A poor diet leads to risk factors affecting the heart and lungs such as obesity, hypertension, heart disease, and chronic lung disease. Inadequate nutrition occurs when nutritional intake does not meet nutritional needs of the body. Without essential nutrients, a patient may experience respiratory muscle wasting resulting in decreased muscle strength and respiratory excursion. Cough efficiency is reduced secondary to respiratory muscle weakness, putting a patient at risk for retention of pulmonary secretions. A patient with chronic lung disease usually requires a diet higher in calories because of the increased work of breathing. A diet with a moderate amount of carbohydrates is recommended to prevent an increase in CO_2 production.

Obesity affects the respiratory and the cardiovascular systems. It leads to a decrease in lung expansion and an increase in oxygen demand to meet metabolic needs. Diets high in fat increase cholesterol and development of plaque in the coronary arteries, placing individuals at risk for CAD. Patients with nutritional alterations are at risk for anemia. There is a reduction in oxygen-carrying capacity if the diet has insufficient iron needed for Hgb and RBC synthesis.

Hydration

Fluid intake is essential for cellular health. It depends on a patient's diet and disease processes that require more or less water. Fluid volume overload or hypervolemia may lead to vascular congestion in patients with heart, kidney, or lung diseases. Dehydration or fluid volume deficit may result in dizziness, fainting, hypotension, a decrease in respiratory secretion production, or a thickening of respiratory secretions making it difficult for a patient to expectorate secretions.

Table 24.2 Changes in the Aging Cardiopulmonary System

Function	Pathophysiological Changes	Key Clinical Findings
HEART		
Muscle contraction	Ventricular wall thickened, collagen increased, and elastin decreased in heart muscle	Signs of decreased cardiac output (edema, shortness of breath, activity intolerance, inability to lie flat for extended time)
Blood flow	Heart valves, especially mitral and aortic valves, become thicker and stiffen	Systolic ejection murmur
Conduction system	SA node becomes fibrotic from calcification; decrease in number of pacemaker cells in SA node	Increased P–R, QRS, and Q–T intervals; decreased amplitude of the QRS complex; tachycardia more poorly tolerated
Arterial vessel compliance	Vessels become calcified; loss of arterial distensibility, decreased elastin in vessel walls, more tortuous vessels	Hypertension, with increase in systolic blood pressure
LUNGS		
Breathing mechanics	Decreased chest wall compliance and loss of elastic recoil Decreased respiratory muscle mass and strength	Prolonged exhalation phase Decreased vital capacity and activity intolerance Decreased ability to clear secretions
Oxygenation	Decreased alveolar surface area because alveoli are more fibrous, and decreased CO_2 diffusion capacity	Decreased PaO_2 Slightly increased $PaCO_2$
Breathing control/breathing pattern	Decreased responsiveness of central and peripheral chemoreceptors to hypoxemia and hypercapnia	Decreased tidal volume Increased respiratory rate
Lung defense mechanisms	Decreased number of cilia Decreased IgA production and humoral and cellular immunity Drier mucous membranes	Decreased airway clearance Increased risk for infection
Sleep and breathing	Decreased respiratory drive Decreased tone of upper airway muscles	Increased risk for aspiration and infection Snoring/obstructive sleep apnea

CO_2, carbon dioxide; *IgA*, immunoglobulin A; *$PaCO_2$*, partial pressure of carbon dioxide; *PaO_2*, partial pressure of oxygen; *SA*, sinoatrial.

Data from Ball J, et al: *Seidel's guide to physical examination*, ed 9, St Louis, 2015, Elsevier; and Touhy T, Jett K: *Gerontological nursing and healthy aging*, ed 5, St Louis, 2018 Elsevier.

Exercise

Exercise increases metabolic activity and oxygen demand of the body. The rate and depth of respiration increase, enabling a person to inhale more oxygen and exhale excess CO_2. A physical exercise program has many benefits (see Chapter 14). People who exercise daily for 30–60 minutes have a lower HR, lower blood pressure, decreased cholesterol, increased blood flow, and greater oxygen extraction by working muscles. The addition of weight training decreases the work of the heart by increasing the efficiency of the other muscles of the body.

Cigarette Smoking

Cigarette smoking is associated with heart disease, COPD, and lung cancer. Inhaled nicotine enables plaque to build up more quickly in the blood vessels, increases the risks for blood clot formation, and causes vasoconstriction in the coronary and peripheral vessels. The risk for lung cancer is 15–30 times greater for a person who smokes than for a nonsmoker. Exposure to secondhand smoke increases the risk for lung cancer in a person who does not smoke and worsens other pulmonary problems such as asthma or COPD (CDC, 2016a).

Substance Abuse

Excessive use of alcohol and other drugs impairs tissue oxygenation. A patient who has chronic substance abuse usually has a poor nutritional intake that often causes a decreased intake of iron-rich foods leading to a decrease in Hgb production. Excessive use of alcohol and drugs such as barbiturates depresses the respiratory center, reducing the rate and depth of respiration and the amount of inhaled oxygen. Substances that are inhaled or smoked directly injure lung tissue, leading to permanent lung damage and impaired oxygenation. I.v. drug use places a person at risk for infections of the heart (endocarditis or myocarditis), blood clots, and transmitted diseases such as human immunodeficiency virus (HIV) and hepatitis.

Stress

Stress is a perceived threat that results in sympathetic stimulation (the fight-or-flight response). It often poses a demand that exceeds a patient's coping ability both physically and emotionally (see Chapter 31). Continuous stress adversely affects a patient's health and well-being. A continuous state of stress increases the metabolic rate and oxygen demand of the body. The body responds to stress by an increased rate and depth of respiration and increased CO. Stressors also alter the normal response to illness and pain. Stress causes an increased release of cortisol, which affects the metabolism of fat and creates a risk for CAD and hypertension. Stressors are also often triggers for asthma attacks. Most people are able to adapt to physical or emotional stressors. Some patients, particularly patients with chronic illnesses or acute life-threatening illnesses, cannot tolerate the oxygen demands associated with stress.

Environmental Factors

The environment also influences oxygenation. The incidence of pulmonary disease is higher in smoggy, urban areas than in rural areas. In addition, a patient's workplace sometimes increases the risks for cardiopulmonary disease. Occupational pollutants include asbestos, talcum powder, dust, and airborne fibers. For example, tunnel workers exposed to dust from blasting, drilling, and rock transport have an increased risk for developing COPD. Construction workers may be at risk for asbestosis from asbestos exposure. This exposure leads to pulmonary fibrosis, a restrictive lung disease, and may lead to lung cancer.

NURSING PROCESS

Assessment

During assessment, thoroughly assess each patient and critically analyze findings to ensure that you make patient-centered clinical decisions for safe patient care.

Nursing History

The nursing history focuses on your patient's ability to meet oxygen needs and control symptoms. Ask questions that help a patient describe symptoms. Box 24.1 gives examples of assessment questions for you to ask your patient with cardiopulmonary conditions.

Risk Factors

Investigate familial, occupational, and environmental risk factors. Review the patient's family history of cardiovascular or lung disease. Document which blood relatives have cardiopulmonary disease, the type of condition, and their present level of health or age at time of death. Other family risk factors to assess include the presence of infectious diseases, particularly tuberculosis (TB). Determine who in the patient's household has the disease and the status of the treatment.

Exposure to certain inhaled environmental substances such as smog, cotton dust, silicon, mold, cockroaches, secondhand smoke, and asbestos is closely linked to respiratory disease. Investigate exposures in the patient's home and workplace. Ask the following questions:

- Are there environmental conditions that affect your breathing where you work?
- Have you recently traveled to countries or areas of the United States where you have been exposed to uncommon respiratory diseases?
- What is/was your occupation? Were you exposed to chemicals or inhalants?

Assess for other risk factors such as exercise habits, presence and frequency of stress, tobacco use, and diet. Ask a patient to record what is eaten over 1 week to assess dietary habits and types of food eaten.

Fatigue

Fatigue is a subjective sensation reported as a loss of endurance. It is a common sign of prolonged exposure to stress and is often an early sign of worsening of an existing chronic cardiopulmonary disease. A visual analog scale is useful to objectively measure fatigue. Have patients rate their fatigue from 0 to 10, with 10 being the worst level of fatigue and 0 being no fatigue. Ask your patients the following questions about their perception of fatigue:

- When did you first notice the fatigue? What makes it get better or worse?
- Was the onset sudden or gradual? Is it related to any time of the day or is it constant throughout the day?
- In what way does the fatigue affect what you want to do?

Pain

Pain originating in the heart does not occur with respiratory variations. It is most often substernal and typically radiates to the left arm and jaw in men. Some women as well as some men have epigastric pain, complaints of indigestion, nausea

BOX 24.1 Nursing Assessment Questions

Nature of Cardiopulmonary Problem

- Tell me the types of breathing problems you are having.
- Describe the problem you are having with your heart. Is there pain? Do you notice abnormal beats?
- Does this problem occur at a specific time during the day, after exercise, or all the time?

Questions to Ask Associated With Breathing

- How has your breathing pattern changed?
- On a scale of 0–10, with 10 being the most severe, rate your shortness of breath.
- What helps your shortness of breath?
- Do you have a cough? Is the coughing increasing? Is it worse at a certain time of day?
- Describe your cough. Is it dry or moist?
- Are you having sputum or phlegm with coughing? What does it look like? Is this different? If so, when did you notice the change?

Questions to Ask Related to Chest Pain

- Are you having any chest pain? Show me where the pain is located. Does it occur with breathing in, breathing out, or both?
- What do you think causes the pain, and how long does it last? Is this a different type of pain? Does it occur with activity?
- On a scale of 0–10, with 0 being no pain and 10 the most severe pain, rate your chest pain at its worst. Is the severity of your pain different today?
- What do you do for this pain? Does it make the pain better?

Questions to Ask Regarding Predisposing Factors

- Have you been around another person who had a cold, flu, or other respiratory illness?
- Tell me the medications you are taking. Are you taking any over-the-counter medications or any supplements? What are these?
- Do you smoke? If so, how much?
- Have you been exposed to secondhand smoke?

Questions to Ask Regarding Effect of Symptoms on Patient

- Tell me how these symptoms affect your daily activities. What effect do these symptoms have on your appetite, sleeping, and activity?

or vomiting, or a choking feeling and dyspnea. Pericardial pain resulting from an inflammation of the pericardial sac is usually nonradiating and often occurs with inspiration or when lying supine. See Chapter 11 for pain assessment.

Pleuritic chest pain is peripheral and usually radiates to the scapular regions. Inspiratory maneuvers such as coughing, yawning, and sighing aggravate pleuritic chest pain. An inflammation or infection in the pleural space usually causes pleuritic chest pain. Patients often describe it as knife-like or sharp, and it increases in intensity with inspiration. Musculoskeletal pain is often present following exercise, rib trauma, and prolonged coughing episodes. Inspiratory movements aggravate the pain and are easily confused with pleuritic chest pain. When assessing pain in patients with cardiopulmonary disease, obtain information specific to cardiac or inspiratory pain (see Box 24.1).

Breathing Patterns

Dyspnea can be a subjective feeling of breathlessness as reported by the patient, or it can be observable labored breathing with shortness of breath (Ball et al., 2015). It is a clinical sign of hypoxia and/or hypoxemia. Dyspnea is associated with symptoms such as exaggerated respiratory effort, use of the accessory muscles of respiration, nasal flaring, and marked increases in the rate and depth of respirations. Collect data about your patient's breathing patterns. Use a visual analog scale to help patients objectively assess their perception of dyspnea (see Box 24.1). This will help to show change in a patient's breathlessness over time.

Dyspnea that occurs when a patient is sleeping is called paroxysmal nocturnal dyspnea (PND). The patient awakens in a panic, feels as if he or she is suffocating, and has a strong need to sit up to relieve the breathlessness. The cause of PND is probably resorption of fluid from dependent body areas when the patient is recumbent or reclining (Lewis et al., 2017).

Orthopnea is an abnormal condition in which a patient has difficulty breathing when lying down and has to use multiple pillows or to sit to breathe. The number of pillows required for sleep (e.g., two or three) quantifies the presence and severity of orthopnea.

Wheezing is not a breathing pattern but is a high-pitched musical sound caused by high-velocity movement of air through a narrowed airway. It is present in asthma, acute bronchitis, or pneumonia. It occurs on inspiration, expiration, or both. Determine any precipitating factors such as respiratory infection, allergens, exercise, or stress.

Cough

Cough is a sudden, audible expulsion of air from the lungs. Coughing is a protective reflex to clear the trachea, bronchi, and lungs of irritants and secretions. Some patients with chronic sinusitis cough only in the early morning, while trying to sleep, or immediately after rising from sleep. This clears the airway of sputum resulting from sinus drainage. Patients with chronic bronchitis generally produce sputum all day, although the body produces greater amounts after rising from a semirecumbent or flat position. A **productive cough** produces sputum that is swallowed or expectorated. Collect data about the type, color, and quantity of sputum.

If a patient reports **hemoptysis** (bloody sputum), determine the source. Is it associated with coughing and bleeding from the upper respiratory tract, from sinus drainage, or from the gastrointestinal tract (hematemesis)? Describe the hemoptysis including amount, color, duration of bleeding, and presence of sputum. When hemoptysis develops, note whether the patient is on anticoagulants.

Respiratory Infections

Determine whether your patient has had a pneumococcal, pertussis, or flu vaccine in the past. Determine whether the patient is on immunomodulators or immunosuppressant therapy or has a chronic lung disease because these patients are at higher risk of developing respiratory infections. Ask about any known exposure to TB and the results of the tuberculin skin test including type of test and date. Some patients with a history of i.v. drug use, blood transfusions, multiple unprotected sex partners, or a homosexual lifestyle are at a higher risk for developing HIV/acquired immunodeficiency syndrome (AIDS) infection. Patients with HIV/AIDS or in other immunocompromised states are at an increased risk of contracting a respiratory infection.

Medication Use

Assess your patient's knowledge and ability to correctly take medication (see Chapter 26). Include a family caregiver in your assessment if the caregiver assists with medication preparation or administration. Review what the patient understands about medication side effects and what or when to report to the health care provider.

Many herbals and over-the-counter (OTC) medications affect the HR and blood pressure and promote blood thinning. For example, the herb ma huang, a naturally occurring ephedrine, increases blood pressure and HR. Patients with cardiopulmonary disease should not use this herb. Patients with asthma should not use ephedrine-containing herbs because they can cause increased bronchospasm and respiratory arrest. Ginseng, garlic capsules, and *Ginkgo biloba* have properties similar to those of aspirin and decrease platelet aggregation, increasing the patient's risk for bleeding.

Illicit drugs often come diluted with talcum powder. This mixture causes pulmonary disorders resulting from the irritant effect of talcum powder on lung tissues.

Older Adult Considerations

The older adult has a wide range of normal HR, from the 40s to more than 100 beats/min (Ball et al., 2015). When assessing older adults, additional assessment areas include functional and cognitive status, caregiver stress, patterns of health and health care, advanced directive and care planning, and the presence of geriatric syndromes (e.g., delirium, falls, dizziness, syncope, urinary incontinence). Other areas of assessment include sexual function, depression, alcoholism, hearing loss, and environmental safety (Touhy and Jett, 2018). Table 24.2 reviews factors that place older adults at increased risk for respiratory infections.

Patient Expectations

Knowing what a patient expects regarding his or her health and disease maintenance determines short-term and long-term needs and goals of care and the interventions needed to achieve the needs and goals. Knowing what a patient expects also helps you find appropriate educational tools and resources for the patient and family to use while at home. Determine what your patient expects from health care providers and other caregivers. Develop trust with patients and family caregivers and encourage them to be active participants in the development of a treatment plan.

Physical Examination

The physical examination includes a detailed, organized, and systematic evaluation of the entire cardiopulmonary system (Tables 24.3–24.5) (see Chapter 7). Be mindful of your patient's limitations such as breathlessness or fatigue. In some cases, you have to complete your assessment in short sections to allow the patient to rest and recover. If your patient is breathless or fatigued, you may ask closed-ended questions with yes or no answers. Focus your initial assessment on your patient's immediate problems (Table 24.6).

Measurement of Oxygen Saturation (Pulse Oximetry)

Pulse oximetry is the indirect measurement of **oxygen saturation** and is the fifth vital sign (see Chapter 6 and Skill 6.4). The pulse oximeter contains a photoelectric sensor with two light-emitting diodes (LEDs) of differing wavelengths that measures the SpO_2 level. SpO_2 stands for peripheral **capillary oxygen saturation**, an estimate of the amount of oxygen in the blood. More specifically, it is

Table 24.3 Inspection of Cardiopulmonary Status

Abnormality	Cause
EYES	
Xanthelasma (yellow lipid lesions in nasal portion of upper or lower eyelid)	Hyperlipidemia; abnormal lipid metabolism
Petechiae on conjunctivae	Bacterial endocarditis or bleeding disorder
SKIN	
Peripheral cyanosis	Vasoconstriction and diminished blood flow; hypoxemia
Central cyanosis	Hypoxemia and/or hypoxia (late sign)
Decreased skin turgor	Dehydration (normal finding in older adults as a result of decreased skin elasticity)
Dependent edema	Heart failure
FINGERTIPS AND NAIL BEDS	
Cyanosis	Decreased cardiac output or hypoxia; sometimes the result of decreased circulation to affected limb or vasoconstriction secondary to cold
Splinter hemorrhages	Bacterial endocarditis
Clubbing of fingertips	Chronic hypoxemia
MOUTH AND LIPS	
Cyanotic mucous membranes	Decreased oxygenation (hypoxia) **Note:** Lips may be more bluish in color in people with darker skin, which is a normal finding
Pursed-lip breathing	Chronic lung disease; increased respiratory effort
Pallor	Anemia
NECK VEINS	
Distention	Heart failure (typically right-sided); fluid overload
NOSE	
Flaring nares	Respiratory distress; dyspnea; hypoxia
Nasal discharge	Color indicates allergy versus infection
CHEST	
Barrel chest	COPD; may be a normal finding in older adults
Breathing pattern	Multiple (see Table 24.4)

COPD, chronic obstructive pulmonary disease.

Data from Ball J, et al: *Seidel's guide to physical examination*, ed 9, St Louis, 2015, Elsevier; and Lewis S, et al: *Medical-surgical nursing: assessment and management of clinical problems*, ed 9, St Louis, 2017, Mosby.

Table 24.4 Assessment of Abnormal Chest Wall Movement

Abnormality	Cause
Asymmetry: Unequal expansion of lungs	Chest wall injury; collapsed lung
Retraction: Visible sinking in soft tissues of chest that lie between and around firmer tissue (e.g., cartilage and bony ribs); retractions have specific beginning point and worsening, with need for increased inspiratory effort; possibly found at intercostal space, infraclavicular space, trachea, and substernally[a]	Any condition that causes increased inspiratory effort (e.g., airway obstruction, asthma, tracheobronchitis)
Paradoxical breathing: Asynchronous breathing; chest contraction during inspiration and expansion during expiration	Flail chest

[a]Infants can experience sternal and substernal retractions with only slight inspiratory effort because of chest pliability.

Table 24.5 Respiratory Patterns

Type/Pattern	Rate	Clinical Significance
Eupnea	12–20 breaths/min	Normal rate in adult
Tachypnea	Greater than 20 breaths/min	Results from anxiety, pain, fever, respiratory infection, or other causes that lead to respiratory distress; can lead to respiratory alkalosis, paresthesia, tetany, and confusion
Bradypnea	Less than 10 breaths/min	Results from sleep, narcotic or sedative drug overdose, or CNS lesion; can lead to respiratory acidosis, disorientation, somnolence, and coma
Apnea	Periods of no respiration lasting greater than 20 s	Sometimes intermittent such as in sleep apnea or prolonged as in a respiratory arrest; sleep apnea can be treated with home CPAP; respiratory arrest needs emergency treatment
Kussmaul	Usually greater than 35 breaths/min	Breaths deep in nature; associated with metabolic acidosis states such as diabetic ketoacidosis
Cheyne–Stokes	Periods of increasing depths of breathing followed by period of apnea	Seen in seriously ill patients, typically with brain injury or drug-associated respiratory distress; may be seen in children and older adults during sleep
Ataxic or Biot	Irregular respirations of varying depths with irregular periods of apnea	Poor prognosis; associated with severe brain injury

CNS, central nervous system; *CPAP*, continuous positive airway pressure.

Adapted from Ball J, et al: *Seidel's guide to physical examination*, ed 9, St Louis, 2015, Mosby.

Table 24.6 Focused Patient Assessment

Factors to Assess	Questions	Physical Assessment
Breathing pattern	When do you become short of breath? When lying down or after activities? Are you able to do your own personal hygiene without getting tired? How far can you walk without getting short of breath? How many pillows do you use to sleep at night?	Observe breathing pattern. Observe the patient perform activities of daily living. Observe for use of pursed-lip breathing. Observe the patient ambulating. Determine distance walked without shortness of breath. Observe the patient's breathing patterns in different positions.
Airway patency	How often do you cough? Do you bring up any mucus when coughing? What does it look like? Is there anything that brings on your cough?	Monitor sputum for color, consistency, amount, and odor.
Chest pain	Do you have any chest pain? Is the pain only since you developed a fever? Is the pain worse when you breathe in?	Patient report of pain score on a visual analog scale of 0–10. Presence of splinting or grimacing, particularly with inspiration or deep breaths.

the percentage of oxygenated Hgb (Hgb containing oxygen) compared with the total amount of Hgb in the blood.

Diagnostic Tests

Diagnostic tests determine adequacy of the cardiac conduction system, myocardial contraction, and blood flow. Tests measure the adequacy of ventilation and oxygenation and visualize structures of the respiratory and cardiac system. Some patients need an ECG, chest radiographic examination, pulse oximetry, laboratory tests (e.g., arterial blood gas levels, complete blood count, sputum analysis, cardiac enzyme levels), cardiac stress test, pulmonary function test, and cardiac catheterization.

TB skin testing is important to determine exposure to TB (CDC, 2016d). Patients from foreign countries often have received bacille Calmette–Guérin (BCG) vaccinations to prevent TB and will have a positive TB skin test. Testing in patients with altered immune function (e.g., older adults, HIV-positive patients, and patients undergoing chemotherapy) is less reliable. Health care providers will often use blood testing instead because it is more reliable in patients who have received BCG vaccinations. Chapter 26 describes the technique and what to evaluate for TB skin testing.

Many patients will have an initial chest radiographic examination if their TB skin test is positive. Repeat chest radiographs are recommended only if a patient develops symptoms such as hemoptysis, weight loss, fatigue, or night sweats. Definitive diagnosis depends on the presence of tubercle bacilli in the patient's sputum.

Nursing Diagnosis

A patient with an altered level of oxygenation often has nursing diagnoses that are associated with conditions of cardiovascular or pulmonary origin. You base each problem-focused or health promotion nursing diagnosis on specific defining characteristics and include the related etiology. For risk diagnoses, base your diagnosis on risk factors (see Chapter 19).

During the assessment process, you collect data that accurately reflect a patient's needs. For example, your objective findings in a patient who comes to the clinic with a diagnosis of pneumonia include nonproductive cough, breathlessness, crackles, tachypnea, shallow respirations, and pleuritic pain. These findings support the problem-focused diagnosis of *Ineffective Airway Clearance related to the presence of tracheobronchial secretions.*

Another example of a nursing diagnosis related to a patient with pneumonia is *Activity Intolerance related to imbalance between oxygen supply and demand*. The objective findings include crackles, nonproductive cough, restlessness, tachycardia, use of accessory muscles, and hypoxemia (PaO_2 less than 60 mm Hg). The subjective findings include the patient stating that he or she feels more short of breath with any sort of activity. Identifying the appropriate related factor, such as an imbalance between oxygen supply and demand, enables you to design nursing interventions (e.g., exercise strategies) to maximize the balance between a patient's oxygen supply and demand.

Possible nursing diagnoses for patients with oxygenation alterations include, but are not limited to, the following:

- *Activity Intolerance*
- *Ineffective Airway Clearance*
- *Ineffective Breathing Pattern*
- *Decreased Cardiac Output*
- *Fatigue*
- *Impaired Gas Exchange*
- *Risk for Infection*
- *Ineffective Peripheral Tissue Perfusion*

Planning

Goals and Outcomes

Patients with impaired oxygenation require patient-centered nursing care plans that are directed toward meeting their actual or potential oxygenation needs. Oxygenation goals for your patient often include having a patent airway, improving oxygenation, and increasing the level of independence and tolerance for activity (see Care Plan given in the subsequent text).

Care Plan

Oxygenation

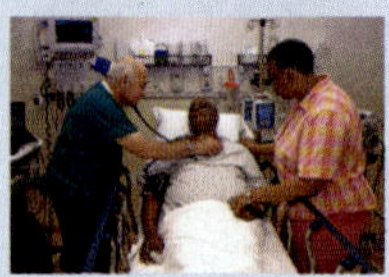

ASSESSMENT

John Smith begins his morning care for Mr King, who is restless and anxious. He complains of difficulty breathing.

ASSESSMENT ACTIVITIES	FINDINGS[a]
Ask Mr King how long he has had difficulty breathing.	He replies, "My breathing has gotten worse over the past week." His vital signs are pulse rate 120 beats/min, temperature 102°F orally, **respiratory rate 36 breaths/min**, blood pressure 110/45 mm Hg, and **SpO_2** of 82% on room air.
Observe patient behaviors.	The patient is **restless** and **is short of breath when talking**.
Auscultate Mr King's lung fields.	On auscultation, there are audible expiratory wheezes, crackles, and **diminished breath sounds** over right lower lobe.
Ask Mr King to produce a sputum sample.	**Sputum** is thick, **copious**, and discolored (yellow-green).

[a]**Defining characteristics/risk factors** are shown in **bold** type.

Nursing diagnosis: Ineffective Airway Clearance related to retained pulmonary secretions

PLANNING

GOALS	EXPECTED OUTCOMES (NOC)[b]
	Respiratory status: Gas exchange
Pulmonary secretions will return to baseline levels within 24–36 h. Mr King's oxygenation status will improve in 36 h.	Mr King's sputum will become less in amount, clear, white, and thinner in consistency within 36 h. Adventitious lung sounds will begin to clear within 24 h. Mr King's respiratory rate will return to normal values. Mr King will clear airway secretions with coughing in 24 h. Mr King's perceptions of dyspnea will improve within 24 h.

[b]Outcome classification labels from Moorhead S, et al, editors: *Nursing outcomes classification (NOC)*, ed 5, St Louis, 2013, Mosby.

INTERVENTIONS (NIC)[c]	RATIONALE
Airway management	
Have Mr King deep breathe and try to perform huff cough every 2 h while awake. If the patient is unable to cough, suction orally or nasopharyngeally.	Helps expectorate sputum; promotes gas exchange.
Elevate the head of the bed 30–45°. Encourage Mr King to change positions frequently and to ambulate and sit in chair, according to early mobility protocol.	Elevating the head of the bed encourages better lung expansion, thereby promoting better gas exchange (Munro and Ruggiero, 2014). Mobilization facilitates expectoration of respiratory secretions (Lewis et al., 2017).

Care Plan—cont'd

Encourage Mr King to increase his fluid intake to at least 2000 mL/24 h if his cardiac condition does not contraindicate it.	Fluids help hydrate the patient and help reduce fever and dry mucous membranes and may help the patient effectively expectorate secretions (Hong and Galvagno, 2013).
Avoid caffeinated beverages and alcohol; recommend water.	Caffeinated and alcoholic beverages promote diuresis and dehydration.

[c]Intervention classification labels from Bulechek GM, et al, editors: *Nursing interventions classification (NIC)*, ed 6, St Louis, 2013, Mosby.

EVALUATION

Nursing Actions	Patient Response/Finding	Achievement of Outcome
Auscultate chest.	Lung sounds are clear.	Outcome met.
Ask Mr King how often he coughs and deep breathes.	Mr King has completed a diary that shows he has been coughing and deep breathing every 2 h while awake 85% of the time.	Mr King is able to clear airways with coughing. Secretions are thin, and there is no evidence of infection. Outcome met.
Check flow sheet for recent vital signs.	Mr King's last set of vital signs shows heart rate 98 beats/min, respiratory rate 20 breaths/min, oral temperature 98.6°F, blood pressure 112/62 mm Hg, and SpO_2 95% on room air.	Mr King's vital signs are within normal limits. Outcome met.

All goals must have measurable outcomes for you to determine whether they have been met. These include objective data such as oxygen saturation levels, laboratory and physical assessment findings, and vital signs. Quantify subjective findings such as the reported degree of breathlessness or pain on visual analog scales.

Patients have more than one nursing diagnosis, and often these diagnoses have an impact on one another. It is important to include the patient and family caregiver in all care planning. Alterations in oxygenation are often chronic problems that affect the patient and family. The patient remains a member of the community despite the illness. Planning with the family and using community resources help patients adapt to activities of daily living.

Setting Priorities

A patient's clinical condition determines which nursing diagnosis takes priority while you care for the patient. For example, a patient who is short of breath and exhibiting signs and symptoms of *Impaired Gas Exchange* while sitting in a chair will not tolerate ambulating in the hallway, and this diagnosis takes priority over *Activity Intolerance*. A patient who reports a pleuritic chest pain score of 7 on a visual analog scale needs treatment of *Acute Pain* before you ask the patient to cough and clear the airways to address the problem of *Ineffective Airway Clearance*.

Collaborative Care

Impaired levels of oxygenation affect all aspects of your patient's life, not just the physical component. Planning care for a patient with a disturbance in oxygenation requires collaboration with other members of the health care team such as physical and occupational therapists and cardiac rehabilitation specialists. The respiratory therapist designs measures to improve breathing and cough control. Base your decision to delegate responsibility to nursing assistive personnel (NAP) on your assessment of the patient and the type of care he or she requires. Consider which tasks are safe to delegate and within the skill set of the NAP and how the patient will feel about the care that you have delegated. The priority is to maintain or improve the patient's oxygenation and meet the patient's needs. You are ultimately responsible for all total patient care.

When planning care for patients with impaired oxygenation, particularly as they transition to home, be sensitive to the needs of both the patient and the family. Chronic illness changes the dynamics of family relationships. Sometimes roles need to change, and the patient and family have difficulty coping. Provide an empathetic ear to both family members and the patient. Help them develop solutions that maintain the dignity of all parties and continue to support the family unit. Case managers or social service workers are often able to help patients and families identify and connect with community resources that offer support.

Implementation

Nursing interventions for patients with oxygenation alterations are diverse. Patients' cultural and religious beliefs may affect the selection of interventions. Health promotion activities may result in healthier lifestyle habits. Symptom management aids in reducing the severity of cardiopulmonary problems. Interventions aimed at improving respiration and ventilation make it easier for patients to breathe.

Health Promotion

Maintaining a patient's optimal level of health reduces the number and severity of cardiopulmonary symptoms. Prevention of disease exacerbations and community-acquired infections is a goal of health promotion. Provide health education to help patients make choices for improving health practices. Consider the following patient education topics: regular blood pressure checkups and taking blood pressure medication as prescribed, following the Dietary Approaches to Stop Hypertension (DASH) diet (NHLBI, 2015) and a proper caloric diet, getting an annual influenza vaccine and a pneumococcal vaccine, smoking cessation, and avoiding secondhand smoke exposure. Individualize patient teaching

BOX 24.2 Care of an Older Adult

Factors Affecting Cardiopulmonary Status

Older adults are at increased risk for developing a cardiopulmonary disorder (CDC, 2015a; Touhy and Jett, 2018). The cardiac and pulmonary systems are closely connected, and often a disturbance in one leads to a disturbance in the other. The following topics must be noted when caring for and educating an older adult:

- Older adults with hypertension have a higher risk of cardiovascular disease such as coronary heart disease, atrial fibrillation, and heart failure (Touhy and Jett, 2018).
- Risk factor modification is important including smoking cessation, weight reduction, a low-cholesterol and low-salt diet, management of hypertension, and exercise.
- Healthy behavior changes sometimes slow or halt the progression of disease in an older adult. However, it is often difficult to get older adults to change long-term unhealthy habits.
- In older adults with underlying pulmonary diseases such as asthma and chronic obstructive pulmonary disease (COPD), mental status changes are often the first sign of worsening respiratory problems (Touhy and Jett, 2018).
- Ensure that educational materials are appropriate for the patient (e.g., large-print handouts for patients with vision disturbances, functioning hearing aids in place in patients with hearing loss).
- Interventions used when caring for older adults with chronic cardiopulmonary illness may need to focus on palliation and not on cure.

to meet the needs of each patient. Older adults have differing needs and respond differently than younger patients (Box 24.2).

Influenza and Pneumococcal Vaccine

Influenza is a viral infection that can cause serious complications in children, older adults, and patients with cardiopulmonary diseases. More than 970,000 patients were admitted to hospitals during the 2014–2015 season because of influenza (CDC, 2015b). The infection can lead to pneumonia and critical conditions requiring hospitalization. CDC recommends annual influenza vaccines for all children 6 months of age and older (CDC, 2016b). People with a history of Guillain–Barré syndrome should speak with their health care provider before receiving the vaccine. Health care providers must assess all other allergies before administering the vaccine.

There are two types of pneumococcal vaccine: PCV13 and PPSV23. Both vaccines protect patients from acquiring pneumococcal disease. PCV13 is recommended for all children younger than 5 years, all adults older than 65 years, patients older than 6 years who are immunocompromised, and adults who are receiving a pneumococcal vaccine for the first time. PPSV23 is recommended for all adults older than 65 years and any person who is immunocompromised between 2 and 64 years of age (CDC, 2016b).

Environmental Modifications

Avoiding exposure to secondhand smoke is important for patients with cardiopulmonary illnesses. Most public places and businesses have adopted a no-smoking policy or offer separate smoking areas. Provide counseling and support so that a patient who lives with secondhand smoke in the home understands its effects. Assess environmental hazards in the workplace. Many health care agency dress codes prohibit the use of perfumes and colognes because they often affect patient breathing patterns and allergies. Discuss risk factors and ways to reduce exposure. For example, pollen is a known trigger for asthma exacerbations. Encourage patients to shut windows and use air filters during times when there are high pollen counts. In infants and children, secondhand smoke and environmental risks (e.g., pollution, cockroach infestation) increase risks for infection and asthma (Hockenberry et al., 2017).

Diet and Exercise

Advise patients to increase their activity levels with a minimum of 10 minutes at a time up to 2 hours and 30 minutes per week (National Heart, Lung, and Blood Institute [NHLBI], 2015). The goal is to achieve a target blood pressure of less than 120/80 mm Hg (Whelton et al., 2018). The risk factors for cardiac disease are lower when total cholesterol is less than 200 mg/dL, HDL is greater than 40 mg/dL in men and greater than 50 mg/dL in women, and LDL is less than 160 mg/dL (Lewis et al., 2017). A patient can reduce his or her blood pressure by 25 points by changing his or her lifestyle. Instruct patients on lifestyle modifications such as exercise and weight reduction by following the DASH diet at http://dashdiet.org/default.asp.

ACUTE CARE

Acute care interventions are directed toward halting the causative pathological processes that affect oxygenation. Nursing interventions also focus on shortening the duration and severity of an illness and preventing complications from illness or treatments such as hospital-acquired infection resulting from invasive procedures.

Dyspnea Management

Dyspnea is difficult to measure and treat, thus requiring individualized treatments for each patient. You will need to treat and stabilize the underlying processes that cause or worsen dyspnea, and then you will administer one or more of the four additional therapies:

1. Medications (e.g., bronchodilators, steroids, mucolytics, antianxiety drugs) to open the airways, decrease inflammation, thin secretions, or decrease anxiety
2. Oxygen therapy, as indicated and ordered, to treat hypoxia
3. Physical techniques (e.g., cardiopulmonary reconditioning, breathing techniques, cough control) to help mobilize secretions and strengthen the muscles used for breathing
4. Psychosocial techniques (e.g., relaxation techniques, biofeedback, meditation) to lessen the sensation of dyspnea

Maintenance of a Patent Airway

The airway is patent when the trachea, bronchi, and large airways are free from obstructions. You use three types of interventions to maintain a patent airway: coughing techniques, suctioning, and insertion of an artificial airway.

Coughing and Deep Breathing Techniques

Directed coughing is a deliberate maneuver that is effective when spontaneous coughing is inadequate. It allows a patient to remove secretions from the upper and lower airways. The normal series of events in a directed cough are deep inhalation, closure of the glottis, active contraction of the expiratory muscles, and glottis opening.

Cascade Cough

With a cascade cough, a patient takes a slow, deep breath and holds it for 2 seconds while contracting the expiratory muscles. Then the patient opens the mouth and performs a series of coughs throughout exhalation, thereby coughing at progressively lowered lung volumes. This technique promotes airway clearance and a patent airway to patients with large volumes of sputum.

Huff Cough

The huff cough is a more natural and gentler cough and is generally effective only for clearing the central airways. Have the patient sit or raise the head of the bed at least 45°. The patient inhales slowly through the mouth while breathing through the diaphragm. The patient then forcefully exhales with his or her mouth open, creating a huff sound or saying the word "Huff." Have the patient repeat the huff process two to three times and then cough and expectorate the sputum. Reinforce to the patient that this type of coughing takes practice, and it can cause a sense of breathlessness when being performed (Lewis et al., 2017).

Quad Cough

The quad cough technique is for patients without abdominal muscle control such as patients with spinal cord injuries. While the patient breathes out with a maximal expiratory effort, the patient or you push inward and upward on the abdominal muscles toward the diaphragm, causing the cough. Evaluate cough effectiveness by the ability to expectorate sputum, a patient's report of swallowed sputum, and clearing of adventitious lung sounds.

Artificial Airways

An artificial airway is for a patient with decreased level of consciousness, airway obstruction, or mechanical ventilation and who is unable to remove tracheobronchial secretions (see Skill 24.1). Patients with artificial airways who are on mechanical ventilation need specific oral hygiene care to prevent ventilator-associated pneumonia (VAP) (see Chapter 16).

Oral Airway

The oral airway (Fig. 24.5), the simplest type of artificial airway, prevents obstruction of the trachea by displacing the tongue into the oropharynx. The oral airway extends from the teeth to the oropharynx, keeping the tongue in the normal position. Determine proper oral airway size by measuring the distance from the corner of the mouth to the angle of the jaw just below the ear. The length is equal to the distance from the flange of the airway to the tip. Use only the correct-size airway. If the airway is too small, the tongue will not stay in the anterior portion of the mouth; if too large, it forces the tongue toward the epiglottis and obstructs the airway.

Insert the airway upside down, then turn the curve of the airway toward the cheek and place it over the tongue. When the airway is in the oropharynx, turn it so that the opening points downward. Correctly placed, the airway moves the tongue forward, away from the oropharynx and the flange. The flat portion of the airway rests against the patient's teeth. Incorrect insertion merely forces the tongue back into the oropharynx.

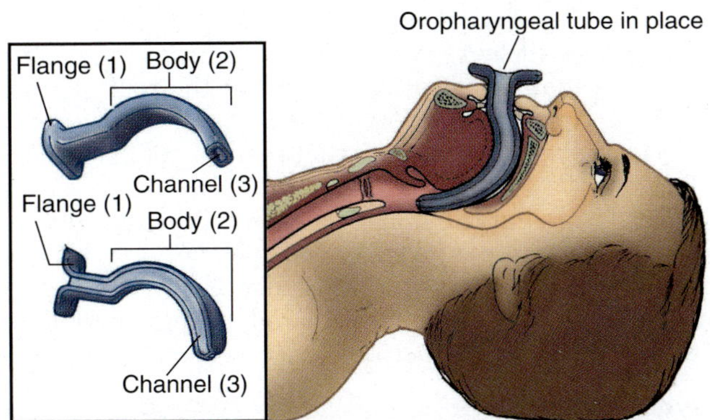

Fig. 24.5 Artificial oral airways. (From Barnes TA: Emergency cardiovascular life support. In Kacmarek RM, et al, eds: *Egan's fundamentals of respiratory care*, ed 10, St Louis, 2013, Mosby.)

Tracheal Airway

An endotracheal or nasotracheal tube is a short-term artificial airway for administering mechanical ventilation. Tracheal tubes are for long-term use. These airways allow easy access to the trachea for deep tracheal suctioning. Because of the artificial airway, a patient no longer has normal humidification of the tracheal mucosa. Ensure that humidity is being supplied to the airway. Humidification is protective and helps reduce the risk for airway plugging. Most patients with tracheal airways cannot speak, and thus it is important to use written or nonverbal communication strategies.

Oxygen Therapy

Some patients require oxygen therapy to keep a healthy level of tissue oxygenation. The goal of **oxygen therapy** is to prevent or relieve hypoxia. Any patient with impaired tissue oxygenation benefits from controlled oxygen administration. Oxygen is not a substitute for other treatments. It is a therapeutic gas that must be prescribed and adjusted only with a health care provider order. Oxygen is a drug with potentially dangerous side effects including the potential to cause hypoventilation in patients with COPD and hypercapnia. Continuously monitor the dosage or concentration. Routinely check the health care provider's orders to verify that the patient is receiving the prescribed oxygen concentration and flow rate. The six rights of medication administration also apply to oxygen administration (see Chapter 26).

Safety Precautions With Oxygen Therapy

Oxygen is a highly combustible gas and fuels fire readily. Although it does not spontaneously burn or cause an explosion, it can easily cause a fire to ignite if it contacts a spark from electrical equipment. With increasing use of outpatient oxygen therapy, patients and health care professionals need to be aware of the dangers of combustion. Follow these oxygen safety precautions:

- Place an "Oxygen in Use" sign on the patient's room door or door of house.

- No smoking should be allowed on the premises.
- Keep oxygen delivery systems 10 feet from any open flames.
- Be sure that electrical equipment in the room is functioning correctly and is grounded.
- Secure oxygen cylinders so that they do not fall over.

Patients discharged home on oxygen therapy need to have an environmental safety assessment (e.g., use of space/kerosene heaters or the presence of smokers who live or visit the home). Patients and family caregivers will also need special discharge instructions.

Oxygen Supply

Within health care settings, oxygen tanks or a permanent wall-piped system supplies oxygen to a patient's bedside. Oxygen tanks are transported on wide-based carriers that allow the tank to be upright at the patient's bedside. Regulators control the amount of oxygen delivered. One common type of oxygen tank has an upright flowmeter with a flow-adjustment valve at the top. A second type is a cylinder indicator with a flow-adjustment handle.

Methods of Oxygen Delivery

Nasal cannula, nasal catheter, face mask (Fig. 24.6), and a mechanical ventilator are ways to deliver oxygen to a patient (Table 24.7; Box 24.3).

Home Oxygen

Home oxygen therapy is indicated in patients whose disease is stable with a PaO_2 of 55 mm Hg or less or an arterial oxygen saturation (SaO_2) of 88%. Patients with a PaO_2 of 55–59 mm Hg and signs of hypoxia qualify for long-term home oxygen therapy (McDonald, 2014). Home oxygen is usually administered by nasal cannula or face mask. If your patient has a permanent tracheostomy, a T tube or tracheostomy collar is necessary to provide humidified air to the airway. Patients requiring home oxygen need extensive teaching to be able to continue oxygen therapy at home efficiently and safely. This teaching includes oxygen safety, regulation of the amount of oxygen, obtaining and troubleshooting equipment, how to use the prescribed home oxygen delivery system, and when to contact local emergency medical services. A case coordinator or social worker usually assists with arranging for a home care nurse and oxygen vendor.

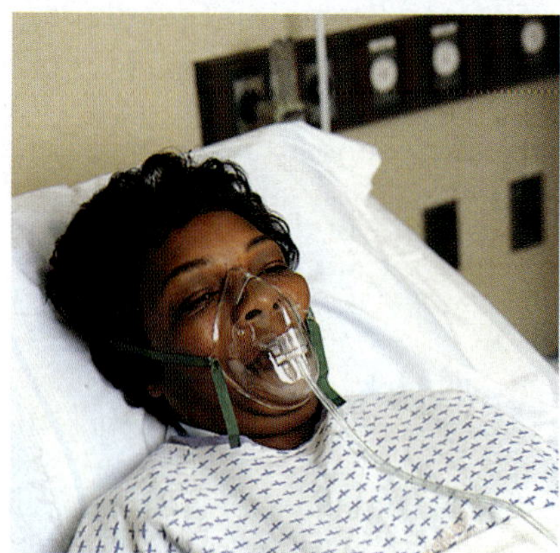

Fig. 24.6 Simple face mask.

Table 24.7 Oxygen Delivery Systems

Delivery System	Flow Rate; FiO_2 Delivered	Advantages	Disadvantages
LOW-FLOW DELIVERY DEVICES			
Nasal cannula	1–6 L/min; 24%–44%	Safe and simple Easily tolerated Effective for low concentrations Does not impede eating or talking Inexpensive Disposable	Unable to use with nasal obstructions Drying to mucous membranes Can dislodge easily May cause skin irritation and breakdown over ears and in nares The patient's breathing pattern (mouth or nasal) affects exact FiO_2
Oxygen-conserving cannula (Oxymizer)	8 L/min; 30%–50%	Indicated for long-term O_2 use in the home Allows increased O_2 concentration and lower flow	Cannula cannot be cleaned More expensive than standard cannula
Simple face mask (see Fig. 24.6)	6–12 L/min; 35%–50%	Useful for short-term therapy such as patient transportation	Contraindicated for patients who retain CO_2 May make the patient feel claustrophobic Therapy interrupted while eating or drinking Increased risk of aspiration
Partial nonrebreather mask[a]	10–15 L/min; 60%–90%	Short-term delivery of increased FiO_2 Easily humidifies O_2 Does not dry mucous membranes	Hot and confining May irritate skin; tight seal is necessary Interferes with eating and talking Bag may twist or kink Should not totally deflate
HIGH-FLOW DELIVERY DEVICES			
Venturi mask	24%–50%	Provides specific amount of O_2 with humidity added Administers constant O_2	Mask and added humidity may irritate skin Therapy interrupted when the patient eats Specific flow rate must be followed
High-flow nasal cannula	Adjustable FiO_2 (0.21–1.0) with modifiable low flow (up to 60 L/min)	Wide range of FiO_2 Can use on adults, children, and infants	FiO_2 dependent on the patient's respiratory pattern and input flow Risk for infection (Messika et al., 2015; Urden et al., 2016).

CO_2, carbon dioxide; *FiO_2*, fraction of inspired oxygen concentration; *O_2*, oxygen.

[a]Reservoir bag should always remain partially inflated. Therefore, flow rate must be high enough to prevent collapse of bag.

BOX 24.3 Procedural Guidelines

Applying a Nasal Cannula or Oxygen Mask

Equipment

Oxygen nasal cannula or mask as ordered by health care provider, oxygen tubing (consider extension tubing), humidifier (if indicated), sterile water for humidifier, face shield as needed for risk of splash, clean gloves if secretions are present, oxygen source, oxygen flowmeter, appropriate "Oxygen in Use" signs, pulse oximeter, and stethoscope. **Note:** When device is used in the home, the medical equipment vendor will supply all the equipment.

Steps

1. Identify the patient by using at least two identifiers (e.g., name and birthday or name and medical record number) according to agency policy. Compare identifiers with information on the patient's MAR or medical record.
2. Review the patient's medical record for medical order for oxygen, noting delivery method, flow rate, duration of oxygen therapy, and parameters for titration of oxygen settings.
3. Obtain the patient's most recent SpO_2 value or most recent arterial blood gas (ABG) results if available.
4. Perform hand hygiene. Assess the patient's respiratory status including symmetry of chest wall expansion, chest wall abnormalities (e.g., kyphosis), temporary conditions (e.g., pregnancy, trauma) affecting ventilation, respiratory rate and depth, sputum production, lung sounds, and signs and symptoms associated with hypoxia. **Note:** Apply face shield if risk of exposure to splashing mucus exists. Apply gloves if the patient has oral or nasal secretions.

Clinical decision point: Excessive amounts of secretions, signs of respiratory distress (increased work of breathing, increased respiratory rate), presence of rhonchi on auscultation, excessive coughing, or decrease in SpO_2 can indicate a need for suctioning.

5. Observe for behavioral changes (e.g., apprehension, anxiety, confusion, decreased ability to concentrate, decreased LOC, fatigue, and dizziness).

Clinical decision point: Patients with sudden changes in their vital signs, LOC, or behavior may be experiencing profound hypoxia. Patients with subtle changes over time may have worsening of a chronic or existing condition or a new medical condition (Lewis et al., 2017).

6. Observe for patent airway and remove secretions by having the patient cough and expectorate mucus or by suctioning. Remove and dispose of gloves and perform hand hygiene.
7. Explain procedure to the patient and family.
8. Gather equipment/supplies.
9. Adjust bed to appropriate height and lower side rail on side nearest you. Check locks on bed wheel.
10. Apply new pair of gloves if the patient has oral or nasal secretions.
11. Attach oxygen delivery device (e.g., cannula, mask) to oxygen tubing, and attach end of tubing to humidified oxygen source adjusted to prescribed flow rate.
    a. Place tips of the cannula into the patient's nares. If tips are curved, they should point downward inside the nostrils. Then loop the cannula tubing up and over the patient's ears. Adjust the lanyard so that the cannula fits snugly but not too tightly without pressure to the patient's nares and ears.
    b. Apply a mask by placing it over the patient's mouth and nose. Then bring the straps over the patient's head and adjust to form a comfortable but tight seal.
12. Maintain sufficient slack on oxygen tubing and secure to the patient's clothes.
13. Observe for proper function of oxygen delivery device.
    a. *Nasal cannula:* Cannula is positioned properly in nares; humidified oxygen flows through tips (see illustration).
    b. *Oxygen-conserving cannula (Oxymizer)* (see illustration): Fit as for nasal cannula. Reservoir is located under the patient's nose or worn as a pendant.
    c. *Nonrebreathing mask* (see illustration): Apply as a regular mask. Contains one-way valves with a reservoir; exhaled air does not enter reservoir bag. Can be combined with a nasal cannula to provide higher FiO_2.
    d. *Simple face mask* (see Fig. 24.6): Select appropriate flow rate.
    e. *Venturi mask* (see illustration): Apply as regular mask. Select appropriate flow rate.
14. Verify setting on flowmeter and oxygen source for proper setup and prescribed flow rate.
15. Check cannula/mask every 8 h or see agency policy. Keep humidifier filled at all times.
16. Post "Oxygen in Use" signs on wall behind bed and at entrance to room.

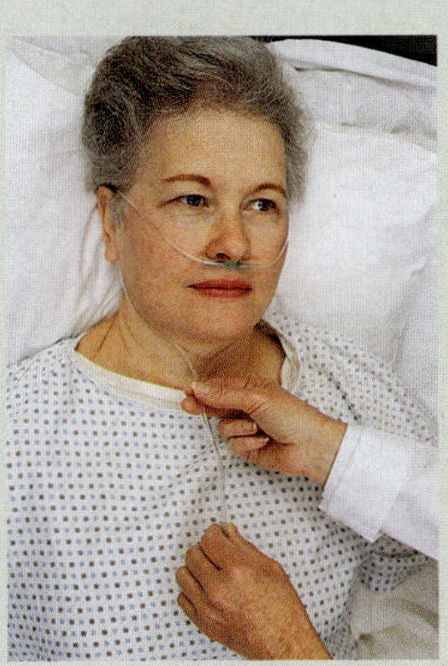

Step 13a Nasal cannula adjusted for proper fit.

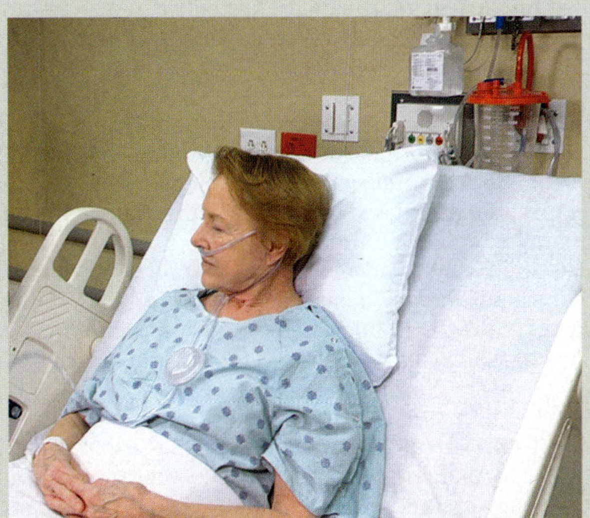

Step 13b Reservoir nasal cannula/Oxymizer. (Copyright © Mosby's Clinical Skills: Essentials Collection.)

BOX 24.3 **Procedural Guidelines—cont'd**

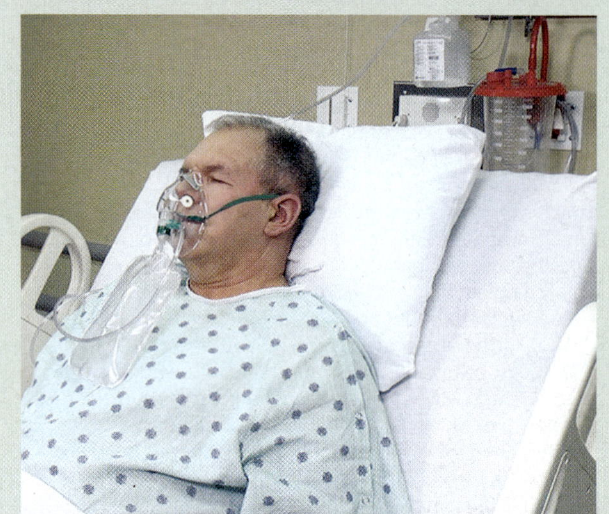

Step 13c Nonrebreathing mask. (Copyright © Mosby's Clinical Skills: Essentials Collection.)

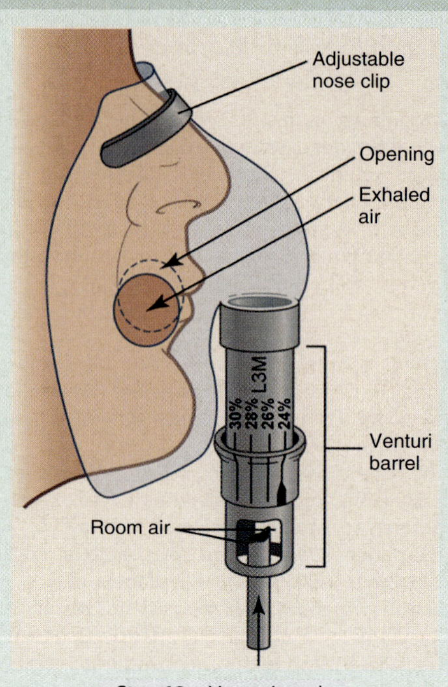

Step 13e Venturi mask.

17. Properly dispose of gloves (if used) and perform hand hygiene.
18. Monitor the patient's response to changes in oxygen flow rate with SpO_2. (**Note:** Monitor arterial blood gases [ABGs] when ordered.)
19. Auscultate lung sounds; observe chest excursion; inspect color of skin; and observe for decreased anxiety, improved LOC and cognitive abilities; decreased fatigue; and absence of dizziness. Measure vital signs.
20. Check adequacy of oxygen flow each shift or as agency policy dictates.
21. Observe the patient's external ears, bridge of nose, nares, and nasal mucous membranes for evidence of skin breakdown.
22. **Use teach back:** "I want to be sure I explained how oxygen will help you. Tell me one benefit of oxygen therapy." Revise your instruction now or develop a plan for revised patient/family caregiver teaching if the patient/family caregiver is not able to teach back correctly.

Mobilization of Pulmonary Secretions

The ability of a patient to mobilize pulmonary secretions out of lung airways is the difference between a short-term illness and a long recovery involving complications.

Hydration

Maintenance of adequate systemic hydration keeps mucociliary clearance normal for removing mucus and cellular debris from the respiratory tract. Excessive coughing to clear secretions is fatiguing and energy depleting. In patients with adequate hydration, pulmonary secretions are thin, white, watery, and easily removable with minimal coughing. Unless contraindicated by a cardiac or renal condition, a fluid intake of 1500–2000 mL/day helps to keep pulmonary secretions thin and easy to expectorate (Lewis et al., 2017).

Humidification

Humidification (adding moisture to the inspired air) is necessary for patients receiving oxygen therapy at a high flow, typically greater than 4 L/min. Oxygen humidification via a nasal cannula or face mask is achieved by bubbling oxygen through water. When using humidity, make sure to use sterile water. Also be sure to change the solution according to agency procedures. Humidification is a source for hospital-acquired infections because the moist environment supports the growth of pathogens.

Nebulization

Nebulization uses the aerosol principle to suspend a maximum number of water drops or particles of the desired size in inspired air. The moisture added to the respiratory system through nebulization improves mucus clearance and is used for administration of medications such as bronchodilators and mucolytic agents.

Incentive Spirometry

Incentive spirometry (IS) encourages voluntary deep breathing by providing visual feedback to patients about their inspiratory volume. It promotes deep inhalation to prevent atelectasis and other pulmonary postoperative complications (AARC, 2011; Cassidy et al., 2013). However, a recent review shows no evidence that IS prevents pulmonary complications following abdominal surgery (do Nascimento et al., 2014). It is effective in increasing lung expansion and thus is commonly used in postoperative care. The AARC (2011) recommends 5–10 breaths per session every hour while awake. Use IS in combination with other pulmonary maneuvers such as deep breathing and coughing, early mobilization, and directed coughing (do Nascimento et al., 2014; Restrepo et al., 2011). Administer pain medications before IS to help a patient breathe deeply.

There are two types of incentive spirometers. Flow-oriented incentive spirometers consist of one or more plastic chambers that contain freely moving colored balls. The patient inhales slowly with an even flow to elevate the balls and keep them floating as long as possible. This allows a maximally sustained inhalation. Volume-oriented IS devices have a bellows that rises to a predetermined volume by an inhaled breath. An achievement light or counter is used to provide feedback. Some devices do not turn the light on unless the bellows is at a minimum desired volume for a specified period of time.

Suctioning Techniques

When coughing does not effectively clear respiratory tract secretions, suctioning is indicated (see Skill 24.1). You need to use sterile technique for orotracheal, nasotracheal, and tracheal suctioning via an artificial airway because the tip of the catheter enters the sterile tracheal airway. The pharynx is considered clean; therefore, oral and nasopharyngeal suctioning requires only clean technique. When suctioning both the oral pharynx and the trachea, always perform nasotracheal and tracheal (sterile) suctioning before suctioning oral pharyngeal (clean) secretions. Suctioning involves the use of a round-tipped, flexible catheter with holes on the sides and end of the catheter. When suctioning, you apply negative pressure (100–150 mm Hg for adults) during catheter withdrawal, never on insertion. Suctioning is indicated when rhonchi, gurgling breath sounds, and diminished breath sounds are audible on auscultation or when visible secretions are present after other methods have failed to remove secretions. There is no evidence to support suctioning on a scheduled basis (Myatt, 2015; Wiegand, 2017).

Oropharyngeal and Nasopharyngeal Suctioning

Use oropharyngeal or nasopharyngeal suctioning to help a patient who is able to cough effectively but is unable to clear secretions by expectorating or swallowing. Use a Yankauer or tonsillar tip suction catheter for oropharyngeal suctioning (Fig. 24.7). The catheter is made of rigid plastic with one large and several small eyelets through which mucus is removed. It is angled to facilitate removal of secretions from the mouth. Use the Yankauer suction catheter when oral secretions are thick and plentiful. Do not use it in the nares because of its size.

Orotracheal and Nasotracheal Suctioning

Orotracheal or nasotracheal suctioning is necessary when a patient is unable to cough well enough to clear the airway but does not have an artificial airway in place. You pass a catheter through the mouth or nose and then into the trachea. The nose is the preferred route because stimulation of the gag reflex is minimal. The procedure is similar to nasopharyngeal suctioning, but the catheter tip enters the trachea.

Tracheal Suctioning

Perform tracheal suctioning through an artificial airway such as a tracheostomy tube or endotracheal tube. The catheter size should be as small as possible to prevent tissue injury. Two tracheal suctioning methods include the use of a single catheter for one-time use and closed suctioning, which includes a multiple-use catheter. The suction catheter in closed suctioning is encased in a plastic sheath (Fig. 24.8). You use closed suctioning most often for patients who require mechanical ventilation because it decreases the patient's risk of having a hypoxic event during suctioning and helps to decrease the patient's risk of developing VAP (Branson et al., 2014). The practice of instilling normal saline into artificial airways to improve secretion removal could be harmful and is not recommended.

Chest Physiotherapy

Chest physiotherapy (CPT) is external chest wall manipulation using postural drainage, percussion, vibration, high-frequency chest wall compression (HFCWC), or all of these for helping patients mobilize pulmonary secretions (Box 24.4). The AARC recommends that CPT be used in patients with cystic fibrosis and other diseases in which there is greater than 30 mL of sputum per day or in patients who have atelectasis on chest X-ray examination (Strickland et al., 2013). It has not been found to be effective in patients with uncomplicated pneumonia, patients with COPD for routine use, patients after surgery, or patients with respiratory muscle weakness (Strickland et al., 2013).

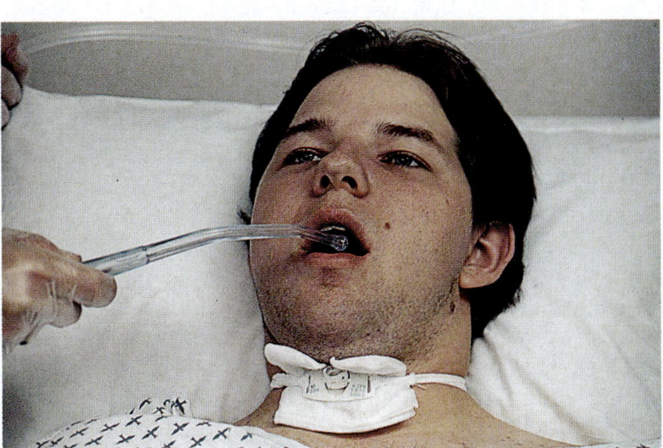

Fig. 24.7 Oropharyngeal suctioning.

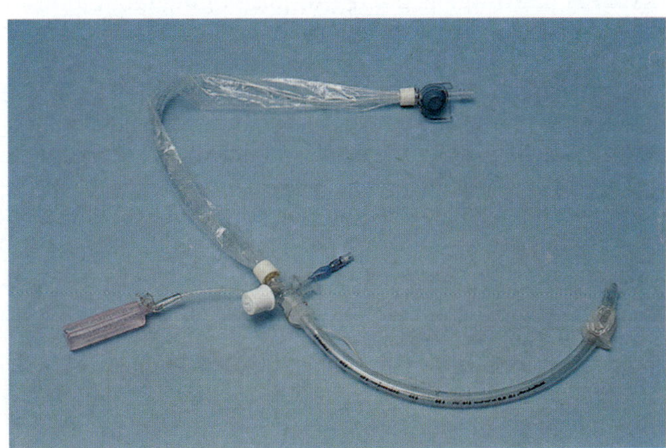

Fig. 24.8 Ballard tracheal care closed suction.

BOX 24.4 Chest Physiotherapy Considerations

Nurses and respiratory therapists collaborate with health care providers to determine whether chest physiotherapy (CPT) is best for a patient. Consultation also determines the position for the patient to assume during the procedure. Follow these guidelines:

- Know a patient's normal range of vital signs. CPT can be physically exhausting, and the activity can affect a patient's vital signs. The degree of change is related to the level of hypoxia, overall cardiopulmonary status, and tolerance of the procedure.
- Know a patient's current medications. Long-term steroid use increases the patient's risk for pathological rib fractures. Anticoagulants and nonsteroidal anti-inflammatory drugs (NSAIDs) increase a patient's risk for bruising. Diuretics and antihypertensives cause fluid and hemodynamic changes.
- Know a patient's medical and surgical history. Conditions such as increased intracranial pressure, spinal cord injuries, abdominal aneurysm resection, severe osteoporosis, and thoracic trauma are contraindications for postural drainage and CPT.
- Know a patient's level of cognitive function. Participation in vibration and controlled cough CPT techniques is dependent on a patient's ability to understand and follow instructions. CPT may result in combative behavior in patients with confusion or delirium.
- Have suction machine equipment available to help clear the airway of secretions.
- Be aware of the patient's exercise tolerance. CPT maneuvers are fatiguing, and patients who are not used to physical activity may have little tolerance for this therapy.

Table 24.8 Positions for Postural Drainage

Lung Segment	Position of Patient
ADULT	
Left and right upper lobes	High Fowler's
Apical Segments	
Right upper lobe—anterior segment	Supine with head elevated
Left upper lobe—anterior segment	Sitting on side of bed Supine with head elevated
Right upper lobe—posterior segment	Side-lying with right side of chest elevated on pillows
Left upper lobe—posterior segment	Side-lying with left side of chest elevated on pillows
Left and right middle lobes—anterior segment	Three-fourths supine position with dependent lung in Trendelenburg's position
Right middle lobe—posterior segment	Prone with thorax and abdomen elevated
Both lower lobes—anterior segments	Supine in Trendelenburg's position
Left lower lobe—lateral segment	Right side-lying in Trendelenburg's position
Right lower lobe—lateral segment	Left side-lying in Trendelenburg's position
Right lower lobe—posterior segment	Prone with right side of chest elevated in Trendelenburg's position
Both lower lobes—posterior segment	Prone in Trendelenburg's position
CHILD	
Sitting on nurse's lap, leaning slightly forward flexed over pillow	
Bilateral—middle anterior segments	Sitting on nurse's lap, leaning against nurse
Bilateral lobes—anterior segments	Lying supine on nurse's lap, back supported with pillow

Postural Drainage

Postural drainage is the use of positioning techniques to drain secretions from specific segments of the lungs and bronchi into the trachea for expectoration (Table 24.8). Because some patients do not require postural drainage of all lung segments, adapt the procedure and position patients based on clinical assessment findings. For example, some patients with left lower lobe bronchiectasis or pneumonia require postural drainage of only the affected region, whereas a patient with cystic fibrosis requires postural drainage of all segments.

Chest Percussion

Chest percussion is the manual external clapping of a patient's chest with cupped hands over the lung segments being drained. A mechanical device can also be used to loosen secretions from the bronchial walls. You perform chest percussion by alternating hand motion against the chest wall (Fig. 24.9). Perform percussion over a single layer of clothing, but not over buttons, snaps, or zippers. The single layer of clothing prevents directly slapping the patient's skin. Thicker or multiple layers of material dampen the percussions. When percussing the lung fields, be careful not to percuss the scapular area, or trauma will occur to the skin and underlying musculoskeletal structures. Percussion is contraindicated in patients with bleeding disorders, osteoporosis, or fractured ribs.

Vibration

Vibration is a gentle shaking pressure applied to the chest wall only during exhalation to shake secretions into larger airways. This pressure can be applied either manually or with a commercially available device. Vibration may be tolerated better than percussion. You use vibration most often with patients with cystic fibrosis. It is not recommended for infants and young children.

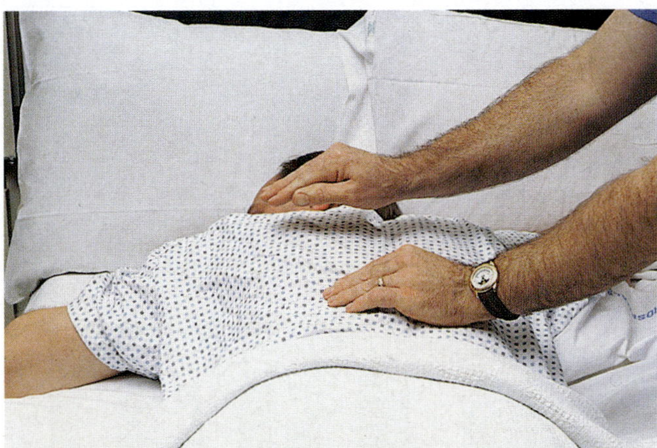

Fig. 24.9 Chest wall percussion alternating hand motion against patient's chest wall.

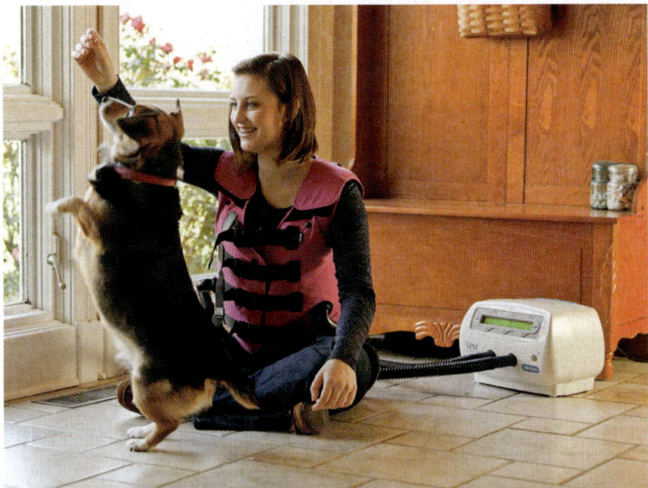

Fig. 24.10 High-frequency chest wall oscillation vest for home use. (Copyright © 2012 Hill-Rom Services, Inc. Reprinted with permission. All rights reserved.)

High-Frequency Chest Wall Compression

HFCWC consists of an inflatable vest that is attached to an air pulse generator. The vest airway clearance system (Fig. 24.10) loosens and removes secretions from the airway by delivering high-frequency, small-volume expiratory pulses to a patient's external chest wall. This therapy benefits patients with neuromuscular disorders, cystic fibrosis, or ineffective cough and airway clearance. HFCWC is also beneficial for patients who produce 25–30 mL of sputum per day because it helps to decrease the viscosity of the mucus, making it easier for a patient to cough and clear the airway (Volsko, 2013).

Chest Tubes

A **chest tube** is a catheter inserted through the rib cage into the pleural space to remove air, fluids, or blood; to prevent air or fluid from reentering the pleural space; or to reestablish normal intrapleural and intrapulmonic pressures.

- Chest tubes are typically 51 cm (20 inches) long and range in size from 12 to 40 F. Large tubes drain blood, whereas smaller tubes drain air.
- Chest tubes are commonly used in patients after cardiac or thoracic surgery or in patients who have a chest trauma to promote lung reexpansion (see Skill 24.2). Once fluid or air is removed, a patient's oxygenation improves (Kane et al., 2013; Myatt, 2015).
  - A **pneumothorax** is a collapse of the lung caused by collection of air or other gas in the pleural space.
    - The gas causes the lung to collapse because it changes the intrapleural pressure from negative to positive, exerting a counterpressure against the lung, making it unable to expand.
    - A pneumothorax is commonly caused by chest trauma resulting in fractured ribs or secondary to chronic disease, or it can occur spontaneously.
    - A patient with a pneumothorax feels sharp pain because atmospheric air irritates the parietal pleura. Dyspnea and tachycardia are common and worsen as the size of the pneumothorax increases.
  - A **tension pneumothorax** is a life-threatening situation that occurs from rupture in the pleura when air accumulates in the pleural space more rapidly than it is removed.
    - Air is trapped in the pleural cavity between the chest wall and the lung. The volume of trapped air increases with each inspiration and is unable to escape with expiration, causing increased pressure on the lung, heart, and blood vessels of the thorax.
    - If left untreated, the lung on the affected side collapses, and the mediastinum shifts to the opposite (unaffected) side leading to tracheal deviation, reduced venous return, and subsequent decrease in CO.
    - Tracheal deviation is a late sign and may be absent in some cases (Zarogoulidis et al., 2014). A large-bore cannula (needle decompression) or chest tube must be placed immediately to release the pressure (Bascom et al., 2016).
  - **Hemothorax** is an accumulation of blood in the pleural space, usually as the result of trauma.
    - It produces a counterpressure and prevents the lung from full expansion. In addition to pain and dyspnea, signs and symptoms of shock develop if blood loss is severe.
    - If it occurs with a pneumothorax, it is called a hemopneumothorax.
  - **Pleural effusions** occur when fluid, in response to infection, inflammation, or cancer, enters the pleural space.
    - Disposable chest drainage systems such as the Thora-Seal (Covidien/Medtronic), Pleur-evac chest drainage system (Teleflex), or Atrium brand systems are one-piece molded plastic units that evacuate any volume of air or fluid with controlled suction (Fig. 24.11).
    - The disposable units are cost-effective and safe. Each unit typically has three chambers: a water-seal chamber to prevent air from being drawn back into the pleural space, a chamber to collect fluid or blood, and a chamber for suction.
    - The suction chamber facilitates removal of chest drainage and trapped air. Suction pressure is measured in centimeters of water and is usually set at −15 to −20 cm H_2O for adults. Children

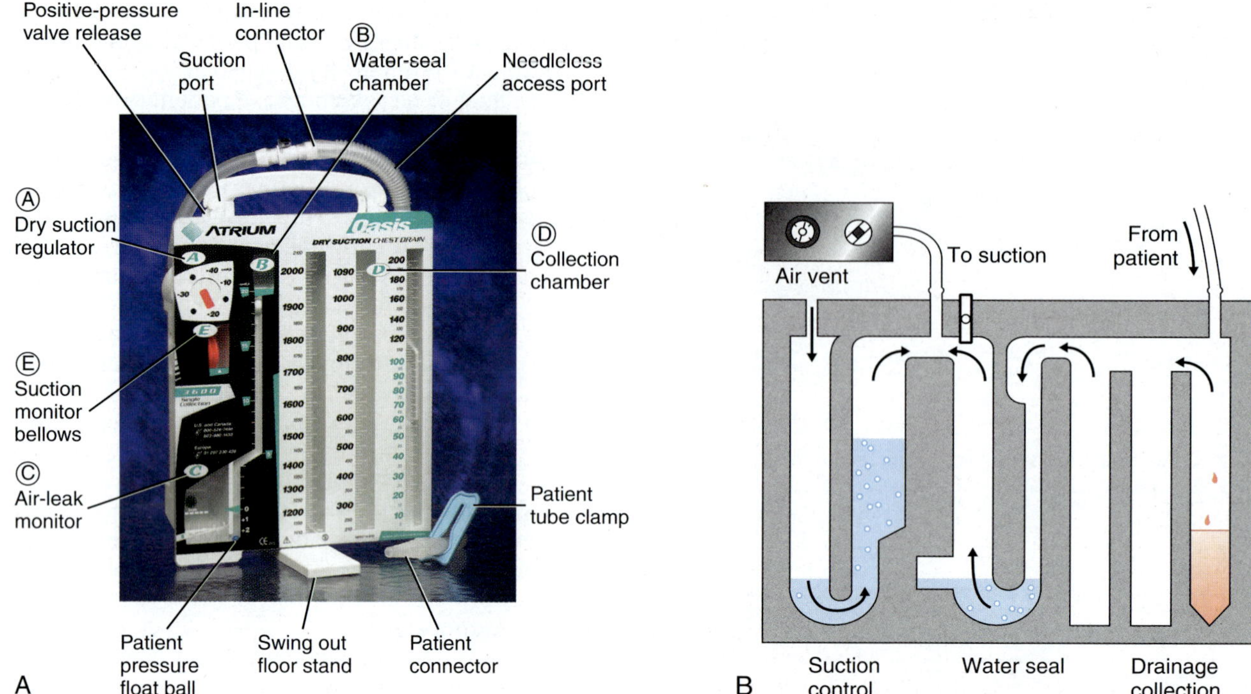

Fig. 24.11 A, Dry suction chest drainage system. **B,** Schematic of drainage device. (**A,** courtesy Atrium Medical Corp.)

may require less pressure. Suction pressure is typically ordered by the health care provider. Your knowledge of the basics of chest tube management and troubleshooting maneuvers reduces a patient's risk for complications.

Special Considerations

Clamping chest tubes is contraindicated when a patient is ambulating or being transported because it may cause a tension pneumothorax (Kane et al., 2013). The health care provider may choose to clamp a tube temporarily to determine whether a patient has fluid or air accumulation. Clamping requires an order, and you must assess the patient frequently. Handle the chest drainage unit carefully and maintain the drainage device below the patient's chest. If the tubing accidentally disconnects from the collection unit, instruct the patient to exhale as much as possible and cough. This maneuver rids the pleural space of as much air as possible. Quickly cleanse the tip of the tubing and reconnect the tubing to the unit.

Chest Tube Removal

A physician, physician's assistant, or nurse practitioner usually removes a chest tube (verify agency policy). Prepare a patient by assessing the need for preremoval analgesia, obtaining the required medication orders, and instructing a patient about the process and what will be requested of him or her. There has been debate about the optimal timing of chest tube removal in relation to the respiratory cycle. Removal at full inspiration maximally expands the lungs and minimizes the potential space between the pleurae. Another recommendation is for chest tube removal at end expiration when the pressure difference between the chest cavity and the atmosphere is the least (Kwiatt et al., 2014). An occlusive dressing is applied immediately after tube removal to maintain a tight seal.

Maintenance or Promotion of Lung Expansion

Nursing interventions to maintain or promote lung expansion include noninvasive techniques such as ambulation, positioning, IS, and chest tube management.

Ambulation

Research shows that after 1 week of bed rest, muscle strength declines by as much as 20%, resulting in an increased oxygen demand, weakened respiratory muscles, and reduced functional status. Early ambulation increases a patient's general strength and lung expansion. Progressive mobilization from dangling the legs off a bed to standing and then walking is safe for all patients, including those who are intubated (Atkins and Kautz, 2014) (see Chapter 14). Support patients in being actively involved in ambulation as soon as possible.

Positioning

Healthy people maintain adequate ventilation and oxygenation by frequent position changes. When a person has restricted mobility, it increases his or her risk for respiratory impairment. Frequent position changes such as every 2 hours are a simple and cost-effective method for reducing a patient's risk for pooled airway secretions and decreased chest wall expansion.

The most effective position for patients with cardiopulmonary disease is the 45° semi-Fowler's position, using gravity to assist in lung expansion and reduce pressure from the abdomen on the diaphragm. Ensure that a patient does not slide down in bed, causing reduced lung expansion. When positioning a patient with unilateral lung disease such as a pneumothorax or atelectasis, position him or her with the healthy lung down. This position promotes better perfusion of the healthy lung and aeration of the diseased lung, improving oxygenation. In the presence of pulmonary abscess or hemorrhage, place the affected lung down to prevent drainage toward the healthy lung.

Noninvasive Ventilation

Noninvasive ventilation (NIV) maintains positive airway pressure and improves alveolar ventilation without the need for an artificial airway. This mechanical ventilator alternative reduces and reverses atelectasis, improves oxygenation, reduces pulmonary edema, and improves cardiac function. Positive airway pressure keeps the alveoli partially inflated, reducing the risk for atelectasis.

Continuous positive airway pressure (CPAP) maintains a steady stream of pressure throughout a patient's breathing cycle. It benefits patients with obstructive sleep apnea. In obstructive sleep apnea, the upper airway collapses during sleep and prevents normal airflow. When the airflow is interrupted, there is a drop in the patient's oxygen saturation, and frequent awakenings occur. CPAP uses continuous positive pressure to keep the airway open and prevent upper airway collapse. The patient breathes more normally, sleeps better, and has markedly reduced snoring. A CPAP setting of 5 cm H_2O provides 5 cm of pressure during inspiration and expiration. The usual CPAP setting is 5–20 cm H_2O. However, there are disadvantages to this device.

Bilevel positive airway pressure (BiPAP) works by providing assistance during inspiration and preventing alveolar closure during expiration. It provides two levels of pressure: inspiratory positive airway pressure (IPAP) and lower expiratory positive airway pressure (EPAP).

The goals of NIV include improved ventilation and sleep, enhanced quality of life, reduction of morbidity, improvement of physical and physiological function, and cost-effectiveness. You prepare family caregivers and patients who are candidates for NIV for discharge by collaborating with a multidisciplinary team.

Restoration of Cardiopulmonary Functioning

The AHA publishes guidelines for cardiopulmonary care and resuscitation every 5 years. It outlines the standards for basic and advanced life support for children and adults (Link et al., 2015). A cardiac arrest is a sudden cessation of CO and circulation. When this occurs, the tissues do not receive oxygen, CO_2 is not transported from tissues, tissue metabolism becomes anaerobic, and metabolic and respiratory acidosis occurs. Permanent heart, brain, and other tissue damage occurs within 4–6 minutes.

Cardiopulmonary Resuscitation

A patient with an absent pulse and respiration is in cardiac arrest and requires immediate **cardiopulmonary resuscitation (CPR)**. CPR is a basic emergency procedure of artificial respiration and manual external cardiac massage. The sequence for CPR is C-A-B: chest compression, early defibrillation, establishing an airway, and rescue breathing (Link et al., 2015). Chest compressions are fast, deep applications of pressure on the lower half of a patient's sternum. While standing to the side of your patient, you place your hands on the lower half of the patient's sternum and push down at least 2 inches (5 cm) and allow the chest to come back up. In some institutions, mechanical chest compression devices are used. Rescue breathing is combined with compressions and consists of performing the head tilt–chin lift maneuver to open the patient's airway and then give the breaths. In acute care agencies, the breaths are typically delivered using a bag-valve-mask device (Lewis et al., 2017).

Defibrillation delivers an electrical current to the myocardium that stops all electrical activity and allows the heart's normal pacemaker to resume its normal electrical activity (Wiegand, 2017). Defibrillation is recommended within 5 minutes for an out-of-hospital sudden cardiac arrest and within 3 minutes for a patient in the hospital. In addition to health care providers, specific lay individuals in public locations with high risk of a witnessed cardiac arrest (e.g., casinos and sporting events) should be trained in using an automated external defibrillator (AED) (AHA, 2015). An AED is a portable device that administers an electrical shock through the chest wall to the heart.

For witnessed sudden collapse of a child or for any adult victim, the recommendation is to activate the emergency response system by using your own mobile phone or the closest available phone, get the AED, and then begin chest compressions. If a child victim is unconscious and no one witnessed the collapse, the rescuer is to deliver chest compressions for 2 minutes and then activate the emergency response system. The rate of compressions for both adults and children is 100–120/min. The rescuer must allow full recoil of the chest after each compression to allow adequate filling of the heart.

The rate of compression varies with age. In children (1–8 years of age) and infants (younger than 1 year but not newborns), the ratio of compressions to breaths is 30:2 for one rescuer and 15:2 for two rescuers. For adults and adolescents, regardless of the number of rescuers, the compressions are 100–120/min at the rate of 30 compressions to 2 breaths (30:2). Continue until an AED is available and ready to analyze rhythm (AHA, 2015).

When a person is choking and has an obstructed airway, perform abdominal thrusts until the person becomes unconscious. Then you perform CPR. You may sweep the mouth and remove the foreign body if you can see it (AHA, 2015).

RESTORATIVE AND CONTINUING CARE

Restorative and continuing care emphasize cardiopulmonary reconditioning as a structured rehabilitation program. **Cardiopulmonary rehabilitation** involves helping a patient achieve and maintain an optimal level of health through controlled physical exercise, nutrition counseling, relaxation and stress management techniques, prescribed medications, and oxygen administration. As physical reconditioning occurs, the patient's physical symptoms, anxiety, depression, or somatic concerns decrease. The patient and the rehabilitation team define the goals of rehabilitation, and patient and family caregiver teaching is individualized according to patient needs (American Association of Cardiovascular and Pulmonary Rehabilitation [AACVPR], 2016).

Respiratory Muscle Training

Respiratory muscle training improves strength and endurance, resulting in improved activity tolerance.

Respiratory muscle training can decrease the presence of debilitating symptoms and prevent respiratory failure in patients with COPD.

Breathing Exercises

Breathing exercises include techniques to improve ventilation and oxygenation. The two basic techniques are pursed-lip breathing and diaphragmatic breathing.

Pursed-lip breathing involves deep inspiration and prolonged expiration through pursed lips to prevent alveolar collapse. Instruct the patient to sit up and then take a deep breath and exhale slowly through pursed lips, as if he or she were whistling. Patients need to gain control of the exhalation phase so that exhalation is longer than inhalation. The patient is usually able to perfect this technique by counting inhalation time and gradually increasing the count during exhalation.

Diaphragmatic breathing, or abdominal breathing, is more difficult and requires a patient to use the diaphragm instead of the chest accessory muscles. The patient concentrates on expanding the diaphragm during controlled inspiration. Teach the patient to place one hand on the chest and one hand on the belly. As the patient inhales the diaphragm descends (belly moves out), and as the patient exhales the diaphragm ascends (belly sinks in). Coach a patient to gently push on the abdomen with the lower hand to gently push on the diaphragm and help the patient exhale air. The exercise is often used with the pursed-lip breathing technique (COPD Foundation, 2016).

Evaluation

Patient Outcomes

You evaluate nursing interventions and therapies by comparing a patient's progress with the goals and desired outcomes of the nursing care plan. For example, your expected outcomes are directed toward improving SaO_2 levels, lung expansion on auscultation, and improved airway clearance as evidenced by improved lung sounds, improved oximetry measurements, and better expectoration of mucus. When measures directed to improve oxygenation are unsuccessful, modify the care plan by revising existing interventions or introducing new ones. For example, in patients who do not clear their airway by deep breathing and coughing, you may need to perform nasotracheal or orotracheal suctioning. Do not hesitate to notify the health care provider about a patient's decline in oxygenation status. Early recognition of a change in cardiopulmonary status and prompt notification help to avoid an emergent situation or the need for CPR.

Patients with chronic cardiopulmonary disease present a nursing challenge, particularly when they present with an acute illness. These patients require interventions that manage both the chronic symptoms and the symptoms associated with acute exacerbations or illness. For example, they may require home oxygen therapy to manage their COPD, but if they have pneumonia, they may have an increased oxygen requirement. Patients with cystic fibrosis, who often require home airway clearance therapy, may need an increase in frequency of their prescribed airway clearance therapy or a change in the therapy that they use. They may need to switch from manual CPT to HFCWC therapy. With chronic diseases, do not think in terms of recovery but rather health maintenance. A measurable outcome for a patient experiencing an acute exacerbation of a chronic illness is a return to baseline functional and cognitive status before this most recent exacerbation. This return of functional status helps to improve the patient's quality of life.

Patient Expectations

Individualize a patient's goals and make sure that they are realistic and incorporate his or her expectations. What you perceive a patient needs can be different from what he or she expects of you and other health care providers. Some patients may want to learn how to cope with chronic disease. Others may simply want to know their prognosis and what will be the course of their illness. Some patients want information about how to perform airway clearance techniques. You must determine in your initial assessment of what a patient perceives is necessary for recovery, such as emotional support, knowledge, or improved self-care abilities. Then during evaluation, determine whether his or her expectations were met. Ask patients to describe whether they believe their expectations were met. Then proceed to evaluate, for example, whether they believe they have the knowledge to better manage their disease. Do they now know more about their condition and ways to promote their health? Measuring achievement of patient expectations offers important evaluation information.

SAFETY GUIDELINES FOR NURSING SKILLS

Ensuring patient safety is an essential role of the professional nurse. To ensure patient safety, communicate clearly with members of the health care team, assess and incorporate the patient's priorities of care and preferences, and use the best evidence when making decisions about your patient's care. When performing the skills in this chapter, remember the following points to ensure safe, individualized care:

- Know a patient's baseline range of vital signs. Patients with sudden changes in their vital signs, level of consciousness, or behavior are possibly experiencing profound hypoxia.
- Test all equipment before use. Have adequate supplies on hand. Verify that suction machine is generating adequate negative suction pressure.
- Perform tracheal suctioning before pharyngeal suctioning whenever possible. The mouth and pharynx contain more bacteria than the trachea. If oral secretions are abundantly present before beginning the procedure, suction the mouth with oral suction device.
- Use caution when suctioning patients with head injuries. Suctioning raises intracranial pressure (ICP). Reduce this risk by hyperventilating before suctioning, which produces hypocarbia that in turn induces vasoconstriction. Vasoconstriction reduces the potential increase in ICP.
- Limit the introduction of a catheter to two times with each suctioning procedure.
- Use caution when suctioning anyone with recent oral or head/neck surgery. Routine suctioning is avoided following tonsillectomy. Do not use or encourage aggressive suctioning and excessive coughing in patients who have undergone throat surgery. These acts can

aggravate the operative site, increasing the risk of infection or bleeding (Hockenberry et al., 2017).

- The routine use of normal saline instillation into the airway before endotracheal and tracheostomy suctioning is not recommended. Normal saline instillation in conjunction with endotracheal suction leads to the spread of microorganisms into the lower respiratory tract and decreases oxygenation saturation (Branson et al., 2014). Current evidence shows that normal saline is not effective in thinning secretions or improving removal of secretions.

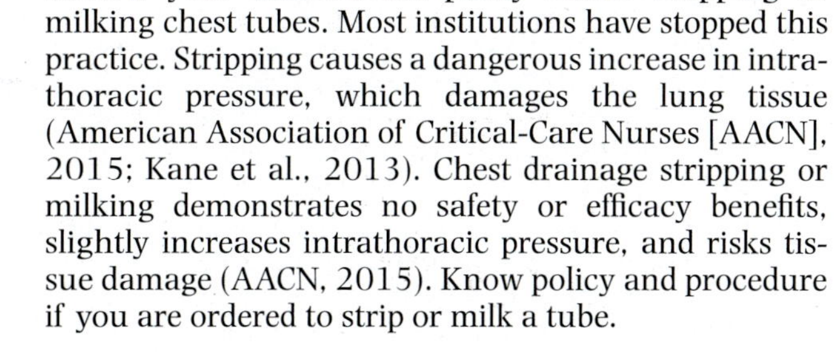

- Review your institutional policy before stripping or milking chest tubes. Most institutions have stopped this practice. Stripping causes a dangerous increase in intrathoracic pressure, which damages the lung tissue (American Association of Critical-Care Nurses [AACN], 2015; Kane et al., 2013). Chest drainage stripping or milking demonstrates no safety or efficacy benefits, slightly increases intrathoracic pressure, and risks tissue damage (AACN, 2015). Know policy and procedure if you are ordered to strip or milk a tube.

SKILL 24.1 SUCTIONING

View Video!

Equipment

- Stethoscope, pulse oximeter, and end-tidal CO_2 detector
- Portable or wall suction machine
- Connecting tubing
- Mask, goggles, gown, or face shield if indicated (have available a manual self-inflating resuscitation bag-valve device/mask with appropriately sized mask and oxygen connecting tubing)

Oropharyngeal (nonsterile) and nasotracheal (sterile) suctioning:

- Oropharyngeal—clean suction catheter or Yankauer catheter, and two clean gloves
- Nasotracheal—sterile suction catheter (12–16 Fr) (smallest diameter preferred), two sterile gloves, and sterile water-soluble lubricant
- Sterile basin with sterile water or normal saline (about 100 mL)
- Clean towel or paper drape

Endotracheal or tracheostomy suctioning:

- A 12- to 16-Fr catheter (no more than half of the internal diameter of artificial airway) (Branson et al., 2014)
- Two sterile gloves or one sterile and one clean glove
- Sterile basin with normal saline (about 100 mL)
- Clean towel or sterile drape

Closed-system or in-line suctioning:

- Closed-system or in-line suction catheter
- Five to 10 mL normal saline in syringe or vials (to cleanse catheter)
- Two clean gloves

STEP	RATIONALE
Assessment	
1. Identify the patient by using at least two identifiers (e.g., name and birthday or name and medical record number) according to agency policy.	Ensures correct patient. Complies with The Joint Commission standards and improves patient safety (TJC, 2018).
2. Review laboratory data for sputum microbiology.	Certain bacteria are easier to transmit or require isolation because of virulence or antibiotic resistance.
3. Review the patient's health care record for factors creating a risk for the patient to be unable to clear airway: history of upper and lower airway obstruction, pulmonary disease, neuromuscular or neurological impairment, anatomical factors that influence upper or lower airway function, recent surgery, head or neck tumors, impaired mobility, decreased level of consciousness, nasal feeding tube, decreased cough or gag reflex, and decreased swallowing ability.	Factors can impair the patient's ability to clear secretions from airway, accumulate secretions, and increase risk for retaining secretions, all requiring suctioning (Urden et al., 2016).
4. Review the patient's health care record for factors that may affect volume and consistency of secretions.	Thickened or copious secretions increase risk for airway obstruction.
a. Fluid balance	Fluid overload increases amount of secretions. Dehydration promotes thicker secretions.
b. Lack of humidity	The environment influences secretion formation and gas exchange. Airway suctioning is needed when the patient cannot clear secretions effectively.
c. Infection (e.g., pneumonia)	Patients are prone to increased secretions that are thicker and sometimes more difficult to expectorate.
5. Perform hand hygiene. Assess for signs and symptoms associated with hypoxia and hypercapnia: decreased SpO_2, increased and irregular pulse, increased respirations and blood pressure, apprehension, anxiety, irritability, lack of concentration, lethargy, decreased level of consciousness (especially sudden change), confusion, dizziness, fatigue, pallor, and cyanosis (very late sign of hypoxia).	Reduces transmission of microorganisms. Physical signs and symptoms resulting from decreased tissue oxygenation. Provides presuction baseline to measure effectiveness of suctioning.

STEP	RATIONALE
6. Assess for signs and symptoms of upper and lower airway obstruction: abnormal respiratory rate, adventitious lung sounds, nasal secretions, gurgling, drooling, restlessness, gastric secretions or vomitus in mouth, and coughing without clearing airway secretions and/or improving adventitious lung sounds.	Physical signs and symptoms result from secretions in upper and lower airways and decreased oxygen to tissues. Presuction assessment provides baseline data to identify need for suctioning and measure effectiveness of suction procedures (Branson et al., 2014).
7. Assess for excessive amounts of secretions or secretions visible in artificial airway, signs of respiratory distress (increased work of breathing, increased respiratory rate), presence of rhonchi on auscultation, excessive coughing, increased peak inspiratory pressures (if patient on mechanical ventilator), sawtooth pattern on ventilator monitor, changes in capnography waveform (if patient on mechanical ventilator), or decrease in the patient's pulse oximeter (Branson et al., 2014).	Perform suctioning only as the patient's condition indicates and not in a scheduled fashion (Lewis et al., 2017; Myatt, 2015).
8. Assess patency of ETT with capnography and/or end-tidal carbon dioxide (CO_2) detector.	ETT may become displaced or blocked by secretions. CO_2 detector is pH sensitive and can identify changes in CO_2 levels resulting from retained secretions (Walsh et al., 2011).
9. For endotracheal suctioning, assess the patient's peak inspiratory pressure on volume-controlled ventilation or tidal volume on pressure-controlled ventilation.	Increased peak inspiratory pressure or decreased tidal volume may indicate airway obstruction (Urden et al., 2016).
Clinical decision point: Assess a patient's vital signs, pulse oximetry, end-tidal CO_2, and respiratory status before and continuously throughout suctioning procedure (Wiegand, 2017).	
10. Identify **contraindications to nasotracheal suctioning** (AARC, 2004): occluded nasal passages; nasal bleeding; epiglottitis or croup; acute head, facial, or neck injury or surgery; coagulopathy or bleeding disorder; irritable airway; laryngospasm or bronchospasm; gastric surgery with high anastomosis; and myocardial infarction.	These conditions are contraindications because passage of a suction catheter through the nasal route traumatizes existing facial trauma and/or surgery, increases nasal bleeding, or causes severe bleeding. In the presence of epiglottitis or croup, laryngospasm, or irritable airway, passage of a suction catheter through the nose causes intractable coughing, hypoxemia, and severe bronchospasm necessitating emergency intubation or tracheostomy. Hypoxemia could worsen cardiac damage in myocardial infarction (AARC, 2004).
11. Assess the patient's understanding of procedure and presence of any apprehension.	Reveals need for instruction or psychosocial support.
Planning	
1. Provide privacy and place pulse oximeter on the patient's finger, if not already in place. Take reading and leave oximeter in place. Prepare bedside environment for patient safety.	Provides continuous SpO_2 value to determine the patient's response to suctioning. Providing privacy and preparing environment ensures a clean and distraction-free area for organizing necessary equipment.
2. Prepare and organize equipment. Place towel across the patient's chest.	Ensures that you have the necessary equipment to implement all the interventions that need to be completed for the patient.
3. Explain to the patient how procedure will help clear airway and relieve breathing difficulty. Explain that temporary coughing, sneezing, gagging, or shortness of breath is normal during procedure.	Encourages cooperation and minimizes risks, anxiety, and pain of procedure.
4. Explain importance of and encourage coughing when catheter is introduced. Have the patient practice coughing if able.	Facilitates secretion removal and reduces frequency and duration of suctioning.
Implementation	
1. Perform hand hygiene and apply appropriate personal protective equipment (PPE) (mask with face shield or goggles; gown if splashing likely).	Reduces transmission of microorganisms.
2. Adjust bed to appropriate height (if not already done) and lower side rail on side nearest you. Check locks on bed wheel.	Minimizes caregiver muscle strain and prevents injury. Prevents the bed from moving.
3. Assist the patient to comfortable position, typically semi-Fowler's or high Fowler's.	Reduces stimulation of gag reflex, promotes patient comfort and secretion drainage, and prevents aspiration.
4. Connect one end of connecting tubing to suction device and place other end in convenient location near the patient. Turn suction device on and set suction pressure to as low a level as possible and yet able to effectively clear secretions. This value is typically between 100 and 120 mm Hg in adults (between 80 and 100 mm Hg in neonates) and should never be more than 180 mm Hg (Branson et al., 2014). Occlude end of suction tubing to check pressure.	Ensures equipment function. Excessive negative pressure damages tracheal mucosa and induces greater hypoxia (Wiegand, 2017).

STEP	RATIONALE
5. If indicated, increase supplemental oxygen therapy to 100% as ordered by health care provider; encourage the patient to deep breathe.	Hyperoxygenation provides some protection from suction-induced decline in oxygenation.
6. Prepare suction catheter for all types of suctioning.	
a. *One-time-use* catheter (open suction technique)	
(1) Using aseptic technique, open suction kit or catheter package. If sterile drape is available, place it across the patient's chest or on bedside table. Do not allow suction catheter to touch any nonsterile surfaces.	Prepares catheter, maintains asepsis, and reduces transmission of microorganisms. Provides sterile surface on which to lay catheter between passes.
(2) Unwrap or open sterile basin and place on bedside table. Be careful not to touch inside of basin. Fill with about 100 mL sterile normal saline solution or water (see illustration).	Saline or water is used to clean tubing after each suction pass.
(3) If performing nasotracheal suctioning, open packet of water-soluble lubricant and apply a small amount onto sterile wrapper or kit without touching it. **Note:** Lubricant is not necessary for artificial airway suctioning.	Water-soluble lubricant helps avoid lipid aspiration pneumonia. Excessive amount of lubricant occludes catheter.
b. losed (in-line) suction catheter	
(1) Using aseptic technique, open suction catheter package and attach closed suction catheter to ventilation circuit by removing swivel adapter and placing closed suction catheter apparatus on ETT or TT. Connect Y on mechanical ventilator circuit to closed suction catheter with flex tubing.	Prepares catheter, maintains asepsis, and reduces transmission of microorganisms.
(2) Connect one end of connecting tubing to suction machine; connect other end to end of closed-system or in-line suction catheter. Check suction pressures.	Many closed-system suction catheters require slightly higher suction pressures (consult manufacturer guidelines).
7. Apply gloves:	
a. Apply clean glove to each hand or dominant hand for oropharyngeal and closed suctioning.	
b. Apply sterile gloves to each hand or nonsterile glove to nondominant hand and sterile glove to dominant hand for nasopharyngeal, nasotracheal, and artificial airway suctioning.	Reduces transmission of microorganisms and maintains sterility of suction catheter.
8. Pick up suction catheter with dominant hand without touching nonsterile surfaces. Pick up connecting tubing with nondominant hand. Secure catheter to tubing (see illustration).	Maintains catheter sterility. Connects catheter to suction.
9. Place tip of catheter into sterile basin and suction a small amount of normal saline solution by occluding suction vent. **Note:** Skip this step with closed suctioning technique.	Ensures equipment function. Lubricates internal catheter and tubing.
10. Suction airway.	
a. **Oropharyngeal suctioning**	
(1) Remove the patient's oxygen mask if present. Nasal cannula may remain in place. Keep oxygen mask near the patient's face.	Allows access to mouth. Reduces chance of hypoxia.

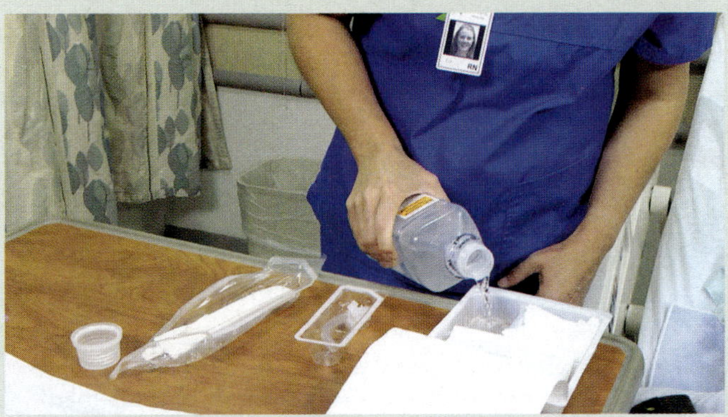

Step 6a2 Pouring sterile saline into tray.

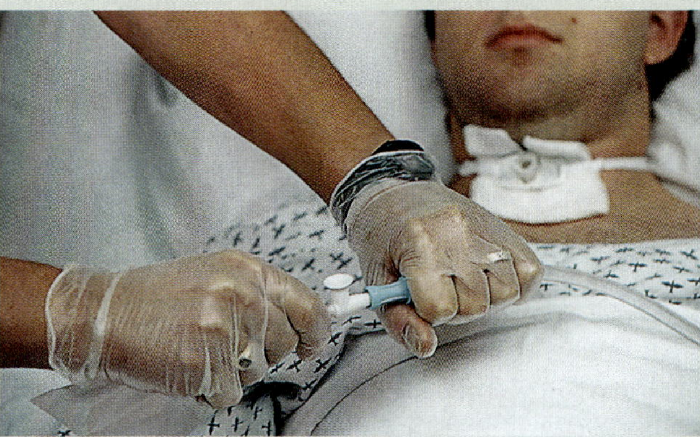

Step 8 Attaching suction catheter to suction tubing.

STEP	RATIONALE
Clinical decision point: Be prepared to quickly reapply supplemental oxygen if SpO_2 value falls below 90% or respiratory distress develops during or at the end of oropharyngeal suctioning. Be prepared to use bag-valve-mask if the patient has serious acute respiratory distress or decline in SpO_2.	
(2) Insert Yankauer catheter into mouth. Then apply suction and move catheter along gum line to pharynx. Suction until secretions have cleared. Encourage the patient to cough. Repeat if needed. Replace oxygen mask if used.	Movement of catheter prevents suction tip from damaging oral mucosal surfaces and causing trauma. Coughing moves secretions from lower airway into mouth and upper airway.
Clinical decision point: Use caution when using a Yankauer tip suction catheter with a patient who had recent oral or head and neck surgery.	
(3) Suction water or saline through catheter until connecting tubing is cleared of secretions.	Rinsing catheter reduces probability of transmission of microorganisms. Clean suction tubing enhances delivery of set suction pressure.
(4) Turn off suction and place catheter in clean, dry area. If the patient is able to suction self, place catheter within his or her reach and leave suction on.	Facilitates prompt removal of airway secretions for future suctioning.
b. **Nasopharyngeal and nasotracheal suctioning**	
(1) Have the patient take deep breaths, if able. Increase oxygen flow rate through cannula or mask if ordered.	Helps to decrease risks of hypoxemia.
(2) For nasotracheal suctioning, lightly coat distal 6–8 cm (2–3 inches) of catheter with water-soluble lubricant.	Lubricates catheter for easier insertion and reduces mucosal trauma.
(3) Remove oxygen delivery device, if applicable, with nondominant hand.	
(a) *Nasopharyngeal:* Without applying suction, have the patient take a deep breath, and use dominant thumb and forefinger to insert catheter following natural course of naris; slightly slant catheter downward and advance to back of pharynx. Do not force through naris. In adults, insert catheter approximately 20 cm (8 inches) into trachea until resistance is met or the patient coughs, and then pull back 1–2 cm (½ inch). In infants and children, the suction catheter must not be passed any further than the suprasternal notch, which is the dip at the front base of the neck (Association of Paediatric Chartered Physiotherapists, 2015) (refer to agency policy). Rule of thumb is to insert catheter distance from tip of nose (or mouth) to angle of mandible.	Application of suction pressure while introducing catheter into nasopharynx increases risk for damage to mucosa and increases risk for hypoxia. Ensure that catheter tip reaches pharynx for suctioning.
Clinical decision point: Do not insert during swallowing or catheter will most likely enter esophagus. Never apply suction during insertion. The patient should cough; if the patient gags or becomes nauseated, catheter is most likely in esophagus and you need to remove it.	
Clinical decision point: If resistance is met during insertion, you may need to try the other naris. Do not force catheter through naris because this will cause mucosal damage.	
(i) Apply intermittent suction for 2 s by placing and releasing nondominant thumb over catheter vent. Then slowly withdraw catheter while rotating it back and forth and applying intermittent suction. Total time should take about 10–15 s.	Intermittent suction for 10–15 s safely removes pharyngeal secretions. Suction time greater than 10–15 s increases risk for suction-induced hypoxemia (Branson et al., 2014).
(b) *Nasotracheal* (without applying suction): Advance catheter using same procedure as nasopharyngeal through the naris. When just above entrance into larynx, have the patient relax and then take a deep breath as you quickly advance catheter into trachea. Advance catheter in an adult approximately 20 cm (8 inches) into trachea (see illustration). The patient will begin to cough; pull back catheter 1–2 cm (1/2 inch) before applying suction. **Note:** In older children, insert 15–20 cm (6–8 inches); in infants and young children, insert 8–14 cm (3–5 1/2 inches).	Inhalation opens glottis and facilitates entrance of catheter tip into trachea for suctioning.
Clinical decision point: Be sure to insert catheter during patient inhalation because epiglottis is open. When using the nasal approach, perform tracheal suctioning before pharyngeal suctioning whenever possible. The mouth and pharynx contain more bacteria than the trachea. If copious oral secretions are present before beginning procedure, first suction mouth with oral suction device such as a Yankauer.	

STEP	RATIONALE

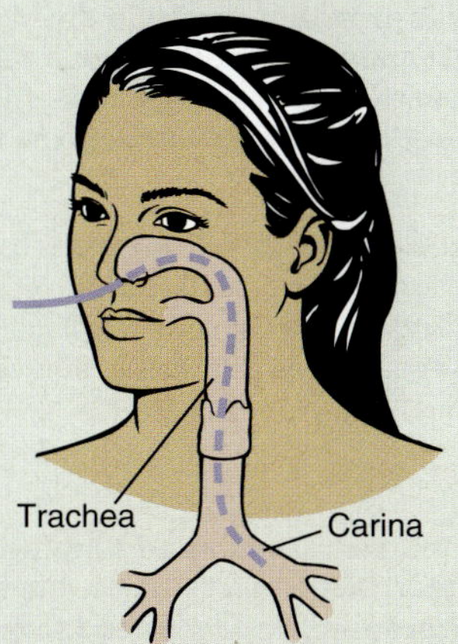

Step 10b(3)(b) Distance of insertion of nasotracheal catheter.

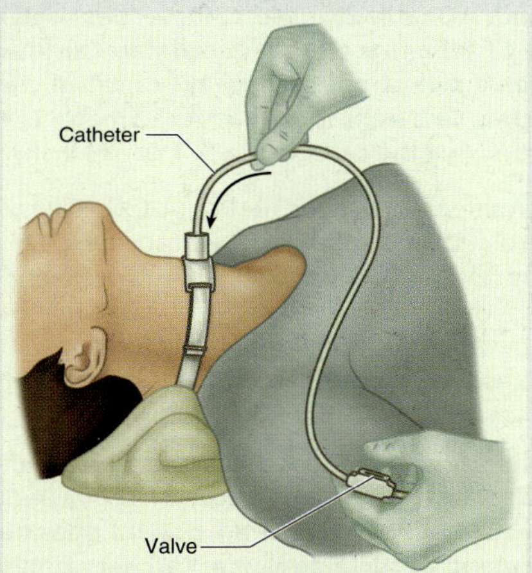

Step 10c(3) Suctioning tracheostomy.

Clinical decision point: When there is difficulty passing catheter, ask the patient to cough or say "ahh" or try to advance catheter during inspiration. Both measures help to open the glottis to permit passage of catheter into the trachea.

STEP	RATIONALE
(i) Positioning option: In some instances, turning the patient's head helps you insert catheter and suction more effectively. If you feel resistance after insertion of catheter, use caution because it has probably hit the carina. Pull catheter back 1–2 cm (0.4–0.8 inch) before applying suction (AARC, 2004).	Turning the patient's head to side elevates bronchial passage on opposite side. Turning head to right helps you suction left mainstem bronchus; turning head to left helps you suction right mainstem bronchus. Suctioning too deep may cause tracheal mucosa trauma.
(ii) Apply intermittent suction for no more than 10–15 s by placing and releasing nondominant thumb over catheter vent. Slowly withdraw catheter while rotating it back and forth between thumb and forefinger.	Suction time greater than 10–15 s increases risk for suction-induced hypoxemia (AARC, 2010; Branson et al., 2014). Intermittent suction and rotation of catheter prevent injury to tracheal mucosa. If catheter "grabs" mucosa, remove thumb to release suction.

Clinical decision point: Monitor the patient's vital signs and oxygen saturation throughout suctioning process. Stop suctioning if there is a 20-beat/min change (increase or decrease) in pulse or if SpO_2 falls below 90% or 5% from baseline.

STEP	RATIONALE
(4) Reapply oxygen delivery device and encourage the patient to take some deep breaths, if able.	Helps to decrease risk of hypoxia. Increases patient comfort.
(5) Rinse catheter and connecting tubing with normal saline or water until cleared.	Secretions that remain in suction catheter or connecting tubing decrease suctioning efficiency.
(6) Assess for need to repeat suctioning. Do not perform more than two passes with catheter. Allow the patient to rest at least 1 min (Wiegand, 2017). Ask the patient to deep breathe and cough.	Observe for alterations in cardiopulmonary status. Suctioning induces hypoxemia, irregular pulse, laryngospasm, and bronchospasm (Wiegand, 2017).
c. **Artificial airway—one-time-use catheter**	
(1) When the patient has artificial airway (e.g., ETT or TT), hyperoxygenate the patient with 100% oxygen for at least 30–60 s before suctioning by either pressing suction hyperoxygenation button on ventilator *or* increasing baseline FiO_2 level on mechanical ventilator. **Note:** Some mechanical ventilators have a button that when pushed delivers 100% oxygen for a few minutes and then resets to previous setting.	Preoxygenation decreases risk of decreased arterial oxygen levels while ventilation or oxygenation is interrupted and volume is lost during suctioning. Some models of resuscitation bags do not deliver 100% oxygen, so this is not the best way to oxygenate a patient (Wiegand, 2017). Consult with respiratory therapist if necessary.
(2) If the patient is receiving mechanical ventilation, open swivel adapter or, if necessary, remove oxygen or humidity delivery device with nondominant hand.	Exposes artificial airway.

Clinical decision point: Suctioning can cause elevations in intracranial pressure (ICP) in patients with head injuries. Reduce this risk by presuction hyperoxygenation, which results in hypocarbia that in turn induces vasoconstriction. Vasoconstriction reduces the potential for increased ICP (Urden et al., 2016).

STEP	RATIONALE
(3) Advise the patient that you are about to begin suctioning. Without applying suction, gently but quickly insert catheter into artificial airway using dominant thumb and forefinger (try to time catheter insertion into artificial airway during inspiration) until you meet resistance or the patient coughs; then pull back 1 cm (0.4 inch) (see illustration) (Wiegand, 2017).	Application of suction pressure while introducing catheter into trachea increases risk for damage to tracheal mucosa and increased hypoxia. Pulling back stimulates cough and removes catheter from mucosal wall so that catheter is not resting against tracheal mucosa during suctioning. Shallow suctioning is recommended to prevent tracheal mucosa trauma (AARC, 2010; Wiegand, 2017).

STEP	RATIONALE
Clinical decision point: If unable to insert catheter past end of ET tube, the catheter is probably caught in the Murphy eye (i.e., side hole at distal end of ET tube that allows for collateral airflow in the event of tracheal mainstem intubation). If this happens, rotate catheter to reposition it away from Murphy eye or withdraw it slightly and reinsert with next inhalation. Usually, the catheter meets resistance at the carina. One indication that the catheter is at the carina is acute onset of coughing because the carina contains many cough receptors. Pull the catheter back 1 cm (½ inch).	
(4) Apply intermittent suction for 10–15 s (AARC, 2010; Branson et al., 2014). Apply intermittent suction by placing and releasing nondominant thumb over vent of catheter; slowly withdraw catheter while rotating it back and forth between dominant thumb and forefinger. Do not use suction for greater than 10–15 s. Encourage the patient to cough. Watch for respiratory distress.	Suction time greater than 10–15 s increases risk for suction-induced hypoxemia (AARC, 2010; Branson et al., 2014). Intermittent suction and rotation of catheter prevents injury to tracheal mucosa. If catheter "grabs" mucosa, remove thumb to release suction.
Clinical decision point: If the patient develops respiratory distress, immediately withdraw catheter and supply additional oxygen and breaths as needed. In an emergency, administer oxygen directly through catheter. Disconnect suction and attach oxygen at prescribed flow rate through catheter. If the patient does not tolerate suctioning procedure, you may need to consider switching to closed (in-line) suctioning or allowing longer recovery times. Notify health care provider if the patient develops significant cardiopulmonary compromise during suctioning (Urden et al., 2016; Wiegand, 2017).	
(5) If the patient is receiving mechanical ventilation, close swivel adapter or replace oxygen delivery device. Hyperoxygenate the patient for 30–60 s.	Reestablishes artificial airway. Helps to decrease risks of hypoxia.
d. **Artificial airway suctioning—closed (in-line)**	
(1) Hyperoxygenate the patient (usually with 100% oxygen) by adjusting FiO_2 setting on ventilator or by using a temporary oxygen enrichment program available on microprocessor ventilators, according to agency policy.	Preoxygenation decreases risk of decreased arterial oxygen levels while ventilation or oxygenation is interrupted and volume is lost during suctioning.
(2) Unlock suction control mechanism on suction catheter if required by manufacturer. Open saline port and attach saline syringe or vial.	Lock prevents catheter from accidentally migrating into airway when not in use. Unlocking catheter allows you to use it. The saline will be necessary to clean catheter between each suction pass.
(3) Pick up suction catheter enclosed in plastic sleeve with dominant hand. While the patient inhales and without applying suction, insert catheter using a repeating maneuver of pushing catheter and sliding (or pulling) plastic sleeve back between thumb and forefinger until resistance is felt or the patient coughs. Then pull back 1 cm (1/2 inch).	Application of suction pressure while introducing catheter into trachea increases risk for damage to tracheal mucosa and increased hypoxia. Pulling back stimulates cough and removes catheter from mucosal wall so that catheter is not resting against tracheal mucosa during suctioning.
(4) Encourage the patient to cough and apply suction by continuously squeezing on suction control mechanism while withdrawing catheter over a period of no longer than 10–15 s.	It is difficult, if not impossible, to apply intermittent pulses of suction to a closed-system catheter. Suctioning for longer periods of time increases risk of complications resulting from hypoxemia.
The following steps pertain to both open and closed tracheal suctioning:	
(5) Rinse catheter and connecting tubing with normal saline until clear. Use continuous suction.	Removes catheter secretions. Secretions left in tubing decrease suctioning efficiency and provide environment for microorganism growth.
(6) Assess the patient's vital signs, cardiopulmonary status, and ventilator measures for secretion clearance. Repeat Steps (1)–(6) once or twice more to clear secretions. Allow adequate time (at least 1 full min) between suction passes.	Suctioning can induce dysrhythmias, hypoxia, and bronchospasm and impair cerebral circulation or adversely affect hemodynamic stability (Wiegand, 2017).
Clinical decision point: Base the number of suction passes on patient assessment and presence of secretions. If secretions persist after two passes, allow the patient more time to rest and recover from these procedures (Wiegand, 2017).	
(7) When pharynx and trachea are sufficiently cleared of secretions, perform oropharyngeal suctioning to clear mouth of secretions. Do not suction nose again after suctioning mouth.	Removes upper airway secretions. More microorganisms generally are present in mouth. Upper airway is considered "clean," and lower airway is considered "sterile." You can use same catheter to suction from sterile to clean areas (e.g., tracheal suctioning to oropharyngeal suctioning) but not from clean to sterile areas.
11. When suctioning is complete, disconnect the one-time-use catheter from connecting tubing. Roll catheter around fingers of dominant hand. Pull glove off inside out so catheter remains coiled in glove. Pull off other glove over first glove in same way. Discard in appropriate receptacle. Turn off suction device. For closed suction catheter, ensure that the catheter is pulled all the way back into sleeve, and if device has a locking mechanism, ensure that mechanism is locked.	Seals contaminants in gloves. Reduces transmission of microorganisms (Wiegand, 2017). Pulling closed suction catheter device back into sleeve ensures that airway is not obstructed.

STEP	RATIONALE
12. Remove towel or drape, place in laundry or appropriate receptacle, and reposition the patient. (Apply clean gloves to continue personal care.)	Reduces transmission of microorganisms. Promotes comfort.
13. If indicated, readjust oxygen to original level because the patient's blood oxygen level should have returned to baseline.	Prevents absorption atelectasis (i.e., tendency for airways to collapse if proximally obstructed by secretions). Prevents oxygen toxicity while allowing the patient time to reoxygenate blood.
14. Discard remainder of normal saline into appropriate receptacle. If basin is disposable, discard into appropriate receptacle. If basin is reusable, rinse it out and place it in soiled utility room.	Reduces transmission of microorganisms.
15. Remove personal protective equipment and discard into appropriate receptacle. Perform hand hygiene.	Reduces transmission of microorganisms.
16. Place unopened suction kit on suction machine table or at head of bed.	Provides immediate access to suction catheter for next procedure.
17. Help the patient to comfortable position and provide oral hygiene as needed. Wash face if secretions are present on the patient's skin.	Prevents skin breakdown. Promotes comfort.
Evaluation	
1. Compare the patient's vital signs, cardiopulmonary assessments, and end-tidal CO_2 ($EtCO_2$) and SpO_2 values before and after suctioning. If on ventilator, compare FiO_2 and tidal volumes and peak inspiratory pressures.	$PetCO_2$ is a noninvasive measurement of a patient's exhaled CO_2, and it can be used to help continuously monitor the amount of CO_2 in patients with artificial airways. Measures identify physiological effects of suction procedure (Wiegand, 2017).
2. Ask the patient whether breathing is easier and whether congestion is decreased.	Provides subjective confirmation that suctioning procedure has relieved airway obstruction.
3. Auscultate lungs and compare the patient's respiratory assessment before and after suctioning.	Provides objective information about any change in lung sounds.
4. Observe character of airway secretions.	Provides data to document presence or absence of respiratory tract infection or thickened secretions.
5. **Use teach back:** "I need to suction your father and I want to be sure that I explained the suctioning procedure and when I need to do this procedure. Please, tell me why I'm having to suction your dad at this time." Revise your instruction now or develop a plan for revised patient/family caregiver teaching if the patient/family caregiver is not able to teach back correctly.	Determines the patient's/family caregiver's level of understanding of instructional topic.

Recording and Reporting

- Record in nurses' notes in electronic health record (EHR), chart, or flow sheets the patient's presuctioning vital signs, cardiopulmonary status, and ventilation measures; need for and type of hyperoxygenation used; amount, consistency, color, and odor of secretions; size of catheter; and route of suctioning.
- Record the patient's response to suctioning and postsuctioning vital signs, cardiopulmonary status, and ventilation measures.
- Document your evaluation of patient/family caregiver learning.
- Report unexpected outcomes.

Unexpected Outcomes and Related Interventions

- The patient has decrease in SpO_2, increased end-tidal CO_2, continued tachypnea, continued increased work of breathing, bronchospasm, and cardiac dysrhythmias.
  - Limit length of suctioning.
  - Determine need for more frequent suctioning, possibly of shorter duration.
  - Determine need for supplemental oxygen or increase in supplemental oxygen. Supply oxygen between suctioning passes as ordered.
  - Notify health care provider.
- Bloody secretions are returned after suctioning.
  - Determine amount of suction pressure used. It may need to be decreased.
  - Ensure that suction is completed correctly using intermittent suction and catheter rotation. Do not apply suction until after catheter has been pulled back 1 cm to prevent applying suction while the catheter is touching the carina.
  - Evaluate suctioning frequency.
- Inability to obtain secretions during suction procedure:
  - Evaluate the patient's fluid status and adequacy of humidification on oxygen delivery device.
  - Assess for signs of infection.
  - Determine need for chest physiotherapy.
  - Notify health care provider.

SKILL 24.2 CARE OF PATIENTS WITH CHEST TUBES

Equipment

- Prescribed chest drainage system with suction source and setup (wall canister or portable):
  - *Water-seal system:* Add sterile water or normal saline (NS) solution to cover lower 2.5 cm (1 inch) of water-seal chamber. Pour sterile water or NS into suction control chamber if suction is to be used (see manufacturer directions).
  - *Waterless system:* Add vial of 30–45 mL sterile sodium chloride or water (for diagnostic air-leak indicator); 20-mL syringe, 21-gauge needle, and antiseptic swab (see manufacturer directions).
  - Dry suction system.
- Suction tubing
- Clean gloves
- Sterile gauze sponges
- Local anesthetic with appropriate-sized syringe and needle, if not an emergent procedure
- Chest tube tray (all items are sterile): knife handle (1), knife blade no. 10 or disposable safety scalpel no. 10, chest tube clamp, small sponge forceps, needle holder, size 3-0 silk sutures, tray liner (sterile field), curved 8-inch Kelly clamps (2), 4 × 4-inch sponges (10), suture scissors, hand towels (3), and sterile gloves
- Dressings: petrolatum (Xeroform) gauze, split chest tube dressings, several 4 × 4-inch gauze dressings, large gauze dressings (2), and 2- or 4-inch tape (see agency procedure)
- Facemask, head cover, face shield, or goggles (as needed)
- Sterile gloves
- Two rubber-tipped hemostats (shodded) for each chest tube (for emergencies)
- A 2.5-cm (1-inch) waterproof adhesive tape or plastic zip ties for securing connections
- Stethoscope, sphygmomanometer, and pulse oximeter

STEP	RATIONALE
Assessment	
1. Identify the patient by using at least two identifiers (e.g., name and birthday or name and medical record number) according to agency policy.	Ensures correct patient. Complies with The Joint Commission standards and improves patient safety (TJC, 2018).
2. Assess the patient for known allergies. Ask the patient whether he or she has had a problem with medications, latex, or anything applied to skin.	Antiseptic solutions are used to clean skin before tube insertion (Kane et al., 2013). Lidocaine is a local anesthetic administered to reduce pain. The chest tube will be held in place with tape and sutures.
3. Review the patient's medication record for anticoagulant therapy or nonsteroidal anti-inflammatory drugs (NSAIDs) including aspirin, warfarin, heparin, or platelet aggregation inhibitors.	Anticoagulants and NSAIDs can increase procedure-related blood loss.
4. Review the patient's hemoglobin and hematocrit levels.	Parameters reflect whether blood loss is occurring, which may affect oxygenation and other vital signs.
5. Perform hand hygiene. Perform a complete respiratory assessment, baseline vital signs, pulse oximetry, and level of cognition.	Reduces transmission of microorganisms. Determines level of respiratory distress. Cognitive changes indicate hypoxia.
a. Assess for signs and symptoms of increased respiratory distress and hypoxia (e.g., decreased breath sounds over affected lungs, cyanosis, asymmetrical chest movements, displaced trachea, shortness of breath, confusion).	Signs and symptoms associated with respiratory distress are related to type and size of pneumothorax, hemothorax, or preexisting illness. Signs of hypoxia are related to inadequate oxygen to tissues (Lewis et al., 2017).
b. Assess for sharp stabbing chest pain or chest pain on inspiration, hypotension, and tachycardia. If possible, ask the patient to rate level of comfort on visual analog scale of 0–10.	Sharp stabbing chest pain, low blood pressure, and increased heart rate may indicate tension pneumothorax. Pneumothorax or hemothorax is painful, particularly with inspiration. In addition, discomfort is associated with presence of chest tube. As a result, patients tend to not cough or change position in an effort to minimize pain (Ball et al., 2015).
6. For patients who have chest tubes in place, observe the following:	
a. Chest tube dressing and site surrounding tube insertion.	Ensures that dressing is intact and occlusive seal remains without air or fluid leaks and that area surrounding insertion site is free of drainage or skin irritation. Leakage of air into tissue manifests as subcutaneous emphysema.
b. Tubing for kinks, dependent loops, or clots.	Maintains a patent, freely draining system, preventing fluid or air accumulation in chest cavity. When tubing is coiled, looped, or clotted, drainage is impeded (Mohammed, 2015).
c. Chest drainage system should be upright and below level of tube insertion.	Upright drainage system facilitates drainage and maintains water seal. If above site of insertion, fluid will drain back into the patient (Lewis et al., 2017; Mohammed, 2015).
7. Determine the patient's and family caregiver's knowledge of procedure and reason for tubes.	Encourages cooperation, minimizes risks and anxiety, and identifies teaching needs.

STEP	RATIONALE
Planning	
1. Provide privacy and prepare bedside environment by removing any items that are not needed for procedure.	Reduces interruptions and provides clean surface areas in the patient environment
2. Prepare and organize equipment and supplies. Place two rubber-tipped hemostats (for each chest tube) in an easily accessible position (e.g., taped to top of the patient's headboard). These should remain with the patient at all times, even during ambulation.	Ensures organized procedure. Chest tubes are double clamped under specific circumstances: (1) to assess for air leak, (2) to empty or quickly change disposable systems, and (3) to assess whether the patient is ready to have tube removed.
3. Explain procedure and continued care of chest tube to the patient and family caregiver.	Encourages cooperation and decreases anxiety.
Implementation	
1. For tube insertion, check agency policy and determine whether informed consent is needed. Complete time-out procedure.	Invasive medical procedures typically require informed consent. Time-out is completed to determine right patient, procedure, and location of insertion or incision site (Kane et al., 2013).
2. Review health care provider's order for chest tube placement.	Insertion of a chest tube requires health care provider order.
3. Perform hand hygiene.	Prevents transmission of microorganisms.
4. Administer premedication such as sedatives or analgesics as ordered 30 min before tube insertion.	Reduces patient anxiety and pain during procedure.
5. Set up water-seal system (or dry system with suction); see manufacturer guidelines.	
a. Remove sterile wrappers and prepare to set up a two- or three-chamber system.	Maintains sterility of system for use under sterile operating room conditions.
b. While maintaining sterility of drainage tubing, stand system upright and add sterile water or NS to appropriate compartments.	Reduces possibility of contamination.
(1) *Two-chamber system (without suction):* Add sterile solution to water-seal chamber, bringing fluid to required level as indicated.	Water-seal chamber acts as one-way valve so that air cannot enter pleural space (Kane et al., 2013).
(2) *Three-chamber system (with suction):* Add sterile solution to water-seal chamber. Add amount of sterile solution prescribed by health care provider to suction control chamber, usually 20 cm H_2O pressure. Connect tubing from suction control chamber to suction source. Tailor length of drainage tube to the patient. **Note:** Suction control chamber vent must not be occluded when using suction (see Fig. 24.11).	Depth of fluid level dictates highest amount of negative pressure that can be present within system. For example, 20 cm of water is approximately 20 cm H_2O pressure. Any additional negative pressure applied to the system is vented into the atmosphere through suction control vent. This safety device prevents damage to pleural tissues from unexpected surge of negative pressure from suction source. After chest tube is inserted, turn up wall or portable suction device until water in suction control bottle exhibits continuous, gentle bubbling (Kane et al., 2013; Mohammed, 2015).
Clinical decision point: Remember when increasing suction that increased bubbling does not result in more suction to the chest cavity but serves only to evaporate the water more quickly.	
(3) *Dry suction system:* Fill water-seal chamber with sterile solution. Adjust suction control dial to prescribed level of suction; suction ranges from −10 to −40 cm H_2O pressure. Suction control chamber vent is never occluded when suction is used. **Note:** On a dry suction system, *do not* obstruct positive-pressure relief valve. This allows air to escape.	Automatic control valve on dry suction control device adjusts to changes in patient air leaks and fluctuation in suction source and vacuum to deliver prescribed amount of suction.
6. Set up waterless system (see manufacturer guidelines).	
a. Remove sterile wrappers and prepare to set up.	Maintains sterility of system for use under sterile operating room conditions.
b. For two-chamber system (without suction), nothing is added or needs to be done to system.	Waterless two-chamber system is ready for connecting to the patient's chest tube after opening wrappers.
c. For three-chamber system (with suction), connect tubing from suction control chamber to suction source.	Suction source provides additional negative pressure to system.
d. Instill 15 mL of sterile water or NS into diagnostic indicator injection port located on top of system.	Allows observation of rise and fall in water in diagnostic air leak window. Constant left-to-right bubbling or rocking is abnormal and indicates air leak. This is not necessary for mediastinal drainage because there is no tidaling. In an emergency, system does not require water for set up.

STEP	RATIONALE
7. Check system patency by: a. Clamping drainage tubing that will connect to the patient's chest tube b. Connecting tubing from float ball chamber to suction source c. Turning on suction to prescribed level	Ensures functioning system.
8. Turn off suction source and unclamp drainage tubing before connecting the patient to system. Suction source is turned on again after the patient is connected.	Having the patient connected to suction when it is initiated could damage pleural tissues from sudden increase in negative pressure. Tubing that is coiled or looped may become clotted and cause tension pneumothorax (Kane et al., 2013).
Clinical decision point: Carefully monitor the patient during procedure for changes in level of sedation. If the patient is too sedated, the patient will lose his or her respiratory drive and could potentially develop hypoxia.	
9. Provide psychological support to the patient (Kane et al., 2013). Reinforce preprocedure explanation, and coach and support throughout insertion of tube(s).	
10. Perform hand hygiene and apply clean gloves and any other PPE if you suspect exposure to fluid spray. Position the patient for tube insertion so that side in which tube is to be inserted is accessible to health care provider.	Reduces transmission of microorganisms. For pneumothorax, place the patient in lateral supine position. For hemothorax, place the patient in semi-Fowler's position (Kane et al., 2013).
11. Assist health care provider with chest tube insertion by providing needed equipment and local anesthetic. Health care provider will anesthetize skin over insertion site, make small skin incision, insert clamped tube, suture it in place, and apply occlusive dressing.	Ensures smooth insertion.
12. Assist health care provider with attaching drainage tube to chest tube; remove clamp. Turn on suction to prescribed level.	Connects drainage system and suction (if ordered) to chest tube.
13. Tape or zip-tie all connections between chest tube and drainage tube. (**Note:** Chest tube is usually taped by health care provider at time of tube placement; check agency policy.)	Secures chest tube to drainage system and reduces risk for air leak that causes breaks in airtight system (Shlamovitz, 2014).
14. Check systems for proper functioning. Health care provider will order chest radiograph.	Verifies intrapleural placement of tube.
15. After tube placement, position the patient in a manner that promotes drainage of fluid or air.	Permits optimum drainage of fluid and/or air. Frequent repositioning promotes better drainage (Lewis et al., 2017).
a. Use semi-Fowler's or high Fowler's position to evacuate air (pneumothorax) (Chotai, 2016).	
b. Use high Fowler's position to drain fluid (hemothorax) (Chotai, 2016).	
16. Check patency of air vents in system.	
a. Water-seal vent must have no occlusion.	Permits displaced air to pass into atmosphere.
b. Suction control chamber vent is not occluded when suction is used.	Provides safety factor of releasing excess negative pressure into atmosphere.
c. Waterless systems have relief valves without caps.	Provides safety factor of releasing excess negative pressure.
17. Position excess tubing horizontally on mattress next to the patient. Secure with clamp provided so that it does not obstruct tubing.	Prevents excess tubing from hanging over edge of mattress in dependent loop. Drainage collected in loop can occlude drainage system, which predisposes the patient to tension pneumothorax (Kane et al., 2013).
18. Adjust tubing to hang in straight line from chest tube to drainage chamber.	Promotes drainage and prevents fluid or blood from accumulating in pleural cavity (Mohammed, 2015).
Clinical decision point: Frequent gentle lifting of drain allows gravity to assist blood and other viscous material to move to drainage bottle. Patients with recent chest surgery or trauma need to have the chest drain lifted based on assessment of the amount of drainage; some patients might need chest tube drains lifted every 5–10 min until drainage volume decreases. However, when coiled or dependent looping of tubing is unavoidable, lift tubing every 15 min at a minimum to promote drainage (Kane et al., 2013).	
19. Be sure that the two rubber-tipped hemostats are accessible to the patient.	Chest tubes are double clamped when air leak is suspected, when there is a need to empty or change systems, or to assess whether the patient is ready for tube removal.
20. Dispose of sharps in proper container, dispose of used supplies, and perform hand hygiene.	Reduces transmission of microorganisms.

STEP	RATIONALE
21. Care of the patient after chest tube insertion	
a. Assess vital signs; oxygen saturation; chest wall movement; skin and mucous membrane color; breath sounds; rate, depth, and ease of respirations; and insertion site every 15 min for the first 2 h and then at least every shift (see agency policy).	Provides immediate information about procedure-related complications such as respiratory distress and leakage.
b. Monitor color, consistency, and amount of chest tube drainage every 15 min for the first 2 h and then hourly (see agency policy). Indicate level of drainage fluid, date, and time on write-on surface of chamber. Be aware of what is normal amount and color of drainage expected for patient condition.	Provides baseline for continuous assessment of type and quantity of drainage. Ensures early detection of complications. Pneumothorax typically has serous drainage with air. Hemothorax will initially have sanguineous drainage that transitions to serosanguineous and then serous. Drainage amounts can vary, but after surgery you can expect 100–300 mL/h for the first few hours and then a decrease to less than 50 mL/h (Kane et al., 2013).
(1) From mediastinal tube, expect less than 100 mL/h immediately after surgery and no more than 500 mL in the first 24 h.	Sudden gush of drainage may result from coughing or changing the patient's position, releasing pooled and/or collected blood rather than indicating active bleeding.
(2) From posterior chest tube, expect between 100 and 300 mL in the first 3 h after insertion, with 500–1000 mL expected in the first 24 h. Drainage is grossly bloody during the first several hours after surgery and then changes to serous (Kane et al., 2013).	Acute bleeding indicates hemorrhage. Health care provider should be notified if there is more than 250 mL of bloody drainage in 1 h (Kane et al., 2013).
(3) From anterior chest tube, expect little or no output from anterior chest tube that is inserted for pneumothorax (Kane et al., 2013).	
c. Observe chest tube dressing and skin around dressing for drainage. Dressing should be occlusive.	Drainage around tube may indicate blockage. Loose dressing increases risk of infection. Some patients may develop subcutaneous emphysema, which is a collection of air under the skin. You will palpate crepitus, or puffed-out skin crackles (Mohammed, 2015).
d. Apply clean gloves. Palpate around tube for swelling and crepitus (subcutaneous emphysema) as noted by crackling.	Indicates presence of air trapping in subcutaneous tissues. Small amounts are commonly absorbed. Large amounts are potentially dangerous. Most occurrences of crepitus are minor (Mao et al., 2015).
Clinical decision point: Some patients may develop subcutaneous emphysema, which is a collection of air under the skin after chest tube placement that can occur if tubing is blocked or kinked. When this occurs, a crepitus (a crackling sensation) is heard on auscultation.	
e. Check tubing to ensure that it is free of kinks and dependent loops.	Promotes drainage.
f. Observe for fluctuation of drainage in tubing during inspiration and expiration (tidaling). Observe for clots or debris in tubing. Assess water-seal chamber for tidaling of water with the patient's inspiration and expiration, and assess level of water.	If fluctuation or tidaling stops, it means that either the lung is fully expanded or the system is obstructed. In a spontaneously breathing patient, fluid rises in water-seal or diagnostic indicator (waterless system) with inspiration and falls with expiration. The opposite occurs in a patient who is mechanically ventilated. This indicates that system is functioning properly (AACN, 2015; Kane et al., 2013).
g. Keep drainage system upright and below level of the patient's chest.	Promotes gravity drainage and prevents backflow of fluid and air into pleural space.
h. Check for air leaks by monitoring bubbling in water-seal chamber. Intermittent bubbling is normal during expiration when air is being evacuated from pleural cavity, but continuous bubbling during both inspiration and expiration indicates leak in system.	Absence of bubbling may indicate that lung is fully expanded in a patient with pneumothorax. Check all connections and locate sources of air leak as described in Table 24.9.
22. Measure any drainage, and document time on surface of drainage system.	Provides assessment for type, quality, and quantity of drainage.
23. In a patient with existing chest tube, apply sterile gloves (per agency policy) and change dressing if loose or saturated.	Check agency policy regarding whether or not dressing change is sterile or clean. Also know health care provider preference for need for petroleum gauze dressing around tube.
24. Remove and dispose of gloves and used supplies, if any, and perform hand hygiene.	Reduces transmission of microorganisms.
25. Assist the patient to comfortable position: semi-Fowler's or Fowler's.	Ensures proper chest tube drainage and facilitates chest wall expansion.

STEP	RATIONALE
Evaluation	
1. Evaluate the patient for decreased respiratory distress and chest pain. Auscultate the patient's lungs and observe chest expansion.	Determines status of lung expansion.
2. Complete all assessment measures in Step 21 and Step 22. Compare with previous findings.	Provides data regarding respiratory status, level of oxygenation, and lung expansion.
Clinical decision point: If no tidaling is present, drainage system could be blocked, the lungs could have reexpanded, or the system is attached to suction. Further investigation is warranted, and critical thinking on your part is needed. If bubbling is increased, an air leak may be present. See Table 24.9 for care of an air leak.	
3. Evaluate the patient's level of comfort on visual analog scale of 0–10, comparing level with comfort before chest tube insertion.	Indicates need for analgesia. Patients with chest tubes typically have pain, which makes it difficult to take deep breaths (Kane et al., 2013).
4. Evaluate the patient's ability to use deep-breathing exercises while maintaining comfort.	Indicates the patient's ability to promote lung expansion and prevent complications.
5. Assess suction control chamber.	
a. *Wet suction system:* Continuous gentle bubbling should be present.	Indicates chamber has appropriate suction and is functioning appropriately. No bubbling indicates that there is no suction, the suction is not high enough, or the air leak is so large that the suction is not high enough to evacuate the leak (Lewis et al., 2017).
b. *Dry suction system (waterless system):* The float ball indicates the amount of suction the patient is receiving.	If the suction the patient is receiving does not match amount ordered, adjust dial to reach prescribed setting.
Clinical decision point: If chest tube drainage suddenly increases or if there is more than 100 mL/h of bloody drainage (except for the first 3 h after surgery), inform health care provider immediately and remain with the patient and assess vital signs, oxygen saturation by pulse oximetry, and cardiopulmonary status. This finding may indicate hemorrhage or perforation of the lung.	
6. **Use teach back:** "I want to be sure I explained why you need a chest tube. Tell me why you have it." Revise your instructions now or develop a plan for revised patient/family caregiver teaching if the patient/family caregiver is not able to teach back correctly.	Determines the patient's/family caregiver's level of understanding of instructional topic.

Table 24.9 Emergency Care With Chest Tubes

Assessment	Intervention
1. Air leak: Can occur at insertion site, at connection between tube and drainage, or within drainage device itself. Continuous bubbling occurs in water-seal chamber and water seal.	Locate leak by using rubber-tipped (shodded) hemostats to clamp tube at different intervals along tube, starting at the patient's chest. If leak stops, the air is coming from the patient—take dressing off, ensure tube is still in place, and notify health care provider. Do not leave chest tube clamped because this can cause collapse of lung, mediastinal shift, and eventual collapse of other lung from buildup of air pressure within pleural cavity. If bubbling continues, clamp tubing inch by inch to determine whether there is a hole in tubing, loose connection, or problem with drainage device. If a leak is found in tubing or drainage device, change it. Use adhesive tape at all connections.
2. Break in chest drainage device.	Place end of chest tube in bottle of sterile saline or water at 2-cm level. Notify health care provider immediately, and change drainage device according to manufacturer instructions.
3. Chest tube dislodgment.	Apply dressing to chest tube site wound using petroleum gauze, dry gauze dressing, and adhesive tape. Notify health care provider immediately and obtain a STAT order for chest radiograph. Prepare for health care provider to insert another chest tube.
4. Tension pneumothorax: Signs and symptoms include the following: ▪ Severe respiratory distress ▪ Low oxygen saturation ▪ Chest pain ▪ Absence of breath sounds on affected side ▪ Tracheal shift to unaffected side ▪ Tachycardia and hypotension	Assess chest tube for clamping or kinking of tubing. Notify health care provider immediately and obtain STAT order for chest X-ray film. Prepare for health care provider to insert another chest tube or perform needle decompression with large-bore needle. Have emergency equipment in the patient's room to prepare for resuscitation if needed. **Note:** Leaving chest tube clamped can cause tension pneumothorax.
5. Drainage suddenly stops.	Assess chest tube for clamping or kinking of tubing. Assess for presence of clots or fibrin within chest tube. Notify health care provider immediately, and obtain order to gently milk chest tube to reestablish chest drainage.
6. Excessive bleeding from chest tube.	Notify health care provider. Assess the patient's vital signs and be prepared for resuscitation. Be prepared for surgical intervention.

Recording and Reporting

- Record in nurses' notes in EHR, chart, or flow sheets relevant respiratory assessments, type of drainage device, amount of suction if used, amount and character of drainage in chamber, and presence or absence of an air leak. Document the integrity of dressing and color and type of drainage. If dressing change is performed, document dressing change with supplies used and wound assessment.
- Record level of patient comfort and pain and vital signs including oxygen saturation.
- Record your evaluation of patient/family caregiver learning.
- Report any unexpected outcomes immediately to nurse in charge and/or health care provider.

Unexpected Outcomes and Related Interventions

- The patient develops respiratory distress, chest pain, decrease in breath sounds, marked cyanosis, asymmetrical chest movements, presence of subcutaneous emphysema around tube insertion site or neck, hypotension, tachycardia, or mediastinal shift.
  - Notify health care provider immediately.
  - Assess vital signs and pulse oximetry.
  - Prepare for chest X-ray.
  - Provide oxygen as ordered.
- Air leak is unrelated to the patient's respirations.
  - Determine source of air leak (see Table 24.9).
  - Notify health care provider.
- Chest tube emergency occurs.
  - See Table 24.9.
  - Observe for mediastinal shift or respiratory distress (medical emergency).
  - Notify health care provider.

KEY POINTS

- The cardiopulmonary system consists of the heart, lungs, airways, and blood vessels, which function to provide oxygen to the tissues and to remove carbon dioxide (CO_2) and waste products from the body.
- Ventilation, diffusion, respiration, and perfusion are processes for providing adequate oxygenation from the alveoli to the blood.
- Cardiac output is determined by the patient's heart rate, strength of contraction, amount of blood in the ventricle, and amount of resistance the heart has to overcome to eject the blood.
- The process of inspiration and expiration is achieved with changes in lung pressures and volumes.
- Respiration is controlled by the central nervous system (CNS) and chemicals within the blood.
- Decreased hemoglobin levels, seen in patients with anemia or acute blood loss, alter a patient's ability to transport oxygen and can cause disturbances in oxygenation.
- Hypoventilation, seen in patients with musculoskeletal abnormalities or nervous system disease, causes CO_2 retention.
- A person's age, nutritional intake, hydration status, level of exercise, exposure to cigarette smoke (including secondhand smoke), substance abuse, environmental factors, and stress all affect the ability to exchange oxygen in the lungs and transport it to the tissues.
- Alterations in cardiac output caused by electrical or mechanical disturbances of the heart can negatively impact a person's ability to deliver oxygen to the tissues.
- Breathing exercises improve ventilation, oxygenation, and sensations of dyspnea.
- Chest physiotherapy, along with postural drainage, aids in mobilizing pulmonary secretions.
- Hydration, humidification, coughing, and suctioning techniques maintain a patent airway.
- Oxygen therapy improves levels of tissue oxygenation and can be delivered via nasal cannula, various types of oxygen masks, or mechanical ventilators via artificial airways.
- Positioning, incentive spirometry, chest tubes, and noninvasive ventilation help to promote lung expansion.
- Cardiopulmonary resuscitation (CPR) is necessary for cardiac arrest, an emergent complication of altered oxygenation and perfusion.

REFERENCES

American Association of Cardiovascular and Pulmonary Rehabilitation (AACVPR). Cardiac rehab patient resources. 2016. Available from: https://www.aacvpr.org/Resources/Resources-for-Patients/Cardiac-Rehab-Patient-Resources.

American Association of Critical-Care Nurses (AACN). Evidence-based care of patients with chest tubes: 2015 AACN NTI ExpoEd. Hudson, NH: Atrium; 2015. Available from: https://chestdrainu.com/wp-content/uploads/2018/09/nti-expoed-slides-chest-drainage-2015.pdf

American Association of Respiratory Care (AARC). AARC clinical practice guideline: nasotracheal suction—2004 revision and update. Respir Care 2004;49:1080.

American Association of Respiratory Care (AARC). AARC clinical practice guideline: endotracheal suctioning of mechanical ventilation patients with artificial airways. Respir Care 2010;55(6):758.

American Association of Respiratory Care (AARC). Clinical practice guideline: incentive spirometry. Respir Care 2011;56(10):1600.

American Heart Association. Highlights of the 2015 American Heart Association guidelines update for CPR and ECC. 2015. Available from: https://www.cercp.org/images/stories/recursos/Guias%202015/Guidelines-RCP-AHA-2015-Full.pdf

Association of Paediatric Chartered Physiotherapists. Guidelines for nasopharyngeal suction of a child or young adult. 2015. Available from: https://apcp.csp.org.uk/system/files/guidelines_for_nasopharyngeal_suction_0_1.pdf

Atkins JR, Kautz DD. Move to improve: progressive mobility in the intensive care unit. Dimens Crit Care Nurs 2014;33(5):275.

Ball J, Dains J, Flynn J, Solomon B, Stewart R. Seidel's guide to physical examination. 9th ed. St. Louis: Elsevier; 2015.

Bascom R. Restoring air-free pleural space in pneumothorax. Medscape 2016. Available from: http://emedicine.medscape.com/article/1959416-overview.

Branson RD, Gomaa D, Rodriquez Jr D. Management of the artificial airway. Respir Care 2014;59(6):974.

Cassidy MR, Rosenkranz P, McCabe K, Rosen JE, McAneny D. I cough: reducing postoperative pulmonary complications with a multidisciplinary patient care program. JAMA Surg 2013;148(8):740.

Centers for Disease Control and Prevention (CDC). Heart disease risk factors. 2015a. Available from: http://www.cdc.gov/heartdisease/risk_factors.htm.

Centers for Disease Control and Prevention (CDC). Estimated influenza illnesses and hospitalizations averted by vaccination—United States, 2014-15 influenza season. 2015b. Available from: http://www.cdc.gov/flu/about/disease/2014-15.htm.

Centers for Disease Control and Prevention (CDC). What are the risk factors for lung cancer? 2016a. Available from: https://www.cdc.gov/cancer/lung/basic_info/risk_factors.htm.

Centers for Disease Control and Prevention (CDC). Get vaccinated. 2016b. Available from: http://www.cdc.gov/flu/consumer/vaccinations.htm.

Centers for Disease Control and Prevention (CDC). Pneumococcal vaccination. 2016c. Available from: http://www.cdc.gov/vaccines/vpd-vac/pneumo/default.htm.

Centers for Disease Control and Prevention (CDC): Tuberculin skin testing. 2016d. Available from: http://www.cdc.gov/tb/publications/factsheets/testing/skintesting.htm.

Chotai P. Tube thoracostomy management. Medscape 2016, Available from: http://emedicine.medscape.com/article/1503275-overview#a6.

COPD Foundation. Breathing exercises and techniques for COPD. 2016. Available from: http://www.copdfoundation.org/What-is-COPD/Living-with-COPD/Breathing-Techniques.aspx.

do Nascimento Junior P, Módolo NS, Andrade S, Guimarães MM, Braz LG, El Dib R. Incentive spirometry for prevention of postoperative pulmonary complications in upper abdominal surgery. Cochrane Database Syst Rev 2014;(2):CD006058.

Giddens J. Concepts for nursing practice. 2nd ed. St. Louis: Elsevier; 2017.

Hong CM, Galvagno SM. Patients with chronic obstructive pulmonary disorder. Med Clin North Am 2013;97(6):1095.

Huether S, McCance K. Understanding pathophysiology. 6th ed. St. Louis: Elsevier; 2017.

Kane CJ, York NL, Minton LA. Chest tubes in the critically ill patient. Dimens Crit Care Nurs 2013;32(3):111.

Kwiatt M, Tarbox A, Seamon MJ, Swaroop M, Cipolla J, Allen C, et al. Thoracostomy tubes: a comprehensive review of complications and related topics. Int J Crit Illn Inj Sci 2014;4(2):143.

Lewis S, Bucher L, Heitkemper M, Harding M, Kwong J. Medical-surgical nursing: assessment and management of clinical problems. 9th ed. St. Louis: Elsevier; 2017.

Link MS, Berkow LC, Kudenchuk PJ, Halperin HR, Hess EP, Moitra VK, et al. Part 7: Adult advanced cardiovascular life support: 2015 American Heart Association guidelines updates for cardiopulmonary resuscitation and emergency cardiovascular care. Circulation 2015;132(Suppl. 2):s444.

MacIntyre N. Tissue hypoxia: implications for the respiratory clinician. Respir Care 2014;59(10):1590.

Mao M, Hughes R, Papadimos TJ, Stawicki SP. Complications of chest tubes: a focused clinical synopsis. Curr Opin Pulm Med 2015;21:376.

Marilyn Hockenberry Cheryl Rodgers David Wilson Wong's Essentials of Pediatric Nursing. Essentials of pediatric nursing. 10th ed. St. Louis: Elsevier; 2017.

McCance KL, Huether SE. Pathophysiology: the biologic basis for disease in adults and children. 7th ed. St. Louis: Mosby Elsevier; 2014.

McDonald C. Oxygen therapy for COPD. J Thorac Dis 2014;6(11):1632.

Messika J, Ben Ahmed K, Gaudry S, Miguel-Montanes R, Rafat C, Sztrymf B, et al. Use of high-flow nasal cannula oxygen therapy in subjects with ARDS: a 1-year observational study. Respir Care 2015;60(2):162.

Mohammed H. Chest tube care in critically ill patient: a comprehensive review. Egypt J Chest Dis Tuberc 2015;64:849.

Mozaffarian D, Benjamin EJ, Go AS, Arnett DK, Blaha MJ, Cushman M, et al. Heart disease and stroke statistics—2016 update. A report from the American Heart Association. 2015. Available from: http://circ.ahajournals.org/content/early/2015/12/16/CIR.0000000000000350.

Munro N, Ruggiero M. Ventilator-associated pneumonia bundle reconstruction for best care. AACN Adv Crit Care 2014;25(2):163.

Myatt R. Nursing care of patient with a temporary tracheotomy. Nurs Stand 2015;29(26):42.

National Heart, Lung, and Blood Institute (NHLBI). How is high blood pressure treated? 2015. Available from: https://www.nhlbi.nih.gov/health/health-topics/topics/hbp/treatment#.

Restrepo RD, Wettstein R, Wittnebel L, Tracy M. Incentive spirometry: 2011. Respir Care 2011;56(10):1600.

Shlamovitz GA. Tube thoracostomy. Medscape 2014. http://emedicine.medscape.com/article/80678-overview#a1.

Strickland SL, Rubin BK, Drescher GS, Haas CF, O'Malley CA, Volsko TA, et al. AARC Clinical practice guideline: effectiveness of nonpharmacologic airway clearance therapies in hospitalized patients. Respir Care 2013; 58(12):2187.

The Joint Commission (TJC). 2018 National Patient Safety Goals. Oakbrook Terrace, IL: The Joint Commission; 2018. Available from: http://www.jointcommission.org/standards_information/npsgs.aspx.

Touhy T, Jett K. Gerontological nursing and healthy aging. 5th ed. St. Louis: Elsevier; 2018.

Urden L, Stacy K, Lough M. Priorities in critical care nursing. 7th ed. St. Louis: Elsevier; 2016.

Volsko TA. Airway clearance therapy: finding the evidence. Respir Care 2013;58(10):1669.

Walsh BK, Crotwell DN, Restrepo RD. Capnography/capnometry during mechanical ventilation: 2011. Respir Care 2011;56(4):503.

Whelton PK, Carey RM, Aronow WS, Casey DE Jr, Collins KJ, Dennison Himmelfarb C, DePalma SM, Gidding S, Jamerson KA, Jones DW, MacLaughlin EJ, Muntner P, Ovbiagele B, Smith SC Jr, Spencer CC, Stafford RS, Taler SJ, Thomas RJ, Williams KA Sr, Williamson JD, Wright JT Jr. 2017 ACC/AHA/AAPA/ABC/ACPM/AGS/APhA/ASH/ASPC/NMA/PCNA Guideline for the Prevention, Detection, Evaluation, and Management of High Blood Pressure in Adults: Executive Summary: A Report of the American College of Cardiology/American Heart Association Task Force on Clinical Practice Guidelines. Hypertension. 2018 Jun;71(6):1269–1324. doi: 10.1161/HYP.0000000000000066. Epub 2017 Nov 13. Erratum in: Hypertension. 2018 Jun;71(6):e136–e139. Erratum in: Hypertension. 2018 Sep;72(3):e33. PMID: 29133354.

Wiegand D. AACN procedure manual for high acuity, progressive, and critical care. 7th ed. St. Louis: Elsevier; 2017.

Zarogoulidis P, Kioumis I, Pitsiou G, Porpodis K, Lampaki S, Papaiwannou A, et al. Pneumothorax: from definition to diagnosis and treatment. J Thorac Dis 2014;6(Suppl. 4):S372.

25 Fluid, Electrolyte, and Acid–Base Balances

OBJECTIVES

- To describe physiological mechanisms that maintain fluid, electrolyte, and acid–base balances.
- To discuss risk factors for fluid, electrolyte, and acid–base imbalances.
- To describe different fluid, electrolyte, and acid–base imbalances.
- To identify appropriate clinical assessments for specific fluid, electrolyte, and acid–base imbalances.
- To discuss appropriate nursing interventions for patients with fluid, electrolyte, and acid–base imbalances.
- To describe purpose and procedures for initiation and maintenance of i.v. therapy.
- To calculate an i.v. flow rate.
- To discuss complications of i.v. therapy and what to do if they occur.
- To describe how to change i.v. solutions, tubing, and dressings.
- To describe the procedure for initiating a blood transfusion and complications of blood therapy.

KEY TERMS

acidosis, p. 601
active transport, p. 594
ADH, p. 596
aldosterone, p. 596
allogeneic transfusion, p. 613
alkalosis, p. 601
angiotensin, p. 596
anions, p. 594
arterial blood gas (ABG), p. 600
autologous transfusion, p. 612
buffers, p. 597
cations, p. 594
clinical dehydration, p. 599
colloid osmotic pressure, p. 595
colloids, p. 607
concentration, p. 598
crystalloids, p. 607
diffusion, p. 594
electrolyte, p. 594
electronic infusion devices (EIDs), p. 608
extracellular fluid volume (ECV) deficit, p. 599
extracellular fluid volume (ECV) excess, p. 599
filtration, p. 595
fluid, p. 594
fluid homeostasis, p. 595
hemolysis, p. 612
hydrostatic pressure, p. 595
hypercalcemia, p. 599
hyperchloremia, p. 599
hyperkalemia, p. 599
hypermagnesemia, p. 599
hypernatremia, p. 599
hypertonic, p. 595
hypocalcemia, p. 599
hypochloremia, p. 599
hypokalemia, p. 599
hypomagnesemia, p. 599
hyponatremia, p. 599
hypotonic, p. 595
hypovolemia, p. 599
infiltration, p. 611
insensible water loss, p. 596
ions, p. 594
isotonic, p. 595
oncotic pressure, p. 595
osmolality, p. 595
osmoreceptors, p. 595
osmosis, p. 594
osmotic pressure, p. 595
parenteral nutrition (PN), p. 607
phlebitis, p. 611
transfusion reaction, p. 613
vascular access device (VAD), p. 607
venipuncture, p. 609

INTRODUCTION

Fluid, electrolyte, and acid–base balances within the body maintain health and function of all body cells, organs, and systems. The body maintains fluid and electrolyte balance by adjusting the intake and output (I&O) of water and electrolytes and their distribution in the body. The body maintains acid–base balance by buffering and excreting acid. Factors that alter these normal processes can cause fluid, electrolyte, or acid–base imbalances. This chapter discusses how the body maintains balance; how imbalances develop and affect patients; and nursing interventions that help patients maintain or restore fluid, electrolyte, and acid–base balance.

Water is the largest single component of the body; 60% of the average man's weight is fluid. The proportion of water is lower in women and older adults and higher in infants (Hall, 2016). The term **fluid** means water that contains dissolved or suspended substances such as glucose, mineral salts, and proteins.

DISTRIBUTION OF BODY FLUIDS

Body fluids are distributed in two major compartments, one containing intracellular fluid (ICF) and the other containing extracellular fluid (ECF) (Fig. 25.1). ICF is inside cells. In adults, the ICF is approximately two-thirds of total body water (Hall, 2016).

ECF is all the fluid outside the cells, approximately one-third of total body water. It is divided into two major compartments plus a minor compartment: intravascular (within blood vessels), interstitial (within tissues), and transcellular (minor). Intravascular fluid is the liquid portion of the blood, the plasma. Interstitial fluid is located between cells and outside the blood vessels. Transcellular fluid is secreted by epithelial cells and includes cerebrospinal, gastrointestinal (GI), peritoneal, and synovial fluids (Hall, 2016).

COMPOSITION OF BODY FLUIDS

Body fluid contains mineral salts that are called electrolytes. An **electrolyte** is a compound that separates into **ions** (charged particles) when dissolved in water. Positively charged ions are **cations**. Major cations within body fluids include sodium (Na^+), potassium (K^+), calcium (Ca^{2+}), and magnesium (Mg^{2+}). Negatively charged ions are **anions**. The three major body fluid anions are chloride (Cl^-), bicarbonate (HCO_3^-), and phosphate (PO_4^{3-} and other forms). Electrolyte concentration is measured in milliequivalents per liter (mEq/L), millimoles per liter (mmol/L), or milligrams per deciliter (mg/dL).

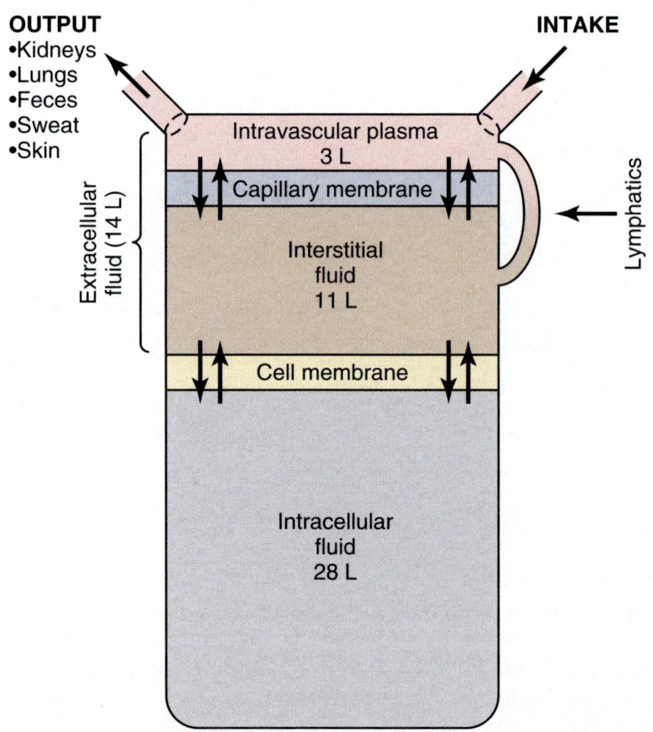

Fig. 25.1 **Body fluid compartments.** (From Hall JE: *Guyton and Hall textbook of medical physiology*, ed 13, Philadelphia, 2016, Elsevier.)

MOVEMENT OF WATER AND ELECTROLYTES

Cell membranes and capillary walls separate the body compartments. Water and electrolytes move between body compartments by processes that allow the compartments to have different electrolyte concentrations while keeping the overall particle concentration (osmolality) equal in all compartments. They move across cell membranes by four processes: active transport, diffusion, osmosis, and filtration.

- **Active transport** moves electrolytes or other substances across cell membranes against a concentration gradient (from an area of low concentration to one of higher concentration).
  - This process requires energy, usually in the form of adenosine triphosphate (ATP). An example of active transport is the sodium–potassium pump that moves sodium ions out of a cell and potassium ions into it, thus keeping the ICF lower in sodium and higher in potassium than the ECF.
- **Diffusion** is passive movement of electrolytes or other particles from an area of higher concentration to one of lower concentration. In other words, the electrolytes move down their concentration gradient until the electrolyte concentration is equal in all areas.
  - Electrolytes cannot diffuse across cell membranes unless the membranes have proteins that serve as ion channels.
  - When ion channels are open, an electrolyte can diffuse across a membrane; when they are closed, no electrolytes pass. Opening and closing of ion channels play an important role in nerve and muscle function.
- **Osmosis** moves water across a semipermeable membrane from a compartment of lower particle concentration to one that has a higher particle concentration (Fig. 25.2).

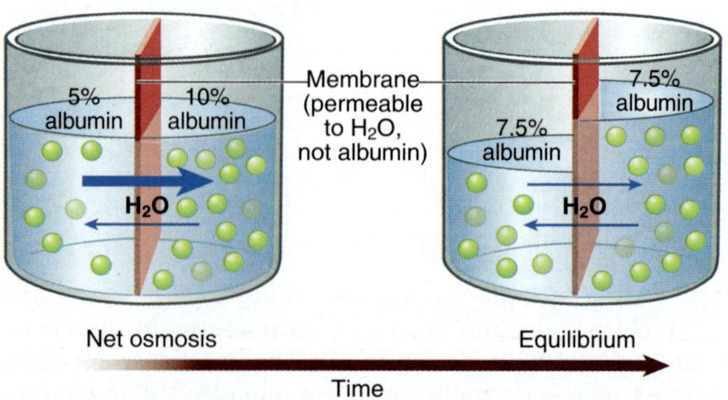

Fig. 25.2 Osmosis moves water through a semipermeable membrane. (From Patton KT, Thibodeau GA: *Anatomy and physiology*, ed 9, St Louis, 2016, Elsevier.)

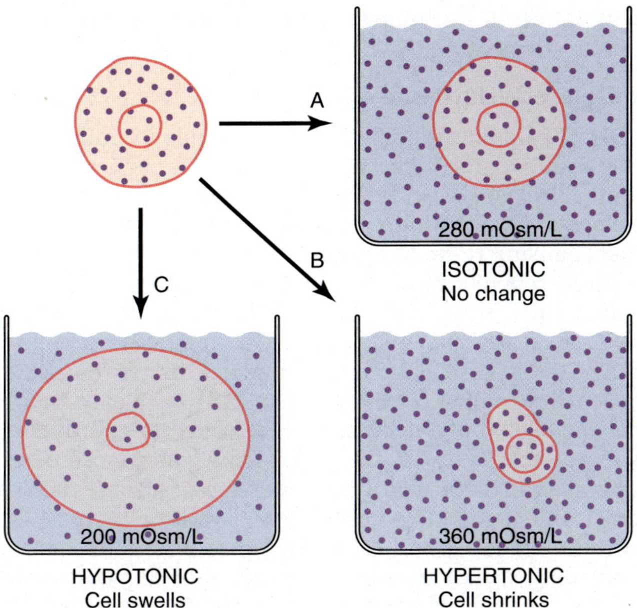

Fig. 25.3 Effects of isotonic **(A)**, hypertonic **(B)**, and hypotonic **(C)** solutions. (From Hall JE: *Guyton and Hall textbook of medical physiology*, ed 13, Philadelphia, 2016, Elsevier.)

- Osmosis equalizes the concentration of particles on each side of a membrane. Cell membranes are known as semipermeable membranes because water crosses them easily but electrolytes do not. The particles in any fluid compartment exert an inward-pulling force called **osmotic pressure**.
- If a semipermeable membrane separates two fluid compartments with different particle concentrations, water is drawn through the membrane to the more concentrated side because it has higher osmotic pressure (inward-pulling force).
- Osmosis continues until the particle concentration is equal in both fluid compartments. This process controls movement of water between the interstitial fluid and the intracellular compartment.
- The **osmolality** of a fluid is a measure of the number of particles per kilogram of water, reported in milliosmoles per kilogram (mOsm/kg). Changes in extracellular osmolality cause rapid shifts of water into or out of cells to equalize the osmolality. Osmosis is a passive process that does not require energy from cells.
- I.v. solutions are hypertonic, isotonic, or hypotonic (Fig. 25.3). Infusion of **hypertonic** i.v. solutions (more concentrated than normal blood) such as 3% sodium chloride pulls fluid from cells by osmosis, causing them to shrink. **Isotonic** solutions such as 0.9% sodium chloride (same osmolality as normal blood) expand the extracellular fluid volume (ECV) of the body without causing water to shift in or out of cells.
- Physiologically **hypotonic** solutions (less concentrated than normal blood after they are infused) such as dextrose 5% in water (D_5W) move water from the extracellular compartment into the cells by osmosis causing them to swell.
- When health care providers write fluid orders for an i.v., they prescribe the type of i.v. fluid that will distribute to specific fluid compartments as needed by each patient's condition.

- **Filtration** is the net effect of several forces that move fluid across a membrane. Fluid moves into and out of capillaries (between the vascular and interstitial spaces) by filtration.
  - **Hydrostatic pressure** is the force of a fluid pressing outward against the walls of its container. Thus, capillary hydrostatic pressure is an outward-pushing force. Capillary hydrostatic pressure is greater at the arterial end of a capillary.
  - **Colloid osmotic pressure**, also known as **oncotic pressure**, is an inward-pulling force caused by the presence of protein molecules. Blood colloid osmotic pressure is greater at the venous end of a capillary.
  - Normally, fluid leaves a capillary at the arterial end (high outward-pushing capillary hydrostatic pressure) carrying oxygen and nutrients to cells; fluid enters the capillary at the venous end (high inward-pulling colloid osmotic pressure) carrying carbon dioxide and other waste products into the blood for disposal.
  - The lymph channels return excess fluid and a few small proteins that entered the interstitial space to the intravascular compartment. Edema occurs when changes in these forces cause fluid to accumulate in the interstitial space.

PHYSIOLOGICAL REGULATION OF FLUID BALANCE

Fluid homeostasis is the dynamic interaction between fluid intake and absorption, fluid distribution, and fluid output (Felver, 2017b). Our daily fluid output consists of hypotonic sodium-containing fluid. To maintain fluid balance, we must have an intake of an equivalent amount of hypotonic sodium-containing fluid (water plus foods with some salt).

Fluid Intake

Fluid intake occurs orally through drinking and eating. Food metabolism creates additional water. Average fluid intake for healthy adults is approximately 2200–2700 mL (Table 25.1), although it varies widely. Other routes of fluid intake that nurses encounter include i.v., GI (tube feedings), rectal (e.g., enemas), and irrigation of body cavities that results in fluid absorption.

Although many people believe that thirst regulates oral fluid intake, habit and social reasons actually account for most fluid intake. Thirst, a conscious desire for water, regulates fluid intake when plasma osmolality increases (osmoreceptor-mediated thirst) or the blood volume decreases (baroreceptor-mediated thirst and angiotensin II–mediated thirst). The thirst-control mechanism is in the hypothalamus of the brain (Hall, 2016). **Osmoreceptors** continually monitor plasma osmolality; when osmolality increases, the hypothalamus stimulates thirst. This thirst mechanism becomes less active in older adults. Dryness of oral mucous membranes also causes thirst. People who can obtain fluid or communicate their thirst to others increase their fluid intake to restore fluid balance.

Table 25.1 Healthy Adult Average Daily Fluid Intake and Output

	Normal (mL/day)	Prolonged, Heavy Exercise
INTAKE		
Fluids ingested		
Oral	1100–1400	280–1100 mL/h
Foods	800–1000	Highly variable
From metabolism	300	16–50 mL/h
Total intake	2200–2700	300–1150 mL/h
OUTPUT		
Skin (insensible and sweat)	500–600	300–2100 mL/h
Insensible: lungs	400	20 mL/h
Feces	100–200	Negligible, unless diarrhea during exercise
Urine	1200–1500	20–1000 mL/h depending on hydration status
Total output	2200–2700	340–3120 mL/h Rehydration with Na^+-containing fluid necessary after prolonged vigorous exercise

Data from Hall JE: *Guyton and Hall textbook of medical physiology*, ed 13, Philadelphia, 2016, Elsevier; American College of Sports Medicine (ACSM): Position stand on exercise and fluid replacement, *Med Sci Sports Exerc* 39(2):377, 2007.

Fluid Distribution

Fluid moves between the vascular and interstitial portions of the ECF (in and out of capillaries) by filtration. It distributes between the extracellular and intracellular compartments by osmosis.

Fluid Output

Fluid output (see Table 25.1) normally occurs through four organs: the skin, lungs, GI tract, and kidneys. When patients are seriously ill, output also occurs abnormally such as through vomiting, wound drainage, and hemorrhage (Felver, 2017b). **Insensible water loss** is not visible; it is continuous and occurs through the skin and lungs. Insensible water output from the lungs changes in response to respiratory rate and depth. Administration of nonhumidified supplemental oxygen increases insensible water loss from the lungs. Output of insensible water also increases with fever (Kamel and Halperin, 2017). Visible perspiration (sweat) is secreted by the sweat glands. Sweat contains sodium chloride and water.

The GI tract plays a vital role in fluid balance. Approximately 3–6 L of fluid moves into the GI tract daily and returns to the ECF. An average healthy adult excretes only 100–200 mL of fluid each day through feces. However, diarrhea causes a large fluid output from the GI tract.

The kidneys are the major regulator of fluid output because they respond to hormones that influence urine production. When healthy people drink more water, they produce more urine to maintain fluid balance. If they drink less water, sweat a lot, or lose fluid by vomiting, their urine volume decreases to maintain fluid balance. These adjustments primarily are the result of the actions of antidiuretic hormone (ADH), aldosterone, and atrial natriuretic peptide (ANP) (Kamel and Halperin, 2017).

Antidiuretic Hormone

ADH regulates osmolality of body fluids by influencing how much water is excreted in urine. The hypothalamus controls release of ADH from the posterior pituitary gland. It circulates to the kidneys where it acts on the collecting ducts causing them to resorb water (Hall, 2016). This antidiuretic effect removes water from the renal tubules and returns it to the blood, diluting the blood. More ADH is released when plasma osmolality increases; increased ADH causes more water resorption and dilutes the plasma back to normal. Conversely, less ADH is released when plasma osmolality decreases; less water is resorbed, so it leaves the body in the urine and plasma osmolality returns to normal. Pain, nausea, stressors, some medications, and severely decreased blood volume increase the secretion of ADH and thus can cause plasma to become more dilute than normal. Ethyl alcohol decreases ADH release, which is why people urinate frequently when they drink alcoholic beverages.

Aldosterone

Aldosterone regulates ECV by influencing how much sodium and water are excreted in urine. The adrenal cortex releases **aldosterone** in response to increased plasma potassium concentration or as the end product of the renin–angiotensin–aldosterone system (RAAS). Renin released by the kidneys acts on the inactive protein angiotensinogen to produce **angiotensin** I, which other enzymes in the lung capillaries convert to angiotensin II. Angiotensin II causes vasoconstriction, which helps regulate blood pressure, and it stimulates the release of aldosterone, which assists fluid homeostasis. Aldosterone circulates to the kidneys where it acts on the distal tubules causing them to resorb sodium and water in isotonic proportions. Removing sodium and water from the renal tubules and returning them to the blood increases ECV. If ECV decreases such as through vomiting and diarrhea, the kidneys release more renin and the RAAS produces more aldosterone to increase sodium and water resorption and restore the ECV. Aldosterone also contributes to electrolyte and acid–base balance by increasing urinary excretion of K^+ and H^+.

Atrial Natriuretic Peptide

ANP is a hormone that opposes the action of aldosterone and promotes vasodilation. It is secreted from the cells of the heart in response to atrial stretching and an increased circulating blood volume. ANP causes sodium and water to be excreted in the urine, decreasing ECV slightly (Hall, 2016).

PHYSIOLOGICAL REGULATION OF ELECTROLYTE BALANCE

Electrolyte homeostasis refers to the relationship between electrolyte intake and absorption, electrolyte distribution, and electrolyte output (Felver, 2017b). To maintain electrolyte balance, electrolyte intake must equal electrolyte output and the electrolyte distribution must be normal.

Sodium Regulation

Normal serum Na^+ concentration ranges from 135 to 145 mEq/L. Sodium is the most abundant cation in ECF but has a smaller concentration inside cells. This unequal distribution is maintained by the Na^+–K^+ pump in cell membranes, which also maintains an unequal K^+ distribution. The concentration of Na^+ in ECF is greatly influenced by the relative amount of water and reflects the osmolality (concentration) of the ECF. Sodium concentration imbalances are water imbalances and are discussed in the section Fluid Imbalances.

Potassium Balance

The normal range for serum K^+ concentration is 3.5–5 mEq/L. In contrast to this small concentration of K^+ in the ECF, K^+ has a high intracellular concentration (Hall, 2016). This maintains the resting membrane potential of cardiac, skeletal, and smooth muscle contraction, allowing for normal muscle function (Kamel and Halperin, 2017). K^+ absorbs easily with dietary intake of food sources such as bananas, spinach, and apricots. Insulin, epinephrine, and alkalosis shift K^+ into cells. Acute and chronic diarrhea increase output of K^+ from the GI tract. Aldosterone facilitates K^+ renal excretion, as does polyuria.

Calcium Balance

Ca^{2+} in blood has two major forms: bound and free. Ca^{2+} bound to albumin and other blood components is inactive. Free (ionized) Ca^{2+} is available for physiological actions. Normal serum total Ca^{2+} levels (bound plus free) are 8.4–10.5 mg/dL. Normal serum ionized Ca^{2+} levels range from 4.5 to 5.3 mg/dL. Most of the calcium in the body is in bone, although intracellular Ca^{2+} has important functions. Ca^{2+} influences the excitability of nerve and muscle cells and is necessary for muscle contraction and blood clotting. Plasma Ca^{2+} concentration is regulated primarily by the actions of parathyroid hormone (shifts Ca^{2+} out of cells) and calcitonin (shifts Ca^{2+} into cells). Vitamin D is necessary to make proteins responsible for dietary Ca^{2+} absorption in the duodenum. Chronic diarrhea and undigested fat increase output of Ca^{2+} in the feces.

Magnesium Balance

Normal plasma concentration of Mg^{2+} ranges from 1.5 to 2.5 mEq/L. Similar to Ca^{2+}, some Mg^{2+} in the blood is bound and inactive. Most of the Mg^{2+} in the body is in bones and inside cells. Mg^{2+} is essential for action of many enzymes and for normal action at neuromuscular junctions. Absorption of dietary Mg^{2+} occurs primarily in the terminal ileum. Chronic diarrhea and undigested fat increase output of Mg^{2+} in the feces. Renal Mg^{2+} excretion increases with a rising blood alcohol.

Chloride Regulation

Normal serum Cl^- concentration ranges from 95 to 105 mEq/L. Cl^- is the major anion in ECF and an important part of gastric hydrochloric acid.

Bicarbonate Regulation

Normal arterial bicarbonate level ranges between 22 and 26 mEq/L; normal venous bicarbonate level is 24–30 mEq/L. Bicarbonate is a base and a key component of the bicarbonate buffering system essential to acid–base balance. The kidneys assist with regulating bicarbonate levels.

Phosphate Balance

Normal serum phosphate level ranges from 2.7 to 4.5 mg/dL. Phosphate exists in three forms ($H_2PO_4^-$, HPO_4^{2-}, and PO_4^{3-}), which are added together in any standard laboratory measurement. Most phosphate in the body is in bone and inside cells. Insulin and epinephrine shift phosphate into cells. Phosphate is needed to produce ATP, the energy source for cellular metabolism. Ca^{2+} and phosphate blood levels are inversely proportional; if one rises, the other falls, except during end-stage renal disease. The GI tract absorbs dietary phosphate easily except in the presence of aluminum or magnesium antacids. Renal excretion is the largest route of phosphate output and decreases greatly with oliguria.

PHYSIOLOGICAL REGULATION OF ACID–BASE BALANCE

Optimal cell function requires a balance between acids and bases. Acids release H^+; bases (alkaline substances) take up H^+. Acid–base homeostasis balances acid production, acid buffering, and acid excretion (Felver, 2017a). Acid–base balance requires acid excretion to be equal to acid production, with acid buffering in blood and renal tubular fluid.

The pH is a measure of fluid acidity or alkalinity. A pH value of 7.0 is neutral, less than 7.0 is acid, and more than 7.0 is alkaline. The greater the concentration of H^+, the more acidic the solution and the lower the pH is; the lower the concentration of H^+ ions, the more alkaline the solution and the higher the pH is. Normal pH range of arterial blood is 7.35–7.45.

Acid Production

Cellular metabolism constantly produces two kinds of acid: carbonic and metabolic. Carbonic acid (H_2CO_3) arises from the carbon dioxide (CO_2) that cells produce. Metabolic acids are all other acids produced by cells that are not carbonic acid such as lactic acid and citric acid.

Acid Buffering

Buffers are pairs of chemicals that work together to maintain normal pH of body fluids.

- If there are too many free H^+ ions, a buffer can take them up so that they no longer are free and cannot decrease the pH.
- If there are not enough free H^+ ions, a buffer can release H^+ to restore a normal pH.
- All body fluids contain buffers. The major buffer in ECF is the bicarbonate buffer system, which buffers metabolic

acids. Other buffers include hemoglobin, protein buffers, and phosphate buffers.

- Buffers normally keep the blood from becoming too acidic when acids produced by cells are circulating to lungs and kidneys for excretion.

Acid Excretion

The body has two acid excretion mechanisms: lungs (excrete carbonic acid) and kidneys (excrete metabolic acids). The lungs excrete carbonic acid in the form of CO_2 and water.

- The chemoreceptors regulate this excretion by altering respiratory rate and depth. Respirations increase when more carbonic acid needs to be excreted, and they decrease (within limits) when the body needs to excrete less carbonic acid.
- The kidneys excrete all acids except carbonic acid by adjusting the amount of H^+ excreted in the urine to maintain acid–base homeostasis (Kamel and Halperin, 2017).

FACTORS AFFECTING AND DISTURBANCES IN FLUID, ELECTROLYTE, AND ACID–BASE BALANCES

Disturbances in fluid, electrolyte, and acid–base balances disrupt normal body processes and often occur together. As a nurse, you need to be familiar with these imbalances and their effects on body functioning.

Fluid Imbalances

Fluid imbalances are isotonic (volume) and/or osmolality (concentration) imbalances (Table 25.2; Fig. 25.4). An isotonic deficit or excess exists when water and sodium are lost or gained in equal proportions, affecting the volume of the ECF. In contrast, an osmolality imbalance is a loss or excess of only water, which affects the **concentration** (osmolality) of the body fluids.

Table 25.2 Fluid Imbalances

Imbalance and Related Causes	Signs and Symptoms
ISOTONIC IMBALANCES—WATER AND SODIUM LOST OR GAINED IN EQUAL OR ISOTONIC PROPORTIONS	
Extracellular fluid volume deficit—body fluids have decreased volume but normal osmolality	
Sodium and water intake less than output, causing isotonic loss Severely decreased oral intake of water and salt Increased GI output: vomiting, diarrhea, laxative overuse, drainage from fistulas or GI drainage tubes Increased renal output: use of diuretics, adrenal insufficiency Loss of blood or plasma: hemorrhage, burns Massive sweating without water and salt intake	*Physical examination:* Sudden weight loss (overnight), postural hypotension, tachycardia, thready pulse, dry mucous membranes, poor skin turgor, slow vein filling, flat neck veins when supine, dark yellow urine *If severe:* Thirst; restlessness; confusion; hypotension; oliguria (urine output **less than** 30 mL/h); cold, clammy skin; hypovolemic shock *Laboratory findings:* Increased hematocrit, increased BUN **more than** 25 mg/dL (hemoconcentration); urine specific gravity usually **more than** 1.030, unless renal cause
Extracellular fluid volume excess—body fluids have increased volume but normal osmolality	
Sodium and water intake greater than output, causing isotonic gain Excessive intake of Na^+-containing isotonic i.v. fluids or oral intake of salty foods and water Renal retention of Na^+ and water: heart failure, cirrhosis, aldosterone or glucocorticoid excess, acute or chronic oliguric renal disease	*Physical examination:* Sudden weight gain (overnight), edema (especially in dependent areas), full neck veins when upright or semiupright, crackles in lungs *If severe:* Confusion, pulmonary edema *Laboratory findings:* Decreased hematocrit, decreased BUN **less than** 10 mg/dL (hemodilution)
OSMOLALITY IMBALANCES	
Hypernatremia (water deficit; hyperosmolar imbalance)—body fluids too concentrated	
Loss of relatively more water than salt ADH deficiency (diabetes insipidus) Osmotic diuresis Large insensible perspiration and respiratory water output without increased water intake **Gain of relatively more salt than water** Administration of salt tablets, tube feedings, or hypertonic parenteral fluids Lack of access to water, deliberate water deprivation, inability to respond to thirst (e.g., immobility, aphasia) Dysfunction of osmoreceptor-driven thirst drive	*Physical examination:* Decreased level of consciousness (confusion, lethargy, coma), perhaps thirst; seizures if develops rapidly or is very severe *Laboratory findings:* Serum sodium level **more than** 145 mEq/L, serum osmolality **more than** 300 mOsm/kg
Hyponatremia (water excess; hypo-osmolar imbalance)—body fluids too dilute	
Gain of relatively more water than salt Excessive ADH (SIADH) Psychogenic polydipsia or forced excessive water intake Excessive i.v. administration of D_5W Use of hypotonic irrigating solutions Tap water enemas **Loss of relatively more salt than water** Replacement of large body fluid output (diarrhea, vomiting) with water but no salt	*Physical examination:* Decreased level of consciousness (confusion, lethargy, coma), seizures if develops rapidly or is very severe *Laboratory findings:* Serum sodium level **less than** 135 mEq/L, serum osmolality **less than** 280 mOsm/kg

Table 25.2 Fluid Imbalances—cont'd

Imbalance and Related Causes	Signs and Symptoms
COMBINED ISOTONIC AND OSMOLALITY IMBALANCE	
Clinical dehydration (ECV deficit plus hypernatremia)—body fluids have decreased volume and are too concentrated	
Sodium and water intake less than output, with loss of relatively more water than salt Most of the causes of ECV deficit (see previous causes) plus poor or no water intake; often with fever causing increased insensible water output	*Physical examination and laboratory findings:* Combination of findings for ECV deficit plus findings for hypernatremia (see previous signs)

ADH, antidiuretic hormone; *BUN*, blood urea nitrogen; *ECV*, extracellular fluid volume; *GI*, gastrointestinal; *D5W*, dextrose 5% in water; *SIADH*, syndrome of inappropriate secretion of ADH.

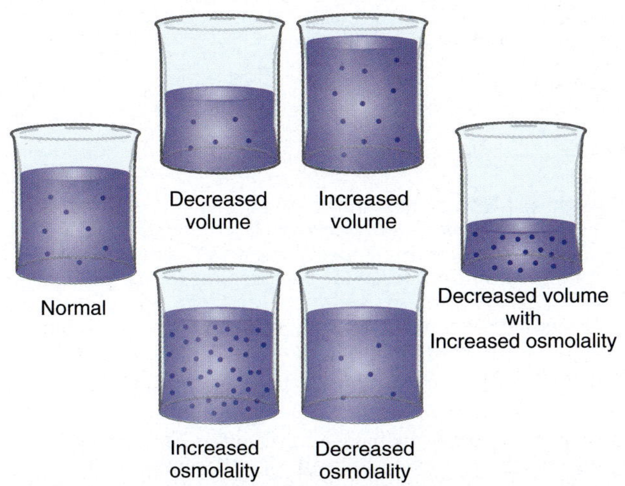

Fig. 25.4 Fluid volume and osmolality imbalances. (From Copstead LC, Banasik JL: *Pathophysiology*, ed 6, St Louis, 2018, Elsevier.)

Extracellular Fluid Volume Imbalances

Extracellular fluid volume ECV excess (**hypervolemia**) is too much isotonic fluid in the extracellular compartment (see Table 25.2). Signs and symptoms come from too much vascular volume and interstitial volume.

- **Edema** is collection of excess fluid in the interstitial space. It may develop if there is an increase in venous hydrostatic pressure, reduction in oncotic pressure, or increase in interstitial oncotic pressure. It may also occur because of an obstruction of lymphatic outflow, which causes decreased shifting of interstitial fluid. Water enters cells by osmosis, causing them to swell. Signs of cerebral dysfunction occur when brain cells swell (see Table 25.2).

  Extracellular fluid volume ECV *deficit* (**hypovolemia**)*, as the name indicates, is too small a volume of isotonic fluid in the vascular and interstitial areas. The term* **hypovolemia** *refers to the decreased vascular volume in ECV deficit (see Table 25.2).*
- **Dehydration:** Water leaves cells by osmosis, and they shrivel. Signs of cerebral dysfunction occur when brain cells shrivel. Hypernatremia often occurs in combination with ECV deficit; the two together are **clinical dehydration** (see Table 25.2).

Electrolyte Imbalances

Sodium Imbalances

- **Hypernatremia** is abnormally high Na^+ concentration in ECF caused by loss of relatively more water than salt or gain of relatively more salt than water (see Table 25.2) (Felver, 2018).
- **Hyponatremia** is abnormally low Na^+ concentration in the ECF, which occurs from gaining relatively more water than salt or losing relatively more salt than water (see Table 25.2) (Felver, 2018).

Potassium Imbalances

- **Hypokalemia**, a common electrolyte imbalance, is an inadequate level of K^+ in the blood. Common causes of hypokalemia involve increased K^+ output not balanced by K^+ intake: diarrhea and use of K^+-wasting diuretics (Table 25.3) (Felver, 2018). Hypokalemia causes muscle weakness and, if severe, cardiac dysrhythmias.
- **Hyperkalemia** is abnormally high blood K^+ concentration. Its causes are increased K^+ intake, shift of K^+ out of cells, and decreased K^+ output. Hyperkalemia produces muscle weakness and dangerous dysrhythmias.

Calcium Imbalances

- **Hypocalcemia** is abnormally low blood concentration of total Ca^{2+} or ionized Ca^{2+}. It usually results from decreased Ca^{2+} intake and absorption or shift of Ca^{2+} into bones or unavailable forms (see Table 25.3) (Felver, 2018). Signs and symptoms are caused by increased neuromuscular excitability.
- **Hypercalcemia** is abnormally high Ca^{2+} concentration in the blood. It often occurs from an underlying disease such as cancer or hyperparathyroidism that causes bone resorption, shifting Ca^{2+} from bones into the ECF. The person may develop pathological fractures from the weak bones that result.

Magnesium Imbalances

- **Hypomagnesemia**, abnormally low blood Mg^{2+} level, often occurs with chronic alcoholism and causes increased neuromuscular excitability (see Table 25.3).
- **Hypermagnesemia**, abnormally high blood Mg^{2+} level, is the result of excess Mg^{2+} intake or decreased Mg^{2+} excretion with oliguric renal disease. It causes decreased neuromuscular excitability.

Chloride Imbalances

- **Hypochloremia** is abnormally low blood chloride level. It frequently is associated with alkalosis and conditions that cause loss of hydrochloric acid (vomiting, nasogastric suction, and gastric fistula drainage). It always occurs with other imbalances and has no unique signs and symptoms.
- **Hyperchloremia** is abnormally high blood chloride level, which occurs with some types of acidosis, some renal conditions, and other electrolyte imbalances. It also has no unique signs and symptoms.

Table 25.3 Electrolyte Imbalances

Imbalance and Related Causes	Signs and Symptoms
HYPOKALEMIA—LOW SERUM POTASSIUM (K^+) CONCENTRATION	
Decreased K^+ intake: Excessive use of K^+-free i.v. solutions **Shift of K^+ into cells:** Alkalosis; treatment of diabetic ketoacidosis with insulin **Increased K^+ output:** Acute or chronic diarrhea, vomiting, or other GI losses; use of potassium-wasting diuretics; aldosterone excess; polyuria; glucocorticoid therapy	*Physical examination:* Bilateral muscle weakness, abdominal distention, decreased bowel sounds, constipation, dysrhythmias *Laboratory findings:* Serum K^+ level **less than** 3.5 mEq/L *ECG abnormalities:* U waves, flattened or inverted T waves; ST segment depression
HYPERKALEMIA—HIGH SERUM POTASSIUM (K^+) CONCENTRATION	
Increased K^+ intake: Iatrogenic administration of large amounts of i.v. K^+; rapid infusion of stored blood; excess ingestion of K^+ salt substitutes **Shift of K^+ out of cells:** Massive cellular damage (e.g., crushing trauma, cytotoxic chemotherapy); insufficient insulin (e.g., diabetic ketoacidosis); some types of acidosis **Decreased K^+ output:** Acute or chronic oliguria (e.g., severe ECV deficit, end-stage renal disease); use of potassium-sparing diuretics; adrenal insufficiency	*Physical examination:* Bilateral muscle weakness, transient abdominal cramps, diarrhea, dysrhythmias; cardiac arrest if severe *Laboratory findings:* Serum potassium level **more than** 5 mEq/L *ECG abnormalities:* Peaked T waves; widened QRS complex; PR prolongation; terminal sine-wave pattern
HYPOCALCEMIA—LOW SERUM CALCIUM (CA^{2+}) CONCENTRATION	
Decreased Ca^{2+} intake and absorption: Calcium-deficient diet; vitamin D deficiency (includes end-stage renal disease); chronic diarrhea, laxative misuse; steatorrhea **Shift of Ca^{2+} into bone or inactive form:** Hypoparathyroidism; rapid administration of citrated blood; hypoalbuminemia; alkalosis; pancreatitis **Increased Ca^{2+} output:** Chronic diarrhea; steatorrhea	*Physical examination:* Numbness and tingling of fingers and circumoral (around mouth) region, positive Chvostek sign (contraction of facial muscles when facial nerve is tapped), hyperactive reflexes, muscle twitching and cramping, carpal and pedal spasms, tetany, seizures, laryngospasm, dysrhythmias *Laboratory findings:* Total serum calcium **less than** 8.4 mg/dL or serum ionized calcium level **less than** 4.5 mg/dL *ECG abnormalities:* Prolonged ST segments
HYPERCALCEMIA—HIGH SERUM CALCIUM (CA^{2+}) CONCENTRATION	
Increased Ca^{2+} intake and absorption: Milk-alkali syndrome **Shift of Ca^{2+} out of bone:** Prolonged immobilization; hyperparathyroidism; bone tumors; nonosseous cancers that secrete bone-resorbing factors **Decreased Ca^{2+}** Use of thiazide diuretics	*Physical examination:* Anorexia, nausea and vomiting, constipation, diminished reflexes, lethargy, decreased level of consciousness, personality change; cardiac arrest if severe *Laboratory findings:* Total serum calcium level **more than** 10.5 mg/dL or serum ionized calcium level **more than** 5.3 mg/dL *ECG abnormalities:* Heart block, shortened ST segments
HYPOMAGNESEMIA—LOW SERUM MAGNESIUM (MG^{2+}) CONCENTRATION	
Decreased Mg^{2+} intake and absorption: Malnutrition; chronic alcoholism; chronic diarrhea, laxative misuse; steatorrhea **Shift of Mg^{2+} into inactive form:** Rapid administration of citrated blood **Increased Mg^{2+} output:** Chronic diarrhea; steatorrhea; other GI losses (e.g., vomiting, nasogastric or fistula drainage); use of thiazide or loop diuretics; aldosterone excess	*Physical examination:* Positive Chvostek sign, hyperactive deep tendon reflexes, muscle twitching and cramping, grimacing, dysphagia, tetany, seizures, insomnia, tachycardia, hypertension, dysrhythmias *Laboratory findings:* Serum magnesium level **less than** 1.5 mEq/L *ECG abnormalities:* Prolonged Q–T interval
HYPERMAGNESEMIA—HIGH SERUM MAGNESIUM (MG^{2+}) CONCENTRATION	
Increased Mg^{2+} intake and absorption: Excessive use of Mg^{2+}-containing laxatives and antacids; parenteral overload of Mg^{2+} **Decreased Mg^{2+} output:** Oliguric end-stage renal disease; adrenal insufficiency	*Physical examination:* Lethargy, hypoactive deep tendon reflexes, bradycardia, hypotension *Acute elevation in Mg^{2+} levels:* Flushing, sensation of warmth *Severe acute hypermagnesemia:* Decreased rate and depth of respirations, dysrhythmias, cardiac arrest *Laboratory findings:* Serum magnesium level **more than** 2.5 mEq/L *ECG abnormalities:* Prolonged P–R interval

ECG, electrocardiogram; *ECV*, extracellular fluid volume; *GI*, gastrointestinal.

FACTORS AFFECTING AND DISTURBANCES IN ACID–BASE BALANCES

Acid–base imbalances disrupt cell function and can be fatal if untreated.

- **Arterial blood gas (ABG)** analysis evaluates acid–base balance and oxygenation. Interpreting ABG levels involves understanding the physiology of six components: pH, $PaCO_2$, PaO_2, SaO_2, base excess, and HCO_3^-. Deviation from normal values indicates that a patient has an acid–base imbalance.
- **pH:** The pH measures H^+ concentration in body fluids. Even a slight change is potentially life threatening. An increase in concentration of H^+ makes a solution more acidic; a decrease makes a solution more alkaline. Normal arterial blood pH value is 7.35–7.45 (acidic is less than 7.35, and alkalotic is greater than 7.45).
- **$PaCO_2$:** $PaCO_2$ is the partial pressure of carbon dioxide in arterial blood and reflects the amount of H_2CO_3 in the blood. Normal range is 35–45 mm Hg. Hyperventilation produces a $PaCO_2$ less than 35 mm Hg. As rate and depth of respiration increase, more CO_2 is exhaled, decreasing the $PaCO_2$. Conversely, hypoventilation produces a $PaCO_2$ greater than 45 mm Hg. As

rate and depth of respiration decrease, less CO_2 is exhaled while cells continue to produce it, which increases the $PaCO_2$.

- **PaO_2**: PaO_2 is the partial pressure of oxygen in arterial blood. Normal range is 80–100 mm Hg. When PaO_2 is within normal range, it has no primary role in acid–base regulation. A PaO_2 less than 60 mm Hg leads to anaerobic metabolism, causing lactic acid production and metabolic acidosis. Hypoxemia can cause hyperventilation leading to respiratory alkalosis.
- **SaO_2**: SaO_2 (oxygen saturation) is the percentage of hemoglobin molecules that are carrying as much oxygen as is possible (saturated). Normal range is 95%–100%. Changes in temperature, pH, and $PaCO_2$ affect SaO_2 levels.
- **Base excess:** Base excess (or deficit) is the amount of blood buffer (hemoglobin and bicarbonate) present in the blood. The normal range is ±2 mmol/L. A higher positive value indicates **alkalosis**, and a lower negative value indicates **acidosis**.
- **Bicarbonate:** Normal range of bicarbonate (HCO_3^-) is 22–26 mEq/L. HCO_3^- is the principal buffer in the ECF. HCO_3^- levels reflect the action of the kidneys in managing metabolic acid. A level less than 22 mEq/L usually indicates metabolic acidosis; a level greater than 26 mEq/L indicates metabolic alkalosis.

Types of Acid–Base Imbalances

Acid–base imbalances are either respiratory or metabolic. The four primary types of acid–base imbalance are respiratory acidosis, respiratory alkalosis, metabolic acidosis, and metabolic alkalosis (Table 25.4). It is possible to have two primary (mixed) acid–base imbalances.

Table 25.4 Acid–Base Imbalances

Imbalance and Related Causes	Signs and Symptoms
RESPIRATORY ACIDOSIS—EXCESSIVE CARBONIC ACID RESULTING FROM ALVEOLAR HYPOVENTILATION	
Impaired gas exchange Type B COPD (chronic bronchitis) or end-stage type A COPD (emphysema) Bacterial pneumonia Airway obstruction Extensive atelectasis (obstruction of small airways often caused by retained mucus) Severe acute asthma episode **Impaired neuromuscular function** Respiratory muscle weakness or paralysis from hypokalemia or neurological dysfunction Respiratory muscle fatigue, respiratory failure Chest wall injury or surgery causing pain with respiration **Dysfunction of brain stem respiratory control** Drug overdose with a respiratory depressant Some types of head injury	*Physical examination:* Headache, light-headedness, decreased level of consciousness (confusion, lethargy, coma), dysrhythmias *Laboratory findings:* Arterial blood gas alterations—pH **less than** 7.35, $PaCO_2$ **more than** 45 mm Hg, bicarbonate level normal (if uncompensated) or **more than** 26 mEq/L (if compensated)
RESPIRATORY ALKALOSIS—DEFICIENT CARBONIC ACID RESULTING FROM ALVEOLAR HYPERVENTILATION	
Hypoxemia from any cause (e.g., initial portion of asthma episode, pneumonia) Acute pain Anxiety, psychological distress, sobbing Inappropriate mechanical ventilator settings Stimulation of brain stem respiratory control (meningitis, gram-negative sepsis, head injury, salicylate overdose)	*Physical examination:* Light-headedness; numbness and tingling of fingers, toes, and circumoral region; tachypnea; excitement and confusion possibly followed by decreased level of consciousness; dysrhythmias *Laboratory findings:* Arterial blood gas alterations—pH **more than** 7.45, $PaCO_2$ **less than** 35 mm Hg, bicarbonate level normal (if short lived or uncompensated) or **less than** 22 mEq/L (if compensated)
METABOLIC ACIDOSIS—EXCESSIVE METABOLIC ACIDS	
Increase of metabolic acids (high anion gap) Ketoacidosis (diabetes, starvation, alcoholism) Hypermetabolic state (severe hyperthyroidism, burns, severe infection) Oliguric renal disease (acute kidney injury, end-stage renal disease) Circulatory shock (lactic acidosis) Ingestion of acid or acid precursors (e.g., methanol, ethylene glycol, boric acid, aspirin overdose) **Loss of bicarbonate (normal anion gap)** Diarrhea Pancreatic fistula or intestinal decompression Renal tubular acidosis	*Physical examination:* Decreased level of consciousness (confusion, lethargy, coma), abdominal pain, dysrhythmias, increased rate and depth of respirations (compensatory hyperventilation) *Laboratory findings:* Arterial blood gas alterations—pH **less than** 7.35, $PaCO_2$ normal (if uncompensated) or **less than** 35 mm Hg (if compensated), bicarbonate level **less than** 22 mEq/L
METABOLIC ALKALOSIS—DEFICIENT METABOLIC ACIDS	
Increase of bicarbonate Excessive administration of sodium bicarbonate Massive blood transfusion (liver converts citrate to bicarbonate) Mild or moderate ECV deficit **Loss of metabolic acid** Excessive vomiting or gastric suctioning Hypokalemia Excess aldosterone	*Physical examination:* Light-headedness; numbness and tingling of fingers, toes, and circumoral region; muscle cramps; possible excitement and confusion followed by decreased level of consciousness; dysrhythmias (may be caused by concurrent hypokalemia) *Laboratory findings:* Arterial blood gas alterations—pH **more than** 7.45, $PaCO_2$ normal (if uncompensated) or **more than** 45 mm Hg (if compensated), bicarbonate level **more than** 26 mEq/L; K^+ level often decreased (below 3.5 mEq/L)

COPD, chronic obstructive pulmonary disease; *ECV*, extracellular fluid volume.
Data from Felver L: Fluid and electrolyte homeostasis and imbalances. In Copstead LC, Banasik JL, editors: *Pathophysiology*, ed 6, St Louis, 2018, Elsevier.

NURSING PROCESS

Assessment

It is important to use knowledge of fluid, electrolyte, and acid–base balance to guide your assessment. By gathering assessment data and using critical thinking skills, nurses identify patients at risk for and patients with imbalances. Thorough assessment enables identification of appropriate nursing diagnoses.

Nursing History

Assessment begins with a patient history, which may reveal risk factors or preexisting conditions that cause or contribute to fluid, electrolyte, and acid–base imbalances. For example, explore a patient's diet history, including normal fluid intake. Determine whether the patient is taking medications that can create electrolyte alterations. Explore these factors with the patient and integrate the information with knowledge of regulation of fluid, electrolyte, and acid–base balances.

Age

Age is an important assessment consideration. Infants and very young children have relatively more body water than older children and adults. They have greater water needs and immature kidneys (Hockenberry et al., 2017). They are at greater risk for **ECV deficit** and hypernatremia because their body water loss is proportionately greater per kilogram of weight. Children aged 2–12 years have less stable regulatory responses to imbalances; therefore, they have a narrow range of tolerance for severe fluid or electrolyte imbalances. Adolescent girls have greater ECV fluctuations because of hormonal changes associated with the menstrual cycle.

Older Adult Considerations

Older adults experience age-related changes that can affect fluid, electrolyte, and acid–base balances. These changes include a reduction in lean muscle mass resulting in a reduction of body water, diminished thirst sensation, and decreased ability to concentrate urine and increase the risk of ECV deficit and hypernatremia (Felver, 2017b; Touhy and Jett, 2014). Kidney changes of normal aging make it more difficult to excrete a large metabolic acid load, increasing the risk for metabolic acidosis. Normal aging changes, chronic diseases, and multiple medications often make maintaining fluid and electrolyte balance a challenge.

Environment

Hot environments increase fluid output through sweating. Sweat is a hypotonic Na^+-containing fluid. Ask patients whether they engage in vigorous physical work or exercise in hot environments. If so, are Na^+-containing fluid replacements available during activity?

Dietary Intake

Assess a patient's normal 24-hour dietary intake of food and fluids. Determine the intake of salt and foods rich in K^+, Ca^{2+}, and Mg^{2+}. Assess recent changes in appetite and ability to chew and swallow, which affect nutritional status and fluid hydration. Also consider a patient's economic situation. Does he or she have the resources to prepare food? Assess whether the patient is on a self-imposed type of diet. Starvation diets or high-fat, no-carbohydrate diets can cause metabolic acidosis.

Lifestyle

Take an alcohol intake history. Ask the patient the number of alcoholic drinks he or she normally consumes in a week. Is the patient a binge drinker? Binge drinking typically occurs after four drinks for women and five drinks for men in about 2 hours (NIAAA, n.d.). Chronic alcohol abuse commonly causes hypomagnesemia, in part because it increases renal Mg^{2+} excretion.

Medications

Obtain a complete list of current medications including over-the-counter (OTC) and herbal preparations to assess risk for fluid, electrolyte, and acid–base imbalances. If your patient takes a medication that causes an electrolyte or acid–base imbalance, assess pertinent laboratory values.

Medical History

A patient's prior medical history provides valuable data about fluid, electrolyte, and acid–base imbalances. When patients have chronic diseases (e.g., cancer, heart failure, oliguric renal disease), review these conditions to understand how they affect fluid, electrolyte, and acid–base balance. Assess duration of the disease and treatment regimens. In addition to chronic health problems, determine whether a patient has a history of recent GI alterations (e.g., diarrhea or vomiting), nasogastric suctioning, or intestinal drainage. Loss of GI fluids predisposes patients to ECV deficit, hypokalemia, and other electrolyte imbalances.

Recent surgery, head injury, respiratory disorders, and burns place patients at high risk for fluid and electrolyte imbalances. The physiological stress response to surgery causes increased secretion of aldosterone, cortisol, and ADH in the first few postoperative days. These changes cause increased ECV, decreased osmolality, and increased K^+ excretion. In otherwise healthy patients, these imbalances resolve without difficulty, but patients with preexisting imbalances or additional risk factors may need treatment.

Physical Assessment

Data gathered through a focused physical assessment validate and extend information gathered in the patient history. Focus your assessment on the areas pertinent to each patient situation. For example, for patients at risk for ECV imbalances, focus your assessment on body weight changes and clinical markers of vascular and interstitial volume. Carefully assess patients' cardiac, respiratory, neuromuscular, and GI status when they are at high risk for electrolyte and acid–base imbalances. Grouping your assessments under these categories helps you know which assessments to prioritize and enables you to assess effectively. Table 25.5 provides a focused assessment of fluid status for a patient.

Daily Weights and Fluid Intake and Output Measurement

Daily weights are an important indicator of fluid status (Felver, 2017b). Each kilogram (2.2 pounds) of weight gained or lost overnight is equal to 1 L of fluid gained or lost. Weigh patients with heart failure or patients who are at high risk for or have ECV excess daily. In a hospital or nursing home setting, obtain the weight at the same time

Table 25.5 Focused Patient Assessment

Factors to Assess	Questions	Physical Assessment
Vital signs and neck veins	Tell me how you feel when you stand up? Do you ever feel light-headed?	Palpate the patient's pulse and auscultate heart rate. Monitor the patient's blood pressure and pulse when supine and then at 1 min after sitting with legs dependent or at 1 min after standing. Observe the patient for light-headedness (unsteady gait). Inspect neck veins when the patient is supine to see whether they are flat or collapsing with inspiration.
I&O	Describe for me how often you are thirsty? How often do you usually urinate?	Monitor the patient's 24-h I&O; note whether having diarrhea fluid. Inspect urine (expect dark yellow color).
Skin, mucous membranes, and daily weight	Is your mouth dry? Has your skin recently been more dry than usual?	Check dryness of mucous membranes between cheek and gum. Inspect the patient's skin; test for turgor over sternum. Obtain a baseline weight and monitor daily.

I&O, intake and output.

each day with the same calibrated scale after a patient voids, if possible. Also have patients wear a gown that weighs the same each time they weigh. In medical clinics and other outpatient centers, use the same scale each time and have patients void beforehand. If you are using a bed scale, always use the same number of linens. Teach patients with heart failure to take and record daily weights at home and to contact their health care provider if weight increases suddenly according to parameters their providers set. Recognizing trends in daily weights is important. Patients who are hospitalized for decompensated heart failure often experience significant increases in daily weights during the week before hospitalization (Wang et al., 2014).

Measuring and recording all liquid I&O during a 24-hour period is an important aspect of fluid balance assessment. Compare 24-hour intake with 24-hour output. The two measures should be approximately equal if the person has normal fluid balance. Recognizing I&O trends is important (e.g., a gradually decreasing fluid output with increased intake may indicate a developing ECV excess).

In most health care settings, I&O measurement is a nursing assessment. Some agencies require a health care provider's order for I&O. Check your agency policies if you want to measure I&O for a patient with compromised fluid status. Fluid intake includes all liquids that a person eats (e.g., gelatin, ice cream, broth), drinks (e.g., juice, coffee, tea, water), or receives through nasogastric or jejunostomy feeding tubes (see Chapter 20). I.v. fluids (continuous and intermittent) and blood components also count as intake. A patient receiving tube feedings may receive numerous liquid medications; water is used to flush the tube before and/or after the medications. During a 24-hour period, these liquids can amount to significant intake; always record them on the I&O record. Patient and family caregiver cooperation is essential for maintaining accurate I&O measurements. Ask alert patients to help measure their oral intake and explain to family members why they should not eat or drink from the patient's meal tray or water pitcher.

Liquid output includes urine, diarrhea, vomitus, gastric suction, and blood and drainage from postsurgical wounds, burns, or other tubes (see Chapters 17, 21, and 22). Record urinary output after each voiding. Instruct patients who are alert and ambulatory to save their urine in a calibrated (graduated) insert that attaches to the rim of a toilet bowl (Fig. 25.5). Teach patients and families the purpose of I&O; tell them to notify a nurse or nursing assistive personnel (NAP) to empty the container with voided fluid, or teach them how to measure and record the result themselves. Patients need good vision and motor skills to perform these assessments. When a patient has an indwelling urinary catheter, drainage tube, or suction, record that output (e.g., at the end of each nursing shift or every hour) as the patient's condition requires.

You can delegate portions of I&O measurement to NAP. Emphasize the importance of accurate measurements, even when available time is limited (McGloin, 2015). In many agencies, NAP can record oral intake but not intake through tubes or i.v. lines; they can record urine, diarrhea, and vomitus output but not drainage through tubes. Work as a team with the NAP to record measurements in the designated location in the electronic health record (EHR) or appropriate paper forms. Accurate I&O evaluates a patient's hydration status.

Laboratory Studies

Review a patient's laboratory test results and compare them with normal ranges to obtain additional data about fluid, electrolyte, and acid–base balances. Box 25.1 and Table 25.6 summarize laboratory data useful for this purpose. The frequency of measurement of electrolyte levels depends on the severity of a patient's illness. Serum electrolyte tests are performed routinely on patients entering a hospital to screen for imbalances and serve as a baseline for future comparisons.

Patient Expectations

Fluid, electrolyte, and acid–base imbalances often accompany serious illness that prevents a review of patient expectations.

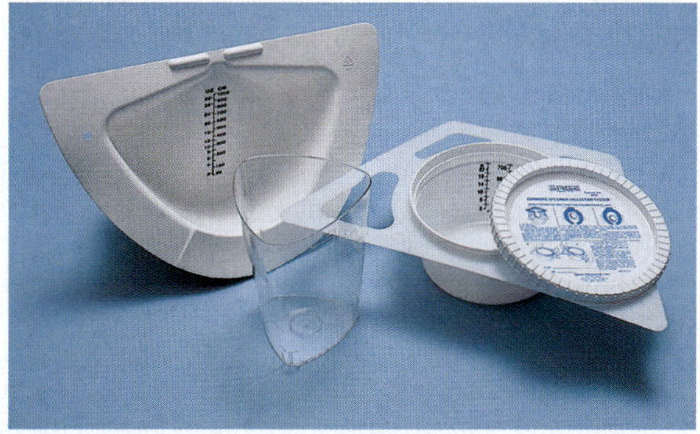

Fig. 25.5 Graduated measuring containers. *Clockwise from top left:* "Hat" receptacle, specimen, and measurement container.

BOX 25.1 Laboratory Data Reflecting Fluid, Electrolyte, and Acid–Base Imbalances

Fluid and Electrolytes

- Alterations in serum sodium, osmolality, potassium, magnesium, calcium, phosphate, and chloride
- Alterations in hematocrit and BUN
- Alterations in urine specific gravity

Metabolic Alkalosis

- pH more than 7.45
- $PaCO_2$ normal or more than 45 mm Hg if lungs are compensating
- HCO_3^- more than 26 mEq/L
- Ionized calcium less than 4.5 mg/dL
- K^+ less than 3.5 mEq/L

Metabolic Acidosis

- pH less than 7.35
- $PaCO_2$ normal or less than 35 mm Hg if lungs are compensating
- HCO_3^- less than 22 mEq/L
- K^+ more than 5 mEq/L

Respiratory Alkalosis

- pH more than 7.45
- $PaCO_2$ less than 35 mm Hg
- HCO_3^- less than 22 mEq/L if kidneys are compensating
- Ionized calcium less than 4.5 mg/dL
- K^+ less than 3.5 mEq/L

Respiratory Acidosis

- pH less than 7.35
- $PaCO_2$ more than 45 mm Hg
- HCO_3^- normal if early respiratory acidosis or more than 26 mEq/L if kidneys are compensating
- K^+ more than 5 mEq/L

BUN, blood urea nitrogen.

Table 25.6 Arterial Blood Gas Assessment

Test	Normal Range for Adults	Significance of Abnormal Findings
pH	7.35–7.45	Increased: Metabolic or respiratory alkalosis Decreased: Metabolic or respiratory acidosis Small changes in pH indicate large changes in H^+ concentration and are clinically important
PaO_2 (mm Hg)	80–100	Decreased: Poor oxygenation of the blood
SaO_2 (%)	95–100	Decreased: Poor oxygenation of the blood
$PaCO_2$ (mm Hg)	35–45	Increased: Respiratory acidosis or compensation for metabolic alkalosis (differentiate with pH) Decreased: Respiratory alkalosis or compensation for metabolic acidosis (differentiate with pH)
Bicarbonate (mEq/L or mmol/L)	22–26	Increased: Metabolic alkalosis or compensation for respiratory acidosis (differentiate with pH) Decreased: Metabolic acidosis or compensation for respiratory alkalosis (differentiate with pH)

Reviewing expectations with patients who are alert may reveal short-term (e.g., provision of comfort from nausea) or long-term (e.g., understanding how to prevent imbalances in the future) needs. Strengthen a patient's trust through competent responses to sudden changes in condition and by keeping patients and/or family caregivers informed so that they become active participants in care.

Nursing Diagnosis

When caring for patients with potential fluid, electrolyte, or acid–base imbalances, use critical thinking to formulate nursing diagnoses. The assessment data that establish the risk for or the actual presence of a nursing diagnosis may be subtle, but patterns and trends emerge after astute assessment. Multiple body systems may be involved, so carefully analyze the defining characteristics or risk factors in clusters. For example, relevant assessment data for the problem-focused nursing diagnosis *Deficient Fluid Volume* include defining characteristics such as insufficient oral intake, sudden weight loss, dry oral mucous membranes, decreased skin turgor, decreased blood pressure, and increased heart rate.

In addition to accurate clustering of assessment data, another part of developing nursing diagnoses is identifying the relevant and accurate causes or related factors for problem-focused and health promotion nursing diagnoses. For example, *Deficient Fluid Volume related to loss of GI fluids from vomiting* requires interventions to manage the patient's vomiting and restore fluid volume (e.g., administer antiemetics, remove sights and odors that induce nausea, and provide i.v. fluid replacement). The same nursing diagnosis with a different related factor such as *Deficient Fluid Volume related to elevated body temperature* requires different interventions (e.g., administer antipyretics and provide oral fluids).

Possible nursing diagnoses for patients with fluid, electrolyte, and acid–base alterations include the following:

- *Decreased Cardiac Output*
- *Acute Confusion*
- *Risk for Electrolyte Imbalance*
- *Deficient Fluid Volume*
- *Excess Fluid Volume*
- *Risk for Imbalanced Fluid Volume*
- *Impaired Gas Exchange*
- *Risk for Injury*

Planning

Goals and Outcomes

During the planning phase, collaborate with each patient to establish goals and expected outcomes for each nursing diagnosis (see Care Plan given in the subsequent text). Make sure that goals are individualized and realistic with measurable outcomes.

Care Plan

Extracellular Fluid Volume Deficit

Assessment

Mrs Susan Reynolds, a 42-year-old married accountant, was admitted yesterday to an acute care unit with a history of nausea, loss of appetite, and diarrhea for 7 days. After obtaining a blood sample for electrolyte levels, complete blood count, and an electrocardiogram (ECG), her health care provider admitted her for observation. Orders include intravenous (i.v.) infusion of 0.9% saline at 125 mL/h, I&O recordings, vital signs every 4 hours, and daily weights.

ASSESSMENT ACTIVITIES	FINDINGS[a]
Ask Mrs Reynolds to describe when her nausea began.	Mrs Reynolds states that she became nauseous after a short business trip, has no appetite, is nauseous, and has had diarrhea for 7 days.
Assess vital signs.	Vital signs: temperature 99.6°F (37.6°C); **pulse, 100 beats/min** and regular; supine **blood pressure (BP), 105/60 mm Hg** with no changes when standing; respirations 18/min and nonlabored; lung sounds clear to auscultation bilaterally.
Assess abdomen and I&O.	Bowel sounds present and hyperactive in all four quadrants. Abdomen soft to palpation. Her 24-h intake was 1850 mL, with output of 2200 mL **(urine output accounted for only 1000 mL)**. She has **dark yellow urine**.
Assess skin, mucous membranes, and daily weight for indicators of extracellular fluid volume (ECV) deficit.	Skin is **dry**, without discoloration, but **turgor is decreased**. Neck veins barely visible when supine. **Dry mucous membranes** between cheek and gum. **Weight** of 143 pounds (65 kg) is **decreased 1 pound** (0.45 kg) since her admission yesterday.
Evaluate laboratory values.	Laboratory result: hematocrit 44% (suggesting hypovolemia); serum K^+ 3.5 mEq/L (low normal because of diarrhea) and Na^+ 140 mEq/L.

[a]Defining characteristics/risk factors are shown in **bold** type.

Nursing diagnosis: Deficient Fluid Volume related to increased fluid output from diarrhea and diuretic

PLANNING

GOAL	EXPECTED OUTCOMES (NOC)[b]
	Fluid Balance
Mrs Reynolds' fluid volume will return to normal by time of discharge.	Urine output equals at least 1400 mL/day in 2 days. Urine color becomes light yellow within 24 h. Heart rate (HR) and BP return to normal in 24 h. Mucous membranes are moist in 24 h. Skin turgor returns to normal within 24 h. Daily weights do not decrease over next 2 days.
Mrs Reynolds will describe how to manage fluid balance at home before hospital discharge.	Mrs Reynolds describes how to replace diarrhea fluid loss. She describes signs and symptoms that indicate the need to increase fluid and sodium intake.
	Electrolyte and Acid–Base Balance
Mrs Reynolds' electrolyte balance will be within normal limits by discharge.	Serum electrolyte levels are within normal limits within 48 h.

[b]Outcomes classification labels from Moorhead S, et al, editors: *Nursing outcomes classification (NOC)*, ed 5, St Louis, 2013, Mosby.

INTERVENTIONS (NIC)[c]	RATIONALE
Fluid/Electrolyte Management	
Administer i.v. fluids (0.9% sodium chloride) at 125 mL/h as prescribed.	Replacement of isotonic fluid restores blood volume; isotonic solutions expand ECV without causing fluid shift into cells.
Provide the patient with additional 480 mL of her favorite noncaffeinated oral fluids at her preferred temperature every 8 h.	Patient-centered care takes individual preferences into account. Cultural preferences regarding temperature of oral fluid when ill influence fluid intake (Abitz, 2016).
Administer bismuth subsalicylate (Pepto-Bismol) as ordered for diarrhea.	Pepto-Bismol is an antidiarrheal that inhibits gastrointestinal secretions, stimulates absorption of fluid and electrolytes, and inhibits intestinal inflammation (Burchum and Rosenthal, 2016).
Maintain accurate I&O measurements.	Documents hydration and fluid balance for directing therapy.
Weigh Mrs Reynolds daily and monitor trends.	Daily weights provide an indication of fluid balance (Felver, 2017b).

[c]Interventions classification labels from Bulechek GM, et al, editors: *Nursing interventions classification (NIC)*, ed 6, St Louis, 2013, Mosby.

Continued

Care Plan—cont'd

EVALUATION

NURSING ACTIONS	PATIENT RESPONSE/FINDING	ACHIEVEMENT OF OUTCOME
Monitor electrolyte levels, daily weights, and I&O trends.	Serum electrolyte levels: K^+ 3.7 mEq/L and Na^+ 140 mEq/L; weight, 143 pounds (65 kg). Mrs Reynolds' 24-h intake is 2800 mL, and output is 2200 mL with 1800 mL urine. Urine is light yellow.	Electrolyte levels within normal range. Daily weight stable. Fluid balance is improving with urine output exceeding stool output.
Assess oral mucous membranes, neck vein fullness, skin turgor, HR, and BP.	Mucous membranes remain dry. Neck veins full when supine. Skin turgor normal. Heart rate 80 beats/min, BP 126/78 mm Hg.	ECV is returning to normal.
Evaluate effectiveness of teaching regarding maintaining fluid and electrolyte balance at home.	Identifies foods and fluids she can eat and drink at home to maintain electrolyte balance.	Mrs Reynolds describes effective home management of fluid and electrolyte balance.

In the acute care setting, a long-term goal is to anticipate the needs of a patient and family to ease the transition to home or long-term care. *For example, Mrs Reynolds likely will be discharged home with new medications or recommendations for a diet that causes less GI upset.* When creating a patient care plan, remember to take into consideration the patient's personal preferences, knowledge and skills of the patient and family caregiver, and available resources.

Setting Priorities

A patient's clinical condition determines which diagnosis takes the greatest priority. Many nursing diagnoses in the area of fluid, electrolyte, and acid–base balance are of highest priority because the consequences for the patient can be serious or life threatening. *For example, in the concept map, Mrs Reynolds has diarrhea, which has created ECV deficit. The nursing diagnosis Deficient Fluid Volume ranks highest priority, requiring intervention to stabilize her status and prevent further complications.* As a patient's status changes, the priority nursing diagnoses also change. For example, the priority nursing diagnosis changes to *Deficient Knowledge* once a patient is well enough to be discharged home. The priority at this time is to ensure that the patient returns safely to the home, which often requires extensive patient and family caregiver education (see Chapter 15).

Collaborative Care

Consult with the patient's health care provider to identify realistic time frames for the goals of care, particularly when a patient's physiological status is unstable. Planning care for a patient requires collaboration with other members of the health care team such as the dietitian or pharmacist. You cannot delegate administration of i.v. medications and/or oxygen therapy to NAP. When a patient is stable, you can delegate daily weights, I&O measurement, and direct physical patient care. Establish a rapport of open communication and teamwork with NAP, as with any member of the interdisciplinary team, to ensure timely and effective administration of care.

Continuity of care is essential as a patient moves from one health care setting to another or to home. Therapeutic regimens established in one setting continue until completed in the next setting. For example, a patient who will continue to monitor I&O at home needs to know how to measure and document fluid I&O. When the patient's discharge has been ordered, it is important to identify which resources are available to promote positive outcomes. Dietitians are a valuable resource for recommending food sources to increase or reduce intake of specific electrolytes. Chapter 20 describes various therapeutic diets (e.g., low Na^+). Pharmacists can provide information about a patient's prescription and OTC medications that may cause electrolyte or acid–base imbalances. The health care provider directs the treatment of any fluid, electrolyte, or acid–base imbalance. Be sure that a patient who will be discharged has the resources for continuing therapeutic regimens to return to a state of optimal functioning. A case manager or social worker might be able to connect patients with those resources.

Implementation

Health Promotion

Health promotion activities focus primarily on patient education. Teach patients and family caregivers how to recognize risk factors for development of imbalances and implement appropriate preventive measures. For example, parents of infants need to understand that GI losses lead quickly to serious fluid imbalances; therefore, when vomiting or diarrhea occurs, they should immediately begin rehydrating with Na^+-containing fluid. People of all ages need to learn to replace body fluid losses with Na^+-containing fluid and water. Encourage patients who have low calcium or vitamin D levels to take daily supplements.

Patients with chronic health alterations need to understand their own risk factors and how to avoid imbalances. For example, patients with oliguric end-stage renal disease often need to restrict intake of fluid, Na^+, K^+, Mg^{2+}, and phosphate. Patients with severe heart failure must limit their intake of liquids and high-sodium foods to prevent fluid retention. Through diet education, patients learn the types of foods to avoid and the daily volume of fluid they are permitted. Know that patients from different cultures may have difficulty with food selection. Be sure to know their likes and dislikes, and try to match appropriate foods with their dietary preferences. Teach patients with chronic diseases and their family caregivers the early signs and symptoms of fluid, electrolyte, and acid–base imbalances for which they are at risk and what to do about them. For example, teach patients with heart failure to measure body weight each day at the same time and inform their health care provider of significant changes in weight from one day to another.

ACUTE CARE

Although patients with fluid, electrolyte, and acid–base imbalances are in all health care settings, it is common to manage them in acute care settings. Acute care nurses conduct frequent and often complex monitoring (e.g., ABG measurement) and administer oral and i.v. fluids and medications to replace fluid and electrolyte deficits or maintain normal balance. They also manage parenteral nutrition (PN) (see Chapter 20) and patients' oxygenation needs (see Chapter 24).

Enteral Replacement of Fluids

Oral replacement of fluids and electrolytes is appropriate when a patient is physiologically stable enough for oral fluids to be replaced rapidly. Oral replacement is contraindicated when a patient has a mechanical obstruction of the GI tract, is at high risk for aspiration, or has impaired swallowing. Patients unable to tolerate solid foods may still be able to ingest fluids. Strategies to encourage fluid intake include offering small sips of fluid frequently, popsicles, and ice chips. If possible, provide each patient's preferred fluids at the preferred temperature. Cultural beliefs regarding appropriate fluid temperature can interfere with fluid intake unless fluid at the preferred temperature is available (Abitz, 2016).

When replacing fluids by mouth in a patient with ECV deficit, choose fluids that contain Na^+ (e.g., Gatorade, salty broth, Pedialyte). Liquids containing lactose or low-Na^+ content are not appropriate when a patient has diarrhea. A feeding tube is used for fluid replacement when a patient's GI tract is healthy but the patient cannot ingest fluids (e.g., after oral surgery or with impaired swallowing) (see Chapter 20).

Restriction of Fluids

Patients who have hyponatremia usually require restricted water intake so their kidneys can resolve the imbalance. Patients who have very severe ECV excess may have both sodium and fluid restrictions. Fluid restriction is difficult for patients, particularly if they take medications that dry the oral mucous membranes or if they breathe through their mouth. Explain why fluids are restricted and ensure that the patient and any family visitors know the amount of fluid permitted orally and understand that ice chips, gelatin, and ice cream are fluids. Allow patients to decide the amount of fluid to drink with each meal, between meals, before bed, and with medications. Unless contraindicated, encourage patients to choose their preferred fluids. Frequently patients on fluid restriction can swallow multiple pills with 30 mL of liquid.

In acute care settings, fluid restrictions often allot half the oral fluids between 7 a.m. and 3 p.m., the period when patients usually are more active, receive two meals, and take most of their oral medications. Offer the remainder of the fluid allowance during the evening and night shifts. Patients on fluid restriction need frequent mouth care to moisten mucous membranes, decrease mucosal drying and cracking, and maintain comfort (see Chapter 16).

Parenteral Replacement of Fluids and Electrolytes

Fluid and electrolytes may be replaced through infusion of fluids intravenously (i.e., directly into veins). Parenteral replacement includes **PN**, i.v. fluid and electrolyte therapy **(crystalloids)**, and blood product **(colloids)** administration. Practice standard body fluid precautions (see Chapter 9) when administering parenteral fluids to minimize your own risk for exposure to blood-borne pathogens. Understand and follow the policy and procedures for parenteral infusions at the agency for which you work.

Parenteral Nutrition

PN is a nutritionally adequate solution consisting of glucose, other nutrients, and electrolytes administered through a central venous catheter. It is the nutritional therapy of choice when a patient's GI tract is nonfunctional (Winkler and Guenter, 2014) (see Chapter 20).

Intravenous Therapy

The goal of i.v. fluid administration is to deliver continuous or intermittent infusion of fluids and medications via the vascular system to correct or prevent fluid and electrolyte imbalances. I.v. fluid therapy requires frequent monitoring to detect ongoing changes in a patient's fluid and electrolyte balance. To provide safe care to patients who require i.v. fluid administration, you need knowledge of the correct solution ordered, the reason it was ordered, the equipment needed, evidence-based procedures required to initiate an infusion, how to regulate the infusion rate and maintain the system, how to identify and correct problems, and how to discontinue the infusion. Whenever you care for a patient who requires i.v. therapy, you need to follow specific standards to decrease the incidence of infection related to the therapy (Box 25.2).

Vascular Access Devices

Vascular access devices (VADs) are catheters or infusion ports designed for repeated access to the vascular system. Peripheral catheters are for short-term use (e.g., to restore fluid volume). Devices for long-term use include central lines, peripherally inserted central catheters (PICCs), and implanted ports. These devices are more effective than peripheral catheters for administering PN, medications, and solutions that are irritating to veins. Nurses need specialized education in the use of these central devices to provide safe care (Wallace and Macy, 2016).

Types of Solutions

Many prepared i.v. solutions are available for use. An i.v. solution is isotonic, hypotonic, or hypertonic. Solutions that contain glucose have a greater tonicity in the i.v. container than their effective concentration in the body because the glucose enters cells rapidly; thus, the rest of the infused fluid determines the effective physiological concentration (Table 25.7).

Equipment

Correct selection and preparation of i.v. equipment ensures safe and quick placement of an i.v. line. Because i.v. fluids infuse directly into the bloodstream, sterile technique is necessary. Organize all equipment at the bedside for efficient

BOX 25.2 Infusion Nurses Society Standards to Decrease Intravascular Infection Related to i.v. Therapy

- Palpate catheter insertion site for tenderness daily through the intact dressing.
- Directly inspect a catheter site if the patient develops tenderness at site, fever without obvious source, or symptoms of local or bloodstream infection.
- Perform hand hygiene before and after palpating, inserting, replacing, or dressing any intravascular device.
- Clean skin site vigorously before venipuncture with an appropriate single-use antiseptic solution.
- Allow site to air-dry before proceeding with procedure: 2% chlorhexidine for 30 s and povidone-iodine for at least 2 min.
- Do not palpate insertion site after skin has been cleaned with single-use antiseptic solution.
- Use a catheter stabilization device that allows visual inspection of access site.
- Change gauze dressings that cover a catheter site every 48 h.
- Leave transparent dressings in place until i.v. tubing is replaced.
- I.v. tubing administration sets can remain sterile for 96 h.
- Replace dressing over peripheral venous catheters when replacing catheter or when dressing becomes damp, loosened, or soiled.
- Clean injection ports with single-use antiseptic solution before accessing system.
- Replace short peripheral catheters and rotate sites based on clinical assessment indicating signs or symptoms of i.v.-related complications.

Modified from Gorski L, et al: Infusion therapy standards of practice, *J Infus Nurs* 39(suppl 1):S1, 2016.

insertion. I.v. equipment includes VADs, tourniquet, clean gloves, dressings, i.v. fluid containers, various types of tubing, and **electronic infusion devices (EIDs)**, also called *i.v. pumps*. Peripheral i.v. catheters are available in a variety of gauges (e.g., 20 and 22 gauge). The gauge indicates the diameter of the catheter. A larger gauge indicates a smaller-diameter catheter.

Use the tubing that is designated for the particular EID that you are using, typically a macrodrip tubing. Macrodrip tubing delivers large drops (standard drop size is 10 or 15 gtt/mL depending on the manufacturer). In contrast, microdrip tubing provides a standard drop size of 60 gtt/mL, which facilitates precise regulation of i.v. fluids at slow rates. Add i.v. extension tubing to increase patient mobility and decrease manipulation and potential contamination of the insertion site.

Peripheral Venipuncture Site

After organizing collected equipment at the bedside, prepare to insert the i.v. catheter by assessing the patient for a venipuncture site. The most common i.v. sites are on the inner arm (Fig. 25.6). You may insert an i.v. in a foot vein in children, but avoid this site in adults because of the danger of thrombophlebitis (Gorski et al., 2016). When assessing patients for potential venipuncture sites, consider conditions that exclude certain sites. For example, because older adults and patients receiving corticosteroids have fragile veins, avoid sites that are easily bumped or moved such as the dorsal surface of the hand (Box 25.3).

Venipuncture is contraindicated in a site that has signs of inflammation, infiltration, or thrombosis. An infected site is red, tender, swollen, and possibly warm to the touch. Avoid

Table 25.7 Intravenous Solutions

Solution	Concentration in i.v. Container and at Tip of VAD	Effective Concentration in Body	Comments
DEXTROSE (GLUCOSE) IN WATER SOLUTIONS			
Dextrose 5% in water (D_5W)	Isotonic	Hypotonic	Isotonic when first enters vein; dextrose enters cells rapidly, leaving free water, which dilutes ECF; most of the water then enters cells by osmosis
Dextrose 10% in water ($D_{10}W$)	Hypertonic	Hypotonic	Hypertonic when first enters vein; dextrose enters cells rapidly, leaving free water, which dilutes ECF; most of the water then enters cells by osmosis
SALINE (SODIUM CHLORIDE [NACL] IN WATER) SOLUTIONS			
0.225% NaCl (quarter NS; 1/4 NS)	Hypotonic	Hypotonic	Expands ECV (vascular and interstitial) and rehydrates cells
0.45% NaCl (half NS; 1/2 NS)	Hypotonic	Hypotonic	Expands ECV (vascular and interstitial) and rehydrates cells
0.9% NaCl (NS)	Isotonic	Isotonic	Expands ECV (vascular and interstitial); does not enter cells
3% or 5% NaCl (hypertonic saline; 3% or 5% NaCl)	Hypertonic	Hypertonic	Draws water from cells into ECF by osmosis
DEXTROSE IN SALINE SOLUTIONS			
Dextrose 5% in 0.45% NaCl (1/2 NS; D_5 0.45% NaCl)	Hypertonic	Hypotonic	Dextrose enters cells rapidly, leaving 0.45% NaCl
Dextrose 5% in 0.9% NaCl (D_5NS; D_5 0.9% NaCl)	Hypertonic	Isotonic	Dextrose enters cells rapidly, leaving 0.9% NaCl
MULTIPLE ELECTROLYTE SOLUTIONS			
LR solution	Isotonic	Isotonic	LR contains Na^+, K^+, Ca^{2+}, Cl^-, and lactate, which liver metabolizes to HCO_3^-; expands ECV (vascular and interstitial); does not enter cells
Dextrose 5% in LR (D_5LR)	Hypertonic	Isotonic	Dextrose enters cells rapidly, leaving LR

ECF, extracellular fluid; *ECV*, extracellular fluid volume; *LR*, lactated Ringer; *NS*, normal saline; *VAD*, vascular access device.

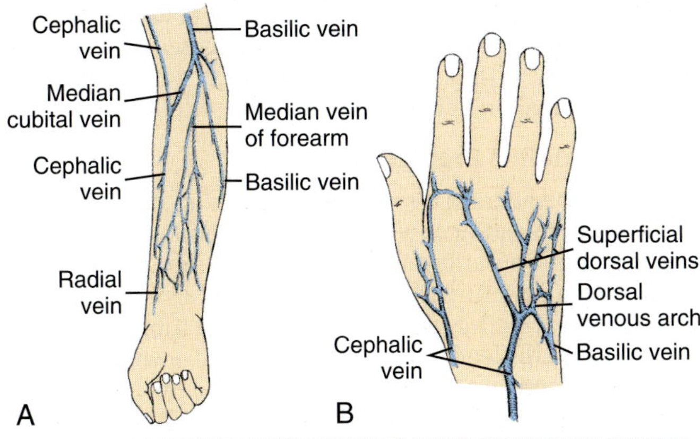

Fig. 25.6 Common i.v. sites. **A,** Inner arm. **B,** Dorsal surface of hand.

BOX 25.3 Care of an Older Adult

Protection of Skin and Veins During i.v. Therapy

- Avoid using a tourniquet when selecting a vein. Position the arm in a dependent position to fill the veins sufficiently for a venipuncture or use a blood pressure cuff for better protection of the older adult's skin. If using a tourniquet, place it over the patient's sleeve.
- Use the smallest-gauge i.v. catheter or needle possible such as 22 or 24 gauge to protect fragile veins. A smaller gauge allows better blood flow to provide increased hemodilution of i.v. fluids or medications (Phillips and Gorski, 2014).
- Avoid placing i.v. in veins that are easily bumped because older adults have less subcutaneous support tissue.
- Avoid the back of the hand, which may compromise a patient's need for independence and mobility.
- Use strict aseptic technique because an older adult patient is more likely to be immunocompromised.
- Do not slap the arm to visualize the patient's veins or use vigorous friction while cleansing the site to prevent tearing fragile skin.
- Decrease the venipuncture insertion angle because of decreased supportive tissue (Phillips and Gorski, 2014).
- Veins roll away from the needle easily as a result of loss of subcutaneous tissue. To stabilize the vein, apply traction to the skin below the projected insertion site (Phillips and Gorski, 2014).
- Secure i.v. site with a catheter stabilization device and a mesh dressing for protection, avoiding excessive use of tape on fragile skin (Touhy and Jett, 2014).
- Use electronic infusion devices or controllers to titrate infusion volume and rate.

using an extremity with a vascular (dialysis) graft or fistula or on the same side as a mastectomy (breast surgery). Initially place i.v. catheters at the most distal point, which allows for the use of proximal sites later if the patient needs a venipuncture site change (Gorski et al., 2016).

Venipuncture accesses a vein by puncture through the skin using a sharp rigid stylet (e.g., metal needle). To collect a blood specimen, the needle has an attached syringe or collection tube. To start an i.v. infusion, you use a stylet partially covered with a plastic catheter (over-the-needle catheter [ONC]). You use aseptic technique to prepare the skin. Only experienced practitioners perform venipuncture on patients with fragile veins (e.g., infants or older adults).

You will use venipuncture to collect a blood specimen, start an i.v. fluid infusion, instill a medication, or inject a tracer for diagnostic examinations. Use intermittent infusion when a patient requires medications only at certain times, in an emergency situation, and to avoid the discomfort of repeated injections. An intermittent infusion involves the same techniques as a continuous i.v. drip, but after you give the complete dose of medication, you disconnect the tubing from the i.v. access device and leave it in place. A continuous infusion of fluids, with or without medications, is achieved over a 24-hour period through use of a VAD. Skill 25.1 describes the technique for initiating peripheral i.v. fluid infusion and incorporates Infusion Nurses Society (INS) standards of practice (Gorski et al., 2016).

Regulating Infusion Flow Rate

After initiating an i.v. infusion and checking it for patency, regulate the rate of infusion according to the health care provider's orders (see Skill 25.2).

The rate of infusion with an i.v. gravity controller depends on the height of the i.v. fluid container, i.v. tubing size, and fluid viscosity. Regardless of the device in use, monitor the patient regularly to verify correct infusion of i.v. fluid and detect complications.

Patency of an i.v. catheter means that fluid flows easily through it. To be patent, the catheter tip needs to be free from clots and be away from the vein wall. A blocked catheter slows or stops the infusion of i.v. fluids. Infiltration (fluid leaking into tissues), a knot or kink in the tubing, external pressure on the tubing, and patient position changes decrease i.v. flow rates. If the i.v. flow decreases or stops, assess the system until you locate the problem. Start your assessment at the catheter insertion site for signs and symptoms of infiltration and phlebitis (Table 25.8).

Maintaining the System

Once a catheter is in place, maintain the integrity of the site and regulate the flow rate accurately to maintain the i.v. system. Agency policies regulate the maintenance of i.v. lines. I.v. line maintenance includes (1) keeping the system sterile and intact; (2) changing i.v. fluid containers, tubing, and contaminated site dressings; (3) assisting a patient with self-care activities (e.g., bathing) so that the i.v. system is not disrupted; and (4) monitoring for complications of i.v. therapy.

Patient safety requires maintaining the integrity of an i.v. line to prevent introduction of microorganisms that can cause infection (Vizcarra et al., 2014). Fig. 25.7 shows potential sites for contamination of a VAD. The procedure for i.v. insertion minimizes contamination during catheter insertion. After insertion, prevent infection through conscientious use of infection control principles, including

Table 25.8 Infusion Nurses Society Phlebitis Scale

Grade	Clinical Criteria
0	No symptoms
1	Erythema at access site with or without pain
2	Pain at access site with erythema and/or edema
3	Pain at access site with erythema, streak formation, palpable venous cord
4	Pain at access site with erythema, streak formation, palpable venous cord greater than 2.5 cm (1 inch) in length, purulent drainage

From Gorski L, et al: Infusion therapy standards of practice, *J Infus Nurs* 39(suppl 1):S1, 2016.

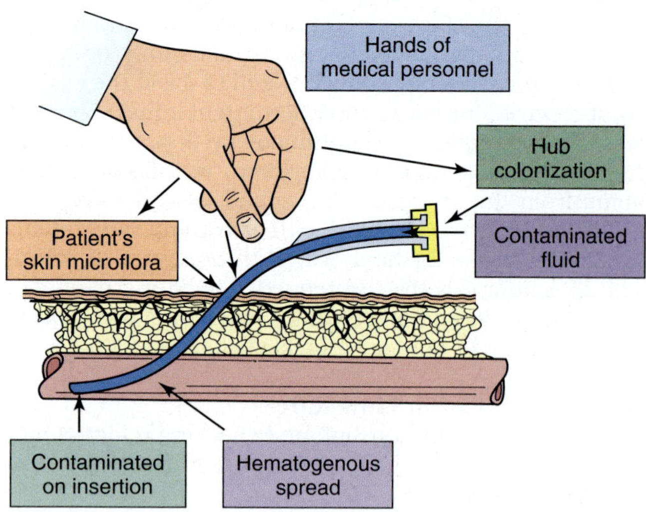

Fig. 25.7 Potential sites for contamination of an intravascular device.

thorough hand hygiene before and after handling any part of the i.v. system and maintaining sterility of the system during tubing and fluid container changes.

Always maintain the integrity of an i.v. system. Never disconnect tubing because it becomes tangled or because it is more convenient to position or move a patient or apply a gown. If a patient needs more room to maneuver, add extension tubing to an i.v. line using aseptic technique. *Never let i.v. tubing touch the floor.* Do not use stopcocks for connecting multiple solutions to a single i.v. site because they are sources of contamination (Gorski et al., 2016). I.v. tubing contains injection ports through which you can insert needleless syringes or other adapters for medication administration. Clean an injection port thoroughly with 2% chlorhexidine (preferred), 70% alcohol, or povidone-iodine, and let it dry before accessing the system (Gorski et al., 2016).

Changing i.v. Fluid Containers, Tubing, and Dressings

Patients receiving i.v. therapy over several days require periodic changing of i.v. fluid containers. Organize your tasks so that you can change solutions before a clot forms in a catheter. Recommended frequency of i.v. tubing change depends on whether it is used for continuous or intermittent infusion. INS standards (Gorski et al., 2016) specify that *continuous* infusion tubing changes should occur *no more frequently than every 96 hours* unless the tubing has been compromised or contaminated, which requires immediate tubing change. In contrast, you should change tubing for *intermittent* infusion every 24 hours because of the increased risk of contamination from opening the i.v. system (Gorski et al., 2016). Blood products and lipids easily promote bacterial growth in tubing. Therefore, change tubing containing blood products every 4 hours and tubing for continuous i.v. lipids every 24 hours (Gorski et al., 2016). Whenever possible, schedule tubing changes when it is time to hang a new i.v. container to decrease risk of infection (see Skill 25.3) (Gorski et al., 2016).

A sterile dressing over an i.v. site reduces the entrance of bacteria into the insertion site. Transparent dressings, the most common type, help secure the VAD, allow continuous visual inspection of the i.v. site, and stay cleaner and drier than gauze dressings. Leave transparent dressings in place until the i.v. tubing is replaced (Gorski et al., 2016). If a gauze dressing is used, change it every 48 hours (Gorski et al., 2016). You change either form of dressing when the i.v. device is removed or when the dressing becomes damp, loosened, or soiled (Gorski et al., 2016). Agency policy may require routine dressing changes in different time frames (see Skill 25.4).

Helping Patients Protect i.v. Integrity

To prevent accidental disruption of an i.v. system, patients often need assistance with hygiene, comfort measures, meals, and ambulation. Bathing and changing gowns are difficult for a patient with an i.v. line in the arm. Teach NAP and patients that they must not disconnect tubing of an i.v. line because this leads to contamination. If available, use a gown with snaps along the top sleeve seam to facilitate gown changes without disturbing the venipuncture site. Change regular gowns by following these steps:

1. Remove the sleeve of the gown from the arm without the i.v. line, maintaining the patient's privacy.
2. Remove the sleeve of the gown from the arm with the i.v. line.
3. Remove the i.v. solution container from its stand and pass it and the tubing through the sleeve. If this involves removing the tubing from an EID, use the roller clamp to slow the infusion to prevent accidental infusion of a large volume of fluid.
4. To apply a gown, place the i.v. solution container and tubing through the sleeve of the clean gown and hang it back on the stand. If the i.v. infusion is controlled by an EID, reassemble, turn on the pump, and open the roller clamp.
5. Place the arm with the i.v. line through the new gown sleeve.
6. Place the arm without the i.v. line through the new gown sleeve.

Mechanical catheter securement devices extend the time that a VAD can be used. Commercial protective devices also prevent accidental dislodgment of an i.v. catheter (Fig. 25.8).

A patient with an arm or a hand infusion is able to walk unless contraindicated. Offer a rolling i.v. pole on wheels. See that the patient has help to get out of bed, if needed, and place the pole next to the involved arm. Teach the patient to hold on to the pole with the involved hand and push it while walking.

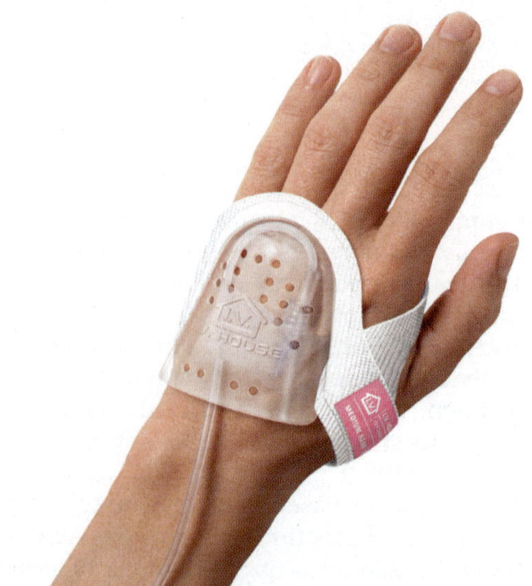

Fig. 25.8 I.V. House protective device. (Courtesy I.V. House, St Louis, MO.)

Check that the i.v. container is at the proper height, there is no tension on the tubing, and the flow rate is correct. Instruct the patient to report any blood in the tubing, stoppage in flow, an EID alarm, or increased discomfort.

Complications of i.v. Therapy

- An **infiltration** occurs when i.v. fluids leak into the subcutaneous tissue around the venipuncture site because the catheter tip no longer is in the vein. When the leakage of i.v. fluids is harmful, causing damage to extravascular tissue, the injury is called an extravasation. Infiltration causes swelling (from increased interstitial fluid), paleness, and coolness (from decreased circulation) around the venipuncture site. The i.v. infusion may slow or stop. Pain may occur, increasing as the infiltration progresses. The INS recommends using an infiltration scale for assessment (Gorski et al., 2016).
- If extravasation occurs, discontinue the infusion and medication immediately. Disconnect the i.v. tubing from the VAD but do not remove the VAD (ONS, 2016) (see agency policy). Certified nurses or a health care provider may attempt to aspirate the residual drug from the i.v. device using a syringe. Later, you will likely remove the VAD. Depending on the solution that extravasates, you may need to administer an antidote. If i.v. therapy still is necessary, insert a new VAD in a vein at a new location. To reduce discomfort, elevate the extremity to promote venous drainage and decrease edema. Apply a warm, moist compress to the site for 15–20 minutes at a time at least four times a day to promote venous return and reduce pain and edema (ONS, 2016).

Certain i.v. medications, especially potassium and some antibiotics, can cause discomfort and burning sensations at the i.v. site. Evaluate the source of discomfort, decrease the infusion rate if allowed, or start a new i.v. line in a larger vein if needed.

Phlebitis is inflammation of a vein. Risk factors include the following:

- Acidic or hypertonic i.v. solutions
- Rapid i.v. rate; irritating i.v. drugs such as potassium chloride (KCl) and vancomycin
- VAD in area of flexion
- Poorly secured catheter
- Poor hand hygiene
- Lack of aseptic technique (Helm et al., 2015)

Signs and symptoms include the following:

- Redness
- Tenderness
- Warmth along the course of the vein starting at the access site
- Possibly a red streak and/or palpable cord along the vein (Gorski et al., 2016)

The INS Phlebitis Scale (see Table 25.8) is easy to use, valid, and reliable (Gorski et al., 2016).

If phlebitis develops, discontinue the i.v. line and insert a new line in another vein. Warm, moist compresses on the site of phlebitis offer some relief to patients (see Chapter 17). Phlebitis is dangerous because blood clots (thrombi) can form, increasing the risk for an embolus (i.e., a clot that becomes dislodged and travels to the lungs). It sometimes damages veins permanently. Although some agencies require routine removal of VADs and site rotation to prevent phlebitis, the INS standards of practice (Gorski et al., 2016) recommend replacing a peripheral VAD only if clinically indicated in adults. Assess the VAD site at least every 4 hours and more frequently with critically ill patients, children, and patients receiving i.v. solutions containing irritating drugs or vasoconstrictors. Avoid routine replacement of peripheral VADs in infants and children (Gorski et al., 2016).

Local infection at a VAD insertion site is possible, showing redness and/or edema and exudate. Before removing a VAD, immediately notify the health care provider to find out whether you need to send the exudate of the catheter tip for a culture. After you take the culture sample, remove the VAD and insert a new one in another site if continued i.v. therapy is necessary. If the health care provider orders antibiotics, do not start them until a blood culture is taken if ordered.

Another complication of i.v. therapy is fluid overload from a too-rapid infusion. Assessment findings depend on the type of solution. Excessive infusion of a sodium-containing isotonic solution causes ECV excess, with shortness of breath and crackles in the lungs. If these clinical signs are present, slow the rate of i.v. infusion, notify the health care provider, raise the head of the bed, provide supplemental oxygen and diuretics as ordered, and monitor the patient's vital signs. Excessive infusion of D_5W causes hyponatremia with confusion, lethargy, and possibly seizures. Whenever your patient has an i.v. running, monitor for the effects of overload of the i.v. fluid.

Discontinuing Peripheral i.v. Access

You discontinue a VAD after the prescribed amount of fluid is infused, when infiltration occurs, if phlebitis is present, or if a clot develops in the catheter. Review the health care provider's order before discontinuing a VAD. Explain to patients the reason for discontinuing an i.v. infusion and that they might feel a burning sensation when the catheter is removed. Perform hand hygiene and apply clean gloves. Close the i.v. tubing roller clamp and turn off the EID (if your patient has one) to prevent spilling i.v. fluid. Remove the i.v. site dressing and any catheter stabilization device. Then remove any tape securing the catheter without using scissors (Gorski et al., 2016). Remove secretions around the skin puncture site by holding the catheter hub and using an antiseptic swab. Allow the skin to dry completely. Place sterile gauze over the venipuncture site and apply light pressure while withdrawing the catheter by pulling away from the insertion site in a slow, steady motion (Fig. 25.9). Keep the catheter hub parallel to the skin during withdrawal. Inspect the catheter end for intactness after removal. Keep gauze in place and apply continuous pressure to the site for 2–3 minutes to control bleeding and minimize hematoma formation (Gorski et al., 2016). If a patient receives anticoagulants or platelet inhibitors, apply steady pressure for 5–10 minutes and assess bleeding. Apply a sterile folded gauze dressing over the removal site and secure it with tape. Then perform hand hygiene. Record the amount of fluid infused and the time the i.v. infusion was discontinued in the medical record. Routinely inspect the site for redness, edema, and tenderness for 48 hours. In some settings, licensed practical nurses (LPNs) discontinue peripheral i.v. infusions (consult agency policy or state Nurse Practice Act).

Blood Replacement

Blood replacement or transfusion is the i.v. administration of whole blood or a blood component such as plasma,

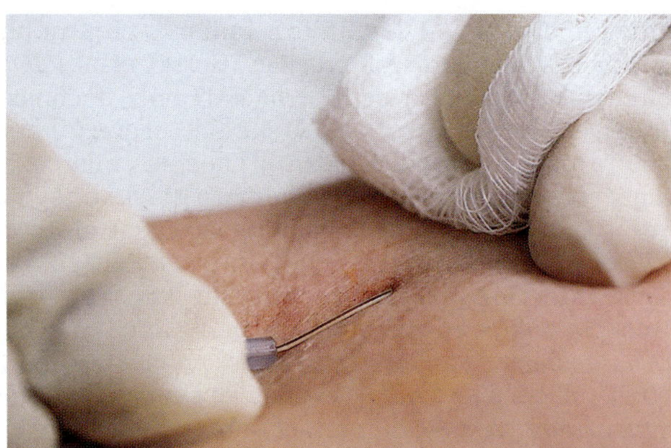

Fig. 25.9 Withdraw i.v. catheter slowly, keeping catheter parallel to vein.

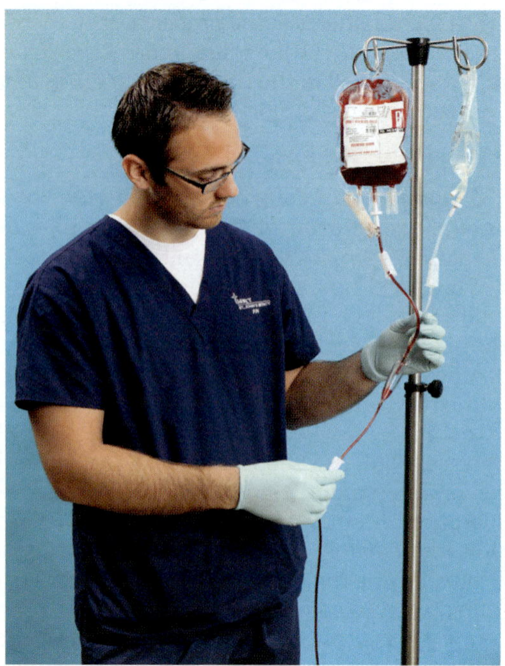

Fig. 25.10 Filling tubing for blood administration.

packed red blood cells (RBCs), or platelets. Blood transfusions (1) increase circulating blood volume after surgery, trauma, or hemorrhage; (2) increase the number of RBCs to maintain hemoglobin levels in patients with severe anemia; and (3) provide selected cellular components as replacement therapy (e.g., clotting factors, platelets, albumin).

Transfusing blood or blood components is a nursing procedure requiring an order from a health care provider. Perform thorough patient assessment before, during, and after a transfusion. Adverse blood transfusion events are included in the public reporting of safety events of a health care institution (NQF, 2016). Before a transfusion, assess the patient to determine whether he or she knows the reason for the blood transfusion and whether he or she has had a previous transfusion or transfusion reaction. Patients who have had a transfusion reaction usually are not at greater risk for a reaction with a subsequent transfusion. However, they usually are anxious about the transfusion, requiring nursing intervention. Before starting a transfusion, explain the procedure and instruct the patient to report any side effects (e.g., chills, light-headedness, or fever) once transfusion begins. Ensure that the patient or representative has signed an informed consent. People from certain cultural backgrounds may refuse blood transfusions or seek alternatives to it (Guinn et al., 2015). Be sensitive to patient preferences.

Because of the danger of transfusion reactions, your pretransfusion assessment includes baseline vital signs (Crookston et al., 2015). These data allow you to determine when changes in vital signs occur as a result of a transfusion reaction. ABO incompatibility is a serious error with transfusions. This error commonly involves misidentification of the patient, unit of blood, or label on the pretransfusion blood sample. For patient safety, follow agency procedure to verify three things: that blood components delivered are the ones that were ordered, that blood delivered is compatible with the patient's blood type listed in the medical record, and that the right patient receives the blood. Many hospitals use bar-code technology to identify patients and verify compatible blood before beginning transfusions. Nurses are responsible for determining that the blood delivered to a patient corresponds to the patient's blood type documented in the medical record. Together two RNs or one RN and one LPN (check agency policy and procedures) must check the label on the blood product against the medical record and the patient's identification number, blood group, and complete name. *If even a minor discrepancy exists, do not give the blood. Notify the blood bank immediately.*

When administering a transfusion, you need an appropriately sized i.v. catheter and special tubing with a 20-micron in-line filter (Fig. 25.10). Adults require a large catheter such as 18 or 20 gauge because blood is more viscous than crystalloid i.v. fluids. Prime the tubing with 0.9% sodium chloride to reduce **hemolysis** (breakdown of RBCs). Start a transfusion slowly to allow for early detection of a transfusion reaction. Maintain the ordered infusion rate, monitor for side effects, assess vital signs, and promptly record all findings. Stay with the patient during the first 15 minutes, the time when a reaction is most likely to occur. After that time period, continue to monitor the patient and obtain vital signs periodically during the transfusion as directed by agency policy. If you suspect a transfusion reaction, *stop* the transfusion immediately and follow the guidelines in Box 25.4.

The transfusion rate usually is specified in the health care provider's orders. Ideally 1 U of whole blood or packed RBCs is transfused in 2 hours. Lengthen the time to 4 hours if a patient is at risk for ECV excess. Beyond 4 hours, there is an increased risk for bacterial contamination of the blood.

When patients have a severe blood loss such as with hemorrhage, they often receive rapid transfusions through a central venous catheter. A blood-warming device is necessary because the tip of the central venous catheter lies in the superior vena cava, above the right atrium. Rapid administration of cold blood can cause cardiac dysrhythmias. Patients who receive large-volume transfusion of citrated blood have high risk of hyperkalemia, hypocalcemia, hypomagnesemia, and metabolic alkalosis (Crookston et al., 2015).

Autologous Transfusion

Autologous transfusion (autotransfusion) is the collection and reinfusion of a patient's own blood. Blood for an autologous transfusion usually is obtained by preoperative donation up to 6 weeks before the scheduled surgery, depending on the type of surgery and ability of the patient to

BOX 25.4 Nursing Interventions for Blood Transfusion Reaction

- *STOP the transfusion immediately*, even when you just suspect a reaction.
- Remove blood component and tubing containing blood product. Replace them with new primed tubing with a container of 0.9% sodium chloride (normal saline). Connect tubing to hub of i.v. catheter.
- **Caution:** Do not turn off the blood and simply turn on the 0.9% (normal saline) that is connected to the Y-tubing infusion set. This would cause blood remaining in the Y-tubing to infuse into the patient. Even a small amount of mismatched blood can cause a major reaction.
- Maintain patent i.v. line using 0.9% normal saline.
- Remain with the patient, observing signs and symptoms and monitoring vital signs every 5 min.
- Immediately notify the health care provider or emergency response team.
- Notify blood bank.
- Prepare to perform CPR and administer emergency drugs such as antihistamines, vasopressors, fluids, and corticosteroids per health care provider's order or protocol.
- Save the blood container, tubing, attached labels, and transfusion record for return to the blood bank.
- Obtain blood and first voided urine specimens per health care provider's order or protocol. **Note:** If the patient is unable to void, insert a catheter to obtain urine specimen.
- Document the transfusion reaction, description, treatment, and outcome.

CPR, cardiopulmonary resuscitation.

maintain an acceptable hematocrit. Blood for autologous transfusion also can be obtained at the time of surgery. After surgery, blood can be salvaged from drainage from chest tubes or joint cavities. Autologous transfusions are safer for patients because they decrease the risk of mismatched blood and exposure to blood-borne infectious agents.

Allogeneic Transfusion

Infusion of a donor's blood into a patient is **allogeneic transfusion**. In the United States, the blood is collected in a donation center and goes through numerous tests to ensure that it is free from infectious agents such as human immunodeficiency virus (HIV), hepatitis B virus (HBV), and hepatitis C virus (HCV) before it is infused. Blood testing positive for infectious agents is discarded; the donor is notified and placed on a list (deferral registry) that prohibits the donor from donating blood again (AABB, 2016).

Transfusion Reactions and Other Adverse Effects

A **transfusion reaction** is an immune system response to a transfusion that ranges from a mild response to severe anaphylactic shock, acute intravascular hemolysis, or acute lung injury, all of which are life threatening. Prompt nursing intervention is essential to maintain a patient's physiological stability (see Box 25.4).

Circulatory overload is a risk when a patient receives massive transfusions for hemorrhagic shock or when a patient with normal intravascular volume receives blood. Older adults and patients with cardiopulmonary diseases have high risk for circulatory overload and need careful monitoring during transfusion.

Another category of adverse transfusion effects is diseases transmitted by blood from infected donors who are asymptomatic. Symptoms of these diseases often arise long after the transfusion. Diseases transmitted through transfusions include malaria, HBV and HCV, HIV infection and acquired immunodeficiency syndrome (AIDS), Chagas disease, West Nile virus infection, and cytomegalovirus infection (Crookston et al., 2015; Custer et al., 2015).

Interventions for Acid–Base Imbalances

Nursing interventions to promote acid–base balance support prescribed medical therapies and aim at reversing the underlying disorder causing the acid–base imbalance while providing for patient safety. Acid–base imbalances often are life threatening and require a rapid nursing response to deliver treatment. Maintain a patent i.v. line and check for changes in prescribed therapies. Give fluid and electrolyte replacements and prescribed drugs promptly. In addition, monitor patients closely for changes in their status. Use protective measures such as bedrails for patients with decreased level of consciousness.

Restorative and Continuing Care

After experiencing acute fluid, electrolyte, or acid–base imbalances, patients often require ongoing maintenance to prevent recurrence. Older adults require special considerations to prevent complications from developing.

Home Intravenous Therapy

I.v. therapy often continues at home for patients requiring long-term hydration, PN, or long-term medication administration. A home i.v. therapy nurse works closely with a patient and family caregivers to ensure that they know how to maintain a sterile i.v. system; how to dispose of sharps and materials exposed to blood safely; techniques for ambulation, hygiene, and other activities of daily living without dislodging the i.v. catheter or disconnecting the system; and how to avoid complications or recognize and report them promptly.

Nutritional Support

Most patients who have electrolyte or acid–base imbalances require ongoing nutritional support. Depending on the type of disorder, you encourage or restrict certain fluids or food. Teach patients or family caregivers who are responsible for meal preparation the nutritional content of foods and how to read the labels of commercially prepared foods.

Medication Safety

Numerous prescription and OTC drugs and supplements contain components or create side effects that alter fluid and electrolyte balance. Patients with chronic disease who receive multiple medications and patients with renal disorders have high risk for fluid and electrolyte imbalances. Apply literacy principles (see Chapter 15), and teach patients and families regarding potential side effects and drug interactions that alter fluid, electrolyte, or acid–base balance. Review all medications with patients and family caregivers, confirm the correct schedule for administering each medication, and encourage the patient to consult the local pharmacist before using an OTC drug or supplement.

Evaluation

Patient Outcomes

Evaluation of a patient's clinical status is important when an acute fluid, electrolyte, or acid–base imbalance exists. You need to recognize the signs and symptoms of impending problems by considering a patient's presenting risk factors and clinical status, effects of the present treatment regimen, and the potential causative agent. Perform an evaluation to determine whether changes have occurred from the patient's baseline or previous patient assessment.

A patient's level of progress determines whether you continue or revise the plan of care. If goals are not met, consult with other members of the health care team to discuss additional methods such as increasing the frequency of an intervention (e.g., provide more fluids to a dehydrated patient), introducing a new therapy (e.g., initiate insertion of an i.v.), or discontinuing a particular therapy. Once a patient meets the outcomes of care, the nursing diagnosis is resolved, and you can focus on other priorities including maintaining normal fluid, electrolyte, and acid–base balance. If an outcome is not met, revise the plan of care as needed.

Patient Expectations

Review with patients how well their major concerns regarding fluid, electrolyte, or acid–base situations were alleviated or addressed. For example, if a patient's concern was feeling uncomfortable with very dry mouth, ask, "How does your mouth feel now?" If a patient's concerns involve having a better understanding of a newly diagnosed problem, evaluate the patient's satisfaction with the education provided. Often a patient's level of satisfaction with care also depends on success in involving family caregivers and friends. If patients have concerns about returning home or to a different care setting, it is important to evaluate how well prepared they feel for the transition from acute care.

SAFETY GUIDELINES FOR NURSING SKILLS

Ensuring patient safety is an essential role of a professional nurse. To ensure patient safety, communicate clearly with members of the health care team, assess and incorporate the patient's priorities of care and preferences, and use the best evidence when making decisions about your patient's care. When performing the skills in this chapter, remember the following points to ensure safe, individualized care:

- Check that you have the necessary information, an order if required, and equipment available for the procedure before beginning.
- Determine whether the patient has latex allergy and use nonlatex items if allergy is present (Gorski et al., 2016).
- Conduct a complete history and physical assessment including vital signs, and review laboratory findings before initiating any solutions or medications. Consider prolonged environmental conditions that affect a patient's fluid status (e.g., exposure to hot, humid weather) leading to fluid and electrolyte imbalances, particularly in infants, older adults, and patients with chronic illnesses.
- Know the indications for prescribed therapy before initiating i.v. therapy. Obtain and review the health care practitioner's order to ensure appropriateness of the prescribed solution or medication for the patient's age, health status, medical diagnosis, allergy status, acuity, VAD type and tip location, dose, frequency, and route of administration (Gorski et al., 2016).
- Use special designated tubing for the specific brand of EID and for blood transfusions and some medications.
- Review the steps of the procedure before entering a patient's room, considering modifications that you may need to make for each specific patient and verifying that the type of i.v. solution is appropriate for the patient.
- Maintain strict aseptic and sterile techniques when manipulating the i.v. system to prevent development of bloodstream infections (Gorski et al., 2016).
- If you contaminate a sterile object during the procedure, do not use it. Use a new sterile one.
- Know and implement the standard precautions for infection control and the Occupational Safety and Health Administration (OSHA) standards for occupational exposure to blood-borne pathogens. Place all disposable blood-contaminated and sharp items in designated puncture-resistant biohazard containers (Gorski et al., 2016).

SKILL 25.1 Initiating Intravenous Therapy

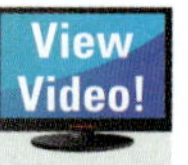

Equipment

- Short peripheral i.v. start kit supplies (available in some agencies): single-use tourniquet, tape, transparent semipermeable membrane (TSM) dressing or sterile gauze and sterile tape, antiseptic solution (chlorhexidine solution preferred, povidone-iodine, or 70% alcohol), 2 × 2–inch gauze pads, and label. **Note:** If kit is not available, gather all equipment separately.
- Appropriate short peripheral i.v. catheter with safety mechanism for venipuncture (Fig. 25.11) (Gorski et al., 2016).
- Clean gloves (latex free for patients with latex allergy; sterile gloves are recommended if palpating the site after skin antisepsis) (Gorski et al., 2016).
- Single-use hair clippers or scissors for hair removal if indicated.
- Short extension tubing with fused needleless connector or separate needleless connector (also called *injection cap, saline lock, heparin lock, i.v. plug, buff cap, buffalo cap, or PRN adapter*).
- Five-milliliter prefilled syringe with preservative-free 0.9% sodium chloride (normal saline [NS]) (Gorski et al., 2016).
- Antiseptic swabs and pads.
- Manufactured catheter stabilization device (if available) and skin protectant swab.
- Prescribed i.v. solution or medication.
- EID (if indicated) and i.v. pole.

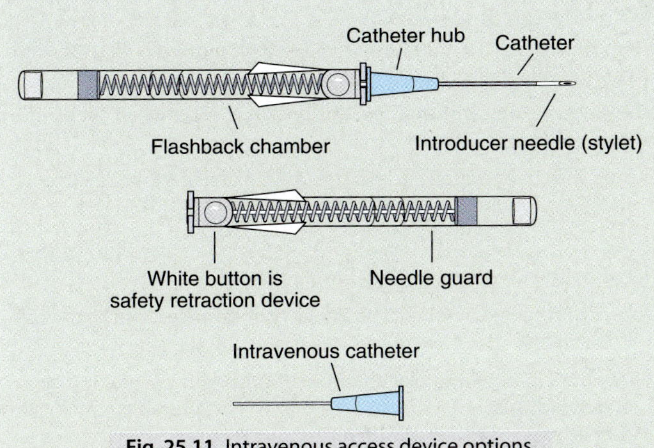

Fig. 25.11 Intravenous access device options.

- I.v. administration set (i.v. tubing), either macrodrip or microdrip, depending on prescribed rate; if using EID, appropriate administration set.
- A 0.2-micron filter for parenteral nutrition solutions that do not contain lipids (fats) (may be incorporated into the infusion set).
- Protective equipment: goggles and mask (optional based on agency policy).
- Vein visualization device (optional based on agency policy).
- Watch with second hand to calculate drip rate.
- Special patient gown with snaps at shoulder seams if available (makes removal with i.v. tubing easier).
- Needle disposal container (*sharps container* or *biohazard container*).
- Stethoscope.

STEP	RATIONALE
Assessment	
1. Identify the patient by using at least two identifiers (e.g., name and birthday or name and medical record number) according to agency policy. Compare identifiers with information on the patient's Medication Administration Record (MAR) or medical record.	Ensures correct patient. Complies with The Joint Commission standards and improves patient safety (TJC, 2018).
2. Review accuracy of health care provider's order: date and time, i.v. solution, route of administration, volume, rate, duration, and signature of ordering health care practitioner (Phillips and Gorski, 2014). Follow the rights of medication administration (see Chapter 26).	Before administering i.v. therapy, a complete order from a health care provider is needed (Gorski et al., 2016).
a. Check approved online database, drug reference book, or pharmacist about i.v. solution composition, purpose, potential incompatibilities, adverse reactions, and side effects.	Ensures safe and correct administration of i.v. therapy and appropriate selection of vascular access device (VAD).
3. Review medical record for the patient's history of allergies, especially to iodine, adhesive, or latex. Confirm with the patient.	Equipment used during VAD insertion may contain substances to which the patient is allergic.
4. Perform hand hygiene. Assess for clinical factors and/or conditions that will respond to or be affected by administration of i.v. solutions.	Provides baseline to determine effectiveness of prescribed therapy. A systems approach is recommended to assess for fluid and electrolyte imbalances (Phillips and Gorski, 2014).
a. Body weight	Rapid changes in body weight can indicate fluid loss or gain (Alexander et al., 2014). A rapid weight gain or loss of 2.2 pounds (1 kg) is equivalent to the gain or loss of 1 L of body water.
b. Clinical markers of vascular volume	
(1) Urine output (decreased, dark yellow with extracellular fluid volume [ECV] deficit)	Kidneys respond to ECV deficit by reducing urine production and concentrating urine. Kidney disease can also cause oliguria.
(2) Vital signs: blood pressure, respirations, pulse, and temperature	Changes in blood pressure may be associated with fluid volume status (e.g., postural hypotension or hypotension seen in ECV deficit). Respirations can be altered in presence of acid–base imbalances. Temperature elevations increase fluid requirements (temperature of 101°F [38.3°C] to 103°F [39.4°C] requires at least 500 mL of fluid replacement within a 24-h period) (Weinstein and Hagle, 2014).
(3) Fullness of neck veins (normally, veins are distended when a person is supine and flat when a person is upright)	Indicator of fluid volume status: flat or collapsing with inhalation when supine with ECV deficit; full when upright or semiupright with ECV excess.
(4) Auscultation of lungs	Crackles or rhonchi in dependent portions of lung may signal fluid buildup caused by ECV excess.
(5) Capillary refill	Indirect measure of tissue perfusion (sluggish with ECV deficit).
c. Clinical markers of interstitial volume	
(1) Skin turgor (pinch skin over sternum or inside of forearm)	Failure of skin to return to normal position after several seconds indicates ECV deficit (Alexander et al., 2014). Not a reliable indicator for older adults (Touhy and Jett, 2014).

STEP	RATIONALE
(2) Dependent edema (pitting or nonpitting)	Edema is not usually apparent until 4.4–8.8 pounds (2–4 kg) of fluid is retained (Phillips and Gorski, 2014).
(3) Oral mucous membrane between cheek and gum	More reliable indicator than dry lips or skin. Dry between cheek and gums indicates ECV deficit.
d. Thirst	Occurs with hypernatremia and severe ECV deficit. Not a reliable indicator for older adults (Phillips and Gorski, 2014).
e. Behavior and level of consciousness	
(1) Restlessness and mild confusion	Occurs with ECV deficit or acid–base imbalance.
(2) Decreased level of consciousness (lethargy, confusion, coma)	Occurs with severe ECV deficit, osmolality imbalances, and acid–base imbalances.
5. Determine whether the patient is to undergo any planned surgeries or procedures.	Allows anticipation and placement of appropriate VAD for infusion and avoids placement in an area that will interfere with medical procedures (Gorski et al., 2016).
6. Assess available laboratory data (e.g., hematocrit, serum electrolytes, arterial blood gases, kidney function [blood urea nitrogen, urine specific gravity, urine osmolality]).	Helps determine priority assessments and establishes baseline for determining whether therapy is effective. Laboratory values are an assessment of hydration status (Alexander et al., 2014).
7. Assess the patient's knowledge of procedure, reason for prescribed therapy, and arm placement preference.	Provides patient-centered care by determining level of emotional support and instruction needed.
Planning	
1. Perform hand hygiene. Collect and organize equipment on clean, clutter-free bedside stand or overbed table.	Reduces transmission of infection. Provides for an organized procedure and reduces contamination of equipment (Gorski et al., 2016).
a. Be sure that you have correct infusion set for EID if being used.	Ensures that the patient receives infusion therapy as prescribed (Gorski et al., 2016).
2. Provide privacy and prepare bedside environment for patient safety.	Providing privacy and preparing the environment before the procedure helps to ensure a clean and distraction-free area.
Implementation	
1. Instruct the patient about rationale for infusion including solution and medications ordered, procedure for initiating an i.v., and signs and symptoms of complications (e.g., redness, pain, tenderness, swelling, bleeding, drainage or leaking from under dressing). Also explain sensation associated with needlestick.	Provides the patient with information about procedure and promotes compliance (Gorski et al., 2016). May help to lessen patient anxiety.
2. Help the patient to comfortable sitting or supine position. Provide adequate lighting.	Promotes comfort and relaxation of the patient. Aids in successful vein location.
3. Perform hand hygiene.	Reduces transmission of infection and contamination of equipment (Gorski et al., 2016).
4. *Option:* Change the patient's gown to more easily removed gown with snaps at shoulder if available.	Use of this gown decreases risk of inadvertently dislodging VAD or administration set when changing gown.
5. Select appropriately sized catheter, and open and prepare sterile packages.	Use the smallest gauge peripheral catheter that will accommodate the prescribed therapy and patient need (Gorski et al., 2016).
6. Prepare short extension tubing with fused needleless connector or separate needleless connector (injection cap) to attach to catheter hub after VAD insertion.	Needleless connectors protect health care workers by eliminating needles and the potential for needlestick injuries when accessing VAD (Gorski et al., 2016).
a. Remove protective cap from needleless connector and attach syringe with 1–3 mL 0.9% sodium chloride (NS), maintaining sterility. Slowly inject enough NS to prime (fill) short extension tubing and connector, removing all air. Leave syringe attached to tubing.	Replaces air with NS, preventing air from entering the patient's vein later during VAD insertion.
b. Maintain sterility of end of connector by reapplying end caps, and set aside for attaching to catheter hub after successful venipuncture.	Prevents touch contamination, which allows microorganisms to enter infusion equipment and bloodstream.

Clinical decision point: Short extension sets may be used on short peripheral catheters to reduce catheter manipulation. For patient safety, all connections should be of Luer-Lok type (Gorski et al., 2016). Many agencies use short extension tubing for continuous infusions and stand-alone saline locks (capped catheters).

STEP	RATIONALE
7. Prepare i.v. tubing and solution for continuous infusion.	
a. Check i.v. solution using rights of medication administration and review the label for name, dosage and concentration, volume, beyond-use and expiration dates, sterility state, and route, rate, and frequency of administration as well as any other special instructions or considerations. If using bar code, scan code on the patient's wristband and then on i.v. fluid container. Be sure that prescribed additives such as potassium and vitamins have been added. Check solution for color, clarity, and expiration date. Check bag for leaks.	Reviewing the label for accuracy reduces the risk for medication errors (Gorski et al., 2016). Bar code system reduces human error (Gorski et al., 2016). Risk for medication errors can be reduced with safe medication practices including the following: ▪ Do not use unlabeled medication syringes unless prepared at the bedside and immediately administered (Gorski et al., 2016). ▪ Do not add medications to infusing containers of i.v. solutions (Gorski et al., 2016). ▪ Do not use solutions that are discolored, contain precipitates, or are expired. Risk for transmission of infection can be reduced with safe medication practices including the following: ▪ Do not use leaking bags because the integrity has been compromised. ▪ Begin administration of any medications compounded outside the pharmacy within 1 h after the start of its preparation (Gorski et al., 2016).
b. Open i.v. infusion set, maintaining sterility. EIDs sometimes have a dedicated administration set.	Prevents touch contamination, which allows microorganisms to enter infusion equipment and bloodstream.
c. Place roller clamp (see illustration A) about 2–5 cm (1–2 inches) below drip chamber of tubing and move roller clamp to "off" position (see illustration B).	Close proximity of roller clamp to drip chamber allows more accurate regulation of flow rate. Moving clamp to "off" prevents accidental spillage of i.v. solution during priming.
d. Remove protective sheath over i.v. tubing port on plastic i.v. solution bag (see illustration) or top of bottle, while maintaining sterility of port.	Provides access for insertion of i.v. tubing spike into solution using sterile technique.
e. Remove protective cover from i.v. tubing spike while maintaining sterility of spike. Insert spike into port of i.v. bag (see illustration). If solution container is a glass bottle, clean rubber stopper on glass-bottled solution with antiseptic swab and insert spike into rubber stopper of i.v. bottle. Bottles require vented tubing.	Flat surface on top of bottled solution may contain contaminants, whereas opening to plastic bag is recessed. Prevents contamination of bottled solution during insertion of spike. If sterility of spike is compromised, discard i.v. tubing and obtain a new one.
f. Compress drip chamber and release, allowing it to fill one-third to one-half full (see illustration).	Creates suction effect; fluid enters drip chamber to prevent air from entering tubing.

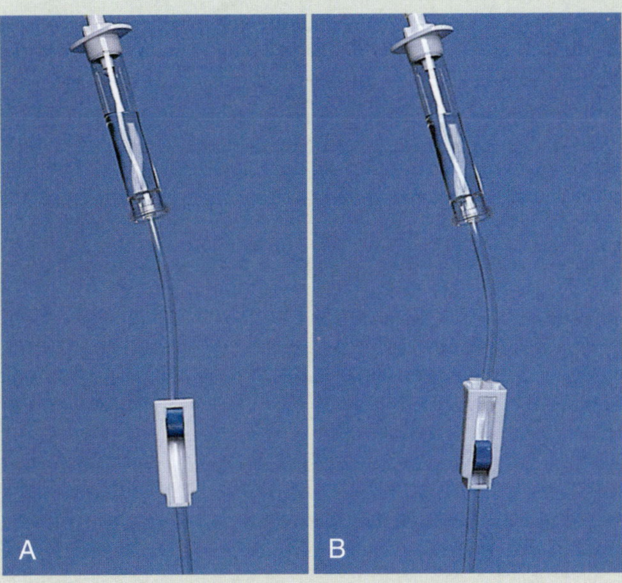

Step 7c **A,** Roller clamp in open position. **B,** Roller clamp in closed position.

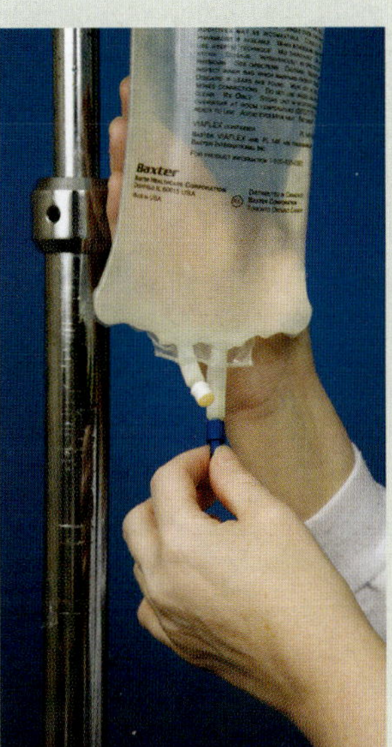

Step 7d Removing protective sheath from i.v. tubing port.

STEP	RATIONALE

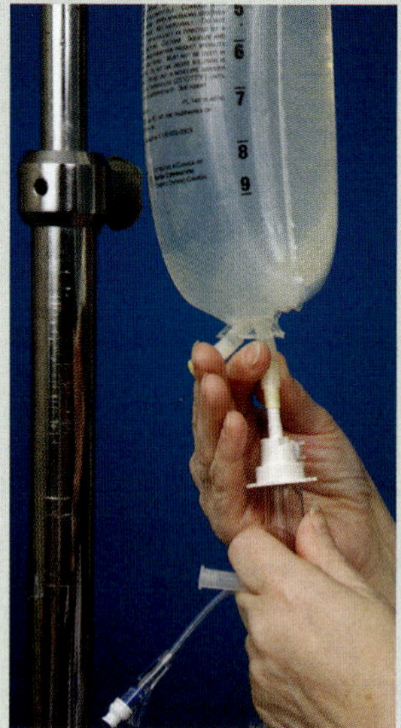
Step 7e Inserting spike into i.v. bag.

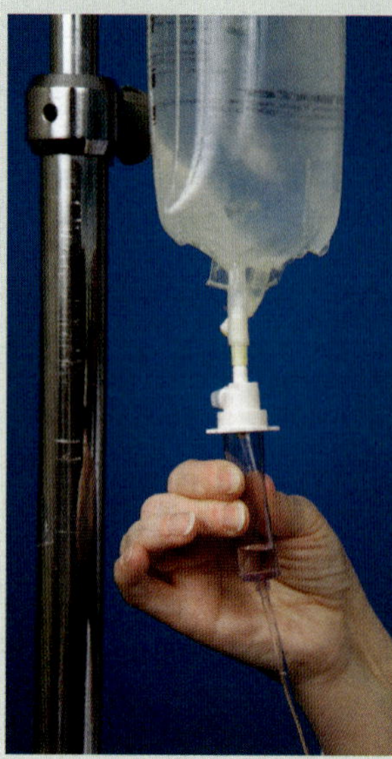
Step 7f Squeezing drip chamber to fill with fluid.

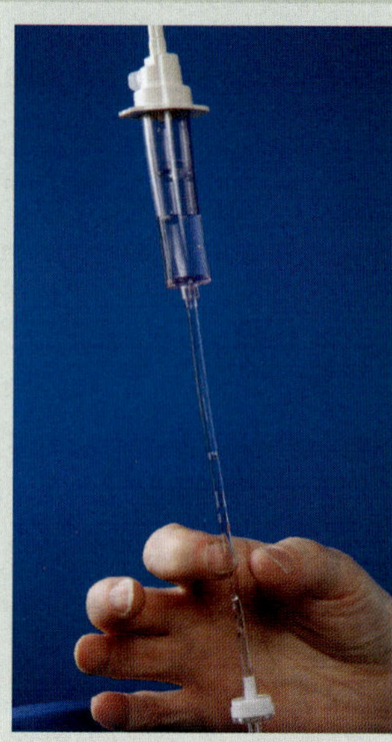
Step 7h Removing air bubbles from tubing.

STEP	RATIONALE
g. Prime air out of i.v. tubing by filling with i.v. solution: Remove protective cover on end of i.v. tubing (some tubing can be primed without removing the protective cover), and slowly open roller clamp to allow fluid to flow from drip chamber to distal end of i.v. tubing. If tubing has a Y connector, invert Y connector when fluid reaches it to displace air. Return roller clamp to "off" position after priming tubing (filled with i.v. fluid). Replace protective cover on distal end of tubing. Label i.v. tubing with date according to agency policy and procedure.	Priming ensures that i.v. tubing is clear of air and filled with i.v. solution before connecting to VAD. Slowly filling tubing decreases turbulence and chance of bubble formation. Closing clamp prevents accidental loss of fluid. Maintains sterility. Labeling i.v. tubing allows for recognition of length of time that tubing has been in use and when to change it.
h. Be certain that i.v. tubing is clear of air and air bubbles. To remove small air bubbles, firmly tap tubing where air bubbles are located. Check entire length of tubing to ensure that all air bubbles are removed (see illustration).	Large air bubbles act as emboli (Cook, 2013).
i. If using optional long extension tubing (not short tubing in Step 6), remove protective cover and attach it to distal end of i.v. tubing, maintaining sterility. Then prime long extension tubing.	Priming removes air from long extension tubing so that it does not enter the patient's vascular system.
j. Insert tubing into EID with power off (if using).	Prepares for administration of infusion.
8. Perform hand hygiene.	Decreases potential risk of microbial contamination and cross-contamination (Gorski et al., 2016).

Clinical decision point: Clean gloves are not necessary to locate vein but must be applied for VAD insertion (Gorski et al., 2016; INS, 2016).

STEP	RATIONALE
9. Apply tourniquet around upper arm about 10–15 cm (4–6 inches) above proposed insertion site (see illustration). Do not apply tourniquet too tightly. Check for presence of pulse distal to the tourniquet.	Tourniquet should be tight enough to impede venous flow while maintaining arterial circulation (Gorski et al., 2016; INS, 2016). If the patient has fragile veins or bruises easily, tourniquet should be applied loosely or not at all to prevent damage to veins and bruising (Gorski et al., 2016).
a. *Option A:* Apply tourniquet on top of a thin layer of clothing such as a gown sleeve to protect fragile or hairy skin.	
b. *Option B:* Blood pressure cuff may be used in place of tourniquet—activate cuff and hold at approximately 50 mm Hg.	Reduces trauma to the skin.
10. Select vein for VAD insertion (see illustration). Veins on dorsal and ventral surfaces of arms (e.g., metacarpal, cephalic, basilic, median) are preferred in adults.	Ensures adequate vein that is easy to puncture and less likely to rupture.
a. Use most distal site in nondominant arm if possible.	Patients with VAD placement in their dominant hand have decreased ability to perform self-care.

STEP	RATIONALE

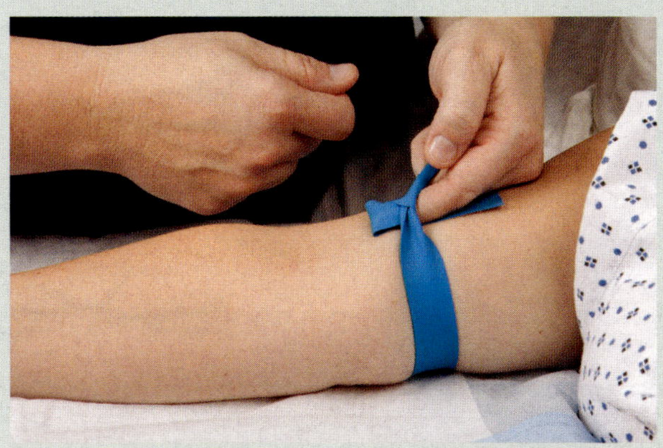

Step 9 Tourniquet placed on arm for initial vein selection.

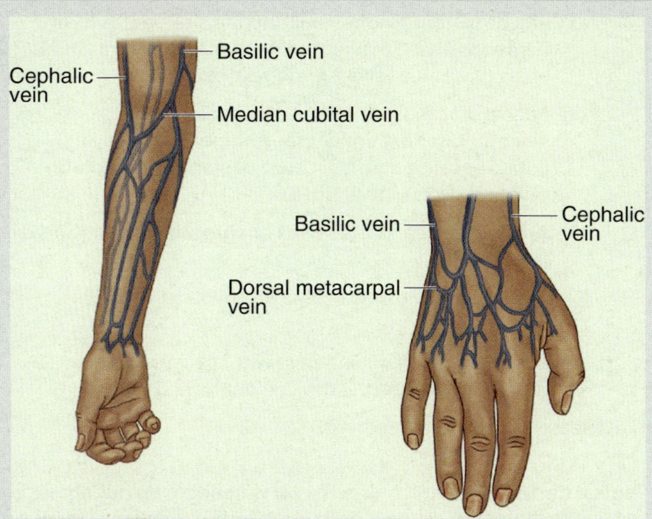

Step 10 Cephalic, basilic, and median cubital veins are best for i.v. placement in adults.

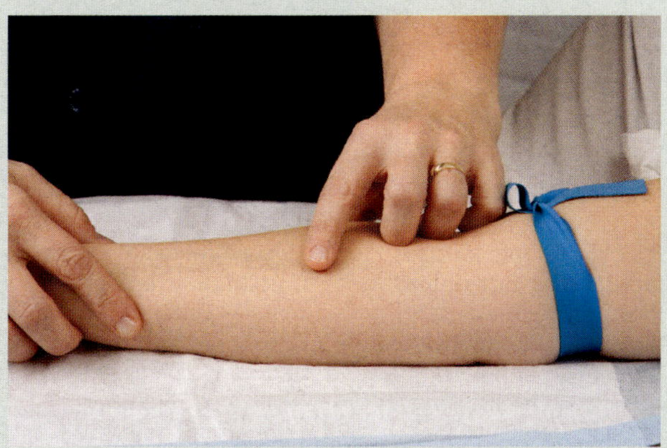

Step 10b Palpate vein.

STEP	RATIONALE
b. With your fingertip, palpate vein at the intended insertion site by pressing downward. Note resilient, soft, bouncy feeling while releasing pressure (see illustration).	Fingertip is more sensitive and better for assessing vein location and condition.
c. Select a well-dilated vein. Methods to improve vascular distention are the following:	Increased volume of blood in vein at venipuncture site makes vein more visible.
(1) Position extremity lower than heart, have the patient slowly open and close fist, and lightly stroke the vein downward.	Use of gravity promotes vascular distention (Gorski et al., 2016).
(2) Apply dry heat to extremity for several minutes.	Dry heat increases successful peripheral catheter insertion (Gorski et al., 2016).

Clinical decision point: Slapping or hard tapping of a vein, especially in older adults, can cause venous constriction and/or bruising and hematoma (Phillips and Gorski, 2014).

11. When selecting a vein

a. Avoid vein selection in the following:

STEP	RATIONALE
(1) Areas with pain on palpation, compromised areas, sites distal to compromised areas (e.g., open wounds, bruising, infection, infiltration, extravasation) (Gorski et al., 2016).	It is difficult to assess for any signs or symptoms of complications if an i.v. device is inserted in an area already compromised.
(2) Upper extremity on the side of breast surgery with axillary node dissection, lymphedema, or after radiation; arteriovenous fistulas or grafts; or affected extremity from a cerebrovascular accident (Gorski et al., 2016).	Increases risk for complications such as infection, lymphedema, or vessel damage.

STEP	RATIONALE
(3) Site distal to previous venipuncture site, sclerosed or hardened veins, previous infiltrations or extravasations, areas of venous valves, or phlebitic vessels.	Such sites cause infiltration around newly placed VAD site and vessel damage.
(4) Fragile dorsal hand veins in older adults. Do not use veins in lower extremities for routine i.v. therapy in adults because of risk of tissue damage and thrombophlebitis (Gorski et al., 2016).	Veins have increased risk for infiltration.
(5) Areas of flexion such as wrist or antecubital area (Gorski et al., 2016).	Veins have increased risk for infiltration, phlebitis, or dislodgment.
(6) Ventral surface of wrist (10–12.5 cm [4–5 inches]).	Venipuncture in the ventral surface of wrist is painful and has potential for nerve damage (Gorski et al., 2016).
b. Choose site that will not interfere with the patient's activities of daily living, use of assist devices, or planned procedures.	Keeps the patient as mobile as possible.
12. Release tourniquet temporarily.	Restores blood flow and prevents venospasm when preparing for venipuncture.

Clinical decision point: If hair removal is needed, do not shave area with a razor. Shaving may increase risk of infection (Gorski et al., 2016). Clip hair with scissors or hair clippers if necessary (explain to the patient).

Clinical decision point: Local anesthetic reduces discomfort associated with placement of a VAD. Topical, transdermal, injectable, or pressure-accelerated local anesthetics can be used to reduce pain and require a health care provider's order. You may apply topical local anesthetic to intended i.v. site 30 min before insertion. Follow manufacturer's recommendations and monitor for allergic reaction (Gorski et al., 2016).

STEP	RATIONALE
13. Perform hand hygiene and apply clean gloves. Wear eye protection and mask (see agency policy) if splash or spray of blood is possible.	Decreases potential risk of microbial contamination and cross-contamination (Gorski et al., 2016).
14. Place adapter end of short extension set (prepared in Step 6) or needleless connector (injection cap) for saline lock nearby in sterile package.	Permits smooth, quick connection of infusion to short peripheral catheter once vein is accessed.
15. If area of insertion is visibly soiled, clean site with antiseptic soap and water and dry. Perform skin antisepsis with chlorhexidine solution using friction in a back-and-forth motion (see illustration) for 30 s and allow to dry completely. If using alcohol or povidone-iodine, clean in concentric circle moving from insertion site outward with the swab. Allow drying time between agents if agents are used in combination (alcohol and povidone-iodine).	Mechanical friction in this pattern allows penetration of antiseptic solution to epidermal layer of the skin (Alexander et al., 2014). Reduces the incidence of catheter-related infections (Alexander et al., 2014). Allow any skin antiseptic agent to fully dry for complete antisepsis; alcoholic chlorhexidine solutions, for at least 30 s; and iodophors, for at least 1.5–2 min (Gorski et al., 2016).

Clinical decision point: If you need to palpate the vein after performing skin antisepsis, use sterile gloves for palpation, or perform skin antisepsis again, as touching cleaned area introduces microorganisms from your finger to site (Gorski et al., 2016; INS, 2016).

STEP	RATIONALE
16. Reapply tourniquet 10–15 cm (4–6 inches) above anticipated insertion site. Check for presence of pulse distal to the tourniquet.	Pressure of tourniquet promotes vein distention. Diminished arterial flow prevents venous filling.
17. Perform venipuncture. Anchor vein below anticipated insertion site by placing thumb over vein 4–5 cm (11/2−2 inches) distal to site (see illustration) and gently stretching skin against direction of insertion. Instruct the patient to relax hand.	Stabilizes vein for needle insertion, prevents vein from rolling, and stretches skin taut decreasing drag during insertion. Some devices require loosening the needle (stylet) from the catheter before venipuncture. Follow manufacturer's directions for use.

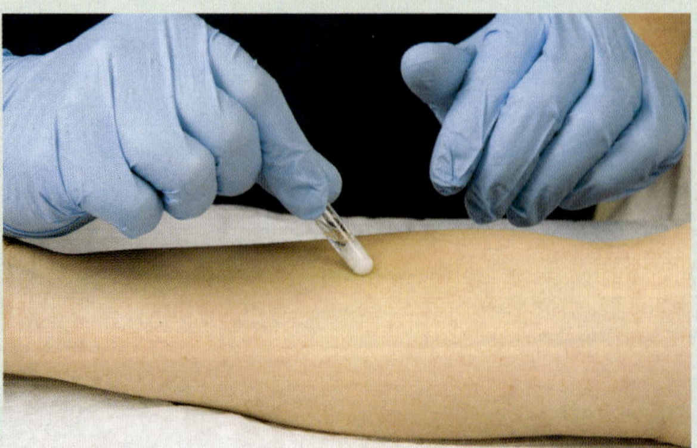

Step 15 Clean site with greater than 0.5% chlorhexidine alcoholic solution.

STEP	RATIONALE

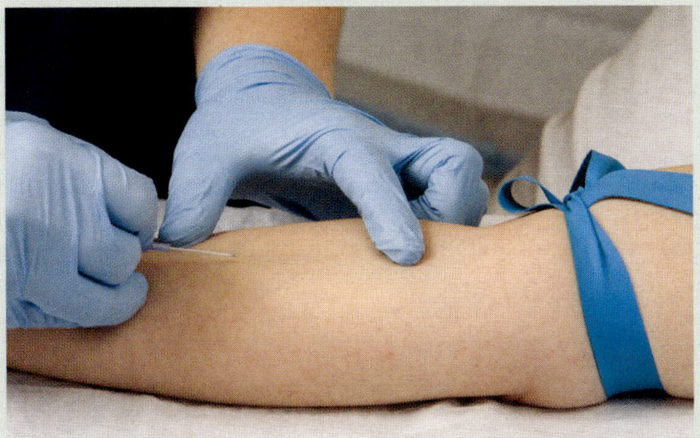

Step 17 Stabilize vein below insertion site.

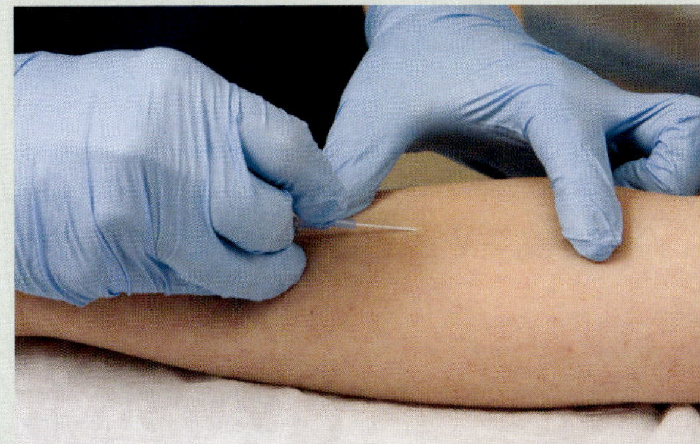

Step 17a Puncture skin with catheter at 10–30° angle.

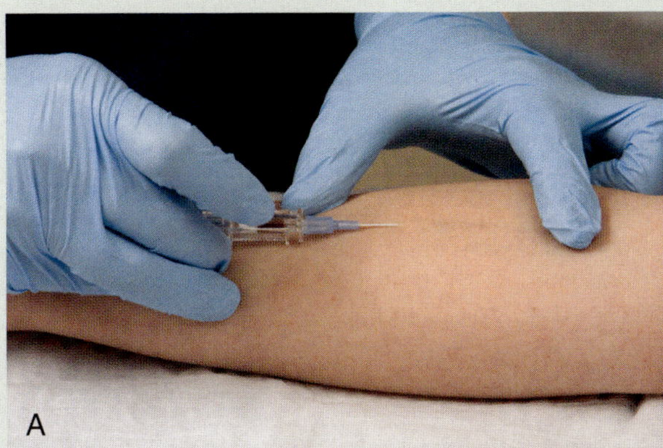

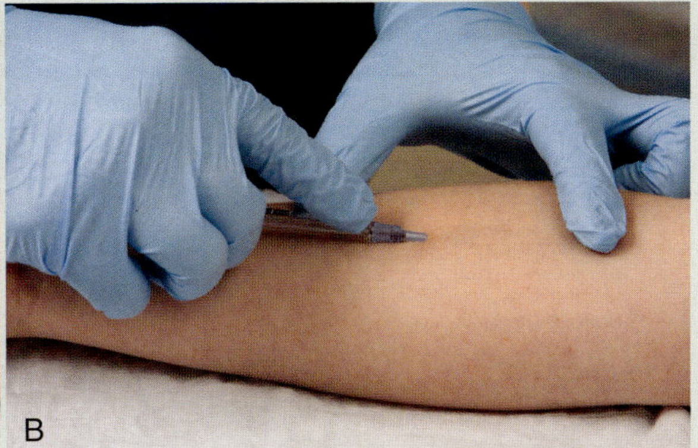

Step 18 A, Observe for blood return in catheter and/or flashback chamber. **B,** Advance catheter into vein until hub rests at venipuncture site.

STEP	RATIONALE
a. Warn the patient of a sharp stick. Hold VAD with the needle bevel up. Align catheter on top of vein at a 10–30° angle. Puncture skin and anterior vein wall (see illustration) (Gorski et al., 2016).	Accessing vein at an angle reduces risk for puncturing posterior vein wall. Superficial veins require a smaller angle. Deeper veins require a greater angle.

Clinical decision point: Use each VAD only once for each insertion attempt.

STEP	RATIONALE
18. Observe for blood return in the catheter or flashback chamber of catheter, indicating that bevel of needle has entered vein (see illustration A). Advance VAD approximately 0.6 cm (1/4 inch) into vein and loosen stylet (needle) of over-the-needle catheter. Continue to hold skin taut while stabilizing VAD, and with the index finger on the push-off tab of the VAD advance the catheter off needle into the vein until hub rests at venipuncture site (see illustration B). Do not push from open catheter hub. *Do not reinsert stylet into catheter once catheter has been advanced into vein.*	Increased venous pressure from tourniquet causes backflow of blood into catheter and/or flashback chamber. Some VADs have a notch in the stylet allowing flash of blood into the catheter. Stabilizing VAD allows for placement of catheter into vein and advancement of catheter off stylet. Advancing entire stylet into vein may penetrate wall of vein, resulting in hematoma. Advancing the catheter with finger on open hub will cause contamination (Gorski et al., 2016). Reinsertion of stylet can cause catheter to shear off with embolization into vein.

Clinical decision point: A single clinician should not make more than two attempts at initiating i.v. access, and total attempts should be limited to no more than four (Gorski et al., 2016).

STEP	RATIONALE
19. Stabilize VAD with nondominant hand and release tourniquet or blood pressure cuff with other hand. While keeping the VAD stable with the index finger, apply gentle but firm pressure with middle finger of nondominant hand 3 cm (11/4 inches) above insertion site. Withdraw stylet from catheter or activate safety device to retract stylet (technique varies by product type; follow manufacturer guidelines).	Permits venous flow and reduces backflow of blood. Digital pressure minimizes blood loss and allows attachment of extension set or needleless connector (INS, 2016).
20. Quickly connect Luer-Lok end of short extension tubing with needleless connector to end of catheter hub. Secure connection. Avoid touching sterile connection ends.	Prompt connection maintains patency of vein, minimizes blood loss, and prevents risk of exposure to blood. Maintains sterility.

STEP	RATIONALE
a. *Option:* I.v. tubing can be attached directly to catheter hub in place of short extension tubing or needleless connector.	
21. Attach prefilled flush syringe of 0.9% sodium chloride to short extension set and aspirate to remove any air and assess blood return. Slowly inject NS from prefilled syringe into VAD (see illustration A). Remove syringe and discard. **Note:** Minimal amount of air should be aspirated if tubing is prepared correctly.	Blood return that is the color and consistency of whole blood confirms placement of catheter in vein (Gorski et al., 2016). Flushing prevents reflux of blood into catheter and occlusion (INS, 2016). Initiates flow of fluid through i.v. catheter, preventing clotting of device. Swelling indicates infiltration, and catheter would need to be removed. Aspirating air prevents air embolism.
a. *Option:* To begin a primary infusion, swab the needleless connector with antiseptic swab and attach the Luer-Lok end of the i.v. tubing to the needleless connector (see illustration B). Fully open roller clamp of i.v. tubing, turn on EID, and begin infusion at correct rate. If using gravity flow instead of EID, adjust roller clamp slowly to regulate rate.	Prevents infusion of large volume of fluid.

Clinical decision point: Needleless connectors protect health care workers and decrease risk for needlestick injuries. They have different internal mechanisms for fluid displacement and vary in the flush–clamp–disconnect sequence to prevent reflux of blood into catheter on disconnection (Gorski et al., 2016). The sequence depends on the type of internal mechanism (Phillips and Gorski, 2014):

- **Neutral displacement devices do not have a specified flush–clamp–disconnect sequence.**
- **For negative-pressure displacement devices, flush, clamp catheter, and then disconnect syringe.**
- **For positive-pressure displacement, flush, disconnect syringe, and then clamp catheter.**

STEP	RATIONALE
22. Observe site for swelling.	Swelling indicates infiltration, which requires immediate removal of catheter.
23. Apply sterile dressing over site.	
a. TSM dressing	
(1) Continue to secure catheter with nondominant hand. Remove adherent backing. Apply one edge of dressing and gently smooth remaining dressing over i.v. insertion site, leaving Luer-Lok connection between tubing and catheter hub uncovered. Gently press dressing to adhere to skin. Remove outer covering and smooth dressing gently over site (see illustration).	Transparent membrane protects catheter insertion site and minimizes risk for infection (Phillips and Gorski, 2014). Allows visualization of insertion site and surrounding area for complications (Gorski et al., 2016). Access to Luer-Lok connection between tubing and catheter hub facilitates changing tubing if necessary.
(2) Place a 2.5-cm (2-inch) piece of tape over Luer-Lok connection (see illustration). **Do not apply tape on top of TSM dressing.**	Removal of tape from TSM dressing can tear dressing and cause catheter dislodgment. Tape on top of TSM dressing prevents moisture from being carried away from skin.
b. Sterile gauze dressing	
(1) Place 5-cm (2-inch) piece of sterile tape over catheter hub (see illustration).	Stabilizes catheter under gauze dressing.

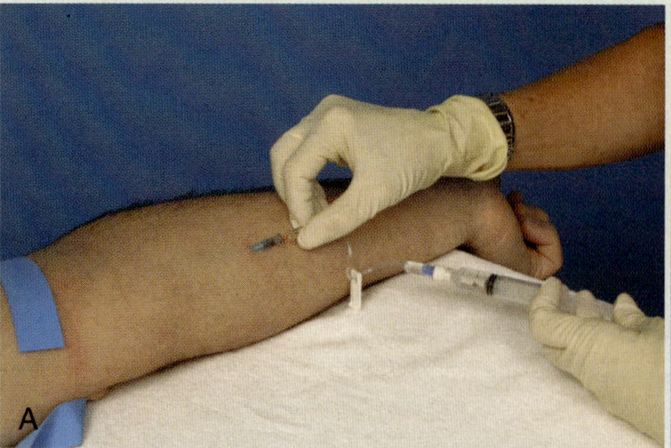

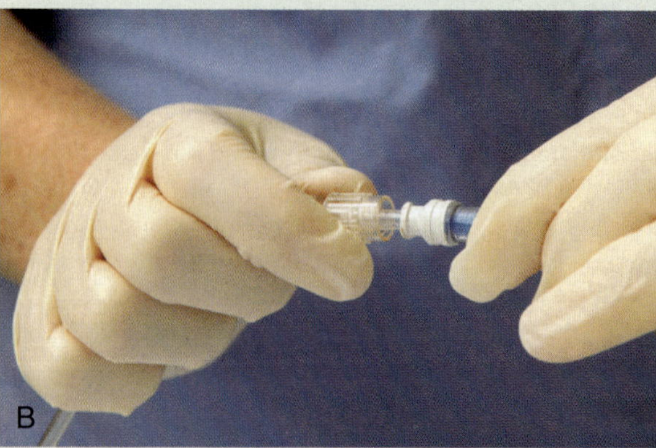

Step 21 A, Flush short extension set after aspirating air and assessing blood return. **B,** Connect i.v. tubing to the short extension set that is attached to the catheter.

STEP	RATIONALE

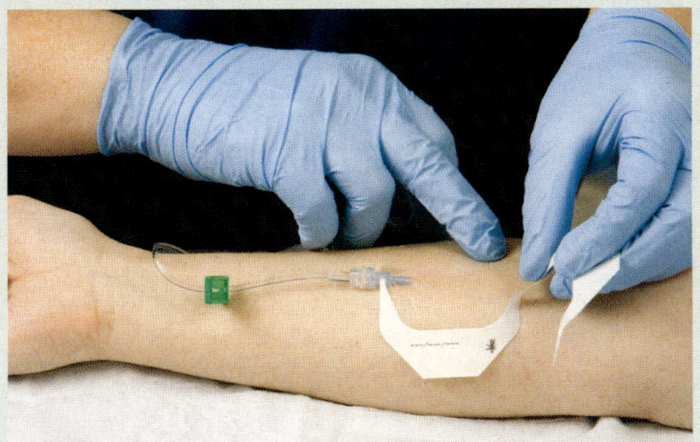

Step 23a(1) Apply transparent semipermeable membrane (TSM) dressing.

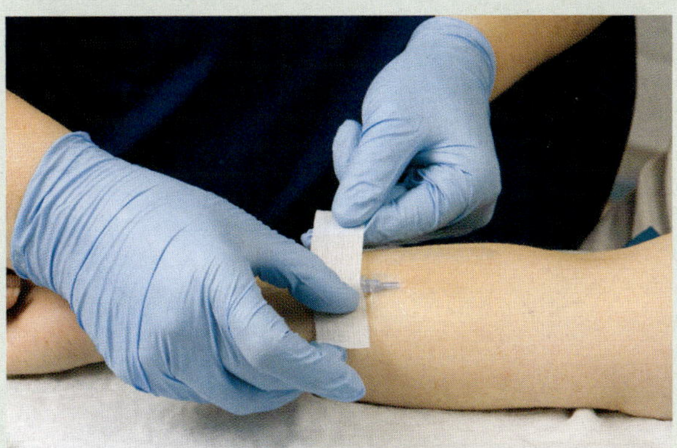

Step 23a(2) Place tape over administration set tubing.

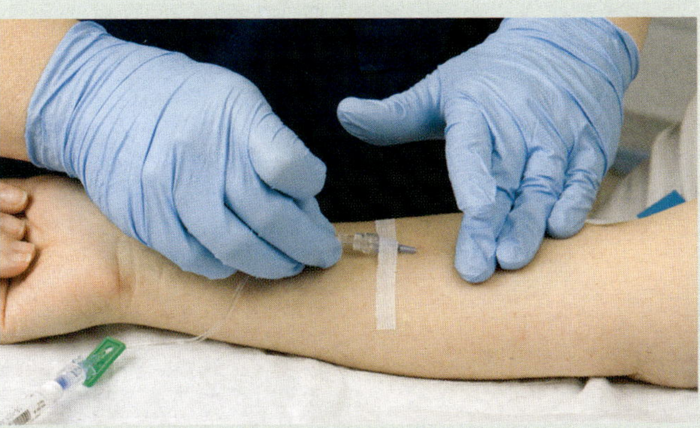

Step 23b(1) Sterile tape over catheter hub.

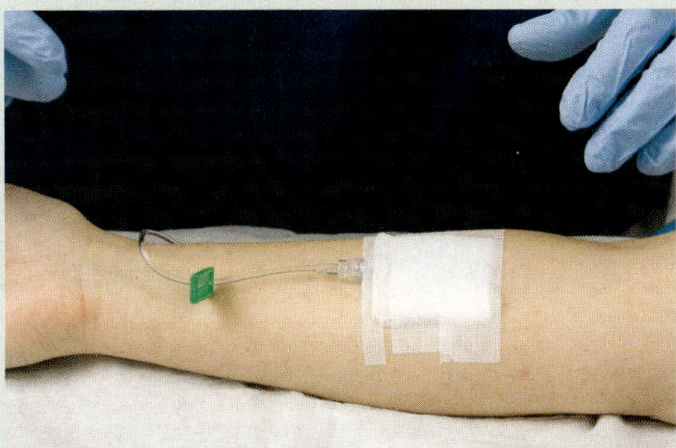

Step 23b(2) Place 2 × 2–inch gauze over insertion site and edge of catheter hub.

STEP	RATIONALE
(2) Place a 2 × 2–inch gauze pad over insertion site and edge of catheter hub. Secure all edges with tape. Do not place tape over insertion site. Do not cover connection between i.v. tubing and catheter hub (see illustration).	Use gauze dressings for site drainage, excessive perspiration, or sensitivity and/or allergic reactions to TSM dressings (Phillips and Gorski, 2014; Gorski et al., 2016).
(3) Fold 2 × 2–inch gauze in half and cover with 1-inch-wide (2.5-cm) tape so that about 1 inch will extend on each side of dressing. Place under Luer-Lok connection (see illustration). Secure Luer-Lok connection and tubing to tape on the folded gauze with a 2.5-cm (1-inch) piece of tape. Avoid applying tape or gauze around arm. Do not use rolled bandages with or without elastic to secure VAD. Taping Luer-Lok connection can be eliminated if an engineered stabilization device is to be used.	Tape on top of gauze makes it easier to access hub and/or tubing junction. Gauze pad elevates hub off skin to prevent pressure area. Prevents back-and-forth motion of catheter. Rolled bandages do not adequately secure VAD, can impair circulation or flow of infusion, and obscure visualization for complications (Gorski et al., 2016).
24. *Option:* Secure i.v. catheter using engineered stabilization device (follow manufacturer's directions; follow agency policy).	Use of engineered stabilization devices that allow visual inspection of an insertion site can reduce risk for VAD complications (i.e., phlebitis, infection, migration) and unintentional loss of access (Gorski et al., 2016).
a. Apply skin protectant to stabilization site and allow to dry completely.	Risk for medical adhesive–related skin injury (MARSI) is increased secondary to age, joint movement, and edema; use of skin protectant can decrease risk (Gorski et al., 2016).
(1) Align anchoring pads with directional arrow pointing to insertion site. Press device retainer over top of Luer-Lok connection while supporting underneath the connection.	
(2) Stabilize catheter and peel off one side of liner and press to adhere to skin. Repeat on other side (see illustration).	
(3) Monitor for MARSI.	Early detection of MARSI is key.

STEP	RATIONALE
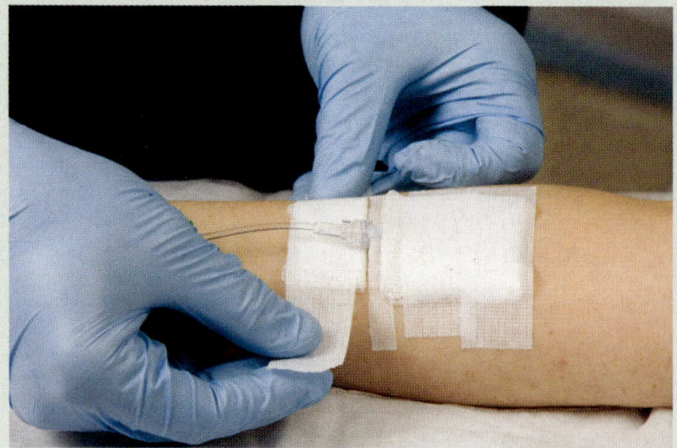 Step 23b(3) Apply folded 2 × 2-inch gauze dressing under tubing junction.	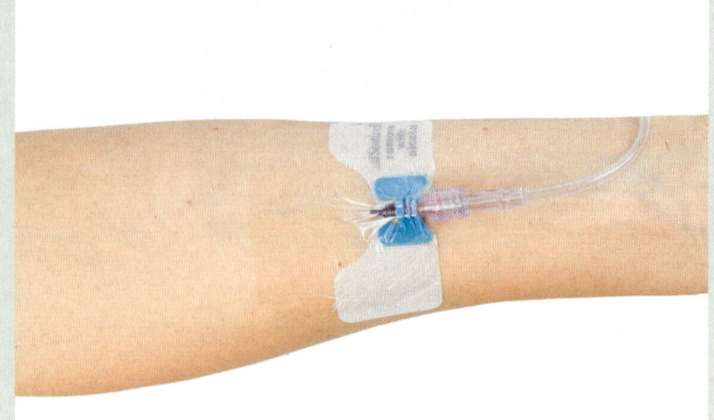 Step 24a(2) Catheter stabilization device in place. (Image courtesy CR Bard, Inc. All rights reserved.)
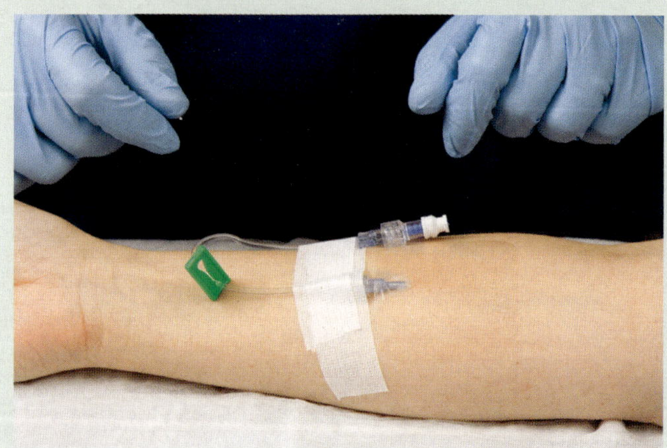 Step 25 Loop and secure tubing.	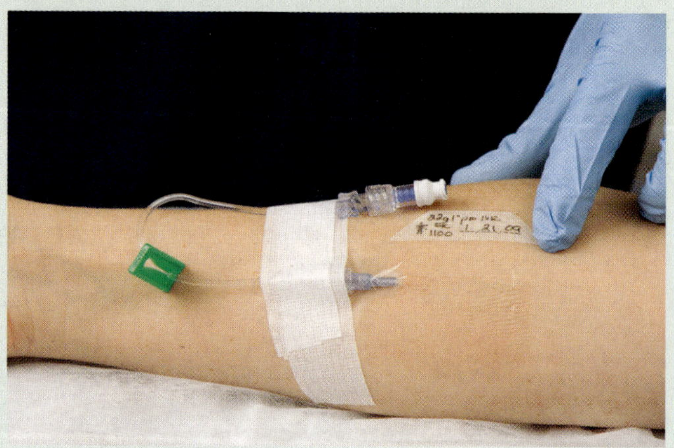 Step 27 Label i.v. dressing.
25. Loop extension or i.v. tubing alongside dressing on arm and secure with second piece of tape directly over tubing (see illustration).	Securing tubing reduces risk for dislodging catheter if i.v. tubing is pulled (i.e., loop comes apart before catheter dislodges).
26. For continuous infusion, verify ordered rate of infusion, and be sure that EID is programmed correctly. If infusing by gravity drip, adjust flow rate to correct drops per minute.	EID maintains correct rate of flow for i.v. solution. Gravity flow fluctuates; thus, it must be checked at intervals for accuracy.
27. Label dressing per agency policy. Include date and time of i.v. insertion, VAD gauge size and length, and your initials (see illustration).	Allows for recognition of type of device and length of time that device has been in place.
28. Dispose of used stylet or other sharps in appropriate sharps container. Discard supplies. Remove gloves and perform hand hygiene.	Reduces transmission of microorganisms; prevents accidental needlestick injuries.
29. Instruct the patient in how to move or turn without dislodging VAD.	Prevents accidental dislodgment of catheter.
Evaluation	
1. Observe the patient every 1–2 h or at established intervals per agency policy and procedure for function, intactness, and patency of i.v. system and for correct infusion rate and accurate type and amount of i.v. solution infused by observing level in i.v. container.	Ensures delivery of prescribed volume over prescribed time and decreases risk for fluid and electrolyte imbalance.
2. Monitor the patient to determine response to therapy (e.g., laboratory values, I&O, weights, vital signs, postprocedure assessments).	Early recognition of complications leads to prompt treatment.

STEP	RATIONALE
3. Observe the patient at established intervals per agency policy and procedure for signs and symptoms of i.v.-related complications by inspecting and gently palpating skin around and above i.v. site over the dressing.	Identifies complications that compromise integrity of VAD or cause inaccurate i.v. solution flow rate.
Clinical decision point: If i.v. is positional, fluid will run slowly or stop, depending on position of the patient's arm; if this continues, you may have to restart i.v.	
4. **Use teach back:** "I want to make sure that I explained problems that can happen with your i.v. site. Tell me what you might feel or observe about the i.v. site that can mean a problem has developed and that you would report." Revise your instruction now or develop a plan for revised patient/family teaching if the patient/family caregiver is unable to teach back correctly.	Determines the patient's and family caregiver's level of understanding of instructional topic.

Recording and Reporting

- Record in nurses' notes in EHR or chart the number of attempts (successful and unsuccessful) and sites of insertion; precise description of insertion site (e.g., cephalic vein on dorsal surface of right lower arm, 2.5 cm [1 inch] above wrist); flow rate; method of infusion (gravity or EID), size and type, length, and brand of catheter; time infusion started; and patient's response to insertion. Use an infusion therapy flow sheet when available.
- If using an EID, document type and rate of infusion and device identification number.
- Record the patient's status, i.v. fluid, amount infused, and integrity and patency of system according to agency policy.
- Record the patient's/family caregiver's knowledge following evaluation of teach back in nurses' notes.
- Report to oncoming nursing staff type of fluid, flow rate, status of VAD, amount of fluid remaining in present solution, expected time to hang subsequent i.v. container, and patient condition.
- Report to health care provider any signs and symptoms of i.v.-related complications.
- Record signs and symptoms of i.v.-related complications including interventions and patient response to treatments.

Unexpected Outcomes and Related Interventions

- Fluid and electrolyte imbalances develop.
  - Notify health care provider.
  - Readjust infusion rate as ordered.
  - Adjust additives in i.v. or type of i.v. fluid as ordered; contact pharmacy.
  - Continue monitoring signs and symptoms of imbalances.
- I.v.-related complications:
  - Infiltration develops at i.v. site.
    - Avoid applying pressure, which can force solution into contact with more tissue causing tissue damage (INS, 2016).
    - Stop infusion and remove i.v. catheter at first sign of infiltration and elevate affected extremity.
    - Use a standard scale for assessing and documenting infiltration (Gorski et al., 2016).
  - Catheter occlusion develops.
    - Determine cause and consider catheter removal.
    - Positional or kinked catheters can be repositioned/readjusted to improve i.v. flow.
    - Remove occluded i.v. catheter. Do not flush occluded catheters, because an embolus can result from dislodging a clot (Alexander et al., 2014).
- Phlebitis, or vein inflammation, develops. Rate of infusion may be altered.
  - Notify health care provider.
  - Determine cause (i.e., chemical, mechanical, bacterial) and consider removal or replacement of VAD.
    - Chemical phlebitis: Apply heat, elevate limb, consider slowing infusion rate, and determine whether catheter removal is necessary (Gorski et al., 2016).
    - Mechanical phlebitis: Apply heat, elevate limb, monitor for 24–48 hours, and consider catheter removal if signs and symptoms persist (Gorski et al., 2016).
    - Bacterial phlebitis: Remove i.v. catheter (Gorski et al., 2016).
  - Document phlebitis using a standardized scale including nursing interventions per agency policy and procedure (see Table 25.8).
- Catheter-related infection with redness, swelling around or above i.v. site, pain, purulent drainage at insertion site, and body temperature elevations (Gorski et al., 2016):
  - Notify health care provider. Obtain order to culture drainage (Gorski et al., 2016).
  - Remove i.v. catheter and culture purulent drainage from around i.v. site (Gorski et al., 2016).
- Hematoma (bleeding under skin) at i.v. site develops.
  - Remove i.v. catheter immediately and apply pressure and a dry sterile dressing.
  - Monitor for additional bleeding.
  - Elevate extremity and monitor for circulatory, neurological, or motor dysfunction (Phillips and Gorski, 2014).
- Nerve injury develops with patient complaints of paresthesia including shock-like pain, tingling or "pins and needles," burning, or numbness on insertion.
  - Notify health care provider of any signs and symptoms of nerve injury (INS, 2016).
  - Immediately stop VAD insertion and remove device if the patient complains of symptoms of paresthesia (Gorski et al., 2016).
  - Continue to monitor neurovascular status (INS, 2016).

SKILL 25.2 Regulating Intravenous Flow Rate

View Video!

Equipment

- Watch with second hand
- Calculator, paper, and pencil
- Tape
- Label
- I.v. solution bag and appropriate administration set
- I.v. administration set: EID *(optional)*
- Clean gloves

STEP	RATIONALE
Assessment	
1. Review accuracy and completeness of health care provider order in the patient's medical record for patient name and correct solution: type, volume, additives, infusion rate, and duration of i.v. therapy. Follow rights of drug administration (see Chapter 26).	Ensures delivery of correct i.v. solution and prescribed volume over prescribed time.
2. Identify the patient by using at least two identifiers (e.g., name and birthday or name and medical record number) according to agency policy. Compare identifiers with information on the patient's MAR or medical record.	Ensures correct patient. Complies with The Joint Commission standards and improves patient safety (TJC, 2018).
3. Identify the patient risk for fluid and electrolyte imbalance, given type of i.v. solution (e.g., neonate, older adult, history of cardiac or renal disease).	Helps prioritize assessments. Volume control needs to be strict. Guides choice of infusion device.
4. Perform hand hygiene and apply clean gloves. Inspect and gently palpate skin around and above i.v. site over dressing. Ask the patient how i.v. site feels. Assess vascular access device (VAD) for patency and signs and symptoms of i.v.-related complications (e.g., infiltration, occlusion of VAD, phlebitis, infection, patient complaints of pain, or leaking under dressing). Remove gloves and perform hand hygiene.	Identifies complications that compromise integrity of VAD and may necessitate replacement of VAD. Reduces transmission of infection.
5. Assess i.v. system for patency from i.v. container to insertion site.	Ensures delivery of prescribed volume over prescribed time.
6. Assess the patient's knowledge of purpose of maintaining prescribed flow rate and how positioning of i.v. site affects flow rate.	Fosters patient participation in maintaining most effective position of arm for optimal flow rate.
Planning	
1. Provide privacy and prepare bedside environment for patient safety.	Providing privacy and preparing the environment before the procedure helps to ensure a clean and distraction-free area for organizing procedure-related equipment.
2. Have a paper and pencil or calculator to calculate flow rate.	Use mathematical calculations to obtain correct rate.
3. Verify with health care provider's order regarding how long each liter of fluid should infuse. If hourly rate (mL/h) is not provided in order, calculate it by dividing volume by hours (see Step 7).	Basis of calculation to ensure infusion of solution over prescribed hourly rate. A volume of 1 L = 1000 mL.

Clinical decision point: It is common for health care providers to write an abbreviated i.v. order such as: "D_5W with 20 mEq KCl 125 mL/h continuous." This order implies that the i.v. should be maintained at this rate until an order has been written for the i.v. to be discontinued or changed to another order.

STEP	RATIONALE
4. If keep vein open (KVO) rate is ordered, check agency policy regarding flow rate of KVO.	Prevents catheter clotting, preserving venous access while infusing a minimal amount of fluid. An order for KVO rate must specify an infusion rate as required by the rights of medication administration. Rates may vary from 0.5 to 30 mL/h based on type of VAD, patient-specific therapy, and method of infusion (gravity or EID).
5. Use hourly rate to program EID or, if gravity-flow infusion, calculate drops per minute (gtt/min).	EID automatically delivers correct minute flow rate. Gravity infusion requires calculation of gtt/min.
6. *For gravity-flow infusion:* Know calibration (drop factor) in drops per milliliter (gtt/mL) of infusion set by agency:	
a. Microdrip: 60 gtt/mL—used to deliver rates less than 100 mL/h	Microdrip tubing universally delivers 60 gtt/mL. Used when small or very precise volumes are to be infused.
b. Macrodrip: 10–15 gtt/mL (depending on manufacturer)—used to deliver rates greater than 100 mL/h	There are different commercial parenteral administration sets for macrodrip tubing. Used when large volumes or fast rates are necessary. Know drip factor for tubing being used.
7. Select one of the following formulas to calculate minute flow rate (drops per minute) based on drop factor of infusion set:	Once you determine hourly rate, these formulas compute the correct flow rate.

STEP	RATIONALE
a. Milliliters per hour/60 min = mL/min Drop factor × mL/min = Drops/min OR b. mL/h × Drop factor/60 min = Drops/min	
Example: Calculate minute flow rate for a bag 1000 mL with 20 mEq KCl at 125 mL/h.	
Microdrip: 125 mL/h × 60 gtt/mL = 7500 gtt/h 7500 gtt/60 min = 125 gtt/min	When using microdrip, milliliters per hour (mL/h) always equals drops per minute (gtt/min).
Macrodrip: 125 mL/h × 15 gtt/mL = 1875 gtt/h 1875 gtt/60 min = 31–32 gtt/min	Multiply volume by drop factor and divide product by time (in minutes).
8. Explain to the patient and family caregiver the purpose of the procedure, what is expected of the patient, and when the patient or family caregiver should alert the nurse about problems with flow rate.	Decreases anxiety and promotes cooperation and compliance with therapy.
Implementation	
1. Perform hand hygiene.	Reduces transmission of microorganisms.
2. **Gravity infusions:** Confirm hourly rate and minute rate based on drop factor of infusion set. Use formula in Planning Step 7 to calculate flow rate.	Confirms calculation of minute flow rate for regulation of gravity infusion.
a. Ensure that i.v. container is at least 76.2 cm (30 inches) above i.v. site for adults. Increase height for more viscous fluids (Alexander et al., 2014).	Pressure caused by gravity is necessary to overcome venous pressure and resistance from tubing and catheter.
b. Slowly open roller clamp on tubing until you can see drops in drip chamber. Hold a watch with second hand at same level as drip chamber and count drip rate for 1 min (see illustration). Adjust roller clamp to increase or decrease rate of infusion.	Regulates flow to prescribed rate.
c. Monitor drip rate at least hourly.	Many factors influence drip rate; frequent monitoring ensures i.v. fluid administration as prescribed.
3. **EID (infusion pump or smart pump):** Follow manufacturer guidelines for setup of EID. Be sure that you are using infusion tubing compatible with EID.	Smart pumps with medication safety software are designed for administration of i.v. fluids that contain medications.
a. Close roller clamp on primed i.v. infusion tubing.	Prevents fluid leakage.
b. Insert compatible infusion tubing into chamber of control mechanism (see manufacturer directions) (see illustration). Roller clamp on i.v. tubing goes between the EID and the patient.	Most EIDs use positive pressure to infuse. Infusion pumps propel fluid through tubing by compressing and milking i.v. tubing.

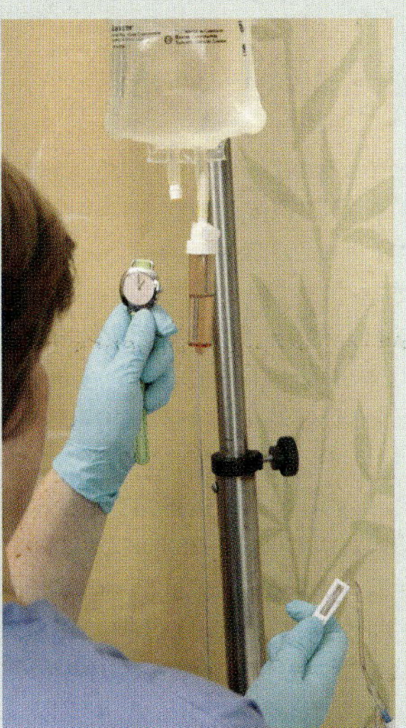

Step 2b Nurse counting drip rate on gravity flow.

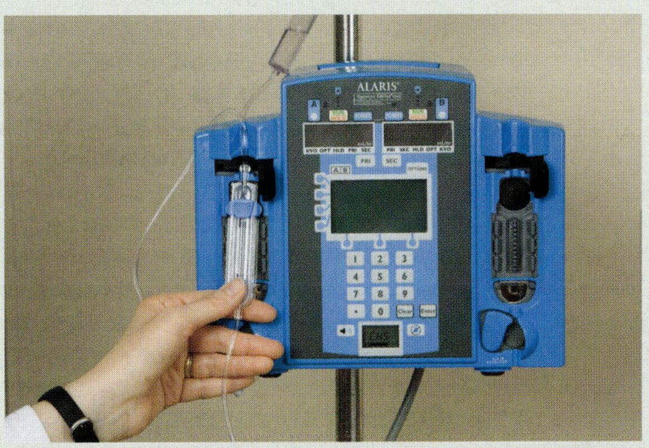

Step 3b Insert i.v. tubing into chamber of control mechanism.

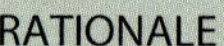

STEP	RATIONALE

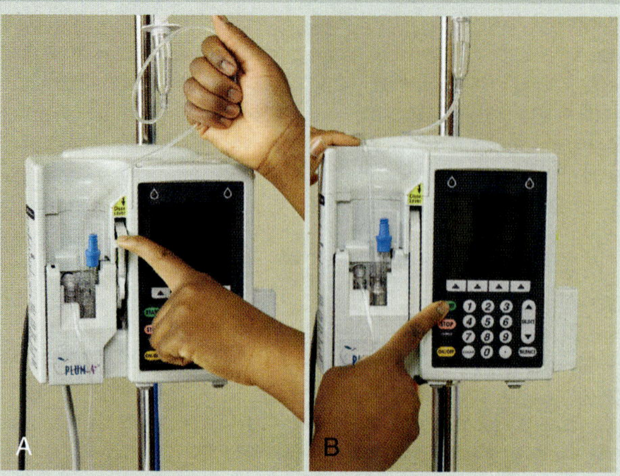

Step 3c **A** and **B,** Select rate and volume to be infused and press start button.

STEP	RATIONALE
c. Secure portion of i.v. tubing through "air in line" alarm system. Close door (see illustration A) and turn on power button, select required drops per minute or volume per hour, close door to control chamber, and press start button (see illustration B). If infusing a medication, access the EID library of medications and set the appropriate rate and dose limits. If smart pump alarms immediately and shuts down, your settings were outside unit parameters.	Ensures safe administration of ordered flow rate or medication dose. Smart pumps require additional information such as patient unit and medication. Computer matches pump setting against a drug database.

Clinical decision point: An anti-free flow safeguard (preventing bolus infusion in the event of machine malfunction or when tubing is removed from machine) is an important element of an EID and is required. Always check and follow manufacturer recommendations for specific device features.

STEP	RATIONALE
d. Open infusion tubing drip regulator completely while EID is in use.	Ensures that pump freely regulates infusion rate.
e. Monitor infusion rate and i.v. site for complications according to agency policy. Use watch to verify rate of infusion, even when using EID.	Flow controllers and pumps do not replace frequent, accurate nursing evaluation. EIDs can continue to infuse i.v. solutions after a complication has developed (Gorski et al., 2016).
f. Assess i.v. system from container to VAD insertion site when alarm signals.	Alarm indicates a situation that requires attention. Empty solution container, tubing kinks, closed clamp, infiltration, clotted catheter, air in the tubing, or low battery can trigger EID alarm.
4. Attach label to i.v. solution container with date and time container was changed (check agency policy).	Provides reference to determine next time for container change.
5. Instruct the patient and family caregiver about the purpose of EID if infusion therapy is delivered by EID; about purpose of alarms; to avoid raising hand or arm, which affects flow rate; and to avoid touching control clamp.	Information allows the patient to protect i.v. site and informs the patient about rationale for not altering control rate.
6. Remove and dispose of any used supplies. Perform hand hygiene.	Prevents transmission of infection.
Evaluation	
1. Observe the patient every 1–2 h or at established intervals per agency policy and procedure for function, intactness, and patency of i.v. system and for correct infusion rate and type and amount of i.v. solution infused.	Ensures delivery of prescribed volume over prescribed time and decreases risk for fluid and electrolyte imbalance.
2. Monitor the patient's response to therapy (e.g., laboratory values, I&O, weights, vital signs, postprocedure assessments).	Provides ongoing evaluation of the patient's fluid status including monitoring for extracellular fluid volume (ECV) excess, ECV deficit, or electrolyte imbalances. Early recognition of complications leads to prompt treatment.
3. Observe the patient at established intervals per agency policy and procedure for signs and symptoms of i.v.-related complications.	Prevents complications that compromise integrity of VAD or cause inaccurate i.v. solution flow rate.
4. **Use teach back:** "I want to be sure that I explained the importance that your i.v. fluids run on time at the rate ordered. Tell me reasons that may cause the pump to alarm to sound and what you would do." Revise your instruction now or develop a plan for revised patient/family caregiver teaching if the patient/family caregiver is unable to teach back correctly.	Determines the patient's/family caregiver's level of understanding of instructional topic.

Recording and Reporting

- Record i.v. solution, rate of infusion in drops per minute (gtt/min) or milliliters per hour (mL/h), and integrity and patency of system in nurses' notes in EHR or chart and on infusion therapy flow sheet according to agency policy.
- Record use of any EID or control device and identification number on that device.
- Record patient response (e.g., laboratory values, I&O, weights, vital signs, postprocedure assessments) to therapy and unexpected outcomes (e.g., signs and symptoms of ECV excess, ECV deficit, or i.v.-related complications).
- Record the patient's/family caregiver's knowledge following evaluation of teach back in nurses' notes.
- At change of shift or when leaving on break, report rate of and volume left in infusion to nurse in charge or next nurse assigned to care for the patient.

Unexpected Outcomes and Related Interventions

- Solution does not infuse at prescribed rate.
  - Sudden infusion of large volume of solution occurs and the patient develops dyspnea; crackles in lung; distended neck veins when upright; and edema, indicating fluid overload (ECV excess).
    - Slow infusion rate: KVO rates must have specific rate ordered by health care provider.
    - Notify health care provider immediately.
    - Place the patient in high-Fowler position.
    - Anticipate new i.v. orders.
    - Anticipate administration of oxygen per order.
    - Administer diuretics if ordered.
  - I.v. solution runs slower than ordered.
    - Check for positional change that affects rate, height of i.v. container, kinking of tubing, or obstruction.
    - Check VAD site for complications.
    - Consult health care provider for new order to provide necessary fluid volume.
- I.v. patency is lost subsequent to i.v. solution container running empty.
  - Discontinue present i.v., and restart new short peripheral catheter in new site.

SKILL 25.3 Changing Intravenous Solution and Tubing

Equipment

- I.v. solution as ordered by health care provider
- Clean gloves
- Antiseptic swabs (chlorhexidine solution [preferred], povidone-iodine, or 70% alcohol)
- Label

Continuous i.v. Infusion

- Microdrip or macrodrip administration set i.v. tubing as appropriate
- Add-on device as necessary (e.g., filters, extension set, needleless connector)
- Tubing label

Intermittent Extension Set

- Three- to 5-mL syringe filled with preservative-free 0.9% sodium chloride (normal saline [NS])
- Short extension tubing (if necessary), injection cap

STEP	RATIONALE
Assessment	
1. Review accuracy and completeness of health care provider's order in the patient's medical record for patient name and correct solution: type, volume, additives, rate, and duration of i.v. therapy. Follow rights of drug administration.	Ensures delivery of correct i.v. solution and prescribed volume over prescribed time (Gorski et al., 2016).
2. Identify the patient by using at least two identifiers (e.g., name and birthday or name and medical record number) according to agency policy. Compare identifiers with information on the patient's MAR or medical record.	Ensures correct patient. Complies with The Joint Commission standards and improves patient safety (TJC, 2018).
3. Note date and time when i.v. tubing and solution were last changed.	Ensures correct timing of tubing changes.
4. Perform hand hygiene and apply clean gloves. Gently palpate skin around and above i.v. site over the dressing. Inspect vascular access site and device (VAD) for patency and signs and symptoms of i.v.-related complications (e.g., infiltration, occlusion of VAD, phlebitis, infection, patient complaints of pain, leaking under dressing).	Identifies complications that compromise integrity of VAD and necessitate replacement of VAD.
5. Check infusion system from the solution container down to the VAD insertion site for integrity including, but not limited to, discoloration, cloudiness, leakage, expiration date, tubing puncture, contamination, or occlusion. Determine compatibility of all i.v. solutions and additives by consulting approved online database, drug reference, or pharmacist. Remove and discard gloves. Perform hand hygiene.	If there has been a break in integrity of the solution container, a new container is needed (Alexander et al., 2014). May indicate need for i.v. tubing change. Incompatibilities cause physical, chemical, and therapeutic changes with adverse patient outcomes (Alexander et al., 2014).

STEP	RATIONALE
6. Check medical record for pertinent laboratory data such as potassium level.	Compare data with baseline to determine ongoing response to i.v. solution administration.
7. Determine the patient's understanding of need for continued i.v. therapy.	Indicates need for any patient education.
Planning	
1. Perform hand hygiene. Collect equipment and assemble at bedside. Have next i.v. solution prepared at least 1 h before needed. If solution is prepared in pharmacy, ensure that it has been delivered to patient care unit. Allow solution to warm to room temperature if it has been refrigerated. Check that solution is correct and properly labeled. Check solution expiration date. Ensure that any light sensitivity restrictions are followed.	Reduces transmission of infection and contamination of equipment (INS, 2016). Proper handling of solutions prevents i.v.-related complications such as occlusion. Checking that solution is correct prevents medication error.
2. Provide privacy and prepare bedside environment for patient safety.	Providing privacy and preparing the environment before the procedure helps to ensure a clean and distraction-free area for organizing procedure-related equipment.
3. Prepare the patient and family caregiver by explaining procedure, its purpose, and what is expected of the patient.	Decreases anxiety and promotes cooperation and compliance with therapy.
Implementation	
1. Changing i.v. fluid container with existing tubing or continuous i.v. infusion	
a. Change solution when fluid remains only in neck of container (approximately 50 mL) or when new type of solution has been ordered.	Prevents waste of solution.
b. Perform hand hygiene.	Reduces transmission of microorganisms.
c. Prepare new solution for changing. If using plastic bag, hang on i.v. pole and remove protective cover from i.v. tubing port. If using glass bottle, remove metal cap and metal and rubber disks.	Permits quick, smooth, and organized change from old to new container.
d. Close roller clamp on existing solution to stop flow rate. Remove i.v. tubing from EID (if used). Then remove old i.v. solution container from i.v. pole. Hold container with tubing port pointing upward.	Prevents solution remaining in drip chamber from emptying while changing solutions. Prevents any solution left in bag from spilling.
e. Quickly remove spike from old solution container and, without touching tip, insert spike into new container (see illustration).	Reduces risk for solution in drip chamber becoming empty and maintains sterility.
Clinical decision point: If spike is contaminated, you will need a new i.v. tubing set. See Step 2.	
f. Check for air in i.v. tubing. If air bubbles have formed, remove them by closing roller clamp, stretching tubing downward, and tapping tubing with finger (bubbles rise in fluid to drip chamber) (see Skill 25.1, Step 7h).	Reduces risk for air entering tubing. Use of an air-eliminating filter also reduces risk.

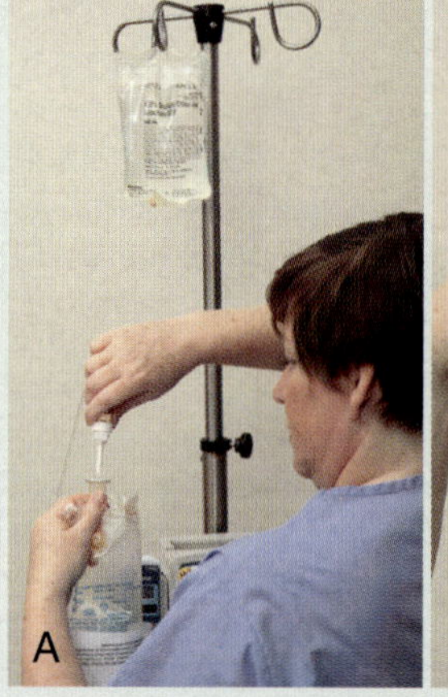

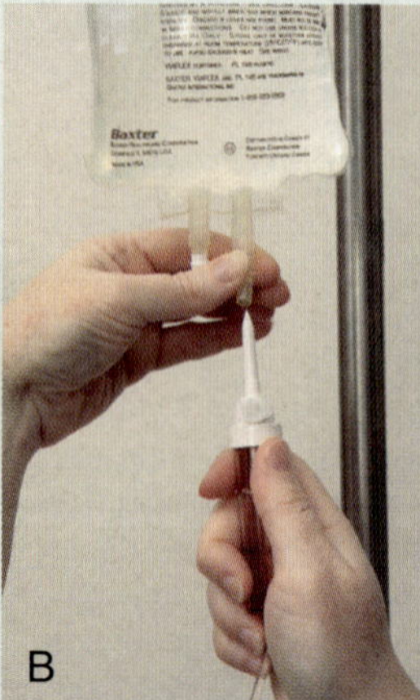

Step 1e **A,** Quickly remove spike from old solution container. **B,** Without touching tip, insert spike into new container.

STEP	RATIONALE
g. Make sure that drip chamber is one-third to one-half full. If drip chamber is too full, level can be decreased by removing bag from i.v. pole, pinching off i.v. tubing below drip chamber, inverting container, squeezing drip chamber (see illustration), releasing and turning solution container upright, and releasing pinch on tubing.	Reduces risk for air entering i.v. tubing. If chamber is completely filled, you cannot observe or regulate drip rate.
h. Reinsert tube into EID if being used. Regulate flow to ordered rate by using roller clamp on i.v. tubing or by programming EID.	Maintains measures to restore fluid balance and deliver i.v. solution as ordered.
i. Place time label on side of container and label with time hung, time of completion, and appropriate hourly intervals. If using plastic bags, mark only on label and not on container.	Provides visual comparison of volume infused compared with prescribed rate of infusion.
j. Instruct the patient in purpose of new i.v. solution, additives, flow rate, potential side effects and what to report.	Informs the patient about purpose for continued i.v. therapy and what to report and protects VAD patency.
k. Discard old i.v. container in appropriate receptacle. Perform hand hygiene.	Reduces transmission of microorganisms.
2. Changing i.v. tubing	
a. Coordinate i.v. tubing changes with solution changes when possible.	Reduces risk of infection by decreasing number of times system is open.
b. Perform hand hygiene.	Reduces transmission of infection and contamination of equipment (Gorski et al., 2016).
c. Open new infusion set and connect add-on pieces (e.g., filters, extension tubing). Keep protective coverings over infusion spike and distal adapter. Place roller clamp about 2–2.5 cm (1–2 inches) below drip chamber and move roller clamp to "off" position. Secure all connections using sterile technique.	Close proximity of roller clamp to drip chamber allows more accurate regulation of flow rate. Securing connections reduces risk later of air emboli and infection. Protective covers reduce entrance of microorganisms. All connections should be of Luer-Lok type (Gorski et al., 2016).
d. Apply clean gloves. If the patient's i.v. cannula hub is not visible, remove i.v. dressing. Do not remove tape securing cannula to skin.	Cannula hub must be visible to provide smooth transition when removing old and inserting new tubing.
e. Prepare i.v. tubing with new i.v. container (see Skill 25.1, Steps 7a–j).	Process ensures sterility of system and filling of tubing.
f. *Prepare i.v. tubing with existing continuous i.v. infusion container.*	
(1) Move roller clamp on new i.v. tubing to "off" position.	Prevents fluid spillage.
(2) Slow rate of infusion through old tubing to keep vein open (KVO) rate, using EID or roller clamp.	Prevents occlusion of VAD.

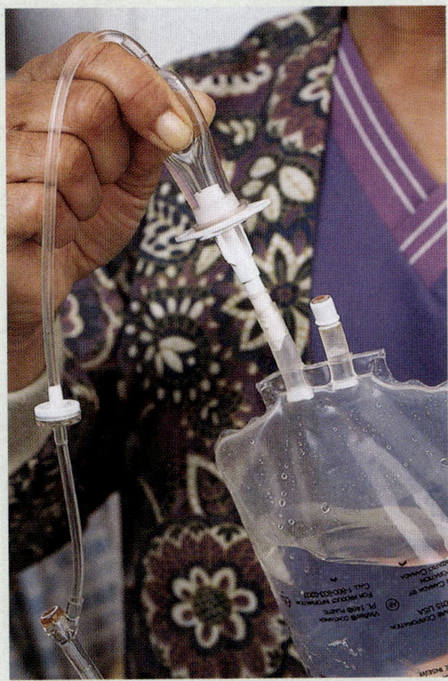

Step 1g Squeeze drip chamber to fill with fluid. Be sure to leave chamber one-third to one-half full.

STEP	RATIONALE
(3) Compress and fill drip chamber of old tubing.	Ensures that drip chamber remains full until new tubing is changed.
(4) Invert container and remove old tubing. Keep spike sterile and upright.	Solution in drip chamber will continue to run and maintain catheter patency.
(5) Insert spike of new infusion tubing into existing solution container. Hang solution bag on i.v. pole, and compress drip chamber on new tubing and release allowing it to fill one-third to one-half full.	Permits drip chamber to fill and promotes rapid, smooth flow of solution through tubing.
(6) Prime air out of i.v. tubing by filling with i.v. solution. Remove protective cover on end of tubing and slowly open roller clamp to allow solution to flow from drip chamber to distal end of i.v. tubing. If tubing has a Y connector, invert Y connector when solution reaches it to displace air. Return roller clamp to "off" position after priming tubing (filled with i.v. solution). Replace protective cover on end of i.v. tubing. Place end of adapter near the patient's i.v. site.	Priming ensures that i.v. tubing is clear of air before connection with VAD and filled with i.v. solution. Slow fill of tubing decreases turbulence and chance of bubble formation. Closing clamp prevents accidental loss of fluid. Maintains sterility. Equipment is positioned for a quick connection of new tubing.
(7) Stop EID or turn roller clamp on old tubing to "off" position.	Prevents fluid spillage.
g. *Prepare extension set or saline lock.*	
(1) If short extension tubing is needed, use sterile technique to connect new injection cap to new extension set or i.v. tubing.	Prepares extension set for connecting with i.v.
(2) Scrub injection cap with antiseptic swab for at least 15 s and allow to dry completely. Attach syringe containing 3–5 mL of NS flush solution and inject through injection cap into extension set.	Ensures effective disinfection (Phillips and Gorski, 2014). Maintains patency of catheter.
h. *Reestablish infusion.*	
(1) Gently disconnect old tubing from extension tubing (or from i.v. catheter hub) and quickly insert Luer-Lok end of new tubing or saline lock into extension tubing connection (or i.v. catheter hub) (see illustrations for example of connecting tubing to short extension set).	Allows smooth transition from old to new tubing, minimizing time system is open.
(2) For continuous infusion, open roller clamp on new tubing and regulate drip rate of gravity infusion by adjusting roller clamp, or remove old tubing from EID, insert new tubing, and then open clamp fully and restart EID at prescribed rate.	Ensures catheter patency and prevents occlusion.
(3) Attach piece of tape or preprinted label with date and time of i.v. tubing change onto tubing below drip chamber.	Provides reference to determine next time for tubing change.
(4) Form loop of tubing and secure it to the patient's arm with strip of tape.	Avoids accidental pulling against site and stabilizes catheter.
i. Remove and discard old i.v. tubing with roller clamp closed. If necessary, apply new i.v. dressing. Remove and dispose of gloves. Perform hand hygiene.	Reduces transmission of microorganisms.
j. Instruct the patient and family caregiver on purpose of new solution, additives, flow rate, potential side effects, how to avoid occluding the tubing, and how to move and turn to prevent contamination of i.v. tubing.	Informs the patient about purpose for continued i.v. therapy and what to report and protects VAD patency. Prevents accidental contamination of i.v. tubing.

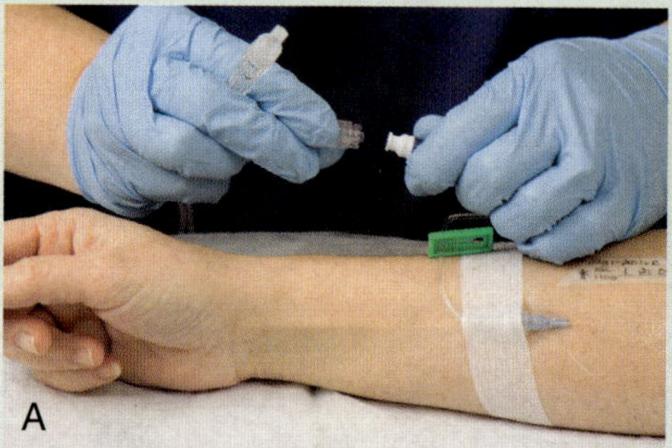

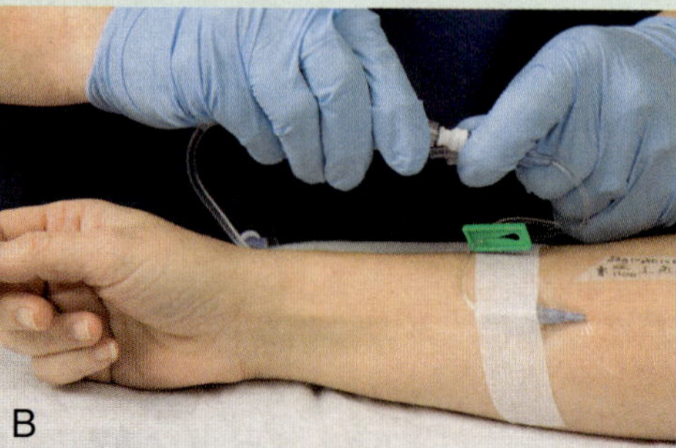

Step 2h(1) A, Disconnect old tubing. **B,** Insert adapter of new tubing.

STEP	RATIONALE
Evaluation	
1. Observe the patient every 1–2 h or at established intervals per agency policy and procedure for function, intactness, and patency of i.v. system; for leaking at connection sites; and for correct infusion rate and type and amount of i.v. solution infused.	Ensures delivery of prescribed volume over prescribed time and decreases risk for fluid and electrolyte imbalance. Ensures that i.v. system is functioning appropriately and minimizes risk of infection secondary to breach in system integrity.
2. Evaluate the patient to determine response to therapy (e.g., laboratory values, I&O, weights, vital signs, postprocedure assessments).	Provides ongoing evaluation of the patient's fluid status.
3. Monitor the patient for signs of extracellular fluid volume (ECV) excess, ECV deficit, or signs and symptoms of electrolyte imbalances.	Early recognition of complications leads to prompt treatment.
4. Evaluate the patient at established intervals per agency policy and procedure for signs and symptoms of i.v.-related complications.	Prevents complications that compromise integrity of VAD or cause inaccurate i.v. solution flow rate.
5. **Use teach back:** "I want to be sure that I explained the problems that can occur with your i.v. Can you tell me what signs and symptoms you would report?" Revise your instruction now or develop a plan for revised patient/family caregiver teaching if the patient/family caregiver is unable to teach back correctly.	Determines the patient's/family caregiver's level of understanding of instructional topic.

Recording and Reporting

- Record on nurse's notes in EHR or chart i.v. solution, rate of infusion, and integrity and patency according to agency policy and procedure.
- Record use of any EID or control device and identification number on that device.
- Record solution and tubing change, type of solution, and volume and rate of infusion on the patient's record. Use infusion therapy flow sheet for parenteral solutions per agency policy.
- Record patient response to therapy and unexpected outcomes (e.g., causes of flow rate inaccuracy).
- Record the patient's/family caregiver's knowledge following evaluation of teach-back in nurses' notes.
- At change of shift or when leaving on break, report changes of solution, infusion rate, and volume left in infusion to nurse in charge or next nurse assigned to care for the patient.

Unexpected Outcomes and Related Interventions

- I.v. fluid infusing is slower than ordered.
  - Check for positional change that affects rate, height of i.v. container, kinking of tubing, or obstruction.
  - Check for patency by opening roller clamp.
  - Check VAD site for complications.
  - Consult health care provider for new order to provide necessary fluid volume.
- Flow rate is incorrect; the patient receives too little or too much solution.
  - Notify health care provider if the patient's anticipated infusion is 100–200 mL less than or greater than anticipated (as per agency policy and procedure).
  - Evaluate the patient for adverse effects of infusion (e.g., ECV excess or ECV deficit).
  - Determine and correct the cause of incorrect flow rate (e.g., change in position, tubing kink, loss of i.v. patency or intactness).
  - Use EID when accurate flow rate is critical.
- Fluid and/or electrolyte imbalances:
  - Notify health care provider.
  - Anticipate orders for changes in i.v. solution or additives.

SKILL 25.4 Changing a Peripheral Intravenous Dressing

Equipment

- Antiseptic swabs (2% chlorhexidine [preferred], povidone-iodine, or 70% alcohol)
- Skin protectant swab *(optional)*
- Adhesive remover *(optional)*
- Clean gloves
- Strips of nonallergenic tape
- Engineered catheter stabilization device or precut strips of sterile tape
- Commercially available i.v. site protection device *(optional)*
- Sterile transparent semipermeable membrane (TSM) dressing *or*
- Sterile 2 × 2– or 4 × 4–inch gauze pad

STEP	RATIONALE
Assessment	
1. Identify the patient by using at least two identifiers (e.g., name and birthday or name and medical record number) according to agency policy. Compare identifiers with information on the patient's MAR or medical record.	Ensures correct patient. Complies with The Joint Commission standards and improves patient safety (TJC, 2018).
2. Determine when dressing was last changed. Dressing should be labeled to include date and time applied, size and type of vascular access device (VAD), and insertion date.	Provides information regarding length of time that present dressing has been in place and allows planning for dressing change.
3. Perform hand hygiene and apply gloves. Observe present dressing for moisture and intactness. Determine whether moisture is from site leakage or external source.	Nonadhering dressing increases risk for insertion site infection or dislodgment of VAD.
4. Inspect and gently palpate skin around and above i.v. site over dressing. Assess VAD for patency and signs and symptoms of i.v.-related complications (e.g., infiltration, occlusion of VAD, phlebitis, infection, patient complaints of pain, leaking under dressing). Remove and discard gloves, and perform hand hygiene.	Identifies complications that compromise integrity of VAD and may necessitate replacement of VAD.
5. Assess the patient's understanding of need for continued i.v. infusion.	Reveals need for patient instruction.
Planning	
1. Provide privacy and prepare bedside environment for patient safety.	Providing privacy and preparing the environment before the procedure helps to ensure a clean and distraction-free area for organizing procedure-related equipment.
2. Perform hand hygiene. Collect equipment and organize on clean, clutter-free bedside stand or overbed table. Apply clean gloves.	Reduces transmission of infection and contamination of equipment (Gorski et al., 2016).
3. Explain procedure and purpose to the patient and family caregiver. Explain that the patient will need to hold affected extremity still.	Decreases anxiety, promotes cooperation, and gives the patient time frame around which to plan personal activities.
Implementation	
1. Perform hand hygiene and apply clean gloves. Remove dressing. a. *For TSM dressing:* Stabilize catheter with nondominant hand (see illustration) and remove dressing by pulling up one corner and gently pulling straight out and parallel to skin. Repeat on all sides until dressing has been removed. b. *For gauze dressing:* Stabilize catheter hub while loosening tape and removing old dressing one layer at a time by pulling toward insertion site. Be cautious if tubing becomes tangled between two layers of dressing.	Technique minimizes discomfort during removal. Use alcohol swab on TSM dressing next to the patient's skin to loosen dressing.
2. Assess VAD insertion site for signs and symptoms of i.v.-related complications. If complication exists, determine whether VAD requires removal. Remove catheter if ordered by health care provider.	Presence of complication may necessitate VAD removal.

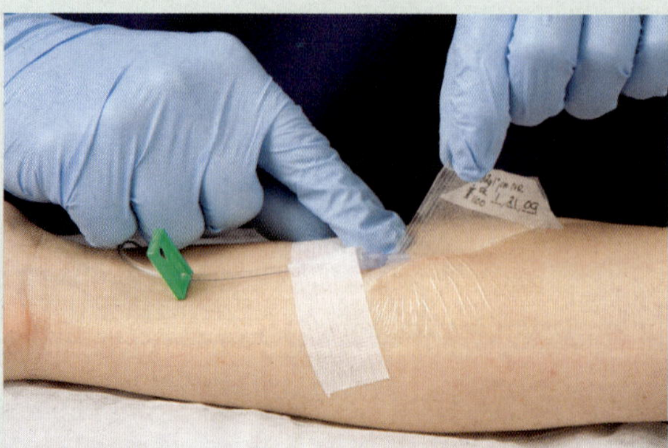

Step 1a Remove transparent semipermeable membrane (TSM) dressing by pulling side laterally.

STEP	RATIONALE

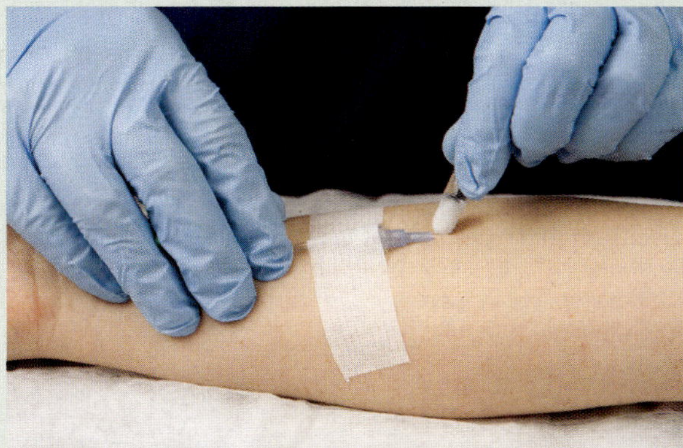

Step 4 Cleanse peripheral site with antiseptic.

STEP	RATIONALE
3. If catheter is to remain in place, assess integrity of engineered stabilization device if used. Continue to stabilize catheter and remove as recommended by manufacturer's directions for use. **Note:** Some stabilization devices are designed to remain in place for the length of time VAD is in as long as adequate stabilization is evident.	Removing stabilization device allows for appropriate skin antisepsis before applying dressing and new stabilization device (Gorski et al., 2016). Stabilization prevents accidental dislodgment of VAD.

Clinical decision point: Keep one finger over catheter at all times until dressing secures catheter hub. If the patient is restless or uncooperative, it is helpful to have another staff member help with procedure.

STEP	RATIONALE
4. While stabilizing i.v., perform skin antisepsis to insertion site with chlorhexidine solution using friction in a back-and-forth motion for 30 s and allow to dry completely. If using alcohol or povidone-iodine, clean in concentric circle moving from insertion site outward with swab (see illustration). Allow antiseptic solution to dry completely.	Reduces incidence of catheter-related infections (Alexander et al., 2014). Allow any skin antiseptic agent to fully dry for complete antisepsis (Gorski et al., 2016).
5. *Optional:* Apply skin protectant to area where you will apply tape or dressing. Allow to dry.	Coats skin with protective solution to maintain skin integrity, prevents irritation from adhesive, and promotes adhesion of dressing.
6. While stabilizing catheter, apply a sterile dressing over site (procedures differ; follow agency policy).	
a. *TSM dressing:* Apply TSM dressing. See Skill 25.1, Step 23a.	Protects catheter insertion site and minimizes risk for infection (Phillips and Gorski, 2014). Allows visualization of insertion site and surrounding area for complications (Gorski et al., 2016).
b. *Sterile gauze dressing:* Apply sterile gauze dressing. See Skill 25.1, Step 23b.	Use only sterile tape under sterile dressing to prevent site contamination. Gauze dressing obscures observation of insertion site and is changed every 2 days (Gorski et al., 2016).
c. *Engineered catheter stabilization device:* Apply catheter stabilization device.	Use of engineered stabilization devices that allow visual inspection of an insertion site can reduce risk for VAD complications (i.e., phlebitis, infection, migration) and unintentional loss of access (Gorski et al., 2016).

Clinical decision point: Because Band-Aids are not occlusive and nonsterile tape increases the risk for insertion site infection, do not use either type over catheter insertion points.

STEP	RATIONALE
7. Remove and discard gloves. Perform hand hygiene.	Prevents transmission of microorganisms.
8. *Optional:* Apply site protection device (e.g., I.V. House UltraDressing).	Reduces risk of VAD dislodgment (Gorski et al., 2016).
9. Anchor extension tubing or i.v. tubing alongside dressing on arm and secure with tape directly over tubing. When using TSM dressing, avoid placing tape over the dressing.	Prevents accidental dislodgment of VAD if tubing is pulled.
10. Label dressing per agency policy. Information on label includes date and time of i.v. insertion, VAD gauge size and length, and your initials.	Communicates type of device and time interval for dressing change and site rotation.
11. Discard equipment and perform hand hygiene.	Reduces transmission of microorganisms.

STEP	RATIONALE
Evaluation	
1. Evaluate function, patency of i.v. system, and flow rate after changing dressing.	Validates that i.v. is patent and functioning correctly. Manipulation of catheter and tubing will affect rate of infusion.
2. Evaluate the patient at established intervals per agency policy and procedure for signs and symptoms of i.v.-related complications.	Identifies complications that compromise integrity of VAD or cause inaccurate i.v. solution flow rate.
3. **Use teach back:** "I want to be sure that I explained reasons that the i.v. dressing may need to be changed. Tell me the problems you would report to the nurse that would require a dressing change." Revise your instruction now or develop a plan for revised patient/family caregiver teaching if the patient/family caregiver is unable to teach back correctly.	Determines the patient's/family caregiver's level of understanding of instructional topic.

Recording and Reporting

- Record in nurse's notes in EHR or chart the time short peripheral dressing was changed, reason for change, type of dressing material used, patency of system, and description of VAD site.
- Record the patient's/family caregiver's knowledge following evaluation of teach back in nurses' notes.
- Report to nurse in charge or oncoming shift nurse that dressing was changed and any significant information about integrity of system.
- Report to health care provider and document any complications, interventions, and patient response to treatment.

Unexpected Outcomes and Related Interventions

- I.v. catheter is accidentally removed or dislodged.
  - Restart new short peripheral i.v. in other extremity or above previous insertion site if continued therapy is necessary.
- I.v. solution is not infusing or runs slower than ordered.
  - Check i.v. catheter for bending, kinking, or dislodgment, as catheter may require replacement.
  - Check for positional i.v. site and reposition catheter, applying new dressing if necessary.
  - Check and adjust height of i.v. container, kinking, or obstruction of i.v. tubing.

KEY POINTS

- Body fluids, consisting of water and the substances dissolved or suspended in it, are distributed in ECF (vascular plus interstitial) and ICF compartments.
- To maintain normal fluid and electrolyte balance, daily intake must equal output, and the fluid and electrolytes must be distributed normally between body fluid compartments.
- Fluid output normally occurs through skin, lungs, GI tract, and kidneys and may occur through abnormal routes in patient populations.
- Patients who are very young or very old; patients whose I&O of fluid and/or electrolytes are not equal; and patients who have various hormone imbalances, chronic diseases, or trauma are at greatest risk for fluid, electrolyte, and acid–base imbalances.
- ECV excess and deficit are abnormal volumes of isotonic sodium-containing fluid, which manifest as sudden changes in body weight and changes in markers of vascular and interstitial volume.
- Osmolality imbalances are abnormal concentrations of body fluids, which manifest as altered serum sodium concentration and altered level of consciousness.
- Treatment for ECV excess is sodium restriction plus fluid restriction if severe; treatment for hyponatremia usually is water restriction.
- Enteral or parenteral administration of appropriate fluids prevents or treats ECV deficit, hypernatremia, and electrolyte deficits.
- Cellular metabolism constantly produces carbonic and metabolic acids; to maintain normal acid–base balance, carbonic acid must be excreted through the lungs, and metabolic acid must be buffered and then excreted through the kidneys.
- Acid–base imbalances are respiratory (excess or deficit of carbonic acid) or metabolic (excess or deficit of metabolic acids), manifested as changes in pH, $PaCO_2$, HCO_3^-, and level of consciousness.
- Initiation and maintenance of i.v. therapy require clinical decision-making, skill, and organized procedures to maintain sterility and patency of the system.
- Nurses monitor for complications of i.v. therapy including infiltration, phlebitis, infection, and overload of the specific i.v. fluid.
- Administration of blood products entails a specific procedure for identification of the patient and the blood product and frequent monitoring during the transfusion for patient safety.
- Risks of blood transfusion include transfusion reactions, circulatory overload, infection, hyperkalemia, hypocalcemia, and hypomagnesemia from rapid administration of blood.
- Nursing interventions for acid–base imbalances support prescribed medical therapies and treat the underlying disorder while providing for patient safety.

REFERENCES

AABB. Blood donation FAQs. 2016. Available from: http://www.aabb.org/tm/donation/Pages/donatefaqs.aspx.

Abitz T. Cultural congruence and infusion nursing practice. J Infus Nurs 2016;39(2):77.

Burchum JR, Rosenthal LD. Lehne's pharmacology for nursing care. 9th ed. St. Louis: Elsevier; 2016.

Cook LS. Infusion-related air embolism. J Infus Nurs 2013;36(1):26.

Crookston KP, Koenig SC, Reyes MD. Transfusion reaction identification and management at the bedside. J Infus Nurs 2015;38(2):104.

Custer B, Kessler D, Vahidnia F, Leparc G, Krysztof DE, Shaz B, et al. Risk factors for retrovirus and hepatitis virus infections in accepted blood donors. Transfusion 2015;55(5):1098.

Felver L. Acid-base balance. In: Giddens JF, editor. Concepts for nursing practice. 2nd ed. St. Louis: Elsevier; 2017a.

Felver L. Fluid and electrolytes. In: Giddens JF, editor. Concepts for nursing practice. 2nd ed. St. Louis: Elsevier; 2017b.

Felver L. Fluid and electrolyte homeostasis and imbalances. In: Copstead LC, Banasik JL, editors. Pathophysiology. 6th ed. St. Louis: Elsevier; 2018.

Gorski L, Hadaway L, Hagle ME, McGoldrick M, Orr M, Doellman D. Infusion therapy standards of practice. J Infus Nurs 2016;39(Suppl. 1):S1.

Guinn NR, Roberson RS, White W, Cowper PA, Broomer B, Milano C, et al. Costs and outcomes after cardiac surgery in patients refusing transfusion compared with those who do not: a case-matched study. Transfusion 2015;55(12):2791.

Hall JE. Guyton and Hall textbook of medical physiology. 13th ed. Philadelphia: Elsevier; 2016.

Helm RE, Klausner JD, Klemperer JD, Flint LM, Huang E. Accepted but unacceptable: peripheral IV catheter failure. J Infus Nurs 2015;38(3):189.

Infusion Nurses Society (INS). Policies and procedures for infusion nursing. 5th ed. Norwood, MA: Infusion Nurses Society; 2016.

Kamel KS, Halperin ML. Fluid, electrolyte, and acid-base physiology: a problem-based approach. 5th ed. St. Louis: Elsevier; 2017.

Kreidieh FY, Moukadem HA, El Saghir NS. Overview, prevention and management of chemotherapy extravasation. World J Clin Oncol. 2016 Feb 10;7(1):87-97. doi: 10.5306/wjco.v7.i1.87. PMID: 26862492; PMCID: PMC4734939.

Marilyn Hockenberry Cheryl Rodgers David Wilson. Essentials of pediatric nursing. 10th ed. St. Louis: Mosby; 2017.

Mary Alexander , Ann M. Corrigan S. , Lisa A Gorski , Lynn Phillips. Core curriculum for infusion nursing. 4th ed. Philadelphia: Lippincott Williams & Wilkins; 2014.

McGloin S. The ins and outs of fluid balance in the acutely ill patient. Br J Nurs 2015;24(1):14.

National Institute on Alcohol Abuse and Alcoholism (NIAAA). Drinking levels defined. n.d. Available from: https://www.niaaa.nih.gov/alcohol-health/overview-alcohol-consumption/moderate-binge-drinking.

National Quality Forum (NQF). Field guide to NQF resources. Washington, DC: 2016. Available from: http://www.qualityforum.org/Field_Guide/List_of_Measures.aspx.

Phillips LD, Gorski L. Manual of I.V. therapeutics: evidence-based practice for infusion therapy. 6th ed. Philadelphia: F.A. Davis; 2014.

The Joint Commission (TJC). 2018 National Patient Safety Goals. Oakbrook Terrace, IL: The Joint Commission; 2018. Available from: https://www.jointcommission.org/standards_information/npsgs.aspx.

Touhy TA, Jett KF. Ebersole and Hess' gerontological nursing and healthy aging. St. Louis: Elsevier; 2014.

Vizcarra C, Cassutt C, Corbitt N, Richardson D, Runde D, Stafford K. Recommendations for improving safety practices with short peripheral catheters. J Infus Nurs 2014;37(2):121.

Wallace MC, Macy DL. Reduction of central line-associated bloodstream infection rates in patients in the adult intensive care unit. J Infus Nurs 2016;39(1):47.

Wang XH, Qiu JB, Ju Y, Chen GC, Yang JH, Pang JH, et al. Reduction of heart failure rehospitalization using a weight management education intervention. J Cardiovasc Nurs 2014;29(6):528.

Weinstein SM, Hagle SM. Plumer's principles and practice of infusion therapy. 9th ed. Philadelphia: Lippincott Williams & Wilkins; 2014.

Winkler M, Guenter P. Long-term home parenteral nutrition: it takes an interdisciplinary approach. J Infus Nurs 2014;37(5):389.

26 Medication Administration

OBJECTIVES

- To identify the characteristics of adverse drug effects.
- To discuss nursing roles and responsibilities in medication administration.
- To describe the physiological mechanism of medication action.
- To compare and contrast the roles of the health care provider, pharmacist, and nurse in medication administration.
- To discuss legal responsibilities in medication administration.
- To differentiate among different types of medication actions.
- To discuss factors that influence medication actions.
- To discuss factors to include in assessing a patient's needs for and response to medication therapy.
- To implement nursing actions to prevent medication errors.
- To describe factors to consider when choosing routes of medication administration.
- To calculate prescribed medication doses correctly.
- To list the six rights of medication administration and apply them in clinical practice.
- To discuss methods used to educate patients and family caregivers about prescribed medications.
- To correctly and safely prepare and administer medications.

KEY TERMS

absorption, p. 640
anaphylactic reactions, p. 643
biotransformation, p. 641
buccal, p. 646
detoxify, p. 641
breath-actuated metered-dose inhalers (BAIs), p. 668
dry powder inhalers (DPIs), p. 668
idiosyncratic reaction, p. 643
infusions, p. 647
injection, p. 641
instillation, p. 646
intradermal (i.d.), p. 646
intramuscular (i.m.), p. 677
intraocular, p. 646
intravenous (i.v.), p. 641
irrigations, p. 647
maintenance medication, p. 670
medication error, p. 655
medication interaction, p. 644
medication reconciliation, p. 656
medication tolerance, p. 644
metric system, p. 647
minimum effective concentration (MEC), p. 644
needles, p. 671
ophthalmic medications, p. 665
oral route, p. 646
parenteral administration, p. 646
peak, p. 644
pharmacokinetics, p. 640
prescriptions, p. 647
pressurized metered-dose inhalers (pMDIs), p. 668
rectal suppositories, p. 668
rescue, p. 670
side effects, p. 640
six rights of medication administration, p. 656
solution, p. 647
subcutaneous, p. 646
sublingual, p. 646
synergistic effect, p. 644
therapeutic effect, p. 642
therapeutic range, p. 644
toxic effects, p. 643
transdermal disk, p. 646
trough, p. 644
verbal order, p. 651
Z-track method, p. 678

INTRODUCTION

Patients with health problems use a variety of methods to restore or maintain their health. One method is the use of medication, a substance used in the diagnosis, treatment, cure, relief, or prevention of health problems. Regardless of where patients receive health care (e.g., hospitals, clinics, home), nurses play an essential role in assessing for factors that place patients at risk when receiving medications and in preparing, administering, and evaluating the effects of medications. Family caregivers, friends, or home care personnel often administer medications when patients cannot perform this task at home. Nurses are also responsible for teaching a patient and family caregiver about medications and their side effects, helping patients adopt practices for adhering to their medication regimen, and evaluating the ability of a patient and family caregiver to administer medications.

Medication administration and evaluation are critical nursing responsibilities, so nurses must understand the actions and effects of all medications they give their patients. To safely and accurately administer medications, you need to have an understanding of the legal aspects of medication administration, pharmacokinetics (the movement of drugs in the human body), life sciences, anatomy, pathophysiology, and mathematics.

THE CENTRAL DRUGS STANDARD CONTROL ORGANIZATION

The Central Drugs Standard Control Organization (CDSCO) is a national regulatory authority of India for the drugs, cosmetics, and device approval and standardization. It is an autonomous organization under the Ministry of Health and Family Welfare, Government of India. The Drugs and Cosmetics Act, 1940 and Rules, 1945, empower the CDSCO for prescribing the standards for drugs; approval of drugs, cosmetics, medical devices, and clinical trials; and quality of imported drugs. The CDSCO also coordinates with state drug authorities for uniform enforcement of the Drugs and Cosmetics Act and Rules of the country.

The Government of India protects the health of citizens by ensuring that medications are safe and effective. The Drugs and Cosmetics Act, 1940, came in force for safe use of drugs throughout the country. Later, the Drugs and Cosmetics Rules, 1945, were implemented under the Drugs and Cosmetics Act, 1940, which provided drug classification under different schedules and guides for the storage, sales, and prescription of different category drugs.

Official publications such as the *Indian Pharmacopeia* (IP) set standards for medication strength, quality, purity, packaging, safety, labeling, and dose form. On July 14, 2010, the Government of India started the Pharmacovigilance Program for India (PvPI) to safeguard public health by validating the safety of products through promoting adverse drug reaction (ADR) reporting. The National Coordinating Centre (NCC) of PvPI is situated at the Indian Pharmacopeia Commission (IPC), Ghaziabad, and there are various regional, zonal, and peripheral centers for smooth and effective reporting of ADR. This program encourages nurses and other health care professionals to report any adverse reaction in which a medication, product, or medical event causes serious harm to a patient. Health care professionals report the incident by completing the ADR form available online or offline to the nearest center. Hospitals and other health care agencies have policies for the proper storage and distribution of controlled substances (Box 26.1).

PHARMACOLOGICAL CONCEPTS

Medication Names

Some medications have three different names: chemical, generic, and trade. The chemical name of a medication gives an exact description of its chemical composition and molecular structure. Nurses rarely use chemical names in clinical practice. The manufacturer who creates the medication gives the generic or nonproprietary name. However, the name requires the CDSCO approval. Each drug has only one generic name. The generic name is not as complex as a chemical name, and it becomes the official name listed in publications such as the *IP*. The trade name, brand name, or proprietary name is the name under which a manufacturer markets a medication. The trade name has the trademark symbol (™) at the upper right of the name, indicating that the manufacturer has trademarked the name of the medication. The following is an example of the different names of a common medication:

- Chemical name: *N*-Acetyl-*para*-aminophenol
- Generic name: Acetaminophen (paracetamol)
- Trade names: Dolo™, Calpol™, Crocin™

Manufacturers create trade names that are easy to pronounce, spell, and remember. Trade names are approved by the CDSCO, India, so that no two trade names are too similar. However, because many companies produce the same medication, similarities in trade names are still often confusing and can result in a medication error. For example, confusing names include Adderall versus Inderal and clonazepam versus lorazepam. Therefore, obtain the exact name and spelling for each medication you administer to your patients. For a full list of medications that are often confused with one another. The recommended, **bolded** tall man (uppercase) letters help nurses recognize the dissimilarities in look-alike drug names.

Classification

Medications with similar characteristics are grouped into classifications. Medication classifications identify the effect a medication has on a body system, the symptoms a medication relieves, or the desired effect of a medication. Sometimes, the

BOX 26.1 Guidelines for Safe Opioid (Narcotic) Administration and Control

- Store all narcotics in a locked, secure cabinet or container (e.g., computerized locked cabinets are preferred).
- Maintain a running count of opioids by counting them whenever dispensing them. If you find a discrepancy, correct the error if possible and report it immediately.
- Use a special inventory record each time a narcotic is dispensed. Records are often kept electronically and provide an accurate ongoing count of narcotics used, wasted, and remaining.
- Use the record to document the patient's name, date, time of medication administration, name of medication, and dosage. Documentation also includes the name of the nurse dispensing and administering the medication.
- A second nurse witnesses disposal of the unused part if a nurse gives only part of a dose of a controlled substance. Ensure that documentation includes the names of the nurses wasting the unused portion of the medication.
- Follow agency policy for appropriate waste of controlled substances. Do not place wasted parts of medications in sharps containers.

last syllables of a generic name indicate the medication classification. For example, the syllables *-olol* at the end of *propranolol* tell you that this medication is in the beta-adrenergic blocker classification. Usually, each class contains more than one medication that health care providers can prescribe for a type of health problem. For example, patients who have asthma often take a variety of medications from the class of beta-2-adrenergic agonists. Other medications are sometimes found in more than one class. For example, aspirin is an analgesic, an antipyretic, and an anti-inflammatory medication.

Medication Forms

Medications come in a variety of forms or preparations. The form of the medication determines its route of administration. The form of a medication is intended to improve its absorption and metabolism. Many medications come in several forms such as tablets, capsules, elixirs, and suppositories. When you administer a medication, be certain to use the proper form (Table 26.1).

PHARMACOKINETICS AS THE BASIS OF MEDICATION ACTIONS

For a medication to be therapeutically useful, it is taken into a patient's body; is absorbed and distributed to cells, tissues, or a specific organ; and alters physiological functions. **Pharmacokinetics** is the study of four major processes: medication absorption, distribution, metabolism, and excretion. You use knowledge of pharmacokinetics when you time medication administration, select the route of administration, and evaluate a patient's response.

Absorption

Absorption is the movement of medication molecules into the blood from the site of medication administration. Factors that affect absorption are the route of administration, ability of the medication to dissolve, blood flow to the site of administration, body surface area (BSA), and lipid solubility of medication.

Table 26.1 Forms of Medication

Form	Description
MEDICATION FORMS COMMONLY PREPARED FOR ADMINISTRATION BY ORAL ROUTE	
Solid Forms	
Caplet	Solid dosage form for oral use; shaped like capsule and coated for ease of swallowing
Capsule	Medication encased in gelatin shell
Tablet	Powdered medication compressed into hard disk or cylinder; in addition to primary medication, contains binders (adhesive to allow powder to stick together), disintegrators (to promote tablet dissolution), lubricants (for ease of manufacturing), and fillers (for convenient tablet size)
Enteric-coated tablet	Coated tablet that does not dissolve in stomach; coatings dissolve in intestine, where medication is absorbed
Liquid Forms	
Elixir	Clear fluid containing water and/or alcohol; often sweetened
Extract	Concentrated medication form made by removing the active part of medication from its other components
Aqueous solution	Substance dissolved in water and syrups
Aqueous suspension	Finely dissolved drug particles dispersed in liquid medium; when suspension is left standing, particles settle to bottom of container
Syrup	Medication dissolved in concentrated sugar solution
OTHER ORAL FORMS AND TERMS ASSOCIATED WITH ORAL PREPARATIONS	
Troche (lozenge)	Flat, round tablets that dissolve in the mouth to release medication; not meant for ingestion
Aerosol	Aqueous medication sprayed and absorbed in the mouth and upper airway; not meant for ingestion
Sustained release	Tablet or capsule that contains small particles of a medication coated with material that requires a varying amount of time to dissolve
MEDICATION FORMS COMMONLY PREPARED FOR ADMINISTRATION BY TOPICAL ROUTE	
Ointment (salve or cream)	Semisolid, externally applied preparation, usually containing one or more medications
Liniment	Usually contains alcohol, oil, or soapy emollient applied to skin
Lotion	Semiliquid suspension that usually protects, cools, or cleanses skin
Paste	Thick ointment; absorbed through skin more slowly than ointment; often used for skin protection
Transdermal disk or patch	Medicated disk or patch absorbed through skin slowly over long period of time (e.g., 24 h)
MEDICATION FORMS COMMONLY PREPARED FOR ADMINISTRATION BY PARENTERAL ROUTE	
Solution	Sterile preparation that contains water with one or more dissolved compounds
Powder	Sterile particles of medication that are dissolved in a sterile liquid (e.g., water, normal saline) before administration
MEDICATION FORMS COMMONLY PREPARED FOR INSTILLATION INTO BODY CAVITIES	
Intraocular disk	Small, flexible, oval (similar to contact lens) consisting of two soft outer layers and a middle layer containing medication; slowly releases medication when moistened by ocular fluid
Suppository	Solid dosage form mixed with gelatin and shaped in form of pellet for insertion into body cavity (rectum or vagina); melts when it reaches body temperature, releasing medication for absorption

Route of Administration

Each route of medication administration has a different rate of absorption. The routes of administration, ranked in order from slowest to fastest, are as follows:

- Topical application to the skin has slow absorption because of the physical makeup of the skin.
- Orally administered medications pass through the gastrointestinal (GI) tract, so the rate of absorption is slow.
- Medications placed on the mucous membranes and respiratory airways are absorbed quickly because these tissues contain many blood vessels.
- Intramuscular (i.m.) and subcutaneous medications absorb more quickly than oral medications, with medications in i.m. injections entering the bloodstream more quickly than medications in subcutaneous injections.
- **Intravenous (i.v.) injection** produces the most rapid absorption because medications are available immediately when they enter the systemic circulation.

Ability of a Medication to Dissolve

The ability of an oral medication to dissolve depends mostly on its form or preparation. The body absorbs solutions and suspensions more readily than tablets or capsules. Acidic medications pass through the gastric mucosa rapidly. Medications that are basic are not absorbed before reaching the small intestine.

Blood Flow to the Site of Administration

The blood supply at the site of administration determines how quickly the body absorbs a drug. Medications are absorbed as blood comes in contact with the site of administration. The richer the blood supply at the site of administration, the faster a medication is absorbed.

Body Surface Area

The size of the surface that a medication comes in contact with affects how quickly the body absorbs the medication. When a medication comes in contact with a large surface area, it is absorbed at a faster rate. This explains why most oral medications are absorbed in the small intestine and not in the stomach (Burchum and Rosenthal, 2016).

Lipid Solubility

Because the cell membrane has a lipid layer, highly lipid-soluble medications cross cell membranes easily and are absorbed quickly. Another factor that often affects medication absorption is whether the stomach contains food. Some oral medications are absorbed more easily when administered between meals. This is because food changes the structure of a medication and sometimes impairs its absorption. When some medications are administered together, they interfere with one another, impairing the absorption of both medications.

To safely administer medications, you need to know the factors that alter or impair absorption of prescribed medications. Use your knowledge and confer with a pharmacist to choose medication administration times that will promote optimal absorption. For example, administer medications as prescribed before or after meals so that the medications will not interact with food. When medications interact with one another, make sure that you avoid giving them at the same time.

Distribution

After a medication is absorbed, it is distributed within the body to tissues and organs and ultimately to its specific site of action. The rate and extent of distribution depend on the physical and chemical properties of the medication and the physiology of the person taking it.

Circulation

Once a medication enters the bloodstream, the blood carries it throughout the tissues and organs of the body. How fast it reaches the intended site depends on the vascularity of the various tissues and organs. Conditions that limit blood flow or blood perfusion inhibit the distribution of a medication. For example, patients with heart failure have impaired circulation, which slows medication delivery to the intended site of action.

Membrane Permeability

Membrane permeability is the ability of tissues and membranes to allow a medication to pass through and enter target cells. To be distributed to an organ, a medication must pass through all of the tissues and biological membranes of that organ. Some membranes serve as barriers to the passage of medications. For example, the blood–brain barrier allows only fat-soluble medications to pass into the brain and cerebrospinal fluid. Thus, CNS infections often require antibiotics to be injected directly into the subarachnoid space in the spinal cord. Some older adults experience adverse effects as a result of the change in the permeability of the blood–brain barrier, with easier passage of fat-soluble medications.

Protein Binding

The degree to which medications bind to serum proteins such as albumin reduces their distribution. Most medications partially bind to albumin, reducing the drug's pharmacological activity. The unbound or "free" medication is its active form. Older adults and patients with liver disease or malnutrition have decreased albumin in the bloodstream. Because more medication is unbound in these patients, they are at risk for an increase in medication activity, toxicity, or both.

Metabolism

After a medication reaches its site of action, it becomes metabolized into a less active or an inactive form that is easier to excrete. **Biotransformation** occurs under the influence of enzymes that **detoxify**, break down, and remove biologically active chemicals. Most biotransformation occurs within the liver, although the lungs, kidneys, blood, and intestines also metabolize medications. The liver is especially important because it oxidizes and transforms many toxic substances. The liver degrades many harmful chemicals before they are distributed to the tissues. If a decrease in liver function occurs such as with aging or liver disease, a medication is usually eliminated more slowly, resulting in its accumulation. Patients are at risk for medication toxicity if organs that metabolize medications are not functioning correctly.

Excretion

After medications are metabolized, they exit the body through the kidneys, liver, bowel, lungs, and exocrine glands. The chemical makeup of a medication determines the organ of excretion. The kidneys are the main organs that excrete medications. Some medications escape metabolism and exit unchanged in the urine. Others undergo biotransformation in the liver before the kidneys excrete them. If renal function declines, a patient is at risk for medication toxicity. If the kidney cannot adequately excrete a medication, it becomes necessary for the health care provider to reduce the dose. Maintaining an adequate fluid intake (50 mL/kg/day) promotes proper medication elimination for an average adult.

Gaseous and volatile compounds such as nitrous oxide and alcohol exit through the lungs. Deep breathing and coughing help patients eliminate anesthetic gases more rapidly after surgery. The exocrine glands excrete lipid-soluble medications. When medications exit through sweat glands, the skin often becomes irritated, requiring you to teach patients good hygiene practices (see Chapter 16).

The GI tract is another route for medication excretion. The liver breaks down medications that enter the hepatic circulation and excretes them into the bile. After chemicals enter the intestines through the biliary tract, the intestines reabsorb them. Factors that increase peristalsis (e.g., laxatives and enemas) accelerate medication excretion through the feces, whereas factors that slow peristalsis (e.g., inactivity and improper diet) often prolong the effects of a medication.

TYPES OF MEDICATION ACTION

A variety of factors affect medication actions (Box 26.2). Understand that patients do not always respond in the same way to each successive dose of a medication. Sometimes, the same medication causes very different responses in different patients.

Therapeutic Effects

Each medication has a **therapeutic effect**, the intended or desired physiological response of a medication. For example, you administer morphine sulfate, an analgesic, to relieve a patient's pain. Sometimes, a single medication has many therapeutic effects. For example, prednisone, a steroid, decreases swelling, inhibits inflammation, reduces allergic responses, and prevents rejection of transplanted organs. Knowing the desired therapeutic effect for each medication allows you to accurately evaluate its desired effect.

Adverse drug effects

Adverse drug effects (ADEs) are unintended, undesirable, and often unpredictable responses to medication. Although ADRs are sometimes seen immediately, they often take weeks or months to develop. Early clinical recognition of ADRs is the important first step in identification. ADRs range from mild (e.g., rashes or photosensitivity to light) to potentially fatal (anaphylaxis). Prompt recognition and reporting of ADRs prevents serious injury to patients. Although some patients such as pregnant women, very young patients, and patients with chronic disorders (e.g., hypertension, epilepsy, heart disease, psychoses) are at a higher risk, assess all your patients for ADRs (Burchum and Rosenthal, 2016). Health care providers report adverse effects to their nearest PvPI center.

BOX 26.2 Factors Influencing Medication Actions

Genetic Differences

- A person's genetic makeup influences drug metabolism. Family members may have similar reactions to the same medication.

Physiological Variables

- Gender, age, body weight, nutritional status, and illnesses influence drug effects.
- Hormonal differences between men and women affect drug metabolism.
- Children usually require lower drug doses than adults.
- Changes accompanying aging influence drug effects.
- There is a direct relationship between the concentration of a medication administered and how quickly it is absorbed by tissues.

Environmental Conditions

- Stress and exposure to heat and cold affect drug actions.
- The setting in which a person takes a drug influences a patient's reaction. For example, when patients are alone or isolated, they may need more pain medication than if they were in a room with other patients.

Psychological Factors

- Attitudes, beliefs about the meaning of a drug, and perceptions of a nurse's behaviors can affect drug actions. Assess these factors in each patient. While administering drugs, demonstrate supportive behaviors and provide relevant instruction.

Diet

- Medication and nutrient interactions alter the action of a drug. For example, mineral oil decreases absorption of fat-soluble vitamins.
- Proper drug metabolism requires healthy nutritional levels.

Side Effects

Every medication has the potential for harm. No medication is totally safe and absolutely free of nontherapeutic effects. **Side effects** are predictable and often unavoidable secondary effects produced at a usual therapeutic drug dose. They either are harmless or cause injury. The intensity of side effects is often dose dependent. If the side effects are serious enough to outweigh the benefits of the therapeutic action of a medication, the health care provider will likely discontinue the medication. Patients commonly stop taking medications because of side effects such as anorexia, nausea, vomiting, dizziness, drowsiness, dry mouth, constipation, and diarrhea. Report any side effect to the health care provider to ensure that it is not incorrectly interpreted as a more serious adverse medication reaction.

Toxic Effects

Toxic effects develop after prolonged intake of a medication or when a medication accumulates in the blood because of impaired metabolism or excretion. Excess amounts of a medication within the body can have lethal effects, depending on the action of the medication. For example, a toxic level of morphine, an opioid, causes severe respiratory depression and death. Antidotes are available to treat specific types of medication toxicity. For example, naloxone, an opioid antagonist, reverses the effects of opioid toxicity.

Idiosyncratic Reactions

An **idiosyncratic reaction** is an unpredictable effect, in which a patient overreacts or underreacts to a medication or has a reaction different from normal. Predicting which patients will have an idiosyncratic response is impossible. For example, lorazepam is an antianxiety medication that may cause agitation and delirium when given to an older adult.

Allergic Reactions

Allergic reactions also are adverse unpredictable responses to a medication. Exposure to an initial dose of a medication causes a patient to become sensitized immunologically. The medication acts as an antigen, which causes antibodies to be produced. With repeated administration, a patient develops an allergic response to the drug, its chemical preservatives, or a metabolite. An allergic reaction ranges from mild to severe, depending on the patient and the medication (Table 26.2). Among the different classes of medications, antibiotics cause a high incidence of allergic reactions. Severe or **anaphylactic reactions**, which are life threatening, are characterized by sudden constriction of bronchiolar muscles, edema of the pharynx and larynx, severe wheezing, and shortness of breath. Some patients become severely hypotensive, necessitating emergency measures.

Hospitalized patients with known drug allergies commonly have their allergy information recorded in a clearly identifiable place. This allows all caregivers to be aware of each patient's allergies. In many health care agencies, this information is recorded in a special section of the electronic health record (EHR), on the front of a patient's hard-copy medical record or chart, in the medication administration record (MAR), or on a specially designed label that is applied to the front of a patient's chart. Patients also receive color-coded allergy identification bands to wear around the wrist. *Always record a patient's allergies in the MAR.* Patients who are cared for in other settings (e.g., home or community clinics) and have a known history of an allergy to a medication or substance should wear an identification bracelet or medal, which alerts all health care providers to the allergies in case a patient is found unconscious or is unable to communicate (Fig. 26.1). Patients commonly list having an allergy to a drug when it is not a true allergy but rather a side effect or ADR. For example, nausea is most often a side effect, whereas hives is a common allergic reaction. It is important to be aware of the difference between a true allergy and a side effect. Ask a patient to describe in detail what type of reactions he or she has experienced.

Table 26.2 Mild Allergic Reactions

Symptom	Description
Urticaria (hives)	Raised, irregularly shaped skin eruptions with varying sizes and shapes; eruptions have reddened margins and pale centers
Rash	Small, raised vesicles that are usually reddened; often distributed over entire body
Pruritus	Itching of skin; accompanies most rashes
Rhinitis	Inflammation of mucous membranes lining nose; causes swelling and clear, watery discharge

Medication Tolerance and Dependence

Medication tolerance occurs over time. It is usually noted clinically when patients receive more and more medication (higher doses) to achieve the same therapeutic effect (Bartlett et al., 2013). Medications that produce tolerance include opium alkaloids (e.g., morphine), nitrates, and ethyl alcohol. Patients hospitalized for acute illnesses usually do not develop tolerance. It may take a month or longer for tolerance to occur.

Medication tolerance is not the same as medication dependence. Two types of medication dependence (addiction) exist: physical or psychological. In psychological dependence, a patient desires the medication for benefit other than the intended effect. Physical dependence is a physiological adaptation to a medication that manifests by intense physical disturbance when the medication is withdrawn. Dependence is rare when patients receive medications for a short time such as for postoperative pain. If a patient is dependent on alcohol, a higher-than-usual medication dose is necessary for the desired effect of the medication.

Nurses and other health care providers play an important role in the care of patients with drug addictions. When patients with addiction are approached by health care providers with disdain and rejection, no matter how subtly, they may reject the care offered. Negative behaviors such as these may result in a missed opportunity for a person who is addicted to learn about important treatments. Incorporating harm reduction strategies and evidence-based interventions in the care of patients with addiction can help them get the care and treatment they need (Bartlett et al., 2013).

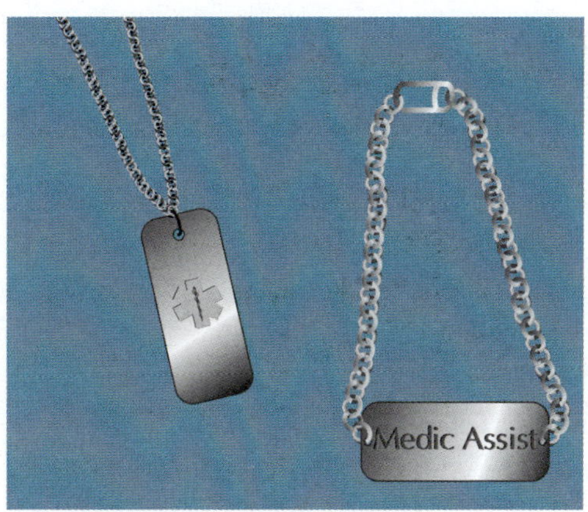

Fig. 26.1 Identification bracelet and medal.

Medication Interactions

In a **medication interaction**, one medication modifies the action of another. Medication interactions are common in individuals who take several medications. Some medications increase or reduce the action of others or alter the way another medication is absorbed, metabolized, or eliminated from the body. In a **synergistic effect**, the combined effect of two medications is greater than the effects when given separately. For example, alcohol is a CNS depressant that has a synergistic effect on antihistamines, antidepressants, barbiturates, and narcotic analgesics.

Sometimes, a medication interaction is desirable. Health care providers order a combination of medications to create an interaction beneficial for the patient. For example, a patient with high blood pressure might take several medications such as diuretics and vasodilators that act together to reduce blood pressure when one medication is not effective.

Medication Dose–Responses

A medication undergoes absorption, distribution, metabolism, and excretion after administration. Medications take time to enter the bloodstream except when administered intravenously. When a medication is prescribed, the goal is a constant blood level within a safe therapeutic range. The **minimum effective concentration (MEC)** is the plasma level of a medication below which the effect of the medication does not occur. The toxic concentration is the level at which toxic effects occur. The safe **therapeutic range** is between the MEC and the toxic concentration (Fig. 26.2). When a medication is administered repeatedly, its serum level fluctuates between doses. The highest level is called the *peak concentration*, and the lowest level is called the *trough concentration*. After peaking, the serum concentration falls progressively. With i.v. infusions, the peak concentration occurs quickly, but the serum level also begins to fall immediately. Some antibiotic doses (e.g., vancomycin or gentamicin) are based on peak and trough serum levels. To determine a peak and trough level, a blood sample is collected 30 minutes before administering the drug (**trough**) and at the time when the drug is expected to reach its peak concentration (**peak**). The results of the blood test reveal whether the drug is reaching its therapeutic blood level.

All medications have a biological half-life, which is the time it takes for excretion processes to lower the serum medication concentration by half. To maintain a therapeutic plateau, a patient needs to receive regular fixed doses. For example, pain medications are most effective for some patients with cancer when they are given around the clock rather than when a patient intermittently complains of pain because the body maintains an almost constant level of pain medication (Burchum and Rosenthal, 2016). After an initial medication dose, the patient receives each successive dose when the previous dose reaches its half-life. The patient and the nurse need to follow regular dosage schedules and administer prescribed doses at correct intervals. Know the following time intervals of medication action to anticipate the effect of a medication:

- *Onset of medication action:* Period of time it takes after you administer a medication for it to produce a therapeutic effect
- *Peak action:* Time it takes for a medication to reach its highest effective peak concentration
- *Trough:* Minimum blood serum concentration of medication reached just before the next scheduled dose
- *Duration of action:* Length of time during which a medication is present in a concentration great enough to produce a therapeutic effect
- *Plateau:* Blood serum concentration reached and maintained after repeated, fixed doses

You and your patient follow prescribed doses and dosage intervals (Table 26.3). Health care agencies usually set schedules for medication administration. However, you can change this schedule based on your knowledge about a medication. For example, you work at an agency where medications ordered once a day are given at 0800 hours. Your patient has a medication ordered once a day that works better when given before bedtime; therefore, you adjust the time to give the medication accordingly. Acute care agencies also follow guidelines from the Institute for Safe Medication Practices (ISMP) to determine safe, effective, and timely administration of medications (Centers for Medicare and Medicaid Services [CMS], 2011; ISMP, 2011a). According to the guidelines, hospitals determine whether medications are time-critical. Medications that are time-critical most likely cause harm or have subtherapeutic effects if they are not administered on time (usually

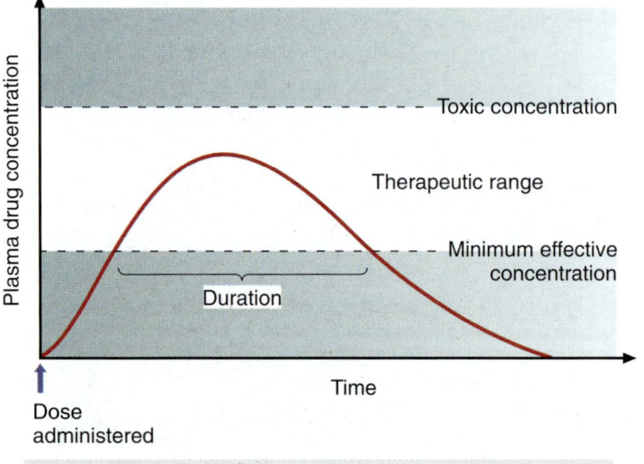

Fig. 26.2 Single-dose time course for an oral medication.

Table 26.3 Common Dosage Administration Schedules

Dosage Schedule	Abbreviation
Before meals	AC, ac
Twice each day	BID, b.i.d.
After meals	PC, pc
Whenever there is a need	prn
Every morning, every a.m.	q am
Every hour	qh
Every day	Daily
Every 4 h	Q4h
Four times per day	QID, q.i.d.
Give immediately	STAT, stat
Three times per day	TID, t.i.d.

30 minutes before or after the scheduled dose). Non-time-critical medications most likely do not cause harm if they are given within 1–2 hours before or after the scheduled time. Thus, you need to administer time-critical medications at a precise time, within 30 minutes before or after their scheduled time. You administer non-time-critical medications within 1–2 hours of their scheduled time. Ensure that you follow your agency medication policies about the timing of medications to ensure that your patients receive their medications at the right time (CMS, 2011; ISMP, 2011a).

When you teach patients about dosage schedules, use familiar language. For example, when teaching a patient about twice-daily medication dosing, instruct him or her to take the medication in the morning and again in the evening.

ROUTES OF ADMINISTRATION

The route prescribed for administering a medication depends on its properties and desired effect and on a patient's physical and mental condition. Because of what you know about each patient, you need to collaborate with a health care provider in determining the best route for a patient's medical condition. Table 26.4 summarizes the factors that influence the choice of administration routes.

Table 26.4 Factors Influencing Choice of Administration Routes

Advantages of Route	Disadvantages/Contraindications
ORAL, BUCCAL, SUBLINGUAL ROUTES	
Convenient and comfortable Economical Easy to administer Often produce local or systemic effects Rarely cause anxiety for the patient	Oral route is avoided when the patient has alterations in GI function (e.g., nausea, vomiting), reduced GI motility (after general anesthesia or bowel inflammation), and surgical resection of GI tract. Oral route is contraindicated in patients unable to swallow (e.g., patients with neuromuscular disorders, esophageal strictures, mouth lesions) and patients who are unconscious, confused, or unable or unwilling to swallow or hold medication under tongue. Oral medications cannot be administered when patients have gastric suction and are contraindicated before some tests or surgery. Oral medications sometimes irritate lining of GI tract, discolor teeth, or have unpleasant taste. Gastric secretions destroy some medications.
PARENTERAL ROUTES (SUBCUTANEOUS, I.M., I.V., I.D.)	
Can be used when oral medications are contraindicated More rapid absorption than with topical or oral routes I.v. infusion provides medication delivery when the patient is critically ill or long-term therapy is necessary; if peripheral perfusion is poor I.v. route preferred to injections	There is risk of introducing infection. Some parenteral medications are expensive. Some patients experience pain from repeated needlesticks. Subcutaneous, i.m., and i.d. routes are avoided in patients with bleeding tendencies. There is risk of tissue damage. I.m. and i.v. routes have higher absorption rates, placing patients at higher risk for reactions. They often cause considerable anxiety in many patients, especially children.
TOPICAL ROUTES	
Skin	
Primarily provides local effect Painless Limited side effects	Patients with skin abrasions are at risk for rapid medication absorption and systemic effects. Medications are absorbed through skin slowly.
Transdermal	
Prolonged systemic effects with limited side effects	Medication leaves oily or pasty substance on skin and sometimes soils clothing.
Mucous Membranes[a]	
Therapeutic effects provided by local application to involved sites Aqueous solutions readily absorbed and capable of causing systemic effects Potential route of administration when oral medications are contraindicated	Mucous membranes are highly sensitive to some medication concentrations. Patients with ruptured eardrum cannot receive ear irrigations. Insertion of rectal and vaginal medication often causes embarrassment. Rectal suppositories are contraindicated if the patient has had rectal surgery or if active rectal bleeding is present.
OTHER ROUTES	
Inhalation	
Provides rapid relief for local respiratory problems Used for introduction of general anesthetic gases	Some local agents cause serious systemic effects.
Intraocular Disk	
Route advantageous because it does not require frequent administration such as with eye drops	Local reactions are possible. Medication is expensive. Patients must be taught to insert and remove disk. Intraocular disks are contraindicated with eye infections.

GI, gastrointestinal; *i.d.*, intradermal; *i.m.*, intramuscular; *i.v.*, intravenous.
[a]Includes eyes, ears, nose, vagina, rectum, and ostomy.

Oral Routes

The **oral route** is the easiest and the most frequent route of medication administration. Medications are given by mouth and swallowed with fluid. Oral medications have a slower onset of action and a more prolonged effect than parenteral medications. Patients generally prefer the oral route.

Sublingual Administration

Sublingual medications (e.g., nitroglycerin, certain enzymes) are readily absorbed when placed under the tongue to dissolve (Fig. 26.3). The area under the tongue is highly vascular, making absorption rapid. Instruct patients not to swallow a **sublingual** medication or drink anything until the medication is completely dissolved to ensure that the medication will produce the desired effect. A sublingual medication may also be ordered if the effects will be lessened during the digestion process. The drug is not metabolized through the liver, and thus a lower dose can be used.

Buccal Administration

A medication is administered by the **buccal** route by placing the solid medication in the mouth against the mucous membranes of the cheek until it dissolves. The cheek is very vascular. Teach patients to alternate cheeks with each subsequent dose to avoid mucosal irritation. Warn patients not to chew or swallow the medication or to take any liquids with it. A buccal medication acts locally on the mucosa or systemically as it is swallowed in a person's saliva.

Parenteral Routes

In **parenteral administration**, you inject a medication into body tissues and not by the GI tract. The four major sites of injection are as follows:

- **Intradermal (i.d.):** Injection into the dermis just under the epidermis
- **Subcutaneous:** Injection into tissues just below the dermis of the skin
- **I.m.:** Injection into a muscle
- **I.v.:** Injection into a vein

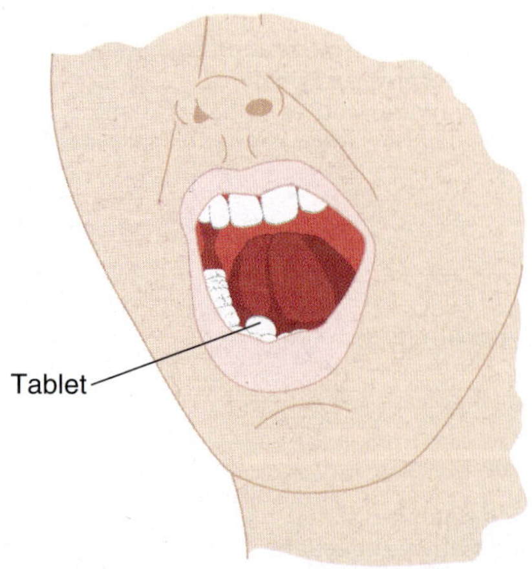

Fig. 26.3 Sublingual administration of tablet.

Health care providers administer some medications into body cavities through other parenteral routes including epidural, intrathecal, intraperitoneal, intrapleural, and intra-arterial. Nurses usually do not administer medications through these routes. Irrespective of whether you actually administer a medication by these less common routes, you remain responsible for the following:

- Monitoring the integrity of the medication delivery system
- Understanding the therapeutic value of the medication
- Evaluating a patient's response to the therapy

Topical Administration

Medications applied to the skin and mucous membranes generally have local effects. You apply topical medications to the skin through one of the following methods:

- Painting or spreading the medication over an area
- Applying moist dressings
- Soaking body parts in a solution
- Giving medicated baths

Systemic effects often occur if a patient's skin is thin or has broken down, the medication concentration is high, or contact with the skin is prolonged. A **transdermal disk** or patch (e.g., nitroglycerin, scopolamine, and estrogens) has systemic effects. The disk secures the medicated ointment to the skin. The nurse may leave a topical application in place for 12 hours to 7 days.

You apply topical medications to mucous membranes by:

- Direct application of a liquid or ointment (e.g., instilling eye drops, gargling, or swabbing the throat)
- Insertion of a medication into a body cavity (e.g., placing a suppository in the rectum or vagina or inserting medicated packing into the vagina)
- Instillation of fluid into a body cavity (e.g., ear drops, nose drops, or bladder and rectal **instillation**); the fluid is retained
- Irrigation of a body cavity (e.g., flushing eye, ear, vagina, bladder, or rectum) with medicated fluid; the fluid is not retained
- Spraying a medication into a body cavity (e.g., instillation into nose and throat)

Inhalation Route

The deeper passages of the respiratory tract provide a large surface area for inhaled medications to be absorbed, resulting in local or systemic effects. You administer inhaled medications into the pulmonary airways via the nasal and oral passages, where medication passes from the pharynx and larynx into the trachea. Medications given by the inhalation route are readily absorbed and work quickly because of the rich vascular alveolar–capillary network in the pulmonary tissue.

Intraocular Route

Intraocular medication delivery involves administering medication into the eye by drops, ointment, or disk. As a patient blinks, eye drops clear rapidly through the tear ducts. To manage this, the drugs used to treat glaucoma, eye injuries, and other conditions come in very high drug concentrations (Bourzac, 2015). These high drug levels increase the chances of systemic side effects once the drops are absorbed. One intraocular route involves inserting a medication disk into a patient's eye. The eye medication disk has two soft outer layers that have medication enclosed in them. You insert the disk into the patient's eye, much like a contact lens. The disk remains in the patient's eye for up to 1 week (Lavik et al., 2011). Research is investigating the development of dissolvable optic disks (Bourzac, 2015).

SYSTEMS OF MEDICATION MEASUREMENT

Safely administering medications requires the ability to compute medication doses accurately and measure medications correctly. A careless mistake in placing a decimal point or adding a zero to a dose can lead to a fatal error. Check every dose carefully before giving a medication.

The health care industry in the United States and internationally uses primarily the metric system as the standard measurement system for medication therapy. Recently, the ISMP recommended that health care providers, pharmacists, and other health care professionals as well as pharmacy computer system and e-prescribing system vendors use only metric measurements in prescription directions (ISMP, 2011b). However, the household system (e.g., cups, teaspoons) may still be used in medication orders, particularly when health care providers write **prescriptions** or orders for medications that are to be taken at home by patients or administered by family caregivers. The ISMP (2011b) recommends that a household measure can be listed in parentheses in an order immediately following the metric measure, as follows: 5 mL (1 teaspoonful). It is also no longer recommended that the apothecary system be used as a system of medication measurement (ISMP, 2011b).

Metric System

As a decimal system, the **metric system** is the most logically organized and safest to use. Metric units are easy to convert and calculate using simple multiplication and division. Each basic unit of measurement is organized into units of 10. Multiplying or dividing by 10 forms secondary units. In multiplication, the decimal point moves to the right; in division, the decimal moves to the left. For example:

$$10\,\text{mg} \times 10 = 100\,\text{mg}$$

$$10\,\text{mg} \div 10 = 1\text{ mg}$$

The basic units of measurement in the metric system are the meter (length), liter (volume), and gram (weight). For medication calculations, only the volume and weight units are used, and lowercase or uppercase letters are used to designate units:

Gram: g or gm
Liter: l or L
Milligram: mg
Milliliter: mL

A system of Latin prefixes designates subdivision of the basic units: deci- (1/10 or 0.1), centi- (1/100 or 0.01), and milli- (1/1000 or 0.001). Greek prefixes designate multiples of the basic units: deka- (10), hecto- (100), and kilo- (1000). Use fractions or multiples of a unit when writing medication doses in metric units. Always give fractions in decimal form:

500 mg or 0.5 g, not 1/2 g
10 mL or 0.01 L, not 1/100 L

Many actual and potential medication errors occur with the use of fractions. For example, 1/4 can look like 14. Follow practice standards when medications are ordered in fractions to prevent medication errors. For example, to make the decimal point more visible, a leading zero is always placed in front of a decimal (e.g., use 0.5, not .5). Do not use a trailing zero (i.e., a zero after a decimal point) because if a health care worker does not see the decimal point, the patient may end up receiving 10 times more medication than that which is prescribed (e.g., use 5 not 5.0) (The Joint Commission [TJC], 2014a). Fractions used to express the number of tablets should appear in the font used for fractions (i.e., 1/2), with a redundant statement in parentheses (one-half) (ISMP, 2010).

Household Measurements

Most people are familiar with household measures, which include liquid measures such as drops, teaspoons, tablespoons, cups, pints, and quarts. Although household measurements are convenient and familiar, they are inaccurate. Dose errors have occurred when household measures are used (ConsumerMedSafety, 2015; ISMP, 2016b). As a result, the ISMP recommends a best practice for all oral liquids that are not commercially available as unit dose products. The liquids should be dispensed by the pharmacy in an oral syringe using metric measurement (ISMP, 2016b). The ISMP also recommends that patients or family caregivers purchase oral liquid dosing devices (oral syringes, cups, droppers) that display the metric scale only. Encourage patients to never use household measuring devices with liquid medicines. Over-the-counter (OTC) liquid medicines currently available almost always come with their own measuring devices (ConsumerMedSafety, 2015).

Solutions

Nurses use solutions of various concentrations for injections, **irrigations**, and **infusions**. A **solution** can be:

- A mass of solid substance dissolved in a known volume of fluid
- A given volume of fluid dissolved in a known volume of another fluid

When a solid is dissolved in a fluid, the concentration is in units of mass per units of volume (e.g., g/L, mg/mL). You also can express a concentration of a solution as a percentage. For example, a 10% solution is 10 g of solid dissolved in 100 mL of solution. A proportion also expresses concentrations. A 1/1000 solution represents a solution containing 1 g of solid in 1000 mL of liquid or 1 mL of liquid mixed with 1000 mL of another liquid.

Clinical Calculations

Often you will not prepare a medication for administration in the unit of measure in which it is ordered and delivered. Pharmaceutical companies package and bottle medications in standard dosages. However, a patient's order may be for a different dosage. For example, a patient is ordered to receive a 2-mg dose of a drug, but the drug is dispensed in 4-mg amounts. Another patient has an order for 1 g of a medication that is available only in milligrams. Accurate drug calculation is essential to administer medications safely. Use your mathematics skills to calculate dosages and mix solutions. You are responsible for converting available units of volume and weight to the desired doses. Know the approximate equivalents in all major measurement systems.

Conversions Within One System

When converting measurements within the metric system, you use division or multiplication. For example, to change milligrams to grams, divide by 1000 or move the decimal three points to the left:

$$1000\,\text{mg} = 1\text{ g}$$

$$350\,\text{mg} = 0.35\text{ g}$$

To convert liters to milliliters, multiply by 1000 or move the decimal three points to the right:

$$1\text{ L} = 1000\text{ mL}$$

$$0.25\text{ L} = 250\text{ mL}$$

To convert units of measurement within the household system, you need to know the equivalent. For example, when converting fluid ounces to quarts, you know that 32 ounces is the equivalent of 1 quart. To convert 8 ounces to a quart measurement, divide 8 by 32 to get the equivalent, 1/4 or 0.25 quart.

Conversion Between Systems

The conversion between measurement systems is becoming less common because of the recommendations for the use of the metric system for liquid medication dosing (ISMP, 2011b). Although health care providers are encouraged to order using the metric system, you may encounter a situation when you calculate the correct dose of a medication by converting weights or volumes from one system of measurement to another. For example, metric units are sometimes converted to equivalent household measures for medication administration at home. To convert from one measurement system to another, always use equivalent measurements. Tables of equivalent measurements are available in all health care agencies. The pharmacist is also a good resource.

Before making a conversion, compare the measurement system available with what was ordered. For example, a health care provider orders 10 mL of guaifenesin for your patient. To provide proper instruction to the patient, you convert "mL" to a common household measurement. By referring to an equivalents table, you determine that 10 mL = 2 tsp. Therefore, you instruct the patient to take 2 tsp of Robitussin.

DOSAGE CALCULATIONS

Dosage calculation methods include the ratio and proportion method, the formula method, and dimensional analysis. Use the method that is the most logical and comfortable for you. Use this same method consistently. Before you begin any calculation, make a mental estimate of the approximate and reasonable dosage. If your estimate does not closely match the answer you calculate, you need to recheck your math before preparing and administering the medication. Many nursing students feel uncomfortable or anxious when they have to do medication calculations. To enhance accuracy and decrease your anxiety, think critically about the steps you go through in calculating medications and practice doing calculations to feel more confident about your math skills.

Most health care agencies require a nurse to double-check calculations with another nurse when high-risk medications are prepared (e.g., heparin, chemotherapeutic drug, or insulin). The ISMP (2013c) recommends that the most effective double check is conducted independently by a second person to reduce the risk of bias that occurs when the person preparing and checking the medication is likely to see what he or she expects to see, even if an error has occurred. Because double checks take considerable time and have not consistently been found to prevent errors, independent double checks should be used only for very selective high-alert medications that most warrant their use (ISMP, 2013c). Consult agency policy regarding double checks of medications. *Always* have another nurse or health care professional double-check your work if the answer to a medication calculation seems unreasonable or inappropriate.

The Ratio and Proportion Method

A ratio indicates the relationship between two numbers. The numbers in a ratio are separated by a colon (:). The colon in the ratio indicates that you need to use division. Think of a ratio as a fraction; the number to the left is the numerator and the number to the right is the denominator. For example, the ratio 1:2 is the same as 1/2. A proportion is an equation that has two ratios of equal value. Write a proportion in one of the following three ways:

Example 1, 1:2 = 5:10
Example 2, 1:2::5:10
Example 3, 1/2 = 5/10

In a proportion, the first and last numbers are called the *extremes*, and the second and third numbers are called the *means*. If you multiply the extremes, you get the same result as if you multiplied the means. For example, in the preceding proportions, if you multiply the means and extremes, you end up with the following equations: $1 \times 10 = 10$ and $2 \times 5 = 10$. Because the numbers in a proportion are in a specific relationship with one another, if you know three of the numbers in the proportion, it is easy to calculate the unknown number. To use this method, you first need to make sure that all terms are in the same unit and system of measurement. After estimating the correct dose in your mind, set up the proportion, labeling all terms in the proportion. Place the ratio that you know (e.g., information on the drug label) first. Put the terms of the ratio in the same sequence (e.g., mg:mL = mg:mL). Cross-multiply the means and the extremes, and then divide both sides by the number before the to obtain the dosage. Always remember to label your answer. If your answer is not close to your estimate, recheck your math.

Example: A health care provider ordered 100 mg of phenytoin to be administered to a patient in a gastric tube. The solution comes in a bottle labeled phenytoin 125 mg/5 mL. Use the following steps to calculate how many milliliters to give:

1. Estimate the answer: The amount you have to give is a little less than the amount that is provided in the solution. Therefore, the patient needs a little less than 5 mL of medication.
2. Set up the proportion:

$$\frac{125\text{ mg}}{5\text{ mL}} = \frac{100\text{ mg}}{x\text{ mL}}$$

3. Cross-multiply the means and the extremes:

$$125x = 100 \times 5$$

4. Divide both sides by the number before x:

$$\frac{125x}{125} = \frac{500}{125}$$

$$x = \frac{500}{125}$$

$$x = 4\text{ mL}$$

5. Compare your estimate from Step 1 with your answer in Step 4: The answer (4 mL) is close to the estimated amount (a little less than 5 mL). Therefore, your answer is correct; prepare and administer 4 mL in the patient's gastric tube.

The Formula Method

When using the formula method to calculate medication dosages, you memorize the formula and substitute information from the medication order into the formula. Estimate what you think the answer should be; then place and label all the information from the medication order into the formula. Ensure that all measures in the formula are in the same units and system of measurement before calculating the dosage. If the measures are not in the same measurement system, convert the numbers to the same system before calculating the dosage. Calculate and label your answer. Compare your answer with your estimated answer; if your estimate is not similar to your answer, recheck your math. Use the following basic formula when using the formula method:

$$\frac{\text{Dose ordered}}{\text{Dose on hand}} \times \text{Amount on hand} = \text{Amount to administer}$$

The dose ordered is the amount of medication prescribed. The dose on hand is the weight or volume of medication available in units supplied by the pharmacy. It is expressed on the medication label as the contents of a tablet or capsule or as the amount of medication dissolved per unit volume of liquid. The amount on hand is the basic unit or quantity of the medication that contains the dose on hand. For solid medications, the amount on hand is usually one capsule or tablet. The amount of liquid on hand depends on the container (e.g., 1 mL or 1 L). The amount to administer is the actual amount of available medication that you will administer. You always express your answer in the same unit as the amount on hand.

Example: Your patient needs to receive meperidine, 50 mg i.m. (dose ordered). The medication is available only in ampules containing 100 mg (dose on hand) in 1 mL (amount on hand). You apply the formula method as follows:

1. Estimate the answer: The medication is a liquid; thus, you need to figure out the answer in milliliters. The amount that you need to give is half of what the dose is, so your answer is going to be about 0.5 mL.
2. Set up the formula:

$$\frac{\text{Dose ordered}}{\text{Dose on hand}} \times \text{Amount on hand} = \text{Amount to administer}$$

$$\frac{50\text{ mg}}{100\text{ mg}} \times 1\text{ mL} = \text{Amount to administer}$$

3. Calculate your answer:

$$\frac{50\text{ mg}}{100\text{ mg}} \times 1\text{ mL} = 0.5\text{ mL}$$

4. Compare your estimate from Step 1 with your answer in Step 3: Both your estimate and your answer are the same; prepare 0.5 mL in a syringe and administer it to your patient.

Dimensional Analysis

Dimensional analysis is also known as the factor-label method or the unit factor method. Because only one equation is needed and the same steps are used in solving every medication problem, you do not have to memorize formulas. Dimensional analysis requires you to use your critical thinking skills. Some nursing students who use dimensional analysis calculate medications more accurately than when they use the formula method (Koohestani and Baghcheghi, 2010). Use the following steps to solve medication problems using dimensional analysis:

1. Identify the unit of measure that you need to administer. For example, if you are giving a pill, you are usually giving a tablet or a capsule; for parenteral or liquid oral medications, the unit is milliliters.
2. Estimate the answer in your mind.
3. Place the name or appropriate abbreviation for x on the left side of the equation (e.g., x tab, x mL).
4. Place available information from the problem in a fraction format on the right side of the equation. Place the abbreviation or unit that matches what you are going to administer (determined in Step 1) in the numerator.
5. Look at the medication order and add other factors into the problem. Set up the numerator so that it matches the unit in the previous denominator.
6. Cancel out like units of measurement on the right side of the equation. You should end up with only one unit left in the equation, and it should match the unit on the left side of the equation.
7. Reduce to the lowest terms if possible and solve the problem or solve for x. Label your answer.
8. Compare your estimate from Step 1 with your answer in Step 2.

Example: A patient's health care provider orders 0.5 g of ampicillin to be given i.m. q8h. You have a vial of ampicillin that says 250 mg/mL. Calculate the dose to administer using dimensional analysis by following these steps:

1. *Identify the unit of measure that you need to administer:* This medication is given intramuscularly, which is a parenteral medication. Therefore, your answer will be in milliliters.
2. *Estimate the answer in your mind:* The medication order of 0.5 g is larger than 250 mg. Because the medication is in a vial of 250 mg in 1 mL, you will need to give more than 1 mL. Based on your knowledge about converting in the metric system, you convert 0.5 g to milligrams by moving the decimal point three places to the right. Therefore, 0.5 g is the same as 500 mg. The number 500 is 2 × 250; thus, the answer is about 2 mL.
3. *Place the name or appropriate abbreviation for x on the left side of the equation:*

$$x \text{ mL} =$$

4. *Place available information from the problem in a fraction format on the right side of the equation:* You are going to administer the medication in milliliters, so place the milliliter in the numerator.

$$x \text{ mL} = \frac{1 \text{ mL}}{250 \text{ mg}}$$

5. Look at the medication order and add other factors into the problem. Set up the numerator so that it matches the unit in the previous denominator: The order is for 0.5 g, and the medication is available in 250-mg vials. You know that 1 g = 1000 mg; add this conversion to your calculation.

$$x \text{ mL} = \frac{1 \text{ mL}}{250 \text{ mg}} \times \frac{1000 \text{ mg}}{1 \text{ g}} = \frac{0.5 \text{ g}}{1}$$

6. Cancel out like units of measurement on the right side of the equation.
7. Reduce to the lowest terms if possible and solve the problem or solve for *x*. Label your answer.

$$x = \frac{1000 \times 0.5}{250}$$

$$x = \frac{500}{250}$$

$$x = 2 \text{ mL}$$

8. *Compare your estimate from Step 1 with your answer in Step 2:* Your answer is 2 mL, which matches the estimate you made in Step 2. Prepare and administer 2 mL of the medication as calculated.

Pediatric Dose Calculations

Children are at high risk for experiencing medication errors. The ISMP (2015d) reported that children are three times more likely than adults to have a harmful medication error or adverse drug reaction because of their size, immature renal and hepatic functions, and inability to communicate symptoms of adverse effects. It is not unusual for a child to receive either the wrong dose or the wrong amount of medication. The risk for medication errors is especially high because medication dosages are often weight-based, and many medications are packaged for adults.

Calculating children's medications dosages requires caution (Hockenberry and Wilson, 2015). Even small discrepancies or errors in medication amounts can negatively affect a child's health status. A child's age, weight, and maturity of body systems affect the ability to metabolize and excrete medications. For example, premature infants have underdeveloped livers and kidneys, which make them especially susceptible to the harmful effects of medications. As children develop out of the newborn period, they metabolize medications more quickly, resulting in the need for more frequent dosing of medications to achieve the desired effect of the medication. It is difficult to evaluate a child's response to medications, especially when he or she cannot communicate with you verbally. For example, a side effect of vancomycin, an antibiotic, is ototoxicity. If a child taking vancomycin cannot talk yet, assessing for ototoxicity is challenging.

Different methods are used to calculate medication dosages for children. Most of the time you use a child's weight to calculate the medication dose. You can use the ratio and proportion method, the formula method, or dimensional analysis to calculate a pediatric dose using body weight. BSA is used in rare situations (e.g., determining chemotherapy doses). If you have to calculate medication doses for a child, refer to a pediatric or pharmacology resource and consult with a patient's health care provider or pharmacist.

ADMINISTERING MEDICATIONS

In addition to nurses, a health care provider and pharmacist also help ensure that the right medication gets to the right patient. You are responsible to know which health care providers are able to prescribe medications. Health care providers who can prescribe medications include physicians, advanced practice nurses, and physician assistants. Practice acts vary by state, and policies vary by agency. Know your Nurse Practice Act (NPA) and agency policies when taking prescriptions and administering medications to protect your patient and yourself. In addition, you are accountable for knowing which medications are prescribed, their therapeutic and nontherapeutic effects, and a patient's needs and abilities related to medication administration. You also are responsible for evaluating the desired effects of a patient's medications.

HEALTH CARE PROVIDER'S ROLE

A health care provider prescribes a patient's medications by writing an order on a form in the patient's medical record, in an order book, or on a legal prescription pad. Medications may also be ordered through computers or handheld electronic devices (e.g., smartphones, tablets). Many health care settings use computerized physician order entry system to enter medication orders. Electronic ordering system requires a health care provider to enter essential information about the medication order, preventing incomplete and illegible orders, enhancing communication, and decreasing medication errors. In a systematic review of the literature, Radley et al. (2013) found that processing a prescription drug order through an electronic prescribing system decreases the likelihood of error on that order by 48%. The researchers also estimated a 12.5% reduction in medication errors, or approximately 17.4 million medication errors averted in the United States in 1 year, up to 2008.

In some situations, a health care provider talks directly with a nurse and gives a **verbal order**. Other times the health care provider gives the nurse an order over the phone; this is known as a *telephone order*. To ensure safety, telephone and verbal orders are given only when written or electronic communication between a health care provider and nurse is not possible (Box 26.3). The National Coordinating Council for Medication Error Reporting and Prevention (NCCMERP, 2015) recommends the following to reduce confusion pertaining to verbal orders and to minimize medication errors:

1. Limit verbal communication of prescription or medication orders to urgent situations where immediate written or electronic communication is not feasible.
2. Health care organizations should establish policies and procedures that do the following:
   - Describe limitations or prohibitions on the use of verbal orders.
   - Provide a mechanism to ensure validity/authenticity of the health care provider.
   - List the elements required for inclusion in a complete verbal order.
   - Describe situations in which verbal orders may be used.
   - List and define the individuals who may send and receive verbal orders.
   - Provide guidelines for clear and effective communication of verbal orders.

BOX 26.3 Guidelines for Telephone and Verbal Orders

- Only authorized staff members receive and record telephone or verbal orders. Institutional policies identify which members are authorized.
- Clearly identify the patient's name, room number, and diagnosis.
- Read back all orders to health care provider (TJC, 2018).
- Use clarification questions to avoid misunderstandings.
- Write "TO" (telephone order) or "VO" (verbal order) and include date and time, name of the patient, and complete order; sign the name of the health care provider and nurse.
- Follow agency policies; some require documentation of the "read-back" or require two nurses to review and sign telephone or verbal orders.
- Health care provider co-signs the order within the time frame required by the agency (usually 24 h; verify agency policy).

A nurse writes an order and the name of the health care provider, signs the order, and follows agency policy to indicate that the order was verified by reading the order back to the health care provider. The health care provider countersigns the order at a later time, usually within 24 hours after making it. Generally, nursing students cannot take medication orders, and verbal orders should be taken only in emergency situations. You cannot give any medication without an order.

Health care providers often use abbreviations when writing orders. The abbreviations indicate dosage frequencies or times, routes of administration, and special information for giving medications (see Table 26.3). Many medication errors occur because of the use of abbreviations. The ISMP maintains a list of abbreviations that are associated with a high incidence of medication errors (ISMP, 2015b) (Table 26.5). *Do not use these abbreviations* when documenting medication orders or other information about medications (TJC, 2016). Abbreviations often vary; check agency policy to determine which abbreviations you can use and what they mean.

Some conditions change the status of a patient's medication orders. For example, surgery automatically cancels all of a patient's preoperative medications. A transfer from a general medical unit to an intensive care unit also cancels

Table 26.5 Prohibited and Error-Prone Abbreviations[a]

The abbreviations, symbols, and dose designations found in this table have been reported to the ISMP through the USP-ISMP Medication Error Reporting Program as being frequently misinterpreted and involved in harmful medication errors. They should NEVER be used when communicating medical information. This includes internal communications, telephone/verbal prescriptions, computer-generated labels, labels for drug storage bins, medication administration records, and pharmacy and health care provider computer order entry screens. The Joint Commission (TJC) has established a National Patient Safety Goal that specifies that certain abbreviations must appear on the Do Not Use list of the accredited organization; they are highlighted with a double asterisk (**). However, we hope that you will consider others beyond the minimum TJC requirements. By using and promoting safe practices and educating one another about hazards, we can better protect our patients.

Abbreviations	Intended Meaning	Misinterpretation	Correction
µg	Microgram	Mistaken as "mg"	Use "mcg"
AD, AS, AU	Right ear, left ear, each ear	Mistaken as OD, OS, OU (right eye, left eye, each eye)	Use "right ear," "left ear," or "each ear"
OD, OS, OU	Right eye, left eye, each eye	Mistaken as AD, AS, AU (right ear, left ear, each ear)	Use "right eye," "left eye," or "each eye"
BT	Bedtime	Mistaken as "BID" (twice daily)	Use "bedtime"
HS	Half-strength	Mistaken as bedtime	Use "half-strength" or "bedtime"
hs	At bedtime, hours of sleep	Mistaken as half-strength	Use "bedtime" or "half-strength"
IU**	International unit	Mistaken as i.v. (intravenous) or 10 (ten)	Use "units"
o.d. or OD	Once daily	Mistaken as "right eye" (OD—oculus dexter), leading to oral liquid medications administered in the eye	Use "daily"

Continued

Table 26.5 Prohibited and Error-Prone Abbreviations[a]—cont'd

Abbreviations	Intended Meaning	Misinterpretation	Correction
Per os	By mouth, orally	The "os" can be mistaken as "left eye" (OS—oculus sinister)	Use "p.o.," "by mouth," or "orally"
q.d. or QD**	Every day	Mistaken as q.i.d., especially if the period after the "q" or the tail of the "q" is misunderstood as an "I"	Use "daily"
qhs	Nightly at bedtime	Mistaken as "qhr" or every hour	Use "nightly"
SC, SQ, sub q	Subcutaneous	SC mistaken as SL (sublingual); SQ mistaken as "5 every"; the "q" in "sub q" has been mistaken as "every" (such as a heparin dose ordered "sub q 2 hours before surgery" misunderstood as every 2 h before surgery)	Use "subcut" or "subcutaneously"
TIW or tiw	3 times a week	Mistaken as "3 times a day" or "twice in a week"	Use "3 times weekly"
U or u**	Unit	Mistaken as the number 0 or 4, causing a 10-fold overdose or greater (e.g., 4 U seen as "40" or 4 u seen as "44"); mistaken as "cc" so dose given in volume instead of units (e.g., 4 u seen as 4 cc)	Use "unit"
Dose Designations and Other Information	**Intended Meaning**	**Misinterpretation**	**Correction**
Trailing zero after decimal point (e.g., 1.0 mg)[b]	1 mg	Mistaken as 10 mg if the decimal point is not seen	Do not use trailing zeros for doses expressed in whole numbers
"Naked" decimal point (e.g., 0.5 mg)**	0.5 mg	Mistaken as 5 mg if the decimal point is not seen	Use zero before a decimal point when the dose is less than a whole unit
Abbreviations such as mg. or mL. with a period following the abbreviation	mg, mL	The period is unnecessary and could be mistaken as the number 1 if written poorly	Use mg, mL, etc., without a terminal period
Drug Name Abbreviations	**Intended Meaning**	**Misinterpretation**	**Correction**
HCl	Hydrochloric acid or hydrochloride	Mistaken as potassium chloride (the "H" is misinterpreted as "K")	Use complete drug name unless expressed as a salt of a drug
HCT	Hydrocortisone	Mistaken as hydrochlorothiazide	Use complete drug name
HCTZ	Hydrochlorothiazide	Mistaken as hydrocortisone (seen as HCT250 mg)	Use complete drug name
$MgSO_4$**	Magnesium sulfate	Mistaken as morphine sulfate	Use complete drug name
MS, MSO_4**	Morphine sulfate	Mistaken as magnesium sulfate	Use complete drug name
PCA	Procainamide	Mistaken as patient-controlled analgesia	Use complete drug name
Stemmed Drug Names	**Intended Meaning**	**Misinterpretation**	**Correction**
"Nitro" drip	Nitroglycerin infusion	Mistaken as sodium nitroprusside infusion	Use complete drug name
Symbols	**Intended Meaning**	**Misinterpretation**	**Correction**
Ð	Dram	Symbol for dram mistaken as "3"	Use metric system
×3d	For 3 days	Mistaken as "3 doses"	Use "for three days"
> and <	Greater than and less than	Mistaken as opposite of intended; mistakenly use incorrect symbol; "<10" mistaken as "40"	Use "greater than" or "less than"
@	At	Mistaken as "2"	Use "at"
&	And	Mistaken as "2"	Use "and"
+	Plus or and	Mistaken as "4"	Use "and"
°	Hour	Mistaken as a zero (e.g., q2° seen as q20)	Use "hr," "h," or "hour"

ISMP, Institute for Safe Medication Practices; *USP*, *United States Pharmacopeia.*
**These abbreviations are included on The Joint Commission's "minimum list" of dangerous abbreviations, acronyms, and symbols that must be included on the "Do Not Use" list of an organization, effective January 1, 2004.
[a]Applies to all orders and medication-related documentation that is handwritten (including free-text computer entry or on preprinted forms).
[b]Exception: A "trailing zero" may be used only where required to show precision of a reported value (such as laboratory test results), in studies that report the size of lesions, or for catheter and tube sizes. A "trailing zero" cannot be used in medication orders or medication-related documentation (Institute for Safe Medication Practices [ISMP], 2013a).
From The Joint Commission (TJC): *Facts About the Official "Do Not Use" List of Abbreviations*, 2016, https://www.jointcommission.org/facts_about_do_not_use_list/. Reprinted with permission.

all of a patient's medication orders, requiring the health care provider to write new orders. When a patient is transferred to another health care agency or to a different unit within a hospital or is discharged, the health care provider reviews the medications, reconciles the list, and writes new orders as indicated.

TYPES OF ORDERS IN ACUTE CARE AGENCIES

Health care providers make five common types of medication orders, based on the frequency and/or urgency of medication administration. As a nurse, it is important to understand the policies and procedures of your agency.

Standing Orders

You carry out a standing order until the health care provider cancels it by another order or until a prescribed number of days elapses. A standing order will sometimes indicate a final date or number of dosages. Many agencies have policies for automatically discontinuing standing orders. The following are examples of standing orders:

Quinapril 20 mg p.o. q12h
Azithromycin, 500 mg p.o. daily for 2 days, and then 500 mg p.o. daily for 7 days

Prn Orders

A health care provider sometimes orders a medication to be given only when a patient requires it for a specific situation, such as pain, nausea, or constipation. This is a prn order. The collection of objective and subjective assessment data and your nursing judgment determine whether a patient needs the medication. Often the health care provider sets minimum intervals for the time of administration. This means that you cannot give the medication any more frequently than when it is prescribed. An example of a prn order is

Magnesium hydroxide 30 mL p.o. prn for constipation

After administering a prn medication, document the assessment data you used to decide to give the medication and the time of medication administration. Frequently evaluate the effectiveness of the medication and record findings in the appropriate record. A prn medication order that includes a range (e.g., morphine sulfate 2–4 mg i.v. push q2–4h prn for pain) is unclear and frequently causes a medication error. If a health care provider writes an order with a range, ensure that the order follows agency policies. An example of a safer range order is the following: Increase morphine dosage 50%−100% if pain is moderate to severe.

When a provider orders multiple prn medications with the same action, the orders must identify the time each medication is to be used and how to use the medications in relation to each other. The following order is an example of a safe prn order for two medications used for treating constipation:

Docusate 100 mg p.o. t.i.d. prn for constipation
Bisacodyl 10 mg suppository rectally daily prn for constipation in addition to docusate if no bowel movement occurs in 2 days

Single (One-Time) Orders

A health care provider often orders a medication to be given only once at a specified time. This is common for preoperative medications or medications given before diagnostic examinations. For example:

Versed 6 mg i.m. on call to OR

STAT Orders

A STAT order means that you give a single dose of a medication immediately and only once. Health care providers usually write STAT orders for emergencies when a patient's condition changes suddenly. For example:

Apresoline 10 mg i.v. push STAT

NOW Orders

A NOW order is more specific than a one-time order and is used when a patient needs a medication quickly but not right away, as in a STAT order. Verify your agency policy to determine how much time you have to administer a NOW medication after it is ordered. Only administer medications ordered NOW one time. For example:

Give vancomycin 1 g i.v. piggyback NOW

Prescriptions

Prescriptions are written for patients who are to take medications at home. The prescription includes more detailed information than a regular hospital medication order because the patient needs to understand how to take a medication and when to refill the prescription if necessary. The parts of a prescription are included in Fig. 26.4.

Pharmacist's Role

Pharmacists prepare and distribute prescribed medications. They work with nurses and other health care providers to evaluate the effectiveness of medication therapy. In the Western world, pharmacists assess the medication plan, make recommendations for revisions, and evaluate a patient's medication-related needs. Pharmacists are responsible for filling prescriptions accurately and for being sure that prescriptions are valid. They rarely mix compounds or solutions except in the case of i.v. medications because most pharmaceutical companies deliver medications in a form ready for use. Pharmacists are responsible for ensuring the dispensation of the right medication, in the right dosage and amount, and with an accurate label. Clinical pharmacists also act as resources and provide information to nurses and health care providers about appropriateness of a medication for a patient's condition and characteristics of medications including actions, side effects, interactions, and incompatibilities.

DISTRIBUTION SYSTEMS

Systems for storing and distributing medications vary. Pharmacists provide the medications, but nurses distribute

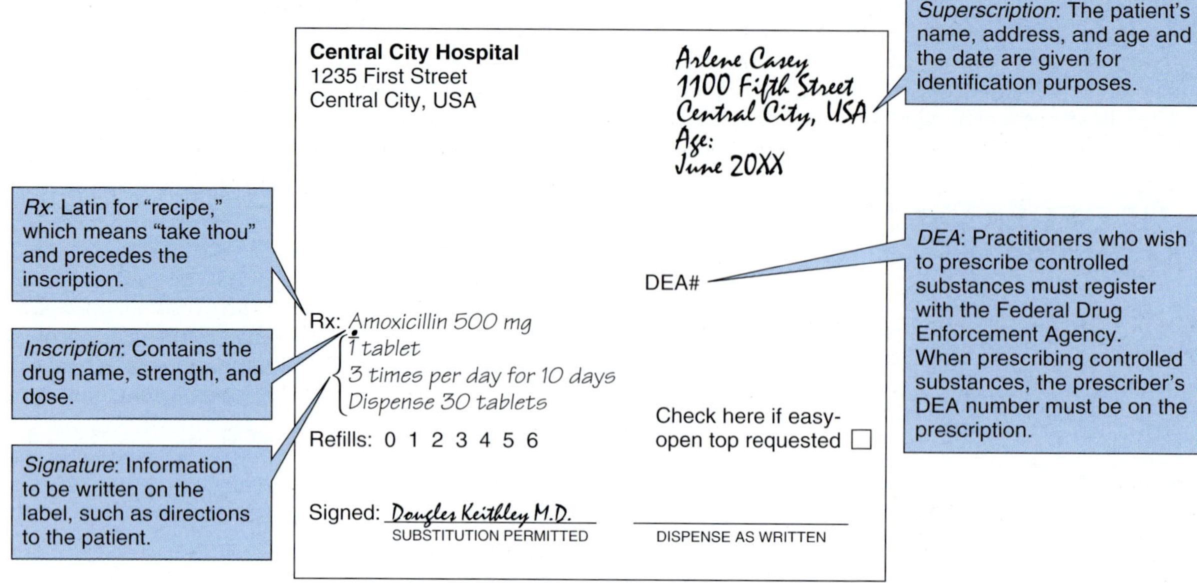

Fig. 26.4 Example of medication prescription.

them to patients. Hospitals have special areas for stocking and dispensing medications such as special medication rooms, portable locked carts, computerized medication cabinets, and individual storage units in patients' rooms. Medication storage areas need to be locked when unattended.

Unit Dose

The unit-dose system uses portable carts containing a drawer with a 24-hour supply of medications for each patient. The unit dose is the ordered dose of medication that a patient receives at one time. Each tablet or capsule is wrapped separately. At a designated time each day, the drawers in the cart are refilled by a pharmacy technician. The cart also contains limited amounts of prn and stock medications for special situations. The unit-dose system is designed to reduce the number of medication errors and saves steps in dispensing medications.

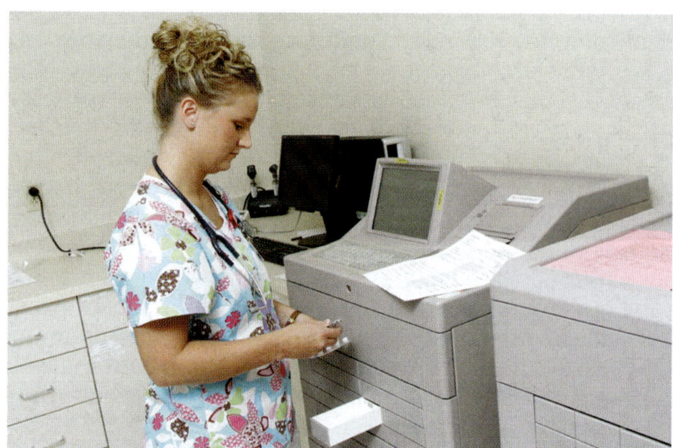

Fig. 26.5 Computer-controlled medication dispensing system.

Automated Medication Dispensing Systems

Automated medication dispensing systems (AMDSs) are used successfully throughout the United States (Fig. 26.5). The systems within a health care agency are networked with one another and with other computer systems in the agency (e.g., the computerized medical record). Research suggests that AMDSs have the potential for reducing nursing time, dispensing and medication errors, and costs in hospital units (Chapuis et al., 2015; Mandrack et al., 2012). AMDSs control the dispensing of all medications including opioids and other controlled substances. Each nurse has a security code that allows access to the system. If your agency uses a system that requires biometric identification, you have to place your finger on a screen to confirm your fingerprint so that you can access the computer. Once logged onto the AMDS, you select the patient's name and medication profile. Then you select the medication, dosage, and route from a list on the computer screen. The system opens the medication drawer or dispenses the medication, records the event, and charges it to the patient. If the system is connected to the patient's medical record, it records information about the medication (e.g., name, dose, and time) and the name of the nurse who retrieved the medication from the AMDS in the patient's medical record. Some systems require nurses to scan bar codes before recording this information in the patient's computerized medical record (Fig. 26.6).

Nurse's Role

When you administer medications to patients, you need knowledge and a set of skills that are unique to nursing. Responsibilities of medication administration include knowing medication therapeutics, assessing a patient for administration, administering medications correctly at the right time, monitoring and evaluating their effects, and assessing a patient's ability to self-administer medications.

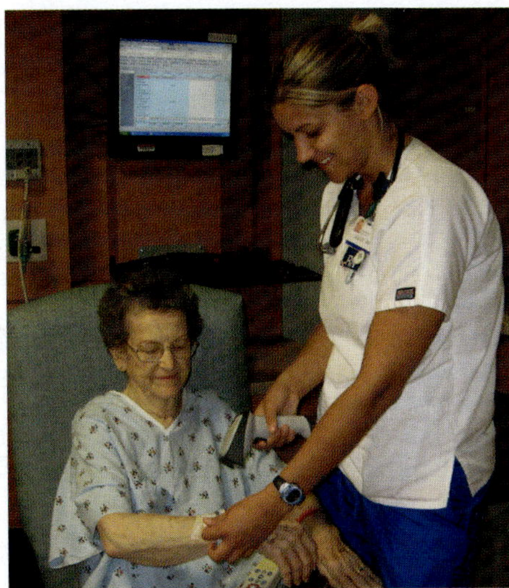

Fig. 26.6 Nurse using bar code scanner during medication administration.

Patient and family caregiver education about proper medication administration and monitoring is an integral part of your role. Never delegate this to nursing assistive personnel (NAP). Use the nursing process to integrate medication therapy into care.

MEDICATION ERRORS

A **medication error** can cause or lead to inappropriate medication use or patient harm. Medication errors include inaccurate prescribing; administering the wrong medication, dose, route, and time interval; administering to the wrong patient; and administering extra doses or failing to administer a medication. A patient death or serious injury because of a medication administration error is a serious reportable event (NQF, 2016), which makes the prevention of medication errors a national priority. The process of administering medications is very complex; thus, it is highly prone to errors. As a nurse, it is essential to be vigilant in prevention of medication errors during preparation and administration (Box 26.4). Advances in technology and informatics help decrease the occurrence of medication errors (Box 26.5).

Medication errors are often related to miscommunication among the members of the health care team, product design, or procedures and systems such as product labeling and distribution. When an error occurs, a patient's safety and well-being become the top priority. As a nurse, assess and examine a patient's condition and notify the health care provider of an incident as soon as possible. Report the incident to the appropriate person in the institution (e.g., manager or supervisor) once the patient is stable.

When a medication error occurs and you are involved, you are responsible for preparing a written occurrence or adverse event report within 24 hours of the incident. The report includes patient identification information; the location and time of the incident; an accurate, factual description of what occurred and what was done; and your signature. The report is not a permanent part of the medical record and should not be referred to in the patient's medical record. This legally protects the health care professional and agency. Agencies use occurrence reports to track incident patterns and initiate quality improvement programs as needed.

Report all medication errors including mistakes that do not cause obvious or immediate harm or near misses. You need to feel comfortable in reporting an error and not fear repercussions from managerial staff (NCCMERP, 2015). Many hospitals have adopted "just culture" environments. A just culture is a learning culture within a health care organization that is constantly improving and oriented toward patient safety and ensures balanced accountability for individuals and the organization responsible for designing and improving systems in the workplace (Boysen, 2013). These organizations create an open, fair, and just culture to learn from errors and then adopt improved systems and processes that minimize risk of human error. Even if patients suffer no harm from

BOX 26.4 Steps to Take to Prevent Medication Errors

- Prepare medications for only one patient at a time.
- Follow the six rights of medication administration.
- Be sure to read labels at least three times (comparing medication administration record [MAR] with label) before administering medication.
- Use at least two patient identifiers.
- Review a patient's allergies whenever administering a medication.
- Do not allow any other activity to interrupt administration of medication to a patient (such as a telephone call, pager, or a discussion with other staff) (Hopkinson and Jennings, 2013).
- Double-check all calculations and other high-risk medication administration processes (such as patient-controlled analgesia) and verify with another nurse.
- Do not interpret illegible handwriting; clarify with health care provider.
- Question unusually large or small doses or any dose outside of the recommended dosage range (or typically prescribed dose).
- Document all medications as soon as they are given.
- When you have made an error, reflect on what went wrong and ask how you could have prevented the error. Complete an adverse event report per institution policy.
- Evaluate the context or situation in which the medication error occurred. This helps to determine whether nurses have the necessary resources for safe medication administration.
- Attend in-service programs that focus on the medications commonly administered.
- Ensure that you are well rested when caring for patients. Nurses make more errors when they are tired (Murphy and While, 2012).
- Involve and educate patients when administering medications. Address patients' concerns about medications before administering them (such as concerns about appearance of medication or side effects).
- Follow established institution policies and procedures when using technology to administer medications (such as automated medication dispensing systems [AMDSs] and bar code scanning). Medication errors occur when nurses "work around" the technology (i.e., override alerts without thinking about them) (Voshall et al., 2013).

BOX 26.5 Informatics and Medication Safety

Medication errors frequently occur when a nurse incorrectly administers medications at a patient's bedside. Innovations in technology and informatics have reduced the number of medication errors in nursing practice:

- Networked computers allow health care providers to see a current list of ordered and discontinued medications.
- Internet and intranet access allows nurses and other health care providers to access current information about medications (e.g., indications, desired effects, adverse effects) and specific agency policies that address medication administration (e.g., how fast to administer an intravenous push [IVP] medication).
- Automated medication dispensing systems (AMDSs), bar coding technology, and electronic medication administration records (MARs) help with medication reconciliation, administration, and documentation.

Application to Nursing Practice

- Actively participate in the evaluation and selection of advanced technologies. Also participate in the development of nursing policies and protocols used for medication administration.
- Always follow agency policies when administering medications.
- Implement agency policies when technology cannot be used (e.g., during downtime or power outages).
- Follow manufacturer guidelines for care of electronic equipment and report problems with technology immediately.

BOX 26.6 Process for Medication Reconciliation

1. **Obtain, verify, document:** Obtain a current comprehensive list of a patient's medications whenever he or she experiences a change in health care setting (e.g., during admission, transfer, discharge). Include all current prescription and over-the-counter (OTC) medications.
2. **Consider and compare:** Review what the patient was taking at home or preadmission and make sure that the list of medications, dosages, and frequencies is accurate. Compare this list with the current ordered medications and treatment plan to ensure accuracy. Include family caregivers in this discussion when appropriate.
3. **Reconcile:** Compare new medication orders with the current list; investigate any discrepancies with the patient's health care provider and document changes.
4. **Communicate:** Ensure that all the patient's health care providers have the most updated list of medications. Communicate and verify changes in medications with the patient.

Data from Gleason KM, et al: *Medications at transitions and clinical handoffs (MATCH) toolkit for medication reconciliation*, Agency for Healthcare Research and Quality, AHRQ Publication No. 11(12)-0059, 2012, http://www.ahrq.gov/professionals/quality-patient-safety/patient-safety-resources/resources/match/match.pdf.

medication errors, agencies benefit from learning why mistakes occurred and what can be done to avoid similar errors in the future.

Medication errors frequently occur when a patient is transferred (e.g., to another health care agency or another unit within the hospital) or discharged. Therefore, reconciling a patient's list of medications during the transfer or discharge process is a National Patient Safety Goal (TJC, 2018). You play an important role in **medication reconciliation** (Box 26.6). It is a process in which you compare the medications that your patient took in the previous setting (e.g., home or another nursing unit) with the current medication orders whenever there is a transition in care (e.g., discharge or transfer) and when a new medication is ordered (Alexander et al., 2012; Infusion Nurses Society [INS], 2016). When a patient leaves that setting for another setting (e.g., skilled care facility or intensive care unit), you communicate the patient's current medications to the health care providers in the new setting. Most health care agencies have computerized or written forms used to facilitate medication reconciliation. Reconciling medications is challenging and requires a great deal of concentration and time. Eliminate distractions and take your time when reconciling your patient's medications. Always clarify information whenever needed by consulting with your patient, the patient's family caregivers, and the interprofessional health care team (e.g., physicians, advanced practice nurses, pharmacists) when reconciling a patient's medications.

SIX RIGHTS OF MEDICATION ADMINISTRATION

Professional standards such as *Nursing: Scope and Standards of Practice* (American Nurses Association [ANA], 2015) apply to medication administration. To prevent medication errors, follow the **six rights of medication administration** consistently every time you administer medications. Many medication errors can be linked in some way to an inconsistency in adhering to these six rights:

1. The right medication
2. The right dose
3. The right patient
4. The right route
5. The right time
6. The right documentation

Right Medication

A medication order is required for every medication that you administer to a patient. Health care providers sometimes write orders in patients' medical records by hand. However, most hospitals and outpatient practices now use some form of computerized prescribing system (AHRQ, 2016). Computerized prescribing systems were originally developed to improve the safety of medication orders, but modern systems now allow electronic ordering of tests, procedures, and consultations. Computerized prescribing systems allow a health care provider to order medications electronically, eliminating the need for written orders and improving medication safety (Radley et al., 2013). Regardless of the way a nurse receives a medication order, the most important step of this first right involves the nurse comparing the health care provider's written orders with the MAR or electronic MAR (eMAR) when it is first ordered. Nurses also verify medication information whenever MARs are created or distributed or when patients transfer from one nursing unit or health care setting to another.

When you have determined that information in a patient's MAR is accurate, use the MAR to prepare and administer medications. When you prepare medications, compare the label of the medication container with the MAR *three times*:

1. Before removing the container from the drawer, compartment, or shelf
2. As the amount of medication ordered is removed from the container
3. At the patient's bedside before administering the medication to the patient

Never prepare medications from unmarked containers or containers with illegible labels (TJC, 2018). When taking unit-dose packaged medications out of the medication dispensing system, compare the label of the medication with the MAR. Finally, compare all medications at the patient's bedside with the patient's MAR, and use at least two identifiers (patient's name verbally or on ID band, patient's date of birth, or medical record number) before giving the patient any medications (TJC, 2018).

Patients who self-administer medications must keep them in their original labeled containers, separate from other medications, to avoid confusion. Many agencies require that nurses administer all medications rather than letting patients self-administer to maintain accuracy and patient safety. Because the nurse who administers the medication is responsible for any related errors, nurses administer only the medications they prepare. You cannot delegate preparation of medication to another person and then administer the medication to the patient. If a patient questions the medication, do not ignore this concern. A patient or a family caregiver familiar with a patient's medications often knows whether a medication differs from those received previously. In most such cases, the patient's medication order has changed. In some cases, however, patient questions reveal an error.

When a patient questions a medication, withhold the medication and recheck it against the health care provider's orders. If a patient refuses a medication, discard it rather than returning it to the original container. Unit-dose medications can be saved if they are not opened. If a patient refuses narcotics, follow proper institution procedure by having someone else witness the "wasted" medication.

Right Dose

The unit-dose system is designed to minimize errors. When you withdraw a medication from a larger volume or strength than needed, or when the health care provider orders a system of measurement that differs from the pharmacy system of measurement, the risk of error increases. When you calculate medication dosages or conversions, you must have another qualified nurse check the calculation. Prepare medications accurately by using standard measurement devices such as graduated cups, syringes, and scaled droppers. Educate patients to use similar measurement devices at home such as measuring spoons with metric calibrations rather than household teaspoons and tablespoons, which are inaccurate.

Splitting pills often leads to medication errors. To ensure patient safety in inpatient settings, pharmacists split the medications, label them, package them, and then send them to the nurse for administration. Because pill splitting is particularly risky in the home care setting, the FDA (2013) developed suggestions to help patients split pills. These suggestions include ensuring that the tablet is designed to be split, using a tablet splitter, not splitting the entire prescription at one time, and determining whether the patient has the motor dexterity or visual acuity to split tablets. If possible, health care providers should avoid ordering medications that require splitting.

Tablets are sometimes crushed and mixed with food. Always clean a crushing device thoroughly before crushing a new tablet. Remnants of previously crushed medications increase the concentration of a medication or cause a patient to receive part of a medication that was not prescribed. Mix crushed medications with very small amounts of food or liquid (such as a single tablespoon). Do not use a patient's favorite foods or liquids because medications alter their taste and reduce the patient's desire for the medication. This is especially a concern for pediatric patients. Not all medications are suitable for crushing. Some medications (such as extended-release capsules) have special coatings to prevent them from being absorbed too quickly. These medications should not be crushed. Refer to the ISMP "Do Not Crush List" available at http://www.ismp.org/tools/donotcrush.pdf (ISMP, 2015c) to ensure that a medication is safe to crush.

Right Patient

A patient getting a drug intended for another patient is a common medication error. There are often two or more patients with the same last name on a patient care unit. Thus, you must be sure that you give the right medication to the right patient. Remembering every patient's name and face is impossible. Before you administer a medication, use at least two patient identifiers (TJC, 2018). Acceptable patient identifiers include the following:

1. A patient's name on an armband
2. A patient stating his or her name or an identification number assigned by a health care agency
3. A patient's date of birth on an armband
4. A patient's social security number
5. A patient's phone number (note that phone numbers can change at any time)

Do not use a patient's room number as an identifier. To identify a patient correctly in an acute care setting, compare the patient identifiers on the MAR with the patient's identification bracelet while at his or her bedside. If an identification bracelet becomes illegible or is missing, get a new one for the patient. Health care settings that are not acute care settings do not require the use of armbands for identification. However, you still need to use a system that verifies the patient's identification with at least two identifiers before administering medications.

Implementing the required identification process requires you to collect patient identifiers reliably when the patient is admitted to a health care agency. Once the identifiers are assigned to a patient (e.g., putting identifiers on an armband and placing the armband on the patient), you use them to match the patient with the MAR, which lists the correct medications.

In addition to using two identifiers, some agencies use bar code medication administration (BCMA) to identify a patient (see Fig. 26.6). This system requires nurses to first scan a personal bar code that is commonly placed on the patient's armband. The nurse then scans a bar code on the single-dose medication package. Finally, the nurse scans the patient's armband again. All this information is stored in a computer for documentation. This system is designed to be in compliance with the six rights of medication administration and to prevent adverse drug effects. Safe use of BCMA requires proper organizational policies, and nurses need to be educated in best practices for BCMA to be most effective. Special care is required for medication administration in children (Box 26.7) and older adults (Box 26.8).

Right Route

Always consult the health care provider if an order does not include a route of administration. Likewise, alert the health care provider immediately if the specified route is not the recommended route. A patient's condition might have changed since the order was written, as in the case of a patient developing nausea and no longer being able to take an oral medication. Medication errors result from use of the wrong route (Teunissen et al., 2013). For example, when nurses prepare an oral medication in a syringe, the risk of administering the medication via the wrong route (such as intravenously) is very high. The ISMP (2011b) recommends that pharmacists, *not nurses*, prepare all oral medications as a unit product to ensure patient safety. Medications prepared commercially are an exception.

The accidental i.v. injection of a liquid designed for oral use produces local complications, such as sterile skin abscess, or systemic effects, such as a fatality. If you work in a setting that requires you to prepare oral medications, use only enteral syringes (e.g., ENFit) when you prepare oral medications. The new ENFit low-dose syringe has a male design feature within the ENFit female connector (syringe tip) that fits inside the fluid lumen of the ENFit male connector on the feeding tube (ISMP, 2015g). Enteral syringes often use a color different from the parenteral syringes and are clearly labeled for oral or enteral use. The ENFit syringe tips will not connect with parenteral medication administration systems (ISMP, 2017). Needles do not attach to enteral syringes, and the syringes cannot be inserted into any type of i.v. line. Label the syringe after preparing the medication and be sure to remove any caps from the tip of an oral syringe before administering the medication. Failure to remove the cap can result in the patient aspirating it, thereby blocking the trachea.

BOX 26.7 Tips for Administering Medications to Children

Oral Medications

- Liquids are safer to swallow than pills to avoid aspiration.
- Use calibrated droppers for administering liquids to infants.
- Offer juice, a soft drink, or frozen juice bar, if allowed, after the child swallows a drug.
- When mixing medications in other foods or liquids, use only a small amount. The child may refuse to take all of a larger mixture.
- Avoid mixing a medication in a child's favorite foods or liquids because the child may later refuse them.
- A plastic, disposable oral syringe is the most accurate device for preparing liquid doses, especially doses less than 10 mL (cups, teaspoons, and droppers are inaccurate).

Injections

- Use caution when selecting intramuscular (i.m.) injection sites. Infants and small children have underdeveloped muscles. Follow agency policy.
- Children are sometimes unpredictable and uncooperative. Make sure that someone (preferably another nurse) is available to restrain a child if needed. If restraint is necessary, have the parent act as a comforter, not restrainer.
- Always awaken a sleeping child before giving an injection.
- Distracting a child with conversation, bubbles, or a toy reduces pain perception.
- If time allows, apply a lidocaine ointment to an injection site before the injection to reduce pain perception during the injection.

BOX 26.8 Medication Administration Safety for Older Adults

- Frequently review a patient's medication history including use of over-the-counter medications, and consult with the health care provider to simplify the drug therapy plan whenever possible (Pasina et al., 2014).
- Keep instructions clear and simple, provide memory aids (e.g., calendar, medication schedule), and ensure that written information about medications is in print large enough for a patient to see (Touhy and Jett, 2014).
- Assess functional status (including vision, hand grasp, fine motor skills) to determine whether a patient will require assistance in taking medications (Touhy and Jett, 2014).
- Some older adults have a greater sensitivity to drugs, especially drugs that act on the central nervous system. Therefore, carefully monitor patients' responses to medications and anticipate dosage adjustments as needed (Touhy and Jett, 2014).
- If a patient has difficulty swallowing a capsule or tablet, ask the health care provider to substitute a liquid medication. If you must give an oral tablet or capsule, instruct the patient to place medication on the front of the tongue and then swallow fluid to help wash it to the back of the throat. If the patient continues to have problems, have him or her try taking medication with a very small amount of semisolid food (e.g., applesauce) (Touhy and Jett, 2014).

Right Time

To administer medications safely, know why a medication is ordered for certain times of day and whether you are allowed to alter the schedule. For example, two medications are ordered, one q8h (every 8 hours) and the other t.i.d. (three times a day). Both medications are scheduled to be administered three times within 24 hours. The health care provider intends for you to give the q8h medication every 8 hours around the clock to maintain therapeutic blood levels of the medication. In contrast, you give the t.i.d. medication at three different times during waking hours. Each agency has a recommended time schedule for medications ordered at frequent intervals. Use your nursing judgment to alter the recommended times if necessary or appropriate.

A health care provider often gives specific instructions for the timing of medication administration. A preoperative medication to be given "on call" means that you give the medication when the operating room staff members notify you that they are coming to pick up a patient for surgery. Give a medication ordered PC (after meals) within half an hour of a meal, when a patient has a full stomach. Give a STAT medication immediately.

Give priority to time-critical medications that must act at certain times and thus must be given at certain times. Hospitals designate medications that are time-critical and medications that are non-time-critical (CMS, 2011; ISMP, 2011a). You administer time-critical medications within 30 minutes before or after their scheduled time around the clock to maintain therapeutic blood levels. Examples of time-critical medications include antibiotics, anticoagulants, insulin, anticonvulsants, and immunosuppressive agents. Give all routinely ordered non-time-critical medications (e.g., laxatives, antihypertensives, vitamin supplements) within 1–2 hours before or after the scheduled time or per agency policy (CMS, 2011; ISMP, 2011a). Researchers found that medication administration time errors are the most common medication error (Teunissen et al., 2013).

Your clinical judgment is required when determining the proper time for administration of some medications. For example, administer a prn sleeping medication when a patient is prepared for bed. In addition, use your judgment when administering prn analgesics. For example, you may need to obtain a STAT order from the health care provider if a patient requires a medication before the prn interval has elapsed. Always document your call to a patient's health care provider to change a medication order.

Before a patient's discharge from a health care agency, evaluate a patient's eligibility for home care, especially if the patient was admitted because of problems with medication self-administration. At home, patients often have to take multiple medications throughout the day. Help plan schedules based on recommended medication intervals and a patient's daily schedule. Use calendars, daily dosage containers, or timers. Involve family caregivers in monitoring medication adherence. In addition, determine whether the medications are adequate or prescribed at therapeutic levels.

Right Documentation

Nurses and other health care providers use documentation to communicate with one another. Many medication errors result from inaccurate documentation. Therefore, always document medications accurately at the time of administration and identify any inaccurate documentation before you give medications. The components of a medication prescription are illustrated in Box 26.9.

BOX 26.9 Components of Medication Orders

A medication order needs to have all of the following parts:

Patient's full name: A patient's full name distinguishes the patient from other people with the same last name. In the acute care setting, patients are sometimes assigned special identification numbers (such as medical record number) to help distinguish patients with the same names. This number is often included with the order.

Date and time that order is written: The day, month, year, and time must be included. Designating the time that an order is written clarifies when certain orders are to start and stop. If a medication error occurs, it is easier to document the incident when this information is available.

Medication name: A health care provider orders a medication by its generic or trade name. Correct spelling is essential to prevent confusion with medications with similar spelling.

Dosage: The amount or strength of the medication is included.

Route of administration: A health care provider uses only accepted abbreviations for medication routes. Accuracy is important to ensure that patients receive medications by the intended route.

Time and frequency of administration: An order will also include the time and frequency of medication administration, which is essential information for anyone filling the order (prescription) or administering the medication including family caregivers. Orders for multiple doses establish a routine schedule for medication administration.

Signature of health care provider: The signature makes an order a legal request.

Before you administer a medication, ensure that the MAR clearly shows the following:

- The patient's full name
- The full name of the ordered medication (without abbreviations of medication names)
- The time the medication is to be administered
- The dosage, route, and frequency of administration

Common problems with medication orders include incomplete information, inaccurate dosage form or strength, illegible order or signature, incorrect placement of decimals, and nonstandard terminology. If you ever have any question about a medication order because it is incomplete, illegible, vague, or not understood, contact the health care provider before you administer the medication. The health care provider is responsible for providing accurate, complete, and understandable medication orders. If you are unable to contact the health care provider or resolve confusion about the medication, follow your agency policy. There is usually a chain-of-command call policy to determine who you need to contact next. Follow this policy until you resolve issues related to your patient's medication orders.

Some medications require you to assess a patient before administration (e.g., taking a blood pressure before administering an antihypertensive medication). Ensure that you document all preassessment data in a patient's medical record before administering the medication. *Record the administration of each medication on the MAR immediately after administration.* Never document that you have given a medication until you have actually given it. Inaccurate documentation, such as forgetting to document giving a medication or documenting an incorrect dose, leads to errors in subsequent decisions about patient care. Consider the following situation: A patient is to receive an antihypertensive medication at 1600 hours, but the nurse who gives the medication fails to document it. The nurse caring for the patient goes home, and you are the patient's new nurse for the day. You notice that the antihypertensive is not documented, so you assume that the previous nurse did not give the medication. You give the patient another dose of the medication. About 2 hours later, the patient develops hypotension, causing him to fall and break a hip when getting out of bed. Accurate documentation and follow-up with the nurse from the previous shift could have confirmed that the antihypertensive was given as ordered and could have prevented this situation.

Document the name of the medication, the dose, the time of administration, and the route in the MAR. Also document the site of any injections you give and the patient's responses to medications, whether positive or negative. Notify the patient's health care provider of any negative responses to medications, and document the time, date, and name of the health care provider who was notified in the patient's medical record. The efforts you make to ensure proper documentation help ensure safe care.

Maintaining Patients' Rights

Another important standard to apply in critically thinking about your approach to medication administration involves patients' rights; because of the potential risks related to medication administration, a patient has the following rights:

- To be informed of the name, purpose, action, and potential undesired effects of a medication
- To refuse a medication regardless of the consequences
- To have qualified nurses or physicians assess a medication history including allergies and use of herbals
- To be properly advised of the experimental nature of medication therapy and give written consent for its use
- To receive labeled medications safely without discomfort in accordance with the six rights of medication administration
- To receive appropriate supportive therapy in relation to medication therapy
- To not receive unnecessary medications
- To be informed if medications are a part of a research study

Know these rights and answer all patient and family questions courteously and professionally. Do not become defensive if a patient refuses medication therapy. Remember that every person of consenting age has a right to refusal.

ORAL ADMINISTRATION

The easiest and best route for administering medications is by mouth (see Skill 26.1). Patients usually can self-administer oral medications. Food sometimes affects absorption. Give medications on an empty stomach if this improves absorption. Likewise, give medications with meals if absorption is improved by food (Burchum and Rosenthal, 2016). Most tablets and capsules must be swallowed and administered with about 60–240 mL of fluid (as allowed).

The oral route is contraindicated in some situations (see Table 26.4). Many medications interact with nutritional and herbal supplements. Learn about these interactions to determine the best time to give oral medications.

An important precaution with any oral preparation is to protect patients from aspiration. Aspiration is the inadvertent entry of food, fluid, or medication into the respiratory tract when it is intended for GI administration. Protect a patient from aspiration by assessing his or her ability to swallow. Box 26.10 presents techniques to protect patients from aspiration. Use an interprofessional approach (such as with a speech therapist, dietitian, and occupational therapist) to determine the best techniques for patients who have difficulty swallowing (see Chapter 20).

Give special consideration when administering oral medications to patients with enteral or small-bore feeding tubes (Box 26.11). Failing to follow current evidence-based recommendations from the American Society for Parenteral and Enteral Nutrition (ASPEN) can result in tube obstruction, reduced medication effectiveness, and increased risk of medication toxicity (Malone, 2014). Tube misconnections continue to cause patient injury because tubes with different functions can be connected with Luer connectors. In response to this issue, the International Organization for Standardization (ISO) (TJC, 2014b) has developed tube

BOX 26.10 Protecting a Patient From Aspiration

- Allow patients to self-administer medications if possible.
- Know and assess for signs of dysphagia (difficulty swallowing): cough, change in voice tone or quality after swallowing, delayed swallowing, incomplete oral clearance or pocketing of food, and regurgitation.
- Assess the patient's ability to swallow and cough by checking for presence of gag reflex and then offering 50 mL of water in 5-mL allotments. Stop if the patient begins to cough.
- Position the patient in an upright seated position at a 90° angle with feet on the floor, hips and knees at 90°, head midline, and back erect if possible and if not contraindicated by his or her condition.
- Usually having the patient slightly flex the head in a chin-down position before swallowing helps prevent aspiration.
- Prepare oral medications in the form that is easiest to swallow.
- If the patient has unilateral weakness, place the medication in the stronger side of the mouth. Turning the head toward the weaker side helps the medication move down the stronger side of the esophagus.
- Give pills one at a time, ensuring that each pill is swallowed properly before the next one is introduced.
- Thicken regular liquids or offer fruit nectars if a patient cannot tolerate thin liquids.
- Some medications can be crushed and mixed with pureed foods if necessary. Refer to a medication reference to identify medications that are safe to crush.
- Avoid straws because they reduce the control a patient has over volume intake, which increases the risk of aspiration.
- Have a patient hold and drink from a cup if possible.
- Time medications to coincide with mealtimes or when a patient is well rested and awake.
- Administer medications using another route if risk of aspiration is severe.

BOX 26.11 Procedural Guidelines

Administering Medications Through a Small-Bore Feeding Tube, Gastrostomy Tube, or Jejunostomy Tube

Equipment

Medication administration record (MAR) (electronic or printed); appropriate medication syringe or 60-mL Asepto syringe for large-bore tubes only; enteral-only connector (ENFit) designed to fit the specific enteral tube (TJC, 2014b) (see illustration); gastric pH test strip (scale of 1–11); graduated container; medication to be administered; pill crusher if medication in tablet form; water or sterile water for immunocompromised patients; clean gloves; stethoscope and pulse oximeter (for evaluation)

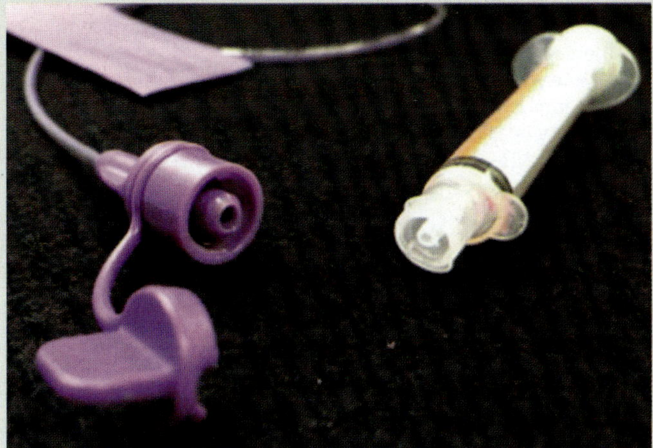

Steps

1. Check accuracy and completeness of each MAR with health care provider's medication order. Check the patient's name, drug name and dosage, route of administration, and time for administration. Clarify incomplete or unclear orders with health care provider before administration.
2. Review pertinent information related to medication including action, purpose, normal dose and route, side effects, time of onset and peak action, and nursing implications.
3. Assess for any contraindications to receiving enteral medications including presence of bowel inflammation, reduced peristalsis, recent gastrointestinal (GI) surgery, and gastric suction that cannot be turned off.
4. Avoid complicated medication schedules that often interrupt enteral feedings. Use alternative routes of medication administration if possible (e.g., transdermal, rectal, i.v.).
   a. Determine where medication is absorbed and ensure that point of absorption is not bypassed by feeding tube. For example, some medications such as antacids are absorbed in stomach, not in jejunum.
   b. Determine whether medication interacts with enteral feeding. If so, hold feeding for at least 30 min before giving medication (see agency policy or consult pharmacist).
5. Assess the patient's medical, medication, and diet history and history of allergies. List drug allergies on each page of MAR and prominently display allergies on the patient's medical record per agency policy. When the patient has allergy, provide allergy bracelet.
6. For a postoperative patient, review postoperative orders for type of enteral tube care.
7. Perform hand hygiene. Gather and review physical assessment data (e.g., bowel sounds, abdominal distention) and laboratory data (e.g., renal and liver function) that may influence drug administration.
8. Check with pharmacy for availability of liquid preparation for the patient's medications. Health care provider may need to change dosage form.
9. Before administration of enteral medications, verify placement of feeding tube (see Chapter 20), and determine that tube is placed in stomach or small intestine correctly.
10. Perform hand hygiene. Collect appropriate equipment and MAR.
11. Prepare medications for instillation into feeding tube (see Skill 26.1). Attend to procedure and avoid distraction. Check label of medication against MAR two times, when removing medication from unit dose or automated medication dispensing system (AMDS) and before leaving medication preparation area. *These are the first and second checks for accuracy.* Fill graduated container with 50–100 mL of tepid water. Use sterile water for immunocompromised or critically ill patients (Allen, 2015; Malone, 2014).

Clinical decision point: Make sure that concentrated liquid medications are thoroughly diluted. Never add crushed medications directly to tube feeding (Guenther and Boullatta, 2013).

   a. *Tablets:* Crush each tablet into a fine powder, using pill-crushing device or two medication cups (see Skill 26.1). Dissolve each tablet in separate cup of 30 mL of warm water.
   b. *Capsules:* Apply clean gloves. Ensure that contents of capsule (granules or gelatin) can be expressed from covering (consult with pharmacist). Open capsule or pierce gel cap with sterile needle and empty contents into 30 mL of warm water (or solution designated by drug company). Gel caps dissolve in warm water, but this may take 15–20 min. Remove and dispose of gloves.
   c. Prepare liquid medication (prepared by pharmacy in appropriate syringe).
   d. Perform hand hygiene.
12. Take medications to the patient at correct time (see agency policy). Consider whether medication is time critical. During administration, apply six rights of medication administration.
13. Identify the patient by using at least two identifiers (e.g., name and birthday or name and medical record number) according to agency policy. Compare identifiers with information on the patient's MAR or medical record.
14. At the patient's bedside, again compare MAR or computer printout with names of medications on medication labels and patient name. Ask the patient whether he or she has allergies. *This is the third check for accuracy.*
15. Explain procedure to the patient and discuss purpose of each medication, action, and possible adverse effects. Allow the patient to ask any questions about medications.
16. Assist the patient to sitting position. Elevate head of bed to minimum of 30° and preferably 45° (unless contraindicated) or sit the patient up in a chair (Malone, 2014).
17. If continuous enteral tube feeding is infusing, adjust infusion pump setting to hold tube feeding.
18. Perform hand hygiene. Apply clean gloves. Check placement of feeding tube (see Chapter 20) by observing gastric contents and checking pH of aspirate contents. *Gastric pH less than 5.0 is a good indicator that tip of tube is correctly placed in stomach.*
19. Check for gastric residual volume (GRV) (see Chapter 20).
20. Irrigate tubing.
   a. Pinch or clamp enteral tube. Draw up 30 mL of water into irrigation syringe. Reinsert tip of syringe into tube, release clamp, and flush tubing. Clamp tube again and remove syringe.
   b. Using appropriate enteral connector, attach to enteral tube.

Clinical decision point: Verify that connector meets the ISO tubing connector standards (TJC, 2014b). Do not attach enteral tubing to a standardized Luer syringe or needleless device (Guenther, 2015; TJC, 2014b).

Continued

BOX 26.11 Procedural Guidelines—cont'd

21. Remove bulb or plunger of syringe and reinsert syringe into tip of feeding tube.
22. Administer dose of first liquid or dissolved medication by pouring into syringe. Allow to flow by gravity.

Clinical decision point: If medication does not flow freely, raise the height of the syringe to increase the rate of flow or try having the patient change position slightly because the end of the feeding tube may be against the gastric mucosa. If these measures do not improve the flow, a gentle push with bulb of Asepto syringe or plunger of the syringe may facilitate flow of fluid.

   a. If giving only one dose of medication, flush tubing with 30–60 mL of water after administration.
   b. To administer more than one medication, give each separately, and flush between medications with 15–30 mL of water.
   c. Follow last dose of medication with 30–60 mL of water.
23. Clamp proximal end of feeding tube if tube feeding is not being administered, and cap end of tube.
24. When continuous tube feeding is being administered by infusion pump, if medications are not compatible with feeding solution, hold feeding for additional 30–60 min (Klang et al., 2013).
25. Help the patient to comfortable position and keep head of bed elevated for 1 h (see agency policy).
26. Dispose of soiled supplies, rinse graduated container and syringe with tap water, remove and dispose of gloves, and perform hand hygiene.
27. Document name of medication, dose, route, and time administered on MAR. Document the patient's response in nurses' notes of MAR in electronic health record (EHR) or chart.
28. Record patient teaching and validation of the patient's understanding on flow sheet or nurses' notes in EHR or chart.
29. Observe the patient for signs of aspiration such as choking, gurgling, gurgling speech, breath sounds, and difficulty breathing.
30. Return within 30 min to evaluate the patient's response to medications.
31. **Use teach back:** "I want to be sure I explained clearly why your father must take his medications through his feeding tube. Tell me why he is receiving his medications through his feeding tube." Revise your instruction now or develop a plan for revised patient/family caregiver teaching if the patient/family caregiver is not able to teach back correctly. Determines the patient's/family caregiver's level of understanding of instructional topic.

connector standards in which the enteral connector will no longer be Luer compatible. A new ISO enteral-only connector (ENFit) is now available to health care agencies, resulting in changes to enteral nutrition practices, policies, procedures, and processes per the new guidelines (ISMP, 2017; TJC, 2014b) (Box 26.12). Before giving a medication by the enteral route, verify that the location of the feeding tube (e.g., stomach or jejunum) is compatible with medication absorption. For example, iron dissolves in the stomach and is mostly absorbed in the duodenum. If it is administered through a jejunal tube, it bypasses the stomach and thus has poor bioavailability. Use only oral syringes, not parenteral syringes, when preparing oral medications for the enteral route to prevent accidental parenteral administration into an i.v. line. In prior adverse events, the inadvertent i.v. administration of an oral product has led to patient harm, including sepsis, emboli, or diffuse intravascular coagulation when injecting an unsterile solution with particulates into a patient's vein (ISMP, 2015f). ENFit connectors are engineered to make it nearly impossible to connect one delivery system to another delivery system that serves a completely different function—for example, accidentally connecting a feeding administration set to a tracheostomy tube, an i.v. tube to an epidural site, or a tube feeding administration to an i.v. line (ISMP, 2017; TJC, 2014b).

When giving oral medications enterally, flush feeding tubes with at least 30 mL of water before and after giving medications. When administering more than one medication, give each medication separately and flush the tube with 15–30 mL of water between medications.

Determine whether you need to give medications on an empty stomach or whether they are compatible with the patient's enteral feeding. If you need to give a medication on an empty stomach or it is not compatible with the feeding (e.g., phenytoin, carbamazepine, warfarin, fluoroquinolones, proton pump inhibitors), give the feeding at least 30 minutes before or 30 minutes after medication administration. Some medications require up to 120 minutes to be absorbed (Guenther and Boullatta, 2013). Verify the time with a drug reference or consult with a pharmacist. Monitor the patient closely for adverse reactions. The risk for drug–drug interactions is high when two or more medications are given via this route because they can interact as soon as they are administered.

BOX 26.12 The Joint Commission Recommendations for ENFit Enteral Tube Connectors

- Trace tubing from the patient to the point of origin:
  - Before connecting or reconnecting any device or infusion.
  - At any care transition such as to a new setting or service.
  - As part of a hand-off process with another health care provider.
- Route tubes and catheters with different purposes in standard directions (e.g., toward the head, toward the feet), and label proximal and distal ends of tubes.
- Use tubing and related equipment only for their intended use.
  - Never use standard Luer syringes for oral medications or enteral feedings.
  - Do not use i.v. tubing or i.v. pumps for enteral feedings.
  - Use distinctly dedicated pumps for i.v. applications.
  - Eliminate the use of temporary adapters on tubing.
  - Do not force a connection and avoid workarounds.
- Use safe practices for high-alert medications.
  - Label the tubing.
  - Do not use tubing with injection port.
  - Use an independent double-check procedure.
- Create a culture of safety and report adverse events.

Adapted from The Joint Commission (TJC): *Sentinel alert event: managing risk during transition to new ISO connector standards*, 2014, https://www.jointcommission.org/sea_issue_53/.

TOPICAL MEDICATION APPLICATIONS

Topical medications are applied locally, most often to intact skin. They come in many forms (see Table 26.1). They are also applied to mucous membranes.

Skin Applications

Because many locally applied medications (e.g., lotions, pastes, and ointments) produce systemic and local effects, apply these medications with gloves and applicators. Use sterile technique if a patient has an open wound. Skin encrustation and dead tissues harbor microorganisms and block contact of medications with the tissues to be treated. Before applying medications, clean the skin thoroughly by washing the area gently with soap and water, soaking the intended site, or locally debriding tissue.

Apply each type of medication according to directions to ensure proper penetration and absorption. When applying ointments or pastes, spread the medication evenly over the involved surface and cover the area well without applying an overly thick layer. Health care providers sometimes order a gauze dressing to be applied over a topical medication to prevent soiling of clothes and accidental wiping away of the medication. Lightly spread lotions and creams onto the surface of the skin. Rubbing often causes irritation. Apply a liniment by rubbing it gently but firmly into the skin. Dust a thin layer of powder over the affected area.

You apply some topical medications in the form of a transdermal patch that remains in place for a longer time (e.g., 12 hours or 7 days). Before applying a new patch, put on disposable clean gloves and remove the old patch. Medication remains on a patch even after it has been used for the recommended time. Nurses and patients have inadvertently left old transdermal patches in place, resulting in a patient receiving an overdose of the medication. For example, patients who use fentanyl transdermal patches for pain management can experience respiratory depression, coma, and death when the patches are not removed. In addition, some people, especially children, have experienced life-threatening harm from accidental exposure to fentanyl patches that were not disposed of properly (FDA, 2012). Many patches are clear, which makes them difficult to see. Therefore, carefully assess a patient's skin and be sure to remove an existing patch before applying a new one. Follow the below-mentioned guidelines to ensure safe administration of transdermal or topical medications:

- When taking a medication history or reconciling medications, specifically ask patients whether they take any medications in the forms of patches, topical creams, or any route other than the oral route.
- When applying a transdermal patch, ask the patient whether he or she currently uses a patch.
- Wear disposable clean gloves when removing and applying transdermal patches.
- If the dressing or patch is difficult to see (e.g., clear), apply a noticeable label to the patch.
- Use the MAR to document the location on the patient's body where the medication was placed.
- Use the MAR to document removal of the patch or medication.
- In most cases, dispose of patches by folding sticky sides of the patch together and disposing in a child-proof container. There are exceptions; a fentanyl patch, an adhesive patch that delivers a potent pain medicine through the skin, comes with instructions to flush used or leftover patches (FDA, 2012). Always read package directions.

MUCOUS MEMBRANE APPLICATIONS

Nasal Instillation

Patients with nasal sinus alterations sometimes receive medications by spray, drops, or tampons (Box 26.13). The most common form of nasal instillation is decongestant spray or drops. These are used to relieve symptoms of sinus

BOX 26.13 Procedural Guidelines

Administering Nasal Instillations

Delegation Considerations

The skill of administering nasal instillations cannot be delegated to nursing assistive personnel (NAP). The nurse instructs the NAP about:

- Potential side effects of medications and to report their occurrence to the nurse
- Reporting any bloody nasal drainage to the nurse

Equipment

Medication administration record (MAR) (electronic or printed); prepared medication with clean dropper or spray container; facial tissue; small pillow *(optional)*; washcloth *(optional)*; clean gloves

Steps

1. Check accuracy and completeness of each MAR with health care provider's medication order. Check the patient's name, drug name and dosage, route (which sinus), and time for administration. Clarify incomplete or unclear orders with health care provider before administration.
2. Review pertinent information related to medication including action, purpose, normal dose and route, side effects, time of onset and peak action, and nursing implications.
3. Assess the patient's medical and medication history and history of allergies. List drug allergies on each page of MAR and prominently display allergies on the patient's medical record per agency policy. When the patient has allergy, provide allergy bracelet.
4. Perform hand hygiene. Use penlight and inspect condition of nose and sinuses (see Chapter 7). Palpate sinuses for pain or tenderness. Note type of drainage if present.
5. Assess the patient's knowledge regarding use of nasal instillations, technique for instillation, and willingness to learn self-administration.
6. Perform hand hygiene. Collect appropriate equipment and MAR.

Continued

BOX 26.13 Procedural Guidelines—cont'd

7. Prepare medications for instillation. Attend to procedure and avoid distraction. Check label of medication against MAR two times (see Skill 26.1). Preparation usually involves checking label when removing nasal drops or sprays out of storage and before leaving preparation area. Check expiration date on container. *These are the first and second checks for accuracy.* Perform hand hygiene.
8. Take medications to the patient at correct time (see agency policy). Consider whether medication is time critical. During administration, apply six rights of medication administration.
9. Identify the patient by using at least two identifiers (e.g., name and birthday or name and medical record number) according to agency policy. Compare identifiers with information on the patient's MAR or medical record.
10. At the patient's bedside, again compare MAR or computer printout with names of medications on medication labels and patient name. Ask the patient whether he or she has allergies. *This is the third check for accuracy.*
11. Explain procedure to the patient and sensations to expect. Discuss purpose of each medication, action, and possible adverse effects. Allow the patient to ask any questions about medications. Patients who self-instill medications may be allowed to give drops under nurse's supervision (check agency policy). Tell patients receiving nasal instillation that they may experience burning or stinging of mucosa or choking sensation as medication trickles into throat.
12. Arrange supplies and medications at bedside. Perform hand hygiene and apply clean gloves (if drainage is present).
13. Gently roll or shake container. Instruct the patient to clear or blow nose gently unless contraindicated (e.g., risk of increased intracranial pressure or nosebleed).
14. Administer nose drops.
    a. Help the patient to supine position and position head properly (American Society of Health-System Pharmacists [ASHP], 2013b).
        (1) For access to posterior pharynx, tilt the patient's head backward.
        (2) For access to ethmoid or sphenoid sinus, tilt head back over edge of bed, or place small pillow under the patient's shoulder and tilt head back (see illustration).
        (3) For access to frontal or maxillary sinus, tilt head back over edge of bed or pillow with head turned toward side to be treated (see illustration).
    b. Support the patient's head with nondominant hand.
    c. Instruct the patient to breathe through mouth.
    d. Hold dropper 1 cm (1/2 inch) above nares and instill prescribed number of drops toward midline of ethmoid bone.
    e. Have the patient remain in supine position for 5 min.
    f. Offer facial tissue to blot runny nose, but caution the patient against blowing nose for several minutes.
15. Administer nasal spray.
    a. Help the patient into upright position with head tilted slightly forward.
    b. Instruct or assist the patient to insert tip of nasal spray into appropriate nares and occlude other nostril with finger. Point spray tip toward side and away from center of nose (ASHP, 2013b).
    c. Have the patient spray medication into nose while inhaling. Help the patient remove nozzle from nose and instruct to breathe out through mouth.
    d. Offer facial tissue to blot runny nose, but caution the patient against blowing nose for several minutes.

Clinical decision point: Some medications are designed for one spray per dose. Examples include calcitonin, desmopressin (DDAVP, Stimate), and sumatriptan. It is essential to ensure that the patient understands the correct number of sprays to use per dose to prevent overdosing.

16. Help the patient to comfortable position after medication is absorbed.
17. Dispose of soiled supplies, remove and dispose of gloves, and perform hand hygiene.
18. Document name of medication, dose, route, and time administered on MAR.
19. Observe the patient for onset of side effects 15–30 min after administration.
20. Ask whether the patient is able to breathe through nose after decongestant administration. It may be necessary to have the patient occlude one nostril at a time and breathe deeply.
21. Reinspect condition of nasal passages between instillations.
22. Ask the patient to describe risks of overuse of decongestants and methods for administration. Feedback ensures that the patient can self-administer medications properly.
23. Have the patient demonstrate self-medication.
24. Record patient response to medication, patient teaching, and validation of patient understanding and self-administration on flow sheet or nurses' notes in electronic health record (EHR) or chart.
25. **Use teach back:** "I want to be sure I explained the importance to not overuse your nasal spray. Explain to me why it is important not to overuse nasal sprays." Revise your instruction now or develop a plan for revised patient/family caregiver teaching if the patient/family caregiver not able to teach back correctly. Determines the patient's/family caregiver's level of understanding of instructional topic.

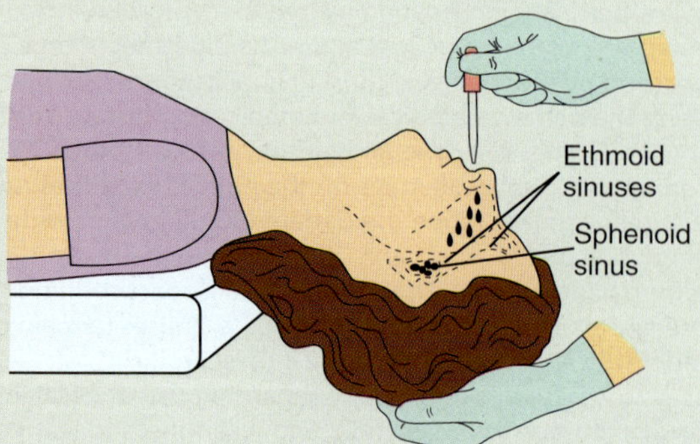

Step 14a(2) Position for instilling nose drops into ethmoid and sphenoid sinus.

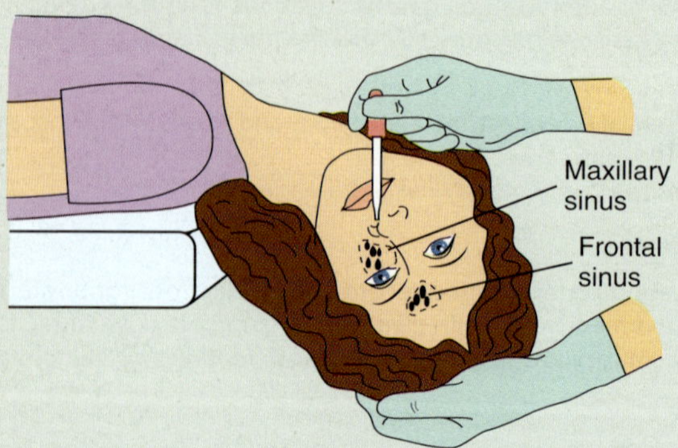

Step 14a(3) Position for instilling nose drops into frontal and maxillary sinus.

congestion and colds. Caution patients to avoid abuse of nasal medications because overuse leads to a rebound effect in which the nasal congestion worsens. When a patient swallows excess decongestant solution, serious systemic effects can develop, especially in children. Saline drops are safer as a decongestant for children than nasal preparations that contain sympathomimetics (such as Afrin or Neo-Synephrine).

Patients can more easily self-administer sprays because they can control the spray and inhale as the medication enters the nasal passages. Always check the nares for irritation in patients who use nasal sprays repeatedly. When a spray is prescribed for a sinus infection, position patients to permit the nasal medication to reach the affected sinus. Severe nosebleeds are usually treated with packing or nasal tampons and are treated with epinephrine to reduce blood flow. A health care provider usually places nasal tampons.

Eye Instillation

Ophthalmic medications in the form of eye drops and ointments are given for eye conditions such as glaucoma and conjunctivitis. Some eye drops are prescribed, and others are available OTC (e.g., Visine or Murine). Many patients who receive eye medications are older adults. Age-related problems including poor vision, hand tremors, and difficulty grasping or manipulating small containers affect the ability of older adults to self-administer eye medications. Educate your patients and family caregivers about the proper techniques for administering eye medications (see Skill 26.2). Evaluate the patient's and family caregiver's ability to self-administer through a return demonstration of the procedure. Showing patients each step of the procedure for instilling eye drops improves their adherence. Apply the following principles when administering eye medications:

1. Avoid instilling any form of eye medication directly onto the cornea. The cornea of the eye has many pain fibers and is very sensitive to anything applied to it.
2. Avoid touching the eyelids or other eye structures with eye droppers or ointment tubes. The risk for transmitting infection from one eye to the other is high.
3. Use eye medication only for a patient's affected eye.
4. Never allow a patient to use another patient's eye medications.

You administer some medications using an intraocular disk (see Skill 26.2). The disk remains in place for up to 1 week. Teach your patient receiving medications in this way to monitor for adverse reactions to the disk and explain methods of insertion and removal.

Ear Instillation

Because internal ear structures are very sensitive to temperature extremes, you must instill ear drops or irrigating solutions at room temperature to prevent vertigo, dizziness, or nausea. Although the structures of the outer ear are not sterile, sterile solutions are used in case the eardrum is ruptured. The entrance of nonsterile solution into the middle ear often results in infection.

If a patient has ear drainage, check with the health care provider to ensure that the patient does not have a ruptured eardrum before instilling the drops. Never occlude or block the ear canal with the dropper or irrigating syringe. Forcing medication into an occluded ear canal creates pressure that injures the eardrum.

Ear irrigations are performed when the external ear canal becomes occluded with cerumen and cannot be removed by more conservative measures such as wax softeners. Typically, an irrigation is performed only when a patient has a hearing deficit, a patient has ear discomfort, or it is necessary to visualize the tympanic membrane. You should not perform an ear irrigation if there is a history of middle ear infection in the last 6 weeks, if the patient has undergone *any* form of ear surgery, or if the patient has a perforation or there is a history of a mucus discharge in the last year. Box 26.14 provides guidelines for administering ear drops and ear irrigations.

BOX 26.14 Procedural Guidelines

Administering Ear Medications

Delegation Considerations

The skill of administering ear medications cannot be delegated to nursing assistive personnel (NAP). The nurse instructs the NAP about:

- Potential side effects of medications and to report their occurrence
- Potential for dizziness or irritation after administration of ear medications

Equipment

Medication administration record (MAR) (electronic or printed)
Drops: Medication bottle with dropper; cotton-tipped applicator; cotton balls; clean gloves if drainage is present
Irrigation: Irrigating solution and syringe; kidney basin; towel

Steps

1. Check accuracy and completeness of each MAR with health care provider's medication order. Check the patient's name, drug name and dosage, route, and time for administration. Clarify incomplete or unclear orders with health care provider before administration.
2. Review pertinent information related to medication including action, purpose, normal dose and route (one or both ears), side effects, time of onset and peak action, and nursing implications.
3. Assess the patient's medical and medication history and history of allergies (including latex). List drug allergies on each page of MAR and prominently display allergies on the patient's medical record per agency policy. When the patient has allergy, provide allergy bracelet.
4. Perform hand hygiene. Assess condition of external ear structures (see Chapter 7). This may be done just before drug instillation (apply clean gloves if drainage is present).
5. Determine whether the patient has any symptoms of ear discomfort or hearing impairment.
6. Assess the patient's level of consciousness (LOC) and ability to follow directions.

Continued

BOX 26.14 Procedural Guidelines—cont'd

7. Assess the patient's knowledge regarding drug therapy and desire to self-administer medication.
8. Assess the patient's ability to manipulate and hold ear dropper.
9. Perform hand hygiene. Collect appropriate equipment and MAR.
10. Prepare medications for instillation. Attend to procedure and avoid distraction. Check label of medication against MAR two times (see Skill 26.1). Preparation usually involves checking label when removing ear drops out of storage and before leaving preparation area. Preparation usually involves taking ear drops out of refrigerator and rewarming to room temperature before administering to the patient. Check expiration date on container. *These are the first and second checks for accuracy.* Perform hand hygiene.
11. Take medications to the patient at correct time (see agency policy). Consider whether medication is time critical. During administration, apply six rights of medication administration.
12. Arrange supplies at bedside.
13. Identify the patient by using at least two identifiers (e.g., name and birthday or name and medical record number) according to agency policy. Compare identifiers with information on the patient's MAR or medical record.
14. At the patient's bedside, again compare MAR or computer printout with names of medications on medication labels and patient name. Ask the patient whether he or she has allergies. *This is the third check for accuracy.*
15. Explain procedure to the patient and sensations to expect. Discuss purpose of each medication, action, and possible adverse effects. Allow the patient to ask any questions about the medications. Patients who self-instill medications may be allowed to give drops under nurse's supervision (check agency policy).
16. Perform hand hygiene (apply clean gloves if drainage present).
17. Administer ear drops.
    a. Position the patient on side (if not contraindicated) with ear to be treated facing up, or the patient may sit in chair or at bedside.
    b. If cerumen or drainage occludes outermost part of ear canal, wipe out gently with cotton-tipped applicator or washcloth. Take care not to force cerumen into canal.
    c. Hold container in the palm of your hands for a few minutes to warm the contents to body temperature. If ear drops are in a cloudy suspension, shake bottle for about 10 s.
    d. Straighten ear canal by pulling pinna up and back to 10-o'clock position (adult or child older than 3 years) or down and back to 6- to 9-o'clock position (child younger than 3 years).
    e. Instill prescribed drops holding dropper 1 cm (1/2 inch) above ear canal. Avoid contact of dropper tip against external ear canal (see illustration).
    f. Ask the patient to remain in side-lying position for a few minutes. Apply gentle massage or pressure to tragus of ear with finger.
    g. If ordered, gently insert part of cotton ball into outermost part of canal. Do not press cotton into canal.
    h. Remove cotton after 15 min. Help the patient to comfortable position after drops are absorbed.
18. Administer ear irrigations.

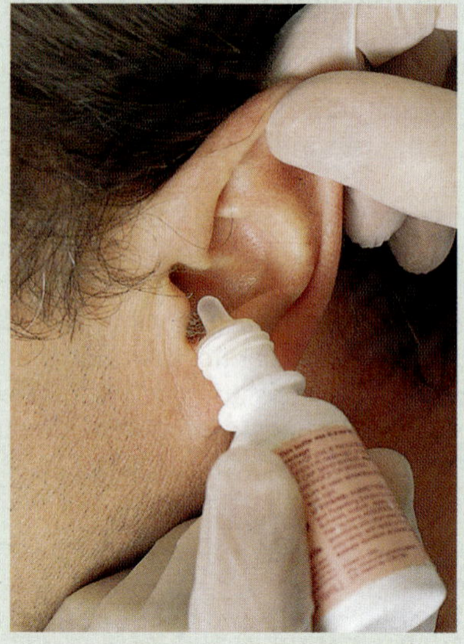

Step 17e Instill prescribed drops holding dropper above ear canal.

    a. Assess tympanic membrane or review medication record for history of eardrum perforation, which contraindicates ear irrigation.
    b. Help the patient into sitting position or lying position with head tilted or turned toward affected ear. Place towel under the patient's head and shoulder and have the patient hold basin under affected ear.
    c. Fill irrigating syringe with solution (approximately 50 mL) at room temperature.
    d. Gently grasp auricle and straighten ear by pulling pinna down and back for children younger than 3 years or upward and outward for adults and children 3 years and older.
    e. Slowly instill irrigating solution by holding tip of syringe 1 cm (1/2 inch) above opening of ear canal. Allow fluid to drain out during instillation. Continue until you use all solution.
19. Clean area and put supplies away.
20. Remove gloves and perform hand hygiene.
21. Record drug, concentration, dose or strength, number of drops, site of application (left, right, or both ears), and time of administration on MAR immediately after administration.
22. Observe response to medication by assessing hearing changes, asking whether symptoms are relieved, and noting any side effects or discomfort felt.
23. Ask the patient to discuss purpose of drug, action, side effects, and technique of administration.
24. Record patient response to medication, patient teaching, and validation of patient understanding and self-administration on flow sheet or nurses' notes in electronic health record (EHR) or chart.
25. **Use teach back:** "I want to be sure I clearly showed you how to give yourself ear drops. Show me how to place ear drops in your ear." Revise your instruction now or develop a plan for revised patient/family caregiver teaching if the patient/family caregiver is not able to teach back correctly.

Vaginal Instillation

Vaginal medications are available as suppositories, foam, jellies, and creams. Solid, oval-shaped suppositories are packaged individually in foil wrappers and are sometimes stored in the refrigerator to prevent them from melting. After a suppository is inserted into the vaginal cavity, body temperature causes it to melt and be distributed and absorbed. Foam, jellies, and creams are administered with an applicator inserter (Box 26.15).

Give a suppository with a gloved hand in accordance with standard precautions (see Chapter 9). Patients often

BOX 26.15 Procedural Guidelines

Administering Vaginal Medications

Delegation Considerations

The skill of administering vaginal medications cannot be delegated to nursing assistive personnel (NAP). The nurse instructs the NAP about:

- Potential side effects of medications and to report their occurrence to the nurse
- Reporting any change in comfort level or new or increased vaginal discharge or bleeding to the nurse

Equipment

Medication administration record (MAR) (electronic or printed); vaginal cream, foam, jelly, tablet, suppository, or irrigating solution; applicators (if needed); clean gloves; tissues; towels and/or washcloths; perineal pad; drape or sheet; water-soluble lubricants; bedpan; irrigation or douche container (if needed); gooseneck lamp (optional)

Steps

1. Review pertinent information related to medication including action, purpose, normal dose and route, side effects, time of onset and peak action, and nursing implications.
2. Assess the patient's medical and medication history and history of allergies. List drug allergies on each page of MAR and prominently display allergies on the patient's medical record per agency policy. When the patient has allergy, provide allergy bracelet.
3. Perform hand hygiene and apply clean gloves. During perineal care, inspect condition of vaginal tissues; note whether drainage is present. Remove gloves and perform hand hygiene.
4. Ask whether the patient is experiencing any symptoms of pruritus, burning, or discomfort.
5. Review the patient's knowledge of medication and readiness to learn (e.g., asks questions about medication, requests education in use of suppository).
6. Assess the patient's ability to manipulate applicator, suppository, or irrigation equipment and to properly position self to insert medication (may be done just before insertion).
7. Perform hand hygiene. Collect appropriate equipment and MAR.
8. Prepare suppository for administration. Attend to procedure and avoid distraction. Check label of medication against MAR two times (see Skill 26.1). Preparation usually involves checking label when removing suppository from refrigerator and before leaving preparation area. Check expiration date on container. *These are the first and second checks for accuracy.* Perform hand hygiene.
9. Take medications to the patient at correct time (see agency policy). Consider whether medication is time critical. During administration, apply six rights of medication administration.
10. Identify the patient by using at least two identifiers (e.g., name and birthday or name and medical record number) according to agency policy. Compare identifiers with information on the patient's MAR or medical record.
11. At the patient's bedside, again compare MAR or computer printout with names of medications on medication labels and patient name. Ask the patient whether he or she has allergies. *This is the third check for accuracy.*
12. Explain procedure to the patient. Be specific if the patient plans to self-administer medication. Discuss purpose of each medication, action, and possible adverse effects. Allow the patient to ask any questions about the medications.
13. Perform hand hygiene. Arrange supplies at bedside and apply clean gloves. Close door or pull curtain.
14. Help the patient lie in dorsal recumbent position. Patients with restricted mobility in knees or hips may lie supine with legs abducted.
15. Keep abdomen and lower extremities draped.
16. Be sure that vaginal orifice is well illuminated by room light. Otherwise, position portable gooseneck lamp.
17. Insert vaginal suppository.
    a. Remove suppository from wrapper and apply liberal amount of water-soluble lubricant to smooth or rounded end. Be sure that suppository is at room temperature. Lubricate gloved index finger of dominant hand.
    b. With nondominant gloved hand, gently separate labial folds in front-to-back direction to expose vaginal orifice.
    c. With dominant gloved hand, insert rounded end of suppository along posterior wall of vaginal canal the entire length of finger (7.5–10 cm [3–4 inches]) (see illustration).
    d. Withdraw finger and wipe away remaining lubricant from around orifice and labia with tissue or cloth.
18. Apply cream or foam.
    a. Fill cream or foam applicator following package directions.
    b. With nondominant gloved hand, gently separate labial folds.
    c. With dominant gloved hand, gently insert applicator approximately 5–7.5 cm (2–3 inches). Push applicator plunger to deposit medication into vagina (see illustration).
    d. Withdraw applicator and place on paper towel. Wipe off residual cream from labia or vaginal orifice with tissue or cloth.
19. Instruct the patient to remain on her back for at least 10 min to prevent loss through vaginal orifice.
20. If using an applicator, wash with soap and warm water, rinse, air dry, and then store for future use.
21. Offer perineal pad when the patient resumes ambulation.
22. Dispose of supplies, remove and dispose of gloves, and perform hand hygiene.
23. Record drug, dosage, route, and actual time and date of administration on MAR immediately after administration, not before. Include initials or signature.

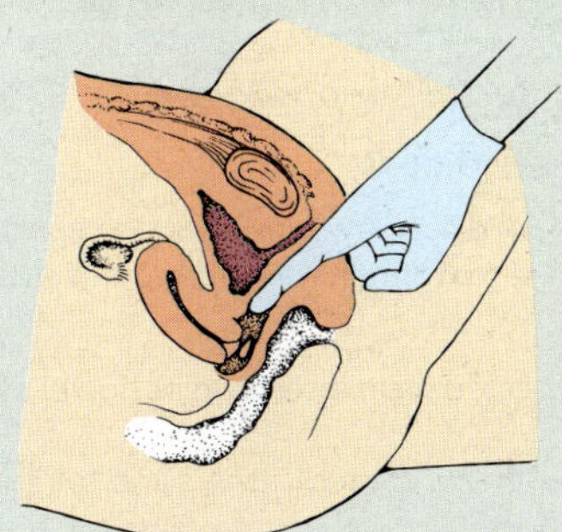

Step 17c Insertion of suppository into vaginal canal.

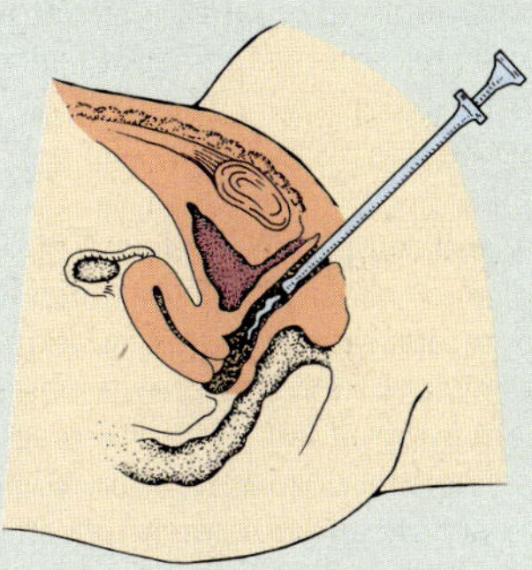

Step 18c Instillation of medication in vaginal canal.

Continued

BOX 26.15 Procedural Guidelines—cont'd

24. Wait 30 min after administration and then perform hand hygiene and apply clean gloves. Inspect condition of vaginal canal and external genitalia. Assess vaginal discharge if present. Remove gloves and perform hand hygiene.
25. Question the patient regarding continued pruritus, burning, discomfort, or discharge.
26. Ask the patient to discuss purpose, action, and side effects of medication.
27. Record patient response to medication, patient teaching, and validation of patient understanding and self-administration of suppository on flow sheet or nurses' notes in electronic health record (EHR) or chart.
28. **Use teach back:** "I want to be sure I explained how to use the vaginal cream applicator. Tell me how you will draw the correct amount of cream into the applicator." Revise your instruction now or develop a plan for revised patient teaching if the patient is not able to teach back correctly.

prefer to administer their own vaginal medications and need privacy. Vaginal medications are often given to treat infection, and vaginal discharge in patients who need vaginal medications usually smells foul. Follow aseptic technique, and offer the patient frequent opportunities to maintain perineal hygiene (see Chapter 16).

Rectal Instillation

Rectal suppositories are thinner and more bullet shaped than vaginal suppositories. The rounded end prevents anal trauma during insertion. Rectal suppositories contain medications that exert local effects, such as promoting defecation, or systemic effects, such as reducing nausea. They are stored in a refrigerator until administered. Sometimes, the rectum must be cleared with a small cleansing enema (see Chapter 22) before a suppository is inserted (Box 26.16).

ADMINISTERING MEDICATIONS BY INHALATION

Medications administered with handheld inhalers are dispersed through an aerosol spray, mist, or powder that penetrates lung airways. The alveolar–capillary network absorbs medications rapidly. **Pressurized metered-dose inhalers (pMDIs)**, **breath-actuated metered-dose inhalers (BAIs)**, and **dry powder inhalers (DPIs)** deliver inhaled medications that produce local effects in the airway such as bronchodilation. Some medications create serious systemic side effects.

pMDIs use a chemical propellant to push the medication out of the inhaler, requiring a patient to apply about 10–20 inHg of pressure to the top of the canister to administer the medication. Children and older adults with

BOX 26.16 Procedural Guidelines

Administering Rectal Suppositories

Delegation Considerations

The skill of rectal medication administration cannot be delegated to nursing assistive personnel (NAP). The nurse instructs the NAP about:

- Reporting expected fecal discharge or bowel movement to the nurse
- Potential side effects of medications and to report their occurrence to the nurse
- Informing nurse of any rectal pain or bleeding

Equipment

Medication administration record (MAR) (electronic or printed); rectal suppository; water-soluble lubricating jelly; clean gloves; tissue; drape

Steps

1. Check accuracy and completeness of each MAR with health care provider's medication order. Check the patient's name, drug name and dosage, route, and time for administration. Clarify incomplete or unclear orders with health care provider before administration.
2. Review pertinent information related to medication, including action, purpose, normal dose and route, side effects, time of onset and peak action, and nursing implications.
3. Review the patient's medical history (e.g., history of rectal surgery or bleeding, cardiac problems), medication history, and history of allergies. List drug allergies on each page of MAR and prominently display allergies on the patient's medical record per agency policy. When the patient has allergy, provide allergy bracelet.
4. Review any presenting signs and symptoms of GI alterations (e.g., constipation or diarrhea).
5. Assess the patient's ability to hold suppository and position self to insert medication.
6. Review the patient's knowledge of purpose of drug therapy and interest in self-administering suppository.
7. Perform hand hygiene. Collect appropriate equipment and MAR.
8. Prepare suppository for administration. Attend to procedure and avoid distraction. Check label of medication against MAR two times (see Skill 26.1). Preparation usually involves checking label when removing suppository out of refrigerator and before leaving preparation area. Check expiration date on container. *These are the first and second checks for accuracy.* Perform hand hygiene.
9. Take medications to the patient at correct time (see agency policy). Consider whether medication is time critical. During administration, apply six rights of medication administration.
10. Identify the patient by using at least two identifiers (e.g., name and birthday or name and medical record number) according to agency policy. Compare identifiers with information on the patient's MAR or medical record.

BOX 26.16 Procedural Guidelines—cont'd

11. At the patient's bedside, again compare MAR or computer printout with names of medications on medication labels and patient name. Ask the patient whether he or she has allergies. *This is the third check for accuracy.*
12. Explain procedure to the patient. Be specific if the patient wishes to self-administer drug. Discuss purpose of each medication, action, and possible adverse effects. Allow the patient to ask any questions about the medications.
13. Perform hand hygiene. Arrange supplies at bedside, and apply clean gloves. Close room curtain or door.
14. Help the patient assume left side-lying Sims position with upper leg flexed upward.
15. If the patient has impairment of mobility, help into lateral position. Obtain help to turn the patient, and use pillows under upper arm and leg.
16. Keep the patient draped with only anal area exposed.
17. Examine condition of anus externally. *Option:* Palpate rectal walls as needed (e.g., if impaction is suspected) (see Chapter 7). If you palpate rectal walls, dispose of gloves by turning them inside out and placing them in proper receptacle if they become soiled. Otherwise, keep gloves on your hands (proceed to Step 19).
18. Perform hand hygiene and apply new pair of clean gloves (if previous gloves were soiled and discarded).
19. Remove suppository from foil wrapper and lubricate rounded end with water-soluble lubricant (see illustration). Lubricate gloved index finger of dominant hand. If the patient has hemorrhoids, use liberal amount of lubricant and touch area gently.
20. Ask the patient to take slow, deep breaths through mouth and relax anal sphincter.
21. Retract the patient's buttocks with nondominant hand. With gloved index finger of dominant hand, insert suppository gently through anus, past internal sphincter, and against rectal wall, 10 cm (4 inches) in adults (see illustration) or 5 cm (2 inches) in infants and children. You should feel rectal sphincter close around your finger.
22. *Option:* A suppository may be given through a colostomy (not ileostomy) if ordered. The patient should lie supine. Use small amount of water-soluble lubricant for insertion.

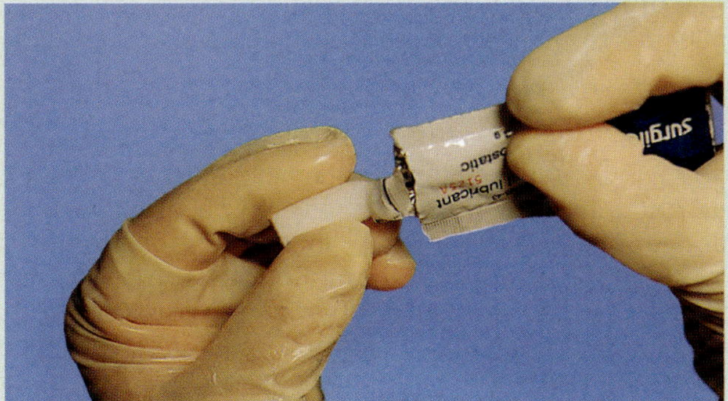

Step 19 Lubricate tip of rectal suppository with water-soluble jelly.

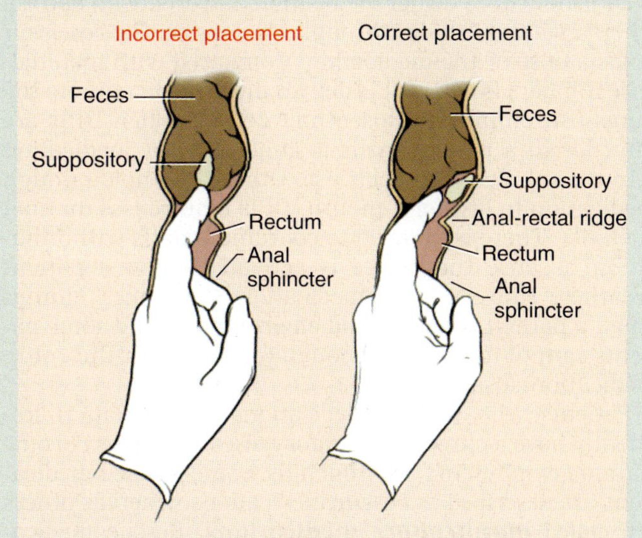

Step 21 Inserting rectal suppository. (From DeWit S: *Fundamental concepts and skills for nursing*, ed 3, Philadelphia, 2009, Saunders.)

23. Withdraw finger and wipe the patient's anal area.
24. Ask the patient to remain flat or on side for 5 min.
25. Discard gloves by turning them inside out and dispose of them and used supplies in appropriate receptacle. Perform hand hygiene.
26. If suppository contains laxative or fecal softener, be sure that nurse call system is in an accessible location so the patient can obtain help to reach bedpan or toilet.
27. If suppository was given for constipation, remind the patient *not* to flush commode after bowel movement so that you can observe characteristics of stool.
28. Record drug, dosage, route, and actual time and date of administration on MAR immediately after administration, not before. Include initials or signature.
29. Return to bedside within 5 min to determine whether suppository was expelled.
30. Ask whether the patient experienced localized anal or rectal discomfort during insertion.
31. Evaluate the patient at time of peak drug effect for relief of symptoms for which medication was prescribed.
32. Record patient response to medication, patient teaching, and validation of patient understanding and self-administration of suppository on flow sheet or nurses' notes in electronic health record (EHR) or chart.
33. **Use teach back:** "I want to be sure I explained clearly to you how to insert a rectal suppository. Describe the steps you will follow to insert the suppository." Revise your instruction now or develop a plan for revised patient/family caregiver teaching if the patient/family caregiver is not able to teach back correctly.

chronic lung diseases often use pMDIs. Because of their diminished hand strength, be sure to assess whether patients have enough strength to use pMDIs.

Sometimes, patients use a spacer with the pMDI. A spacer is a tube 10.16–20.32 cm (4–8 inches) long that attaches to the pMDI and allows the particles of medication to slow down and break into smaller pieces. This helps the medication get deeper into the lungs and enhances absorption. Spacers are helpful when a patient has difficulty coordinating the steps or coordinating inhalation with the steps involved in self-administering inhaled medications. Patients who do not use their spacers correctly do not receive the full effect of the medication. BAIs and DPIs do not use spacers. BAIs release medication when a patient raises a lever and inhales. A BAI is a good choice for patients who have difficulty using pMDIs because the BAI eliminates the need for hand–breath coordination (Ari and Restrepo, 2012).

DPIs hold dry powder medication and create an aerosol when a patient inhales through a reservoir. The reservoir holds a dose of the medication. Compared with metered-dose inhalers (MDIs), DPIs deliver more medication to the lungs (Burchum and Rosenthal, 2016). When DPIs are unit dosed, a patient loads a single dose of medication into the inhaler with each use. Other DPIs hold enough medication to last for a month. DPIs require less manual dexterity. There is no need to coordinate puffs with inhalation because the device is activated when a patient breathes. However, the medication sometimes clumps when a patient is in a humid environment, and some patients cannot inspire fast enough to administer the entire medication dosage.

Patients who receive medications by inhalation frequently have a chronic respiratory disease such as chronic asthma, emphysema, or bronchitis. Some inhaled medications are described as ***rescue*** medications, whereas others are called ***maintenance* medications**. Rescue medications are short-acting; patients take them to relieve acute respiratory distress immediately. Patients need to be cautioned not to overuse rescue medications. If respiratory distress increases, instruct the patient to contact his or her health care provider and not to overuse the rescue mediations. The patient may need an adjustment of the maintenance medication.

Patients take maintenance medications on a daily schedule to prevent acute respiratory distress; their effects start within hours of administration and last for a longer period of time than rescue inhalers. Some inhalers combine rescue and maintenance medications. Proper use of inhalers improves patient outcomes and decreases mortality associated with chronic airway diseases. However, current evidence shows that many patients do not use their inhalers correctly. Thus, teach your patients about safe and effective use of these inhalers and verify that they can use an inhaler even if they have been using one for a long time (see Skill 26.3) (Ari and Restrepo, 2012).

Help your patients determine when inhalers are empty and need to be replaced. Do not float the pMDI in water to determine how much medication is left because the container floats even if it is empty. Devices that attach onto the MDI and count down the number of remaining doses are available for MDIs. Some DPIs have an indicator that shows how many doses are left. However, these are not always accurate. Therefore, the best way to calculate how long medication in an inhaler will last is to divide the number of doses in the container by the number of doses that your patient takes per day. For example, your patient is to take albuterol, a beta-adrenergic agonist bronchodilator. The ordered dose is two puffs four times a day (q.i.d.). The canister has 200 puffs. You complete the following calculations to determine how long the MDI will last:

$$2 \text{ puffs} \times 4 \text{ times a day} = 8 \text{ puffs per day}$$

$$200 \text{ puffs}/8 \text{ puffs per day} = 25 \text{ days}$$

Therefore, the canister will last 25 days. To ensure that the patient does not run out of medication, teach the patient to refill the medication at least 7–10 days before it runs out.

ADMINISTERING MEDICATIONS BY IRRIGATIONS

Some medications irrigate or wash a body cavity and are delivered through a stream of solution. Irrigations most often use sterile water, saline, or antiseptic solutions on the eye, ear, throat, vagina, and urinary tract. Use aseptic technique if there is a break in the skin or mucosa. Use clean technique when the cavity to be irrigated is not sterile, as in the case of the ear canal or vagina. Irrigations are used to:

- Cleanse an area
- Instill a medication
- Apply heat or cold to injured tissue (see Chapter 17)

PARENTERAL ADMINISTRATION OF MEDICATIONS

Parenteral administration of medications involves the injection of a medication into body tissues. A needle piercing the skin carries a risk of infection. This is an invasive procedure that is performed with the following aseptic techniques:

- Draw up medication quickly to avoid contaminating solutions. Do not allow ampules to stand open.
- Avoid letting a needle touch contaminated surfaces (e.g., outer edges of ampule or vial, outer surface of needle cap).
- Avoid touching length of plunger or inner part of barrel. Keep tip of syringe covered with cap or needle.
- Prepare skin by washing with soap and water if soiled. Use friction and a circular motion when cleaning with an antiseptic swab. Swab from center of site and move outward in a 5-cm (2-inch) radius.

Each type of injection requires certain skills to ensure that the medication reaches the proper location. The effects of a parenteral medication occur rapidly, depending on the rate of medication absorption. You must closely observe a patient's response to parenteral medications.

Equipment

You will administer parenteral medications by using a needle and a syringe, available in a variety of sizes. Each size is designed to deliver a certain volume of a medication to a specific type of tissue. Determine the appropriate size of syringe, length and gauge of needle, volume of solution, and medication route based on the quantity and type of medication prescribed and the body size of a patient. Most syringes come with needleless systems or safety needles that help prevent needlestick injuries.

Syringes

A syringe has a cylindrical barrel with a close-fitting plunger and a tip designed to fit the hub of a hypodermic needle. Syringes are single use, disposable, and either Luer-Lok or non-Luer-Lok (Fig. 26.7). The designation of a Luer-Lok or non-Luer-Lok syringe depends on the design of the syringe tip. Syringe tips are packaged separately, in a paper wrapper or rigid plastic container. Syringes come with or without a sterile needle and with a needleless sharp with

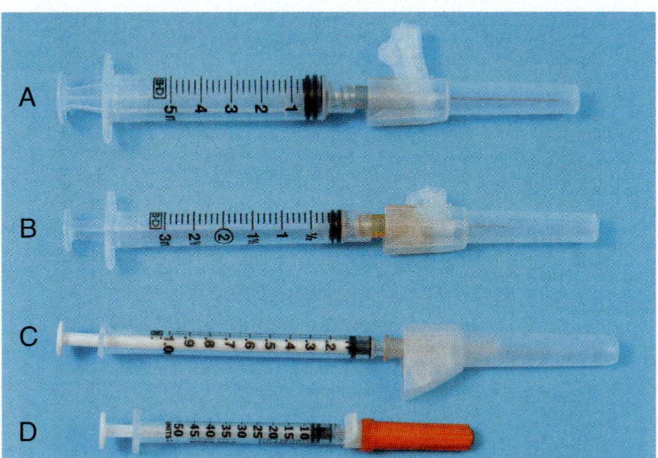

Fig. 26.7 Types of syringes. **A,** 5-mL syringe. **B,** 3-mL syringe. **C,** Tuberculin syringe marked in 0.01 (hundredths) for doses less than 1 mL. **D,** Insulin syringe marked in units (50).

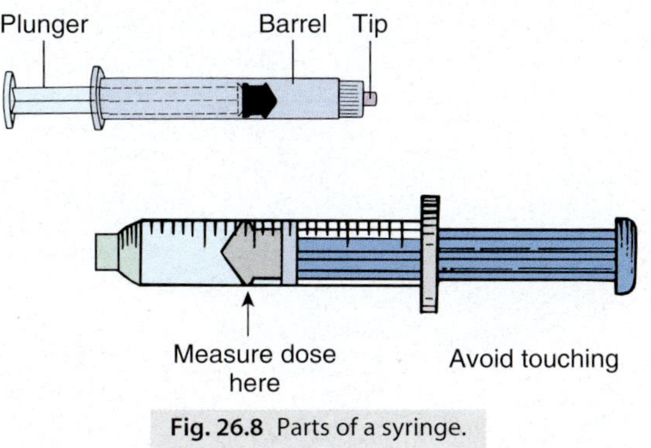

Fig. 26.8 Parts of a syringe.

engineered sharps injury protection (SESIP) device. The parts of a syringe are shown in Fig. 26.8. Non-Luer-Lok syringes use needles or needleless devices that slip onto the tip. Luer-Lok syringes (see Fig. 26.7A and B) use standard needles or needleless devices that are twisted onto the tip and lock themselves in place. The Luer-Lok design prevents the accidental removal of a needle from the syringe.

Syringes come in a variety of sizes ranging in capacity from 0.5 to 60 mL. When you select a syringe, choose the smallest syringe size possible to improve accuracy of medication preparation. In addition, avoid injecting a large volume of fluid into tissues. A 1- to 3-mL syringe is usually adequate for a subcutaneous or i.m. injection. Larger volumes result in pain and discomfort for a patient. Syringes are most commonly marked in a scale of tenths of a milliliter. You use tuberculin (TB) syringes to prepare small amounts of medications for i.d. and subcutaneous injections (see Fig. 26.7C). Insulin syringes (see Fig. 26.7D) hold 0.3–1 mL; low-dose insulin syringes (30 units per 0.3 mL or 50 units per 0.5 mL) hold 0.3–0.5 mL. All insulin syringes come with preattached needles and are calibrated in units. Most insulin syringes are U-100s, designed for use with U-100-strength insulin. Each 1 mL of solution contains 100 units of insulin.

To fill a syringe, pull the plunger outward while the needle tip remains immersed in the prepared solution. To maintain sterility, touch the outside of the syringe barrel and the handle of the plunger only.

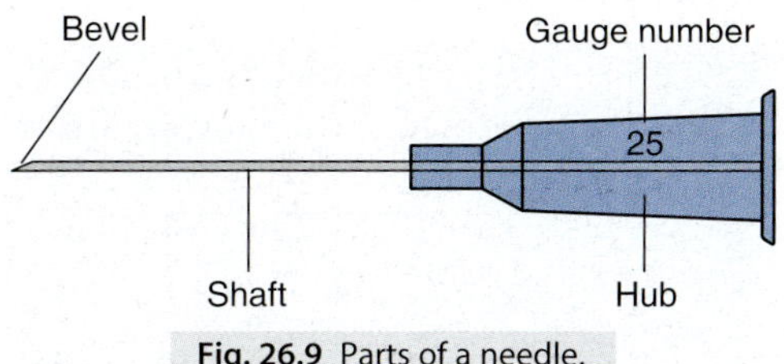

Fig. 26.9 Parts of a needle.

Use larger syringes to administer some i.v. medications and irrigate drainage tubes. Some syringes are packaged with their needle attached, and some syringes require you to change the needle based on the viscosity of the medication, route of administration, and size of the patient. Before use, carefully examine the syringe to determine the measurement scale and ensure that you use the correct syringe for preparing the ordered medication.

Needles

Some **needles** come attached to syringes. Others come packaged individually to allow flexibility in selecting the right needle for a patient. Needles are disposable, and most are made of stainless steel. A needle has three parts: the hub, which fits onto the tip of a syringe; the shaft, which connects to the hub; and the bevel, or slanted tip (Fig. 26.9). When injected into tissue, the bevel creates a narrow slit that quickly closes when you remove the needle. This prevents leakage of medication, blood, or serum. Long, beveled tips are sharp and narrow, which minimizes discomfort when entering tissue used for subcutaneous and i.m. injections. The needle hub, shaft, and bevel must remain sterile at all times. To prevent contamination, use gentle force to place the needle onto the syringe with the cap intact. Some needles come with filters for preparation of medications. Never use a filter to administer a medication.

Needles vary in length from 1/4 to 3 inches (Fig. 26.10). Choose the needle length according to a patient's size and weight and the type of tissue into which the medication is to be injected. Current evidence suggests that i.m. needle length should be based on the patient's weight (Davidson and Rourke, 2013). There should be a 5-mm depth of muscle penetration to achieve an i.m. injection (Hibberd et al., 2015). A child or slender adult generally requires a shorter needle. Use longer needles (1–1½ inches) (25–38 mm) for i.m. injections and a shorter needle (3/8–5/8 inch) (9–16 mm) for subcutaneous injections. Needles also vary in gauge or circumference. As the needle gauge becomes smaller, the needle diameter becomes larger. The selection of a gauge depends on the viscosity of fluid to be injected or infused.

Disposable Injection Units

Single-dose, prefilled, disposable syringes are available for some medications. You do not need to prepare the medication dose except perhaps to expel unneeded portions of medication or air. However, it is important to check the medication and concentration carefully because prefilled syringes appear very similar. Prefilled unit-dose systems such as Tubex and Carpuject injection systems include reusable plastic syringe holders and disposable, prefilled,

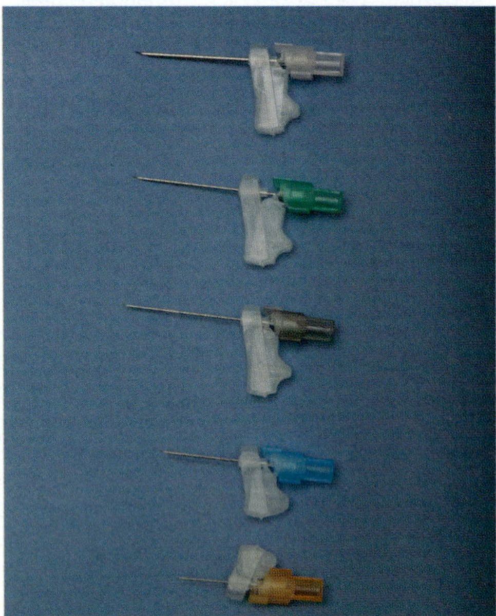

Fig. 26.10 Hypodermic needles (top to bottom): 18 gauge, 1½-inch length; 21 gauge, 1½-inch length; 22 gauge, 1½-inch length; 23 gauge, 1-inch length; and 25 gauge, 5/8-inch length.

sterile, glass cartridge units (Fig. 26.11A). To assemble a prefilled system, place the cartridge, barrel first, into the plastic syringe holder (Fig. 26.11B). Following manufacturer instructions, turn the plunger rod to the left (counterclockwise) (see Fig. 26.11C) and then lock to the right (clockwise) until it "clicks." Finally, remove the needle guard and advance the plunger (see Fig. 26.11D) to expel air and excess medication as with a regular syringe. The cartridge may be used with SESIP needles. After giving the medication, dispose of the glass cartridge safely in a puncture-proof and leak-proof container. This design reduces the risk for needlestick injury.

Preparing an Injection From an Ampule

Ampules contain single doses of medication in a liquid. They are available in several sizes, from 1 to 10 mL or more (Fig. 26.12A). An ampule consists of glass with a constricted neck that you snap off to access the medication. A colored ring around the neck indicates where the ampule is scored so that you can break it easily. Carefully aspirate the medication into a syringe (see Skill 26.4) with a filter needle. Use a filter needle to prevent particulate matter such as small glass fragments from entering the syringe (Alexander et al., 2014). Replace the filter needle with an appropriate-size needle or a needleless access device before administering the injection.

Preparing an Injection From a Vial

A vial is a single-dose or multidose container with a rubber seal at the top (see Fig. 26.12B). A metal cap protects the seal until it is ready for use. Vials contain liquid or dry forms of medications. Medications that are unstable in solution are packaged dry. The vial label specifies the solvent or diluent, usually sterile normal saline or sterile distilled water,

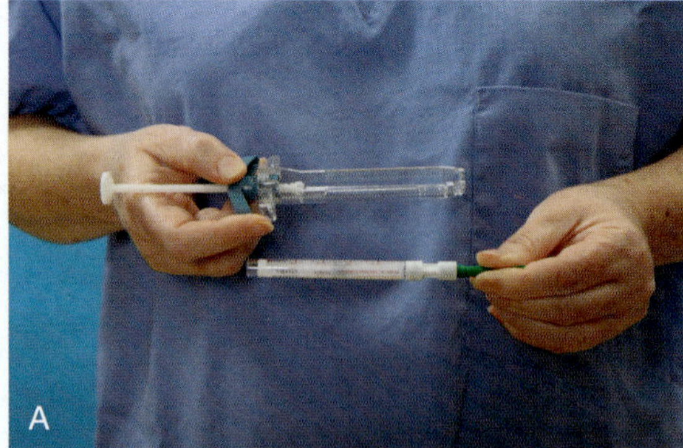

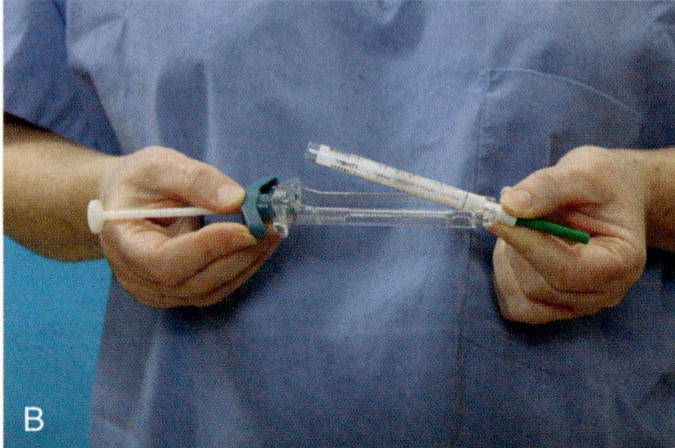

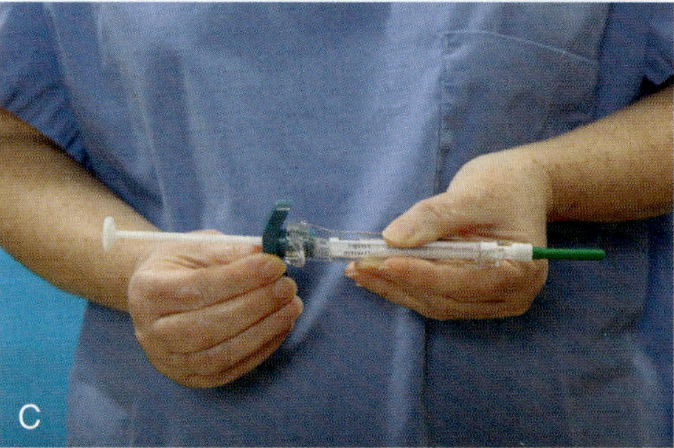

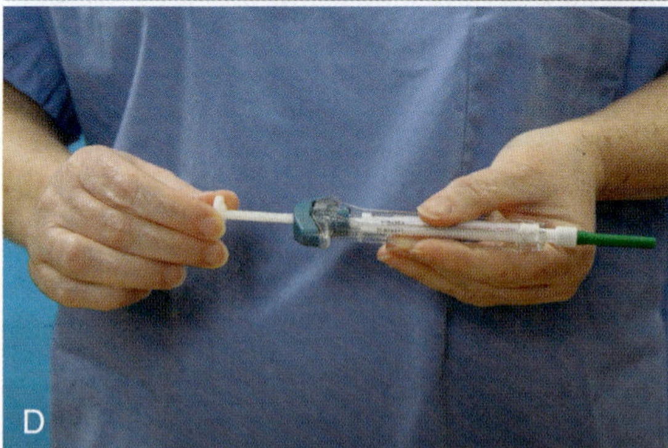

Fig. 26.11 **A,** Carpuject syringe and prefilled sterile cartridge with needle. **B,** Assembling Carpuject. **C,** Cartridge slides into syringe barrel, turns, and locks at needle end. **D,** Plunger screws into cartridge end. Expel excess medication to obtain accurate dose (not pictured).

used to dissolve the medication and the amount of diluent needed to prepare a desired concentration.

In contrast to the ampule, the vial is a closed system, and air must be injected into the vial to permit easy withdrawal of the solution. Failure to inject air when withdrawing creates a vacuum within the vial that makes withdrawal difficult. If you are concerned about drawing up parts of the rubber stopper or other particles into the syringe, use a filter needle when preparing medications from vials (Alexander et al., 2014).

Some vials contain powder, which is mixed with a diluent during preparation and before injection (see Skill 26.4). After you mix multidose vials, make a label that includes the date and time of mixing and the concentration of medication per milliliter. Some multidose vials require refrigeration after the contents have been reconstituted.

Mixing Medications

If two medications are compatible, you may mix them in one injection if the total dose is within accepted limits. This prevents a patient from having to receive more than one injection at a time. Most patient care units have charts that list common compatible medications. If you have any doubts about medication compatibilities, consult a pharmacist or a medication reference.

Mixing Medications From a Vial and an Ampule

When you mix medication from both a vial and an ampule, prepare the medication from the vial first. Using the same syringe and filter needle, next withdraw medication from the ampule. This technique prepares the medications in this order so it is not necessary to add air to withdraw medication from an ampule.

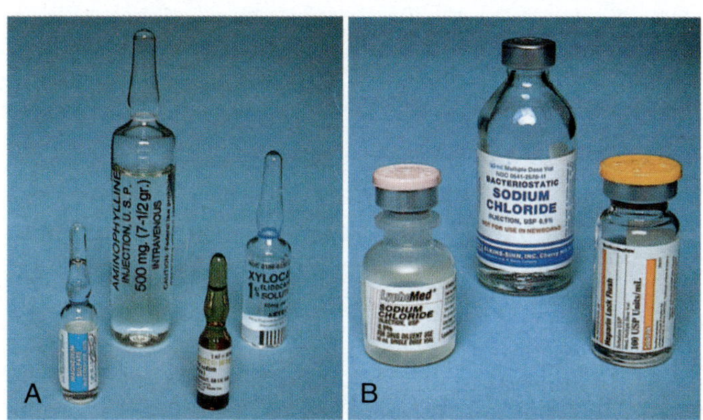

Fig. 26.12 A, Medication in ampules. **B,** Medication in vials. Rubber top must be cleansed with alcohol when vial is opened or reused.

Mixing Medications From Two Vials

Apply the following principles when mixing medications from two vials:

1. Do not contaminate one medication with another.
2. Ensure that the final dose is accurate.
3. Maintain aseptic technique.

Use only one syringe with an attached needle or needleless access device to mix medications from two vials. Aspirate the volume of air equivalent to the first medication dose (vial A) into the syringe. Then inject the air into vial A (Fig. 26.13A), making sure that the needle does not touch the solution. Withdraw the needle and aspirate air equivalent to the dose of the second medication (vial B). Inject the volume of air into vial B (Fig. 26.13B). Immediately withdraw the medication from vial B into the syringe and insert the needle back into vial A, being careful not to push the plunger and expel the medication within the syringe into the vial. Withdraw the desired amount of medication from vial A into the syringe (Fig. 26.13C). After you withdraw the necessary amount, withdraw the needle and apply a new safety needle or needleless access device suitable for injection.

INSULIN PREPARATION

Insulin is the hormone used to treat diabetes mellitus. You must administer it by subcutaneous injection because the GI tract breaks down and destroys an oral form of insulin. Most patients with diabetes mellitus who require insulin injections learn to administer their own injections. In the United States and Canada, health care providers usually prescribe insulin in concentrations of 100 units per milliliter of solution. This is called *U-100 insulin*. Insulin is also commercially available in concentrations of 50 and 500 units per milliliter of solution, or *U-50* and *U-500 insulin*. U-500 insulin is five times as strong as U-100 insulin and is used only in rare cases in which patients are very resistant to insulin.

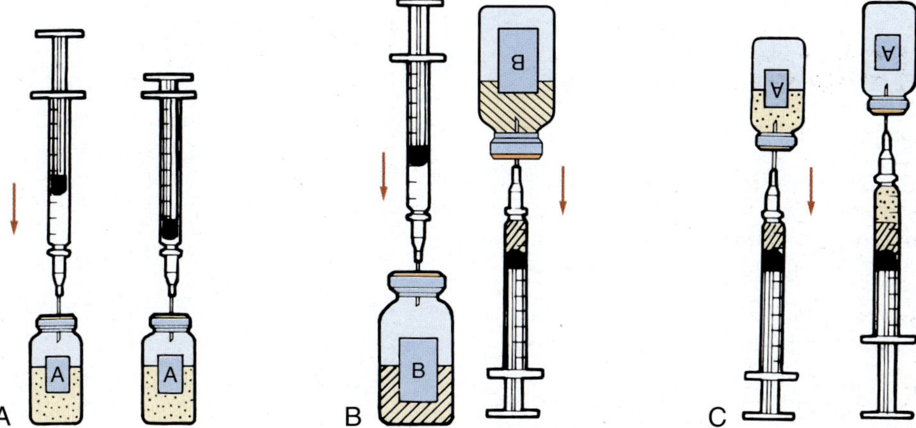

Fig. 26.13 Steps in mixing medications from two vials.

When preparing insulin, use the correct syringe that corresponds to the unit concentration ordered. For example, use a 100-unit insulin syringe or insulin pen to prepare U-100 insulin. Because no syringe is currently available for preparing U-500 insulin, many medication errors result with this kind of insulin. To prevent errors, ensure that the order for U-500 specifies units and volume (e.g., 150 units, 0.3 mL of U-500 insulin), and use TB syringes to draw up the doses (ISMP, 2013a). Verify every injection you prepare with another nurse before administering it. Additional safety measures common with U-500 insulin include the following:

- Listing the insulin as being concentrated in computerized medication dispensing systems
- Making health care providers and pharmacists verify that a patient is to receive U-500 insulin when it is ordered
- Stocking only U-500 insulin on patient care units when it is ordered for a specific patient (ISMP, 2013a)

Insulin is classified by rate of action including rapid-acting, short-acting, intermediate-acting, and long-acting. To provide safe and effective care, you must know the onset, peak, and duration for your patients' ordered insulin doses. Refer to a medication reference or consult with a pharmacist if you are unsure of this information. Regular insulin is the only type of insulin that can be given intravenously.

A patient with diabetes mellitus sometimes requires more than one type of insulin. For example, a patient receiving a short-acting (regular) and an intermediate-acting Neutral Protamine Hagedorn (NPH) insulin receives greater sustained control of blood glucose levels over 24 hours. The timing of insulin injections attempts to imitate the normal pattern of insulin release from the pancreas. Some insulins come in a stable premixed solution (e.g., 70/30 insulin is 70% NPH [intermediate] and 30% regular), eliminating the need to mix the insulins in a syringe. Other patients use an insulin pen. The insulin pen contains multiple doses and enables a patient to select the dose, avoiding the need to use a syringe.

Research shows that various types of a patient's blood cells can enter an insulin pen after an injection. Several US health care organizations recently reported that the same insulin pen was inadvertently used on multiple patients. This exposed the patients to blood-borne illnesses (such as human immunodeficiency virus [HIV], hepatitis B virus, and hepatitis C virus). Thus, the ISMP recommends that insulin pens be used only at home and that inpatient settings such as hospitals stop using them whenever possible (ISMP, 2013b).

Insulin is ordered as a specific dose at specific times of the day. Thus, timely administration is critical. Correction insulin, also known as sliding-scale insulin, is a dose of insulin based on a patient's blood glucose level. The term *correction insulin* is preferred because it indicates that small doses of rapid-acting or short-acting insulin are used to correct a patient's elevated blood sugar. Reliance on correction insulin is unlikely to achieve long-term glucose control. Thus, it should be ordered only temporarily (American Diabetes Association [ADA], 2015). An example of a correction insulin order follows:

Give regular U-100 insulin subcutaneously:
Two units for glucose 150–200 mg/dL
Four units for glucose 201–275 mg/dL
Call for dosage for glucose greater than 275 mg/dL

In the case of a patient's blood glucose being 201 mg/dL following lunch, the nurse would refer to the correction insulin order and administer 4 units of regular insulin to the patient.

Before preparing an insulin dose, gently roll all cloudy insulin preparations between the palms of your hands to resuspend the insulin (Diggle, 2014). Do not shake insulin vials. Shaking causes bubbles to form. Bubbles take up space in the syringe and alter the dose. If the patient requires more than one type of insulin to manage his or her diabetes, you may mix two different types of insulin into one syringe *if* they are compatible (Box 26.17). If regular and intermediate-acting insulins are ordered, prepare the

BOX 26.17 Procedural Guidelines

Mixing Two Types of Insulin in One Syringe

Delegation Considerations

The skill of mixing two kinds of insulin in one syringe cannot be delegated to nursing assistive personnel (NAP).

Equipment

Medication administration record (MAR) (electronic or printed); insulin vials; insulin syringe; antiseptic swab

Steps

1. Check accuracy and completeness of each MAR with health care provider's medication order. Check the patient's name, drug name and dosage, route of administration, and time for administration. Clarify incomplete or unclear orders with health care provider before administration.
2. Review medication and medical history (e.g., type of diabetes, reason for elevated blood sugars) and allergies to medications, food, and latex.
3. Verify insulin labels carefully against MAR before preparing the dose to ensure that you give the correct type of insulin. *This is the first accuracy check.*
4. Perform hand hygiene.
5. If the patient takes insulin that is cloudy, roll the bottle of insulin between the hands to resuspend the insulin preparation.
6. Wipe off tops of both insulin vials with alcohol swabs and allow to dry.
7. Verify insulin dosages against MAR a second time. *This is the second accuracy check.*
8. If mixing rapid-acting or short-acting insulin with intermediate-acting insulin, take insulin syringe and aspirate volume of air equivalent to dose to be withdrawn from intermediate-acting insulin first. If two intermediate-acting insulins are mixed, it makes no difference which vial you prepare first.
9. Insert needle and inject air into vial of intermediate-acting insulin. Do not let the tip of the needle touch the insulin.
10. Remove the syringe from the vial of intermediate-acting insulin without aspirating medication.
11. With the same syringe, inject air equal to the dose of rapid-acting or short-acting insulin into the vial and withdraw the correct dose into the syringe.

BOX 26.17 **Procedural Guidelines—cont'd**

12. Remove the syringe from the rapid-acting or short-acting insulin and get rid of air bubbles to ensure accurate dosing.
13. After verifying insulin dosages with MAR a third time, show insulin prepared in syringe to another nurse to verify that you prepared correct dosage of insulin. *This is the third accuracy check.* Determine which point on syringe scale combined units of insulin measure by adding the number of units of both insulins together (e.g., 5 units regular + 10 units NPH = 15 units total).
14. Place the needle of the syringe back into the vial of intermediate-acting insulin. Be careful not to push plunger and inject insulin in syringe into the vial.
15. Invert the vial and carefully withdraw the desired amount of insulin into syringe.
16. Withdraw needle and check fluid level in syringe. Keep needle of prepared syringe sheathed or capped until ready to administer medication. Show another nurse the syringe to verify that you prepared the correct dose.
17. Dispose of soiled supplies in proper receptacle. Place empty vials in puncture-proof and leak-proof container and perform hand hygiene.
18. Because rapid-acting or short-acting insulin binds with intermediate-acting insulin, which reduces the action of the faster-acting insulin, administer mixture within 5 min of preparing it.

Modified from American Diabetes Association (ADA): *Insulin and other injectables*, 2013, http://www.diabetes.org/living-with-diabetes/treatment-and-care/medication/insulin; and Dunning T: *Care of people with diabetes: a manual of nursing practice*, ed 4, Hoboken, NJ, 2013, Wiley-Blackwell.

regular insulin first to prevent it from becoming contaminated with the intermediate-acting insulin (Diggle, 2014). Use the following principles when mixing insulins (Diggle, 2014; Novo Nordisk, 2015; Weinstock, 2015):

- Patients whose blood glucose levels are well controlled on a mixed-insulin dose need to maintain their individual routine when preparing and administering their insulin.
- Do not mix insulin with any other medications or diluents unless approved by the health care provider.
- Never mix insulin glargine (Lantus) or insulin detemir (Levemir) with other types of insulin.
- Inject rapid-acting insulins mixed with NPH insulin within 15 minutes before a meal.
- Verify insulin doses with another nurse while you are preparing the injection.

ADMINISTERING INJECTIONS

Each injection route differs with the type of tissues the medication enters. The characteristics of the tissues affect the rate of medication absorption, affecting the onset of medication action. Before injecting a medication, know the volume of the medication to administer, the characteristics and viscosity of the medication, and the location of anatomical structures underlying injection sites (see Skill 26.5).

If you administer injections incorrectly, negative patient outcomes result. For example, a rare condition is reported to result from an incorrect injection technique into the deltoid muscle, shoulder injury related to vaccine administration (SIRVA). SIRVA is thought to occur as a result of unintentional injection of a vaccine antigen into tissues and structures underlying the deltoid muscle or trauma from the needle into and around the underlying shoulder bursa. Failure to consider anatomical landmarks when selecting an injection may result in nerve or bone damage during needle insertion. Inability to maintain stability of the needle and syringe unit can result in pain and tissue damage. If you fail to aspirate the syringe before injecting an i.m. medication, the medication may be accidentally injected directly into an artery or vein. Injecting too large a volume of medication for the site selected causes extreme pain and results in local tissue damage.

Many patients, particularly children, fear injections. Patients with serious or chronic illness often are given several injections daily. Minimize discomfort in the following ways:

- Use a sharp-beveled needle in the smallest suitable length and gauge.
- Position a patient comfortably to reduce muscular tension.
- Use anatomical landmarks to select the proper injection site.
- Apply a vapocoolant spray (e.g., Fluori-Methane spray or ethyl chloride) or topical anesthetic (e.g., eutectic mixture of local anesthetics [EMLA] cream) to the injection site before giving the medication when possible.
- Divert the patient's attention from the injection by asking open-ended questions.
- Insert the needle quickly and smoothly to minimize tissue pulling.
- Hold the syringe steady while the needle remains in tissues.
- Inject the medication slowly and steadily.

Subcutaneous Injections

Subcutaneous injections involve injecting medication into the loose connective tissue underlying the dermis. Subcutaneous tissue does not contain as many blood vessels as muscles, and thus medications are absorbed more slowly than with i.m. injections. Physical exercise or application of hot or cold compresses influences the rate of drug absorption by altering local blood flow to tissues. Any condition that impairs blood flow is a contraindication for subcutaneous injections.

Because subcutaneous tissue contains pain receptors, patients often experience slight discomfort. Injection into blood vessels is rare; thus, you do not need to aspirate when giving subcutaneous injections (Lilley et al., 2016). Subcutaneous tissue is sensitive to irritating solutions and large volumes of medications. Thus, you administer only small volumes (0.5–1.5 mL) of water-soluble medications subcutaneously to adults. In children, you give smaller volumes up to 0.5 mL (Hockenberry and Wilson, 2015). Examples of subcutaneous medications include epinephrine, insulin, allergy medications, opioids, and heparin.

The best subcutaneous injection sites include the outer posterior aspect of the upper arms, the abdomen from below the costal margins to the iliac crests, and the anterior aspects of the thighs (Fig. 26.14). These areas are easily accessible and are large enough to allow rotating multiple injections within each anatomic location. Site rotation prevents the formation of lipohypertrophy or lipoatrophy in the skin. Choose an injection site that is free of skin lesions, bony prominences, and large underlying muscles or nerves.

The site most frequently recommended for heparin injections is the right or left side of the abdomen, at least 5 cm (2 inches) away from the umbilicus (Fig. 26.15). The administration of low-molecular-weight heparin (LMWH) (e.g., enoxaparin) requires special considerations. Administer LMWH in its prefilled syringe with the attached needle, and do not expel the air bubble in the syringe before giving the medication. Some evidence supports a slower injection rate of 30 seconds to reduce bruising and pain (Akbari Sari et al., 2014; Sanofi-Aventis, 2014).

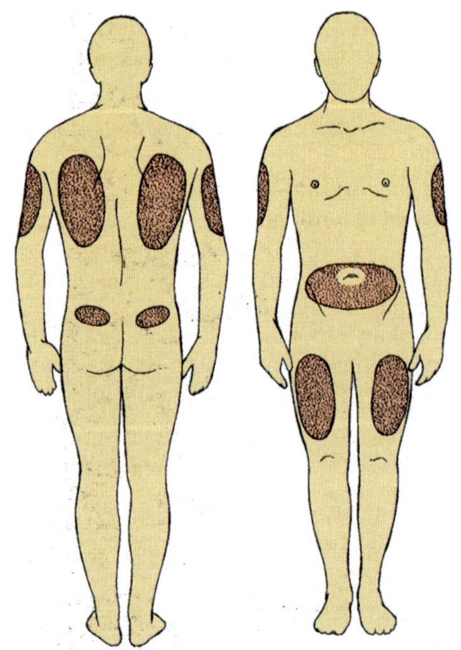

Fig. 26.14 Sites recommended for subcutaneous injections.

Recommended sites for insulin injection include the abdomen, upper arm, anterior and lateral parts of the thigh, and buttocks. Rotating injections within the same body part (intrasite rotation) produces consistency in the absorption of the insulin. For example, if a patient receives morning insulin in the right arm, give the next injection in a different place in the same arm, at least 2.5 cm (1 inch) away from the previous site (Frid et al., 2016). Do not reuse injection sites for at least 1 month. The rate of insulin absorption varies based on the site. The abdomen has the fastest absorption, followed by the arms, thighs, and buttocks (Weinstock, 2015).

A patient's body weight and adipose tissue indicate the depth of the subcutaneous layer. Therefore, choose the needle length and angle of insertion on the basis of a patient's weight and an estimation of the amount of subcutaneous tissue (Ogston-Tuck, 2014a). Nurses typically use a 25-gauge, 16-mm (5/8-inch) needle inserted at a 45° angle for injections (Fig. 26.16) or a 12-mm (1/2-inch) needle inserted at a 90° angle to administer subcutaneous medications to a normal-size adult patient (except with insulin; see next paragraph). Some children require only a 12-mm

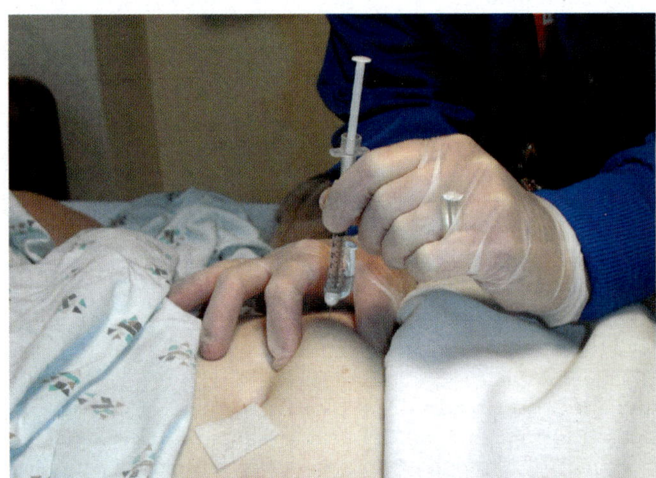

Fig. 26.15 Giving subcutaneous heparin in abdomen.

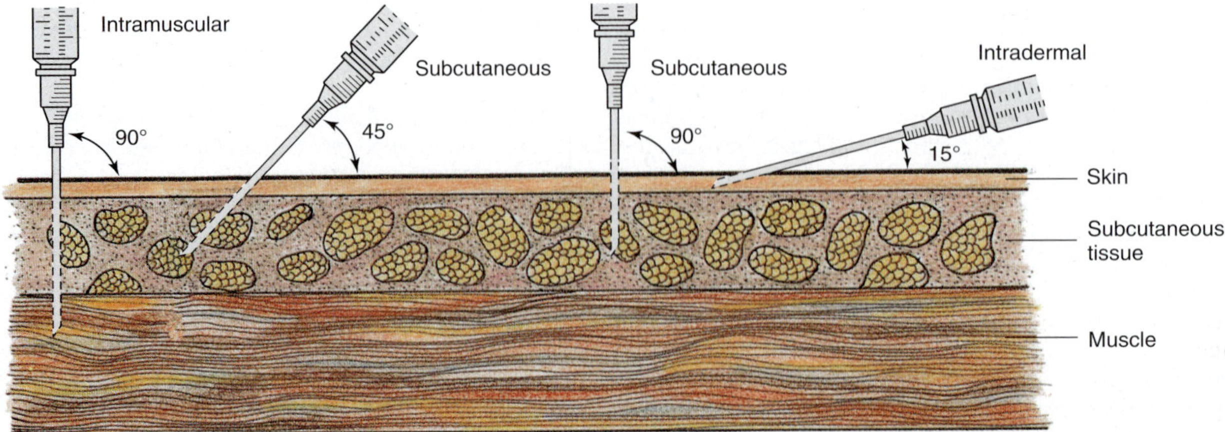

Fig. 26.16 Comparison of angles of insertion for intramuscular (90°), subcutaneous (45° and 90°), and intradermal (15°) injections.

(1/2-inch) needle. If the patient is obese, pinch the tissue and use a needle long enough to insert through fatty tissue at the base of the skinfold. Thin patients often do not have sufficient tissue for subcutaneous injections; the upper abdomen is usually the best site in this case. To ensure that a subcutaneous medication reaches the subcutaneous tissue, follow this rule: If you can grasp 5 cm (2 inches) of tissue, insert the needle at a 90° angle; if you can grasp only 2.5 cm (1 inch) of tissue, insert the needle at a 45° angle.

Research in insulin administration now shows that insulin needles that are 5/16 inch (8 mm) or longer often enter the muscles of men and people with a body mass index (BMI) of 25 or less. Shorter (3/16-inch or 4- to 5-mm) needles were associated with less pain, adequate control of blood sugars, and minimal leakage of medication (Diggle, 2014; Hirsch et al., 2012). Thus, when administering insulin, you should use 3/16-inch (4- to 5-mm) needles administered at a 90° angle to reduce pain and achieve adequate control of blood sugars with minimal adverse effects for people of all BMIs including children (American Association of Diabetes Educators [AADR], 2013).

Frequently patients who self-administer insulin at home reuse needles because of financial limitations. In a systematic review of the current scientific literature, there is no clear evidence to suggest for or against reuse of needles in the home setting for subcutaneous insulin injection (Frid et al., 2016; Zabaleta-Del-Olmo et al., 2016) with regard to patient safety. A few studies have found that reused needles cause more discomfort. The practice of reusing needles is very common among people with diabetes mellitus; thus, the researchers recommend further research.

Several different devices are available for administration of subcutaneous injections. *Injection pens* allow patients to self-administer medications (e.g., epinephrine, insulin, or interferon) subcutaneously (Fig. 26.17). Injection pens are a convenient delivery method using prefilled, disposable cartridges. The patient pinches the skin, inserts the needle, and injects a predetermined medication dose. Teaching is essential to ensure that patients use the correct injection technique and deliver the correct dose of medication. Reinforce to patients and family caregivers that insulin pens are used by only one patient and are not shared (Frid et al., 2016). In addition, teach patients the importance of priming the pen before use. Priming involves pointing the pen needle up in the air, dialing one or two units (see package directions) on the pen, and then pressing the plunger fully with the thumb repeatedly until a drop appears. This clears the needle of air and ensures that a full dose is ready. The disadvantages to this device include increased risk for needlestick injury and user's lack of knowledge and skill in administration technique (Ogston-Tuck, 2014a). The needle-free injection system administers medications without the use of needles. Needle-free injections use a precise, narrow stream of liquid to penetrate the skin with the medication into the subcutaneous tissue (Fig. 26.18). Another option for subcutaneous injection is the *subcutaneous injection device* (e.g., Insuflon) (Fig. 26.19). You insert the device into the subcutaneous tissue. You then remove the needle, leaving the cannula in the tissue to provide an avenue for administering medications for up to 3 days without having to puncture the skin with each injection.

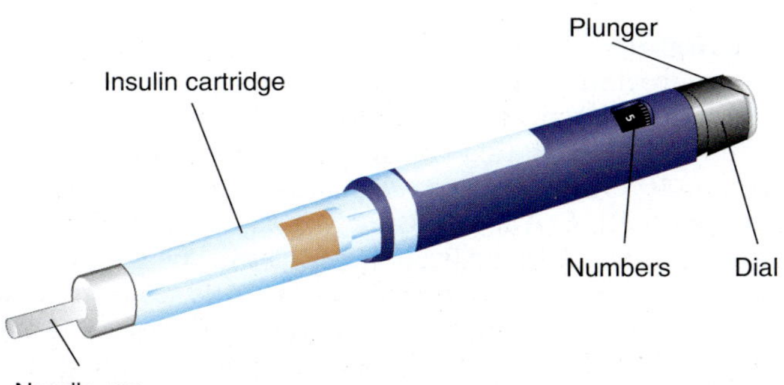

Fig. 26.17 Insulin injection pen. (From Lewis SL, et al: *Medical-surgical nursing: assessment and management of clinical problems*, ed 8, St Louis, 2011, Mosby.)

Intramuscular Injections

The **intramuscular (IM)** i.m. injection route deposits medication into deep muscle tissue, which has a rich blood supply, allowing medication to absorb faster than by the subcutaneous route. However, there is a risk for injecting drugs directly into blood vessels. Any factor that interferes with local tissue blood flow affects the rate and extent of i.m. drug absorption. In addition, if a medication is not injected correctly into a muscle, complications can arise such as abscess, hematoma, ecchymosis, pain, and vascular and nerve injury (Kara Yilmaz and Karaman, 2015; Kaya et al., 2015; Nicoll and Hesby, 2002). Therefore,

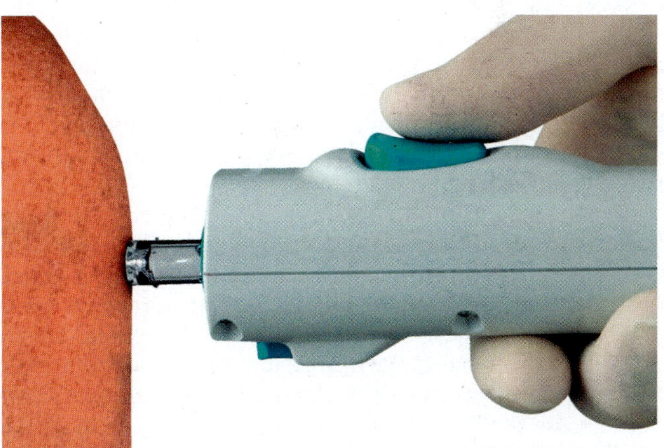

Fig. 26.18 Jet injection system is held perpendicular to skin. (Image courtesy Pharmajet. All rights reserved.)

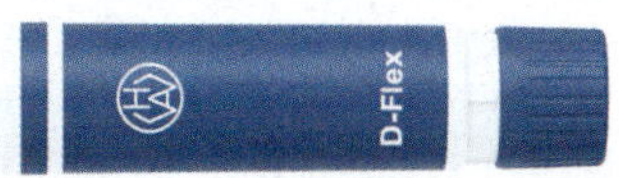

Fig. 26.19 Subcutaneous device. (D-Flex™ is a trademark of Haselmeier AG)

whenever administering a medication by the i.m. route, first verify that the injection is justified (Nicoll and Hesby, 2002; World Health Organization [WHO], 2015). Some medications such as hepatitis B and tetanus, diphtheria, and pertussis (Tdap) immunizations are given only intramuscularly.

The viscosity of a medication, injection site, patient's weight, and amount of adipose tissue influence needle gauge and length selection. Use a longer and heavier-gauge needle to pass through subcutaneous tissue and penetrate deep muscle tissue (see Skill 26.5). A patient's BMI and the amount of adipose tissue affect the choice of needle. Many needles available in health care settings are not long enough to reach the muscle, especially in female patients and patients who are obese (Bhalla et al., 2013; Dayananda et al., 2014; Palma and Strohfus, 2013). Because most health care agencies have needles that range in length from only 3/8 to 1½ inches (9 to 38 mm), investigate other medication routes, especially when i.m. injections are ordered for female patients who are obese.

The angle of insertion for an i.m. injection is 90° (see Fig. 26.16). Muscle is less sensitive to irritating and viscous medications. An adult patient who is well developed tolerates 2–5 mL of medication in a larger muscle without severe muscle discomfort (Nicoll and Hesby, 2002; Hopkins and Arias, 2013). Larger volumes of medication (4–5 mL), however, are unlikely to be absorbed properly. Children, older adults, and patients who are thin tolerate only 2 mL of an i.m. injection. Do not give more than 1 mL to small children and older infants, and do not give more than 0.5 mL to younger infants (Hockenberry and Wilson, 2015).

Assess a muscle before giving an injection. Properly identify the site for the i.m. injection by palpating bony landmarks, and be aware of the potential complications associated with each site. The site needs to be free of tenderness because repeated injections in the same muscle cause severe discomfort. With the patient relaxed, palpate the muscle to rule out hardened lesions. Minimize discomfort during an injection by helping a patient assume a position that reduces muscle strain. Other interventions such as distraction and application of ice or pressure to an i.m. site reduce pain during an injection.

Rotate i.m. injection sites to decrease the risk for tissue hypertrophy. Emaciated or atrophied muscles absorb medication poorly; avoid their use when possible. The **Z-track method**, a technique for pulling the skin during an injection, is recommended for i.m. injections (Nicoll and Hesby, 2002). It prevents leakage of medication into subcutaneous tissues, seals medication in the muscle, and minimizes irritation. To use the Z-track method, attach the appropriate-size needle to the syringe and select an i.m. site, preferably in a large, deep muscle such as the ventrogluteal. Pull the overlying skin and subcutaneous tissues approximately 2.5–3.5 cm (1–1½ inches) laterally to the side with the ulnar side of the nondominant hand. Hold the skin in this position until you have administered the injection (Fig. 26.20A). After cleaning a site, inject the needle deeply into the muscle. Aspirate the injection and if no blood is returned on aspiration, inject the medication slowly into the muscle. To reduce injection site discomfort, there is no longer any need to aspirate after the needle is injected when *administering vaccines* (CDC, 2015). It is the nurses' responsibility to follow agency

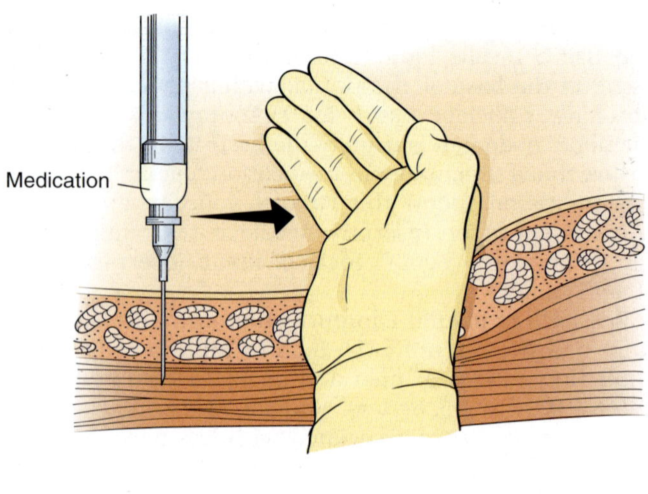

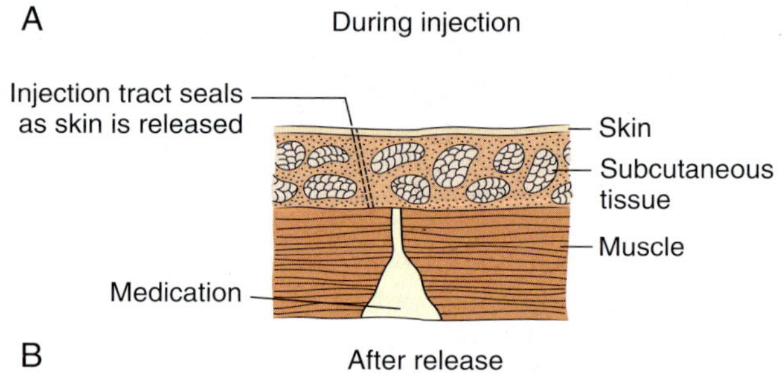

Fig. 26.20 Z-track method of injection prevents deposit of medication into sensitive tissues.

policy for aspiration when giving vaccines. Keep the needle inserted for 10 seconds to allow the medication to disperse evenly. Release the skin after withdrawing the needle. This leaves a zigzag path that seals the needle track wherever tissue planes slide across one another see (Fig. 26.20B). The medication is sealed in the muscle tissue.

Injection Sites

When selecting an i.m. site, consider the following:

- Is the area free of infection or necrosis?
- Are there local areas of bruising or abrasions?
- What are the locations of underlying bones, nerves, and major blood vessels?
- What volume of medication is to be administered?
- Can you position a patient anatomically and comfortably so as to access the site?

Ventrogluteal Muscle

The ventrogluteal muscle is the preferred and safest site for all adults, children, and infants, especially for large-volume, viscous, and irritating medications (Hockenberry and Wilson, 2015; Hopkins and Arias, 2013; Kara Yilmaz and Karaman, 2015; Yapucu Günes et al., 2016). The site involves the gluteus medius where the thickness of subcutaneous tissue is less than that of other injection sites and there are relatively fewer nerves and blood vessels (Kara Yilmaz and Karaman, 2015). Furthermore, in this site, the muscles are large and well established, and it is easy to find the muscle limit points (Kara Yilmaz and Karaman, 2015).

The ventrogluteal site is recommended for volumes greater than 2 mL (Hopkins and Arias, 2013; Nicoll and

Hesby, 2002). Research shows that injuries such as fibrosis, nerve damage, abscess, tissue necrosis, muscle contraction, gangrene, and pain are associated with all the common i.m. sites *except* the ventrogluteal site (Hopkins and Arias, 2013).

One way to locate the ventrogluteal muscle is to use the "V" method (Kara Yilmaz and Karaman, 2015). You position a patient in a supine or lateral position with the knee and hip flexed to relax the muscle. Use your right hand for the left hip and your left hand for the right hip. For example, if you are administering the injection into the patient's left hip, place the palm of your right hand over the greater trochanter of the patient's hip with your wrist perpendicular to the femur. Then move your thumb toward the patient's groin and your index finger toward the anterior superior iliac spine. Extend or open your middle finger back along the iliac crest toward the patient's buttock. The index finger, the middle finger, and the iliac crest form a V-shaped triangle with the injection site in the center of the triangle (Fig. 26.21) (Kara Yilmaz and Karaman, 2015; Kilic et al., 2014).

There has been some evidence to suggest that the "V" technique is not always reliable because of differences in hand structure of nurses and body structure of patients, especially when a patient is obese (Kara Yilmaz and Karaman, 2015). Thus, the "G" method or geometric method is another option for selecting the correct ventrogluteal site. With a patient in the side-lying position, you reference three bony prominences and draw imaginary lines between the ends of the bones (Kara Yilmaz and Karaman, 2015). You imagine lines drawn from the patient's greater trochanter to the iliac crest and then to the anterior superior iliac spine and from the greater trochanter to the anterior superior iliac spine. Thus, a triangle is created by the imaginary lines. After that, draw median lines from every corner of the triangle to the opposite side. As shown in Fig. 26.22, the convergence point of the three median lines is the center for the triangle, the needle entry point for i.m. injections (deMeneses and Marques, 2007; Kaya et al., 2015). In a study by deMeneses and Marques (2007), the G method was found to be 100% reliable in determining the ventrogluteal site in i.m. injections.

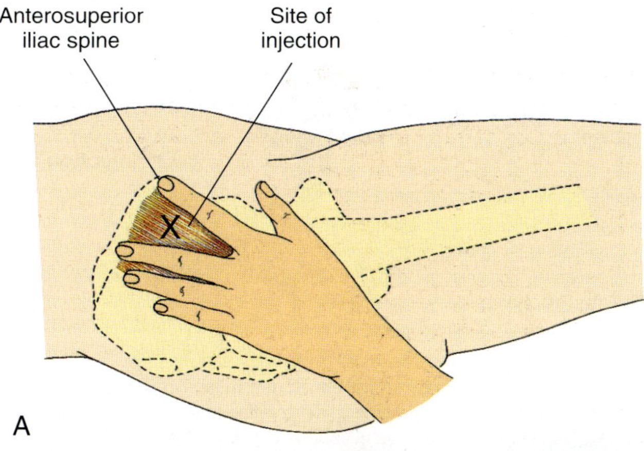

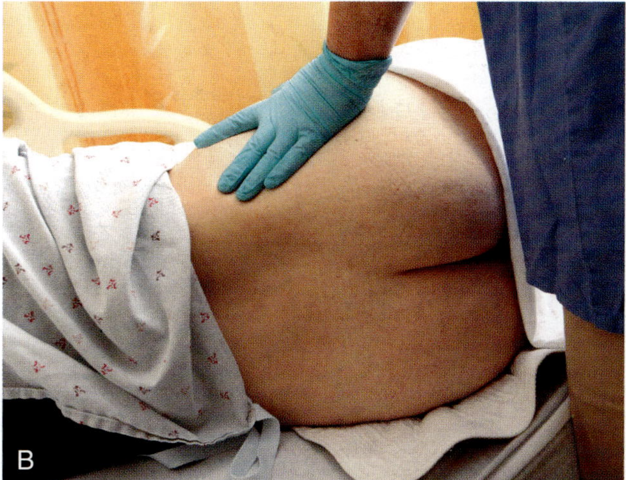

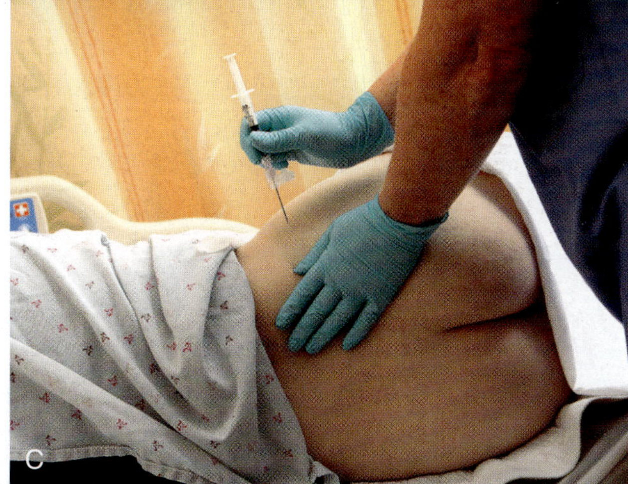

Fig. 26.21 A, Landmarks for "V" ventrogluteal injection site. **B,** Locating ventrogluteal site in patient. **C,** Giving intramuscular injection in ventrogluteal muscle using Z-track method.

Vastus Lateralis Muscle

The vastus lateralis muscle is another injection site for adults and children. The muscle is thick and well developed, is located on the anterior lateral aspect of the thigh, and extends in an adult from a hand breadth above the knee to a hand breadth below the greater trochanter of the femur (Fig. 26.23A and B). Use the middle third of the muscle for injection. The width of the muscle usually extends from the midline of the thigh to the midline of the outer side of the thigh. With young children or cachectic patients, grasping the body of the muscle during injection helps to ensure that the medication is deposited in muscle tissue. To help relax the muscle, ask the patient to lie flat with the knee slightly flexed or in a sitting position. The vastus lateralis site is often used for infants, toddlers, and children receiving biologicals (e.g., immunoglobulins, vaccines, or toxoids) (Nicoll and Hesby, 2002).

Deltoid Muscle

Although the deltoid site is easily accessible, this muscle is not well developed in many adults. This site has a potential for injury because the axillary, radial, brachial, and ulnar nerves and the brachial artery lie within the upper arm under the triceps and along the humerus (Barnes et al., 2012; Imran and Hayley, 2013). Use this site for small medication volumes (2 mL or less), as in the case of immunizations (e.g., hepatitis B, flu shot) or when other sites are inaccessible because of dressings or casts (Davidson and Rourke, 2013; Hopkins and Arias, 2013; Nicoll and Hesby, 2002).

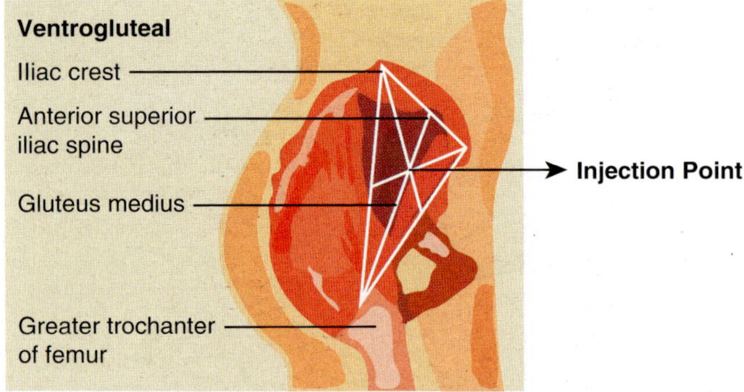

Fig. 26.22 Determination of intramuscular injection site according to the G method. (From Kaya N, et al: The reliability of site determination methods in ventrogluteal area injection: a cross-sectional study, *Int J Nurs Stud* 52:355, 2015.)

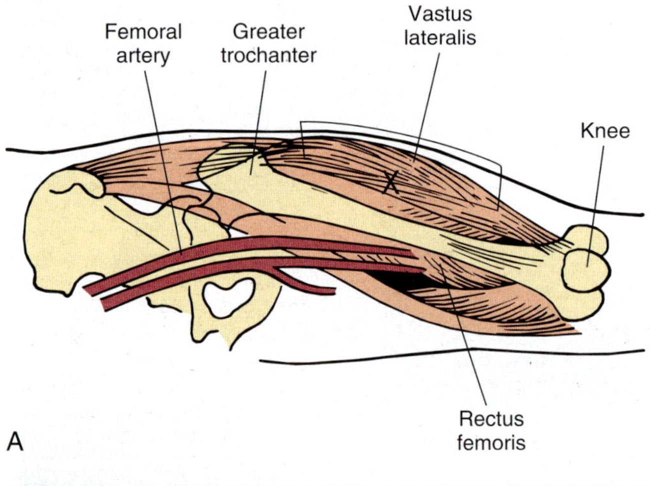

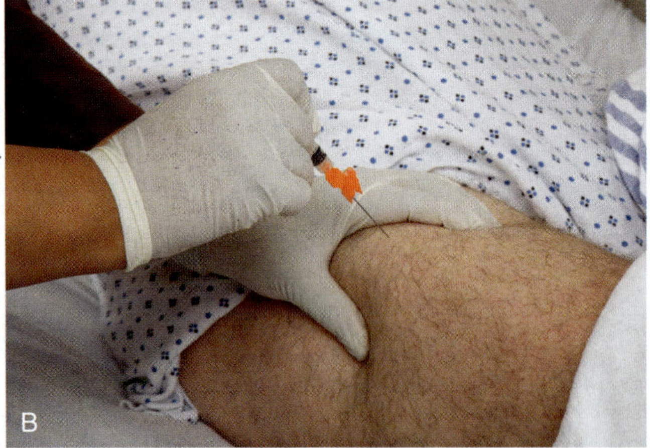

Fig. 26.23 A, Landmarks for vastus lateralis site. **B,** Giving intramuscular injection in vastus lateralis muscle.

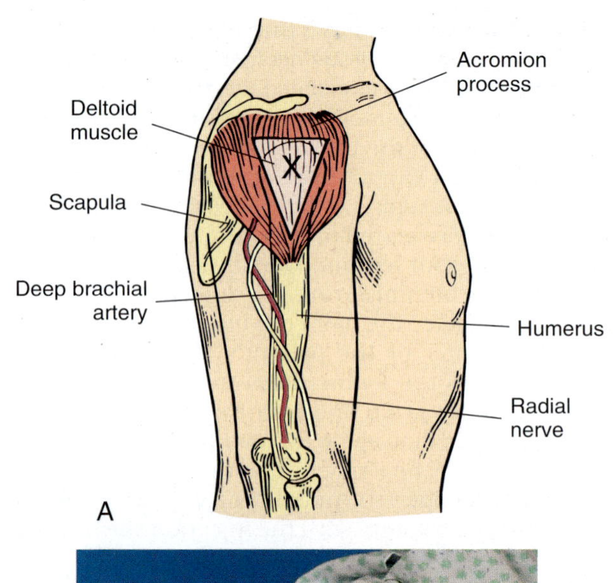

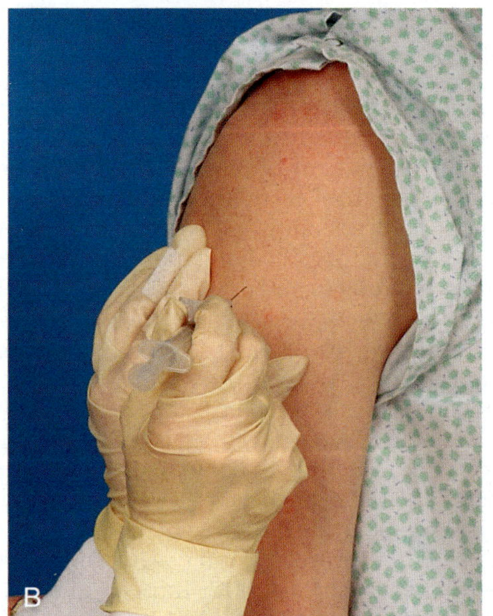

Fig. 26.24 A, Landmarks for deltoid site. **B,** Giving intramuscular injection in deltoid muscle.

Carefully assess the condition of the deltoid muscle, consult medication references for suitability of the medication, and carefully locate the injection site using anatomical landmarks (Fig. 26.24A). To locate the muscle, fully expose the patient's upper arm and shoulder. Do not roll up a tight-fitting sleeve. Have the patient relax the arm at the side and flex the elbow. The patient may sit, stand, or lie down (Fig. 26.24B). Palpate the lower edge of the acromion process, which forms the base of a triangle in line with the midpoint of the lateral aspect of the upper arm. The injection site is in the center of the triangle, about 3–5 cm (1–2 inches) below the acromion process. You also can locate the site by placing four fingers across the deltoid muscle, with the top finger along the acromion process. The injection site is then three finger widths below the acromion process.

Intradermal Injections

I.d. injections are used for skin testing (e.g., tuberculosis screening and allergy tests). Because such medications are potent, you inject them into the dermis, where blood supply is reduced and drug absorption occurs slowly. A patient may have an anaphylactic reaction if the medication enters the circulation too rapidly. For patients with a history of multiple allergies, a health care provider will perform skin testing using i.d. injections. Skin testing often requires you to visually inspect the test site. Therefore, make sure that the i.d. site is free of lesions and injuries and is relatively hairless. The inner forearm and upper back are ideal locations.

To administer an i.d. injection, use a TB or small syringe with a short (3/8- to 5/8-inch [3- to 16-mm]), fine-gauge (25–27) needle. The angle of insertion for an i.d. injection is 5–15° (see Fig. 26.16). Inject only small amounts of medication (0.01–0.1 mL) intradermally. Administer amounts only up to 0.1 mL to children (Hockenberry and Wilson, 2015). If a bleb does not appear or if the site bleeds after needle withdrawal, the medication may have entered subcutaneous tissues. In this situation, skin test results will not be valid.

SAFETY IN ADMINISTERING MEDICATIONS BY INJECTION

Needleless Devices

There is of statistics on national data on risk of occupational exposure to blood-borne pathogens such as HIV and hepatitis B virus in India; wherein, needlestick injury is reported as higher as .30% healthcare professionals. In the case of parenteral injections, an exposure is defined as a percutaneous injury (e.g., needlestick or cut with a sharp object) (CDC, 2013). Needlestick injuries often occur when health care workers do the following:

- Recap needles
- Mishandle i.v. lines and needles
- Leave needles at a patient's bedside

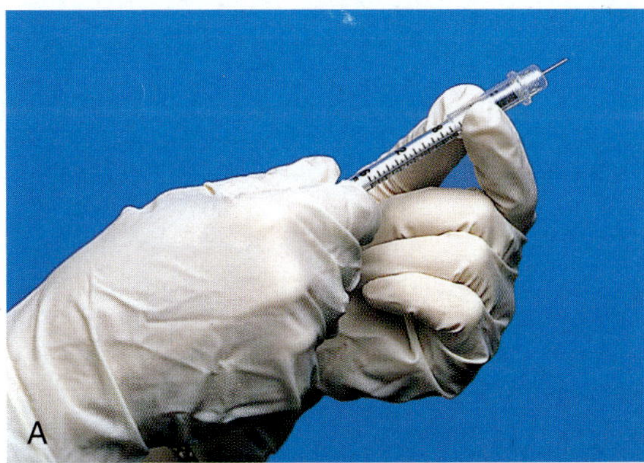

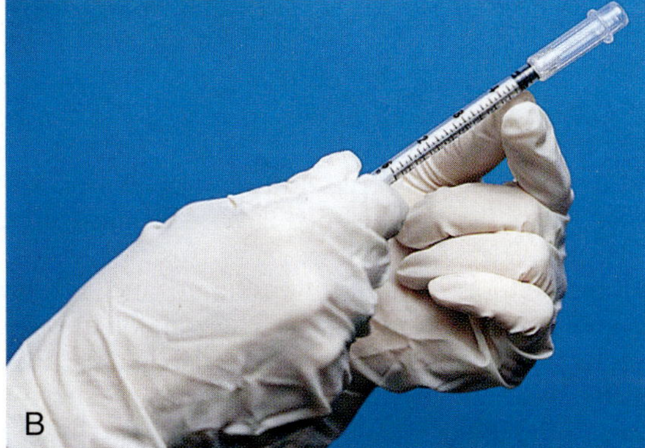

Fig. 26.25 Needle with plastic guard to prevent needlesticks. **A,** Position of guard before injection. **B,** After injection, a nurse locks guard in place, covering needle.

Exposure to blood-borne pathogens is one of the deadliest daily hazards to which nurses are exposed. Most needlestick injuries can be prevented with the use of safe engineering controls such as sharps disposal containers, rubber dams, self-sheathing needles, and needleless devices (CDC, 2013).

Safety syringes have a sheath or guard that covers a needle immediately after it is withdrawn from the skin (Fig. 26.25). This feature eliminates the chance for a needlestick injury. The syringe and sheath are discarded together in a sharps container. Needleless devices used for injections include a blunt cannula attached to a syringe. Use needleless devices for injections when available. Always dispose of needles and other instruments considered sharps into clearly marked appropriate containers (Fig. 27.26). Containers must be clearly visible to health care workers in the area where sharps are used. Additionally, they need to be puncture-proof, leak-proof, durable during installation and transport, and of an appropriate size and shape. The closure should be secure and minimize exposure during use (CDC, 2010). Never force a needle into a full needle disposal receptacle. Receptacles should be emptied when they are two-thirds full. Never place used needles and syringes in a wastebasket, in your pocket, on a patient's meal tray, or at the patient's bedside. Box 26.18 summarizes the recommendations for the prevention of needlestick injuries.

Intravenous Administration

Nurses administer medications intravenously by:

1. Infusion of large-volume i.v. fluid containers that contain medications mixed by the pharmacy
2. Injection of a bolus or small volume of medication through an existing i.v. infusion line or intermittent venous access (heparin or saline lock)
3. "Piggyback" infusion of a solution containing the prescribed medication and a small volume of i.v. fluid through an existing i.v. line

In all three methods, the patient has either an existing i.v. infusion running continuously or an i.v. access site for intermittent infusions. Most policies and procedures list

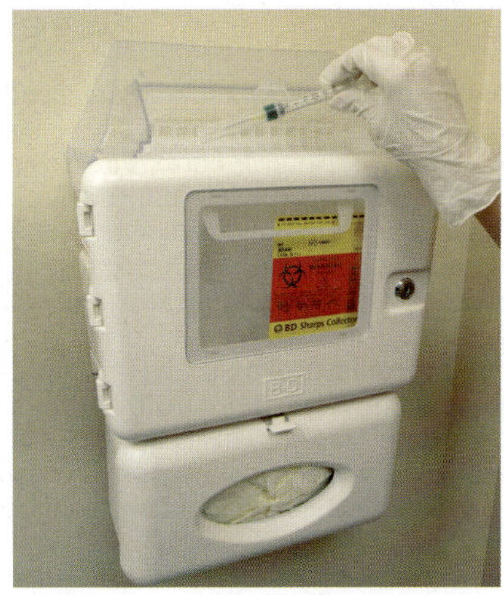

Fig. 26.26 Sharps disposal using only one hand.

BOX 26.18 Recommendations for Prevention of Needlestick Injuries

- Avoid using needles when effective needleless systems or sharps with engineered sharps injury protection (SESIP) safety devices are available.
- Do not recap any needle after medication administration.
- Plan safe handling and disposal of needles before beginning a procedure.
- Immediately dispose of needles, needleless systems, and SESIP devices into puncture-proof, leak-proof sharps disposal containers.
- Maintain a sharps injury log that includes the following: type and brand of device involved in incident, location of incident (e.g., department or work area), description of incident, and a way to protect privacy of the employees who have had sharps injuries.
- Attend educational programs on blood-borne pathogens and follow recommendations for infection prevention, including receiving the hepatitis B vaccine.
- Participate in the selection and evaluation of SESIP devices with safety features within your institution whenever possible.

Data from Occupational Safety and Health Administration (OSHA): Bloodborne pathogens and needlestick injuries, *Fed Reg* 77(64):19934, 2012, https://www.osha.gov/FedReg_osha_pdf/FED20120403.pdf.

the people who may give i.v. medications, the types of medications, and the patient care units in which they can be given. These policies are based on the medication, capability, and availability of staff and the type of monitoring equipment available. Chapter 25 describes the technique for performing venipuncture and establishing continuous i.v. fluid infusions.

When you administer i.v. medications, observe patients closely for symptoms of adverse reactions. After a medication enters the bloodstream, it begins to act immediately, and there is no way to stop its action. Thus, take special care to avoid errors in dose calculation and preparation. Carefully follow the six rights of safe medication administration and know the desired action and side effects of every medication you give. If the medication has an antidote, make sure that it is available during administration. There are situations where it is recommended to do an independent double check of a medication dosage, especially high-risk medications given intravenously. The ISMP (2013c) describes how to do an independent double check:

- A double check must be conducted independently by a second person.
- Two people must *separately* check each component of the work process. For example, a pharmacist calculates a dose, prepares a syringe of medication, and compares the product with the order; then a nurse *independently* checks the order, calculates the dose, and compares the results with the dispensed product for verification.
- Two people are unlikely to make the same mistake if they work independently. It is not effective to hold up a syringe and a vial and say, "This is 5 units of insulin; can you check it?" The person asking for the double check must not influence the individual checking the product in any way.
- Use a double check only for very selective high-risk tasks or high-alert medications *(not all)* that most warrant their use (see agency policy) (Box 26.19). High-alert medications are defined as medications that are the most likely to cause significant patient harm, even when used correctly.
- Fewer double checks performed strategically at the most vulnerable points of the medication use process are more effective than too many.

BOX 26.19 Evidence-Based Practice

PICO Question: What guidelines should RNs follow in the safe administration of high-alert medications?

Summary of Evidence

High-alert medications (e.g., insulin, anticoagulants, opioids) are medications that are the most likely to cause significant patient harm, even when used correctly (Pfoh et al., 2013). These medications are more likely to be associated with harm because of narrow therapeutic ranges (increasing the potential for a prescribing error). Drugs with a narrow therapeutic range are dangerous because small changes in dosage or blood drug levels can lead to dose-dependent or blood concentration–dependent critical therapeutic failures or adverse drug effects (Anderson and Townsend, 2015). High-alert medications also cause more significant harm when an error does occur because of the significant nature of the potential adverse effects such as bleeding or hypoglycemia (Pfoh et al., 2013). The Joint Commission (2014a) requires hospitals to develop an up-to-date list of high-alert medications, to have a process for managing high-alert medications, and to implement that process. The Institute for Safe Medication Practices (2014) routinely updates a list of high-alert medications (https://www.ismp.org/tools/institutionalhighAlert.asp).

Application to Nursing Practice

- Hospitals should form multidisciplinary pharmacy and therapeutics committee teams with nurses and pharmacists working together to identify issues contributing to high-alert medication errors.
- Nurses should perform independent double checks for high-alert medications (ISMP, 2014).
- Other strategies include improving access to information about high-alert drugs; limiting physical access to high-alert medications; using auxiliary labels and automated alerts; and standardizing ordering, storage, preparation, and administration of these drugs (ISMP, 2014).
- Errors may be avoided by reducing interruptions from patients' families, transporters, physicians, and telephone calls. Limit communication during medication administration by screening telephone calls and placing removable warning signs on medication carts during medication administration (Pfoh et al., 2013).

Administering medications by the i.v. route has advantages. It is the best route in emergencies when a fast-acting medication must be delivered quickly. The i.v. route is also best when the patient needs medications at constant therapeutic blood levels.

Some medications are highly alkaline and irritating to muscle and subcutaneous tissue. These medications cause less discomfort when given intravenously. Because i.v. medications are immediately available to the bloodstream after they are administered, you must verify the rate of administration with a medication reference or a pharmacist before giving these medications to ensure that you give them safely over the appropriate amount of time. Patients experience severe adverse reactions if i.v. medications are administered too quickly.

Large-Volume Infusions

In the past, nurses often mixed medications into large volumes of i.v. fluids (500–1000 mL). However, safety standards and scientific evidence no longer support this practice (INS, 2016). Many patient safety risks such as incorrect calculation, poor aseptic technique, incorrect labeling, pump programming errors, lack of medication knowledge, and mix-up with another medication occur when nurses have to prepare medications in i.v. containers on patient care units. Box 26.20 summarizes current best practices for preparation and administration of i.v. medications.

Pharmacies prepare medications in large volumes (500 or 1000 mL) of compatible i.v. fluids such as normal saline or lactated Ringer solution. Vitamins and potassium chloride are two types of medications often added to i.v. fluids. Continuous infusion carries a risk: If the i.v. fluid is infused too rapidly, the patient is at risk for medication overdose and circulatory fluid overload.

Nurses mix medications into i.v. fluids *only* in emergencies. A nurse *never* prepares high-alert medications (such as heparin, dopamine, dobutamine, nitroglycerin, potassium, antibiotics, or magnesium) on a patient care unit. Check with a pharmacist to confirm medication and dose before mixing a medication in an i.v. container. If a pharmacist confirms that you need to prepare the medication, ask another nurse to verify your medication calculations and add medications *only* to new i.v. bags. *Do not* add medications to i.v. bags that are already hanging because you have no way to know the exact concentration of the medication. Always have an experienced nurse watch you during the entire procedure to ensure that you prepare the medication safely.

Administer the medication to the patient at the prescribed rate (see Chapter 25). When you administer medications in large i.v. infusions, regulate the i.v. rate according to the health care provider's order. Monitor patients closely for adverse reactions to the medication and fluid volume overload. Also, check the site often for infiltration and phlebitis.

BOX 26.20 Best Practices for Administration of Intravenous Solutions and Medications

- Use standardized concentrations and dosages of medication.
- Use standardized procedures for ordering, preparing, and administering i.v. medications.
- Use technology (e.g., bar code, smart pump with dose-error reduction software), when available, to verify medications before administration.
- Administer solutions and medications prepared and dispensed from the pharmacy or as commercially prepared solutions and medications in accordance with the *United States Pharmacopeia* (USP).
- Never prepare high-alert medications (e.g., heparin, dopamine, dobutamine, nitroglycerin, potassium, antibiotics, or magnesium) on a patient care unit.
- Use standardized infusion concentrations of high-alert medications.
- Standardize storage of i.v. medications.
- Use the mnemonic CATS PRRR to help remember safety checks for administering i.v. medications: *C*, compatibilities; *A*, allergies; *T*, tubing correct; *S*, site checked; *P*, pump safety checked; *R*, right rate; *R*, release clamps; *R*, return and reassess the patient.
- Use standardized label practices: Patient name in bold, generic drug name, and patient-specific dose.

Adapted from Infusion Nurses Society: Infusion nursing standards of practice, *J Intraven Nurs* 39(1S), 2016; Institute for Safe Medication Practices (ISMP): *Guidelines for standard order sets*, 2010, available at http://www.ismp.org/tools/guidelines/StandardOrderSets.pdf; Institute for Safe Medication Practices (ISMP): *Principles of designing a medication label for intravenous piggyback medication for patient specific, inpatient use*, 2015, http://www.ismp.org/Tools/guidelines/labelFormats/Piggyback.asp; and The Joint Commission: *2017 National Patient Safety Goals hospital program*, 2017, http://www.jointcommission.org/standards_information/npsgs.aspx.

Intravenous Bolus

An i.v. bolus introduces a concentrated dose of a medication directly into the systemic circulation (see Skill 26.6). Because a bolus requires only a small amount of fluid to deliver a medication, it is especially useful in patients who have fluid restrictions. The i.v. bolus, or "push," is the most dangerous method for administering medications because there is no time to correct errors. A bolus may cause irritation to the lining of blood vessels.

Before you administer a bolus, confirm placement of the i.v. line. Never give a medication intravenously if the insertion site appears swollen or edematous or the i.v. fluid cannot flow at the proper rate. Accidental injection of a medication into the tissues around a vein causes pain, sloughing of tissues, and abscesses, depending on the composition of the medication. Medications that carry a risk of adverse effects if administered too quickly into a vein should be diluted and administered as a piggyback or via an infusion pump.

Determine the rate of administration of an i.v. bolus medication by the amount of medication that can be given each minute. For example, if a patient is to receive 4 mL of a medication over 2 minutes, give 2 mL of the i.v. bolus medication every minute. Refer to a pharmacy reference to look up each medication to determine its recommended concentration and rate of administration. The ISMP (2015e) recommends avoiding terms such as "i.v. push," "IVP," or "bolus" in orders with drugs that require administration over 1 minute or longer. Use more descriptive terms such as "i.v. over 5 minutes." Consider the purpose for which a medication is prescribed and any potential adverse effects related to the rate or route of administration.

Volume-Controlled Infusions

Another method of administering i.v. medications is through small amounts (50–100 mL) of compatible i.v. fluids. The fluid is within a secondary fluid container separate from the primary fluid bag. The container connects directly to the primary i.v. line or to separate tubing that inserts into the primary line (see Skill 26.7). There are three types of containers: piggyback sets, volume-control administration sets (such as Volutrol or Pediatrol), and syringe pumps. Volume-controlled infusion has several advantages:

- It reduces the risk of rapid-dose infusion by i.v. push. Medications are diluted and infused over longer time intervals (e.g., 30–60 minutes).

- It allows for administration of medications (such as antibiotics) that are stable for a limited time in solution.
- It allows for control of i.v. fluid intake.

A piggyback is a small (25- to 250-mL) i.v. bag or bottle connected to a short tubing line that connects to the *upper* Y-port of a primary infusion line or to an intermittent venous access device such as a saline lock. The label on the medication follows the ISMP i.v. piggyback medication label format (Fig. 26.27) (ISMP, 2016c).

The piggyback tubing is a microdrip or macrodrip system (see Chapter 25). The set is called a *piggyback* because the small bag or bottle is set *higher* than the primary infusion bag or bottle. In the piggyback setup, the main line does not infuse when a compatible piggybacked medication is infusing. The port of the primary i.v. line contains a back-check valve that automatically stops the flow of the primary infusion once the piggyback infusion flows. After the piggyback solution infuses and the solution within the tubing falls below the level of the primary infusion drip chamber, the back-check valve opens, and the primary infusion starts to flow again.

Volume-control administration (such as with Buretrol) sets are small (150-mL) containers that attach just below the primary infusion bag or bottle. The set is attached and filled in a manner similar to that used with a regular i.v. infusion. Follow package directions for priming sets.

A syringe pump is battery operated and allows medications to be given in very small amounts of fluid (5–60 mL) within controlled infusion times using standard syringes.

Intermittent Venous Access

An intermittent venous access (commonly called a *saline lock*) is an i.v. catheter capped off on the end with a small chamber covered by a rubber diaphragm or a specially designed cap. Special rubber-seal injection caps usually accept needleless safety devices (see Chapter 25). The advantages of intermittent venous access include cost savings resulting from the omission of continuous i.v. therapy and saving a nurse's time by eliminating constant monitoring of flow rates. Intermittent venous access allows increased patient mobility, safety, and comfort.

Before you administer an i.v. bolus or volume-controlled medications, assess the patency of the line and placement of the i.v. catheter. After the medication has been administered through an intermittent venous access, the access must be flushed with a solution to keep it patent. Normal saline generally is an effective flush solution for peripheral catheters. Some agencies require the use of heparin. Follow agency policies for the care and maintenance of the i.v. site.

Administration of Intravenous Therapy in the Home

Patients sometimes need i.v. medication therapy at home. Common infusions that patients receive include antibiotics, chemotherapy, total parenteral nutrition, and analgesics. Most patients receive home i.v. therapy through a long-term central venous catheter (CVC) (see Chapter 25). Home health nurses assess patients' responses to the medication, monitor the CVC site, and teach patients and family caregivers how to administer infusions and medications and maintain the CVC.

Carefully assess patients and family caregivers to determine their ability to manage i.v. therapy at home. Begin instruction on i.v. care as soon as you know that a patient will have i.v. therapy at home. Patients and families must learn to recognize problems such as signs of infections related to i.v. therapy, symptoms of ADRs, and steps to take when these problems occur. Patients also need to know when to notify the home care nurse or health care provider. Plan to teach patients and family caregivers how to maintain i.v. administration equipment including the infusion pump.

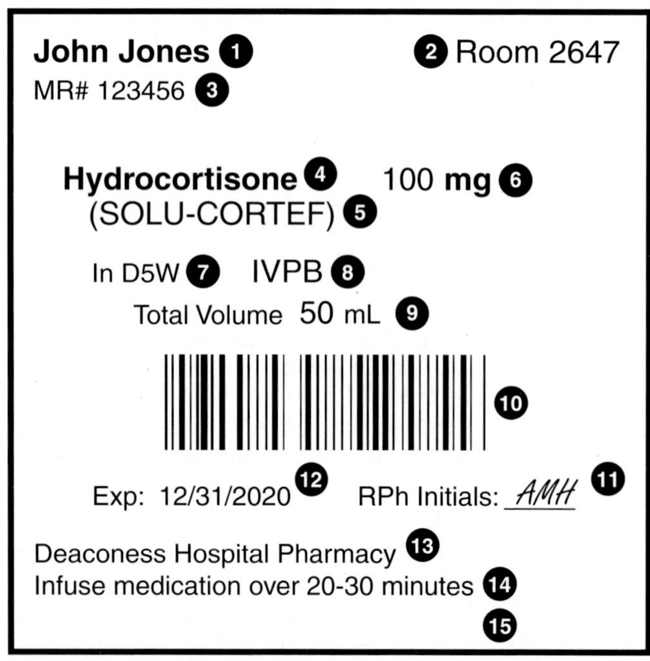

1. **Patient name**
2. Location
3. Second identifier (Date of birth, Financial #, Encounter #, Medical record #)
4. **Generic name**
5. BRAND name
6. **Patient dose**
7. Diluent
8. Route
9. Total volume
10. Bar code
11. Initials as needed
12. Expiration date as needed, in MM/DD/YYYY format
13. Pharmacy information if required
14. Comments
15. Other information as required by state or federal law

Fig. 26.27 I.v. piggyback medication label following Institute for Safe Medication Practices safe labeling guidelines.

SAFETY GUIDELINES FOR NURSING SKILLS

Ensuring patient safety is an essential role of the professional nurse. To ensure patient safety, communicate clearly with members of the health care team, assess and incorporate the patient's priorities of care and preferences, and use the best evidence when making decisions about your patient's care. When you perform the skills covered in this chapter, remember the following points to ensure safe, individualized patient care:

- Be vigilant during the entire process of medication preparation and administration, and make sure that your patients receive the appropriate medications. Know why your patient is receiving each medication; know what you need to do before, during, and after medication administration; and evaluate the effectiveness of the medication and assess for adverse effects.
- Use strict aseptic technique during medication preparation and administration.
- Take care of yourself. Ensure that you are as healthy as possible to enable yourself to think as clearly and critically as possible. Healthy behaviors help you better process information and make safe decisions during medication administration.
- Prepare medications in areas that are free from distractions. No-interruption zones (NIZs) are recommended (Yoder et al., 2015). NIZs are created by placing red tape or tile borders on the floor around medication carts. Nurses standing in these zones are not to be interrupted.
- Always verify that medications have not expired.
- Use at least two patient identifiers before administering medications to your patients.
- Clarify unclear orders and ask for help whenever you are uncertain about a medication order or calculation. Consult with your peers, pharmacists, and other health care providers.
- Use technology (e.g., bar scanning, eMARs) that your institution uses when preparing and giving medications. Follow all policies related to the use of the technology and do not use work-arounds. Nurses who use work-arounds fail to follow institution protocols, policies, or procedures during medication administration in an attempt to administer medications to patients more quickly.
- Follow standards set by your state's NPA and guidelines established by your health care agency before delegating medication administration. Licensed practical nurses (LPNs) or licensed vocational nurses (LVNs) usually can administer medications via the oral (p.o.), subcutaneous, i.m., and i.d. routes. Some states also allow certified medical assistants (CMAs) to administer some types of medications (e.g., oral medications) in some health care settings (e.g., long-term care facilities).
- Follow safety guidelines to prevent needlestick injuries. Use engineering devices, and dispose of all sharps in safety containers.

SKILL 26.1 Administering Oral Medications

Equipment

- Automated, computer-controlled drug dispensing system or medication cart
- Oral syringe dispensed by pharmacy (liquid medications only)
- Disposable medication cups (for holding tablets and/or capsules)
- Glass of water, juice, or preferred liquid and drinking straw
- Device for crushing or splitting tablets *(optional)*
- Paper towels
- MAR (electronic or printed)
- Clean gloves (if handling an oral medication)

STEP	RATIONALE
Assessment	
1. Check accuracy and completeness of each MAR with health care provider's medication order. Check the patient's name and drug name, dosage, and route and time of administration. Clarify incomplete or unclear orders with health care provider before administration.	The order sheet is the most reliable source and only legal record of medications that the patient is to receive. Ensures that the patient receives correct medications (Mandrack et al., 2012). Illegible MARs are a source of medication errors (Alassaad et al., 2013).
2. Review pertinent information related to medication including action, purpose, normal dose and route, side effects, time of onset and peak action, and nursing implications.	Allows you to anticipate effects of drug while observing the patient's response.
3. Assess for any contraindications to the patient receiving oral medication including being on NPO status, inability to swallow, nausea/vomiting, bowel inflammation, reduced peristalsis, recent gastrointestinal (GI) surgery, gastric suction, and decreased level of consciousness (LOC). Notify health care provider if any contraindications are present.	Alterations in GI function can interfere with drug absorption, distribution, and excretion. Giving oral medications to patients with impaired swallowing or decreased LOC increases their risk for aspiration (Park et al., 2013). Patients with GI suction do not experience actions of oral medications because the medications are suctioned from the GI tract before they are absorbed.

STEP	RATIONALE
4. Assess the patient's medical, medication, and diet history and history of allergies. List any drug allergies on each page of the MAR and prominently display on the patient's medical record. When allergies are present, the patient should wear an allergy bracelet.	These factors influence how certain drugs act. Information reveals previous problems with medication administration. Allergy alert helps prevent adverse events.
5. Perform hand hygiene. Gather and review physical assessment findings including the patient's weight (in metric units), vital signs, and laboratory data that influence drug administration such as results of renal and liver function studies.	Many medication doses are based on a patient's weight (ISMP, 2016b). Physical examination findings or laboratory data may contraindicate drug administration. Renal and liver function status affects metabolism and excretion (Burchum and Rosenthal, 2016).
6. Assess risk for aspiration using a dysphagia screening tool if available (see Chapter 20). Protect the patient from aspiration by assessing swallowing ability.	Aspiration occurs when food, fluid, or medication intended for GI administration is inadvertently administered into the respiratory tract. Patients with altered ability to swallow are at higher risk for aspiration (Park et al., 2013).
7. Assess the patient's symptoms before initiating medication therapy.	Provides information to evaluate desired effect of medication.
8. Assess the patient's and family caregiver's knowledge regarding health and medication use, medication schedule, and ability to prepare medications.	Determines the patient's and caregiver's need for medication education and guidance to achieve drug adherence.
9. Assess the patient's preference for fluids and determine whether medications can be given with these fluids. Maintain fluid restrictions as prescribed.	Some fluids interfere with medication absorption (e.g., dairy products affect tetracycline). Offering fluids during drug administration is an excellent way to increase the patient's fluid intake. Fluids ease swallowing and facilitate absorption from the GI tract. However, if fluid restrictions exist, skillful planning of fluid intake must coordinate with medication times and type of medications.
Planning	
1. Perform hand hygiene. Collect appropriate equipment and MAR.	Promotes time management and efficiency when preparing medications for all patients.
2. Plan preparation to avoid interruptions. Create a quiet environment. Do not take phone calls or talk with others. Follow agency no-interruption zone policy.	Interruptions contribute to medication errors (see Box 26.4) (Beyea, 2014; Yoder et al., 2015).
Implementation	
1. Prepare medications.	
a. Perform hand hygiene.	Reduces transfer of microorganisms.
b. Arrange medication tray and cups in medication preparation area or move medication cart to position outside the patient's room.	Organization of equipment saves time and reduces error.
c. Log on to automated dispensing system (ADS) or unlock medicine drawer or cart.	Medications are safeguarded when locked in cabinet, cart, or ADS.
d. Prepare medications for *one patient at a time.* Follow the six rights of medication administration. Keep all pages of MARs or computer printouts for one patient together or look at only one patient's medication administration computer screen.	Prevents preparation errors.
e. Select correct medication from ADS, unit-dose drawer, or stock supply. Compare name of medication on label with MAR or computer printout (see illustration). Exit ADS after removing drug.	Reading label and comparing it against transcribed order reduces errors. Exiting ADS ensures that no one else can remove medications using your identity. *This is the first check for accuracy.*

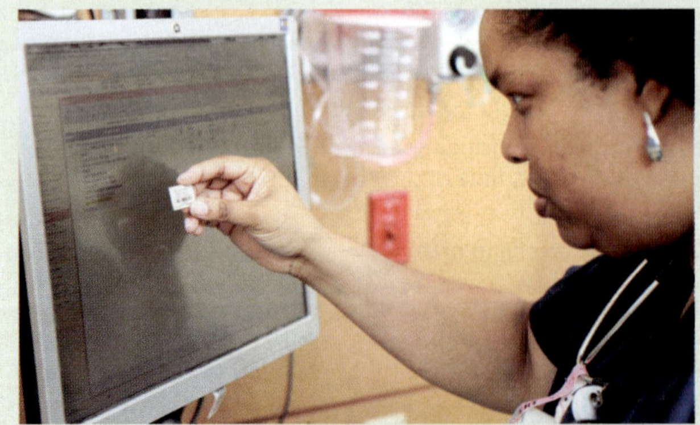

Step 1e Check label of medication with patient's MAR.

STEP	RATIONALE
f. Check or calculate drug dose as necessary. Double-check any calculation. Check expiration date on all medications and return outdated medication to pharmacy.	Double-checking pharmacy calculations reduces risk for error. Agency policy may require you to check calculations of certain medications such as insulin with another nurse (Kim and Bates, 2013). Expired medications may be inactive or harmful to the patient.
g. If preparing a controlled substance, check record for previous medication count and compare current count with supply available. Controlled drugs may be stored in computerized locked cart.	Controlled substance laws require nurses to carefully monitor and count dispensed controlled drugs (e.g., opioids).
h. Prepare solid forms of oral medications.	
(1) To prepare unit-dose tablets or capsules, place packaged tablet or capsule directly into medication cup without removing wrapper. Administer medications only from containers with labels that are clearly marked.	Wrappers maintain cleanliness and identify drug name and dose, which can facilitate teaching.
(2) When using a blister pack, "pop" medications through foil or paper backing into a medication cup (see illustration).	Packs provide a 1-month supply, with each "blister" usually containing a single dose.
(3) If it is necessary to give half the dose of medication, pharmacy should split, label, package, and send medication to unit. If you must split medication, use clean, gloved hand to cut with clean pill-cutting device. Only cut tablets that are prescored by the manufacturer (line traverses the center of the tablet).	Reduces contamination of tablet. In health care agencies, only pharmacy should split tablets to ensure patient safety (FDA, 2013). If a tablet is FDA-approved to be split, this information will be printed in the "HOW SUPPLIED" section of the professional label insert.
(4) Place all tablets or capsules that the patient will receive in one medicine cup except for those requiring preadministration assessments (e.g., pulse rate or blood pressure). Place these in separate additional cup with wrapper intact.	Keeping medications that require preadministration assessments separate from others serves as a reminder and makes it easier to withhold drugs as necessary.
(5) If the patient has difficulty swallowing and liquid medications are not an option, use a pill-crushing device (see illustration). Clean device before using. If a device is not available, place medicine in between two cups, and grind and crush. Mix ground tablet in small amount (teaspoon) of soft food (custard or applesauce).	Large tablets are often difficult to swallow. Ground tablet mixed with palatable soft food is usually easier to swallow.
Clinical decision point: Not all medications can be safely crushed. Consult with a pharmacist or the ISMP Do Not Crush List (ISMP, 2015c).	
i. Prepare liquids.	
(1) Unit-dose container with correct amount of medication: Gently shake the container. Administer medication packaged in a single-dose cup directly from the single-dose cup. Do not pour medicine into another cup.	Using unit-dose container with correct dosage of medication provides most accurate dose of medication (ISMP, 2016b). Shaking container ensures that medication is mixed before administration.
(2) Unit-dose oral syringe (see illustration): Be sure to use only oral syringes marked "Oral Use Only" dispensed by the pharmacy.	Ensure that all oral liquids that are not commercially available as unit-dose products are dispensed by the pharmacy in an oral syringe (ISMP, 2016b).

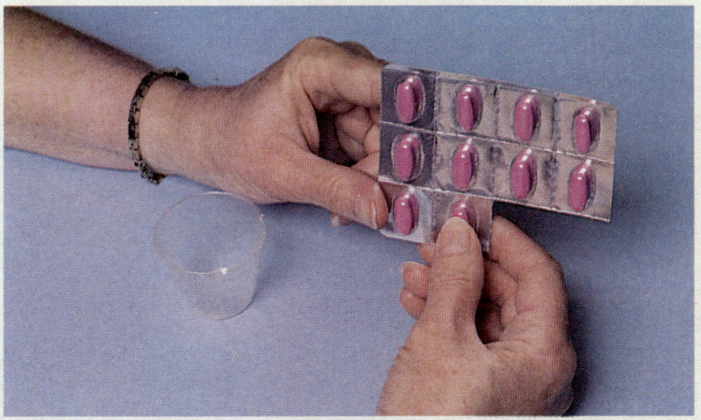

Step 1h(2) Place tablet from blister pack into medicine cup without removing wrapper.

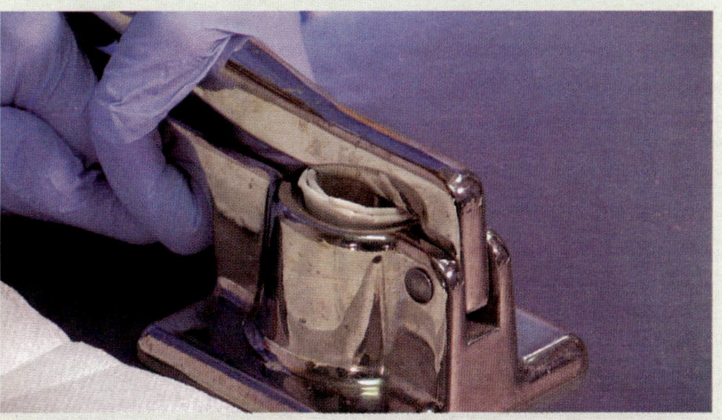

Step 1h(5) Pill-crushing device.

STEP	RATIONALE

Clinical decision point: Based on current best practice (ISMP, 2016b; Paparella, 2014), liquid medications that are not available or are not in correct dose in a unit-dose container should be dispensed by the pharmacy in special oral syringes marked "Oral Use Only." These syringes do not connect to any type of parenteral (e.g., i.v.) tubing. Additionally, current evidence shows that liquid measuring devices on patient care units result in inaccurate dosing. Having oral medications prepared in the pharmacy ensures accurate dosing and prevents parenteral administration of oral medications.

STEP	RATIONALE
j. Return stock containers or unused unit-dose medications to shelf or drawer. Label medication cups and poured medications with the patient's name before leaving medication preparation area. Do not leave drugs unattended. Perform hand hygiene.	Ensures that correct medications are prepared for the correct patient.
k. Before going to the patient's room, compare the patient's name and name of medication on label of prepared drugs with MAR.	Reading labels a second time reduces errors. *This is the second check for accuracy.*
2. Administer medications.	
a. Take medication to the patient at correct time (see agency policy). Medications that require exact timing include STAT doses, first-time or loading doses, and one-time doses. Give time-critical scheduled medications at exact time ordered (no later than 30 min before or after scheduled dose). Given non-time-critical scheduled medications within a range of 1 or 2 h of scheduled dose (ISMP, 2011a). During administration, apply six rights of medication administration.	Hospitals must adopt medication administration policy and procedure for timing of medication administration that considers the nature of prescribed medication, specific clinical application, and patient needs (CMS, 2011; ISMP, 2011a). Time-critical scheduled medications are those for which early or delayed administration of maintenance doses may cause harm or result in substantial suboptimal therapy or pharmacological effect. Non-time-critical medications are those for which early or delayed administration should not cause harm or result in substantial suboptimal therapy or pharmacological effect (CMS, 2011; ISMP, 2011a).
b. Identify the patient by using at least two identifiers (e.g., name and birthday or name and medical record number) according to agency policy. Compare identifiers with information on the patient's MAR or medical record.	Ensures correct patient. Complies with The Joint Commission Standards and improves patient safety (TJC, 2018).
c. At the patient's bedside, again compare MAR or computer printout with name of medication on medication label and patient name. Ask the patient whether he or she has allergies.	*This is the third check for accuracy* and ensures that the patient receives correct medication. Confirms the patient's allergy history.
d. Explain the purpose of each medication, action, and most common possible adverse effects. Allow sufficient time for the patient to ask questions. Include family caregiver if appropriate.	The patient has the right to be informed, and patient and family caregiver understanding of each medication improves adherence with drug therapy.
e. Perform hand hygiene. Perform necessary preadministration assessment (e.g., blood pressure, pulse) for specific medications. Ask the patient again whether he or she has allergies.	Reduces transmission of microorganisms. Determines whether specific medications should be withheld at that time. Confirms the patient's allergy history.

Clinical decision point: If the patient expresses concern regarding accuracy of a medication, do not give the medication. Explore the patient's concern and verify health care provider's order before administering. Listening to the patient's concerns may prevent a medication error.

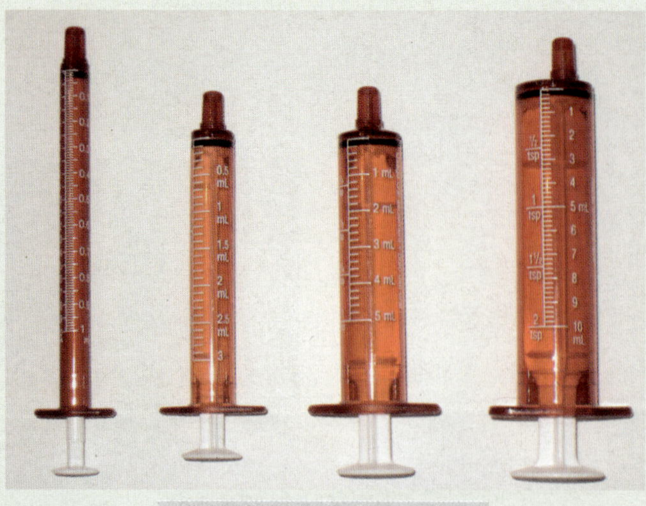

Step 1i(2) Unit-dose oral syringe.

STEP	RATIONALE
f. Assist the patient to sitting or Fowler's position. Use side-lying position if the patient is unable to sit. Have the patient stay in this position for 30 min after administration.	Decreases risk for aspiration during swallowing.
g. For tablets: The patient may wish to hold solid medication in hand or cup before placing in mouth. Offer water or preferred liquid to help the patient swallow medication.	The patient can become familiar with medications by seeing each drug. Choice of fluid can improve fluid intake.
h. For orally disintegrating formulations (tablets or strips): Remove medication from packet just before use. Do not push tablet through foil. Place medication on top of the patient's tongue. Caution against chewing it.	Orally disintegrating formulations begin to dissolve when placed on tongue. Water is not needed. Careful removal from packaging is necessary because tablets and strips are thin and fragile.
i. For sublingually administered medications: Have the patient place medication under tongue and allow it to dissolve completely. Caution the patient against swallowing tablet or saliva.	Drug is absorbed through blood vessels of undersurface of tongue. If swallowed, drug is destroyed by gastric juices or rapidly detoxified by liver, preventing therapeutic blood level.
j. For buccal administered medications: Have the patient place medication in mouth against mucous membranes of cheek and gums until it dissolves.	Buccal medications act locally or systemically as they are swallowed in saliva.
Clinical decision point: Avoid administering anything by mouth until orally disintegrating buccal or sublingual medication is completely dissolved.	
k. For powdered medications: Mix with liquids at bedside and give to the patient to drink.	When prepared in advance, powdered drugs thicken and some even harden, making swallowing difficult.
l. For crushed medications mixed with food: Give each medication separately in teaspoon of food.	Ensures that the patient swallows all of medicine. *Never mix medication in a meal serving of food.*
m. For lozenges: Caution the patient against chewing or swallowing lozenges.	Lozenges act through slow absorption through oral mucosa, not gastric mucosa.
n. For effervescent medications: Add tablet or powder to a glass of water. Administer immediately after dissolving.	Effervescence improves unpleasant taste and often relieves GI problems.
o. If the patient is unable to hold medications, place medication cup or oral syringe to lips and gently introduce each drug into mouth. Give a tablet or capsule one at a time. Inject a liquid slowly. A spoon can also be used to place a pill in the patient's mouth. Do not rush or force medications.	Administering a single-dose tablet, capsule, or oral syringe dose eases swallowing and decreases risk for aspiration.
Clinical decision point: If tablet or capsule falls to the floor, it becomes contaminated; discard it and repeat preparation.	
p. Stay until the patient swallows each medication completely or takes it by the prescribed route. Ask the patient to open mouth if uncertain whether medication has been swallowed.	Ensures that the patient receives ordered dose. If left unattended, the patient may not take dose or may save drugs, causing health risks.
q. For highly acidic medications (e.g., aspirin), offer the patient a nonfat snack (e.g., crackers) if not contraindicated by his or her condition.	Reduces gastric irritation. Fat content of foods may delay drug absorption.
r. Help the patient return to position of comfort.	Maintains the patient's comfort.
s. Dispose of soiled supplies and perform hand hygiene. Return cart to medication room if used. Clean work area.	Reduces spread of microorganisms.
3. Replenish stock such as cups and straws, and return cart to medication room and clean work area.	Enhances efficiency and reduces transfer of microorganisms.
Evaluation	
1. Return within an appropriate time to evaluate the patient's response to medications including therapeutic effects, side effects or allergy, and adverse reactions.	Evaluates therapeutic benefit of drug and helps to detect onset of side effects or allergic reactions. Sublingual medications act in 15 min; most oral medications act in 30–60 min.
2. Ask the patient or family caregiver to identify drug name and explain purpose, action, dose schedule, and potential side effects.	Determines level of knowledge gained by the patient and family caregiver.
3. **Use teach back:** "I want to be sure I showed you how to use your sublingual nitroglycerin. For this dose, show me where you will place the tablet in your mouth." Revise your instruction now or develop a plan for revised patient/family caregiver teaching if the patient/family caregiver is not able to teach back correctly.	Determines the patient's/family caregiver's level of understanding of instructional topic.

Recording and Reporting

- Record drug, dose, route, and time administered on the patient's MAR immediately after administration, not before. Include initials or signature.
- Record patient response to medication, instruction (including teach back), and validation of understanding on flow sheet or nurses' notes in EHR or chart.
- If you do not give the drug, record reason on flow sheet or nurses' notes in EHR or chart, and follow agency policy for noting withheld doses.
- Report adverse effects and patient response and/or withheld drugs to nurse in charge or health care provider. Depending on medication, immediate notification of health care provider may be required.

Unexpected Outcomes and Related Interventions

- The patient exhibits adverse effects (e.g., side effect, toxic effect, allergic reaction).
    - Notify health care provider and pharmacy.
    - Withhold further doses.
    - Assess vital signs.
    - Symptoms such as urticaria, rash, pruritus, rhinitis, and wheezing may indicate an allergic reaction and need for emergency medications.
    - Add allergy information to the patient's medical record.
- The patient refuses medication.
    - Assess reason for the patient refusing medication.
    - Provide further instruction.
    - Do not force the patient to take medications.
    - Notify health care provider.
- The patient is unable to explain drug information.
    - Further assess the patient's or family caregiver's knowledge of medications and guidelines for drug safety.
    - Further instruction or different approach to instruction is necessary.

SKILL 26.2 Administering Eye (Ophthalmic) Medications

Equipment

- Appropriate medication (eye drops with sterile eye dropper, ointment tube)
- Clean gloves
- MAR (electronic or printed)

Eye Drops/Ointment Only

- Cotton ball or tissue
- Washbasin filled with warm water and washcloth
- Eye patch and tape *(optional)*

STEP	RATIONALE
Assessment	
1. Check accuracy and completeness of each MAR with health care provider's medication order. Check the patient's name, drug name and dosage, route, and time for administration. Clarify incomplete or unclear orders with health care provider before administration.	The order sheet is the most reliable source and only legal record of medications that the patient is to receive. Ensures that the patient receives correct medications (Mandrack et al., 2012). Illegible MARs are a source of medication errors (Alassaad et al., 2013).
2. Review pertinent information related to medication including action, purpose, normal dose and route, side effects, time of onset and peak action, and nursing implications.	Allows you to anticipate effects of drug while observing the patient's response.
3. Assess the patient's medical and medication history and history of allergies. List any drug allergies on each page of the MAR and prominently display on the patient's medical record. When allergies are present, the patient should wear an allergy bracelet.	Factors influence how certain drugs act. Reveals the patient's need for medication. Allergy alert prevents adverse event.
4. Perform hand hygiene. Assess condition of external eye structures (see Chapter 7). This may be done just before drug instillation (if drainage is present, apply clean gloves).	Provides baseline to determine whether local response to medications occurs. Also indicates need to clean eye before drug application.
5. Determine whether the patient has any symptoms of eye discomfort or visual impairment.	Certain eye medications act to either lessen or increase these symptoms. Provides baseline for evaluation of medication effect.
6. Assess the patient's level of consciousness (LOC) and ability to follow directions.	If the patient becomes restless or combative during procedure, greater risk for accidental eye injury exists.
7. Assess the patient's and family caregiver's knowledge regarding drug therapy and the patient's desire to self-administer medication.	Indicates need for health teaching. Motivation influences teaching approach.
8. Assess the patient's ability to manipulate and hold dropper or ocular disk.	Reflects the patient's ability to learn to self-administer drug.

STEP	RATIONALE
Planning	
1. Perform hand hygiene. Collect appropriate equipment and MAR.	Reduces transmission of microorganisms. Promotes time management and efficiency when preparing medications for all patients.
2. Plan preparation to avoid interruptions. Create a quiet environment. Do not take phone calls or talk with others. Follow agency no-interruption zone policy.	Distractions and interruptions contribute to medication errors (see Box 26.4) (Beyea, 2014; Yoder et al., 2015).
Implementation	
1. Prepare medications for one patient at a time. Attend to procedure and avoid distraction. Check label of medication against MAR two times, when removing medication from unit dose or AMDS and before leaving medication preparation area (see Skill 26.1). Prepare eye drops by taking container out of refrigerator and rewarming to room temperature before administering to the patient. Check expiration date on container. Perform hand hygiene.	Warming eye drops reduces eye irritation. *These are the first and second checks for accuracy.* Process ensures that right patient receives right medication.
2. Take medication to the patient at correct time (see agency policy). Medications that require exact timing include STAT doses, first-time or loading doses, and one-time doses. Give time-critical scheduled medications at exact time ordered (no later than 30 min before or after scheduled dose). Give non-time-critical scheduled medications within a range of 1 or 2 h of scheduled dose (ISMP, 2011a). During administration, apply six rights of medication administration.	Hospitals must adopt medication administration policy and procedure for timing of medication administration that considers nature of prescribed medication, specific clinical application, and patient needs (CMS, 2011; ISMP, 2011a). Time-critical scheduled medications are those for which early or delayed administration of maintenance doses may cause harm or result in substantial suboptimal therapy or pharmacological effect. Non-time-critical medications are those for which early or delayed administration should not cause harm or result in substantial suboptimal therapy or pharmacological effect (CMS, 2011; ISMP, 2011a).
3. Identify the patient by using at least two identifiers (e.g., name and birthday or name and medical record number) according to agency policy. Compare identifiers with information on the patient's MAR or medical record.	Ensures correct patient. Complies with The Joint Commission Standards and improves patient safety (TJC, 2018).
4. At the patient's bedside, again compare MAR or computer printout with names of medications on medication labels and patient name. Ask the patient whether he or she has allergies.	*This is the third check for accuracy* and ensures that the patient receives correct medication. Confirms the patient's allergy history.
5. Discuss purpose of each medication, action, and possible adverse effects. Allow the patient to ask any questions about the drugs. Patients who self-instill medications may be allowed to give drops under nurse's supervision (check agency policy).	The patient has the right to be informed, and the patient's understanding of each medication improves adherence to drug therapy.
6. Tell patients receiving eye drops (e.g., mydriatics) that vision will be blurred temporarily and sensitivity to light may occur.	May relieve anxiety.
Clinical decision point: Instruct and reinforce that the patient should not drive or operate machinery or perform any activity that requires clear vision until vision and sensitivity to light return to normal.	
7. Instill eye medications.	
a. Apply clean gloves. Ask the patient to lie supine or sit back in chair with head slightly hyperextended, looking up.	Position provides easy access to eye for medication instillation and minimizes drainage of medication into tear duct.
Clinical decision point: Do not hyperextend the neck of a patient with cervical spine injury.	
b. If drainage or crusting is present along eyelid margins or inner canthus, gently wash away. Soak any dried crusts with warm, damp washcloth or cotton ball over eye for several minutes. Always wipe clean from inner to outer canthus. Remove gloves and perform hand hygiene.	Soaking allows easy removal of crusts without applying pressure to eye. Cleaning from inner to outer canthus avoids entrance of microorganisms into lacrimal duct (Burchum and Rosenthal, 2016).
c. Explain there might be temporary burning sensation from drops.	Corneas are highly sensitive.
d. Instill eye drops.	
(1) Hold clean cotton ball or tissue in nondominant hand on the patient's cheekbone just below lower eyelid.	Cotton or tissue absorbs medication that escapes eye.
(2) With tissue or cotton ball resting below lower lid, gently press downward with thumb or forefinger against bony orbit, exposing conjunctival sac. Never press directly against the patient's eyeball.	Prevents pressure and trauma to eyeball and prevents fingers from touching eye.

STEP	RATIONALE
(3) Ask the patient to look at ceiling. Rest dominant hand on the patient's forehead; hold filled medication eye dropper approximately 1–2 cm (0.5–1.0 inch) above conjunctival sac (see illustration).	Action moves cornea up and away from conjunctival sac and reduces blink reflex. Prevents accidental contact of eye dropper with eye and reduces risk of injury and transfer of microorganisms to dropper (ophthalmic medications are sterile).
(4) Drop prescribed number of drops into conjunctival sac.	Conjunctival sac normally holds one or two drops. Provides even distribution of medication across eye.
(5) If the patient blinks or closes eye, causing drops to land on outer lid margins, repeat procedure.	Drops must enter conjunctival sac to achieve therapeutic effect.
(6) When administering drops that have systemic effects, apply gentle pressure to the patient's nasolacrimal duct with clean tissue for 30–60 s over each eye, one at a time. Avoid pressure directly against the patient's eyeball.	Prevents overflow of medication into nasal and pharyngeal passages. Prevents absorption into systemic circulation (American Society of Health-System Pharmacists [ASHP], 2013a).
(7) After instilling drops, ask the patient to close eyes gently.	Helps distribute medication. Squinting or squeezing eyelids forces medication from conjunctival sac (ASHP, 2013a).
e. Instill ophthalmic ointment.	
(1) Holding applicator above lower lid margin, apply thin ribbon of ointment evenly along inner edge of lower eyelid on conjunctiva (see illustration) from inner to outer canthus.	Distributes medication evenly across eye and lid margin.
(2) Have the patient close eye and rub lid lightly in circular motion with cotton ball if not contraindicated. Avoid placing pressure directly against the patient's eyeball.	Further distributes medication without traumatizing eye.
(3) If excess medication is on eyelid, gently wipe it from inner to outer canthus.	Promotes comfort and prevents trauma to eye.
(4) If the patient needs an eye patch, place it over affected eye so that entire eye is covered. Tape securely without applying pressure to eye.	Clean eye patch reduces risk of infection.
8. After administering eye medications, remove and dispose of gloves and soiled supplies; perform hand hygiene.	Reduces spread of microorganisms.
Evaluation	
1. Observe response to medication by assessing visual changes, asking whether symptoms are relieved, and noting any side effects or discomfort felt.	Evaluates effects of medication.
2. Ask the patient to discuss purpose of drug, action, side effects, and technique of administration.	Determines the patient's level of understanding.
3. **Use teach back:** "I want to be sure I explained to you clearly how to give yourself eye drops. Show me how to insert your drops into your left eye." Revise your instruction now or develop a plan for revised patient/family caregiver teaching if the patient/family caregiver is not able to teach back correctly.	Determines the patient's/family caregiver's level of understanding of instructional topic.

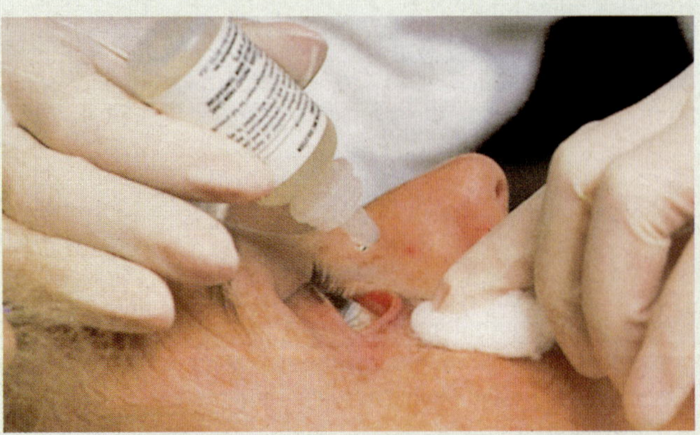

Step 7d(3) Hold eye dropper above conjunctival sac.

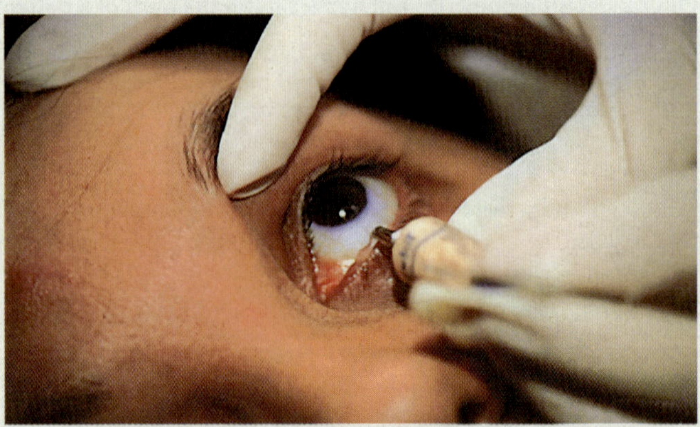

Step 7e(1) Apply ointment along lower eyelid.

Recording and Reporting

- Record drug, concentration, dose or strength, number of drops, site of application (left, right, or both eyes), and time of administration on MAR immediately after administration, not before. Include initials or signature.
- Record objective data related to tissues involved (e.g., redness, drainage, irritation), any subjective data (e.g., pain, itching, altered vision), and the patient's response to medications. Note any side effects experienced on flow sheet or nurses' notes in EHR or chart.
- Record patient teaching and validation of understanding on flow sheet or nurses' notes in EHR or chart. Report adverse effects and patient response and/or withheld drugs to nurse in charge or health care provider.

Unexpected Outcomes and Related Interventions

- The patient complains of burning or pain or experiences local side effects (e.g., headache, bloodshot eyes, local eye irritation). Both drug concentration and patient's sensitivity influence chances of side effects developing.
  - Notify health care provider for possible adjustment in medication type and dosage.
- The patient experiences systemic effects from drops (e.g., increased heart rate and blood pressure from epinephrine, decreased heart rate and blood pressure from timolol).
  - Notify health care provider immediately.
  - Remain with the patient. Assess vital signs.
  - Withhold further doses.
- The patient is unable to explain drug information or steps for taking eye drops and/or has trouble manipulating dropper.
  - Repeat instructions and include family caregiver as appropriate. Include return demonstration.

SKILL 26.3 Using Metered-Dose or Dry Powder Inhalers

Equipment

- Inhaler device with medication canister (metered-dose inhaler [MDI] or dry powder inhaler [DPI])
- Spacer device, such as AeroChamber or InspirEase *(optional for MDI)*
- Facial tissues *(optional)*
- Stethoscope
- MAR (electronic or printed)
- Peak flowmeter *(optional)*

STEP	RATIONALE
Assessment	
1. Check accuracy and completeness of each MAR with health care provider's medication order. Check the patient's name, drug name and dosage, route, and time for administration. Clarify incomplete or unclear orders with health care provider before administration.	The order sheet is the most reliable source and only legal record of medications that the patient is to receive. Ensures that the patient receives correct medications (Mandrack et al., 2012). Illegible MARs are a source of medication errors (Alassaad et al., 2013).
2. Review pertinent information related to medication including action, purpose, normal dose and route, side effects, time of onset and peak action, and nursing implications.	Allows you to anticipate effects of drug while observing the patient's response.
3. Assess the patient's medical and medication history and history of allergies. List any drug allergies on each page of MAR and prominently display on the patient's medical record. When allergies are present, the patient should wear an allergy bracelet.	Factors influence how certain drugs act. Reveals the patient's need for medication. Allergy alert helps prevent adverse events.
4. Perform hand hygiene. Assess the patient's respiratory pattern and auscultate breath sounds.	Reduces transmission of infection. Establishes baseline of airway status for comparison during and after treatment.
5. Measure the patient's peak expiratory flow rate using a peak flowmeter. Have the patient measure if the patient does so at home. Use the patient's peak flowmeter if available (see Chapter 24).	A peak flowmeter is used to measure air flow or peak expiratory flow rate and aids in monitoring airway status of patients with chronic asthma (American Academy of Allergy, Asthma and Immunology [AAAAI], 2016).
6. Assess the patient's symptoms before initiating medication therapy.	Provides information to evaluate desired effect of medication.
7. Assess the patient's ability to hold, manipulate, and depress canister and inhaler.	Any impairment of grasp or presence of hand tremors interferes with the patient's ability to depress canister within inhaler. Spacer device is often necessary with an MDI.
8. If the patient was previously instructed in self-administration, have the patient demonstrate how to use the device.	Patients who have adequate understanding of how to use an inhaler often forget the procedure. Ongoing assessment of inhaler technique identifies areas for further education and reinforcement (Ari and Restrepo, 2012).

STEP	RATIONALE
9. Assess the patient's readiness and ability to learn and use inhaler. Determine type of device the patient prefers, considering portability, access to obtain, and cost. Ask questions about medication and its availability; is patient alert and participative in own care; is patient fatigued, in pain, or in respiratory distress?	When selecting an aerosol delivery device, consider several factors such as drug availability and administration time, patient age and ability to use device correctly, portability of device, convenience in both outpatient and inpatient settings, costs, and physician and patient preference (Barrons et al., 2015; Bonini and Usmani, 2015). In some situations, mental or physical limitations affect the patient's ability to learn and methods used for instruction.
10. Assess the patient's knowledge and understanding of disease and purpose and action of prescribed medications.	Knowledge of disease is essential for the patient to realistically understand when to use inhaler.
Planning	
1. Perform hand hygiene. Collect appropriate equipment and MAR.	Reduces transmission of microorganisms. Promotes time management and efficiency when preparing medications for all patients.
2. Plan preparation to avoid interruptions. Create a quiet environment. Do not take phone calls or talk with others. Follow agency no-interruption zone policy.	Interruptions contribute to medication errors (see Box 26.4) (Beyea, 2014; Yoder et al., 2015).
Implementation	
1. Prepare medications for inhalation. Attend to procedure and avoid distraction. Check label of medication against MAR two times, when removing inhaler from unit dose or AMDS and before leaving medication preparation area (see Skill 26.1). Preparation usually involves taking inhaler device out of storage and into patient room. Check expiration date on container. Perform hand hygiene.	*These are the first and second checks for accuracy.* Process ensures that right patient receives right medication.
2. Take medication to the patient at correct time (see agency policy). Medications that require exact timing include STAT doses, first-time or loading doses, and one-time doses. Give time-critical scheduled medications at exact time ordered (no later than 30 min before or after scheduled dose). Give non-time-critical scheduled medications within a range of 1 or 2 h of scheduled dose (ISMP, 2011a). During administration, apply six rights of medication administration.	Hospitals must adopt medication administration policy and procedure for timing of medication administration that considers nature of prescribed medication, specific clinical application, and patient needs (CMS, 2011; ISMP, 2011a). Time-critical scheduled medications are those for which early or delayed administration of maintenance doses may cause harm or result in substantial suboptimal therapy or pharmacological effect. Non-time-critical medications are those for which early or delayed administration should not cause harm or result in substantial suboptimal therapy or pharmacological effect (CMS, 2011; ISMP, 2011a).
3. Identify the patient by using at least two identifiers (e.g., name and birthday or name and medical record number) according to agency policy. Compare identifiers with information on the patient's MAR or medical record.	Ensures correct patient. Complies with The Joint Commission Standards and improves patient safety (TJC, 2018).
4. At the patient's bedside, again compare MAR or computer printout with names of medications on medication labels and patient name. Ask the patient whether he or she has allergies.	*This is the third check for accuracy* and ensures that the patient receives correct medication. Confirms the patient's allergy history.
5. Help the patient sit comfortably in chair.	The patient is more likely to remain receptive to nurse's explanations in a comfortable position, and it is easier to use inhaler.
6. Discuss purpose of each medication, action, and possible adverse effects. Allow the patient to ask any questions about the drugs. Warn about overuse of inhaler and side effects.	The patient has the right to be informed, and the patient's understanding of each medication improves adherence to drug therapy.
7. Explain procedure to the patient. Be specific if the patient wishes to self-administer drug. Allow adequate time for the patient to manipulate inhaler, canister, or spacer device (if appropriate). Explain where and how to set up at home.	The patient must be familiar with how to use equipment.
8. Explain and demonstrate steps for administering MDI without spacer.	Simple one-on-one instruction and demonstration of step-by-step administration allows the patient to ask questions at any point during procedure and increases patient adherence to inhaler use (Ari and Restrepo, 2012).
a. Insert MDI canister into holder. Then remove mouthpiece cover from inhaler.	
Clinical decision point: If dirt or foreign objects are in mouthpiece, clean before using inhaler to avoid inhalation of unwanted material. Clinical decision point: If MDI is new or has not been used for several days, push a "test spray" into the air to prime the device before using. This ensures that the MDI is patent and the metal canister is positioned properly.	
b. Shake inhaler well five or six times.	Aerosolizes fine particles of medication.

STEP	RATIONALE
c. Have the patient hold inhaler in dominant hand.	Easier position to activate device.
d. Instruct the patient to position inhaler in one of the following two ways:	
(1) Have the patient close mouth around mouthpiece with opening toward back of throat, closing lips tightly around it (see illustration). This is the most common method.	Proper positioning of inhaler is essential to administering medication correctly.
(2) Position mouthpiece 2–4 cm (about 1–2 inches) in front of widely opened mouth (see illustration), with opening of inhaler toward back of throat. Lips should not touch inhaler.	Directs aerosol spray toward airway. This is best way to deliver medication without a spacer.
e. With inhaler positioned correctly, be sure that the patient holds inhaler with thumb at mouthpiece and index finger and middle finger at the top. *This is a three-point or lateral hand position.*	MDIs are easier to activate when patients use a three-point or lateral hand position to activate canister (Burchum and Rosenthal, 2016).
f. Instruct the patient to tilt head back slightly and inhale slowly and deeply through mouth for 3–5 s while depressing canister fully.	Medication is distributed to airways during inhalation.
g. Have the patient hold breath for as long as comfortable, up to 10 s.	Allows aerosol spray droplets to reach deeper branches of airways.
h. Have the patient remove MDI from mouth and then exhale slowly through nose or pursed lips.	Keeps small airways open during exhalation.
9. Explain and demonstrate steps to administer MDI using spacer device.	Simple one-on-one instruction and demonstration of step-by-step administration allows the patient to ask questions at any point during procedure and increases patient adherence to inhaler use (Ari and Restrepo, 2012).
a. Remove mouthpiece cover from MDI and mouthpiece of spacer device.	Inhaler fits into end of spacer device.
b. Shake inhaler well five or six times.	Aerosolizes fine particles of medication.
c. Insert MDI into end of spacer device.	Spacer device traps medication released from MDI; the patient then inhales drug from device. Spacer reduces hand–breath coordination difficulty, thus improving delivery of correct dose of inhaled medication (Barrons et al., 2015).
d. Instruct the patient to place spacer device mouthpiece in mouth and close lips. Do not insert beyond raised lip on mouthpiece. Avoid covering small exhalation slots with the lips.	Medication should not escape through mouth.
e. Have the patient take a deep breath, exhale, and then breathe normally through spacer device mouthpiece (see illustration).	Allows the patient to empty lungs and relax before delivering medication.
f. Instruct the patient to depress medication canister one time, spraying one puff into spacer device.	Spacer contains fine spray and allows the patient to inhale more medication. This increases drug delivery and deposition of medication on oropharyngeal mucosa (Burchum and Rosenthal, 2016).

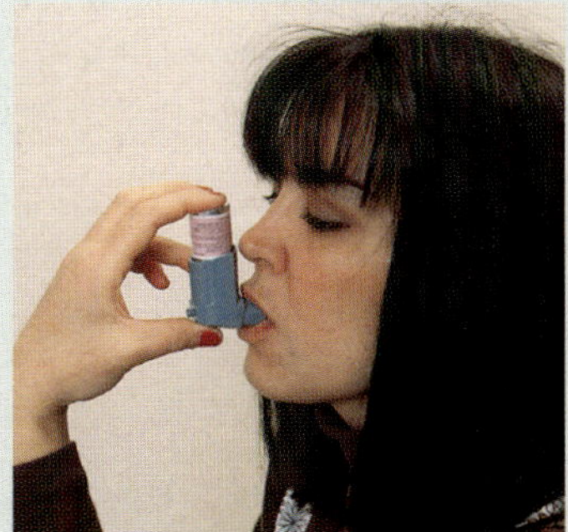

Step 8d(1) One technique for use of inhaler. Patient opens lips and places inhaler in mouth with opening aimed toward back of throat.

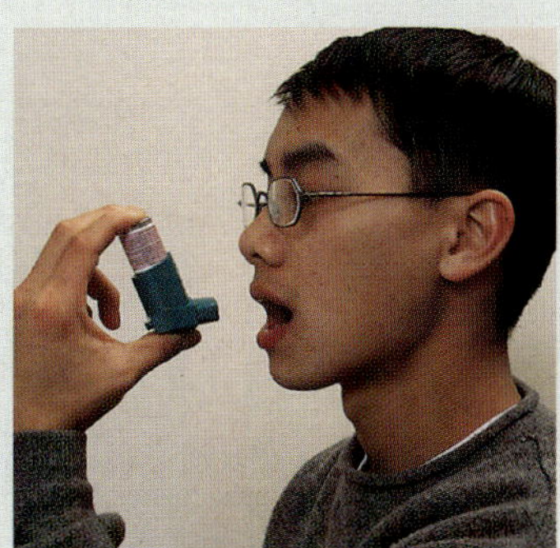

Step 8d(2) One technique for use of inhaler. Patient positions mouthpiece 1–2 inches from mouth.

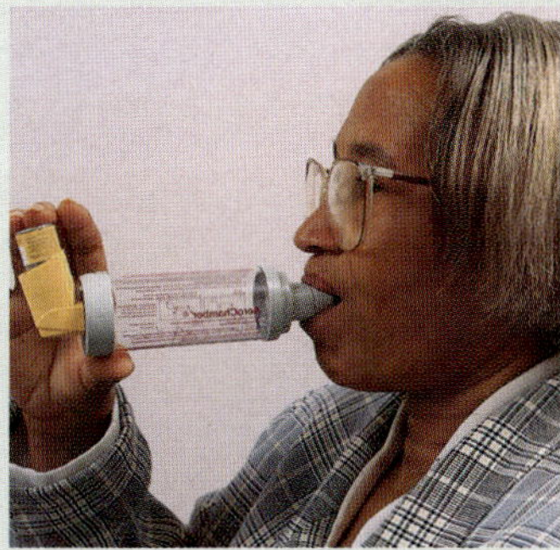

Step 9e Have patient place mouthpiece in mouth and close lips, being careful to keep exhalation slots exposed.

STEP	RATIONALE
g. Have the patient breathe slowly and fully through mouth for 5 s.	Ensures that particles of medication are distributed to deeper airways.
h. Instruct the patient to hold full breath for 10 s.	Ensures full drug distribution through airways.
i. Have the patient remove MDI and spacer and then exhale.	
10. Explain steps to administer DPI or breath-activated MDI.	
a. If DPI has an external counter, note number indicated.	Determines doses remaining.
b. Remove mouthpiece cover. *Do not shake* inhaler.	
c. Prepare medication. Some DPIs require loading medication before administration, some require rotation of a lever to load medication or insertion of a capsule, and some require insertion of a disk into inhaler device. Follow manufacturer's specific instructions.	Primes inhaler, ensuring that medication is delivered to the patient effectively.
d. Have the patient take a breath and exhale away from the inhaler.	Prevents loss of powder.
e. Have the patient position mouthpiece of DPI between lips and inhale quickly and deeply through mouth (see illustration).	Keeps medication from escaping through mouth. Forceful inhalation creates an aerosol.
f. Have the patient hold breath for 5–10 s and then exhale.	Distributes medication.
11. Instruct the patient to wait 20–30 s between inhalations (if same medication) or 2–5 min between inhalations (if different medications). Be sure that the patient inhales correct number of prescribed puffs.	Drugs must be inhaled sequentially. Always administer bronchodilators before steroids so that dilators can open airway passages (Burchum and Rosenthal, 2016).
12. Instruct the patient to not repeat inhalations before next scheduled dose.	Drugs are prescribed at intervals during day to provide constant drug levels and minimize side effects. Beta-adrenergic MDIs are ordered on an "as-needed" basis or regularly every 4–6 h.
13. Warn patients that they may feel gagging sensation in throat caused by droplets of medication on pharynx or tongue.	This occurs when medication is sprayed and inhaled incorrectly.
14. About 2 min after last dose, instruct the patient to rinse mouth with warm water and spit water out.	Steroids may alter normal flora of oral mucosa and lead to development of fungal infection. Rinsing out the mouth reduces the risk of fungal infection and risk (Ari and Restrepo, 2012).
15. Instruct the patient on how to clean the inhaler.	Removes residual medication and reduces spread of microorganisms.
a. Once a day remove MDI canister and cap from the mouthpiece. Do not wash the canister or immerse it in water. Run warm tap water through the top and bottom of the plastic mouthpiece for 30–60 s. Make sure that inhaler is completely dry before reusing. Do not get valve mechanism of canister wet.	Water damages valve mechanism of canister. Accumulation of medication around mouthpiece interferes with proper drug distribution during use.
b. Instruct the patient to clean the mouthpiece of MDI and spacer twice a week with a mild dishwashing soap, rinse thoroughly, and dry completely before storage.	Provides better antimicrobial removal. Pressurized MDIs are potential reservoirs for bacteria (Borovina et al., 2012).
16. Help the patient to comfortable position, and perform hand hygiene.	Reduces spread of microorganisms and promotes patient comfort.

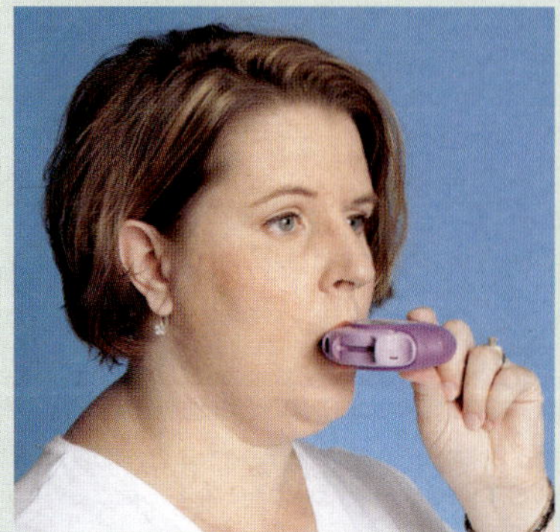

Step 10e Have patient place mouthpiece of dry powder inhaler between lips.

STEP	RATIONALE
Evaluation	
1. Auscultate patient lungs, listen for abnormal breath sounds, and obtain peak flow measures if ordered.	Determines patient response to medication.
2. Have the patient explain and demonstrate steps in use and cleaning of inhaler.	Return demonstration provides feedback for measuring patient's learning.
3. Ask the patient to explain drug schedule and dose of medication.	Improves likelihood of adherence to therapy.
4. Ask the patient to describe side effects of medication and criteria for calling health care provider.	Allows the patient to recognize signs of overuse and need to seek medical support when drugs are ineffective.
5. **Use teach back:** "I want to be sure I showed you how to use your inhaler. For this dose, show me how you take a dose of your medicine." Revise your instruction now or develop a plan for revised patient/family caregiver teaching if the patient/ family caregiver is not able to teach back correctly.	Determines the patient's/family caregiver's level of understanding of instructional topic.

Recording and Reporting

- Record drug administered, dose or strength, route, number of inhalations, and actual time administered on MAR immediately after administration, not before. Include initials or signature.
- Record on flow sheet or nurses' notes in HER or chart the patient's response to inhaled medication (e.g., breath sounds, peak flow rate), evidence of side effects (e.g., arrhythmia, feelings of anxiety), and the patient's ability to use inhaler.
- Record patient teaching and validation of understanding on flow sheet or nurses' notes in EHR or chart.
- Report adverse effects and patient response and/or withheld drugs to nurse in charge or health care provider.

Unexpected Outcomes and Related Interventions

- The patient's respirations are rapid and shallow; breath sounds indicate wheezing.
  - Evaluate vital signs and respiratory status.
  - Notify health care provider.
  - Reassess type of medication and/or delivery method.
- The patient needs bronchodilator more than every 4 hours (may indicate respiratory problem).
  - Reassess type of medication and delivery methods needed with health care provider.
- The patient experiences cardiac dysrhythmias (lightheadedness, syncope), especially if receiving beta-adrenergic medications.
  - Withhold all further doses of medication.
  - Evaluate cardiac and pulmonary status (see Chapter 7).
  - Notify health care provider for reassessment of type of medication and delivery method.

SKILL 26.4 Preparing Injections from Vials and Ampules

Equipment

Medication in an Ampule

- Syringe, needle, and filter needle
- Small sterile gauze pad or unopened alcohol swab

Medication in a Vial

- Syringe and two needles
- Needles:
  - Needleless blunt-tip vial access cannula or needle (with safety sheath) for drawing up medication (if needed)
  - Filter needle if indicated
- Small, sterile gauze pad or alcohol swab
- Diluent (e.g., 0.9% sodium chloride or sterile water if indicated)

Both

- MAR or computer printout
- Sharps with engineered sharps injury protection (SESIP) safety needle for injection
- Medication in vial or ampule
- Puncture-proof container for disposal of syringes, needles, and glass

STEP	RATIONALE
Assessment	
1. Check accuracy and completeness of each MAR or computer printout with health care provider's written medication order. Check the patient's name, medication name and dosage, route of administration, and time of administration. Recopy or reprint any part of MAR that is difficult to read.	The order sheet is the most reliable source and only legal record of medications that the patient is to receive. Ensures that the patient receives correct medications (Mandrack et al., 2012). Illegible MARs are a source of medication errors (Alassaad et al., 2013).

STEP	RATIONALE
2. Assess the patient's medical and medication history and history of allergies. List any drug allergies on each page of MAR and prominently display on the patient's medical record. When allergies are present, the patient should wear an allergy bracelet.	Determines need for medication or possible contraindications for medication administration. Allergy alert helps prevent adverse events.
3. Review medication reference information for action, purpose, side effects, and nursing implications.	Allows you to administer drug properly and monitor the patient's response.
4. Assess the patient's body build, muscle size, and weight if giving subcutaneous or i.m. medication.	Determines type and size of syringe and needle for injection.
Planning	
1. Perform hand hygiene. Collect appropriate equipment and MAR.	Reduces transmission of microorganisms. Ensures organized procedure.
2. Follow agency's no-interruption zone (NIZ) policy. Prepare medications for one patient at a time. Keep all pages of MARs or computer printouts for one patient together or look at only one patient's electronic MAR at a time.	Preventing distractions reduces medication preparation errors. Use NIZ when possible (Beyea, 2014; Yoder et al., 2015).
Implementation	
1. Prepare medication.	
a. If using a medication cart, move it outside the patient's room.	Organization of equipment saves time and reduces error.
b. Unlock medication drawer or cart or log onto computerized medication dispensing system.	Medications are safeguarded when locked in cabinet, cart, or computerized medication dispensing system.
c. Select correct drug from stock supply or unit-dose drawer. Compare label of medication with MAR computer printout or computer screen.	Reading label and comparing it with transcribed order reduces errors. *This is the first check for accuracy.*
d. Check expiration date on each vial or ampule, one at a time.	Medications used past their expiration date are sometimes inactive, less effective, or harmful to patients.
e. Calculate drug dose as necessary. Double-check calculation. Ask another nurse to check calculations if needed.	Double-checking may help reduce error especially for high-risk medications.
f. If preparing a controlled substance, check record for previous drug count and compare with supply available.	Controlled substance laws require careful monitoring of dispensed narcotics.
g. Do not leave drugs unattended.	Nurse is responsible for safekeeping of drugs.
2. Prepare ampule.	
a. Tap top of ampule lightly and quickly with finger until fluid moves from its neck (see illustration).	Dislodges any fluid that collects above neck of ampule. All solution moves into lower chamber.
b. Place small gauze pad around neck of ampule (see illustration).	Protects fingers from trauma as glass tip is broken off. Do not use opened alcohol swab to wrap around top of ampule because alcohol may leak into ampule.

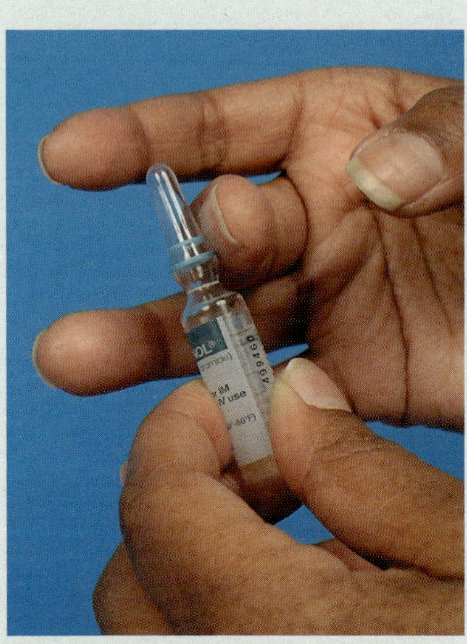

Step 2a Tapping ampule moves fluid down ampule neck.

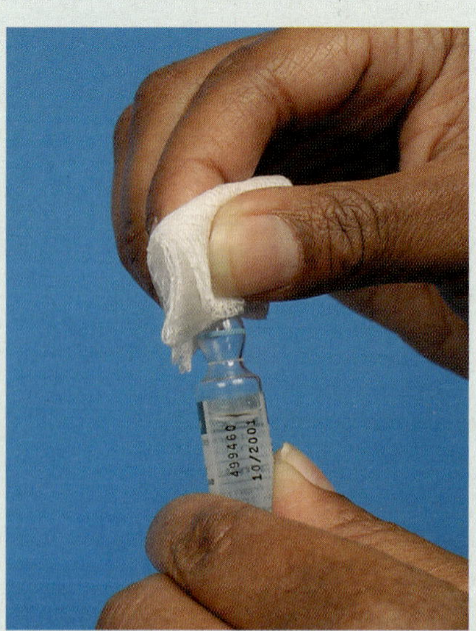

Step 2b Gauze pad placed around neck of ampule protects fingers.

STEP	RATIONALE
c. Snap neck of ampule quickly and firmly away from hands (see illustration).	Protects your fingers and face from shattering glass.
d. Draw up medication quickly, using filter needle long enough to reach bottom of ampule to access medication.	System is open to airborne contaminants. Filter needles filter out any fragments of glass (Alexander et al., 2014).
e. Hold ampule upside down or set it on flat surface. Insert filter needle into center of ampule opening. Do not allow needle tip or shaft to touch rim of ampule.	Broken rim of ampule is considered contaminated. When ampule is inverted, solution dribbles out if needle tip or shaft touches rim of ampule.
f. Aspirate medication into syringe by gently pulling back on plunger (see illustrations).	Withdrawal of plunger creates negative pressure within syringe barrel, which pulls fluid into syringe.
g. Keep needle tip under surface of liquid. Tip ampule to bring all fluid within reach of needle.	Prevents aspiration of air bubbles.
h. If you aspirate air bubbles, do not expel air into ampule.	Air pressure forces fluid out of ampule, and medication will be lost.
i. To expel excess air bubbles, remove needle from ampule. Hold syringe vertically with needle pointing up. Tap side of syringe to cause bubbles to rise toward needle. Draw back slightly on plunger and push plunger upward to eject air. Do not eject fluid.	Withdrawing plunger too far removes it from barrel. Holding syringe vertically allows fluid to settle in bottom of barrel. Pulling back on plunger allows fluid within needle to enter barrel so that fluid is not expelled. You then expel air at top of barrel and within needle.
j. If syringe contains excess fluid, use sink for disposal. Hold syringe vertically with needle tip up and slanted slightly toward sink. Slowly eject excess fluid into sink. Recheck fluid level in syringe by holding it vertically.	Safely disperses excess medication into sink. Position of needle allows you to expel medication without having it flow down needle shaft. Rechecking fluid level ensures proper dose.
k. Cover needle with its safety sheath or cap. Replace filter needle with regular SESIP needle.	Minimizes needlesticks. Filter needles cannot be used for injection.
3. Prepare vial containing a solution.	
a. Remove cap covering top of unused vial to expose sterile rubber seal. If a multidose vial has been used before, the cap is already removed and does not require cleansing. Firmly and briskly wipe surface of rubber seal with alcohol swab. Allow it to dry.	Vial comes packaged with cap that cannot be replaced after seal removal. Not all drug manufacturers guarantee that rubber seals of unused vials are sterile. Swabbing with alcohol reduces transmission of microorganisms. Allowing alcohol to dry prevents alcohol from coating needle and mixing with medication.
b. Pick up syringe and remove needle cap or cap covering the needleless vial access device (see illustration). Pull back on plunger to draw amount of air into syringe equivalent to volume of medication to be aspirated from vial.	Injecting air into vial prevents buildup of negative pressure in vial when aspirating medication.

Clinical decision point: Some medications and agencies require use of a filter needle when preparing medications from vials. Check agency policy or medication reference. If you use a filter needle to aspirate medication, you need to change it to a regular SESIP needle of the appropriate size to administer medication (Alexander et al., 2014).

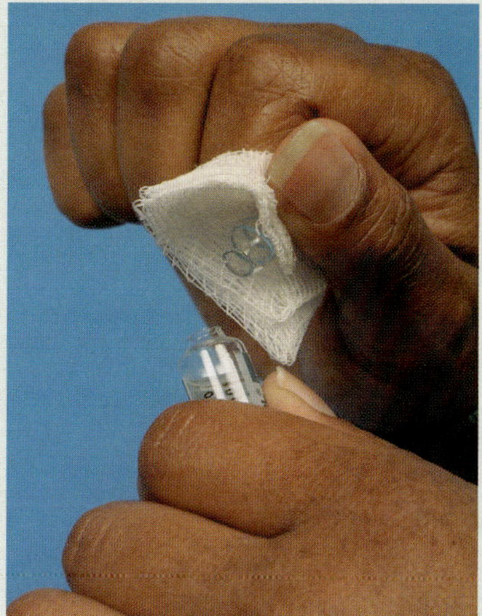

Step 2c Snapping neck away from hands.

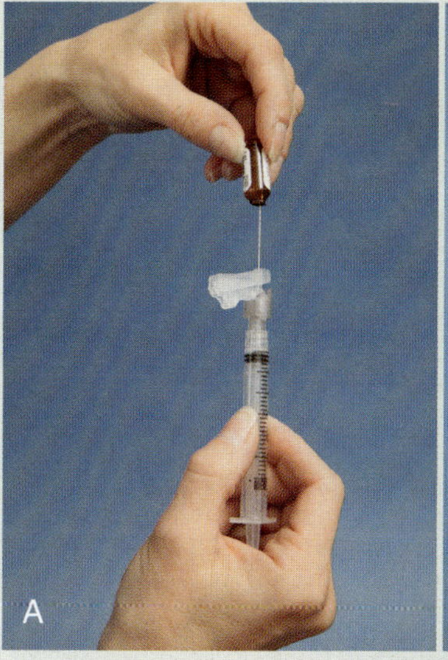

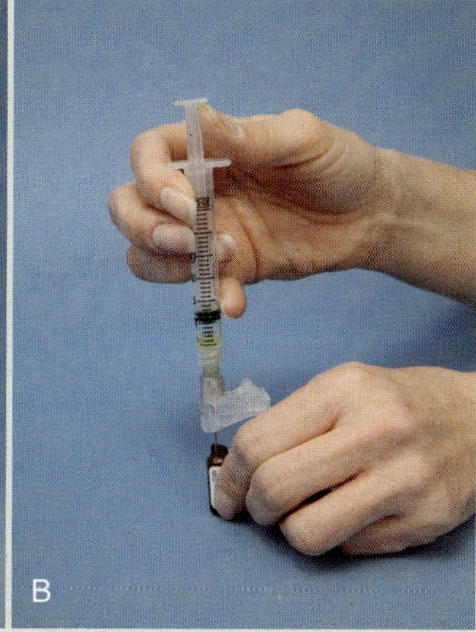

Step 2f A, Medication aspirated with ampule inverted. **B,** Medication aspirated with ampule on flat surface.

STEP	RATIONALE

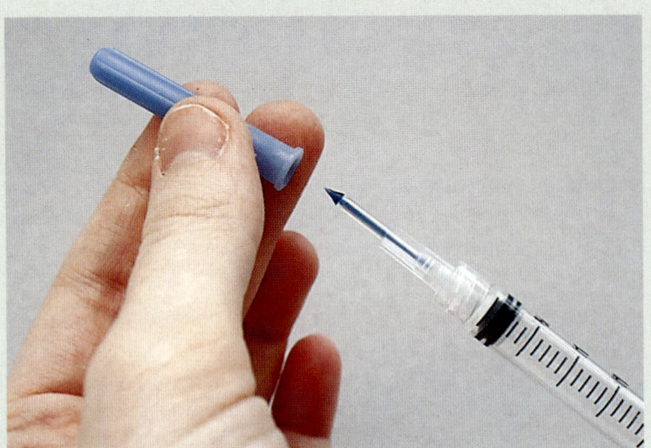

Step 3b Syringe with needless vial adapter.

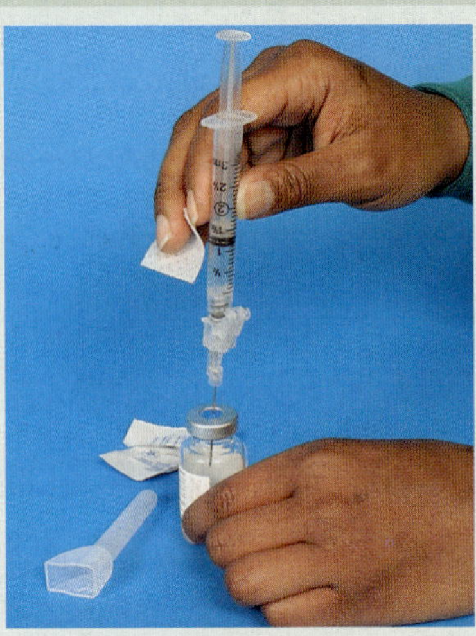

Step 3c Insert safety needle through center of vial diaphragm (with vial setting flat on table).

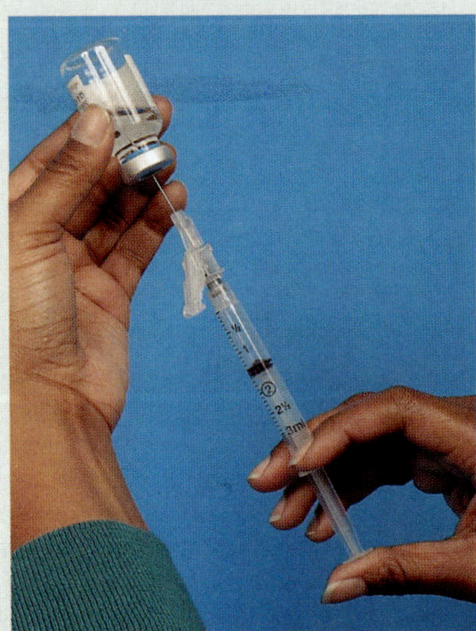

Step 3g Fluid withdrawn from vial.

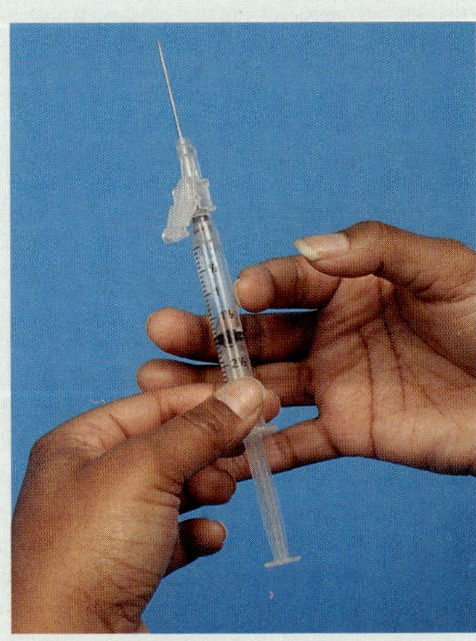

Step 3h Hold syringe upright; tap barrel to dislodge air bubbles.

STEP	RATIONALE
c. With vial on flat surface, insert tip of needle or needleless vial access device through center of rubber seal (see illustration). Apply pressure to tip of needle during insertion.	Center of seal is thinner and easier to penetrate. Using firm pressure prevents dislodging rubber particles that could enter vial or needle.
d. Inject air into air space of vial, holding on to plunger. Hold plunger firmly; plunger is sometimes forced backward by air pressure within vial.	Injection of air creates vacuum needed to get medication to flow into syringe. Injecting into air space of vial prevents formation of bubbles and an inaccurate dose.
e. Invert vial while keeping firm hold on syringe and plunger. Hold vial between thumb and middle fingers of nondominant hand. Grasp end of syringe barrel and plunger with thumb and forefinger of dominant hand to counteract pressure in vial.	Inverting vial allows fluid to settle in lower half of container. Position of hands prevents forceful movement of plunger and permits easy manipulation of syringe.
f. Keep tip of needle or needleless device below fluid level.	Prevents aspiration of air.
g. Allow air pressure from vial to fill syringe gradually with medication. If necessary, pull back slightly on plunger to obtain correct amount of medication (see illustration).	Positive pressure within vial forces fluid into syringe.
h. When you obtain desired volume, position needle or needleless device into air space of vial; tap side of syringe barrel gently to dislodge any air bubbles (see illustration). Eject any air remaining at top of syringe into vial.	Forcefully striking barrel while needle is inserted in vial may bend needle. Accumulation of air displaces medication and causes dose errors.

STEP	RATIONALE
i. Remove needle or needleless access device from vial by pulling back on barrel of syringe.	Pulling plunger rather than barrel causes plunger to separate from barrel, resulting in loss of medication.
j. Hold syringe at eye level at 90° angle to ensure correct volume and absence of air bubbles. Remove any remaining air by tapping barrel to dislodge any air bubbles. Draw back slightly on plunger; then push it upward to eject air. Do not eject fluid. Recheck volume of medication.	Holding syringe vertically allows fluid to settle in bottom of barrel. Tapping dislodges air to top of barrel. Pulling back on plunger allows fluid within needle to enter barrel so that you do not expel fluid. You then expel air at top of barrel and within needle.
Clinical decision point: When preparing medication from single-dose vial, do not assume that volume listed on label is total volume in vial. Some manufacturers provide small amount of extra liquid, expecting loss during preparation. Be sure to draw up only desired volume.	
k. If you need to inject medication into the patient's tissue, change needle with regular SESIP to appropriate gauge and length according to route of medication administration.	Inserting needle through rubber stopper dulls beveled tip. New needle is sharper and, because no fluid is along shaft, does not track medication through tissues. Filter needles cannot be used for injection.
l. Cover needle with its safety sheath or cap.	Minimizes needlesticks.
m. For multidose vial, make label that includes date of opening, concentration of drug (per milliliter), and your initials.	Ensures that nurses will prepare future doses correctly. You discard some drugs within a certain time frame after mixing.
4. Prepare vial containing powder (reconstituting medications).	
a. Remove cap covering vial of powdered medication and cap covering vial of proper diluent. Firmly swab both rubber seals with alcohol swab and allow alcohol to dry.	Allowing alcohol to dry prevents it from coating needle and mixing with medication.
b. Draw up manufacturer's suggestion for volume and type of diluent into syringe.	Prepares diluent for injection into vial containing powdered medication.
c. Insert tip of needle or needleless device through center of rubber seal of vial of powdered medication. Inject diluent into vial. Remove needle.	Diluent begins to dissolve and reconstitute medication.
d. Mix medication thoroughly. Roll in palms. Do not shake.	Ensures proper dispersal of medication throughout solution and prevents formation of air bubbles.
e. Reconstituted medication in vial is ready to be drawn into new syringe. Read label carefully to determine dose after reconstitution.	Once you add diluent, concentration of medication (mg/mL) determines dose you give. Reading medication label carefully decreases medication errors.
f. Draw up reconstituted medication into syringe. Insert needleless device/needle into vial. Do not add air.	Prepares medication for administration.
Clinical decision point: Some agencies require that you verify dose of certain medications (e.g., insulin and heparin) for accuracy with another nurse. Check guidelines before administering medication.	
5. Compare label of medication with MAR, computer screen, or computer printout.	*This is the second check for accuracy.*
6. Dispose of soiled supplies. Place broken ampule and/or used vials and used needle or needleless device in puncture-proof and leak-proof container. Clean work area, and perform hand hygiene.	Proper disposal of glass and needle prevents accidental injury to staff. Controls transmission of infection.
Evaluation	
1. Just before administering drug to the patient, compare MAR with label of prepared drug and compare dose in syringe with desired dose.	Ensures that dose is accurate. *This is the third check for accuracy.*

Unexpected Outcomes and Related Interventions

- Air bubbles remain in syringe.
  - Expel air from syringe and add medication to it until you prepare correct dose.
- Incorrect dose of medication is prepared.
  - Discard prepared dose.
  - Prepare correct new dose.

SKILL 26.5 Administering Injections

Equipment

Proper-size syringe and SESIP needle:

- Subcutaneous: Syringe (1–3 mL) and needle (25–27 gauge, 1/8–5/8 inch):
  - Immunizations: 23- to 25-gauge, 5/8-inch needle (CDC, 2015)
  - Subcutaneous U-100 insulin: Insulin syringe (1 mL) with preattached needle (28–31 gauge, 5/16–3/16 inch)
  - Subcutaneous U-500 insulin: 1 mL tuberculin (TB) syringe with needle (25–27 gauge, 1/2–5/8 inch)
- Intramuscular (i.m.): Syringe 2–3 mL for adult, 0.5–1 mL for infants and small children (21- to 23-gauge, 1- to 1½-inch needle):
  - Needle length corresponding to site of injection, age, gender, and size of patient. Refer to following guidelines; length needed may vary outside of these guidelines for patients who are smaller or larger than average.

Needle Length for Immunizations[a]

Site	Child (inch)	Adult (inch)
Ventrogluteal	1/2–1	1½
Vastus lateralis	5/8–1	5/8–1
Deltoid	1/2–1	1–1½

Male Gender	Female Gender	Needle Length (inch)
Less than 130 pounds	Less than 130 pounds	5/8–1
130–152 pounds	130–152 pounds	1
153–260 pounds	153–200 pounds	1–1½
Greater than 260 pounds	Greater than 200 pounds	1½

[a]Based on CDC (2015) guidelines.

  - Needle gauge often depends on length of needle; administer biologicals and medication in aqueous solution with a 20- to 25-gauge needle. Use 18- to 21-gauge needles for medications in oil-based solutions.
- I.d.: 1-mL TB syringe with preattached 25- or 27-gauge, 1/8- to 5/8-inch needle
- All injections:
  - Small gauze pad *(optional)*
  - Alcohol swab
  - Medication vial or ampule
  - Clean gloves
  - MAR or computer printout
  - Puncture-proof container for sharps

STEP	RATIONALE
Assessment	
1. Check accuracy and completeness of MAR or computer printout with health care provider's original medication order. Check the patient's name, medication name and dosage, route of administration, and time of administration. Recopy or reprint any part of MAR that is difficult to read.	The order sheet is the most reliable source and only legal record of medications that the patient is to receive. Ensures that the patient receives correct medications (Mandrack et al., 2012). Illegible MARs are a source of medication errors (Alassaad et al., 2013).
2. Assess the patient's medical and medication history and history of allergies. List any drug allergies on each page of the MAR and prominently display on the patient's medical record. When allergies are present, the patient should wear an allergy bracelet.	Determines need for medication or possible contraindications for medication administration. Allergy alert helps prevent adverse events.
3. Review medication reference information for medication action, purpose, normal dose, side effects, time and peak of onset, and nursing implications. In the case of an i.d. injection, review expected reaction and/or anticipated effects when testing skin with specific allergen and appropriate time to read site.	Allows you to administer medication safely and monitor the patient's response to therapy. Type of reaction to an immunization depends on the patient's ability to mount a cell-mediated immune response. Knowledge of expected and adverse reactions to skin testing helps you determine for which symptoms to monitor, how frequently, and when to reassess the patient.
4. Assess for contraindication to injections: ■ I.d. injections—reduced local tissue perfusion. Assess for history of severe adverse reactions or necrosis that occurred after previous i.d. injection. ■ Subcutaneous injection—circulatory shock or reduced local tissue perfusion. ■ I.m. injection—muscle atrophy, reduced blood flow, or circulatory shock.	Decreased tissue perfusion reduces absorption of subcutaneous and i.d. medications and affects drug distribution of subcutaneous medication. Prior history of severe reactions increases risk for future severe reactions. Factors interfering with blood flow to muscles impair i.m. drug absorption.
5. Assess the patient's knowledge of purpose and expected response to medication or skin testing.	Patients need to know when to return for follow-up reading of skin test and when and how to report any reaction. Poses implications for patient education.
6. Assess the patient's symptoms before initiating medication therapy.	Provides information to evaluate desired effect of medication.

STEP	RATIONALE
7. For subcutaneous insulin or heparin, assess relevant laboratory results (e.g., blood glucose, partial thromboplastin time).	Provides baseline for measuring drug response.
8. Observe the patient's previous verbal and nonverbal responses to injection.	Anticipating the patient's anxiety allows you to use distraction to reduce pain awareness.
9. Check date of expiration for medication.	Dose potency increases or decreases when outdated.
Planning	
1. Perform hand hygiene. Collect appropriate equipment and MAR.	Reduces transmission of microorganisms. Ensures organized procedure.
2. Follow agency no-interruption zone (NIZ) policy. Prepare medications for one patient at a time. Keep all pages of MARs or computer printouts for one patient together or look at only one patient's electronic MAR at a time.	Preventing distractions reduces medication preparation errors. Use NIZ when possible (Beyea, 2014; Yoder et al., 2015).
Implementation	
1. Prepare medication for one patient at a time using aseptic technique. Attend to preparation and avoid distraction. Check label of medication carefully with MAR or computer printout two times, when removing medication from unit dose or AMDS and before leaving medication preparation area (see Skill 26.4). Perform hand hygiene.	Reduces transmission of microorganisms. Ensures that medication is sterile. *These are the first and second checks for accuracy* and ensure that correct medication is administered.
2. Take medication to the patient at correct time (see agency policy). Medications that require exact timing include STAT doses, first-time or loading doses, and one-time doses. Give time-critical scheduled medications at exact time ordered (no later than 30 min before or after scheduled dose). Give non-time-critical scheduled medications within a range of 1 or 2 h of scheduled dose (ISMP, 2011a). During administration, apply six rights of medication administration.	Hospitals must adopt medication administration policy and procedure for timing of medication administration that considers nature of the prescribed medication, specific clinical application, and patient needs (CMS, 2011; ISMP, 2011a). Time-critical scheduled medications are those for which early or delayed administration of maintenance doses may cause harm or result in substantial suboptimal therapy or pharmacological effect. Non-time-critical medications are those for which early or delayed administration should not cause harm or result in substantial suboptimal therapy or pharmacological effect (CMS, 2011; ISMP, 2011a).
3. Close room curtain or door.	Provides privacy.
4. Identify the patient by using at least two identifiers (e.g., name and birthday or name and medical record number) according to agency policy. Compare identifiers with information on the patient's MAR or medical record.	Ensures correct patient. Complies with The Joint Commission standards and improves patient safety (TJC, 2018).
5. At the patient's bedside, again compare MAR or computer printout with names of medications on medication labels and patient name. Ask the patient whether he or she has allergies.	*This is the third check for accuracy* and ensures that the patient receives correct medication. Confirms the patient's allergy history.
6. Discuss purpose of each medication and/or skin test, action, and possible adverse effects. Allow the patient to ask any questions. Tell the patient that injection will cause slight burning or sting. An i.d. injection will create a small bleb on the skin.	The patient has the right to be informed, and the patient's understanding of each medication improves adherence to drug therapy. Helps minimize the patient's anxiety.
7. Perform hand hygiene and apply clean gloves. Keep sheet or gown draped over body parts not requiring exposure.	Reduces transmission of infection.
8. Select appropriate injection site. Inspect skin surface over sites for bruises, inflammation, or edema. ▪ I.d.: Note lesions or discolorations of skin. If possible, select site three to four finger widths below antecubital space and one hand width above wrist. If you cannot use forearm, inspect upper back. If necessary, use sites appropriate for subcutaneous injections. ▪ Subcutaneous: Do not use an area that is bruised or has signs associated with infection. Palpate sites and avoid those with masses or tenderness. Be sure that needle is correct size by grasping skinfold at site with thumb and forefinger. Measure fold from top to bottom. Make sure that needle is one-half length of fold. When administering insulin or heparin, use abdominal injection sites first, followed by thigh injection site. Choose site on right or left side of abdomen at least 5 cm (2 inches) away from umbilicus. ▪ I.m.: Note integrity and size of muscle. Palpate for tenderness or hardness. Avoid these areas. If the patient receives frequent injections, rotate sites. Use ventrogluteal if possible.	Injection sites need to be free of abnormalities that interfere with medication absorption. An i.d. injection site is free of discoloration or hair so that you can see results of skin test and interpret them correctly (WHO, 2015). Injection sites are free of abnormalities that interfere with drug absorption. Subcutaneous sites used repeatedly become hardened from lipohypertrophy (increased growth in fatty tissue). You can mistakenly give subcutaneous injections in muscle, especially in abdomen and thigh sites. Appropriate size of needle ensures that you inject medication into subcutaneous tissue (Hirsch et al., 2012; Ogston-Tuck, 2014a). Injecting low-molecular-weight heparin on side of abdomen helps decrease pain and bruising at injection site (Sanofi-Aventis, 2014).

STEP	RATIONALE
9. Help the patient into comfortable position. ▪ I.d.: Have the patient extend elbow and support it and forearm on flat surface. ▪ Subcutaneous: Have the patient relax arm, leg, or abdomen, depending on site selection. ▪ I.m.: Position the patient depending on chosen site (e.g., sit, lie flat, on side, or prone).	Stabilizes injection site for easy accessibility. Relaxation of site minimizes discomfort. Reduces strain on muscle and minimizes injection discomfort.
10. Relocate site using anatomical landmarks. For subcutaneous insulin, rotate site within an anatomical area (e.g., abdomen) and systematically rotate sites within that area.	Injection into correct anatomical site prevents injury to nerves, bone, and blood vessels. Rotating injection sites within an anatomical site maintains consistency in day-to-day insulin absorption.
11. Clean site with antiseptic swab. Apply swab at center of site and rotate outward in circular direction for about 5 cm (2 inches) (see illustration).	Mechanical action of swab removes secretions containing microorganisms.
▪ *Option for i.m. injection:* Apply eutectic mixture of local anesthetics (EMLA) cream on injection site at least 1 h before i.m. injection or use vapocoolant spray (e.g., ethyl chloride) just before injection.	Decreases pain at injection site.
12. Hold swab or gauze between third and fourth fingers of nondominant hand.	Swab or gauze remains readily accessible for use when withdrawing needle after injection.
13. Remove needle cap from needle by pulling it straight off.	Preventing needle from touching sides of cap prevents contamination.
14. Hold syringe between thumb and forefinger of dominant hand: ▪ I.d.: Hold syringe with bevel of needle pointing up. ▪ Subcutaneous and i.m.: Hold as dart, palm down (see illustration).	Smooth injection requires proper manipulation of syringe parts. With bevel up, you are less likely to deposit medication into i.d. tissues below dermis.
15. Administer injection.	
a. **I.d.**	
(1) With nondominant hand, stretch skin over site with forefinger or thumb.	Needle pierces tight skin more easily.
(2) With needle almost against the patient's skin, insert it slowly at 5–15° angle until resistance is felt. Advance needle through epidermis to approximately 3 mm (1/8 inch) below skin surface. You will see bulge of needle tip through skin.	Ensures that needle tip is in dermis. You obtain inaccurate results if you do not inject needle at correct angle and depth (WHO, 2015).
(3) Inject medication slowly. Normally, you feel resistance. If not, needle is too deep; remove and begin again.	Slow injection minimizes discomfort at site. Dermal layer is tight and does not expand easily when you inject solution.
Clinical decision point: It is not necessary to aspirate an i.d. injection because dermis is relatively avascular.	
(4) While injecting medication, note that small bleb (approximately 6 mm [1/4 inch]) resembling mosquito bite appears on skin surface (see illustration).	Bleb indicates that you deposited medication in dermis.

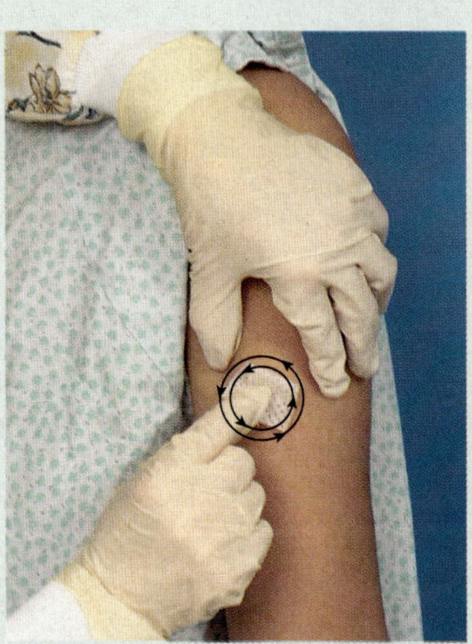

Step 11 Clean site using circular motion.

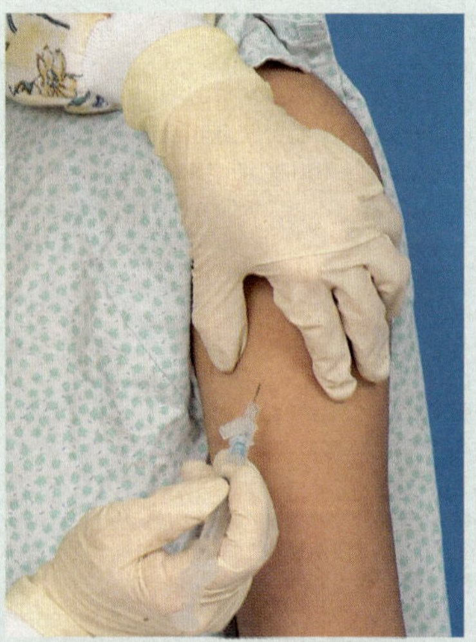

Step 14 Hold syringe as if grasping a dart.

STEP	RATIONALE

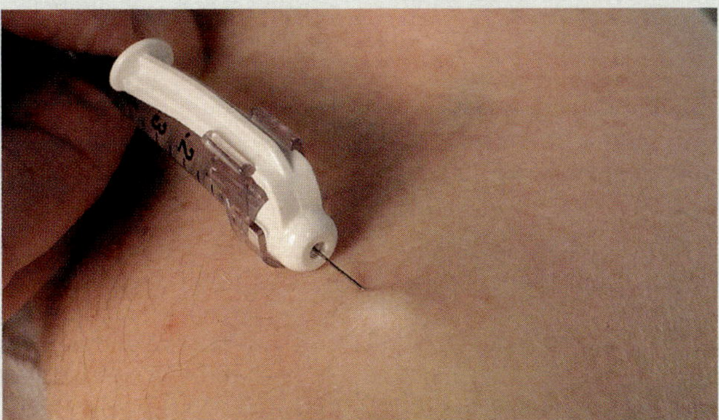
Step 15a(4) Intradermal injection creates small bleb.

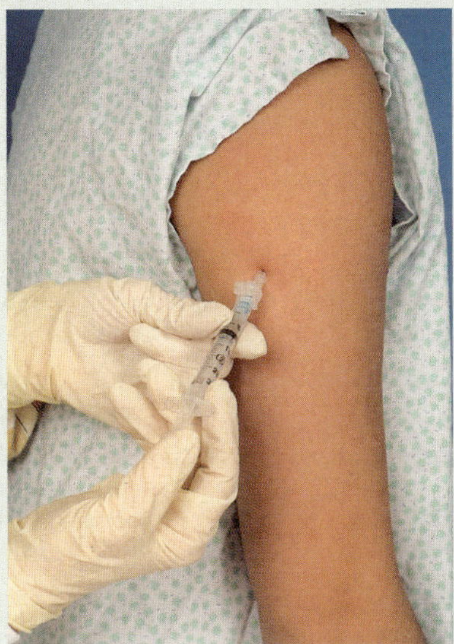
Step 15b(4) Inject medication slowly.

b. **Subcutaneous**

STEP	RATIONALE
(1) For an average-size patient, hold skin across injection site or pinch skin with nondominant hand.	Needle penetrates tight skin more easily than loose skin. Pinching elevates subcutaneous tissue and desensitizes area.
(2) Inject needle quickly and firmly at 45–90° angle (see figure 26.15). Release skin if pinched. *Option:* When using injection pen or giving heparin, continue to pinch skin while injecting medicine.	Quick, firm insertion minimizes discomfort. (Injecting medication into compressed tissue irritates nerve fibers.) Correct angle prevents accidental injection into muscle.
(3) For an obese patient, pinch skin at site and inject needle at 90° angle below tissue fold.	Obese patients have fatty layer of tissue above subcutaneous layer.
(4) After needle enters site, grasp lower end of syringe barrel with nondominant hand to stabilize it. Move dominant hand to end of plunger and slowly inject medication over several seconds (see illustration). When giving heparin, inject over 30 s (Akbari Sari et al., 2014; Sanofi-Aventis, 2014). Avoid moving syringe.	Movement of syringe may displace needle and cause discomfort. Slow injection of medication minimizes discomfort.

Clinical decision point: Aspiration after injecting a subcutaneous medication is not necessary. Piercing a blood vessel in a subcutaneous injection is very rare. Aspiration after injecting heparin and insulin is not recommended (Lilley et al., 2016).

c. **I.m.**

STEP	RATIONALE
(1) Position ulnar side of nondominant hand just below site and pull skin laterally approximately 2.5–3.5 cm (1–1½ inches) (see Fig. 26.20). Hold position until medication is injected. With dominant hand, inject needle quickly at 90° angle into muscle (see Fig. 26.16).	Z-track creates zigzag path through tissues that seals needle track to avoid tracking medication. A quick dart-like injection reduces discomfort. Use Z-track for all i.m. injections (Hopkins and Arias, 2013; Nicoll and Hesby, 2002; Ogston-Tuck, 2014b).

STEP	RATIONALE
(2) *Option:* If the patient's muscle mass is small, grasp body of muscle between thumb and forefingers.	Ensures that medication reaches muscle mass (CDC, 2015; Hockenberry and Wilson, 2015).
(3) After needle pierces skin, while still pulling on skin with nondominant hand, grasp lower end of syringe barrel with fingers of nondominant hand to stabilize it. Move dominant hand to end of plunger. Avoid moving syringe.	Smooth manipulation of syringe reduces discomfort from needle movement. Skin remains pulled until after medication is injected to ensure Z-track administration.
(4) Pull back on plunger 5–10 s. If no blood appears, inject medication slowly at rate of 1 mL/10 s (Nicoll and Hesby, 2002).	Aspiration of blood into syringe indicates possible placement into a vein. Aspiration of blood into syringe indicates i.v. placement of needle. Slow injection rate reduces pain and tissue trauma and reduces chance of leakage of medication back through needle track (Hockenberry and Wilson, 2015; Nicoll and Hesby, 2002).
Clinical decision point: The Centers for Disease Control and Prevention (CDC, 2015) no longer recommends aspiration when administering an immunization. For all other i.m. injections, if blood appears in syringe, remove needle, dispose of medication and syringe properly, and prepare another dose of medication for injection to prevent injection of medication directly into the bloodstream.	
(5) Once medication is injected, wait 10 s, and then smoothly and steadily withdraw needle, release skin, and apply gauze gently over site.	Allows time for medication to absorb into muscle before removing syringe. Dry gauze minimizes discomfort associated with alcohol on nonintact skin.
16. Apply gentle pressure to site. Do not massage site. Apply bandage if needed.	Massage damages underlying tissue.
17. Help the patient to comfortable position.	Gives the patient sense of well-being.
18. Discard uncapped needle or needle enclosed in safety shield and attached syringe into puncture-proof and leak-proof receptacle (see Fig. 26.26).	Prevents injury to patients and health care personnel. Recapping needles increases risk for needlestick injury (OSHA, n.d.).
19. Remove gloves and perform hand hygiene.	Reduces transmission of microorganisms.
20. Stay with the patient for several minutes and observe for any allergic reactions.	Dyspnea, wheezing, and circulatory collapse are signs of severe anaphylactic reaction and are likely to occur immediately after injection.
Evaluation	
1. Return to room in 15–30 min and ask whether the patient feels any acute pain, burning, numbness, or tingling at injection site.	After an i.d. injection, continued discomfort could indicate injury to underlying tissues. Continued discomfort after a subcutaneous or i.m. injection may indicate injury to underlying bones or nerves.
2. After an i.d. injection, ask the patient to discuss implications of skin testing and signs of hypersensitivity.	The patient's ability to recognize signs of skin testing helps to ensure timely reporting of results.
3. Inspect i.d. bleb. *Optional:* Use skin pencil and draw circle around perimeter of injection site. Read TB test site at 48–72 h; look for induration (hard, dense, raised area) of skin around injection site of: ▪ 15 mm or more in patients with no known risk factors for tuberculosis ▪ 10 mm or more in patients who are recent immigrants; injection drug users; residents and employees of high-risk settings; patients with certain chronic illnesses; children younger than 4 years; and infants, children, and adolescents exposed to high-risk adults ▪ 5 mm or more in patients who are human immunodeficiency virus (HIV) positive, have fibrotic changes on chest X-ray film consistent with previous tuberculosis infection, have had organ transplants, or are immunosuppressed	Determines whether reaction to antigen occurs; indication positive for tuberculosis or tested allergens. Site must be read at various intervals to determine test results. Pencil marks make site easy to find. You determine results of skin testing at various times, based on type of medication used or type of skin testing completed. Manufacturer directions determine when to read test results.
4. Inspect subcutaneous or i.m. site; note any bruising or induration. Apply warm compress to site if bruising or induration noted.	Bruising or induration indicates complication associated with injection. Document findings and notify health care provider.
5. Observe the patient's response to medication at times that correlate with onset, peak, and duration of medication. Review laboratory results as appropriate (e.g., blood glucose, partial thromboplastin time).	Adverse effects of parenteral medications develop rapidly. Evaluate effect of medication on basis of onset, peak, and duration of action.

STEP	RATIONALE
6. **Use teach back:** "I want to be sure I explained to you the purpose of your TB injection. Explain for me why you are receiving the injection and what to look for on your skin tomorrow." Revise your instruction now or develop a plan for revised patient/family caregiver teaching if the patient/family caregiver is not unable to teach back correctly.	Determines the patient's/family caregiver's level of understanding of instructional topic.

Recording and Reporting

- Record drug, dose, route, site, time, and date on MAR in EHR or chart immediately after administration, not before. Correctly sign MAR according to agency policy.
- Record area of i.d. injection and appearance of skin in EHR or chart.
- Record patient teaching, validation of understanding, and the patient's response to medication in EHR or chart.
- Report any undesirable effects from medication to the patient's health care provider, and document adverse effects in record.

Unexpected Outcomes and Related Interventions

- The patient complains of localized pain or continued burning at injection site, indicating potential injury to nerve or vessels.
  - Assess injection site.
  - Notify the patient's health care provider.
- Raised, reddened, or hard zone (induration) forms around i.d. test site.
  - Notify the patient's health care provider.
  - Document sensitivity to injected allergen or positive test if tuberculin skin testing was completed.
- During i.m. injection, blood is aspirated.
  - Immediately stop injection and remove needle.
  - Prepare new syringe of medication for administration.
- The patient displays adverse reaction with signs of urticaria, eczema, pruritus, wheezing, and dyspnea.
  - Follow agency policy or guidelines for appropriate response to allergic reactions (e.g., administration of antihistamine such as diphenhydramine or epinephrine).
  - Notify the patient's health care provider immediately.
  - Add allergy information to the patient's record.

SKILL 26.6 Administering Medications by Intravenous Bolus

Equipment

- Watch with second hand
- Clean gloves
- Antiseptic swab
- Medication in vial or ampule
- Proper-size syringes for medication and saline flush with needleless device or SESIP needle (21- to 25-gauge)
- I.v. lock: Vial of normal saline flush solution (saline recommended [Alexander et al., 2014]); if institution continues to use heparin flush, the most common concentration is 10 units/mL; check institution policy
- MAR or computer printout
- Puncture-proof container for sharps

STEP	RATIONALE
Assessment	
1. Compare accuracy and completeness of each MAR or computer printout with health care provider's written medication order. Check the patient's name, medication name and dosage, route of administration, and time of administration. Recopy or reprint any portion of MAR that is difficult to read.	The order sheet is the most reliable source and only legal record of medications that the patient is to receive. Ensures that the patient receives correct medications (Mandrack et al., 2012). Illegible MARs are a source of medication errors (Alassaad et al., 2013).
Clinical decision point: Some i.v. medications can be pushed safely only when monitoring a patient continuously for dysrhythmias, blood pressure changes, or other adverse effects. Therefore, some medications can be pushed only in specific patient care units. Confirm agency guidelines.	
2. Assess the patient's medical and medication history and history of allergies. List any drug allergies on each page of the MAR and prominently display on the patient's medical record. When allergies are present, the patient should wear an allergy bracelet.	Determines need for medication or possible contraindications for medication administration. I.v. bolus delivers medication rapidly. Allergic response is immediate.

STEP	RATIONALE
3. Review medication reference information for medication action, purpose, side effects, normal dose, time of peak onset, how slowly to give medication, and nursing implications such as need to dilute medication or administer it through a filter.	Knowledge of medication allows you to give it safely and monitor the patient's response to therapy.
4. If you give medication through an existing i.v. line, determine compatibility of medication with i.v. fluids and any additives within i.v. solution.	I.v. medication is not always compatible with i.v. solution and/or additives, and a new site may be needed.
5. Assess the patient's symptoms before initiating medication therapy.	Provides information to evaluate desired effects of medication.
6. Perform hand hygiene. (Apply clean gloves if there is a risk of contracting body fluids.) Assess condition of i.v. needle insertion site for signs of infiltration or phlebitis.	Reduces transmission of microorganisms. Do not administer medication if site is edematous or inflamed.
7. Assess patency of the patient's existing i.v. infusion line or saline lock.	For medication to reach venous circulation effectively, i.v. line must be patent, and fluids must infuse easily.
8. Assess the patient's understanding of purpose of drug therapy.	Poses implications for education.
Planning	
1. Perform hand hygiene. Collect appropriate equipment and MAR.	Reduces transmission of microorganisms. Ensures organized procedure.
2. Follow agency's no-interruption zone (NIZ) policy. Prepare medications for one patient at a time. Keep all pages of MARs or computer printouts for one patient together or look at only one patient's electronic MAR at a time.	Preventing distractions reduces medication preparation errors. Use NIZ when possible (Beyea, 2014; Yoder et al., 2015).
Implementation	
1. Prepare medication for one patient at a time using aseptic technique. Attend to preparation and avoid distraction. Keep all pages of MARs or computer printouts for one patient together or look at only one patient's electronic MAR at a time. Check label of medication against MAR two times, when removing medication from unit dose or AMDS and before leaving medication preparation area (see Skill 26.4 when preparing i.v. medication). Perform hand hygiene.	Reduces transmission of microorganisms. Ensures that medication is sterile. *These are the first and second checks for accuracy* and ensure that correct medication is administered.
Clinical decision point: Some i.v. medications require dilution before administration. Verify with agency policy or pharmacy if dilution is permitted. If a small amount of medication is given (e.g., less than 1 mL), dilute medication in small amount (e.g., 5 mL) of normal saline or sterile water so the medication does not collect in the "dead spaces" (e.g., Y-site injection port, i.v. cap) of the i.v. delivery system.	
2. Take medication to the patient at correct time (see institution policy). Medications that require exact timing include STAT doses, first-time or loading doses, and one-time doses. Give time-critical scheduled medications at exact time ordered (no more than 30 min before or after scheduled dose). Give non-time-critical scheduled medications within a range of 1 or 2 h of scheduled dose (ISMP, 2011a). During administration, apply six rights of medication administration.	Hospitals must adopt medication administration policy and procedure for timing of medication administration that considers nature of the prescribed medication, specific clinical application, and patient needs (CMS, 2011; ISMP, 2011a). Time-critical scheduled medications are those for which administration of maintenance doses more than 30 min before or after the scheduled dose may cause harm or result in substantial suboptimal therapy or pharmacological effect. Non-time-critical medications are those for which early or delayed administration within a specified range of either 1 or 2 h should not cause harm or result in substantial suboptimal therapy or pharmacological effect (CMS, 2011; ISMP, 2011a).
3. Close room curtain or door.	Provides privacy.
4. Identify the patient by using at least two identifiers (e.g., name and birthday or name and medical record number) according to agency policy. Compare identifiers with information on the patient's MAR or medical record.	Ensures correct patient. Complies with The Joint Commission standards and improves patient safety (TJC, 2018).
5. At the patient's bedside, again compare MAR or computer printout with names of medications on medication labels and patient name. Ask the patient whether he or she has allergies.	*This is the third check for accuracy* and ensures that the patient receives correct medication. Confirms the patient's allergy history.
6. Discuss purpose of each medication, action, and possible adverse effects. Allow the patient to ask questions. Explain that you will give medication through existing i.v. line. Encourage the patient to report any discomfort at i.v. site.	Keeps the patient informed of planned therapies, minimizing anxiety. Patients who report pain at i.v. site help detect i.v. infiltrations early, lessening damage to surrounding tissues.

STEP	RATIONALE
7. Perform hand hygiene and apply clean gloves.	Reduces transmission of infection.
8. I.v. push (existing i.v. line):	
a. Select injection port of i.v. tubing closest to the patient. Use needleless injection port.	Follows provisions of Needle Safety and Prevention Act of 2001 (OSHA, n.d.).

Clinical decision point: Never administer i.v. medications through tubing that is infusing blood, blood products, or parenteral nutrition solutions.

STEP	RATIONALE
b. Clean injection port with antiseptic swab. Allow to dry.	Prevents transfer of microorganisms during blunt cannula insertion.
c. Connect syringe to i.v. line: Insert needleless tip of syringe containing drug through center of port (see illustration).	Prevents introduction of microorganisms. Prevents damage to port diaphragm and possible leakage from site.
d. Occlude i.v. line by pinching tubing just above injection port (see illustration). Pull back gently on plunger of syringe to aspirate for blood return.	Final check ensures that medication is being delivered into bloodstream.

Clinical decision point: In some cases, especially with smaller gauge i.v. needles, blood return is not aspirated even if i.v. line is patent. If i.v. site does not show signs of infiltration and i.v. fluid is infusing without difficulty, give i.v. push.

STEP	RATIONALE
e. Release tubing and inject medication within amount of time recommended by institution policy, pharmacist, or medication reference manual. Use watch to time administrations (see illustration). You can pinch i.v. line while pushing medication and release it when not pushing medication. Allow i.v. fluids to infuse when not pushing medication.	Ensures safe medication infusion. Rapid injection of i.v. drug can be fatal. Allowing i.v. fluids to infuse while pushing i.v. drug enables medication to be delivered to the patient at prescribed rate.

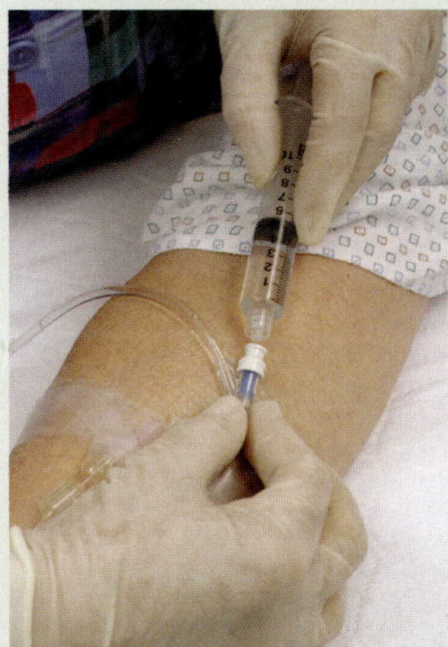

Step 8c Connecting syringe to i.v. line with blunt needleless cannula tip.

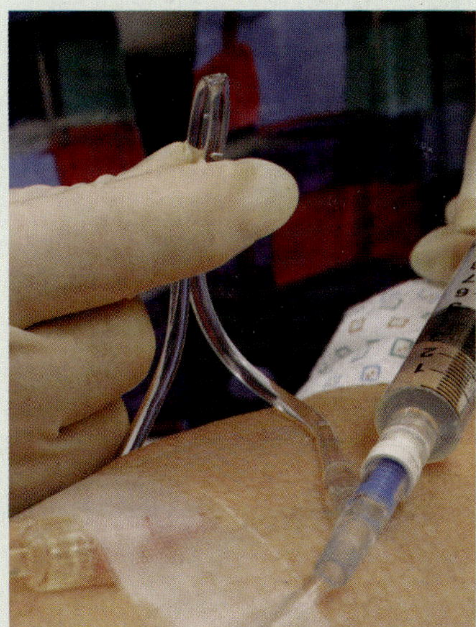

Step 8d I.v. line pinched above injection port allowing to aspirate for blood return.

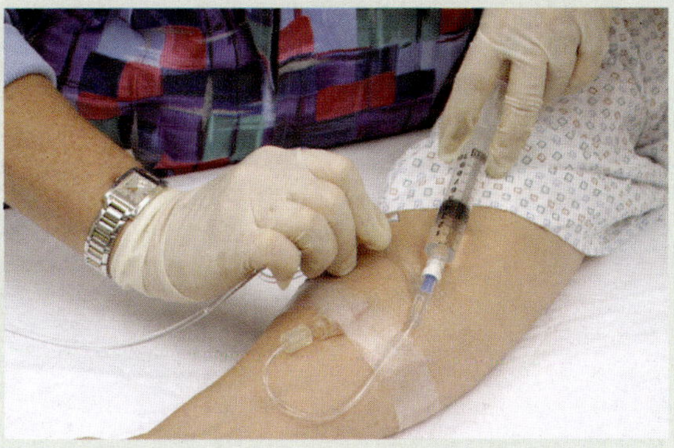

Step 8e Using watch to time an i.v. push medication.

STEP	RATIONALE
f. After injecting medication, withdraw syringe and recheck i.v. fluid infusion rate.	Injection of bolus may alter rate of fluid infusion. Rapid fluid infusion can cause circulatory fluid overload.
g. If i.v. medication is incompatible with i.v. fluids, stop i.v. fluids, clamp i.v. line, and flush with 10 mL of normal saline or sterile water (see institution policy). Then give i.v. bolus over appropriate amount of time and flush with another 10 mL of normal saline or sterile water at *same rate* as medication was administered. Restart i.v. fluids at prescribed rate.	Allows i.v. bolus to be administered without risks associated with i.v. incompatibilities. Ensure that institution guidelines permit flushing lines with incompatible medications. A new site may be needed.
h. If i.v. line that is currently hanging is a medication, disconnect it and administer i.v. push medication as outlined in Step 9. Verify institution policy for stopping i.v. fluids or continuous i.v. medications. If unable to stop i.v. infusion, start new i.v. site and administer medication using i.v. push (i.v. lock) method.	Avoids giving the patient sudden bolus of medication in existing i.v. line.
9. I.v. push (i.v. lock):	
a. Prepare two syringes filled with 2–3 mL of normal saline (0.9%).	Normal saline is effective in keeping i.v. locks patent, is compatible with wide range of medications (Patidar et al., 2014), and does not carry risk of thrombocytopenia with heparin.
b. Administer medication.	
(1) Clean lock injection port with antiseptic swab.	Prevents transfer of microorganisms during needle insertion.
(2) Insert needleless tip of syringe with normal saline 0.9% through center of injection port of i.v. lock (see illustrations).	
(3) Pull back gently on syringe plunger and check for blood return.	Indicates whether needle or catheter is in vein.
(4) Flush i.v. site with normal saline by pushing slowly on plunger.	Clears needle and reservoir of blood. Flushing without difficulty indicates patent i.v. line.
Clinical decision point: Carefully observe the area of skin above the i.v. catheter. Note any puffiness or swelling as i.v. site is flushed, which could indicate infiltration into the vein, requiring removal of catheter.	
(5) Remove saline-filled syringe.	
(6) Clean injection port with antiseptic swab.	Prevents transmission of microorganisms.
(7) Insert needleless tip of syringe containing prepared medication through injection port of i.v. lock.	Allows administration of medication.
(8) Inject medication within amount of time recommended by institution policy, pharmacist, or medication reference manual. Use watch to time administration.	Many medication errors are associated with i.v. pushes that are administered too quickly. Following guidelines for i.v. push rates promotes patient safety.
(9) After administering bolus, withdraw syringe.	
(10) Clean injection port with antiseptic swab.	Prevents transmission of microorganisms.
(11) Flush injection port by attaching syringe with normal saline and inject flush at same rate that medication was delivered. Remove syringe.	Flushing i.v. line with saline prevents occlusion of i.v. access device and ensures that all medication is delivered. Flushing i.v. site at same rate as medication ensures that any medication remaining within i.v. needle is delivered at the correct rate.

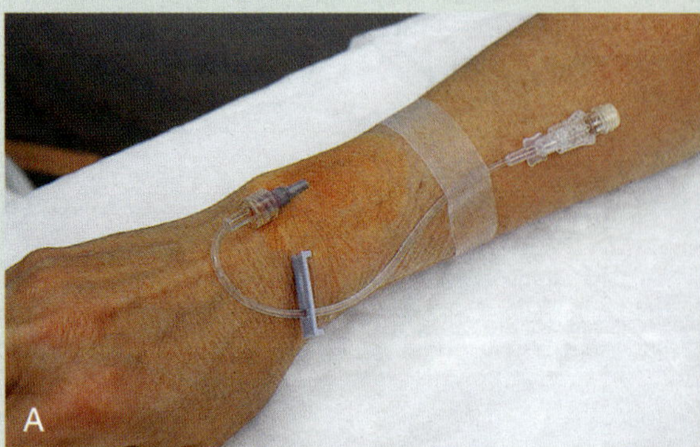

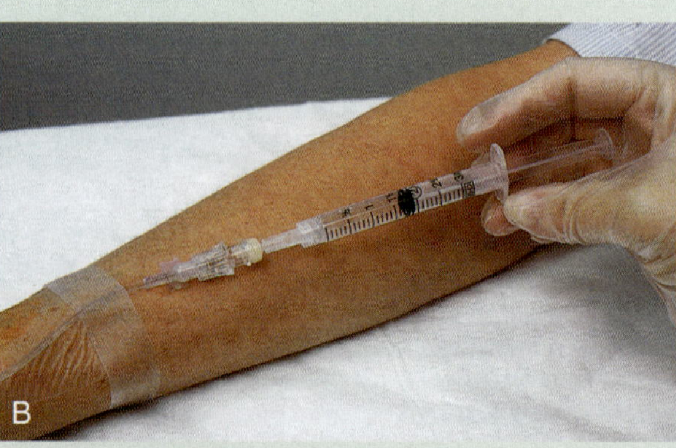

Step 9b(2) A, I.v. catheter with saline lock adapter. **B,** Syringe inserted into injection port.

STEP	RATIONALE
10. Dispose of SESIP-covered needles and syringes in puncture-proof and leak-proof container.	Prevents accidental needlestick injuries and follows CDC guidelines for disposal of sharps (OSHA, n.d.).
11. Stay with the patient for several minutes and observe for any allergic reactions.	Dyspnea, wheezing, and circulatory collapse are signs of anaphylactic reaction.
12. Remove gloves and perform hand hygiene.	Reduces transmission of microorganisms.
Evaluation	
1. Observe the patient closely for adverse reactions during administration and for several minutes thereafter.	I.v. medications act rapidly.
2. Observe i.v. site during injection for sudden swelling and for 48 h after i.v. push.	Swelling indicates infiltration into tissues surrounding vein. Signs of infiltration may not occur for 48 h.
3. Evaluate the patient's status after giving medication to evaluate effectiveness of the medication.	Some i.v. bolus medications can cause rapid changes in the patient's physiological status. Some medications require careful monitoring and assessment and possibly future laboratory testing (e.g., vasopressors and antiarrhythmics, which require blood pressure and heart rate monitoring, and heparin, which requires laboratory studies after administration to determine therapeutic levels).
4. **Use teach back:** "I want to be sure I explained to you why you are receiving this medication I am giving you in your i.v. Tell me in your own words what this medication is for and what we expect it will do for you." Revise your instruction now or develop a plan for revised patient/family caregiver teaching if the patient/family caregiver is not able to teach back correctly	Determines the patient's/family caregiver's level of understanding of instructional topic.

Recording and Reporting

- Immediately record medication administration including drug, dose, route, time instilled, and date and time administered on MAR in EHR or chart. Include initials or signature.
- Record patient teaching and validation of understanding on flow sheet or nurses' notes in EHR or chart.
- Record the patient's medication response in nurses' notes.
- Report any adverse reactions to the patient's health care provider. The patient's response sometimes indicates need for additional medical therapy.

Unexpected Outcomes and Related Interventions

- The patient develops adverse reaction to medication.
  - Stop delivering medication immediately and follow institution policy or guidelines for appropriate response to allergic reaction and reporting of adverse drug effects.
  - Notify the patient's health care provider of adverse effects immediately. Add allergy information to the patient's record.
- I.v. site shows symptoms of infiltration or phlebitis.
  - Stop i.v. infusion immediately or discontinue access device and restart in another site.
  - Determine how much damage i.v. medication can produce in subcutaneous tissue.
  - Provide i.v. extravasation care as indicated by institution policy.

SKILL 26.7 Administering Intravenous Medications by Piggyback, Intermittent Infusion Sets, and Mini-Infusion Pumps

Equipment

- Adhesive tape *(optional)*
- Antiseptic swab
- Clean gloves
- I.v. pole
- MAR or computer printout
- Puncture-proof container for sharps

Piggyback or Mini-Infusion Pump

- Medication prepared in 50- to 250-mL labeled infusion bag or syringe
- Prefilled syringe of normal saline flush solution (for saline lock only)
- Short microdrip, macrodrip, or mini-infusion i.v. tubing set with blunt-ended (needleless) cannula attachment
- Needleless device
- Mini-infusion pump if indicated

Volume-Control Administration Set

- Volutrol or Buretrol
- Infusion tubing with needleless system attachment
- Syringe (1–20 mL)
- Vial or ampule of ordered medication

STEP	RATIONALE
Assessment	
1. Check accuracy and completeness of each MAR or computer printout with health care provider's written medication order. Check the patient's name, medication name and dosage, route of administration, and time of administration. Recopy or reprint any portion of MAR that is difficult to read.	The order sheet is the most reliable source and only legal record of medications that the patient is to receive. Ensures that the patient receives correct medications (Mandrack et al., 2012). Illegible MARs are a source of medication errors (Alassaad et al., 2013).
2. Assess the patient's medical and medication history and history of allergies. List any drug allergies on each page of the MAR and prominently display on the patient's medical record. When allergies are present, the patient should wear an allergy bracelet.	Determines need for medication or possible contraindications for medication administration. I.v. administration delivers medication rapidly and can cause rapid allergic response.
3. Review medication reference information for medication action, purpose, normal dose, side effects, time and peak of onset, how slowly to give medication, and nursing implications (e.g., need to dilute medication, administer through filter).	Allows you to administer medication safely and monitor the patient's response to therapy.
4. If you give medication through existing i.v. line, determine compatibility of medication with i.v. fluids and any additional additives within i.v. solution.	I.v. medication is sometimes not compatible with i.v. solution and/or additives.
Clinical decision point: Never administer i.v. medications through tubing that is infusing blood, blood products, or parenteral nutrition solutions.	
5. Perform hand hygiene. Assess condition of i.v. needle insertion site for signs of infiltration or phlebitis.	Do not administer medication if site is edematous or inflamed.
6. Assess patency and placement of the patient's existing i.v. infusion line or saline lock (see Chapter 25).	For medication to reach venous circulation effectively, i.v. line must be patent, and fluids must infuse easily.
Clinical decision point: If the patient's i.v. site is saline locked, clean the port with alcohol and assess the patency of the i.v. line by flushing it with 2–3 mL of sterile sodium chloride.	
7. Assess the patient's symptoms before initiating medication therapy.	Provides information to evaluate desired effects of medication.
8. Assess the patient's knowledge of medication.	Poses implications for education.
Planning	
1. Perform hand hygiene. Collect appropriate equipment and MAR.	Reduces transmission of microorganisms. Ensures organized procedure.
2. Follow agency's no-interruption zone (NIZ) policy. Prepare medications for one patient at a time. Keep all pages of MARs or computer printouts for one patient together or look at only one patient's electronic MAR at a time.	Preventing distractions reduces medication preparation errors. Use NIZ when possible (Beyea, 2014; Yoder et al., 2015).
Implementation	
1. Prepare medications for one patient at a time using aseptic technique. Attend to the procedure and avoid distraction. Check label of medication against MAR two times, when removing medication from unit dose or AMDS and before leaving medication preparation area (see Skill 26.4). Pharmacy prepares piggyback and prefilled syringes. You will prepare medication for a volume administration set. Perform hand hygiene.	Reduces transmission of microorganisms. Ensures that medication is sterile. *These are the first and second checks for accuracy* and ensure that correct medication is administered.
2. Take medication to the patient at correct time (see agency policy). Medications that require exact timing include STAT doses, first-time or loading doses, and one-time doses. Give time-critical scheduled medications at exact time ordered (no later than 30 min before or after scheduled dose). Give non-time-critical scheduled medications within a range of 1 or 2 h of scheduled dose (ISMP, 2011a). During administration, apply six rights of medication administration.	Hospitals must adopt medication administration policy and procedure for timing of medication administration that considers nature of the prescribed medication, specific clinical application, and patient needs (CMS, 2011; ISMP, 2011a). Time-critical scheduled medications are those for which early or delayed administration of maintenance doses may cause harm or result in substantial suboptimal therapy or pharmacological effect. Non-time-critical medications are those for which early or delayed administration should not cause harm or result in substantial suboptimal therapy or pharmacological effect (CMS, 2011; ISMP, 2011a).
3. Close room curtain or door.	Provides privacy.
4. Identify the patient by using at least two identifiers (e.g., name and birthday or name and medical record number) according to agency policy. Compare identifiers with information on the patient's MAR or medical record.	Ensures correct patient. Complies with The Joint Commission standards and improves patient safety (TJC, 2018).

STEP	RATIONALE
5. At the patient's bedside, again compare MAR or computer printout with names of medications on medication labels and patient name. Ask the patient whether he or she has allergies.	*This is the third check for accuracy* and ensures that the patient receives correct medication. Confirms the patient's allergy history.
6. Discuss purpose of each medication, action, and possible adverse effects. Allow the patient to ask any questions. Explain that you will give medication through existing i.v. line. Encourage the patient to report symptoms of discomfort at site.	Keeping the patient informed of planned therapies minimizes anxiety. Patients who report pain at i.v. site help detect i.v. infiltrations early, lessening damage to surrounding tissues.
7. Perform hand hygiene and apply clean gloves. Administer drug infusion.	Reduces transmission of infection.
a. **Piggyback infusion**	
(1) Connect infusion tubing to medication bag (see Chapter 25). Fill tubing by opening regulator flow clamp. Once tubing is full, close clamp and cap end of tubing.	Filling infusion tubing with solution and freeing air bubbles prevent air embolus.
(2) Hang piggyback (see illustration) medication bag above level of primary fluid bag. (Use hook to lower main bag.)	Height of fluid bag affects rate of flow to the patient.
(3) Connect tubing of piggyback infusion to appropriate connector on upper Y-port of primary infusion line.	Connection allows i.v. medication to enter main i.v. line.
(a) Needleless system: Wipe off needleless port of main i.v. line with alcohol swab, allow to dry, and insert cannula tip of piggyback infusion tubing (see illustrations).	Use needleless connections to prevent accidental needlestick injuries (INS, 2016; OSHA, n.d.).

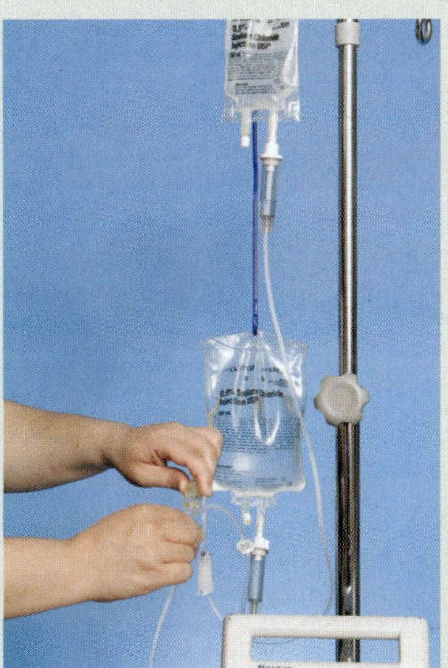

Step 7a(2) Small-volume minibag for piggyback infusion.

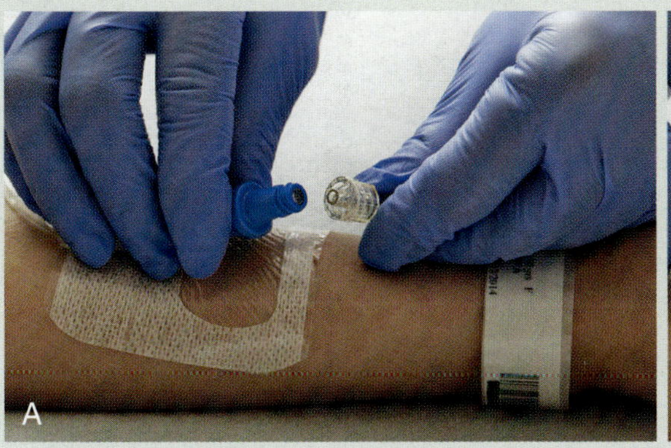

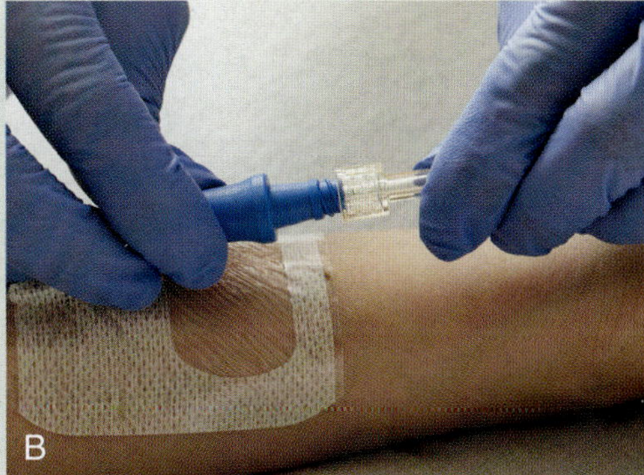

Step 7a(3)(a) A, Needless lock cannula system. **B,** Blunt-ended cannula inserts into port and locks.

STEP	RATIONALE
(4) *Option:* Normal saline lock—follow steps to flush and prepare a saline lock (see Chapter 25). Wipe off port with alcohol swab, let dry, and insert tip of piggyback infusion tubing via needleless access.	Flushing of lock ensures patency.
(5) Regulate flow rate of medication solution by adjusting regulator clamp or i.v. pump infusion rate. Infusion times vary. Refer to medication reference or agency policy for safe flow rate.	Provides slow, safe, intermittent infusion of medication and maintains therapeutic blood levels.
(6) Once medication has infused:	
(a) Continuous infusion: Check flow rate of primary infusion. Primary infusion automatically begins after piggyback solution is empty.	Back-check valve on piggyback prevents flow of primary infusion until medication infuses. Checking flow rate ensures proper administration of i.v. fluids.
(b) Normal saline lock: Disconnect tubing, clean port with alcohol, and flush i.v. line with 2–3 mL of sterile 0.9% sodium chloride. Maintain sterility of i.v. tubing between intermittent infusions.	
(7) Regulate continuous main infusion line to ordered rate.	Infusion of piggyback sometimes interferes with main line infusion rate.
(8) Leave i.v. piggyback and tubing in place for future drug administration (see agency policy) or discard in puncture-proof and leak-proof container.	Establishment of secondary line produces route for microorganisms to enter main line. Repeated changes in tubing increase risk for infection transmission.
b. **Volume-control administration set (e.g., Volutrol)**	
(1) Fill Volutrol with desired amount of i.v. fluid (50–100 mL) by opening clamp between Volutrol and main i.v. bag (see illustration).	Small volume of fluid dilutes i.v. medication and reduces risk of fluid infusing too rapidly.
(2) Close clamp and check to be sure that clamp on air vent Volutrol chamber is open.	Prevents additional leakage of fluid into Volutrol. Air vent allows fluid in Volutrol to exit at regulated rate.
(3) Clean injection port on top of Volutrol with antiseptic swab.	Prevents introduction of microorganisms during needle insertion.
(4) Remove needle cap or sheath and insert needleless syringe or syringe needle through port and inject medication (see illustration). Gently rotate Volutrol between hands.	Rotating mixes medication with solution to ensure equal distribution in Volutrol.

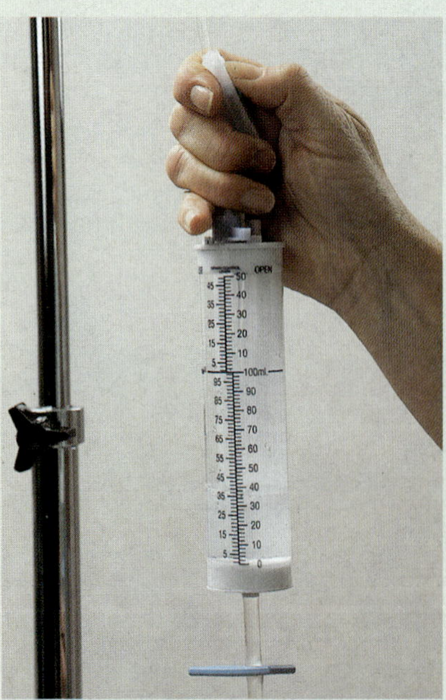

Step 7b(1) Fill volume-control administration device.

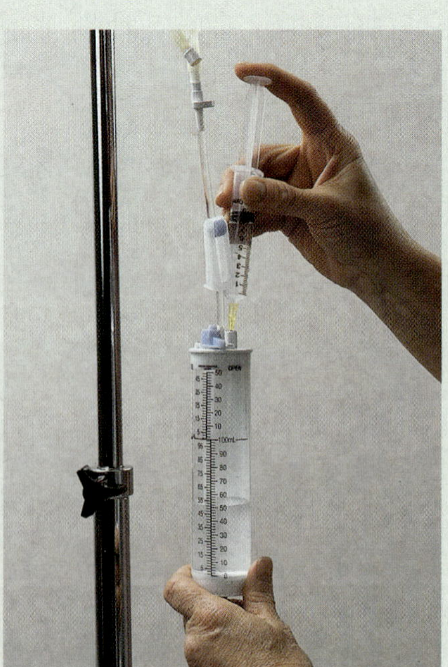

Step 7b(4) Medication injected into device.

STEP	RATIONALE
(5) Regulate i.v. infusion rate to allow medication to infuse in time recommended by agency policy, pharmacist, or medication reference manual.	For optimal therapeutic effect, medication should infuse in prescribed time interval.
(6) Label Volutrol with name of medication, dosage, total volume including diluent, and time of administration following ISMP (2015h) safe medication label format.	Alerts nurses to medication being infused. Prevents other medications from being added to Volutrol.
(7) If the patient is receiving continuous i.v. infusion, check infusion rate after Volutrol infusion is complete.	Ensures appropriate rate of administration.
(8) Dispose of uncapped needle or needle enclosed in safety shield and syringe in puncture-proof and leak-proof container. Discard supplies in appropriate container. Perform hand hygiene.	Prevents accidental needlesticks (OSHA, n.d.). Reduces transmission of microorganisms.
c. **Mini-infusion pump administration**	
(1) Connect prefilled syringe to mini-infusion pump tubing; remove end cap of tubing.	Special tubing designed to fit syringe delivers medication to main i.v. line.
(2) Carefully apply pressure to syringe plunger, allowing tubing to fill with medication.	Ensures that tubing is free of air bubbles to prevent air embolus.
(3) Place syringe into mini-infusion pump (follow product directions) and hang on i.v. pole. Be sure that syringe is secured (see illustration).	Secure placement is needed for proper infusion.
(4) Connect end of mini-infusion pump tubing to main i.v. line or saline lock.	Establishes route for i.v. medication to enter main i.v. line.
(a) Existing i.v. line: Wipe off needleless port on main i.v. line with alcohol swab, allow to dry, and insert tip of mini-infusion pump tubing through center of port.	Needleless connections reduce risk for accidental needlestick injuries (OSHA, n.d.).
(b) Normal saline lock: Follow steps to flush and prepare saline lock (see Chapter 25). Wipe off port with alcohol swab, allow to dry, and insert tip of mini-infusion tubing.	Flushing of lock ensures patency.
(5) Set pump to deliver medication within time recommended by agency policy, pharmacist, or medication reference manual. Press button on pump to begin infusion.	Pump automatically delivers medication at safe, constant rate based on volume in syringe.
(6) Once medication has infused:	
(a) Main i.v. infusion: Check flow rate. Infusion automatically begins to flow once pump stops. Regulate infusion to desired rate as needed.	Maintains patent primary i.v. fluids.
(b) Normal saline lock: Disconnect tubing, clean port with alcohol, and flush i.v. line with 2–3 mL of sterile 0.9% sodium chloride. Maintain sterility of i.v. tubing between intermittent infusions.	

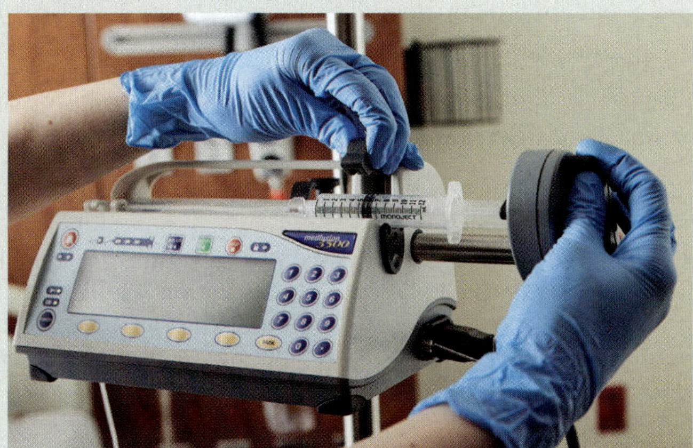

Step 7c(3) Ensure that syringe is secure after placing it into mini-infusion pump.

STEP	RATIONALE
8. Dispose of uncapped needles or needle enclosed in safety shield and syringes in puncture-proof and leak-proof container. Discard supplies in appropriate container. Remove and dispose of gloves, and perform hand hygiene.	Prevents accidental needlesticks (OSHA, n.d.). Reduces transmission of microorganisms.
9. Stay with the patient for several minutes and observe for any allergic reactions.	Dyspnea, wheezing, and circulatory collapse are signs of severe anaphylactic reaction.
Evaluation	
1. Observe the patient for signs or symptoms of adverse reaction.	I.v. medications act rapidly.
2. During infusion, periodically check infusion rate and condition of i.v. site.	I.v. must remain patent for proper drug administration. Infiltration of i.v. site requires discontinuing infusion.
3. Ask the patient to explain purpose and side effects of medication.	Evaluates the patient's understanding of instruction.
4. **Use teach back:** "I want to be sure I explained to you the reason for this i.v. medication. Can you explain to me why you are receiving the medication and what to report to the nurse?" Revise your instruction now or develop a plan for revised patient/family caregiver teaching if the patient/family caregiver is not able to teach back correctly.	Determines the patient's/family caregiver's level of understanding of instructional topic.

Recording and Reporting

- Immediately record medication, dose, route, infusion rate, and date and time administered on MAR in EHR or chart. Include initials or signature.
- Record volume of fluid in medication bag or Volutrol on intake and output (I&O) form.
- Record patient teaching and validation of understanding on flow sheet or nurses' notes in EHR or chart.
- Report any adverse reactions to the patient's health care provider.

Unexpected Outcomes and Related Interventions

- The patient develops adverse or allergic reaction to medication.
  - Stop medication infusion immediately.
  - Follow agency policy or guidelines for appropriate response to allergic reaction (e.g., administration of antihistamine such as diphenhydramine or epinephrine) and reporting of adverse medication reactions.
  - Notify the patient's health care provider of adverse effects immediately.
  - Add allergy information to the patient's record per agency policy.
- Medication does not infuse over established time frame.
  - Determine reason (e.g., improper calculation of flow rate, poor positioning of i.v. needle at insertion site, infiltration).
  - Take corrective action as indicated.
- I.v. site shows signs of infiltration or phlebitis (see Chapter 25).
  - Stop i.v. infusion and discontinue access device.
  - Treat i.v. site as indicated by agency policy.
  - Insert new i.v. catheter if therapy continues.
  - For infiltration, determine how harmful i.v. medication is to subcutaneous tissue. Provide i.v. extravasation care (e.g., injecting phentolamine around i.v. infiltration site) as indicated by agency policy or consult pharmacist to determine appropriate follow-up care.

KEY POINTS

- Application of knowledge about the four major pharmacokinetic processes—medication absorption, distribution, metabolism, and excretion—allows you to better time medication administration, select the route of administration, and evaluate a patient's response.
- Prompt recognition and reporting of adverse drug effects prevents serious patient injury.
- Hospitalized patients with known drug allergies have their allergy information recorded in a clearly identifiable place to inform all caregivers.
- When a medication is prescribed, the goal is a constant blood level within a safe therapeutic range.
- Medications that are time-critical most likely cause harm or have subtherapeutic effects if they are not administered on time (usually 30 minutes before or after scheduled dose).
- The route prescribed for administering a medication depends on its properties and desired effect and on a patient's physical and mental condition.
- Metric units are easy to convert and calculate using simple multiplication and division with each basic unit of measurement organized into units of 10.
- Responsibilities of medication administration include knowing medication therapeutics, assessing a patient for administration, calculating doses, administering medications using the six rights of medication administration, monitoring and evaluating medication effects, and assessing a patient's ability to self-administer medications.
- The six rights of medication administration are the right medication, right dose, right patient, right route, right time, and right documentation.
- Before administering medications, perform a physical assessment to reveal physical findings for any indications or contraindications for medication therapy.
- Factors contributing to medication nonadherence in older adults include depression, problems with cognitive or functional abilities, dislike for medication side

effects, a busy and active lifestyle, and inability to afford medications.

- Collaboration with patients and family caregivers is essential, particularly if patients will require assistance with self-administration and if medication regimens are complicated.
- For patient safety, it is essential that you refer to the MAR each time you prepare a medication and have it available at the patient's bedside when administering medications.
- Distractions may cause a medication error. They include a page, phone call, and request from a colleague or patient that draws away, disturbs, or diverts attention from a current desired task or forces attention on a new task at least temporarily.
- An important precaution with any oral preparation is to protect patients from aspiration.
- Rotate i.m. injection sites to decrease the risk for tissue hypertrophy, and use the Z-track method for administration.

REFERENCES

Agency for Healthcare Research and Quality (AHRQ). Computerized provider order entry. 2016. Available from: https://psnet.ahrq.gov/primers/primer/6/computerized-provider-order-entry.

Akbari Sari A, Janani L, Mohammady M, Nedjat S. Slow versus fast subcutaneous heparin injections for prevention of bruising and site-pain intensity. Cochrane Database Syst Rev 2014;(7):CD008077.

Alassaad A, Gillespie U, Bertilsson M, Melhus H, Hammarlund-Udenaes M. Prescription and transcription errors in multidose-dispensed medications on discharge from hospital: an observational and interventional study. J Eval Clin Pract 2013;19(1):185.

American Academy of Allergy, Asthma and Immunology (AAAAI). Peak flow meter. 2016. Available from: https://aaaai.execinc.com/store/product.asp?productid=104.

American Association of Diabetes Educators (AADR). Teaching injection technique to people with diabetes. 2013. Available from: https://www.diabeteseducator.org/docs/default-source/legacy-docs/_resources/pdf/research/injectioneducationpracticeguide.pdf?sfvrsn=2.

American Diabetes Association (ADA). Diabetes care in the hospital, nursing home, and skilled nursing facility. Diabetes Care 2015; 38(S1):S80. Available from: http://care.diabetesjournals.org/content/38/Supplement_1/S80.full.

American Nurses Association (ANA). Nursing: scope and standards of practice. 3rd ed. Silver Spring, MD: The Association; 2015.

American Society of Health-System Pharmacists (ASHP). How to use eye drops properly. 2013a. Available from: http://www.safemedication.com/safemed/MedicationTipsTools/HowtoAdminister/HowtoUseEyeDropsProperly.aspx.

American Society of Health-System Pharmacists (ASHP). How to use nose drops properly. 2013b. Available from: http://www.safemedication.com/safemed/MedicationTipsTools/HowtoAdminister/HowtoUseNoseDropsProperly.aspx.

Anderson P, Townsend T. Preventing high-alert medication errors in hospital patients. Am Nurse Today 2015;10(5). Available from: https://www.americannursetoday.com/preventing-high-alert-medication-errors.

Ari A, Restrepo RD. Aerosol delivery device selection for spontaneously breathing patients. Respir Care 2012;57(4):613.

Barnes MG, Ledford C, Hogan K. A "needling" problem: shoulder injury related to vaccine administration. J Am Board Fam Med 2012;25:919.

Barrons R, Wheeler J, Woods JA. Opportunities for inhaler device selection in elderly patients with asthma or COPD. Patient Intell 2015;7:53. Available from: https://www.dovepress.com/opportunities-for-inhaler-device-selection-in-elderly-patients-with-as-peer-reviewed-article-PI.

Bartlett R, Brown L, Shattell M, Wright T, Lewallen L. Harm reduction: compassionate care of persons with addictions. Medsurg Nurs 2013; 22(6):349.

Beyea S. Interruptions and distractions in health care: improved safety with mindfulness. Agency for Healthcare Research and Quality. 2014. Available from: https://psnet.ahrq.gov/perspective/interruptions-and-distractions-health-care-improved-safety-mindfulness.

Bhalla MC, Gable BD, Frey JA, Reichenbach MR, Wilber ST. Predictors of epinephrine autoinjector needle length inadequacy. Am J Emerg Med 2013;31(12):1671.

Bonini M, Usmani OS. The importance of inhaler devices in the treatment of COPD. COPD Res Pract 2015;1:9. Available from: https://copdrp.biomedcentral.com/articles/10.1186/s40749-015-0011-0.

Borovina LR, Tremellen KE, Walker MP, Hawley TM, Horgan AR, Grant GD, et al. The microbial contamination of pressurised metered-dose inhalers anonymously sourced from the South-East Queensland Australia community population. Int J Pharm Pract 2012;20(2):129.

Bourzac K. Dissolving disks deliver drugs to the eye. Chemical and Engineering News; February 5, 2015. Available from: http://cen.acs.org/articles/93/web/2015/02/Dissolving-Disks-Deliver-Drugs-Eye.html.

Boysen PG. Just culture: a foundation for balanced accountability and patient safety. Ochsner J 2013;13(3):400.

Burchum J, Rosenthal L. Lehne's pharmacology for nursing care. 9th ed. St. Louis: Saunders; 2016.

Centers for Disease Control and Prevention (CDC). Stop sticks campaign. 2010. Available from: https://www.cdc.gov/nora/councils/hcsa/stopsticks/default.html.

Centers for Disease Control and Prevention (CDC). Vaccine administration. 2015. Available from: http://www.cdc.gov/vaccines/pubs/pinkbook/vac-admin.html.

Centers for Medicare and Medicaid Services (CMS). Updated guidance on medication administration, Hospital Appendix A of the State Operations Manual (SOM). 2011. Available from: https://www.cms.gov/Regulations-and-Guidance/Guidance/Manuals/downloads/som107ap_a_hospitals.pdf.

Chapuis C, Bedouch P, Detavernier M, Durand M, Francony G, Lavagne P, et al. Automated drug dispensing systems in the intensive care unit: a financial analysis. Crit Care 2015;19:318.

ConsumerMedSafety. Tips for measuring liquid medicines safely. 2015. http://www.consumermedsafety.org/tools-and-resources/medication-safety-tools-and-resources/taking-your-medicine-safely/measure-liquid-medications.

Davidson K, Rourke L. Teaching best evidence: deltoid intramuscular injection technique. J Nurs Educ Pract 2013;3(7):122.

Dayananda L, Belaval VV, Raina A, Chandana R. Intended intramuscular gluteal injections: are they truly intramuscular? J Postgrad Med 2014;60(2):175.

deMeneses AS, Marques IR. A proposal for a geometrical delimitation model for ventro-gluteal injection. Rev Bras Enferm 2007;60(5):552.

Diggle D. Are you FIT for purpose? The importance of getting injection technique right. J Diabetes Nurs 2014;18:50.

Food and Drug Administration (FDA). FDA reminds the public about the potential for life-threatening harm from accidental exposure to fentanyl transdermal systems ("patches"). 2012. Available from: https://www.fda.gov/drugs/ensuring-safe-use-medicine/best-practices-tablet-splitting#:~:text=If%20your%20healthcare%20professional%20asks,before%20splitting%20the%20next%20tablet.

Food and Drug Administration (FDA). Best practices for tablet splitting. 2013. Available from: http://www.fda.gov/Drugs/ResourcesForYou/Consumers/BuyingUsingMedicineSafely/EnsuringSafeUseofMedicine/ucm184666.htm.

Frid AH, Kreugel G, Grassi G, Halimi S, Hicks D, Hirsch LJ, et al. New insulin delivery recommendations. Mayo Clin Proc 2016;91(9):1231.

Guenther P. New enteral connectors: raising awareness. Nutr Clin Pract 2015;29:612.

Guenther P, Boullatta J. Drug administration by enteral feeding tube. Nursing 2013;43(12):26.

Haynes J. WATER CONTENT OF STERILE AND NON-STERILE BOLL WEEVILS AS INFLUENCED BY FEEDING INCREASED LEVELS OF SUCROSE OR COTTON SQUARES. Journal of Entomological Science. 1988;23(2):155–160.

Hibberd P. Approach to immunizations in healthy adults. UpToDate; 2015. Available from: https://www.uptodate.com/contents/immunizations-in-adults-with-.

Hirsch LJ, Gibney MA, Li L, Bérubé J. Glycemic control, reported pain and leakage with a 4 mm × 32 G pen needle in obese and non-obese adults with diabetes: a post hoc analysis. Curr Med Res Opin 2012; 28(8):1305.

Hockenberry MJ, Wilson D. Wong's nursing care of infants and children. 10th ed. St. Louis: Mosby; 2015.

Hopkins U, Arias CY. Large-volume i.m. injections: a review of best practices. Oncol Nurse Advis 2013. http://www.oncologynurseadvisor.com/chemotherapy/large-volume-im-injections-a-review-of-best-practices/article/281208/.

Hopkinson SG, Jennings BM. Interruptions during nurses' work: a state-of-the-science review. Res Nurs Health 2013;36(1):38.

Imran M, Hayley D. Injection-induced axillary nerve injury after a drive-through flu shot. Clin Geriatr 2013;21(12).

Infusion Nurses Society (INS). Infusion therapy standards of practice. J Infus Nurs 2016;39(Suppl. 1):S1.

Institute for Safe Medication Practices (ISMP). ISMP's guidelines for standard order sets. 2010. Available from: http://www.ismp.org/tools/guidelines/standardordersets.pdf.

Institute for Safe Medication Practices (ISMP). Acute care guidelines for timely administration of scheduled medications. 2011a. Available from: http://www.ismp.org/Tools/guidelines/acutecare/tasm.pdf.

Institute for Safe Medication Practices (ISMP). ISMP statement on use of metric measurements to prevent errors with oral liquids. 2011b. Available from: https://www.ismp.org/pressroom/PR20110808.pdf.

Institute for Safe Medication Practices (ISMP). As U-500 insulin safety concerns mount, it's time to rethink safe use of strengths above U-100. 2013a. Available from: https://www.ismp.org/newsletters/acutecare/showarticle.aspx?id=62.

Institute for Safe Medication Practices (ISMP). Ongoing concern about insulin pen reuse shows hospitals need to consider transitioning away from them. 2013b. Available from: http://www.ismp.org/newsletters/acutecare/showarticle.aspx?id=41.

Institute for Safe Medication Practices (ISMP). Independent double checks: undervalued and misused: selective use of this strategy can play an important role in medication safety. 2013c. Available from: https://www.ismp.org/newsletters/acutecare/showarticle.aspx?id=51.

Institute for Safe Medication Practices (ISMP). List of high-alert medications in acute care settings. 2014. Available from: https://www.ismp.org/tools/institutionalhighAlert.asp.

Institute for Safe Medication Practices (ISMP). ISMP's list of error-prone abbreviations, symbols, and dose designations. 2015b. Available from: https://www.ismp.org/tools/errorproneabbreviations.pdf.

Institute for Safe Medication Practices (ISMP). Oral dosage forms that should not be crushed. 2015c. Available from: http://www.ismp.org/tools/donotcrush.pdf.

Institute for Safe Medication Practices (ISMP). Results of pediatric medication safety survey (part 2): comparing data subsets points out areas for improvement. 2015d. Available from: https://www.ismp.org/newsletters/acutecare/showarticle.aspx?id=112.

Institute for Safe Medication Practices (ISMP). ISMP safe practice guidelines for adult i.v. push medications. 2015e. Available from: http://www.ismp.org/Tools/guidelines/IVSummitPush/IVPushMedGuidelines.Pdf.

Institute for Safe Medication Practices (ISMP). Acute Care: ISMP Medication safety alert, A successful ENFit launch still won't stop all incidents of oral medications given intravenously 2015f ;20(16):1–4. Available from: http://www.ismp.org/newsletters/acutecare/showarticle.aspx?id=115.

Institute for Safe Medication Practices (ISMP). Principles of designing a medication label for intravenous piggyback medication for patient-specific inpatient use. 2015h. Available from: https://www.ismp.org/resources?field_resource_type_target_id%5B0%5D=33&field_resource_type_target_id%5B1%5D=33&field_resource_type_target_id%5B2%5D=33#resources—resources_list.

Institute for Safe Medication Practices (ISMP). 2016-2017 targeted medication safety best practices for hospitals. 2016b. Available from": http://www.ismp.org/tools/bestpractices/TMSBP-for-hospitals.pdf.

Institute for Safe Medication Practices (ISMP). Principles of designing a medication label for intravenous piggyback medication for patient specific inpatient use. 2016c. Available from: https://www.ismp.org/sites/default/files/attachments/2017-11/ISMP97-Guidelines-071415-3.%20FINAL.pdf.

Institute for Safe Medication Practices (ISMP). Acute Care ISMP Medication Safety Alert. Transition adapters for ENFit syringes can defeat the purpose of ENFit itself. ISMP 2017;22(19):1. Available from: https://www.ismp.org/newsletters/acutecare/currentissue.aspx.

Kara Yilmaz D, Karaman D. Using ventrogluteal site in intramuscular injections is a priority or an alternative? Int J Caring Sci 2015;8(2):507.

Kaya N, Salmaslıoğlu A, Terzi B, Turan N, Acunaş B. The reliability of site determination methods in ventrogluteal area injection: a cross-sectional study. Int J Nurs Stud 2015;52:355.

Kilic E, Kalay R, Kilic C. Comparing applications of intramuscular injections to dorsogluteal or ventrogluteal regions. J Exp Integr Med 2014;4(3):171.

Kim J, Bates DW. Medication administration errors by nurses: adherence to guidelines. J Clin Nurs 2013;22(3/4):590.

Klang M, McLymont V, Ng N. Osmolality, pH, and compatibility of selected oral liquid medications with an enteral nutrition product. JPEN J Parenter Enteral Nutr 2013;37:689.

Koohestani H, Baghcheghi N. Comparing the effects of two educational methods of intravenous drug rate calculations on rapid and sustained learning of nursing students: formula method and dimensional analysis method. Nurse Educ Pract 2010;10(4):233.

Lavik E, Kuehn MH, Kwon YH. Novel drug delivery systems for glaucoma. Eye (Lond) 2011;25(5):578.

Lilley LL, Collins RS, Snyder J. Pharmacology and the nursing process. 8th ed. St. Louis: Mosby; 2016.

Making Health Care Safer II. Content last reviewed April 2018. Agency for Healthcare Research and Quality, Rockville, MD. https://www.ahrq.gov/research/findings/evidence-based-reports/ptsafetytabb.html

Malone A. Clinical guidelines from the American Society for Parenteral and Enteral Nutrition: best practices recommendations for patient care. J Infus Nurs 2014;37(3):179.

Mandrack M, Cohen MR, Featherling J, Gellner L, Judd K, Kienle PC, et al. Nursing best practices using automated dispensing cabinets: nurses' key role in improving medication safety. Medsurg Nurs 2012;21(3):134.

Mary Alexander, Ann M. Corrigan S., Lisa A Gorski and Lynn Phillips. Core curriculum for infusion nursing. 4th ed. Philadelphia: Williams & Wilkins; 2014.

Moczygemba LR, Gatewood SB, Kennedy AK, Osborn RD, Alexander AJ, Matzke GR, Goode JV. Medication reconciliation campaign in a clinic for homeless patients. Am J Health Syst Pharm. 2012 Apr 1;69(7):558, 560–2.

Murphy M, While A. Medication administration practices among children's nurses: a survey. Br J Nurs 2012;21(15):928.

National Coordinating Council for Medication Error Reporting and Prevention (NCCMERP). Recommendations to reduce medication errors associated with verbal medication orders and prescriptions. 2015. Available from: http://www.nccmerp.org/recommendations-reduce-medication-errors-associated-verbal-medication-orders-and-prescriptions.

National Quality Forum (NQF). Serious reportable events. 2016. Available from: http://www.qualityforum.org/Topics/SREs/Serious_Reportable_Events.aspx.

Nicoll L, Hesby A. Intramuscular injection: an integrative research review and guideline for evidence-based practice. Appl Nurs Res 2002;16(2):159.

Novo Nordisk. Levemir. 2015. Available from: http://www.levemir.com/.

Occupational Safety and Health Administration (OSHA). Bloodborne pathogens and needlestick prevention. n.d. Available from: https://www.osha.gov/SLTC/bloodbornepathogens/index.html.

Ogston-Tuck S. Subcutaneous injection technique: an evidence based approach. Nurs Stand 2014a;29(3):53.

Ogston-Tuck S. Intramuscular injection technique: an evidence based approach. Nurs Stand 2014b;29(4):55.

Palma S, Strohfus P. Are i.m. injections i.m. in obese and overweight females? A study in injection technique. Appl Nurs Res 2013;26(4):e1.

Paparella S. Adopt the 2014-2015 targeted best practices for medication safety. J Emerg Nurs 2014;40(3):263.

Park YH, Han HR, Oh BM, Lee J, Park JA, Yu SJ, et al. Prevalence and associated factors of dysphagia in nursing home residents. Geriatr Nurs 2013;34(3):212.

Pasina L, Brucato AL, Falcone C, Cucchi E, Bresciani A, Sottocorno M, et al. Medication non-adherence among elderly patients newly discharged and receiving polypharmacy. Drugs Aging 2014;31(4):283.

Pérez-Diaz C, Calixto OJ, Faccini-Martínez ÁA, Bravo-Ojeda JS, Botero-García CA, Uribe-Pardo E, Mantilla-Florez YF, Benitez F, Duran A, Osorio J. Occupational exposure to blood borne pathogens among healthcare workers: a cross-sectional study of a registry in Colombia. J Occup Med Toxicol. 2015 Dec 16;10:45. doi: 10.1186/s12995-015-0088-z. PMID: 26677395; PMCID: PMC4681124.

Radley DC, Wasserman MR, Olsho LE, Shoemaker SJ, Spranca MD, Bradshaw B. Reduction in medication errors in hospitals due to adoption of computerized provider order entry systems. J Am Med Inform Assoc 2013;20(3):470.

Ruth S Weinstock. General principles of insulin therapy in diabetes mellitus. UpToDate; 2015. Available from: http://www.uptodate.com/contents/general-principles-of-insulin-therapy-in-diabetes-mellitus.

Sanofi-Aventis. Lovenox subcutaneous injection. 2014. Available from: https://www.lovenox.com/patient-self-injection-video.

Sharma SK, Mudgal SK, Gaur R, Sharma R, Sharma M, Thakur K. Heparin flush vs. normal saline flush to maintain the patency of central venous catheter among adult patients: A systematic review and meta-analysis. J Family Med Prim Care 2019; 8(9):2779–92.

Teunissen R, Bos J, Pot H, Pluim M, Kramers C. Clinical relevance of and risk factors associated with medication administration time errors. Am J Health Syst Pharm 2013;70(12):1052.

The Joint Commission (TJC). Revisions to the medication management standards regarding sample medications. July 2014a. Available from:

http://www.jointcommission.org/assets/1/6/SampleMedications_HAP.pdf.

The Joint Commission (TJC). Sentinel event alert 53: managing risk during transition to new ISO tubing connector standards. 2014b. Available from: https://www.jointcommission.org/sea_issue_53/.

The Joint Commission (TJC). Facts about the official "do not use" list of abbreviations. 2016. Available from: https://www.jointcommission.org/facts_about_do_not_use_list/.

The Joint Commission (TJC). 2018 National Patient Safety Goals. Oakbrook Terrace, IL: The Joint Commission; 2018. Available from: http://www.jointcommission.org/standards_information/npsgs.aspx.

Touhy TA, Jett KF. Ebersole and Hess' gerontological nursing and healthy aging. 4th ed. St. Louis: Elsevier; 2014.

Voshall B, Piscotty R, Lawrence J, Targosz M. Barcode medication administration work-arounds: a systematic review and implications for nurse executives. J Nurs Adm. 2013 Oct;43(10):530–5.

World Health Organization (WHO). Injection safety. 2015. Available from: https://www.who.int/infection-prevention/campaigns/injections/global-campaign/en/.

Yapucu Gūnes Ü, Ceylan B, Bayındır P. Is the ventrogluteal site suitable for intramuscular injections in children under the age of three? J Adv Nurs 2016;72(1):127.

Yoder M, Schadewald D, Dietrich K. The effect of a safe zone on nurse interruptions, distractions, and medication administration errors. J Infus Nurs 2015;38(2):140.

Zabaleta-Del-Olmo E, Vlacho B, Jodar-Fernández L, Urpí-Fernández AM, Lumillo-Gutiérrez I, Agudo-Ugena J, et al. Safety of the reuse of needles for subcutaneous insulin injection: a systematic review and meta-analysis. Int J Nurs Stud 2016;60:121.

27 Sensory Needs

OBJECTIVES

- To differentiate the processes of reception, perception, and reaction to sensory stimuli.
- To compare the relationship of sensory function with an individual's level of wellness.
- To discuss common causes and effects of sensory alterations.
- To discuss common sensory changes that occur with aging.
- To identify factors to assess in determining a patient's sensory status.
- To describe behaviors indicating sensory alterations.
- To develop a plan of care for patients with sensory deficits.
- To describe nursing interventions with rationales that promote effective communication with patients who have sensory alterations.
- To describe conditions in the health care agency or patient's home that you adjust to promote meaningful sensory stimulation.
- To discuss ways to maintain a safe environment for patients with sensory alterations.
- To discuss the causes and pathophysiology of unconsciousness.
- To describe nursing interventions in health care facility to manage unconscious patients.

KEY TERMS

accommodation, p. 722
age-related macular degeneration, p. 723
auditory, p. 720
cataracts, p. 722
diabetic retinopathy, p. 723
glaucoma, p. 723
gustatory, p. 720
Meniere disease, p. 723
olfactory, p. 720
ototoxic, p. 722
presbycusis, p. 722
presbyopia, p. 722
proprioception, p. 720
refractive errors, p. 722
sensory deficits, p. 722
sensory deprivation, p. 722
sensory overload, p. 722
tactile, p. 720
tinnitus, p. 722

INTRODUCTION

People are unique because they are able to sense a variety of stimuli in their environment. Stimulation comes from many sources inside and outside of the body, particularly through the senses of sight **(visual)**, hearing **(auditory)**, touch **(tactile)**, smell **(olfactory)**, and taste **(gustatory)**. Additional senses include pressure, pain, temperature, vibration, and position **(proprioception)** (Meiner, 2015). People learn about the environment from healthy sensory organs. Patients need to adapt to their environment when their sensory function is altered. As a nurse, you will learn to recognize when patients are at risk for developing sensory problems and help meet their needs when they have sensory alterations. Your nursing care helps patients learn to alter their environment for improved safety.

NORMAL SENSATION

The nervous system continually receives thousands of bits of information from sensory nerve organs, relays the information through appropriate neurological channels, and integrates the information into a meaningful response. Sensory stimuli reach the sensory organs to elicit an immediate reaction or store information in the brain for future use. The nervous system must be intact for sensory stimuli to reach appropriate brain centers and for an individual to perceive the sensation. After interpreting the significance of a sensation, the person is then able to react to the stimulus. Table 27.1 summarizes normal hearing and vision.

COMPONENTS OF SENSORY EXPERIENCE

Reception, perception, and reaction are the three components of any sensory experience.

Reception

Reception begins with stimulation of a nerve cell called a *receptor*, which is usually for only one type of stimulus such as light, touch, taste, or sound. In the case of special senses, the receptors are grouped close together or located

Table 27.1 Normal Hearing and Vision

Function	Anatomy and Physiology
EAR	
Transmits to brain a pattern of all sounds received from the environment, the relative intensity of these sounds, and the direction from which they originate	Two ears provide stereophonic hearing to judge sound direction. The external ear canal shelters the eardrum and maintains relatively constant temperature and humidity to maintain elasticity. The middle ear is an air-containing space between the eardrum and the oval window. It contains three small bones (ossicles). The eardrum and ossicles transfer sound to the fluid-filled inner ear. Movement of the stapes in the oval window creates vibrations in the fluid that bathes the membranous labyrinth, which contains the end organs of hearing and balance. The union of the vestibular (balance) and cochlear (hearing) parts of the labyrinth explains the combination of hearing and balance symptoms that occur with inner ear disorders. Vibration of the eardrum transmits through the bony ossicles. Vibrations at the oval window transmit in perilymph within the inner ear to stimulate hair cells that send impulses along the eighth cranial nerve to the brain.
EYE	
Transmits a pattern of light to the brain that is reflected from solid objects in the environment and becomes transformed into color and hue	Light rays enter the convex cornea and begin to converge. An adjustment of light rays occurs as they pass through the pupil and lens. Change in the shape of the lens focuses light on the retina. The retina has a pigmented layer of cells to enhance visual acuity. The sensory retina contains the rods and cones (i.e., photoreceptor cells sensitive to stimulation from light). Photoreceptor cells send electrical potentials by way of the optic nerve to the brain.

in specialized organs such as the taste buds of the tongue or the retina of the eye. When a nerve impulse is created, it travels along pathways to the spinal cord or directly to the brain. For example, sound waves stimulate hair cell receptors within the organ of Corti in the ear, which causes impulses to travel along the eighth cranial nerve to the acoustic area of the temporal lobe. Sensory nerve pathways usually cross over to send stimuli to opposite sides of the brain.

Perception

The actual perception or awareness of unique sensations depends on the receiving region of the cerebral cortex, where specialized neurons interpret the quality and nature of sensory stimuli. When a person becomes conscious of a stimulus and receives the information, perception takes place. Perception includes integration and interpretation of stimuli on the basis of the person's experiences. A person's level of consciousness influences perception and interpretation of stimuli. Any factors lowering consciousness impair sensory perception. If sensation is incomplete such as blurred vision or if past experience is inadequate for understanding stimuli such as pain, the person can react inappropriately to the sensory stimulus.

Reaction

It is impossible to react to all stimuli entering the nervous system. The brain prevents sensory bombardment by discarding or storing sensory information. A person usually reacts to stimuli that are most meaningful or significant at the time. After continued reception of the same stimulus, a person stops responding, and the sensory experience goes unnoticed. For example, a person concentrating on reading a good book is not aware of background music. This adaptability phenomenon occurs with most sensory stimuli except for those of pain.

The balance between sensory stimuli entering the brain and those actually reaching a person's conscious awareness maintains a person's well-being. If an individual attempts to react to every stimulus within the environment or if the variety and quality of stimuli are insufficient, sensory alterations occur.

AROUSAL MECHANISM

Arousal is a state of physiological and mental wakefulness or sense of organs stimulated to a point of optimum perception and coherent performance of cognitive and behavioral activities. Arousal mechanism involves activation of the ascending reticular activating system (ARAS) in the brain, which leads to a state of wakefulness, and stimulation of the autonomic nervous system and endocrinal system that manifests sensory alertness, raised blood pressure, pulse, perspiration, and readiness to respond to the external world.

Arousal or wakefulness is regulated by ARAS, which is mainly controlled by five neurotransmitters in the brain stem and cortex, that is, dopamine, histamine, norepinephrine, acetylcholine, and serotonin. The release of these neurotransmitters leads to increased cortical activity, and thereby a state of alertness. It is essential to understand the arousal mechanism because it is responsible for regulating consciousness, alertness, attention, information processing, and motivational behaviors such as mobility, pursuit of nutrition, fight-or-flight response, and sexual activities. Hans Eysenck believed that the basic personality an individual has also largely depends on the state of arousal. An optimum state of arousal and alertness is required for an appropriate level of consciousness and engagement in coherent cognitive and behavioral response to the external world. A suboptimal or higher state of arousal may cause hindrance in appropriate perception and response to external stimuli.

BOX 27.1 Factors That Influence Sensory Function

Age

Infants

- Binocular vision begins at 6 weeks and is well established by 4 months. During the second year of life, infants discriminate shapes, objects, and colors.
- Neonates respond to loud noises. Within a year, infants visually locate the source of noises.
- Newborns react to strong odors such as alcohol and vinegar by turning their heads. They can identify their own mother's milk.

Children

- **Refractive errors** are the most common types of visual disorders in children and are treated with corrective lenses.
- Serious visual impairment affects a child's ability to play and socialize.
- Children are usually frightened and confused by a sudden or progressive loss of sight. Parents and children need support to help them adjust to a disability (Hockenberry and Wilson, 2015).

Adults

- Visual changes include **presbyopia** and the need for glasses for reading (ages 40–50). In addition, the cornea, which helps with light refraction to the retina, becomes flatter and thicker. These aging changes lead to astigmatism.
- Pigment is lost from the iris; collagen fibers build up in the anterior chamber, which increases the risk for glaucoma by decreasing the resorption of intraocular fluid.

Older Adults

- Atrophy of the cerumen glands causes thicker and dryer cerumen, which is more difficult to remove and may completely obstruct the auditory canal (Touhy and Jett, 2014).
- Obstructive hearing loss is reversible, but changes in the structure and function of the inner ear that occur as older adults grow older are not.
- Age-related hearing changes include **presbycusis**, characterized by decreased hearing acuity, speech intelligibility, and pitch discrimination. Low-pitched sounds are easiest to hear, but it is difficult to hear conversation over background noise. It is also difficult to discriminate consonants (*f, s, th, ch, sh, b, p, k,* and *t*). Speech sounds are distorted, and there is a delayed reception and reaction to speech.
- Visual changes include reduced visual fields, increased glare sensitivity, impaired night vision, reduced **accommodation**, reduced depth perception, and reduced color discrimination. Symptoms occur because the pupils in the older adult take longer to dilate and constrict secondary to weaker iris muscles. Color vision decreases because the retina is duller and the lens yellows. Older adults may require three times as much light to see things as they did when they were in young adulthood (Touhy and Jett, 2014).
- Olfactory changes begin around age 50 and include a loss of cells in the olfactory bulb of the brain and a decrease in the number of sensory cells in the nasal lining. Reduced sensitivity to odors is common.
- A small decrease in the number of taste cells occurs with aging, beginning around age 60. Reduced sour, salty, and bitter taste discrimination is common. The ability to detect sweet tastes seems to remain intact (Touhy and Jett, 2014).
- Proprioceptive changes include increased difficulty with balance, spatial orientation, and coordination. These changes make it difficult to avoid obstacles and prevent an accident from happening when fast action is necessary. The automatic response to protect and brace oneself when falling is slower.
- Tactile changes are common including declining sensitivity to pain, pressure, and temperature secondary to peripheral vascular disease and neuropathies.

Medications

- **Ototoxic** medications such as analgesics, antibiotics, or diuretics affect hearing acuity, balance, or both, with the most common symptom being **tinnitus** (ringing in the ears). Ototoxicity causes a progressive or continuing hearing loss that in many patients goes unnoticed until the ability to understand speech is affected (Cone et al., 2016). Hearing loss is not always permanent, depending on the extent of damage and the length of time that the drug is given. Patients with renal failure have an increased sensitivity to ototoxic drugs.

Environment

- Excessive environmental stimuli result in sensory overload marked by confusion, disorientation, and inability to make decisions. Restricted environmental stimulation leads to sensory deprivation. Poor quality of environment worsens sensory impairment.

Preexisting Illnesses

- Disorders such as peripheral vascular disease and stroke alter peripheral tissue perfusion and affect tactile information. Diabetic neuropathy is a common complication of diabetes and can result in retinal edema, detachment, and blindness (Meiner, 2015).

Smoking

- Chronic tobacco use atrophies the taste buds and affects olfactory function.

Noise Levels

- Constant exposure to high noise levels causes hearing loss.

FACTORS AFFECTING SENSORY FUNCTION

Many factors influence the capacity to receive or perceive sensations (Box 27.1). You manage all of these conditions or situations when delivering patient care.

TYPES OF SENSORY ALTERATIONS

In your nursing experience, you care for patients with a variety of sensory problems such as **sensory deficits**, **sensory deprivation**, and **sensory overload**. When patients have more than one sensory alteration, their ability to function and relate within the environment becomes impaired.

Sensory Deficits

A sensory deficit occurs when problems with sensory reception or perception exist (Box 27.2). Patients are not able to receive certain stimuli (e.g., light and sound), or stimuli are distorted (e.g., blurred vision because of **cataracts** and abnormal taste sensation because of xerostomia) (NEI, 2015). A sudden sensory loss can be caused by injury or as a side effect to medications. When a deficit is chronic or develops

BOX 27.2 Common Sensory Deficits

Visual

- Presbyopia: Gradual decline in ability of the lens to accommodate or to focus on close objects. Reduces ability to see near objects clearly.
- Cataract: Clouding of the lens in the eye that interferes with passage of light through the lens and reduces the light that reaches the retina. Cataracts usually develop gradually and often result in cloudy or blurry vision, glare, double vision, and poor night vision (National Eye Institute [NEI], 2015).
- Dry eyes: Result when tear glands produce too few tears, resulting in itching, burning, or reduced vision.
- Glaucoma: A slowly progressive increase in intraocular pressure that causes progressive pressure against the optic nerve. At first, vision stays normal, and there is no pain. If left untreated, there may be a loss of peripheral (side) vision (Touhy and Jett, 2014).
- Diabetic retinopathy: Pathological changes of the blood vessels of the retina secondary to increased pressure, resulting in hemorrhage, macular edema, and reduced vision or vision loss.
- Age-related macular degeneration: Occurs when the macula (specialized portion of the retina responsible for central vision) degenerates as a result of aging and loses its ability to function efficiently. An early sign includes distortion that causes edges or lines to appear wavy. The disease causes the progressive loss of central vision. Peripheral vision remains intact (Touhy and Jett, 2014).

Hearing

- Presbycusis: A common progressive hearing disorder in older adults (see Box 27.1).
- Cerumen accumulation: Buildup and hardening of earwax in the external auditory canal causes conduction deafness.

Balance

- Dizziness and disequilibrium: Common condition in older adults, usually resulting from vestibular dysfunction and precipitated by change in position of the head to the rest of the body.
- **Meniere disease:** Caused by pressure in the inner ear as a result of excessive fluid. Cause of the excessive fluid is unknown. Diagnosis is based on medical history interview, physical examination, and clinical symptoms of vertigo, tinnitus, and a full feeling or pressure in the affected ear (Meiner, 2015).

Taste

- Xerostomia: Decrease in salivary production that leads to thicker mucus and a dry mouth. Interferes with the ability to eat and leads to appetite and nutritional problems.

Neurological

- Peripheral neuropathy: Most commonly associated with diabetes. Other causes include alcoholism, peripheral vascular disease, traumatic injury, medication effects, infections, and immune system diseases. Characterized by symptoms that include numbness and tingling of the affected area and stumbling gait.
- Hemiplegia: Caused by a thrombus, hemorrhage, or embolus affecting a blood vessel leading to or within the brain. Creates altered proprioception with marked incoordination and imbalance. Loss of sensation and motor function in extremities controlled by the affected area of the brain also occurs.

gradually, a patient learns to rely on the unaffected senses. Some senses become more acute to compensate for an alteration. For example, a patient who is blind develops an acute sense of hearing and learns to use a cane to adapt to visual challenges, whereas a patient who cannot hear "bluffs" his or her way through a conversation instead of admitting that he or she did not hear what was said.

Sensory deficits such as low vision and blindness are very common forms of disability. Four major diseases that frequently cause impaired vision in Americans 40 years of age and older are **age-related macular degeneration**, **glaucoma**, cataracts, and **diabetic retinopathy** (Touhy and Jett, 2016). Sensory deficits frequently cause patients to change their behaviors in adaptive or maladaptive ways. For example, some patients withdraw socially to cope with the loss (Touhy and Jett, 2014).

Sensory Deprivation

Sensory deprivation occurs when an inadequate quality or quantity of stimuli impairs perception. It has different causes such as reduced sensory input (hearing loss), confusion, and a restricted environment (bed rest). Sensory deprivation sometimes produces cognitive changes such as the inability to solve problems, poor task performance, and disorientation. It also can cause affective changes (e.g., boredom, restlessness, increased anxiety, emotional lability) and/or perceptual changes (e.g., reduced attention span, disorganized visual and motor coordination, confusion of sleeping and waking states).

Children often become more anxious, displaying restlessness, difficulty with problem solving, and depression when they experience sensory deprivation (Hockenberry and Wilson, 2015). In adults, the symptoms of sensory deprivation are similar to those of psychological illness, confusion, severe electrolyte imbalance, or the influence of psychotropic drugs. Thus, accurate diagnosis of sensory deprivation is crucial.

Sensory Overload

When a person receives multiple sensory stimuli, the brain has difficulty distinguishing the stimuli, leading to sensory overload. A person with sensory overload no longer perceives the environment in a way that makes sense. Overload prevents a meaningful response to stimuli. As a result, thoughts race, attention moves in many directions, and restlessness occurs. The patient demonstrates panic, confusion, and aggressiveness. The patient may have loss of sleep or altered sleeping patterns (daytime drowsiness). Sensory overload causes a state similar to that of sensory deprivation.

Patients of all ages who are acutely ill easily develop sensory overload in the health care environment. Constant pain; noise from equipment; and nursing activities of turning, repositioning, and administering treatments overwhelm patients with stimuli. Some patients such as patients in critical care settings are at a greater risk for sensory overload than others. Behavioral changes are easily confused with mood swings or disorientation. Constant reorientation

BOX 27.3 Communication Methods for Patients With Aphasia, Artificial Airway, and Hearing Impairment

- **Patients with aphasia**
  - Listen to the patient and provide sufficient time for him or her to communicate.
  - Do not shout or speak loudly (hearing loss is not the problem).
  - If the patient has problems with comprehension, use simple, short questions and facial gestures to give additional clues.
  - Speak of things familiar and of interest to the patient.
  - If the patient has problems with speaking, ask questions that require simple yes or no answers or blinking of the eyes. Offer pictures or a communication board so the patient can point.
  - Speak slowly and give the patient time to understand; be calm and patient; do not pressure or tire him or her.
  - Avoid patronizing and childish phrases.
- **Patients with an artificial airway**
  - Use pictures, objects, or word cards so the patient can point.
  - Offer a pad and pencil or Magic Slate for the patient to write messages.
  - Do not shout or speak loudly.
  - Give the patient time to write messages because patients tire easily.
  - Provide an artificial voice box (vibrator) for the patient with a laryngectomy to use to speak.
- **Patients with hearing impairment**
  - Get the patient's attention. Do not startle him or her when entering the room. Do not approach the patient from behind. Be sure that he or she knows that you want to speak.
  - Face the patient and stand or sit on the same level. Be sure that your face and lips are illuminated to promote lip reading. Keep hands away from mouth.
  - Be sure that the environment is not noisy.
  - Be sure that patients keep eyeglasses clean so they are able to see your gestures and face.
  - If the patient wears a hearing aid, make sure that it is in place and working.
  - Speak slowly and articulate clearly. Sometimes people with hearing loss take longer to process verbal messages.
  - Use a normal tone of voice and inflections of speech. Do not speak with something in your mouth.
  - When you are not understood, rephrase rather than repeat the conversation.
  - Use visible expressions. Speak with your hands, face, and eyes.
  - Do not shout. Loud sounds are usually higher pitched and often impede hearing by accentuating vowel sounds and concealing consonants. If you need to raise your voice, speak in lower tones.
  - Talk toward the patient's best or normal ear.
  - Use written information to enhance the spoken word.
  - Do not restrict the hands of a patient who is deaf. Never have intravenous lines in both of the patient's hands if the preferred method of communication is sign language.
  - Avoid eating, chewing, or smoking while speaking.
  - Avoid speaking from another room or while walking away.

and control of excessive stimuli become an important part of a patient's care.

PROMOTING COMMUNICATION IN PATIENTS WITH SENSORY IMPAIRMENT

Patients with aphasia, artificial airway, and hearing impairment require special techniques, tools, and strategies for communication. In acute care hospitals or long-term care facilities, nurses often care for patients with artificial airways (such as an endotracheal tube). The placement of an endotracheal tube prevents a patient from speaking. In other instance, a nurse may be caring for a patient with stroke, who cannot speak, and a patient having congenital or acquired impartment. In this case, the nurse uses special communication methods to facilitate his or her ability to express needs. The patient is sometimes completely alert and able to hear and see the nurse normally. Giving him or her time to convey any needs or requests is very important. Use creative communication techniques (e.g., a communication board or electronic tablet) to foster and strengthen a patient's interactions with health care personnel, family, and friends. The special techniques and strategies to be used for the promotion of meaningful communication in patients with aphasia, artificial airway, and hearing impairment are illustrated in Box 27.3. Furthermore, introduction of stimulus into the care setting also may help in improved communication (see Box 27.4) and nurses may use special techniques to beat the loneliness of old age patients to facilitate communication (see Box 27.5). While serving the food to a visually impaired patient, the nurse may arrange food on a plate and orient the patient to placement based on numbers of time on a clock face (see Fig. 27.1).

BOX 27.4 Introducing Stimuli Into the Care Setting

Visual

- Open the drapes to the patient's room.
- Raise the head of the bed and draw back dividing curtains or partitions.
- Provide attractive decorations on tables or cabinets such as fresh flowers, plants, a picture, or greeting cards.
- Provide audiobooks and large-print reading material.

Auditory

- Sit down and speak with the patient. Make the conversation meaningful.
- Turn on a radio with the type of music the patient enjoys. A favorite radio or television program is stimulating.

Taste and Smell

- Provide attractive, taste-appealing meals. Be sure that tableware and glasses are clean. Make sure that warm foods are served warm and cold foods are served cold.
- Provide a variety of textures, aromas, and flavors to enhance the patient's appetite.

BOX 27.5 Care of an Older Adult

Therapies to Reduce Loneliness

- Spend time with a person in silence or conversation.
- When it is acceptable to a patient, use physical contact such as holding a hand or embracing a shoulder to convey caring.
- Help older adults maintain contact with people important to them.
- Recommend alterations in living arrangements if physical isolation is a factor.
- Provide information about support groups or groups that provide assistive services.
- Link a person with organizations attuned to the social needs of older adults.
- Introduce the idea of bringing a companion such as a pet into the home when appropriate.

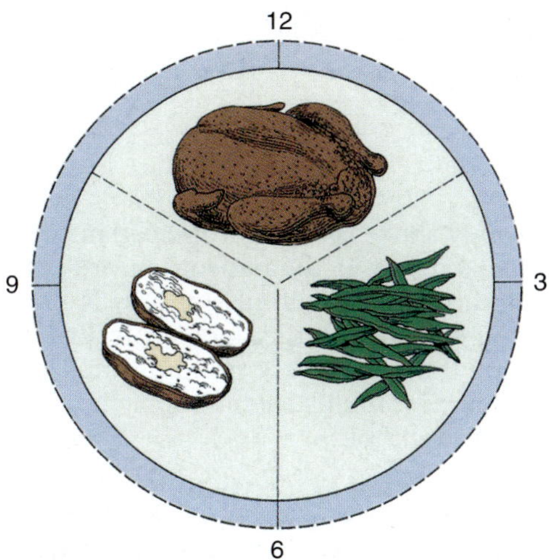

Fig. 27.1 Arrange food on a plate and orient patient to placement based on numbers on a clock face.

CARE OF UNCONSCIOUS PATIENTS

Meaning and Definition of Unconsciousness

Unconsciousness or decreased level of consciousness is a physiological condition in which the person usually is unresponsive to sensory stimulus and lacks awareness of self and the surroundings. Many central nervous system diseases and alterations of other body systems' functions can result in a decreased level of consciousness or unconsciousness. There are multiple causes of a decreased level of consciousness, including central nervous system lesions and metabolic causes. The depth and duration of unconsciousness or decreased level of consciousness encompasses a wide range of manifestations that include fainting and sudden loss of consciousness, and finally it leads to enhanced depressive states of consciousness that lasts for weeks or months. The term coma is reserved for a clinical condition in which the state of unconsciousness is sustained for a prolonged period, from hours to months. The pathophysiological basis for coma is direct structural injury or physiological dysfunction in cerebral hemispheres, the brain stem, or both hemispheres and brain stem. Coma is typically a transient state evolving toward the recovery of consciousness, persistent vegetative state, or brain death.

Unconsciousness is a state in which a person is not able to maintain an awareness of self and his or her surroundings. It means a complete or near-complete lack of responsiveness to the person and other surrounding stimuli (Hickey JV, 2009).

Causes and Risk Factors of Unconsciousness

A depressed level of consciousness or unconsciousness may occur because of:

- Damage, due to injury or disease, of the brain structure that is responsible for maintaining consciousness
- Metabolic problems or alterations that have a toxic effect on the brain such as hypoxia, ischemia, hypoglycemia, or vitamin deficiency; uremic or hepatic coma; electrolyte imbalances; alteration in the endocrine function; and use of sedatives and other drugs
- Alteration in the physiology of brain structures because of injuries or disease (e.g., seizures, cerebral edema)

As a nurse, we can remember "A-E-I-O-U" and "TIPSS" to learn the major causative factors of decreased level of consciousness or unconsciousness (Hickey JV, 2009):

A-E-I-O-U: A—**a**lcohol; E—**e**pilepsy or **e**xposure (heat stroke, hypothermia); I—**i**nsulin; O—**o**pium or **o**verdose or **o**xygen deficiency; U—**u**remia

TIPSS: T—**t**umor; I—**i**njury; P—**p**sychiatric or **p**oisoning; S—**s**troke; S—**s**epsis

Pathophysiology of Unconsciousness

The pathophysiology of unconsciousness is presented in the following flowchart 27.1:

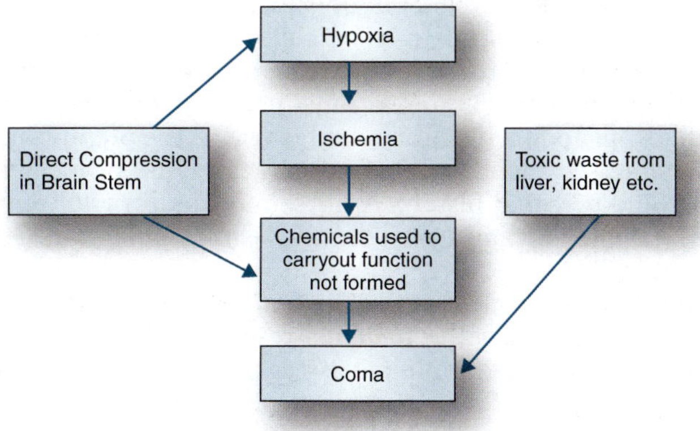

Flowchart 27.1 Pathophysiology of unconsciousness.

Stages of Unconsciousness

There is neither standard taxonomy to define or label LOC nor internationally common acceptance agreement regarding the accurate clinical presentation of the different stages of unconsciousness. So, no accurate and common term is present for providing information regarding a person from one health care professional to another. From extensive literature review, stages of consciousness are given as follows (Hickey JV, 2009):

- **Full consciousness:** A person is oriented to time, place, and person; aware and awake; and able to understand and express ideas in either verbal or written forms.
- **Confusion:** A person is disoriented to time, place, or person; is restless and irritable; has less attention span; has difficulty in memory and following commands; and shows difficulty in normal perception of stimuli.
- **Lethargy:** A person is not oriented to time, place, and person; and has very slow and sluggish speech, mental functions, and motor activities; but responds properly to painful stimuli.
- **Obtundation:** A person is in a state of severe drowsiness and may be aroused with moderate stimuli; verbally responses with a word or two; and is responsive to painful stimuli.
- **Stupor:** A person has minimum spontaneous movement and lies quietly; is usually unresponsive and only vigorous and repeated stimuli will arouse the person; may present incomprehensible sounds; and is responsive to painful stimuli.
- **Coma:** A person is unarousable with eyes closed and is unresponsive to bodily or environmental stimuli.

ASSESSMENT AND MANAGEMENT OF PATIENTS WITH UNCONSCIOUSNESS

Assessment

In this phase, you assess each client thoroughly and critically think about findings to make sure that your patient-centered clinical decisions are safe for the patient. Subjective data about unconscious patients or patients with a decreased level of consciousness can be collected from the family members or any other significant persons who are familiar with the patient. The nurse must collect appropriate and detailed history, which includes history of the present and past illnesses, identification of risk factors, use of medication, and personal history. A nurse must assess vital signs (see Chapter 6) and carry out physical examination (see Chapter 7).

As a nurse, you can assess the LOC by applying stimulation and observing the patient's response. We can apply auditory and tactile stimuli to assess the level of consciousness and procedures carried out depend on which type of stimulus is attempted (Hickey JV, 2009).

- **Auditory stimuli:** First, auditory stimulus should be applied and normal speaking voice is used. If the person responds, then the nurse can ask questions to assess orientation about time, place, or person and response to questions. If the person is unresponsive to a normal speaking voice, then the nurse may attempt with a louder voice. If the person responses to a loud voice, then the nurse can ask questions to assess orientation.
- **Tactile stimuli:** Apply tactile stimulation if a person is unresponsive to auditory stimulation. Initially, you should gently shake the arm of the patient while calling the patient's name. If the patient is unresponsive after the initial attempt, a painful stimulus is used. Painful stimuli can be applied either by a central stimulus such as pinching the trapezius or pectoralis major muscle or by a peripheral stimulus such as applying firm pressure to the nail beds or toes.

The **Glasgow Coma Scale** (GCS) is a quick, standard, and widely used tool to assess the level of consciousness. The scale is categorized into three domains: (1) eye opening, (2) best verbal response, and (3) best motor response. The highest GCS score is 15, which indicates that the patient is conscious and oriented to time, place, or person, whereas the lowest possible score is 3, indicative of deep coma. A GCS score of 8 or less is indicative of unconsciousness. An unconscious or comatose patient needs a high standard of nursing care and is usually required to be in the intensive care unit (Box 27.6).

BOX 27.6 Glasgow Coma Scale

Eye Opening

4: Opens eyes spontaneously
3: Opens eyes in response to voice
2: Opens eyes in response to painful stimuli
1: Lack of response

Best Verbal Response

5: Oriented to time, place, and person
4: Confused, conversing but disoriented to one or more spheres
3: Speaks only in words or phrases that make little or no meaning
2: Incomprehensible sounds
1: Lack of sound even with painful stimuli

Best Motor Response

6: Can obey a command
5: Localizes to painful stimuli
4: Flexion withdrawal
3: Abnormal flexion; flexes elbows and wrists while extending lower legs to pain
2: Abnormal extension; extends upper and lower extremities to pain
1: Lack of response

Acute Care Management

Meticulous nursing care has a direct impact on patient outcomes. Clinical reasoning, based on a systematic ongoing assessment of all body systems, alerts the nurse to signs and symptoms of complications. The nurse should implement preventive strategies as well as treatment protocols according to the best practices related to optimal outcomes. Ongoing assessment is the basis for identifying patient, nursing, and collaborative problems (Stevens R, 2006).

Respiratory Management

- **Airway patency:** Maintaining a patent airway for an unconscious patient or a patient with impaired cough reflex is the highest priority. Patients with a decreased level of consciousness are at a high risk for aspiration, and, therefore, suctioning will be necessary. If there is evidence of inability to protect the airway, the health care professional may insert an endotracheal tube on an emergency basis to prevent aspiration and the risk of aspiration-related infection. If the decreased level of consciousness is prolonged and the patient continues to require an artificial airway, a tracheotomy tube will be inserted.

- **Positioning:** The nurse should provide the lateral recumbent position to the patient if it is not contraindicated. This position promotes drainage of secretions, facilitates respirations, prevents pooling of secretions, and prevents the tongue from obstructing the airway. Change the patient position from side to side every 2 hours to prevent pooling of secretions. The head of the bed should be elevated 30° and turned to the side to facilitate drainage of secretions when lying in bed.
- **Suctioning:** When needed, oropharyngeal or tracheal suctioning may be necessary to clear the airway of mucus, blood, or other drainage. Suctioning is limited to 8–10 seconds and catheter insertion is limited to only three times to prevent hypoxia. Keep the patient oxygenated (using an Ambu bag) with 100% oxygen before and after suctioning to control hypoxemia (see Chapter 24 and Skill 24.1).
- **Others:** A consultation with the respiratory therapist is beneficial. Chest physical therapy may be recommended. It consists of percussion and vibration, oropharyngeal stimulation of coughing, suctioning, and possible use of bronchodilators or mucolytic agents to facilitate movement of secretions (see Chapter 24 and Box 24.4).

Cardiac Management

Appropriate nursing interventions and nursing management are necessary to maintain cardiovascular function properly in the unconscious patients. These interventions include the following:

- Change the patient position periodically, usually every 1–2 hours.
- When the patient is in the lateral recumbent position, use a pillow to separate the upper leg from the lower leg. It will prevent the formation of a pressure ulcer on the lower leg.
- Use thigh-high elastic stockings and sequential compression air boots to facilitate blood return to the heart and minimize venous stasis.
- Assess the patient for clinical manifestations of deep vein thrombosis or thrombophlebitis (i.e., comparison of leg circumference, distal pulses, and Homan sign).
- Periodically, sit the patient in a chair, if at all possible; this alters intravascular pressure and stimulates the orthostatic neurovascular reflexes.
- Review the patient's hemodynamic profile and trends over time.
- Maintain blood pressure within the desired range.
- Evaluate lower extremity Doppler studies.

The nurse must assess the risk factors for the development of venous thromboembolism. These include advanced age, known malignancy, presence of a neurological deficit, or a previous DVT.

Gastrointestinal Management

An institution-approved bowel program (e.g., stool softeners, bulk-forming, mild laxatives) should be initiated and follow-up of patients should be ensured. If it is needed to administer the drugs, use a feeding tube, gastrostomy, or jejunostomy tube (see Chapter 20). If constipation or diarrhea is a diagnosis, a nurse should understand the following points:

- Constipation may increase intra-abdominal pressure, which may lead to intracranial hypertension.
- A medication that stimulates peristalsis may be added, such as metoclopramide (Reglan).
- If the patient develops diarrhea, the following points should be kept in mind:
  - Review the amount, type, and rate of enteral feeding ordered; feeding intolerance, especially to lactose, may be present.
  - Discuss with the clinical dietitian to decide dietary alternatives (e.g., change the feeding to one of increased bulk or slow the rate of administration).
  - Consider an infectious process such as from pseudomembranous colitis if diarrhea is severe and ongoing.
  - Ongoing drug therapy, especially antibiotics, can cause diarrhea. Consult with primary care physician for discontinuing a highly suspected drug or changing it to another drug.
  - Consider adjusting the dosage, route, and frequency of the drug.
  - Discuss with physician to add drug therapy to decrease peristalsis and control diarrhea and follow it.

Gastric aspirations and stool should be assessed for occult blood. A nurse should understand that assessing gastrointestinal (GI) bleeding is necessary in the neurological patients because GI bleeding is very common in these patients. The nurse should also be aware about other risk factors for GI bleeding, such as use of dexamethasone, which may irritate the GI tract.

An unconscious patient with neurological problems may develop gastric ulcer, which is called a Cushing's ulcer. All patients should be on a GI prophylaxis drug regimen to prevent gastric ulcers. Proton pump inhibitors and histamine-2 receptor antagonists are the usual drug groups used for prophylaxis. Follow the institutional protocol ordered by the physician.

Genitourinary Management

Urinary problems in patients with a decreased level of consciousness must be managed with different nursing interventions. At the time of admission, physicians usually insert an indwelling catheter (see Chapter 21). An indwelling catheter may be needed to monitor urinary output, and keep the patient dry and comfortable. The evidence supports that urinary tract infection is associated with urinary catheters. Therefore, a nurse must assess risk and benefits of inserting and maintaining a urinary catheter.

- If an indwelling catheter is needed, remove it as soon as possible.
- A condom catheter may be an alternative option for a male patient.

- An alternative to continuous urinary drainage is an intermittent catheterization program, useful in both genders.
- For some patients, absorbent incontinence pads that are changed frequently may be chosen to avoid the risk of infection from a catheter.
- Assess the condition of the skin. If areas of skin breakdown already exist, being wet for even a short time could increase that breakdown.

Skin Care

Evidence-based practice guidelines are available to predict, prevent, and treat pressure ulcers. Follow your institutional evidence-based practice guidelines to prevent pressure ulcers (see Chapter 17).

- Keep the skin clean and dry; provide frequent skin care.
- Male patients should be shaved daily. If the patient is receiving anticoagulation therapy, an electric razor should be used.
- Trophic skin changes, such as dryness, can occur with some neurological conditions; lubricate the skin with lotion to prevent skin breakdown.
- Provide periodic skin care.
- Change the patient's position every 1–2 hours; be sure that bony prominent and other vulnerable areas are positioned and protected properly to prevent pressure ulcers.
- Do not use donut appliances, which simply reposition areas of breakdown.
- When moving the patient, turn and lift rather than pull, which results in shearing and friction on skin.
- Provide a special bed to prevent skin breakdown in high-risk patients.
- Provide the nasogastric and endotracheal tube care daily to prevent skin breakdown from the tube.

Mouth Care

Follow research-based best-practice protocols for mouth care (see Chapter 16):

- Assess the oral cavity daily or as per institutional policy.
- Routinely brush teeth to prevent the formation of dental plaque.
- Perform oral care every 2–4 hours or as needed to promote healing and maintenance of the oral cavity.
- Use alcohol-free antiseptics to prevent or reduce microorganism load.
- Suction the mouth and pharynx as per protocol to remove secretions and minimize the risk of aspiration.
- Apply a water-based moisturizer to the lips and oral mucosa.
- Avoid the use of lemon glycerin swabs, which have no moisturizing properties, irritate the oral mucosa, decalcify teeth, and dry the mucous membrane from the citric acid and glycerin.

Eye Care

- Assess the eyes for signs of edema, ecchymosis, eye drainage, irritation, or abrasions.
- Cleanse eyes to remove exudate with cotton balls and saline; the eyes should then be lubricated with methylcellulose or normal saline drops four times daily or as per institutional guidelines. The unconscious patient cannot blink periodically to cleanse and lubricate the eyes. Corneal drying or injury to the eye can lead to corneal ulceration and blindness. Many clinicians advice taping of the eyelids to prevent corneal abrasions. Application of an eye patch or eye shield may be helpful to prevent the eye injury (see Chapter 16).

Scalp and Hair Care

The scalp and hair require attention (see Chapter 16):

- Inspect the scalp for abrasions, pressure ulcers (especially in the occiput region), and edema.
- Treat any bruised or broken area.
- Patients with head injury may have hair that is matted with blood, dirt, or glass; remove by combing and washing the hair, if not contraindicated, as per institutional procedure guidelines.
- Comb the hair; long hair can be braided or pulled to the side with an elastic band.

Fingernails and Toenails

An unconscious patient may clench the fists, thereby digging the nails into the hands and causing injury. File and clip fingernails and toenails to protect the patient from injury (see Chapter 16).

Musculoskeletal Management

The following nursing interventions are useful for maintaining musculoskeletal function in patients with a decreased level of consciousness:

- Position the patient in a neutral side-lying position and maintain the patient's body alignment properly using pillows, rolls, and other equipment (e.g., positioning boots, splints, and trochanter rolls) as needed.
- Although the side-lying position is most often used, the dorsal position with the patient lying on his or her back is also useful. The same principles apply for alignment.
- The head is in neutral position aligned with the spine.
- The arms are slightly flexed at the elbows with the hands resting at the sides on pillows with the fingers extended over the pillows.
- The hips are aligned with the head. Place a pillow between the legs to prevent internal rotation, adduction, and inversion of the upper leg.
- The knees are positioned in slight flexion, often supported by a pillow for each leg. Care must be taken to prevent pressure on the peroneal nerve at the fibula head.

Prevention of Nosocomial Infections

- An unconscious patient is always at a high risk for infection for various reasons. Serious illnesses, often involving multiple body systems, challenge the body's immune system. Major or minor surgeries and invasive procedures (e.g., central lines and urinary catheters) can cause infection. Moreover, the use of corticosteroids may result in opportunistic infections.

- Make sure to follow the Centers for Disease Control and Prevention (CDC) recommendations for body substance isolation.
- Body substance isolation means the use of gloves when contact with body fluids, secretions, and blood is anticipated. Gloves are removed and properly disposed of between procedures and patients.
- When it is anticipated that contact with a patient could result in splashing of clothing, the skin, or face of the caregiver with secretions, blood, or body fluids, use personal protective equipment that includes gloves, a plastic apron, a mask, and goggles.
- Proper disposal of contaminated material will isolate the infectious material. The most effective method to prevent spread of infectious agents continues to be hand washing.

Environmental Safety

A safe and therapeutic care environment contributes to healing and recovery. The care environment is important for all patients, but particularly for those with depressed states of consciousness who are completely dependent on others for survival. A restorative care environment provides for the physical, psychological, spiritual, and other needs of the patient. Providing physical space that is clean, safe from hazards, and pleasing aesthetically increases the comfort levels of both patients and their families. Patient safety is of paramount importance; using National Patient Safety goals is a priority for all health care providers. A culture of patient safety is one that encourages clinicians, patients, and others to be vigilant in identifying potential or actual errors. Creating an environment for re-establishment of sleep–wakefulness cycles and other circadian rhythms is often challenging. Hospital settings are often very noisy because of the use of technology with monitors and alarms as well as the sounds created by the care providers, family, and patients. Newer architectural designs provide for therapeutic environments with control of temperature, light, sound, and air quality. However, it is the vigilant staff that implements the common sense measure of a controlled environment to support the balance for patient care and rest. Strategic timing of nursing interventions allows for adequate time for restful sleep. Promoting undisturbed sleep may facilitate recovery from illness. The sleep/rest periods should not be filled with nursing activity.

Psychosocial Considerations

Although unconscious patients appear to be completely unaware of their surroundings, it is not possible to determine whether they are aware of any stimulus in the immediate surroundings. Many patients have regained consciousness and given accurate accounts of what happened and what was said to them when they were supposedly unconscious; therefore, it is important to maintain a positive attitude in the presence of these patients and assume that some stimuli do penetrate the complexities of unconsciousness. Stimuli can be provided by playing the radio, touching the patient, and talking. In providing care, patients should be told what you will be doing. In addition, orient the patient to person, place, time, and the environment (weather and so forth).

Caring for patients with a decreased level of consciousness includes caring for the patient and the caregivers. Caregivers of these patients have been reported to experience a range of emotional reactions including shock, grief, anxiety, guilt, depression, and hostility toward caregivers. Caregivers may feel unexpected role changes such as assuming the role of primary caregiver or becoming the only wage earner of the family while concurrently having lost a main source of emotional support.

COMPLICATIONS OF UNCONSCIOUSNESS

An unconscious patient may develop several complications; some of the most common complications are listed as follows:

- Atelectasis/pneumonia (aspiration, bacterial pneumonia)
- Deep vein thrombosis/pulmonary embolism
- Ventilator dependency
- Tracheal ulceration or necrosis
- Anemia
- Pressure ulcers (decubitus ulcers)
- Acute urinary retention
- Paralytic ileus
- Gastric ulcer
- Electrolyte imbalance
- Negative nitrogen balance
- Peripheral nerve impairment/neuropathies
- Corneal ulceration
- Stress fractures and contractures
- Osteoporosis
- Joint dislocation
- Pain

KEY POINTS

- Sensory perception depends on the region in the cerebral cortex where specialized brain cells interpret the quality and nature of sensory stimuli.
- Because a patient learns to rely on unaffected senses after a sensory loss, you design interventions to preserve function of these senses.
- Aging results in a gradual decline of acuity in all senses.
- Environmental stimuli in a hospital such as in an intensive care unit place a patient at risk for sensory overload.
- The extent of support from family members and significant others influences the quality of sensory experiences.
- Assessment of sensory function includes a physical examination and measurement of functional abilities.
- The presence of cerumen in the external auditory canal is a common cause of hearing loss in older adults.
- Sensory losses create loneliness and impair the ability to socialize.
- An assessment of the environment includes identifying hazards, sources of meaningful stimulation, and the amount of stimuli.

- The care plan for patients with sensory alterations includes participation by family members.
- Patients with visual impairments need to learn boundaries within the environment to ambulate safely.
- Patients with existing hearing deficits are able to learn alternative ways to communicate.
- Nursing care for patients with sensory alterations includes using stronger sensory stimuli, compensating with other senses, and modifying the environment to maximize remaining sensory function.
- To prevent sensory overload, control stimuli, orient the patient to the environment, and promote rest by minimizing interruptions.
- Safety is a top concern when setting priorities for patients who experience sensory deprivation.
- Decreased level of consciousness or unconsciousness is related to problems of body system that affect the central nervous system.
- Management of adequate oxygenation is the highest priority when determining the goals and interventions.

REFERENCES

American Academy of Ophthalmology (AAO). Frequency of ocular examinations. San Francisco, CA: American Academy of Ophthalmology; 2015.

Centers for Disease Control and Prevention (CDC). Eye safety. 2013. Available from: https://www.cdc.gov/niosh/topics/eye/.

Centers for Disease Control and Prevention (CDC). Noise and hearing loss prevention. 2016. Available from: https://www.cdc.gov/niosh/topics/noise/reducenoiseexposure/noisecontrols.html.

Cone B, Dorn P, Konrad-Martin D, Lister J, Ortiz C, Schairer K. Ototoxic medications (medication effects). 2016. Available from: http://www.asha.org/public/hearing/Ototoxic-Medications/.

Contrera KJ, Wallhagen MI, Mamo SK, Oh ES, Lin FR. Hearing loss health care for older adults. J Am Board Fam Med 2016;29(3):394.

Crews JE, Chou CF, Zhang X, Zack MM, Saaddine JB. Health-related quality of life among people aged ≥ 65 years with self-reported visual impairment: findings from the 2006-2010 behavioral risk factor surveillance system. Ophthalmic Epidemiol 2014;21(5):287.

Fillary J, Chaplin H, Jones G, Thompson A, Holme A, Wilson P. Noise at night in hospital general wards: a mapping of the literature. Br J Nurs 2015;24(10):536.

Heine C, Browning C. Dual sensory loss in older adults: a systematic review. Gerontologist 2015;55(5):913.

Hickey JV. The Clinical practice of neurological and neurosurgical nursing. 6th ed. Philadelphia: Wolters Kluwer Health; 2009.

Hockenberry MJ, Wilson D. Wong's nursing care of infants and children. 10th ed. St. Louis: Mosby; 2015.

Konkani A, Oakley B, Penprase B. Reducing hospital ICU noise: a behavior-based approach. J Healthc Eng 2014;5(2):229.

Maidl CA, Leske JS, Garcia AE. The influence of "quiet time" for patients in critical care. Clin Nurs Res 2014;23(5):544.

McAndrew NS, Leske J, Guttormson J, Kelber ST, Moore K, Dabrowski S. Quiet time for mechanically ventilated patients in the medical intensive care unit. Intensive Crit Care Nurs 2016;35(22):22.

Meiner SE. Gerontologic nursing. 5th ed. St. Louis: Mosby; 2015.

National Eye Institute (NEI). Facts about cataract. 2015. Available from: https://nei.nih.gov/health/cataract/cataract_facts.

National Institute of Deafness and Other Communication Disorders (NIDCD). Hearing loss and older adults. 2016. Available from: https://www.nidcd.nih.gov/health/hearing-loss-older-adults.

Occupational Safety and Health Administration (OSHA). Eye and face protection. n.d. Available from: https://www.osha.gov/SLTC/eyefaceprotection/standards.html.

Riemer HC, Mates J, Ryan L, Schleder BJ. Decreased stress levels in nurses: a benefit of quiet time. Am J Crit Care 2015;24(5):396.

Rosen T, Mack KA, Noonan RK. Slipping and tripping: fall injuries in adults associated with rugs and carpets. J Inj Violence Res 2013;5(1):61.

Stevens R, Anish B. Approach to the comatose patient. Crit Care Med 2006;34(1):31-41.

Tainter CR, Levine AR, Quraishi SA, Butterly AD, Stahl DL, Eikermann M, et al. Noise levels in surgical ICUs are consistently above recommended standards. Crit Care Med 2016;44(1):147.

The Joint Commission (TJC). 2017 Hospital accreditation standards. Oakbrook, IL: The Joint Commission; 2017.

Touhy TA, Jett A. Ebersole & Hess' Gerontological nursing and healthy aging. 4th ed. St. Louis: Mosby; 2014.

Touhy TA, Jett A. Ebersole & Hess' Toward health aging: human needs and nursing response. 9th ed. St. Louis: Mosby; 2016.

Varma R, Vajaranant TS, Burkemper B, Wu S, Torres M, Hsu C, et al. Visual impairment and blindness in adults in the United States: demographic and geographic variations from 2015 to 2050. JAMA Ophthalmol 2016;134(7):802.

World Health Organization (WHO). Visual impairment and blindness. 2014. Available from: http://www.who.int/mediacentre/factsheets/fs282/en/.

28 Care of Terminally Ill, Death, and Dying

OBJECTIVES

- To define loss and grief.
- To explain five categories of loss, that is, perceived loss, necessary loss, maturational loss, actual loss, and situational loss.
- To understand the difference between grief, bereavement, and mourning.
- To compare different types of grief, that is, normal, anticipatory, complicated, and disenfranchised grief.
- To describe factors that influence a person's response to loss and grief including human development, psychological perspectives of grief, and nature of loss.
- To understand the concept of grief and mourning with the help of various theories, that is, Kübler-Ross' theory, Bowlby's theory, Worden's theory, Rando's theory, and postmodern theory.
- To identify nursing interventions for helping patients in coping with loss, death, and grief.
- To explain the concept of death and dying with an explanation of signs of impending death and a dying patient's bill of rights.
- To discuss principles of palliative and hospice care.
- To identify ways to educate and involve family caregivers in providing palliative care.
- To understand the importance of communication, spiritual well-being, and peaceful environment during grief period.
- To enumerate the physiological changes after death.
- To understand the role of a nurse in death declaration and death certification.
- To define autopsy and embalming along with its indications.
- To demonstrate skills of counseling and supporting for the grieving family and advance directives.
- To discuss about DNR order, euthanasia, and organ donation and its importance.

KEY TERMS

acceptance, p. 734
actual loss, p. 732
anger, p. 734
anticipatory grief, p. 733
autopsy, p. 739
bargaining, p. 734
bereavement, p. 732
complicated grief, p. 733
death, p. 735
denial, p. 734
depression, p. 734
disenfranchised grief, p. 733
disorganization and despair, p. 734
grief, p. 732
hope, p. 736
hospice care, p. 735
maturational losses, p. 732
mourning, p. 732
necessary losses, p. 732
normal or uncomplicated grief, p. 733
numbing, p. 734
palliative care, p. 735
perceived loss, p. 732
postmortem care, p. 740
reorganization, p. 734
reminiscence, p. 734
resilience, p. 735
situational loss, p. 732
yearning and searching, p. 734

INTRODUCTION

Grief and loss affect a person's health physically, psychologically, socially, and spiritually. Patients at the end of life need knowledge, compassion, and expert nursing care as they live with illnesses that cannot be cured and come to the end of their lives. As a result, care at the end of life is enhanced when nurses provide holistic, patient-centered and family-centered care (Dobrina et al., 2016). Situations that involve loss and grief can also bring out stress, fear, and uncertainty in caregivers (Coelho et al., 2015). Fortunately, nursing knowledge regarding the care of people who are grieving and dying has expanded in the last decade for patients and family caregivers (Barrere and Durkin, 2014).

LOSS

Throughout our lives from birth to death, we form attachments and suffer losses. We become independent from our parents, leave home to attend school, begin careers, and form new lifelong relationships. Growing up is natural and positive, yet throughout life we experience **necessary losses**. Often, losses are replaced by something different or better. For example, a person leaves behind family members to begin college but makes new friends and begins a meaningful career. Other necessary losses, such as death of a loved one, challenge a person's sense of security and coping skills.

How we perceive loss depends on what we value. Our family, friends, society, culture, and faith traditions shape our priorities and help us determine what matters most in life. A person experiences loss when a meaningful object, person, body part or function, emotion, or idea is no longer present. There are several types of loss (Table 28.1). People experience an **actual loss** when they can no longer touch, hear, see, or have near them valued people or objects. Examples include the loss of a body part, pet, friend, life partner, or job. People feel grief when a valued object becomes worn out, lost, stolen, or destroyed by disaster. A child often grieves after losing a favorite toy. A **perceived loss** is uniquely experienced by a grieving person and is often less obvious to others. It is very real to the person who has had the loss. For example, a person perceives that she is less loved by her parents and experiences a loss of self-esteem. Other people often misunderstand perceived losses.

People experience **maturational losses** as they go through a lifetime of normal developmental processes. For example, when a child goes to school for the first time, he or she spends less time with his or her parents, leading to a change in the parent–child relationship. Grieving maturational losses help a person cope with the change. A **situational loss** occurs as a result of an unpredictable life event. It often involves multiple losses. For example, a divorce begins with the loss of a life companion but often leads to financial strain, changes in living arrangements, less contact with one's children, and loss of friends who were part of the couple's married life.

How an individual interprets the meaning of any loss and the type of loss influence how that person grieves. People respond to loss differently. For some people, the loss of a possession or pet causes the same level of grief as the loss of a person. The value that people place on an absent object or changed social status influences their emotional response to the loss.

People experience multiple losses when they become ill or need to be hospitalized. They often lose their privacy, modesty, sense of safety, and control over body functions and daily routines. Chronic, debilitating illness often adds financial concerns, requires job changes, threatens independence, forces changes in lifestyle, and challenges family relationships.

Death is the ultimate loss. Although death is a part of life, its mysterious, uncertain character often produces anxiety and fear (Momtaz et al., 2015). Death ends relationships with family and friends and separates people from the physical presence of those important to them. Persons at the end of life and their caregivers often experience sorrow, uncertainty, fear, or physical and spiritual challenges throughout the dying process. Death can also lead to personal growth and a meaningful reprioritization of life. Close friends and caregivers of a dying person are reminded of their own mortality. Most people do not want to become dependent on others at the end of life, yet they do not want to die alone.

Facing death often brings out emotions such as guilt, anger, sadness, and fear. Some family members and family caregivers, fearful of the intensity of the experience, withdraw at a time when the dying person most needs their love and support. A person's basic beliefs and values, culture, and spirituality and the quality of emotional support influence the way a person and family approach dying. They need individually designed, compassionate end-of-life care.

Table 28.1 Types of Loss

Definition	Implications of Loss
Loss of external objects (e.g., misplacement, theft, destruction by nature)	Extent of grieving depends on object's value, sentiment attached to it, and its usefulness.
Loss of a known environment (e.g., moving from a neighborhood, hospitalization, a new job, moving to a long-term care facility)	Loss occurs through maturational or situational events and with injury or illness. Loneliness in an unfamiliar setting threatens self-esteem and makes grieving difficult.
Loss of a significant other (e.g., divorce; loss of a family member, friend, trusted nurse, or pet; family rifts)	Significant others meet a person's need for psychological safety, love and belonging, and self-esteem.
Loss of an aspect of self (e.g., body part, psychological or physiological function, job; financial uncertainty)	Illness, injury, or developmental changes result in a loss that causes changes in body image, self-concept, and level of independence.
Loss of life (e.g., death of family member, friend, or acquaintance; own death)	Loss of a life creates grief for those left behind. Persons facing death often fear pain and loss of control or independence.

GRIEF, BEREAVEMENT, AND MOURNING

Grief is the emotional response to a loss. People grieve in different ways, based on their experiences, cultural expectations, and spiritual beliefs (Schonfeld et al., 2015; Wienclaw, 2016) (see Chapters 32 and 33). Grief involves **mourning**, the conscious and unconscious behaviors associated with loss. **Bereavement** includes grief and mourning, the inner feelings and outward behaviors of a survivor. Many theorists describe the grief process that occurs with any loss. The following classic grief theories describe general psychological and behavioral characteristics and patterns (Harris and Winokuer, 2016). Theories provide a framework for nurses to plan nursing care for individuals experiencing grief. Grieving is an individual experience, and an individual may not go through all the steps or patterns described in grief theories (Wienclaw, 2016).

Types of Grief

Normal Grief

Normal or uncomplicated grief consists of commonly expected emotional and behavioral reactions to a loss (e.g., resentment, sorrow, anger, crying, loneliness, temporary withdrawal from activities). When persons feel supported and valued as they grieve, they often come to view the experience later as growth producing and positive.

Anticipatory Grief

The process of "letting go" before an actual loss or death has occurred is called **anticipatory grief**. For example, after a person and family members accept the reality of a terminal diagnosis, they begin saying goodbye and complete life affairs before death occurs. After a prolonged dying process, a patient's family members often do not respond with shock and disbelief at the time of death, and feelings of sadness mingle with some relief that the suffering is over. There are risks associated with anticipatory grieving. On one hand, some family members begin withdrawing emotionally from the patient as a self-protective mechanism, leaving the patient with less support as death approaches. On the other hand, if a person thought to be near death survives longer than anticipated, others can have difficulty reconnecting or feel resentful that the stressors associated with anticipating a death continue.

Complicated Grief

Complicated grief happens when a person has difficulty progressing through the loss experience. The person does not accept the reality of the loss, and the intense feelings associated with acute grief do not go away (Sierra Hernandez et al., 2016). A person experiencing complicated grief feels strain in relationships and finds it hard to go forward in life. Characteristics of complicated grief include intense yearning for the loss; intrusive thoughts of the death; and disturbing emotions of anger, avoidance, or disbelief (Guldin, 2014; Waller et al., 2016).

Disenfranchised Grief

Individuals experience disenfranchised grief when they cannot openly acknowledge a loss or receive full social support from others. This type of grieving is difficult for others to understand. **Disenfranchised grief** occurs in situations in which others view a person's loss as insignificant or invalid. For example, a grieving woman does not experience support from her parents when experiencing the loss of her ex-husband. People often experience disenfranchised grief when a loss is deeply private or secretly experienced (e.g., early miscarriage or death of a family member as a result of alcoholism).

FACTORS INFLUENCING LOSS AND GRIEF

Human Development

A person's age and stage of development affect the ability to understand loss. Expressions of grief evolve as individuals mature. For example, toddlers cannot understand the permanence of death but feel anxiety over loss of objects and separation from parents. Although school-age children are able to understand the significance of loss more completely, they see their loss as a challenge to their emerging identity or self-concept. Adolescents do understand the significance of loss. For some adolescents, coping with the loss of a parent or sibling is often difficult. Some adolescents have problems with school, withdraw from family and/or friends, or increase risk-taking behaviors. Young adults, who are just beginning their independent lives, find the loss of a parent or sibling life-changing. Young adulthood is a time when adult relationships with parents or siblings begin, and they grieve for the loss of the past and new relationship. Middle-age adults often use grief experiences to re-examine or reprioritize their lives. Older adults anticipate grief as they encounter declining physical function or life opportunities, give up employment or social status, or lose loved ones.

Psychological Perspectives of Grief and Loss

Individuals respond to loss by using their usual coping strategies. Sometimes when people experience multiple losses or lose something of great significance, their usual coping strategies are inadequate. At the end of life, people often find new coping mechanisms and new resources to maintain control and stability (Bell Meisenhelder et al., 2016; Rodrigo, 2014) (see Chapter 31).

Socioeconomic Status

Socioeconomic status influences access to resources and support for coping with loss. Generally, people feel greater burden from a loss when they lack financial, educational, or occupational resources. For example, a person with limited financial resources is unable to replace a home lost in a fire or afford the medical care needed to manage a newly diagnosed disease.

Nature of Personal Relationships

If you gain information about the quality and meaning of a relationship that a person had with the deceased, you will better understand a person's grief. If the two people were close and well connected, the surviving person often finds it very difficult to cope with the loss. If there was conflict or abuse in the relationship, the survivor often feels guilt, remorse, regret, or relief.

Nature of the Loss

The visibility of a loss influences the amount of support a person receives. For example, a family who loses a home in a tornado gets strong support from the community, whereas a family in the same community who loses an early-term pregnancy experiences less support. Many people empathize with the first very public loss. In the case of a private loss, fewer people know about it or appreciate its significance. People respond differently to sudden, unexpected, or stigmatized deaths (e.g., suicide) than to anticipated or seemingly inevitable losses. Individuals who lose a family member from suicide often express guilt and self-blame for not intervening before the death (Honeycutt and Praetorius, 2016).

Culture and Ethnicity

Patient-centered, culturally competent care focuses on respecting individual differences including cultural and religious responses to grief and loss. Cultural belief systems provide the structures and interpretations that people need to cope with change, loss, illness, or death. For example, in Western societies, many people grieve privately and restrain their emotions. In other cultures, it is acceptable to have public demonstrations of grief that communicate the significance of their loss to others. Although members of a cultural or religious group often share similar beliefs, each person still responds in his or her own unique way. Gain knowledge and appreciation of values and beliefs as they apply to each individual's culture (Schonfeld et al., 2015).

Spiritual Beliefs

People use their faith in a higher power, a community of friends, their sources of hope and meaning in life, and religious rituals and practices to cope with life challenges and grief (Finocchiaro, 2016; Van Hook, 2016) (see Chapter 32). Regardless of their beliefs, all people have a need for love, meaning, and purpose. A loss often provokes questions related to spiritual values and the meaning of life. Spirituality may help patients buffer the stress of chronic illness and other life challenges (Rafferty et al., 2015; Van Hook, 2016).

THEORIES OF GRIEF AND MOURNING

Theories of loss, death, grief, or mourning help you understand common shared feelings and behaviors. Use these theories to develop individualized interventions based on a patient's experiences.

Kübler-Ross' Five Stages of Grief

Kübler-Ross' classic theory (1969) identifies five responses to loss: denial, anger, bargaining, depression, and acceptance. Individuals in the **denial** stage act as though nothing has changed. They cannot believe or understand that a loss has occurred. In the **anger** stage, a person resists the loss, is angry about the situation, and sometimes becomes angry with God. During **bargaining**, the individual postpones awareness of the loss and tries to prevent it from happening by making deals or promises. A person realizes the full significance of the loss during the **depression** stage. When depressed, the person feels overwhelmingly lonely or sad and withdraws from interactions with others. During the stage of **acceptance**, the individual begins to accept the reality and inevitability of loss and looks to the future.

Bowlby's Four Phases of Mourning

Attachment, the foundation of Bowlby's four phases of mourning (1980), is an instinctive behavior that leads to the development of lifelong bonds of affection between children and their primary caregivers. In the **numbing** phase, a person has periods of extremely intense emotion and reports feeling "stunned" or "unreal." The **yearning and searching** phase evokes emotional outbursts, tearful sobbing, and acute distress. To move forward, people need to experience this painful phase of grief. Common physical symptoms include tightness in the chest and throat, shortness of breath, a feeling of weakness and lethargy, insomnia, and loss of appetite. During the phase of **disorganization and despair**, an individual spends much time thinking about how and why the loss occurred. The person often expresses anger at anyone he or she believes to be responsible. Gradually this phase gives way to an acceptance that the loss is permanent. During the final phase of **reorganization**, the person accepts unaccustomed roles, acquires new skills, and builds new relationships.

Worden's Four Tasks of Mourning

The four tasks of mourning theory (Worden, 1982) describe how individuals help themselves through mourning and ask others for help. Although the time needed varies from person to person, moving through Worden's tasks typically takes at least 1 year.

- *Task I: Accept the reality of the loss.* People experience a period of disbelief and surprise that a loss has happened, even when a death is expected. In this phase, people realize that a person or object is gone and will not return.
- *Task II: Work through the pain of grief.* It is impossible to experience a loss without some degree of emotional pain. Individuals who deny or suppress the pain often prolong their grief.
- *Task III: Adjust to the environment in which the deceased is missing.* A person does not realize the full impact of a loss for at least 3 months. After the first few weeks after a death, visitors and friends become less attentive, and a person experiences the full impact of the loss. Adjustment happens as a person takes on roles formerly filled by the deceased and participates in new activities.
- *Task IV: Emotionally relocate the deceased and move on with life.* People who move on with life do not forget the deceased or devalue the relationship but begin the difficult task of giving the deceased a less central place in their emotional life. Eventually a person is able to love other people without loving the deceased person less.

Rando's R Process Model

Rando's model of mourning (1993) is specific to the Western society. Mourning is an action-oriented process involving recognizing the loss, reacting to the pain of separation, reminiscence, relinquishing old attachments, and readjusting to life after loss. Reminiscence is an important activity in grief and mourning. In **reminiscence**, a person recollects and re-experiences the deceased and the relationship by mentally or verbally reliving and remembering the person and past experiences.

Postmodern Grief Theories

The phase and task theories described in the previous sections often have limited empirical evidence and may not consider cultural differences (Harris and Winokuer, 2016). Recent studies about grief focus on the multiple ways that people react to loss based on their personal, cultural, and social circumstances. Research suggests that people do not grieve in predictable, linear stages, and they do not necessarily complete the grieving tasks (Hall, 2014). Instead, they move back and forth between stages, experience phases in an overlapping manner, or do not exhibit typical emotions (e.g., depression or anger) or grief behaviors. People rarely "get over" a significant loss but instead learn to live with loss. They can experience distress associated with the loss for a lifetime. People who demonstrate **resilience** accept their loss over time and return to their preloss level of functioning. Because people experience grief differently, you need to listen as people tell their stories and engage them as their story unfolds (Harris and Winokuer, 2016).

DEATH AND DYING

There are legal responsibilities for nurses to assume when caring for patients during the process of death and dying. Carefully document all events that occur, including patient status, any interventions or supportive care measures delivered, and the patient's response while caring for a dying patient. There are two standards for the determination of death: **cardiopulmonary death** and **brain death** (Uniform Determination of Death Act, 1980). The cardiopulmonary standard requires failure of a patient's circulatory and respiratory functions. The brain death standard requires irreversible failure of all functions of the entire brain including the brainstem. The reason for the development of the two definitions is to set the legal standard for determining death in all situations. The definitions are helpful to health care providers when there is a question of whether to continue life support or when the discussion of organ donation is appropriate.

Signs of Impending Death

Most people exhibit some signs and symptoms of grief in situations of serious illness, loss, or impending death. Your assessment becomes more specific as you begin to observe behaviors, listen to patients' conversations, and identify sign of impending death (Box 28.1).

Dying Patient's Rights

The use of appropriate standards guides you during the assessment phase of the nursing process so that you gather the data most pertinent to the patient's situation. Professional standards include bioethical principles, and the "right to die" peacefully is a part of fundamental right to life as enshrined under Article 21 of the Constitution of India; the End-of-Life Nursing Consortium basic and advanced curricula for end-of-life care (American Association of Colleges of Nursing, 2016), the Hospice and Palliative Nurses Association (HPNA) standards of practice for clinical education (HPNA, 2015), and *Palliative Nursing: Scope and Standards of Practice* (2014) by the American Nurses Association (ANA) and HPNA are available. The National Institute on Aging (NIA, 2015) offers guidelines for the care of older adults at the end of life.

BOX 28.1 Signs of Impending Death

- Minimal intake of food or water
- Increased sleeping and decreased consciousness
- Disorientation and restlessness
- Decreased urinary output and/or incontinence
- Cool hands and feet
- Noisy breathing
- Irregular breathing patterns with long pauses
- At the time of death, you will note:
  - Absence of breathing and heartbeat
  - Bowel and bladder release
  - Unresponsiveness
  - Eyes fixed on a certain spot
  - Dilated pupils

CARE OF DYING PATIENT

Palliative Care

Interventions for patients with serious chronic illnesses or patients near the end of life are based on a philosophy of total care called *palliative care*. **Palliative care** is practiced in any setting and focuses on the prevention, reduction, or relief of physical, emotional, social, and spiritual symptoms of disease or treatment at the end of life when cure is no longer possible. People of any age or diagnosis receive palliative care at any time and in any setting. Expert palliative care involves an interdisciplinary team composed of health care professionals (i.e., nurses, social workers, spiritual care professionals, nutritionists, physicians, psychologists, and pharmacists). Therapists who use complementary healing interventions (e.g., massage, music, healing touch, or aromatherapy) also work with palliative care teams (Nyatanga, 2015). The World Health Organization (WHO, 2016) summarizes palliative care philosophy and practice as follows:

- Affirms life and regards dying as a normal process
- Neither hastens nor postpones death
- Provides relief from pain and other distressing symptoms
- Integrates psychological and spiritual aspects of patient care
- Offers a support system to help patients live as actively as possible until death
- Offers a support system to help families cope during the patient's illness and their own bereavement
- Enhances the quality of life
- Uses a team approach to meet the needs of patients and families

Above all, palliative care ensures that patients with advanced chronic illness or patients near death receive care that is as free of avoidable pain and suffering as possible; is consistent with patient and family wishes; and is consistent with clinical, cultural, and ethical standards.

Hospice Care

Hospice care provides services for patients who are at the end of life. Many people do not know about this option for care and depend on you to explain hospice services and care philosophy to them. Patients who meet the criteria for hospice care no longer receive treatment to cure their disease and are terminally ill (Harrison and Connor, 2016). Hospice teams provide physical, emotional, and spiritual care for

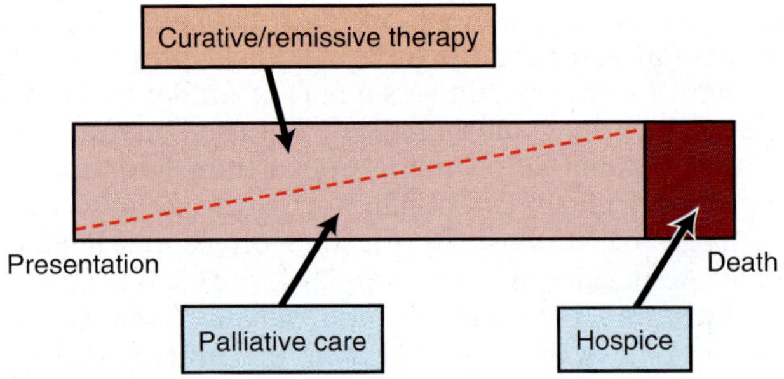

Fig. 28.1 **Continuum of palliative and hospice care.** (From Emanuel L, et al: Education in palliative and end of life care (EPEC) curriculum: the EPEC Project, Chicago, 2003, Northwestern University Press.)

patients, family caregivers, and family members in many settings (i.e., home, hospital, or extended care facilities). Hospice care focuses exclusively on palliative care interventions to relieve the symptoms and burdens of illness or treatment and help patients live as fully as possible until death. Nurses base hospice care on a patient's goals and support patient and family preferences for maintaining comfort and a high quality of life. Hospice programs are built on the following core beliefs and services:

- Patient and family as the unit of care
- Coordinated home care with access to inpatient and nursing home beds when needed
- Symptom management
- Provision of an interdisciplinary care team
- Medical and nursing services available at all times
- Bereavement follow-up after a patient's death
- Use of trained volunteers for visitation and respite support

For a patient to receive home hospice care, a family caregiver must be living in the home. The family caregiver receives support from professional and volunteer hospice team members who are available 24 hours a day. If a patient receiving home hospice care goes to the hospital for the management of acute symptoms, a nurse can use a hospice-to-hospital hand-off tool to communicate a patient's status and care goals to promote patient safety (Darrah and O'Connor, 2016). Fig. 28.1 illustrates the relationship between palliative care and hospice.

Communicate Therapeutically

A trusting nurse–patient relationship enables you to support patients in grief and to provide palliative care. Trust develops as you relate to patients and family members with an open, nonassuming communication style (Harris and Winokuer, 2016). Open-ended questions invite patients to expand on their thoughts and tell their stories. Closed-ended questions usually lead patients to give short answers (yes or no).

Use active listening, learn to be comfortable with silence, and use prompts (e.g., "go on" or "tell me more") to encourage continued conversation. Verbally empathize with the patient's grief and build a trusting relationship by offering your caring presence using intentional, meaningful touch (Bezemer and Kress, 2014; Harris and Winokuer, 2016).

Some people do not want to talk about their feelings of loss or grief with others. Do not take a person's inability or lack of desire to communicate with you personally. Some people cope with stress and loss by talking things out, whereas others need to process their loss privately before they can talk to others. Cultural or gender expectations also influence the degree to which people talk about their loss. If patients do not want to share feelings or concerns, convey a willingness to be available if they want to talk later. When you are respectful of patients' personal or cultural values and their need for dignity, respect, and privacy, a therapeutic relationship will develop.

Grief brings out intense feelings such as anger, denial, depression, or guilt. People often become demanding and accusing and take out their anger on family or caregivers. Recall that denial, anger, and depression are normal reactions to loss. Reflect on how you react to people who exhibit intense feelings or negative behaviors. If you show fear or disappointment when people express intense emotions, they do not find it easy to confide in you. Offer support by saying, "I can see this is very upsetting to you. I just want you to know I am available to talk if you want." Avoid creating barriers to communication such as denying a patient's grief, offering false reassurance, or offering unsolicited advice (see Chapter 4).

Do not avoid a topic that a patient who is dying wishes to discuss. When you sense that patients want to talk, find the time to listen. In a busy acute care setting, you need to reprioritize your responsibilities so that you can talk to your patients when they are ready. Respond to questions openly and honestly. Provide information to help patients understand their condition, consider the benefits and burdens of treatment choices, and clarify their personal values and goals.

Promote Hope and Spiritual Well-Being

Hope, a concept relevant to the human spirit, is the anticipation of a continued good or an improvement or lessening of something unpleasant. It energizes and comforts people and enhances their coping skills as they face personal challenges. To help patients feel more hopeful, remind them of their strengths and reinforce their expressions of courage, positive thinking, and realistic goal setting. Patients feel more hopeful when they have a sense of control. In a recent qualitative study, patients diagnosed with terminal cancer identified the importance of their family involvement and sense of hope for the future. The study results suggest that nurses can ease a patient's suffering by respecting the patient's sense of hope and encouraging family involvement in care (Nilmanat et al., 2015). Offer information to patients about their illness, correct misinformation, and clarify patients' perceptions. Patients can behave in hopeful ways also. Help them practice healthy behaviors (e.g., enjoying meals, talking with friends, and getting rest) and suggest that they develop a workable schedule for each day. People give hope to one another. Encourage patients to nurture important relationships. When people have strong relationships and a sense of emotional connectedness to others, they know that help is available. Nurses connect with patients to foster hope (Nilmanat et al., 2015).

Facilitate Mourning

Nursing interventions often help people acknowledge the reality of their loss. Discuss how and when the loss or illness occurred, under what circumstances, and other similar topics to help make the event more real and place it in perspective. Support efforts to live in the face of disability or in cases when the family must face being without the deceased person. Ask the people involved to identify and prioritize concerns and then facilitate the development of a plan to address their concerns. Encourage them to rely on their support network of family members, friends, professionals, and community resources. Suggest that they begin by reaching out to others in welcoming groups (e.g., religious communities or volunteer activities).

- Reinforce the understanding that people grieve differently and that feelings change or resolve over time. Some people have "anniversary reactions" (heightened or renewed feelings of loss or grief) months or years after a loss. They worry that they are losing ground when signs of grief reappear after a period of relative calm. Offer reassurance that anniversary reactions are common and encourage pleasant reminiscence.
- Provide continuing support. Patients and their families need to talk about their loved one and need support long after their loss. If you see the patients or family caregivers after an extended time, it is appropriate to ask them how they are doing after the loss. This gives them the opportunity to talk and lets them know that their loved one is remembered.

Manage Symptoms

Expert palliative care focuses primarily on managing the distress caused by unwanted symptoms of disease or side effects of treatments. Worry or fear concerning symptoms heightens a patient's perception of distress. Assess the character of a patient's symptoms carefully and individualize therapies. See Chapter 11 for a detailed discussion of both pharmacological and nonpharmacological pain management strategies, which are essential to achieve high-level palliative care. Patients at the end of life commonly experience other physical symptoms (e.g., dyspnea, fatigue, urinary incontinence, or nausea), psychological symptoms (e.g., anxiety, fear, or depression), social symptoms (e.g., loneliness, isolation, or loss of community), and spiritual symptoms (e.g., hopelessness, despair, or loss of meaning). A comprehensive care plan addresses symptoms identified by a patient as most distressing (Matzo and Sherman, 2015). See Table 28.2 for a summary of nursing implications of commonly experienced symptoms.

Table 28.2 Managing Symptoms in Terminally Ill Patients

Symptoms	Characteristics or Causes	Nursing Implications
Pain	Pain can be related to the disease process, medical interventions, chronic conditions, prolonged bed rest, or pressure injuries.	Address pain reports promptly; provide medication as ordered and multiple nonpharmacological measures such as massage, repositioning, relaxation, guided imagery, or reiki (Kisvetrová et al., 2016) (see Chapter 11).
Discomfort	Discomfort can result from any source of physical irritation (e.g., dehydration, immobility) that causes pressure injuries and pain.	Provide thorough skin care including daily baths; lubrication of skin; and dry, clean bed linens to reduce irritants (see Chapter 16).
	As patients approach death, they breathe through the mouth, the tongue becomes dry, and lips become dry and cracked.	Provide oral care at least every 2–4 h. Use soft toothbrushes or foam swabs dipped in water for frequent mouth care. Apply a light film of petroleum jelly to lips and tongue (see Chapter 16).
	Blinking reflexes diminish near death; eyes often remain open, causing drying of cornea.	Gently remove crusts from eyelid margins. Use artificial tears to reduce corneal drying (see Chapter 16).
Fatigue	Increased metabolic demands, disease progression, pain, and declining heart function cause weakness and fatigue.	Help the patient to identify valued or desired tasks; conserve energy for only those tasks. Help with activities of daily living.
	Exhaustion phase of general adaptation syndrome causes energy depletion.	Plan frequent rest periods in a quiet environment and pace nursing care activities.
Nausea	Occurs as a side effect of medications or disease progression, or as a result of severe pain.	Give antiemetic: provide oral care at least every 2–4 h; offer clear liquids and ice chips; avoid liquids that cause stomach acidity such as coffee, milk, and citrus juice (Moradian and Howell, 2015).
Constipation	Opioid medications and immobility slow peristalsis. Lack of bulk in diet or reduced fluid intake occurs as appetite decreases.	Increase fluid and fiber intake if possible. Administer prophylactic stool softeners (Huang et al., 2015).
Diarrhea	Diarrhea results from some disease processes and side effects of medications.	Assess for fecal impaction. Confer with health care provider to change medication if possible. Provide low-residue diet.
Urinary incontinence	Incontinence results from disease progression and decreased level of consciousness.	Protect skin from irritation or breakdown (see Chapter 17). Change linens frequently. Use indwelling urinary catheter or condom catheters if indicated (Farrington et al., 2014).
Decreased appetite	Decreased blood flow to intestines at the end of life causes anorexia. Nausea and vomiting decrease appetite.	Give patients whatever food or fluids they enjoy. Offer frequent, small meals, small portions, and/or snacks rather than large meals. Do not force people to eat. Offer small portions of desired foods or home-cooked meals if the patient prefers (Ní Bhuachalla et al., 2016).

Continued

Table 28.2 Managing Symptoms in Terminally Ill Patients—cont'd

Symptoms	Characteristics or Causes	Nursing Implications
Dyspnea or shortness of breath	Disease progression involves lung tissue (e.g., pneumonia, pulmonary edema). Anemia reduces oxygen-carrying capacity. Anxiety increases oxygen demands. Fever increases oxygen demands.	Provide ordered treatments for the underlying cause. Maximize lung expansion and ease of breathing (e.g., position the patient upright, provide supplemental oxygen if ordered; decrease anxiety or fever). Give medications (e.g., bronchodilators, anxiolytics, inhaled steroids, opioids) to suppress cough and ease breathing (Maeda and Hayakawa, 2016). Provide antipyretics as ordered.
Anxiety	Anxiety has physical causes such as shortness of breath, pain, fear of death, spiritual concerns, and relationship concerns.	Give anxiolytics as ordered (Thekdi et al., 2015). Offer self as healing presence and provide information to decrease uncertainty (Hawthorn, 2015). Discuss spiritual or relational issues causing anxiety or fear (Finocchiaro, 2016). Collaborate with spiritual care professionals. Discuss feelings/reasons associated with the anxiety.

Maintain Dignity and Self-Esteem

You enhance patients' self-esteem by helping them maintain a pleasing physical appearance. Cleanliness, absence of body odors, attractive clothing, and personal grooming often elevate a patient's mood. Demonstrate respect, patience, and willingness when helping patients with toileting and bathing, especially as they become increasingly dependent on caregivers. Patients experience added grief and embarrassment when they can no longer tend to their basic needs. Include patients in making care decisions (e.g., how to perform personal hygiene, diet preferences, and timing of activities). Inform patients in advance about activities and their anticipated effects. Provide privacy while giving care and give patients and family members quiet, uninterrupted time together.

Prevent Feelings of Abandonment and Isolation

Many people fear dying alone. In hospitals or extended care facilities, answer patients' nurse call system promptly and assure them that caregivers are available throughout the day and night. Be readily available to answer questions or interpret changes in a patient's condition. Offer your comforting presence and use gentle touch when providing care (Fig. 28.2). Unless family members need privacy or are remaining with the patient around the clock, avoid placing patients in a private room. Patients who are actively dying often feel a sense of involvement and companionship when sharing a room and have more opportunities to interact with staff and visitors.

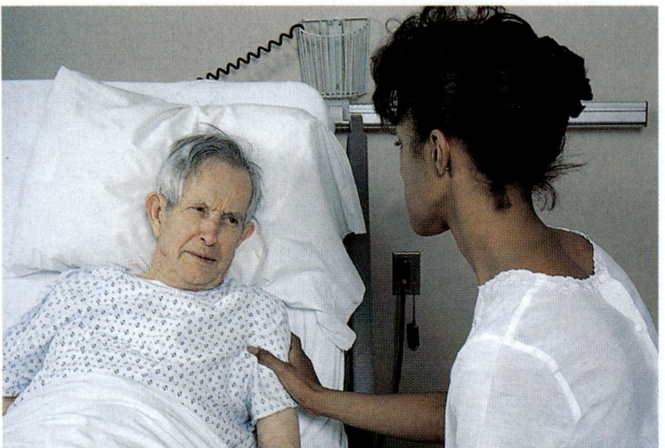

Fig. 28.2 Offer your calm, comforting presence, and use gentle touch when providing care.

Family members who are having difficulty accepting a patient's impending death sometimes avoid visits. When family members visit, reassure them that their presence is important, encourage interaction, and offer information about what the patient was talking about or has recently experienced. Encourage family members to discuss normal family activities, reminisce about enjoyable times, and ask about the patient's concerns. Suggest simple and appropriate tasks for family members to perform (e.g., offering help with meals, simple hygiene or comfort activities, or filling out a menu).

Some people feel lonely or fearful at night and want a family member to stay with them. In acute care settings or extended care facilities, allow visitors to remain with a patient who is dying and relax other visiting restrictions (e.g., visits from children and number of visitors) to accommodate the patient's circumstances. Know how to contact family members so that they can be notified at any time if a patient wants to see them or if the patient's condition changes. Older adults often have a smaller support group and age-related needs at the end of life (Box 28.2).

Provide a Comfortable and Peaceful Environment

Promote patient comfort by repositioning, keeping bed linens dry, and controlling environmental temperature and noise. Keep the patient's immediate surroundings pleasant and clean. Open curtains so that patients can experience the natural changes from day to night. Remove sources of unpleasant odors (e.g., stale food and used bedpans or emesis basins) promptly. Pictures, cherished objects, cards from friends and family, or plants create a comforting and familiar environment for patients and family members (Regan et al., 2014). Offer the patient frequent body massage if desired and provide opportunities for patients to hear their favorite music (Clements-Cortes, 2016; Nyatanga, 2015; Pische, 2015). A comfortable environment often helps patients relax, promotes sleep, and minimizes severity of symptoms.

BOX 28.2 **Care of an Older Adult**

Family Caregiver Concerns

- Older adults exhibit resilience. Others around them can learn from their courage and ability to respond to life challenges graciously, accepting life with integrity and wholeness (Boman et al., 2015).
- Older adults are at risk for complicated grieving secondary to multiple losses, potential for cognitive impairment, or decreased physical abilities. Other risks include depression, loneliness, and accompanying functional decline.
- Pain is often underreported and undertreated in older adults, particularly in patients with dementia or cognitive impairments.
- Side effects of pain medications are often more pronounced in older adults (Paladini et al., 2015).
- Older adults benefit from the same therapeutic techniques as persons in other age groups and have opportunities for growth and development through their loss experiences (Boman et al., 2015).
- Older adults are likely to be cared for across multiple health care settings, increasing the risk of fragmentation of care from one setting to another (Brown and Bub, 2016).

BOX 28.3 **Physiological Changes After Death**

1. Immediate changes
   a. Cessation of nervous system functions
   b. Cessation of respiration
   c. Cessation of circulation or heartbeat
2. Early changes
   a. Facial pallor: In postmortem, there is cessation of blood circulation; therefore, blood comes in big vessels from capillaries or small vessels, so face looks pale.
   b. Loss of skin elasticity: This is because of loss of skin muscle tone.
   c. Primary relaxation of muscles: In postmortem condition, muscles lose their tone and become flaccid, joints loosen, and chest becomes flattened.
   d. Algor mortis/cooling of the dead body: It is the condition or process in which body cools after death. Body temperature falls only if the surrounding environmental temperature is less than the body temperature.
   e. Livor mortis/postmortem staining: It is the bluish or reddish purple discoloration that appears at the undersurface of skin of the dependent areas of the body.
   f. Rigor mortis or postmortem rigidity: It is the condition in which muscles of a dead body become rigid or stiff.
   g. Changes in the eyes: With death, eyelids close, cornea becomes hazy, corneal and pupillary reflexes are lost, and pupil becomes dilated.
3. Late changes
   a. Putrefaction: It is the process in which complex organic body tissues are converted into simpler ones because of autolysis and action of saprophytic organisms.

Physiological Changes After Death

After death, there are various physiochemical processes that may lead to various changes in the body after death. Depending on the sequence of presence, the changes in the body after death are categorized into three categories: immediate, early, and late changes (Box 28.3).

Death Declaration, Certification

Usually, a physician must make a declaration of the death of a person when specific criteria are fulfilled. There are two standards for the determination of death: cardiopulmonary death (irreversible cessation of heartbeat and breathing) and brain death (irreversible cessation of brain functions). It is important to note that the patient must be assessed for minimum 5 minutes before declaring that patient dead. The criteria for declaring legal death are given as follows:

- There is no breath or heart sounds (more than 1 minute).
- There is no palpable pulse (more than 1 minute).
- Pupils are fixed, dilated, and unreactive to light.
- There is no response to painful stimulus.
- There is no reflex.
- There is a flat brain wave or ECG.

Death Certificate

After declaration of death, a competent authority issues a legal document that states the date, time, fact, reason, and other necessary information about the death of the person. It is mandatory to register the death within 21 days.

Autopsy

Autopsy is the surgical dissection of a body after death to determine the cause of death or how the person died or to contribute to the knowledge of the disease.

An autopsy requires consent by a patient before his or her death or by a close family member at the time of the patient's death (Autopsy Consent, 1998). The priority for giving consent for autopsies is (1) the patient, in writing before death; (2) durable power of attorney for health care (if named); (3) surviving spouse; and (4) surviving child, parent, brother, or sister in the order named. State statutes specify that you need to notify the coroner when there are reasonable grounds to believe that a patient died as a result of violence, homicide, suicide, accident, or death occurring in any unusual or suspicious manner. You also notify the coroner or medical examiner if a patient's death is unforeseen and sudden and a health care provider has not seen the patient in a certain amount of time (determined by state law). In these "coroner's cases," an autopsy is typically performed.

Embalming

Embalming is the procedure in which an embalmer treats a human with chemicals after his/her death for delaying decomposition. The three main purposes of embalming are sanitization, presentation, and preservation of the dead body. The embalming process usually involves four categories: arterial embalming, cavity embalming, hypodermic embalming, and surface embalming.

Last Office/Care of Dead Body

Nurses coordinate all aspects of care surrounding a patient's death. If a hospitalized patient dies while in a semiprivate room, transfer the other patient temporarily to another room to provide privacy for the deceased patient and family and avoid exposing the roommate to the stressors related to

BOX 28.4 Care of the Body After Death

Health Care Provider Responsibilities

1. Confirm the time of death and take appropriate actions.
2. Determine the need for autopsy and order autopsy if indicated.
3. A staff member educated in making requests for organ and tissue donation discusses with the family the donation options.

Nurse Responsibilities

1. Perform hand hygiene and apply clean gloves.
2. Provide care with dignity and sensitivity to the patient and family members. Place the patient in a supine position and elevate the head of the bed 30° or elevate with pillows to prevent discoloration of the face as you prepare for and complete postmortem care.
3. Check orders for any specimens to be collected or special postmortem instructions such as autopsy or retrieval of donated tissues.
4. Ask family members whether and how they would like to help care for the body. Make arrangements for a member of the professional staff (e.g., spiritual care provider) to stay with family members if they do not wish to participate in body care. Ask family members whether they have any special requests for body preparation (e.g., shaving, a special gown, Bible or rosary with the body).
5. Ask the family about shaving male facial hair. Some cultures or religions prohibit shaving facial hair or cutting hair.
6. Remove all catheters, tubes, or indwelling devices from the patient's body except in the case of autopsy. In that case, leave medical devices in place. Remove medical equipment, supplies, and dirty linens from the room to create a clean, natural environment.
7. Bathe the body thoroughly, keeping the head of the bed elevated; apply clean sheets.
8. Brush and comb the patient's hair. Apply the patient's hairpiece, if possible, for natural appearance.
9. Position according to protocol. Close eyes gently by holding eyelids down briefly. Some cultural groups prefer that the eyes remain open. Dentures remain in the mouth to maintain facial alignment.
10. Cover the body with a clean sheet up to the chin with arms outside covers if possible.
11. Lower the lighting and reduce unpleasant odors as able.
12. Dispose of supplies, remove gloves, and perform hand hygiene.
13. Give family members an opportunity to view the body and accompany them to the bedside. Some will not want to view their dead loved one; assure them that either choice is acceptable.
14. Encourage the family to say goodbye with words and touch.
15. Do not rush the process of family visitation and body viewing. Once the family is more comfortable, *ask* whether they would like to be left alone. Tell them how to find you easily.
16. Ask which personal belongings remain with or on the body. Give remaining personal items to a family member and document a description of the item and the date and time you transferred the belongings to the family's possession.
17. Do not throw away any personal belongings left behind by the family. Call a family member to describe the items and arrange for someone to retrieve the items they want to keep.
18. Apply name tags to the body according to agency protocol, usually on the right big toe and/or outside a shroud before transporting the body. Clearly mark the outside of the shroud if the body presents an isolation or contamination risk.
19. Document all care and any observations of injury to the skin in the nursing notes.
20. Remain sensitive to other hospitalized patients or visitors when transporting the body. Cover the body with a clean sheet and avoid moving it past groups of visitors when transporting it to the morgue or funeral home.
21. Follow all agency protocols and policies and comply with national or state laws regarding end-of-life issues.

postmortem care. Use postmortem care guidelines to make the body appear as natural and comfortable as possible.

After a patient's death, shift your care to surviving family members. Make all appropriate resources available to them. They may want their family priest, minister, or rabbi to be with them; or they may appreciate the presence of the spiritual care staff at the health care agency. Social workers and counselors also offer valuable support. Remember that this is a very stressful but important event in the family's history. Do all you can to calmly and smoothly facilitate family members' requests, attend to their needs, and ask them about their preferences. Some family members prefer to be left alone and are unable to talk about the event until they have processed it privately.

Document all the activities surrounding a death carefully to provide an accurate record of the final events of a patient's life. Sometimes your summary of activities is used for risk management or legal investigations. Include in your documentation the time and date of death, the name of the health care provider who pronounces the death, organ or tissue donation status (e.g., request made and donation decision), preparation of the body, medical devices left in or on the body, valuables or belongings left with the patient (e.g., dentures, glasses, or wedding ring) or given to the family (e.g., clothing, mail, or photographs), time of discharge, and destination of the body (e.g., morgue at the agency or funeral home). Become familiar with the policies and procedures for postmortem care used in your agency and be sure that your care and documentation reflect those guidelines.

A nurse assumes responsibility for **postmortem care** (i.e., care of the body after death) (Box 28.4). Give postmortem care with dignity and sensitivity and in a manner consistent with a patient's religious or cultural beliefs. Because a body undergoes many physical changes after death, provide postmortem care as soon as possible to prevent tissue damage or disfigurement of body parts. For example, immediately after death, elevate the head of the bed to 30° or place the patient's head on pillows to prevent pooling of blood, which can discolor the face.

COUNSELING AND SUPPORTING GRIEVING FAMILY

When a patient chooses to be at home at the end of life, family members become primary caregivers. Caring for a person dying at home is often rewarding yet physically exhausting and emotionally and spiritually stressful (Jaffray et al., 2016). Family caregivers benefit from education regarding the physical, emotional, and spiritual issues that often arise through each phase of the dying process

BOX 28.5 Patient Teaching

Preparing the Dying Patient's Family

Nurse establishes a teaching plan for Mr Manjeet and Mrs Rama to help them learn how to perform palliative care interventions.

Outcome

At the end of the teaching session, Mr Manjeet and Mrs Rama demonstrate ways to help Mrs Manjeet with activities of daily living, pain management, and mobility safety.

Teaching Strategies

- Describe and demonstrate techniques for helping a person experiencing fatigue to eat safely and select easily chewed and swallowed foods.
- Demonstrate bathing, mouth care, and other hygiene measures and allow the family to perform a return demonstration.
- Show video on simple transfer techniques and use of walker to prevent injury to themselves and the patient. Observe family members practice the techniques.
- Describe ways the family can promote the patient's comfort (e.g., frequent rest periods, giving massage, repositioning).
- Discuss medication purposes and side effects.
- Discuss ways to assess fatigue, bowel and bladder symptoms, and shortness of breath.
- Demonstrate how to assess pain, record pain intensity, and give medications.
- Teach the family to recognize signs and symptoms of impending death and who to call in an emergency and when death occurs.
- Invite questions from the family and provide information as needed.

Evaluation

- Use the principles of teach back to evaluate patient/family caregiver learning:
  - "Mr Manjeet and Mrs Rama, tell me what we discussed about the purpose and dosage of pain medications and how frequently you can administer them to Mr Manjeet."
  - "Mr Manjeet and Mrs Rama, tell me how you can use hospice services and who you will call when Mr Manjeet dies."

(Box 28.5). They also need information about home care services, hospice, and community service resources. Hospice programs offer respite care for family caregivers to temporarily relieve them of their duties so that they can get needed rest and rejuvenation. In some cases, families need assistance and support in making the difficult decision about nursing home placement.

Provide family members with a description of common symptoms the patient will likely experience, the signs and symptoms of impending death, and the implications for care (Box 28.2). Encourage family members to talk openly with their loved one to give everyone a chance to discuss lingering concerns or requests. Family members often appreciate the opportunity to share their concerns with you in private. As death approaches, encourage the use of silent vigil at the patient's bedside, touch, and verbal reassurances that the person is loved and not alone. After death, help family caregivers notify the funeral home, other family members, and friends who were not present at the bedside; arrange for safe transportation of the body; and gather the patient's belongings.

ADVANCE DIRECTIVES

You may encounter legal issues associated with caring for patients who are terminally ill, severely debilitated, or in a persistent vegetative state (permanently comatose). One of these legal issues involves the right to refuse medical treatment and the withholding of food and nutrition. The doctrine of informed consent is the basis of the right to refuse treatment. The Supreme Court has held that a competent person has the right to refuse medical treatment, including lifesaving food and nutrition.

Advance directives include living wills and durable powers of attorney for health care. **Living wills** are documents that provide instructions about a patient's wishes in certain situations, including withholding or withdrawing life-sustaining procedures in patients who are terminally ill. If a patient has executed a durable **power of attorney for health care**, the document designates an individual, also known as a **health care proxy** or a **surrogate**, who can give consent for health care treatment when the patient is no longer able. State law may designate a surrogate decision maker such as a spouse, who acts as a substitute when no documented preference exists. Each state providing for living wills or advance directives has its own requirements for executing them. In general, you need two witnesses who are not relatives or health care providers when a patient signs the document. Only a competent patient can revoke advance directives. Health care providers who ignore valid living wills, advance directives, or the directions of a health care power of attorney may be subject to civil liability. The Patient Self-Determination Act (1991) requires health care institutions to inquire about the presence of advance directives, give patients information on advance directives, and document whether a patient states that he or she has an advance directive.

DO NOT RESUSCITATE / INTUBATE (DNR/DNI)

In addition to the patient's refusal of treatment, a nurse frequently encounters a DNR or "no code" DNR order.

If a health care provider has documented in the progress notes that a patient is deteriorating and the health care provider and the patient have made the decision not to administer cardiopulmonary resuscitation, the health care provider should enter a DNR order. Health care providers need to regularly review DNR orders in case a patient's condition warrants a change. Be familiar with the policies of your institution and procedures concerning DNR orders, as there may be specific regulations about nurses entering telephone orders for DNR status.

EUTHANASIA

Euthanasia is derived from two Greek words: "*eu*," which means good or well, and "*Thanatos*," which means death. Therefore, euthanasia is a practice of ending a life intentionally for providing relief from pain and suffering. Euthanasia is defined as "the painless killing of a patient suffering from an incurable and painful disease or in an irreversible coma." Passive euthanasia is legalized in India since March 9, 2018, with a special judgment by the Supreme Court of India. The passive euthanasia is an act of withdrawal of life support to a person in a permanent vegetative state for the peaceful end of life.

ORGAN DONATION

Provide a private area for the family to discuss organ donation if this is an option. Professionals educated in organ procurement and transplant procedures (e.g., transplant coordinators, social workers, or spiritual care providers) make the first contact with family members regarding requests for donation of organs or tissues. They consider the family's personal, religious, and cultural needs and discuss which tissues or organs are suitable for transplant; offer a description of the process, costs, and impact of donation on funeral plans; and answer family members' questions. For example, many people do not understand "brain death." For their loved one to donate major organs (e.g., heart, lungs, and liver), the body must be kept in a good functional condition so the organs do not become damaged before donation. The patient remains on a ventilator until his or her organs are removed. Family members often believe that the person is still alive because his or her heart is still beating. Be available to reinforce explanations of the organ retrieval process during this most stressful, tragic time. Nonvital tissues such as corneas, skin, long bones, and middle ear bones can be removed at the time of death without maintaining vital functions. If the patient left no communication regarding his or her preferences for organ donation, family members make that decision with support and conversation. Review your state laws regarding organ retrieval and the formal consent process.

KEY POINTS

- The type and meaning of a loss influence how a person experiences and expresses grief.
- Individuals move back and forth through the phases or tasks of grieving, experience them simultaneously over a period of time, or do not experience them at all.
- A person's age, developmental stage, beliefs, roles, culture, relationships, and socioeconomic status influence reactions to loss and expressions of grief.
- When assessing patients experiencing grief or loss, do not make assumptions about how you think they feel. Ask them to share their experience in their own words and tell their stories.
- Therapeutic communication fosters the development of trust and provides an opportunity for patients and family members to talk about their concerns.
- Nursing care of a patient who is grieving or at the end of life focuses on enhancing a patient's sense of identity, dignity, and self-esteem and maintaining the highest possible quality of life.
- Patients of any age or diagnosis benefit from palliative care at any time in the course of their illness.
- Palliative and hospice care principles include involving patients and family caregivers in developing the plan of care; helping patients make informed choices; providing relief for physical, emotional, or spiritual symptoms; and offering support from an interdisciplinary team.
- Provide education and opportunities for family caregivers who want to be involved in end-of-life care.
- Provide care of a body after death and care for surviving family members with respect and sensitivity for their preferences and culture and/or religion and based on evidence-based protocols and standards.
- Nurses benefit from acknowledging and attending to their own grief when caring for patients at the end of life and their family members.

REFERENCES

American Association of Colleges of Nursing [AACN]. ELNEC fact sheet. 2016. Available from: http://www.aacn.nche.edu/elnec/about/fact-sheet.

American Nurses Association [ANA], Hospice and Palliative Nurses Association [HPNA]. Palliative nursing: scope and standards of practice. Silver Spring MD: Author; 2014.

Barrere C, Durkin A. Finding the right words: the experience of new nurses after ELNEC education integration into a BSN curriculum. Medsurg Nurs 2014;23(1):35.

Bezemer J, Kress G. Touch: a resource for making meaning. Aust J Lang Literacy 2014;37(2):78.

Boman E, Häggblom A, Lundman B, Nygren B, Fischer RS. Inner strength as identified in narratives of elderly women: a focus group interview study. ANS Adv Nurs Sci 2015;38(1):10.

Bowlby J. Attachment and loss, vol 3, Loss, sadness, and depression. New York: Basic Books; 1980.

Brown H, Bub L. Care transitions across the continuum: improving geriatric competence. Geriatr Nurs 2016;37(1):69.

Clements-Cortes A. Development and efficacy of music therapy techniques within palliative care. Complement Ther Clin Pract 2016;23:125.

Coelho A, Delalibera M, Barbosa A, Lawlor P. Prolonged grief in palliative family caregivers: a pilot study in a Portuguese sample. Omega (Westport) 2015;72(2):151.

Darrah N, O'Connor N. Toward safer transitions: a curriculum to teach and assess hospital-to-hospice handoffs. J Pain Symptom Manage 2016;51(6):961.

Dobrina R, Vianello C, Tenze M, Palese A. Mutual needs and wishes of cancer patients and their family caregivers during the last week of life: a descriptive phenomenological study. J Holist Nurs 2016;34(1):32.

Farrington N, Fader M, Richardson A, Prieto J, Bush H. Indwelling urinary catheter use at the end of life: a retrospective audit. Br J Nurs 2014;23(9):S10.

Finocchiaro D. Supporting the patient's spiritual needs at the end of life. Nursing 2016;46(5):58.

Guldin M. Complicated grief—a challenge in bereavement support in palliative care: an update of the field. Prog Palliat Care 2014;22(3):138.

Hall C. Bereavement theory: recent developments in our understanding of grief and bereavement. Bereave Care 2014;33(1):9.

Harris DL, Winokuer HR. Principles and practices of grief counseling. 3rd ed. New York: Springer; 2016.

Harrison K, Connor S. First Medicare demonstration of concurrent provision of curative and hospice services for end-of-life care. Am J Public Health 2016;106(8):1405.

Hawthorn M. The importance of communication in sustaining hope at the end of life. Br J Nurs 2015;24(13):702.

Honeycutt A, Praetorius R. Survivors of suicide. Illn Crises Loss 2016;24(2):104.

Hospice and Palliative Nurses Association (HPNA). HPNA standards for clinical education of hospice and palliative nurses. 2015. Available from: https://journals.lww.com/jhpn/fulltext/2015/04000/hospice_and_palliative_nurses_association.9.aspx.

Huang TT, Yang SD, Tsai YH, Chin YF, Wang BH, Tsay PK. Effectiveness of individualized intervention on older residents with constipation in nursing home: a randomized controlled trial. J Clin Nurs 2015;24:3449.

Jaffray L, Bridgman H, Stephens M, Skinner T. Evaluating the effects of mindfulness-based interventions for informal palliative caregivers: a systematic literature review. Palliat Med 2016;30(2):118.

Kisvetrová H, Školoudík D, Joanovič E, Konečná J, Mikšová Z. Dying care interventions in the intensive care unit. J Nurs Scholarsh 2016;48(2):142.

Kübler-Ross E. On death and dying. New York: Macmillan; 1969.

Maeda T, Hayakawa T. Combined effect of opioids and corticosteroids for alleviating dyspnea in terminal cancer patients: a retrospective review. J Pain Palliat Care Pharmacother 2016;30(2):106.

Matzo M, Sherman D. The interprofessional practice of palliative care nursing. Palliative care nursing: quality care to the end of life. 4th ed. New York: Springer; 2015.

Meisenhelder JB, D'Ambra C, Jabaley T. Spiritual coping at the end of life. J Hosp Palliat Nurs 2016;18(1):66.

Momtaz YA, Haron SA, Ibrahim R, Hamid TA. Spousal death anxiety in old age. Omega (Westport) 2015;72(1):69.

Moradian S, Howell D. Prevention and management of chemotherapy-induced nausea and vomiting. Int J Palliat Nurs 2015;21:216.

National Institute on Aging (NIA). End of life: helping with comfort and care. 2015. Available from: https://www.nia.nih.gov/health/providing-comfort-end-life.

Ní Bhuachalla É, Connor AO, Healy J, Dwyer F, Ryan AM. Good nutrition for cancer recovery—a nutritional resource for the treatment of cancer-induced weight loss. Nutr Bull 2016;41(2):151.

Nilmanat K, Promnoi C, Phungrassami T, Chailungka P, Tulathamkit K, Noo-urai P, et al. Moving beyond suffering: the experiences of Thai persons with advanced cancer. Cancer Nurs 2015;38(3):224.

Nyatanga B. Using complementary therapies in palliative care. Br J Community Nurs 2015;20(4):203.

Paladini A, Fusco M, Coaccioli S, Skaper SD, Varrassi G. Chronic pain in the elderly: the case for new therapeutic strategies. Pain Physician 2015;18(5):E864.

Pische K. Integrative and holistic oncology nursing. Beginnings 2015;35(3):19.

Rafferty K, et al. Spirituality, religion, and health: the role of communication, appraisals, and coping for individuals living with chronic illness. J Relig Health 2015;54(5):1880.

Rando T. Treatment of complicated mourning. Champaign, IL: Research Press; 1993.

Regan A, Tapley M, Jolley D. Improving end of life care for people with dementia. Nurs Stand 2014;28(48):39.

Rodrigo L. A rare kind of light at the end of a rare kind of tunnel: trauma of a life-altering, chronic, degenerative disease and its redemption. J Loss Trauma 2014;19(6):584.

Schonfeld D, Quackenbush M, Demaria T. Grief across cultures: awareness for schools. NASN Sch Nurse 2015;30(6):350.

Sierra Hernandez CA, Piper WE, Ogrodniczuk JS, Joyce AS, Weideman R. Use of referential language in short-term group psychotherapy for complicated grief. Group Dyn 2016;20(1):10.

Thekdi SM, Trinidad A, Roth A. Psychopharmacology in cancer. Curr Psychiatry Rep 2015;20(15):522.

Van Hook MY. Spirituality as a potential resource for coping with trauma. SWC 2016;43(1):13.

Waller A, Turon H, Mansfield E, Clark K, Hobden B, Sanson-Fisher R. Assisting the bereaved: a systematic review of the evidence for grief counselling. Palliat Med 2016;30(2):133.

Wienclaw R. Grief and bereavement. Grief Bereave Res Starters Sociol 2016;3:1.

Worden JW. Grief counseling and grief therapy. New York: Springer; 1982.

World Health Organization (WHO). Palliative care. 2016. Available from: http://www.who.int/ncds/management/palliative-care/introduction/en/.

29 Self-Concept

OBJECTIVES

After reading this chapter, the student should be able to:

- Explain the components of self-concept.
- Describe the components of self-concept as each relates to Erikson's developmental stages.
- Identify stressors that affect self-concept and self-esteem.
- Discuss the ways in which your self-concept and nursing actions affect your patient's self-concept and self-esteem.
- Apply the nursing process to promote a patient's self-concept.

KEY TERMS

body image, p. 745
identity, p. 744
role performance, p. 746
self-concept, p. 744
self-esteem, p. 746

INTRODUCTION

Self-concept is your subjective view of who you are. Self-concept, or how you *think* about yourself, directly affects self-esteem, or how you *feel* about or value yourself. Classic research conducted by Franken (1994) noted that self-concept is, perhaps, the basis for all motivated behavior. One's self-concept gives rise to possible selves, and it is possible selves that create the motivation for behavior. Because self-concept is related to self-esteem, Franken (1994) further notes that people who have strong self-esteem have a clearly differentiated self-concept. When people know themselves, they can maximize outcomes because they know what they can and cannot do.

What you think and how you feel about yourself affect the way in which you care for yourself physically and emotionally. Self-concept influences the way in which you care for others. You need to have knowledge of factors that affect self-concept and self-esteem. Be aware of differences in self-concept and self-esteem across age, gender, ethnicity, socioeconomic status, and other cultural variables to individualize your approach to patient care (see Chapter 33).

DEVELOPMENT OF SELF-CONCEPT

The development of self-concept is a complex process that involves many factors. It begins at birth and continues throughout life. Erikson's psychosocial theory of development describes key tasks that individuals face at various stages of development (Erikson, 1963). Each stage builds on the tasks of the previous stage. Completing each developmental stage successfully leads to a solid sense of self.

Use Erikson's theory to identify the stage of psychosocial development of a patient based first on the patient's biological age and then adjusted based on any significant life events. You apply this knowledge when you assess a patient's psychosocial development stage by determining how the patient is handling the developmental tasks of that stage. Adolescence is a particularly critical developmental period when many variables including school, family, and friends affect self-concept and self-esteem (Forsén Mantilla et al., 2014). Awareness of lifelong developmental tasks (Box 29.1) will allow you to select individualized nursing actions tailored to your patient's needs.

COMPONENTS OF SELF-CONCEPT

A positive self-concept gives a sense of meaning and wholeness to a person. Nurses care for patients who experience threats to the various components of self-concept including identity, body image, role performance, and self-esteem. Sexuality also influences self-concept. Likewise, identity, body image, role performance, and self-esteem affect sexual health. Although overlap exists among concepts, this chapter presents each one separately.

Identity

Identity involves the internal sense of individuality, wholeness, and consistency of a person over time and in different

BOX 29.1 Erikson's Developmental Tasks and Impact on Self-Concept and Sexuality

Trust versus Mistrust (Birth to 18 Months)

- Develops trust from consistency in caregiving and nurturing interactions with caregivers
- Distinguishes self from environment

Autonomy versus Shame and Doubt (18 Months to 3 Years)

- Begins to communicate likes and dislikes
- Increasingly independent in thoughts and actions
- Appreciates body appearance and function (including dressing, feeding, talking, and walking)

Initiative versus Guilt (3–5 Years)

- Takes initiative
- Identifies with a gender
- Enhances self-awareness
- Increases language skills including identification of feelings

Industry versus Inferiority (6–12 Years)

- Incorporates feedback from peers and teachers
- Increases self-esteem with new skill mastery (e.g., reading, math, sports, music)
- Sexual identity strengthens
- Aware of strengths and limitations

Identity versus Role Confusion (12–18 Years)

- Accepts body changes and maturation
- Examines attitudes, values, and beliefs; establishes goals for the future
- Feels positive about expanded sense of self

Intimacy versus Isolation (18–35 Years)

- Has intimate relationships with family and significant others
- Has stable, positive feelings about self
- Experiences successful role transitions and increased responsibilities

Generativity versus Self-Absorption (35–55 or 65 Years)

- Able to accept changes in appearance and physical endurance
- Reassesses life goals
- Shows contentment with aging

Ego Integrity versus Despair (55 or 65 Years to Death)

- Feels positive about one's life and its meaning
- Interested in providing a legacy for the next generation

situations. It implies being distinct and separate from others. Being "oneself" or living an authentic life is the basis of true identity. Children learn culturally accepted values, behaviors, and roles through identification and modeling. They often gain an identity from self-observations and from what individuals tell them. An individual first identifies with parenting figures and later with other role models such as teachers or peers. Relationships with parents, teachers, and peers have unique and combined effects on young children's general, academic, and social self-concept (Verschueren et al., 2012). To form an identity, a child must be able to bring together learned behaviors and expectations into a coherent, consistent, and unique whole (Erikson, 1963).

The achievement of identity is necessary for intimate relationships because individuals express identity in relationships with others (Stuart, 2013). Sexuality is a part of identity, and its focus differs across the life span. For example, as an adult ages, the focus shifts from procreation to companionship, physical and emotional intimacy, and pleasure seeking (Touhy and Jett, 2014). Gender identity is a person's private view of maleness or femaleness; gender role is the masculine or feminine behavior exhibited. This image and its meaning depend on culturally determined values (see Chapter 3).

Cultural Differences in Identity

Cultural identity develops from identification and socialization within an established group and through the experience of integrating the response of individuals outside the group into one's self-concept. Differences in cultural identity (e.g., Mexican American or Cuban American, homosexual or heterosexual) exist through identification with traditions, customs, and rituals within one's cultural group (e.g., Hispanic, Latino, gender identity). When cultural identity is central to self-concept and is positive, cultural pride and self-esteem tend to be strong (Rhea and Thatcher, 2013). An individual who experiences discrimination, prejudice, or environmental stressors such as low-income or high-crime neighborhoods often conceptualizes himself or herself differently than an individual who experiences better living conditions.

Body Image

Body image involves attitudes related to the perception of the body including physical appearance, femininity and masculinity, youthfulness, health, and strength. These views are not always the same, as the person's actual physical structure or appearance is ever changing. The way others view a person's body and the feedback offered are also influential. For example, a husband who is controlling and violent tells his wife that she is fat and ugly and that no one else would want her. Over the years of marriage, she incorporates this criticism into her self-concept.

Cultural and societal attitudes and values influence body image and sexuality. Some cultures are more accepting of individuals who are slightly overweight because this body type represents being healthy and prosperous. Racial and ethnic backgrounds play an integral role in body satisfaction and the differences among groups. Race, gender, and the social environment (family, peers, media) also affect a person's body image, particularly in adolescence. For example, identification and pride in ethnic background can act as a partial buffer against advertisements, magazines, television, and movies depicting the thin-ideal white image and help vulnerable teenage girls feel more comfortable with themselves and their appearance (Schooler and Daniels, 2014). Furthermore, body image is more favorable in cultures in which people describe more reasonable views about physical appearance, report less social pressure for thinness, and have less tendency to base self-esteem on body image. Body art such as tattoos and piercings is increasingly common among all ages of individuals and has become a popular way to express individuality, which is part of one's body image.

Body image depends only partly on the reality of the body. When physical changes occur, individuals may or may not incorporate these changes into their body image. For example, a patient who experiences significant weight loss may not perceive himself or herself as thin and tells you that there is still a "fat person" inside. Body image issues are often associated with negative self-concept and self-esteem. Most men and women experience some degree of body dissatisfaction, which often affects body image and overall self-concept.

Normal developmental changes such as puberty and aging have a more obvious effect on body image than on other aspects of self-concept. Hormonal changes during puberty and menopause in later adulthood influence body image. The development of secondary sex characteristics and changes in body fat distribution have a tremendous impact on the self-concept of an adolescent. Changes associated with aging (e.g., wrinkles; graying hair; decrease in visual acuity, hearing, and mobility) affect body image in older adults.

Role Performance

Role performance is the way in which a person views his or her ability to carry out significant roles. Common roles include mother or father, wife or husband, daughter or son, sister or brother, employee or employer, and nurse or patient. For example, stating, "I am a good father" or "I am a caring and competent nurse" reflects a positive self-concept and self-esteem. Each role involves meeting certain expectations.

Self-Esteem

Self-esteem is an individual's overall sense of personal worth or value. It is positive when one feels capable, worthwhile, and competent. Once established, basic feelings about the self tend to be constant, even though sometimes fluctuation exists. A situational crisis such as a hospitalization often temporarily affects one's self-esteem.

Self-evaluation is an ongoing mental process. A positive sense of self-worth, or self-esteem, is important for determining how an individual functions in the world. A person's ability to contribute in a meaningful way to society often affects self-concept and self-esteem. Some individuals who are chronically ill feel a sense of worthlessness. Your acceptance of a patient as an individual with worth and dignity helps to maintain and improve the patient's self-esteem.

FACTORS INFLUENCING SELF-CONCEPT

A self-concept stressor is any real or perceived change that threatens identity, body image, or role performance. An individual's perception of the stressor is the most important factor in determining his or her response. The ability to reestablish balance following a stressor is related to numerous factors, including the number of stressors, duration of the stressor, and health status (see Chapter 31). Stressors challenge a person's adaptive capacities. Changes that occur in physical, spiritual, emotional, sexual, familial, and sociocultural health affect self-concept. Being able to successfully adapt to stressors is likely to lead to a positive sense of self, whereas failure to adapt often leads to a negative self-concept.

Any change in health is a stressor that potentially affects self-concept. A physical change in the body sometimes leads to an altered body image, affecting identity and self-esteem. Chronic illnesses often alter role performance, which change an individual's identity and self-esteem. An essential process in the adjustment to loss is the development of a new self-concept. A loss of a partner can lead to a loss of identity and a lower self-esteem. Unlike the loss in self-esteem shown in vulnerable older adults, the resiliency demonstrated in some older adults may reflect more sophisticated cognitive strategies to manage losses.

The stressors created as a result of a crisis also affect a person's health. If the resulting identity confusion, disturbed body image, low self-esteem, or role conflict is not relieved, illness can result. For example, the diagnosis of cancer places additional demands on a person's established living pattern. It changes his or her appraisal of and satisfaction with the current level of physical, emotional, and social functioning. Assess self-esteem, effectiveness of coping strategies, and social support in all patients. During self-concept crises, supportive and educative resources are valuable in helping a person learn new ways of coping with and responding to the stressful event or situation to maintain or enhance self-concept.

Identity Stressors

Stressors throughout life affect an individual's identity; identity is particularly vulnerable during adolescence, which is a time of great change. Adolescents are trying to adjust to the physical, emotional, and mental changes of increasing maturity, which can result in insecurity and anxiety. For example, an adolescent who wants to be identified as part of the popular crowd at school develops a poor self-concept if not included in that group. Although social media and social networking sites (e.g., Facebook, Instagram, Snapchat, Twitter, YouTube) provide opportunities to connect with others and to feel included in groups, individuals who are ignored (e.g., messages unread or unopened) or are the recipient of mean posts are at risk for negative self-concept responses. A decline in self-concept occurs in people who are bullied and cyberbullied on social media. Low self-esteem is associated with individuals who commit peer aggression including cyberbullying (Toledano et al., 2015). Family and cultural factors can influence self-concept resulting in negative health practices such as cigarette smoking, at-risk drinking or drug use, and unsafe sexual practices. Promoting a change in a patient's self-concept demands an evidence-based approach supported by the entire health care team.

An adult generally has a stable identity and thus a more developed self-concept than an adolescent. Once a person has established his or her identity, the mature adult is better able to handle stressors such as marriage, divorce, menopause, aging, and retirement. Job satisfaction and overall performance in adulthood are also linked to self-esteem. Self-enhancing opportunities such as exploring new ideas, solving problems in creative ways, and learning new skills predict job satisfaction and commitment as well as promote self-concept clarity and self-esteem (McIntyre et al., 2014). Sometimes, when individuals lose a job, their sense of self diminishes, they lose motivation to be socially active, and they may even become depressed. If a person's identity is tied to a job, retirement can alter the person's self-perceptions and self-care practices. Some people at retirement begin to reevaluate their identities and accomplishments. Many older people are working past the traditional retirement age or change careers after retirement. Some do so because of a financial need, whereas others have a desire to remain involved and productive. Sometimes, loss of a significant other leads a person to reexamine aspects of his or her identity.

Body Image Stressors

Changes in the appearance or function of a body part require a body image adjustment. An individual's perception of the change and the relative importance placed on body image in the individual's self-concept affect the significance of the loss or change. For example, if a woman considers her breasts key to her femininity, a mastectomy negatively affects her body image. Changes in the appearance of the body such as an amputation, facial disfigurement, or burns are obvious stressors affecting body image. Surgical procedures, potentially undetected by others, have a significant impact on an individual. Elective changes such as breast augmentation or reduction also affect body image. Chronic illnesses such as heart and lung disease involve a change in function (less tolerant of exercise) in which the body no longer performs at an optimal level. Physical changes associated with aging or treatment for medical conditions can also negatively affect body image. In addition, the effects of pregnancy, significant weight gain or loss, medication management of an illness, and radiation therapy all change body image. Negative body image sometimes leads to adverse health outcomes.

Many people associate success with a specific body part or function. For example, some athletes consider their bodies and physical activities to be the focus of personal success. Their adaptation and rehabilitation is often affected if an injury prevents future participation in athletics. Body image changes require reevaluation of long-accepted self-perceptions and alterations in lifestyle.

Role Performance Stressors

Throughout life, a person undergoes many role changes. Normal changes associated with maturation result in changes in role performance. For example, when a couple has a child, both the man and the woman need to adjust to new parenting roles and changes in their personal relationship. When a middle-aged woman with young children assumes responsibility for the care of her older parents, she adapts to the increased demands of this new role. Acute and chronic illnesses alter a person's ability to carry out various roles, which affects self-esteem and identity.

All people must adapt to changes that occur with aging. Role performance changes associated with retirement differ for men and women. Many women have adjusted to several different roles throughout their lifetime and are more likely than men to have developed friendships that are not work related. Adjusting to changes in role performance has an impact on the marital relationship. Changes in role performance after the loss of a spouse or partner also affect self-concept. A widow who has never paid bills or who needs to learn to cook needs help to change roles.

Self-Esteem Stressors

Individuals with high self-esteem are generally better able to cope with demands and stressors than individuals with low self-esteem. Low self-worth contributes to feeling unfulfilled and misunderstood and results in depression and anxiety. Illness, surgery, or injuries that change lifestyle patterns also influence feelings of self-worth. Chronic illnesses such as diabetes, arthritis, and heart disease that interfere with the ability to engage in activities contributing to feelings of worth or success affect self-esteem. Self-esteem and health behaviors are intertwined. Self-concept guides health behaviors and influences health-related actions (Thomas and Moring, 2014).

Self-esteem stressors vary with developmental stages and differ across the life span. A child's self-worth lessens if the child feels unable to meet his or her parents' expectations or if his or her parents harshly criticize or inconsistently discipline him or her. The self-esteem of an adolescent is also vulnerable because he or she expends so much energy worrying about appearance, searching for identity, and being overly concerned about what others think. At-risk behaviors and stressors such as smoking, hazardous alcohol consumption, and unprotected sexual activities often signal self-esteem disturbances in adolescents. Stressors affecting the self-esteem of an adult include failures at work and in relationships, and stressors in older adults include retirement and the death of friends. Box 29.2 discusses ways to promote self-concept, self-esteem, and healthy sexuality in older adults.

Family Effect on Self-Concept Development

The family plays a key role in creating and maintaining the self-concepts of its members. Children develop a basic sense

BOX 29.2 Care of an Older Adult

Promoting Self-Concept and Self-Esteem

It is important to understand how self-concept and self-esteem change across the life span. Although self-concept is sometimes negatively affected in older adults as a result of a number of life changes, sexuality remains important to the older adult's well-being (Haesler et al., 2016). However, in some individuals, aging promotes improved coping strategies that protect against the declining feelings of self-esteem despite the physical and emotional changes associated with aging (Touhy and Jett, 2016). Nursing interventions aimed at enhancing self-concept and self-esteem in older adults are essential, particularly during experiences of illness, injury, or disability (Haesler et al., 2016):

- Clarify what the life changes mean and the impact on self-concept for the older adult (Touhy and Jett, 2016).
- Be alert to preoccupation with physical complaints. Assess complaints thoroughly; if no physical explanation exists, encourage the older adult to verbalize needs (e.g., fear, insecurity, loneliness) in a nonphysical way (Touhy and Jett, 2016).
- Identify positive coping mechanisms.
- Reinforce positive coping strategies and support and teach new strategies (Stuart, 2013).
- Encourage reminiscence through the review of old photographs and use of storytelling (Chan et al., 2014).
- Communicate that the older adult is worthwhile by actively listening to and accepting the older adult's feelings, being respectful, and praising healthy behaviors (Touhy and Jett, 2016).
- Reinforce the older adult's self-care and efforts at independence, and provide additional time to complete self-care tasks (Touhy and Jett, 2016).

of who they are from their family caregivers. A child also gains accepted norms for thinking, feeling, and behaving from family members. Sometimes, well-meaning parents cultivate negative self-concepts in children. Some literature suggests that parents are the most important influences on a child's development, yet variations in parenting approach depend on the culture. Specifically, a child's positive self-esteem and school achievement are fostered by parents who respond in a firm, consistent, and warm manner. High parental support and parental monitoring are related to greater self-esteem and lower risk behaviors. Parents who are harsh, inconsistent, or have low self-esteem themselves often behave in ways that foster negative self-concepts in their children. Positive communication and social support foster self-esteem and well-being in adolescence. To reverse a patient's negative self-concept, first assess the family's style of relating. Family and cultural factors sometimes influence negative health practices such as excessive drinking. Self-concept change demands an evidence-based practice approach supported by the entire health care team.

Nurse's Effect on Patient's Self-Concept

Your acceptance of a patient with an altered self-concept can promote positive change. Often this simply involves sitting with a patient and forming a therapeutic relationship. When a patient's physical appearance has changed, it is likely that both the patient and the family look to nurses and observe their verbal and nonverbal responses and reactions to the changed appearance. You need to remain aware of your own feelings, ideas, values, expectations, and judgments. Self-awareness is critical in understanding and accepting others. Nurses derive their self-concepts and professional identity from their public image; work environment; education; and professional, social, and cultural values (Ten Hoeve et al., 2014). They need to assess and clarify the following self-concept issues about themselves:

- Thoughts and feelings about lifestyle, health, and illness
- Awareness of how their own nonverbal communication affects patients and families
- Personal values and expectations and how these affect patients
- Ability to convey a nonjudgmental attitude toward patients and families
- Preconceived attitudes toward cultural differences in self-concept and self-esteem

Some patients with a change in body appearance or function are extremely sensitive to the verbal and nonverbal responses of the health care team. A positive, matter-of-fact approach to care provides a model for the patient and family to follow. For example, when you observe a positive change in a patient's behavior, note it and allow the patient to establish its meaning. Nurses have a significant effect on patients by conveying genuine interest and acceptance. Including self-concept issues in the planning and delivery of care can influence patient outcomes positively. Building a trusting nurse–patient relationship that incorporates both the patient and the family in the decision-making process enhances self-concept and self-esteem. You can individualize your approach by highlighting a patient's unique needs and incorporating alternative health care practices or methods of spiritual expression into the plan of care. It is important that health care providers understand the degree to which self-esteem and sexuality affect patient outcomes.

Your nursing care significantly affects a patient's body image. For example, the body image of a woman following a mastectomy is positively influenced by showing acceptance of the mastectomy scar. On the other hand, a nurse who has a shocked or disgusted facial expression contributes to the woman developing a negative body image. Patients closely watch the reactions of others to their wounds and scars, and it is very important to be aware of your responses toward the patient. Statements such as "This wound is healing nicely" or "This tissue looks healthy" are affirmations for the body image of the patient. Nonverbal behaviors convey the level of caring that exists for a patient and affect self-esteem. Anticipate personal reactions, acknowledge them, and focus on the patient instead of the unpleasant task or situation. Nurses who put themselves in the patient's situation incorporate measures to ease embarrassment, frustration, anger, and denial.

Preventive measures, early identification, and appropriate treatment minimize the intensity of self-esteem stressors and the potential effects for a patient and his or her family. Learn to design specific self-concept interventions to fit a patient's profile of risk factors. It is essential to assess a patient's perception of a problem and work collaboratively to resolve self-concept issues. Interventions designed to promote active living and healthy eating may be beneficial for preventing childhood obesity, improving self-esteem, preventing chronic diseases, and improving health outcomes in adulthood.

QSEN: Building Competency in Patient-Centered Care

You are a third-year nursing student who feels insecure in the clinical setting. You are caring for Mrs Johnson who had a bilateral mastectomy. This is your first time caring for this type of patient, and you hope that your clinical instructor will not ask you questions about your patient because you "forget" everything when your assigned faculty approaches; you feel embarrassed that you sometimes "hide" or "look busy" to avoid interacting with your instructor. You wonder, "How can I attend to my patient's physical care and self-concept and self-esteem issues when I can't even deal with my own?" Which actions must you take to improve your self-esteem and self-concept as a student nurse?

NURSING MANAGEMENT

Assessment

When assessing self-concept and self-esteem, focus on all components (identity, body image, and role performance) and on behaviors suggestive of altered self-concept or self-esteem (Box 29.3). Also, assess for actual and potential self-concept stressors (see Fig. 29.1). Determining a patient's current and past coping patterns is also important. If a patient shows mood changes such as depression, a mental

BOX 29.3 **Behaviors Suggestive of Altered Self-Concept**

- Avoidance of eye contact
- Slumped posture
- Unkempt appearance
- Overly apologetic
- Hesitant speech and/or withdrawn
- Overly critical or angry
- Frequent or inappropriate crying
- Negative self-evaluation
- Excessively dependent
- Hesitant to express views or opinions
- Lack of interest in what is happening
- Passive attitude
- Difficulty making decisions

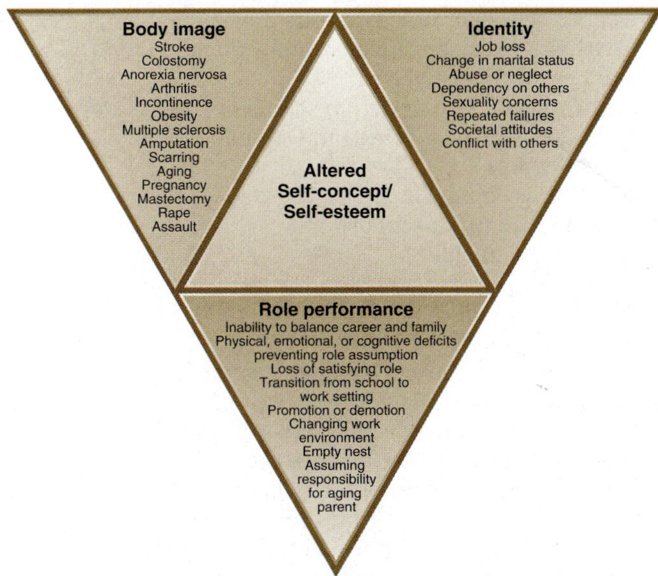

Fig. 29.1 Common stressors that influence self-concept.

status examination may also be helpful (see Chapter 3). In addition to direct questioning, you effectively gather much of the data regarding self-concept by observing a patient's nonverbal behavior and paying attention to what he or she says. Take note of the way patients talk about the people in their lives because this provides clues to both stressful and supportive relationships. It also suggests key patient roles and obligations.

Apply your knowledge of developmental stages (see Box 29.1) to determine what aspects of self-concept are likely to be important to the patient, and inquire about these aspects of the person's life. For example, ask a 67-year-old male patient about his life now that retirement is approaching and what is now most important to him. Spend time asking a school-age patient how he or she has adjusted to transferring to a new school and whether he or she has been able to make friends. Conversations with individual patients will likely provide data relating to role performance, identity, self-esteem, stressors, and coping patterns. At appropriate times, specific questions are useful (Table 29.1).

Bullying is very common in schools and any other locations in which children gather and interact. In the case of school-age children and adolescents, assess for signs of bullying (Johns Hopkins, n.d.; Youth Connection, 2005):

- Damaged or missing clothing and belongings
- Unexplained cuts, bruises, or torn clothes
- Lack of friends
- Frequent claims of having lost pocket money, possessions, packed lunches, or snacks

Table 29.1 Focused Patient Assessment

Factors to Assess	Questions	Physical Assessment
Identity	How would you describe yourself?	Note verbal and nonverbal responses. Watch for hesitant speech, poor eye contact, and slumped posture. Derogatory answers (e.g., "I don't know; there's not too much worth mentioning") raise concern and need further assessment.
Body image	Which aspects of your appearance do you like? Describe any aspects of your appearance that you would like to change.	Determine the patient's ability to identify something positive about appearance or body functions (e.g., "People have always told me I have nice eyes" or "I'm strong"). People who do not identify positive characteristics often have negative body image and poor self-esteem.
Self-esteem	Tell me about the things you do that make you feel good about yourself. How do you feel about yourself? If you were to describe yourself to someone else, which characteristics would you use?	Observe verbal and nonverbal responses. With prompting, most patients can identify something favorable. Statements about not having any strengths or not being able to do anything well raise concern and require additional assessment.
Role performance	Tell me about your primary roles (e.g., partner, parent, friend, sister, professional role, volunteer). How effective are you at carrying out each of these roles? Do you have any barriers to fulfilling your roles?	Listen for the number of primary roles identified. Many primary roles will put the patient at risk for role conflicts and role overload. Patients who do not think that these roles are met adequately may be experiencing alterations in self-concept.
Sexuality	How has your illness, medication, or surgery affected your sex life? Are your needs for intimacy being met? Do you have any concerns about your sexual functioning?	Identify concerns about sexual functioning (e.g., erectile dysfunction in men, changes in vaginal lubrication in women) or overall change in sex drive. Determine whether the patient is hesitant to bring up issues of sexuality.

- Fear of school or of leaving the house
- Avoidance of places, friends, family members, or activities adolescents once enjoyed
- Unusual routes to and from school or the bus stop
- Poor appetite, headaches, and stomachaches
- Mood swings
- Trouble sleeping
- Lack of interest in schoolwork
- Talk about suicide
- Uncharacteristic aggression toward younger siblings or family members

Depending on the environment, some young people—such as LGBTQ+ youth, youth with disabilities, and socially isolated youth—may be at an increased risk of being bullied (American Society for the Positive Care of Children, 2017). Ask parents (when appropriate) whether they have noticed any of the behaviors that may indicate bullying.

Your nursing assessment includes consideration of previous coping behaviors; the nature, number, and intensity of stressors; and a patient's internal and external resources. Knowing how a patient has dealt with self-concept stressors in the past provides insight into his or her style of coping. Not all patients address issues in the same way, but often a person uses a familiar coping pattern for newly encountered stressors. As you identify previous coping patterns, it is useful to determine whether these patterns contributed to healthy functioning or created more problems. For example, the use of drugs or alcohol during times of stress often creates additional stressors (see Chapter 31).

Valuable assessment data often evolve from conversations with family and significant others. Sometimes, significant others have insights into a person's way of dealing with stressors and knowledge about what is important to the person's self-concept. The way in which a loved one talks about a patient including his or her nonverbal behaviors provides information about what kind of support is available for the patient. Ask patients whether they feel comfortable when they are relating to their partner and whether there is openness in the interaction.

BOX 29.4 Patient-Centered Care

Self-Concept and Impact on Adolescent Drinking Behaviors

Low self-concept may precede or perhaps even motivate adolescent drinking. Because many teens engage in behaviors that increase the potential for morbidity and mortality, helping youth develop a healthy self-concept may prevent health risk behaviors including teen drinking (Kann et al., 2016). The 2015 Centers for Disease Control and Prevention Youth Risk Behavior Survey found that among high school students, during the past 30 days, 33% of underage teens drank some amount of alcohol, 18% binge drank, 8% drove after drinking alcohol, and 20% knowingly rode with a driver who had been drinking alcohol (Kann et al., 2016). Identifying risk and protective factors is important when creating drinking prevention programs. Enhancing opportunities to learn communication skills and engage in alternative behaviors may reduce drinking as an adolescent risk behavior.

Implications for Practice

- Include stress management and self-esteem improvement in drinking prevention interventions.
- Assess for effective adolescent coping strategies such as effective communication, conflict resolution, and stress management.
- Family members, peers, teachers, and health care providers should instill adolescents' ethnic pride, which promotes self-concept and encourages protective factors against risk behaviors such as drinking.
- Address family, social, and behavioral factors during preadolescence and adolescence.
- Identify risk factors for early drug and alcohol use, including genetic predisposition, family environment, and ethnic identity.

Nursing Interventions

Health Promotion

Collaborate with patients and family caregivers to help develop healthy lifestyle behaviors that contribute to a positive self-concept. Interventions that support adaptation to stress such as proper nutrition (see Chapter 31), regular exercise within a patient's capabilities, adequate sleep and rest (see Chapter 10), stress-reducing practices (see Chapter 31), elimination of stressors, or risk reduction contribute to a healthy self-concept. A patient-centered approach to care is important to support patients who engage in high-risk behaviors and who have alterations in self-concept (Box 29.4). You are in a unique position to identify lifestyle practices that place a patient's self-concept at risk or are suggestive of altered self-concept. For example, a college student visits an outpatient clinic with complaints of being unable to sleep and anxiety attacks. In gathering the patient history, you learn of lifestyle practices such as too little rest, many life changes occurring simultaneously, irregular menstrual cycles, and excessive use of alcohol. These data suggest actual or potential self-concept disturbances. You then talk with the patient to determine how she views the various lifestyle elements, to facilitate her insight into behaviors, and to make appropriate referrals or provide needed health teaching.

Acute Care

In the acute care setting, you are likely to encounter patients who are experiencing potential threats to their self-concept because of the nature of the treatment and diagnostic procedures. Threats to a patient's self-concept result in anxiety and/or fear. You need to address numerous new stressors with your patient including a new diagnosis and the need to make changes in lifestyle after hospitalization. In the acute care setting, there is often more than one stressor, increasing the overall stress level for patients and their families.

You also care for patients who are faced with the need to adapt to an altered body image because of surgery or other physical change. Often a visit by someone who has experienced similar changes and adapted to them is helpful. The timing of such a visit is important. Because it is often difficult to address these needs while in an acute care setting, appropriate follow-up and referrals including home care and information about support groups are essential. Be sensitive to a patient's level of acceptance of the change. Forcing confrontation with the change before a patient is ready delays the patient's acceptance. Signs that a patient is receptive to such a visit include the patient's asking questions related to how to manage an aspect of what has happened or looking at the changed area. As the patient expresses readiness to integrate the body change into his or her self-concept, you either let him or her know about groups that are available or ask whether he or she wants you to make the initial contact. In addition, respond to the change with acceptance to model acceptance for both the patient and the family.

Restorative and Continuing Care

Home care or restorative care environments provide opportunities to work with a patient to attain a more positive self-concept. Interventions designed to help a patient reach the goal of adapting to changes in self-concept or attaining a positive self-concept are based on the premise that a patient first develops insight and self-awareness concerning problems and stressors and then acts to solve the problems and cope with the stressors. You incorporate this approach into patient teaching for alterations in self-concept including situational low-self-esteem, which is sometimes present in the home care setting. Increase a patient's self-awareness by establishing a trusting relationship that allows the patient to openly explore thoughts and feelings. A priority nursing intervention is the expert use of communication skills to clarify the expectations of the patient and family as interventions are implemented. Open exploration makes the situation less threatening for the patient and encourages behaviors that expand self-awareness. Encourage the patient's self-exploration by accepting his or her thoughts and feelings, helping him or her to clarify interactions with others, and being empathetic. Also facilitate self-expression, and stress the patient's self-responsibility.

Promoting a patient's self-evaluation involves helping the patient define problems clearly and identify positive and negative coping mechanisms. Work closely with each patient to help analyze adaptive and maladaptive responses, consider alternatives, and discuss outcomes. Design opportunities that result in success, reinforce the patient's skills and strengths, and help the patient obtain needed assistance.

Teach patients to move away from ineffective coping mechanisms and develop successful coping strategies. Offering support when patients attempt to adopt health-promoting behaviors motivates patients to continue efforts at promoting health. Promoting adaptive, flexible coping is essential to intervening in self-concept alterations. Patients who are experiencing threats to or alterations in self-concept often benefit from collaboration with mental health and community resources to promote increased awareness. Knowledge of available community resources allows you to make appropriate referrals.

Establishing a therapeutic relationship is critical to successfully intervening with patients who have alterations in self-concept, whether care is focused on health promotion, dealing with an acute process, or addressing restorative care. To support the development of a positive self-concept in a patient, convey genuine caring for the patient. Then and only then do you establish a partnership with the patient to address underlying problems.

KEY POINTS

- Self-concept is an integrated set of conscious and unconscious attitudes and perceptions about the self.
- Components of self-concept are identity, body image, and role performance. Self-esteem and self-concept are closely related components.
- Each developmental stage involves factors that are important to the development of a healthy, positive self-concept.
- Identity is particularly vulnerable during adolescence.
- Body image is the mental picture of one's body and is not necessarily consistent with a person's actual body structure or appearance.
- Body image stressors include changes in physical appearance, structure, or functioning caused by normal developmental changes or illness.
- Self-esteem is the emotional appraisal of self-concept and reflects the overall sense of being capable, worthwhile, and competent.
- Self-esteem stressors include developmental and relationship changes, illness (particularly chronic illness involving changes in what were normal activities), surgery, accidents, and the responses of other individuals to changes resulting from these events.
- The nurse's self-concept and nursing actions often influence a patient's self-concept.
- Planning and implementing nursing interventions for self-concept disturbance involve expanding the patient's self-awareness, encouraging self-exploration, aiding in self-evaluation, helping formulate goals regarding adaptation, and helping the patient achieve these goals.

REFERENCES

American SPCC Bullying Statistics. Bullying Statistics: American Society for the Positive Care of Children; 2018 https://anannkefoundation.org/bullying-statistics-american-society-for-the-positive-care-of-children/.

Chan MF, Leong KS, Heng BL, Mathew BK, Khan SB, Lourdusamy SS, et al. Reducing depression among community-dwelling older adults using life-story review: a pilot study. Geriatr Nurs 2014;35(2):105.

Erikson E. Childhood and society. 2nd ed. New York: WW Norton; 1963.

Forsén Mantilla E, Bergsten K, Birgegård A. Self-image and eating disorder symptoms in normal and clinical adolescents. Eat Behav 2014;15:125.

Franken R. Human motivation. 3rd ed. Pacific Grove, CA: Brooks/Cole Publishing; 1994.

Haesler E, Bauer M, Fetherstonhaugh D. Sexuality, sexual health and older people: a systematic review of research on the knowledge and attitudes of health professionals. Nurse Educ Today 2016:40:57.

Johns Hopkins Bloomberg School of Public Health. The teen years explained: bullying. n.d. Available from: http://www.jhsph.edu/research/centers-and-institutes/center-for-adolescent-health/_includes/_pre-redesign/Bullying_HQP.pdf.

Kann L, McManus T, Harris WA, Shanklin SL, Flint KH, Hawkins J, et al. Youth risk behavior surveillance—United States, 2015. MMWR Surveill Summ 2016;65(6):1.

McIntyre K, Mattingly BA, Lewandowski Jr GW, Simpson A. Workplace self-expansion: implications for job satisfaction, commitment, self-concept clarity, and self-esteem among the employed and unemployed. Basic Appl Soc Psych 2014;36:59.

Rhea DJ, Thatcher WG: Ethnicity, ethnic identity, self-esteem, and at-risk eating disordered differences of urban adolescent females, *Eat Disord* 21: 223, 2013.

Schooler D, Daniels EA. "I am not a skinny toothpick and proud of it." Latina adolescents' ethnic identity and responses to mainstream media images. Body Image 2014;11:11.

Stuart GW. Principles and practice of psychiatric nursing. 10th ed. St. Louis: Mosby; 2013.

Thomas JJ, Moring JC. Development of a revised generalized health-related self-concept inventory. Am J Health Behav 2014;38(4):614.

Toledano S, Werch BL, Wiens BA. Domain-specific self-concept in relation to traditional and cyber peer aggression. J Sch Violence 2015;14:405.

Ten Hoeve Y, et al: The nursing profession: public image, self-concept and professional identity: a discussion paper, *J AdvNurs* 70(2):295, 2014.

Touhy TA, Jett KF: *Ebersole and Hess' Gerontological nursing and healthy aging*, ed 4, St Louis, 2014, Elsevier.

Touhy TA, Jett K. Ebersole and Hess' toward healthy aging: human needs and nursing response. 9th ed. St. Louis: Elsevier; 2016.

Verschueren K, et al: Relationships with mother, teacher, and peers: unique and joint effects on young children's self-concept, *Attach Hum Dev* 14(3):233, 2012.

Youth Connection. Institute for youth development. 2005. Available from: www.youthdevelopment.org.

30 Sexuality

OBJECTIVES

After reading this chapter, the student should be able to:

- Explain the basic concept of sexuality.
- Describe key concepts of sexual development across the life span.
- Discuss the factors affecting sexuality.
- Assess a patient's sexuality.
- Formulate appropriate nursing diagnoses for patients with alterations in sexuality.
- Identify patient risk factors in the area of sexual health.
- Identify and describe nursing interventions to promote sexual health.
- Evaluate patient outcomes related to sexual health needs.
- Identify health care providers and community resources available to help patients resolve sexual concerns that are outside the nurse's level of expertise.
- Use critical thinking skills when helping patients meet their sexual needs.

KEY TERMS

bisexual, p. 754
climacteric, p. 760
condom, p. 758
contraception, p. 756
diaphragm, p. 758
dyspareunia, p. 754
gay, p. 754
gender identity, p. 753
gender roles, p. 753
hypoactive sexual desire disorder, p. 757
infertility, p. 757
lesbian, p. 754
perimenopausal, p. 754
sexual dysfunction, p. 757
sexual health, p. 755
sexual orientation, p. 753
sexuality, p. 753
sterilization, p. 758
transgender, p. 754
tubal ligation, p. 758
vasectomy, p. 758

INTRODUCTION

Sexuality is part of a person's personality and is important for overall health. Even though discussion of sexual topics has increased over the years, many adults lack knowledge regarding **sexuality**. Although patients may be hesitant to bring up their concerns, they often share their feelings when a nurse addresses sexuality in a relaxed, matter-of-fact manner. To feel comfortable addressing sexuality, nurses need therapeutic communication skills and to be knowledgeable about sexual functioning, issues, and assessment. Many values and issues surround sexuality. Religious teachings, cultural influences on **gender roles**, beliefs about **sexual orientation**, and social and environmental climates influence the value systems for both patients and health care providers.

Sexuality has many definitions. Expression of an individual's sexuality is influenced by interaction among biological, sociological, psychological, spiritual, economic, political, religious, and cultural factors (WHO, n.d.). In addition, values, attitudes, behaviors, relationships with others, and the need to establish emotional closeness with others influence sexuality.

SEXUAL DEVELOPMENT THROUGHOUT LIFE

Sexuality changes as a person grows and develops. Each stage of development brings changes in sexual functioning and the role of sexuality in relationships.

Infancy and Early Childhood

The first 3 years of life are crucial in the development of **gender identity** (Edelman and Mandle, 2014). The child identifies with the parent of the same sex and develops a complementary relationship with the parent of the opposite sex. Children become aware of differences between the sexes, begin to perceive that they are either male or female, and interpret the behaviors of others as behavior appropriate for a female or a male.

School-Age Years

During the school years, parents, educators, and peer groups serve as role models and teachers about how men and women act with and relate to one another. School-age children generally have questions regarding the physical and emotional aspects of sex. They need accurate information from home and school about changes in their bodies and emotions during this period and what to expect as they move into puberty (Edelman and Mandle, 2014). Knowledge about normal emotional and physical changes associated with puberty decreases anxiety as these changes begin to happen.

Puberty/Adolescence

The emotional changes during puberty and adolescence are as dramatic as the physical ones. Adolescents function within a powerful peer group, with the almost constant anxiety of "Am I normal?" and "Will I be accepted?" (Fig. 30.1). They face many decisions and need accurate information on topics such as body changes, sexual activity, emotional responses within intimate sexual relationships, sexually transmitted infections (STIs), contraception, and pregnancy. Adolescence is often a time when individuals explore their primary sexual orientation (Hockenberry and Wilson, 2015; Pascoe, 2013).

Adolescents may identify with a sexual minority group such as **lesbian**, **gay**, **bisexual**, or **transgender** (LGBT) (Young-Bruehl, 2010). A transgender individual's self-recognition as a male or female is in conflict with his or her biological sex characteristics or what is culturally determined as belonging to a male or female (Olson et al., 2011; Rosenthal, 2014). Transgender patients may pursue treatments or modification procedures to promote physical characteristics consistent with their gender identification (Rosenthal, 2014). Adolescents often face significant stress related to sexual identity and benefit from education about sexuality issues (Doty et al., 2010; Johnson and Amella, 2014; Lim et al., 2014). LGBT individuals are at a higher risk for depression; suicide; and abuse of tobacco, alcohol, and drugs than the general population.

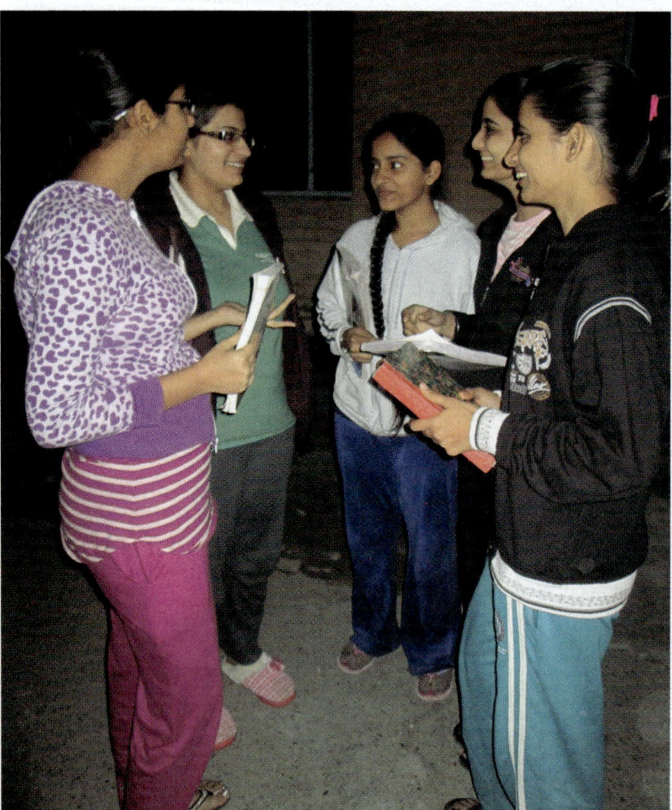

Fig. 30.1 Adolescents function within a powerful network of peers as they explore their sexual identity.

In the United States, almost 50% of high school students report that they have had sexual intercourse at least one time, and 15% of high school students had had four or more sexual partners (CDC, 2014d; Kann et al., 2014). Adolescents who engage in risky sexual behaviors experience negative health outcomes such as STIs and unintended pregnancy (Dunne et al., 2014; Scott et al., 2011). In addition, the pattern of risk-taking behavior tends to be established and continue throughout life. Parents need to understand the importance of providing factual information, sharing their values, and promoting sound decision-making skills. They need to know that, even with the best guidance and information, adolescents make their own decisions and need to be held accountable for them. Support from peers, family, school counselors, clergy, nurses, and other health professionals is important during this time.

Young Adulthood

Although young adults have matured physically, they continue to explore and mature emotionally in relationships. Intimacy and sexuality are issues for all young adults whether they are in a sexual relationship, choose to abstain from sex, remain single by choice, are homosexual, or are widowed. People are sexually healthy in numerous ways. Sexual activity is often defined as a basic need, and healthy sexual desire is channeled into forms of intimacy throughout a lifetime. At times, young adults require support and education or therapy to achieve mutually satisfying sexual relationships.

Middle Adulthood

Changes in physical appearance in middle adulthood sometimes lead to concerns about sexual attractiveness. In addition, actual physical changes related to aging affect sexual functioning. Decreasing levels of estrogen in **perimenopausal** woman lead to diminished vaginal lubrication and decreased vaginal elasticity. Both of these changes often lead to **dyspareunia**, or the occurrence of pain during intercourse. Decreasing levels of estrogen may also result in a decreased desire for sexual activity. As men age, they are likely to experience changes such as an increase in the postejaculatory refractory period and delayed ejaculation. Anticipatory guidance regarding these normal changes, using vaginal lubrication, and creating time for caressing and tenderness ease concerns regarding sexual functioning. Some aging adults also need to adjust to the impact of chronic illness, medications, aches, pains, and other health concerns about sexuality.

Later in the adult years, some individuals have to adjust to the social and emotional changes associated with children moving away from home. This results in either a time of renewed intimacy between partners or a time when formerly intimate partners realize that they no longer care for one another or have common interests. In either case, when children leave home, intimate relationships usually change.

Older Adulthood

Sexuality in older adults is an important aspect of health that often is overlooked by health care providers. Studies show a positive correlation between sexual activity and physical health in older adults (Lindau and Gavrilova, 2010; Stewart and Graham, 2013). Research indicates that many older adults are more sexuality active than previously thought and engage in high-risk sexual encounters, resulting in a steady increase of human immunodeficiency virus (HIV) and STI rates over the past 12 years (Box 30.1).

Factors that determine sexual activity in older adults include present health status, medications, past and present life satisfaction, and the status of marital or intimate relationships. For example, many older women are widowed or divorced and lack available sexual partners, which accounts for their decline in sexual activity. Nurses working with older adults need to assess the sexuality of their patients and sexual interest and functioning, and plan accordingly (Ayaz, 2013; Buttaro et al., 2014). It is essential to maintain a nonjudgmental attitude and convey that sexual activity is normal in later years. Emphasize that it is not essential to maintaining quality of life, especially when patients have decided not to remain sexually active.

To be effective in promoting sexual health, nurses need to understand the normal sexual changes that occur as people age. The excitement phase prolongs in both men and women, and it usually takes longer for them to reach orgasm. The refractory time following orgasm is also longer. Both genders experience a reduced availability of sex hormones. Men often have erections that are less firm and shorter acting. Women usually do not have difficulty maintaining sexual function unless they have a medical condition that impairs their sexual activity. Typically, the infrequency of sex in older women is related to the age, health, and sexual function of their partner. Women continue to experience changes related to menopause, and those with problems related to urinary incontinence often experience embarrassment during intercourse. Couples who have physically disabling conditions often need information about which positions are more comfortable when having sexual intercourse.

BOX 30.1 Focus on Older Adults

- Sexuality and continued interest in sex throughout middle and late life are usually associated with good physical health (Bach et al., 2013).
- Physiological changes with aging that influence sexual response are multifactorial and related to changes in circulation, hormones, and neurological pathways (Horstman et al., 2012).
- Pathological issues with the aging sexual response are often related to illnesses and side effects from medications (Bach et al., 2013; Buttaro et al., 2014; Syme, 2014).
- Older adults are often reluctant to discuss sexual problems with health care providers (Buttaro et al., 2014).
- Older adults who live in extended care facilities often lose their privacy and experience a decline in physical and cognitive abilities that affects their sexual expression. People who live in assisted living facilities have more privacy and are often able to live as couples (Katz, 2013; Syme, 2014).
- As the population ages and remains healthy, increasing numbers of older lesbian, gay, bisexual, and transgender (LGBT) people remain sexually active (CDC, 2013b)
- Increased availability of treatments for male and female sexual dysfunction contributes to continued sexual activity throughout the life span (Stewart and Graham, 2013).
- Older sexually active adults are at risk for contracting sexually transmitted infections. Because the risk of pregnancy is not an issue, older adults often do not recognize the need for protected sex when becoming active with new and/or multiple partners (Johnson, 2013; Stewart and Graham, 2013).

SEXUAL ORIENTATION

Sexual orientation describes the predominant pattern of a person's sexual attraction over time. Many stereotypical myths remain about people who are LGBT. Current evidence indicates that they experience decreased access to health care and do not readily seek preventive care (Lim et al., 2014; Williamson, 2010). Nonjudgmental nurses who have a solid knowledge base help to discourage these myths and provide nursing care that includes attention to the person's sexual orientation.

SEXUAL HEALTH

Sexuality differs from *sexual health*. According to WHO (n.d.), **sexual health** is "a state of physical, emotional, mental, and social well-being in relation to sexuality; it is not merely the absence of disease, dysfunction, or infirmity." People who are sexually healthy have a positive and respectful approach to sexuality and sexual relationships. They also have a potential for having pleasurable and safe sexual experiences that are free from coercion, discrimination, and violence.

FACTORS INFLUENCING SEXUALITY

Use critical thinking skills and basic nursing knowledge when addressing patients' sexual health needs. Draw from the following areas of nursing knowledge: sociocultural dimensions of sexuality, decisional issues, and alterations in sexual health.

Sociocultural Dimensions of Sexuality

People assign different meanings to sexuality on the basis of their culture, gender, education, socioeconomic status, and religion (Giger, 2013). Society plays a powerful role in shaping sexual values and attitudes and supporting specific expression of sexuality in its members.

Each cultural and social group has its own set of rules and norms that guide sexual behavior, sexual health, and the willingness to discuss this private part of life. For example, cultural norms influence how people find partners,

BOX 30.2 Cultural Aspects of Care

All sexually active individuals are at risk for HIV; however, some cultures have higher infection rates. The majority of HIV cases result from heterosexual activity. Cultural-specific norms and values that contribute to sexual risk behaviors include gender roles, religion, and sexual communication patterns. Health care providers need to consider cultural values and their influence on sexual practices when working with the Latino population.

Implications for Patient-Centered Care

- Establish a therapeutic relationship with a patient/family before discussing sexual health.
- Provide both males and females written and verbal information in English and Spanish, or in their native language, regarding contraception, sexually transmitted infections (STIs), and HIV testing and management options.
- Target adolescents by expanding education on STIs, HIV, and contraception in middle- and high-school curriculum.
- Promote gender neutrality by addressing assertive communication and negotiation strategies among females.
- Increase HIV testing at community clinics and offer combined laboratory work for STIs and HIV to promote acceptance (CDC 2010).
- Promote cultural-specific bilingual multimedia and community education about HIV risk reduction strategies (CDC 2010).

whom they choose as partners, how they relate to one another, how often they have sex, and what they do when they have sex. Personal beliefs enable certain practices and prohibit others (Box 30.2).

Impact of Pregnancy and Menstruation on Sexuality

Sexual interest and activity of women and their partners vary during pregnancy and menstruation. Some cultures encourage sexual intercourse or male–female contact during menstruation and pregnancy, but others strictly forbid it. For example, in the Hindu culture, a woman avoids worship, cooking, and other members of the family during menstruation. Research has found no physiological contraindication to intercourse during menstruation or during most pregnancies. Female sexual interest tends to fluctuate during pregnancy, with increased interest during the second trimester and often decreased interest during the first and third trimesters. There is often a decrease in libido during the first trimester because of nausea, fatigue, and breast tenderness. During the second trimester, blood flow to the pelvic area increases to supply the placenta, resulting in increased sexual enjoyment and libido. During the third trimester, the increased abdominal size often makes finding a comfortable position difficult (Link, 2012).

Discussing Sexual Issues

Sexuality is a significant part of each person's being, yet sexual assessment and interventions are not always included in health care (Ayaz, 2013; Ivarsson et al., 2010; Sobecki et al., 2012; Steinke et al., 2013). The area of sexuality is often emotionally charged for nurses and patients. Sometimes, nurses avoid discussing sexual issues with patients because they lack information or have different values than their patients. Nurses who have difficulty discussing topics related to sexuality need to explore their discomfort and develop a plan to address it. If you are uncomfortable with topics related to sexuality, the patient is unlikely to share sexual concerns with you. You need to be aware of your personal beliefs before discussing sexuality with your patients.

Decisional Issues

Individuals make many decisions about their sexuality. Some nurses help patients make decisions about contraception and abortion.

Contraception

Decisions patients make regarding contraception have far-reaching effects on their lives. Pregnancy, whether planned or unplanned, significantly affects the life of the mother and father and often their support network. Effects are physical, interpersonal, social, financial, and societal. The choice to use contraception is multifaceted and not completely understood. Factors that affect the effectiveness of contraception include the type of method used, the couple's understanding of the method, the consistency of use, and compliance with the requirements of the chosen method. Choice of contraception method varies in relation to the age, ethnicity, marital status, income, education, sexual orientation, and previous pregnancies of the woman (Casey and Gomez-Lobo, 2013; Godfrey et al., 2011; Jones et al., 2012). Mobile apps are available to help patients and health professionals monitor reproductive health (e.g., to remind you when to take oral contraceptives, to replace your transdermal patch or vaginal ring, or when your most fertile time is occurring). Some examples of women's health apps include Clue, Period Tracker, Glow, Glow Nurture, Ovia Fertility, and iBreastCheck (Garcia, 2014).

Abortion

Half of all pregnancies in the United States are unplanned; unintended pregnancy rates are highest among low-income women, women aged 18–24 and more than 40, cohabiting women, and minority women (Finer and Zolna, 2014). Approximately 40% of unintended pregnancies end in abortion. Abortions have been performed since ancient times. The safety and availability of abortions in the United States improved after the 1973 Supreme Court decision *Roe v. Wade*, which established the right of every woman to have an abortion. They are safer and less costly when performed in the early weeks of pregnancy.

Abortion is a hotly debated issue. Women and their partners who face an unwanted pregnancy may consider it. If caring for a patient contemplating abortion, provide an environment in which the patient is able to discuss the issue openly, allowing exploration of various options with an unwanted pregnancy. Discuss religious, social, and personal issues in a nonjudgmental manner with patients. Reasons for choosing an abortion vary and include terminating an unwanted pregnancy or aborting a fetus known to have birth defects. When a woman chooses abortion as a way of dealing with an unwanted pregnancy, the woman and often her partner experience a sense of loss, grief, and/or guilt.

Be aware of personal values related to abortion. As a nurse, you are entitled to your personal views. You should not be forced to participate in counseling or procedures contrary to your beliefs and values. It is essential to choose specialties or places of employment where personal values are not compromised and the care of a patient in need of health care is not jeopardized.

Alterations in Sexual Health

Infertility

Infertility is the inability to conceive after 1 year of unprotected intercourse. A couple who wants to conceive but is unable to has special needs. Some experience a sense of failure and think that their bodies are defective. Sometimes, the desire to become pregnant grows until it permeates most waking moments. Some individuals become preoccupied with creating just the right circumstances for conception. With advances in reproductive technology, infertile couples face many choices that involve religious and ethical values and financial limitations.

Choices for the infertile couple include pursuit of adoption, medical assistance with fertilization, or adapting to the probability of remaining childless. Organizations such as RESOLVE: The National Organization of Infertility, a national support group for couples with infertility, or international adoption groups provide couples with support and offer referral sources.

Sexual Abuse

Sexual abuse is a widespread health problem. Abuse crosses all gender, socioeconomic, age, and ethnic groups. Most often it is at the hands of a former intimate partner or family member. Sexual abuse has far-ranging effects on physical and psychological functioning (Edelman and Mandle, 2014). Sometimes, it begins, continues, or even intensifies during pregnancy. Cues that raise a question of possible sexual abuse include extreme jealousy and refusal to leave a woman's presence. The overall appearance is sometimes that of a very concerned and caring husband or boyfriend, when the underlying reason for this behavior is very different.

Nurses are in an ideal position to assess occurrences of sexual violence, help patients confront these stressors, and educate individuals regarding community services. They are mandated reporters and must report suspected abuse to the proper authorities. When you suspect or recognize abuse, mobilize support for the victim and the family. When abuse is suspected, remember to *not* ask the potential victim about any abusive behaviors in the presence of the suspected abuser. Provide privacy for the abuse victim and obtain information in a protective environment. When there is abuse, all family members usually require therapy to promote healthy interactions and relationships.

Rape victims often need to work through the crisis before feeling comfortable with intimate expressions of affection. The partner needs to know how to help and support the victim. Children who have been molested sexually need to understand that they are not at fault for the incident. The parents need to understand that their response is critical to how the child reacts and adapts.

Sexual Dysfunction

Sexual dysfunction, the absence of complete sexual functioning, is common. The incidence of sexual dysfunction in the general population is estimated to be as high as 40% in men and 60%–80% in women (Buttaro et al., 2014; Touhy and Jett, 2014). It is more prevalent in men and women with poor emotional and physical health. Sometimes, the exact cause cannot be determined.

The incidence of erectile dysfunction (ED) increases with age but can occur in men younger than 40 (Capogrosso et al., 2013; Syme, 2014). Risk factors are similar to those for heart disease (i.e., diabetes mellitus, hyperlipidemia, hypertension, hypothyroidism, chronic renal failure, smoking, obesity, alcohol abuse, and lack of exercise). The etiology of ED is often multifactorial. Neurogenic problems, medications, or endocrine or psychogenic factors can cause it. An age-related decrease in testosterone often results in decreased tone of the erectile tissues.

One of the most common problems affecting women of all ages is **hypoactive sexual desire disorder** (HSDD) (Buster, 2013; Buttaro et al., 2014; Kingsberg, 2011; Rosen et al., 2012). Biological, organic, or psychosocial factors can contribute to the incidence of HSDD. Chronic medical conditions such as breast or gynecological cancers and hormonal fluctuations, pain, or depression and anxiety can contribute to a decreased interest in sexual intimacy (Bach et al., 2013).

Personal and Emotional Conflicts

Ideally sex is a natural, spontaneous act that passes easily through a number of recognizable physiological stages and ends in one or more orgasms. In reality, this sequence of events is more the exception than the rule. You will care for patients who have problems with one or more of the stages of sexual activity, including the feeling of wanting sex, the physiological processes and emotions of having sex, and the feelings experienced after sex. For example, some women and men who are taking antidepressants report that their ability to reach orgasm is affected negatively.

PREVENTION OF SEXUALLY TRANSMITTED INFECTIONS AND UNWANTED PREGNANCY

Human Immunodeficiency Virus Infection

HIV infection is a blood-borne pathogen and is present in most body fluids. It is sometimes spread through sexual contact. Transmission occurs when there is an exchange of body fluid. Primary routes of transmission include contaminated intravenous (i.v.) needles, anal intercourse, vaginal intercourse, oral-genital sex, and transfusion of blood and blood products.

The natural history of HIV progresses in three stages. The primary infection stage lasts for about a month after contracting the virus. During this time, the person often experiences flu-like symptoms. Then he or she enters the clinical latency phase; at this time, there are no symptoms of infection. HIV antibodies appear in the blood about 6 weeks to 3 months after infection. If left untreated, people who are infected with HIV live about 10 years. The last stage, acquired immunodeficiency syndrome (AIDS), happens when a person begins to show symptoms of the disease. AIDS is a serious, debilitating, and eventually fatal disease. Highly active antiretroviral therapy (HAART) and having an experienced HIV clinician greatly increase the survival time of people who live with HIV/AIDS (Marrazzo and Cates, 2011).

Human Papillomavirus Infection

Human papillomavirus (HPV) is the most common STI in the United States, with approximately 14 million new infections every year (CDC, 2014b). Most HPV infections are asymptomatic and self-limiting. However, certain types can cause cervical cancer in women and anogenital cancers and genital warts in both men and women. HPV is spread through direct contact with warts, semen, and other body fluids from others who have the disease. The textured warts often have a cauliflower appearance and are most common on the penis and scrotum in men and the vagina and cervix in women. A vaccine that protects both men and woman against nine types of HPV that most commonly cause health concerns is now available (ACOG, 2015; CDC, 2015b) (Box 28.2).

Chlamydia

The bacteria *Chlamydia trachomatis* causes chlamydia. It is the most commonly reported infectious disease in the United States, affecting about 3 million Americans each year (CDC, 2014c). Chlamydia is spread by contact with fluids from the infected site. The infection can be transmitted during the birthing process and cause conjunctivitis and pneumonia in newborn babies. It frequently infects the cervix and, if left untreated, can cause PID, ectopic pregnancy, and infertility from damage to the female reproductive organs. Most people do not realize that they are infected with chlamydia because it causes few symptoms (CDC, 2015a). For this reason, the CDC recommends annual screening for all sexually active women up to age 25. High-risk populations are people who have multiple sex partners or are infected with other STIs and men who have sex with men.

Contraception

Numerous contraceptive options are available to sexually active couples nowadays. They provide varying levels of protection against unwanted pregnancies. Some methods do not require a prescription, whereas others require a prescription or some other type of intervention from a health care provider. Methods that are effective for contraception do not always reduce the risk of STIs. For example, the pill and intrauterine contraceptive device (IUD) are effective as birth control but not for protection from STIs. A latex condom should be used during each act of intercourse to reduce the risk of STIs. Effectiveness varies with each contraceptive method and the consistency of use. Unplanned pregnancies occur because contraceptives are not used, are used inconsistently, or are used improperly (Schwartz and Gabelnick, 2011; Trussell and Guthrie, 2011).

Nonprescription Contraceptive Methods

Nonprescription methods for contraception include abstinence, barrier methods, and timing of intercourse with regard to a woman's ovulation cycle. Although abstinence from sexual intercourse is 100% effective, it is often difficult for both men and women to use consistently. Any act of unprotected intercourse potentially results in pregnancy and exposure to STIs.

Barrier methods include over-the-counter spermicidal products and condoms. Spermicidal products (e.g., creams, jellies, foams, and sponges) are put into the vagina before intercourse to create a spermicidal barrier between the uterus and the ejaculated sperm. A latex **condom** is a thin rubber sheath that fits over the penis to prevent entrance of sperm into the vagina. A diaphragm is a barrier method, which must be used with a spermicide with each sexual encounter. Vaginal spermicides and condoms are most effective when instructions are followed carefully; their combined use is more effective in preventing pregnancy than the use of either one alone (Cates and Harwood, 2011).

Nonprescription methods of contraception based on the physiological changes of the menstrual cycle include the rhythm, basal body temperature, cervical mucus, and fertility awareness methods. Couples who use these methods need to understand the reproductive cycle of the woman's body and the subtle signs and signals that her body gives during the cycle. To prevent pregnancy, couples abstain from sexual intercourse during designated fertile periods.

Methods That Require a Health Care Provider's Intervention

Contraceptive methods that require the intervention of a health care provider include hormonal contraception, IUDs, the diaphragm, the cervical cap, and **sterilization**. Hormonal contraception is available in several forms: oral contraceptive pills, vaginal contraceptive rings, hormonal injections, subdermal implant, transdermal skin patches, and IUDs. Hormonal contraception alters the hormonal environment to prevent ovulation, thicken cervical mucus, and thin the lining of the uterus.

An IUD is a plastic device inserted by a health care provider into the uterus through the cervical opening. IUDs contain either copper or progesterone. The primary mechanism by which both types of IUDs prevent pregnancy is to stop the sperm from fertilizing an egg (Dean and Schwarz, 2011; Murphy, 2011). The release of progesterone may also increase cervical mucus thickness and alter the lining of the uterus.

The **diaphragm** is a round, rubber dome that has a flexible spring around the edge. It is used with a contraceptive cream or jelly and is inserted in the vagina so it provides a contraceptive barrier over the cervical opening. The woman needs to be refitted after a significant change in weight (10-pound gain or loss) or pregnancy. The cervical cap functions like the diaphragm; however, it covers only the cervix. It may be left in place longer, and some perceive it as more comfortable than the diaphragm.

Sterilization is the most effective contraception method other than abstinence. Female sterilization, or **tubal ligation**, involves cutting, tying, or otherwise ligating the fallopian tubes. In male sterilization, or **vasectomy**, the vas deferens, which carries the sperm away from the testicles, is cut and tied. Both a tubal ligation and a vasectomy usually are considered permanent surgical procedures.

DEALING WITH INAPPROPRIATE SEXUAL BEHAVIOR

Apply the nursing process and use a critical thinking approach in your care of patients. The nursing process provides a clinical decision-making approach to help you develop and implement an individualized plan of care. Assess all relevant factors, including physical, psychological, social, and cultural, to determine a patient's sexual well-being. The nursing role in addressing sexual concerns ranges from ongoing assessment to providing information, counseling, and referral. Keep in mind that nurses are not expected to have answers to all sexual issues and concerns identified.

Assessment

During the assessment process, thoroughly assess each patient and critically analyze findings to ensure that you make patient-centered clinical decisions required for safe nursing care.

Factors Affecting Sexuality

In gathering a sexual history, consider physical, functional, relationship, lifestyle, developmental, and self-esteem factors that influence sexual functioning. Sexual desire varies among individuals; some people want and enjoy sex every day, whereas others want sex only once a month, and still others have no sexual desire and are quite comfortable with that fact. Sexual desire becomes an issue if the person wants to satisfy it more often, if he or she believes that it is necessary to measure up to some cultural norm, or if there is a discrepancy between the sexual desires of the partners in a relationship.

Sexual Health History

Most patients want to know how medications, treatments, and surgical procedures influence their sexual relationship even though they often do not ask questions. With experience, nurses recognize that most patients welcome the opportunity to talk about their sexuality, especially when they are experiencing difficulties. The PLISSIT model provides an approach that nurses can use to assess sexuality in patients (Ayaz, 2013) (Box 30.3).

Incorporate assessment questions related to sexuality in the nursing history (Box 30.4).

In light of the prevalence of intimate partner violence, questions relating to abusive relationships are important. Address these questions in private. Recognizing both subjective and objective signs and symptoms of abuse in children and adults helps to identify this too-common problem (Table 30.1).

BOX 30.3 PLISSIT Assessment of Sexuality

Permission to discuss sexuality issues
Limited **I**nformation related to sexual health problems being experienced
Specific **S**uggestions—only when the nurse is clear about the problem
Intensive **T**herapy—referral to professional with advanced training if necessary

Modified from Annon JS: The PLISSIT model: a proposed conceptual scheme for the behavioral treatment of sexual problems, *J Sex Educ Ther* 2(2):1, 1976.

BOX 30.4 Nursing Assessment Questions

- Are you sexually active?
- With whom do you have sex: men, women, or both?
- How many sexual partners do you have (or have you ever had)?
- How do you feel about the sexual aspects of your life?
- Have you noticed any changes in the way you feel about yourself?
- How has your illness, medication, or surgery affected your sex life?
- It is not unusual for people with your condition to be experiencing some sexual changes. Have you noticed any changes, or do you have any concerns?
- Are you in a relationship in which someone is hurting you?
- Has anyone ever forced you to have sex against your will?
- Tell me what you know about safe sex practices, use of contraceptives, or prevention of sexually transmitted infections.
- Tell me the safe sex practices that you follow.

Table 30.1 Signs and Symptoms That Indicate Possible Current Sexual Abuse or a History of Sexual Abuse

Types of Findings	Symptoms Often Found in Children	Symptoms Often Found in Adults
Injuries and/or physical signs	Bruises, bleeding, soreness, infection, or irritation of external genitalia, anus, mouth, or throat Sexually transmitted infections Recurrent urinary tract infections Unintended pregnancy Chronic pain Difficulty walking or sitting Unusual odor in genital area Penile discharge Torn, stained, or bloody underclothing	Welts, bruising, swelling, scars, burns, or lacerations on arms, legs, breasts, or abdomen Wounds that do not match the patient's "story" Multiple bruises in various stages of healing Vaginal or rectal bleeding Fractures of face, nose, ribs, or arms Trauma to labia, vagina, cervix, or anus Vomiting or abdominal tenderness
Behavior, nonverbal and/or vague somatic complaints	Physical aggression Sexual acting out Excessive masturbation Expressions of low self-esteem Poor school performance Poor peer relationships Sleep disturbances Social withdrawal and excessive daydreaming Running away from home Substance abuse or suicide attempts	Facial grimacing Absence of facial response or flat affect Anxiety Depression Panic attacks Difficulty sleeping Anorexia Slow, unsteady gait

Data from Hockenberry MJ, Wilson D: *Wong's nursing care of infants and children*, ed 10, St Louis, 2015, Elsevier; Touhy TA, Jett K: *Ebersole & Hess' Gerontological nursing and healthy aging*, ed 4, St Louis, 2014, Elsevier.

Sexual Dysfunction

Many illnesses, injuries, medications, and aging changes have a negative effect on sexual health. Sexual dysfunction is either temporary or permanent. Apply knowledge about conditions and medications that frequently cause sexual dysfunction while assessing a patient's risks.

Physical Assessment

The physical examination is important in evaluating the cause of sexual concerns or problems and usually provides the best opportunity to teach an individual about sexuality. In examining a woman's breasts and the external and internal genitalia, a nurse has the opportunity to assess the woman's reaction, answer questions, and provide information about the examination of anatomical and physiological structures. For example, a nurse teaches a woman how to perform breast self-examination during physical assessment (see Chapter 7). During physical assessment of the genitalia, he or she teaches men how to perform testicular self-examination (see Chapter 7). Knowledge of normal scrotal anatomical structures helps men detect signs of testicular cancer. Instruct both men and women on signs and symptoms of STIs during the examination when patients' histories suggest risks for them.

Health Promotion

Helping patients maintain or gain sexual health involves consideration of factors that influence sexual satisfaction. Educate patients about sexual health, including measures for contraception, safe sex practices, and prevention of STIs. Regular breast self-examinations, mammograms, and Papanicolaou (Pap) smears are important sexual health measures for women; testicular self-examinations are important for men. Offer the nine-valent HPV vaccine to males and females who are between 11 and 26 years of age (ACOG, 2015; CDC, 2015b). The vaccine is safe for girls as young as 9 years old and is recommended for females ages 11–26 if they have not already completed the three required injections. Booster doses currently are not recommended. The vaccine is most effective if administered before sexual activity or exposure (ACOG, 2015).

Exploring an individual's values, discussing levels of satisfaction, and providing sex education require therapeutic communication skills. Structure the environment and timing to provide privacy, comfort, and uninterrupted time (Ayaz, 2013). For example, when discussing methods of contraception with a woman, provide education in a private area with the patient fully dressed rather than in the examination room when the patient is only partially clothed.

Topics of education vary and often are related to a patient's developmental level. For example, a nurse talks to school-age children regarding the appearance of breast buds or pubic hair. When discussing sexual health with patients of childbearing age, always consider a patient's cultural and religious beliefs regarding contraception. The discussion includes the desire for children, usual sexual practices, and acceptable methods of contraception. Review all methods of contraception to allow patients to make informed decisions.

Major developmental crises (e.g., puberty, **climacteric**, or menopause) prompt education about sexuality. Situational crises such as a life change with pregnancy, illness, divorce, extreme financial stress, placement of a spouse in a nursing home, or loss and grief affect sexuality. Effects sometimes last for days, months, or years and are often minimized when the individual is prepared for possible changes in sexual functioning.

Demonstrate recognition, acceptance, and respect for an older adult's sexuality by displaying a willingness to openly discuss sex and sexuality-related concerns. Strategies that enhance sexual functioning include the following (Bach et al., 2013; Buttaro et al., 2014):

- Avoid alcohol (in excess) and tobacco.
- Eat well-balanced meals.
- Plan sexual activity for times when the couple feels rested.
- Take pain medication if needed before sexual intercourse.
- Use pillows and alternate positioning to enhance comfort.
- Encourage touch, kissing, hugging, and other tactile stimulation.
- Communicate concerns and fears with partner and health care provider.

Individuals who have more than one sex partner or whose partner has other sexual experiences need to learn about safe sex practices. Provide information about STI symptoms and transmission, use of condoms, and risky sexual activities (e.g., trauma from penile-anal sex). To prevent HIV infection, teach patients to avoid having multiple sex partners and use condoms to reduce the risk of HIV/AIDS. Role play is useful in helping a person learn to say no or negotiate with a partner to use a condom. Also teach patients to avoid the use of i.v. drugs. If people do use i.v. drugs, tell them to avoid sharing needles with others and to always use new needles. When discussing safe sex, consider patients' physical and emotional health.

Encourage patients to have regular health and screening examinations to maintain sexual health. Often asymptomatic STIs are diagnosed during a physical examination with appropriate laboratory work. Annual health examinations provide an opportunity to discuss contraception and safe sex practices. However, some people do not seek annual health examinations routinely. For example, Arab women frequently do not have breast examinations, mammograms, and cervical cancer screening because of religious and cultural beliefs about modesty (Cohen and Azaiza, 2010). Develop a therapeutic relationship with patients and provide culturally sensitive education that is written at an appropriate reading level (see Chapter 15). Barriers to reproductive health services include cultural beliefs, low socioeconomic status, and low health literacy (Hall et al., 2012). The Affordable Health Care Act offers increased access to health care for previously uninsured individuals (USDHHS, 2012).

Acute Care

Illness and surgery create situational stressors that often affect a person's sexuality. During periods of illness, individuals experience major physical changes, the effects of drugs or treatments, the emotional stress of a prognosis, concern about future functioning, and separation from significant others. Never assume that sexual functioning is not a concern merely because of an individual's age or severity of prognosis. After identifying concerns, address them in the context of his or her value system.

When a patient identifies sexual concerns, initiate discussion and education appropriately. Refer to appropriate outpatient resources. Help patients anticipate how their illness or disease will change over time and the adjustments that will be necessary to achieve sexual fulfillment.

Restorative and Continuing Care

You need to establish relationships with couples to encourage honest and open discussions about sexual health during restorative or continuing care. Address needs by taking a sexual health history and implementing a basic model such as PLISSIT to provide options for patients (see Box 30.3). Assessment and management of sexual concerns are important when promoting sexual intimacy and providing closeness and closure between partners at the end of life.

In the home environment, it is important to provide information on how an illness limits sexual activity and give ideas for adapting or facilitating sexual activity. Interventions range from giving permission for a partner to lie in bed and hold a patient to coordinating nursing care and medications to provide opportunity for privacy and intimacy. Often nurses help individuals create an environment that is comfortable for sexual activity in the home. This sometimes involves making recommendations for ways to arrange the bedroom to accommodate physical limitations. For example, some individuals who are in a wheelchair prefer being able to move the chair close to the side of the bed at an angle that allows for more ease in touching and caressing. Suggestions regarding how to accommodate barriers such as Foley catheters or drainage tubes contribute to sexual activity.

In the long-term care setting, facilities need to make proper arrangements for privacy during residents' sexual experiences (Katz, 2013). The ideal situation is to set up a pleasant room that is used for a variety of activities that the resident is able to reserve for private visits with a spouse or partner. If this is not possible, make arrangements for the roommate of a patient to be somewhere else to allow a couple time alone. Never leave patients alone in a situation in which they can injure themselves.

KEY POINTS

- Sexuality is related to all dimensions of health, is a part of each individual's identity, and includes biological sex, gender identity, gender role, and sexual partner preference.
- Attitudes toward sexuality vary widely. Religious beliefs, society values, the media, the family, and other factors all influence it.
- Nurses' attitudes toward sexuality vary and often differ from those of patients; be sensitive to patients' sexual preferences and needs.
- Sexual development begins in infancy and involves some level of sexual behavior or growth in all developmental stages.
- The physiological sexual response changes with aging, but aging does not lead to diminished sexuality.
- Sexual health contributes to an individual's sense of self-worth and positive interpersonal relationships.
- Sexual dysfunctions result from varied and complex etiologies.
- Interventions for sexual dysfunctions depend on the condition and the patient; they often include giving information, teaching specific exercises, improving communication between partners, and referral to a knowledgeable professional.
- Sexual biases, comfort with touching genitalia, desire for future fertility, financial status, ability to plan sexual contact, and ability to communicate with the sex partner all affect the choice and use of effective contraceptive methods.
- Include a brief review of sexuality whenever assessing a patient's level of wellness.
- Most nursing interventions that enhance sexual health require providing education.
- Evaluate patient satisfaction with outcomes of care by talking with patients regarding satisfaction with sexual functioning and through observations of nonverbal behaviors that suggest clients' discomfort.

REFERENCES

American College of Obstetricians and Gynecologists (ACOG). Committee Opinion: human papillomavirus vaccination, Number 641. September 2015. https://www.acog.org/clinical/clinical-guidance/committee-opinion/articles/2020/08/human-papillomavirus-vaccination.

Ayaz S: Sexuality and nursing process: a literature review, Sex Disabil 32: 3, 2013.

Bach LE, et al: The association of physical and mental health with sexual activity in older adults in a retirement community, J Sex Med 10: 2671, 2013.

Buster J. Managing female sexual dysfunction. Fertil Steril 2013;100(4):905.

Buttaro TM, Koeniger-Donohue R, Hawkins J. Sexuality and quality of life in aging: implications for practice. J Nurse Pract 2014;10(7):480.

Capogrosso P, et al: One out of four with newly diagnosed erectile dysfunction is a young man-worrisome picture from the everyday clinical practice, J Sex Med 10: 1833, 2013.

Casey F, Gomez-Lobo V. Disparities in contraceptive access and provision. Semin Reprod Med 2013;31(5):347.

Cates W, Harwood B. Vaginal Barriers and spermicides. New York: Ardent Media; 2011. [Google Scholar] Hatcher RA, Trussell J, Nelson AL, Cates W, Kowal D, Policar M, editors. Contraceptive Technology: Twentieth Revised Edition.

Centers for Disease Control and Prevention (CDC). Estimated lifetime risk for diagnosis of HIV infection among Hispanics/Latinos—37 states and Puerto Rico, 2007. MMWR Morb Mortal Wkly Rep. 2010 Oct 15;59(40):1297–301.

Centers for Disease Control and Prevention (CDC). The state of aging and health in America. 2013b. Available from: http://www.cdc.gov/aging/pdf/state-aging-health-in-america-2013.pdf. Accessed October 2015.

Centers for Disease Control and Prevention (CDC). Genital HPV infection fact sheet. 2014b. Available from: http://www.cdc.gov/std/HPV/STDFact-HPV.htm. Accessed October 2015.

Centers for Disease Control and Prevention (CDC). Chlamydia: CDC fact sheet. 2014c. Available from: http://www.cdc.gov/std/chlamydia/STDFact-chlamydia-detailed.htm. Accessed October 2015.

Centers for Disease Control and Prevention (CDC). Adolescent and school health: sexual risk behavior: HIV, STD, & teen pregnancy prevention. 2014d. Available from: http://www.cdc.gov/HealthyYouth/sexualbehaviors/. Accessed October 2015.

Centers for Disease Control and Prevention (CDC). Chlamydial infections—2015 STD treatment guidelines. 2015a. Available from: http://www.cdc.gov/std/tg2015/chlamydia.htm. Accessed October 2015.

Centers for Disease Control and Prevention (CDC). Vaccine information statement (interim) HPV vaccine (gardasil-9) (04/15/2015). 2015b.

Available from: http://www.cdc.gov/vaccines/hcp/vis/vis-statements/hpv-gardasil-9.html. Accessed October 2015.

Cohen M, Azaiza F: Increasing breast examinations among Arab women using a tailored culture-based intervention, Behav Med 36: 92, 2010.

Dean G, Schwarz EB, editors. Intrauterine contraception. New York: Ardent Media; 2011. [Google Scholar] Hatcher RA, Trussell J, Nelson AL, Cates W, Kowal D, Policar M, editors. Contraceptive Technology: Twentieth Revised Edition.

Doty ND, et al: Sexuality-related social support among lesbian, gay, and bisexual youth, J Youth Adolesc 39: 1134, 2010.

Dunne A, et al: Adolescents, sexually transmitted infections, and education using social media: a review of the literature, J Nurse Pract 10 (6): 401, 2014.

Finer LB, Zolna MR. Shifts in intended and unintended pregnancies in the United States, 2001-2008. Am J Public Health 2014;104(S1):S43.

Garcia P. 6 Women's health apps we keep hearing about. 2014. Available from: http://www.vogue.com/946793/period-fertility-pregnancy-health-apps-for-women/. Accessed October 2015.

Giger JN. Transcultural nursing. 6th ed. St. Louis: Mosby; 2013.

Godfrey NP, et al: Contraceptive methods and use by women age 35 and over: a qualitative study of perspectives, BMC Womens Health 11 (1): 5, 2011.

Hall KS, et al: Determinants of and disparities in reproductive health service use among adolescent and young adult women in the United States, 2002-2008, Am J Public Health 102 (2): 359, 2012.

Hockenberry MJ, Wilson D. Wong's nursing care of infants and children. 10th ed. St. Louis: Mosby; 2015.

Horstman AM, Dillon EL, Urban RJ, Sheffield-Moore M. The role of androgens and estrogens on healthy aging and longevity. J Gerontol A Biol Sci Med Sci 2012;67(11):1140.

Ivarsson V, et al: Health professionals' views on sexual information following MI, Br J Nurs 19 (16): 1052, 2010.

Johnson BK. Sexually transmitted infections and older adults. J Gerontol Nurs 2013;39(11):53.

Johnson MJ, Amella EJ: Isolation of lesbian, gay, bisexual and transgender youth: a dimensional concept analysis, J AdvNurs 70 (3): 523, 2014.

Jones J, et al. Current contraceptive use in the United States, 2006–2010, and changes in patterns of use since 1995, Hyattsville, MD, 2012, National Center for Health Statistics. National health statistics reports No 60.

Kann L, Kinchen S, Shanklin SL, Flint KH, Kawkins J, Harris WA, et al. Youth risk behavior surveillance—United States, 2013. MMWR Suppl 2014;63(4):1.

Katz A. Sexuality in nursing care facilities. Am J Nurs 2013;113(3):53.

Kingsberg SA. Hypoactive sexual desire disorder: understanding the impact on midlife women. Female Patient 2011;36(3):39.

Lim FA, Brown DV Jr, Justin Kim SM. Addressing health care disparities in the lesbian, gay, bisexual, and transgender population: a review of best practices. Am J Nurs 2014;114(6):24.

Lindau ST, Gavrilova N: Sex, health and years of sexually active life gained due to good health: evidence from two US population-based cross-sectional surveys of aging, Br Med J 340: c810, 2010.

Link DG. Nursing care of the family during pregnancy. In: Lowdermilk D, Alden KR, Cashion MC, Perry SE, editor. Maternity and women's health care. 10th ed. St. Louis: Elsevier; 2012. p. 329.

Marrazzo JM, Cates W. Reproductive tract infections, including HIV and other sexually transmitted infections. New York: Ardent Media; 2011. [Google Scholar] Hatcher RA, Trussell J, Nelson AL, Cates W, Kowal D, Policar M, editors. Contraceptive Technology: Twentieth Revised Edition.

Murphy PA. Contraception and reproductive health. In: King TL, Brucker MC, editors. Pharmacology for women's health. Sudbury, MA: Jones & Bartlett; 2011.

Olson J, Forbes C, Belzer M. Management of the transgender adolescent. Arch Pediatr Adolesc Med 2011;165(2):171.

Pascoe BHM. Sexuality. In: Giddens JF, editor. Concepts of nursing practice. St. Louis: Elsevier; 2013.

Rosen RC, et al: Sexual desire problems in women seeking healthcare: a novel study design for ascertaining prevalence of hypoactive sexual desire disorder in clinic-based samples of US women, *J Women's Health* 215: 505, 2012.

Rosenthal SM. Approach to the patient: transgender youth: endocrine considerations. J Clin Endocrinol Metab 2014;99(12):4379.

Schwartz J, Gabelnick HL. Contraceptive research and development. New York: Ardent Media; 2011. [Google Scholar] Hatcher RA, Trussell J, Nelson AL, Cates W, Kowal D, Policar M, editors. Contraceptive Technology: Twentieth Revised Edition.

Steinke EE, Jaarsma T, Barnason SA, Byrne M, Doherty S, Dougherty CM, et al. Sexual counselling for individuals with cardiovascular disease and their partners: a consensus document from the American Heart Association and the ESC Council on cardiovascular nursing and allied professions (CCNAP). Eur Heart J 2013;34(41):3217.

Stewart A, Graham S. Sexual risk behavior among older adults. MMWR Recomm Rep 2013;52(RR-12):1.

Syme ML. The evolving context of older adult sexual behavior and its benefits. J Am Soc Aging 2014;38(1):35.

Touhy TA, Jett KF. Ebersole& Hess' gerontological nursing and healthy aging. 4th ed. St. Louis: Elsevier; 2014.

Trussell J, Guthrie KA. Choosing a contraceptive: efficacy, safety, and personal considerations. New York: Ardent Media; 2011. [Google Scholar] Hatcher RA, Trussell J, Nelson AL, Cates W, Kowal D, Policar M, editors. Contraceptive Technology: Twentieth Revised Edition.

U.S. Department of Health and Human Services (USDHHS). Read the law: the affordable care act, section by section. Washington, DC: US Department of Health and Human Services; 2012. Available from: http://www.hhs.gov/healthcare/rights/law/index.html. Accessed October 2015.

Williamson C. Providing care to transgender persons: a clinical approach to primary care, hormones, and HIV management. J Assoc Nurses AIDS Care 2010;21(3):221.

World Health Organization (WHO). Gender and human rights: sexual health. n.d. Available from: http://www.who.int/reproductivehealth/topics/gender_rights/sexual_health/en/. Accessed October 2015.

Young-Bruehl E. Sexual diversity in cosmopolitan perspective. Stud Gend Sex 2010;11:1.

31 *Stress and Adaptation*

OBJECTIVES

After reading this chapter, the student should be able to:

- Define the concept of stress and the importance of identifying stressors.
- Explain how stress and coping relate to the concept of health.
- Enumerate different types of stressors experienced by an individual throughout his or her lifetime.
- Discuss stress adaptation model and phases of general adaptation syndrome and local adaptation syndrome.
- Describe the coping mechanisms with illustrations of examples and strategies that can be used to manage stress.
- Explain the factors influencing stress and coping including maturational, situational, and sociocultural factors.
- Identify the effects that compassion fatigue can have in the health care workplace.
- Discuss how the stress can be managed with different techniques such as problem solving, optimism, and mindfulness.
- Understand the integration of nursing theory and role of stress including Neuman's system model and Pander's health promotion model.
- Elaborate recreational diversion therapies used in dealing with stress with a focus on the types, forms, steps, and examples of therapies used in a particular disease condition.
- Understand the importance of nursing process in managing stress and develop a care plan for a patient experiencing stress.
- Explain and demonstrate the implementation of techniques for health promotion including building resilience, regular exercise, MBSR, and assertive training.
- Discuss how acute and restorative care can be used in crisis intervention.

KEY TERMS

adventitious crises, p. 764
appraisal, p. 768
compassion fatigue, p. 770
coping, p. 764
crisis, p. 764
crisis intervention, p. 772
developmental crises, p. 764
endorphins, p. 770
flashbacks, p. 764
general adaptation syndrome (GAS), p. 765
homeostasis, p. 765
neuroendocrine stress response, p. 765
post-traumatic stress disorder (PTSD), p. 764
primary appraisal, p. 768
secondary appraisal, p. 768
situational crises, p. 764
stress, p. 764
stress management, p. 770
stressor, p. 763

INTRODUCTION

It is important to become familiar with stress to effectively assess and treat your patients and families suffering from the impact of stress. In the presence of a physical and/or mental illness, stress affects the entire family, and both the family's and the patient's health care needs must be considered in the plan of care. Equally important, health care professionals also experience stressful events in the course of clinical practice and their own lives. Nurses need to recognize the signs and symptoms of stress in the form of compassion fatigue and understand stress management techniques to aid personal coping and design stress management interventions for patients and families.

Responding to stress within the environment involves physiological and psychological processes. Stress is the disruption of body homeostasis (Miller and Callaghan, 2002). A **stressor** is any tension-producing event, such as an alarm sounding, angry patients confronting their nurses, or being informed that an emergent situation is leading to multiple admissions to your work unit. Our response to stress has the potential to adversely affect our

BOX 31.1 Factors Influencing the Response to Stressors

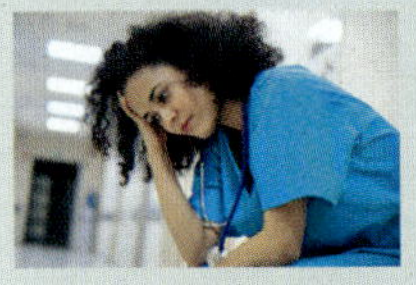
Copyright © gpointstudio/ iStock/Thinkstock.

Aspects of a Stressor That Influence the Stress Response

As Becky interviews Rachael, she learns more about Rachael's stressors and how she perceives them.

Intensity

Rachael experiences pressures at work and home. This combination of stressors creates continuous intensity.

Scope

Rachael's stress is affecting all aspects of her life, both at work and at home, day and night.

Duration

Rachael has felt the effects of stress for about 6 weeks. She has problems sleeping and feels overwhelmed and hopeless.

Number and Nature of Other Stressors Present

Rachael has multiple stressors. She has stress at home from being a caregiver of three children as well as her husband, who has physical limitations resulting from recent illnesses. There is stress from being the sole financial provider and stress at work with low staffing and low staff and patient satisfaction scores.

Predictability

Rachael is unable to anticipate or control the stressor of her husband's illness or the poor satisfaction scores.

Characteristics of the Individual That Influence the Stress Response

Level of Personal Control

Rachael feels no control over patient and staff satisfaction at work or her husband's disability.

Feelings of Competence

Rachael questions her competence at work with the lower satisfaction scores and staff leaving to work elsewhere.

Cognitive Appraisal

Rachael is telling herself that she is a failure, and she is afraid of losing her job. She is afraid of not being able to support her family. Her identity as a nurse and her image of nursing conflict with the events in her life.

Availability of Social Supports

Rachael does not report having the support of other people who could help reduce her stress.

health. When an event is perceived as a threat, exceeding our ability to immediately deal with it, **stress** results. An important part of determining whether an event leads to stress lies in the meaning that we attach to the event; this is appraisal. **Appraisal** is how a person interprets the impact of the stressor. During appraisal, a person evaluates the meaning of an event (Is it a threat or not?) and considers the available resources to help manage the stressor. This can occur very quickly (e.g., finding shelter when a storm siren and sudden gusts of winds develop) or with more reflection (e.g., addressing repeated disagreements between a work group).

Coping refers to strategies or practices that help people deal with stress (Box 31.1). Depending on the immediacy and degree of stress and the presence of other factors such as social support, coping may or may not be effective. When coping is ineffective, a degree of crisis may result. An important part of nursing is helping to promote positive adaptation in patients and families as well as in members of the health care team. This requires the ability to recognize stress in others and an awareness of how people respond to stress. To intervene effectively, you first need to be able to successfully assess for the presence of stress and the patterns of coping used by yourself and others. Stressful events will occur in the course of your clinical practice that can affect your performance as a nurse. Thus, an understanding of stress and coping is an important part of nursing.

TYPES OF STRESS

Stress arises from work, social, and family stressors that can be either chronic or acute. Examples include daily hassles, dysfunctional relationships, emotional trauma, and crisis. One person looks at a stimulus and sees it as a challenge, leading to mastery and growth. Another sees the same stimulus as a threat, leading to stress and a potential sense of loss. An individual with family responsibilities and a full-time job outside the home and who experiences a job loss or a chronic illness can experience chronic stress. Chronic stress occurs in stable conditions and from stressful roles. Living with a long-term illness produces chronic stress. Conversely, time-limited events that threaten a person for a relatively brief period (e.g., death of a family member or friend) provoke acute stress.

Post-traumatic stress disorder (PTSD) is a mental health problem that some people develop after experiencing or witnessing a life-threatening event, such as military combat, physical assault, or a natural disaster. The person responds with a sense of intense fear or helplessness. There are four types of PTSD symptoms: (1) reliving the event (bad memories, nightmares), (2) avoiding situations that remind the person of the event, (3) having more negative beliefs and feelings about oneself or the world, and (4) hyperarousal (anxiety, irritability, trouble sleeping). Some people with PTSD experience **flashbacks**, or recurrent and intrusive recollections of the event. Depression and PTSD commonly occur together, and both are associated with self-destructive behaviors such as suicide attempts and substance abuse (Stevens et al., 2013).

A **crisis** implies that a person is facing a turning point in life. This means that previous ways of coping are not effective. There are three types of crises: (1) maturational or **developmental crises**, (2) **situational crises**, and (3) **adventitious crises** (Varcarolis, 2017). A new developmental stage such as marriage, birth of a child, or retirement requires new coping styles. Developmental crises occur as a person moves through the stages of life. External sources such as a job change, a motor vehicle crash, a death, or a severe illness provoke situational crises. An adventitious or social crisis is a rare and unexpected tragedy that may affect an entire community or population, such as a major natural disaster, man-made disaster, or violent crime.

Patient-centered care provides an important context for any crisis intervention (Gillespie and Gates, 2013). The vital questions for a person in crisis are the following: "What does this mean to you?" "How does it affect your life?" What causes extreme stress for one person is not always stressful to another. The perception of the event, situational supports, and coping mechanisms all influence return of equilibrium. A person either grows or regresses as a result of a crisis, depending on how he or she manages the situation (Gillespie and Gates, 2013; Varcarolis, 2017).

STRESS ADAPTATION

Hans Selye, a Vienna-born endocrinologist, was the first scientist to single out the physical side effects of stress. While conducting experiments related to hormone production, Selye noticed that his subjects showed a similar set of side effects regardless of the type of life-threatening stimulus that researchers presented. Selye termed this collection of responses the **general adaptation syndrome (GAS)**, a three-stage set of physiological processes that prepare, or adapt, the body for danger so that an individual is more likely to survive when faced with a threat (Waude, 2016).

General Adaptation Syndrome

Selye (1993) identified the three stages to the stress response as (1) initial alarm, (2) resistance as a person attempts to compensate for changes induced by the alarm stage, and (3) a state of exhaustion if the person cannot adapt successfully during the stage of resistance or if stress remains unrelieved. When stress reaches chronic and harmful levels, negative consequences follow. Selye's initial theory has evolved as scientists have learned more about the physiological responses to stress.

Neuroendocrine Stress Response

When there is a stressor within our environment, our sensory system is the first to play a role in the stress response. When someone confronts an oncoming car or hears an alarm, the eyes or ears (or both) send the information to the amygdala, an area of the brain that processes emotions (Harvard Medical School, 2016). The amygdala interprets the sensory images and sounds and, when it perceives danger, instantly sends a distress signal to the hypothalamus, which is the command center for responding to stress. When stress is perceived, the hypothalamus activates one of the following two systems: (1) the hypothalamic–pituitary–adrenal (HPA) axis, and (2) the sympathetic nervous system (SNS) (Miller & O'Callaghan, 2002; Smith & Vale, 2006). This results in a series of neural and endocrine adaptations known as the **neuroendocrine stress response**. A cascade of events allows the two systems to make the necessary physiological and metabolic changes required to maintain homeostasis. The effects of stress are both immediate and long-term (Fig. 31.1), with each response resulting in different physiological reactions from the two systems (Table 31.1).

Fight or Flight—Alarm

In the alarm stage described by Selye (1993), the hypothalamus communicates with the rest of the body through the autonomic nervous system so that a person has the energy to fight or flee. The autonomic nervous system has two components: the SNS and the parasympathetic nervous system. The SNS functions like a gas pedal in a car for triggering the fight-or-flight response (Harvard Medical School, 2016), giving the body a burst of energy so that it can respond to perceived dangers. The parasympathetic nervous system acts like a brake to promote the "rest and digest" response that calms down the body after the danger has passed (Harvard Medical School, 2016).

When there is an initial perceived stressor, the hypothalamus activates the SNS for a short-term response by stimulating the release of epinephrine and norepinephrine from the adrenal gland. The response prepares a person for action by increasing heart and respiratory rates, dilating the bronchioles, diverting blood from the intestines to the brain and striated muscles, and increasing blood pressure and blood glucose levels. As a result, extra oxygen is sent to the brain, increasing a person's alertness and causing sight, hearing, and other senses to become sharper (Harvard Medical School, 2016). The release of glucose and fats from temporary storage sites in the body supply energy to all parts of the body. The physiological fight-or-flight response happens so quickly that people aren't aware of it. This is why a person can jump out of the way of an incoming car before even thinking about what he or she is doing.

Long-Term Stress Response—Resistance

After the initial surge of epinephrine subsides, the hypothalamus activates the HPA axis to keep the SNS activated (the gas pedal is still pressed down) (Harvard Medical School, 2016). The HPA axis responds to a stressor primarily through the synthesis and/or release of three key hormones: corticotropin-releasing factor (CRF), adrenocorticotropic hormone (ACTH), and the glucocorticoid hormone cortisol (Miller & O'Callaghan, 2002) (see Fig. 31.1). If the brain continues to perceive something as a threat, the hypothalamus releases CRF, which travels to the pituitary gland and triggers the release of ACTH. ACTH then travels to the adrenal glands, prompting the release of cortisol and vasopressin. Cortisol increases blood glucose, enhances the use of glucose by the brain, and increases the availability of substances for tissue repair. Vasopressin increases resorption of water by the kidneys and causes vasoconstriction, raising blood pressure. Thus, the body stays revved up and on high alert. Cortisol will be released for several hours after encountering a stressor.

Once a certain blood concentration of cortisol is reached, the "protection" against stress is met and the cortisol exerts negative feedback to the hypothalamic release of CRF and the pituitary release of ACTH. At this point, systemic homeostasis returns (Alschuler, 2016). **Homeostasis** is a state of physiological balance in which the body has a chance to recover from the physiological activation experienced during stress. As cortisol levels fall, the parasympathetic nervous system acts as a "brake" to dampen the stress response (Harvard Medical School, 2016). Over time the body may experience an excessive state of activation that cannot be inhibited by the parasympathetic system. Alternatively, the ability of the parasympathetic system to respond to stress may be reduced. This pattern of response reflects the stages of resistance.

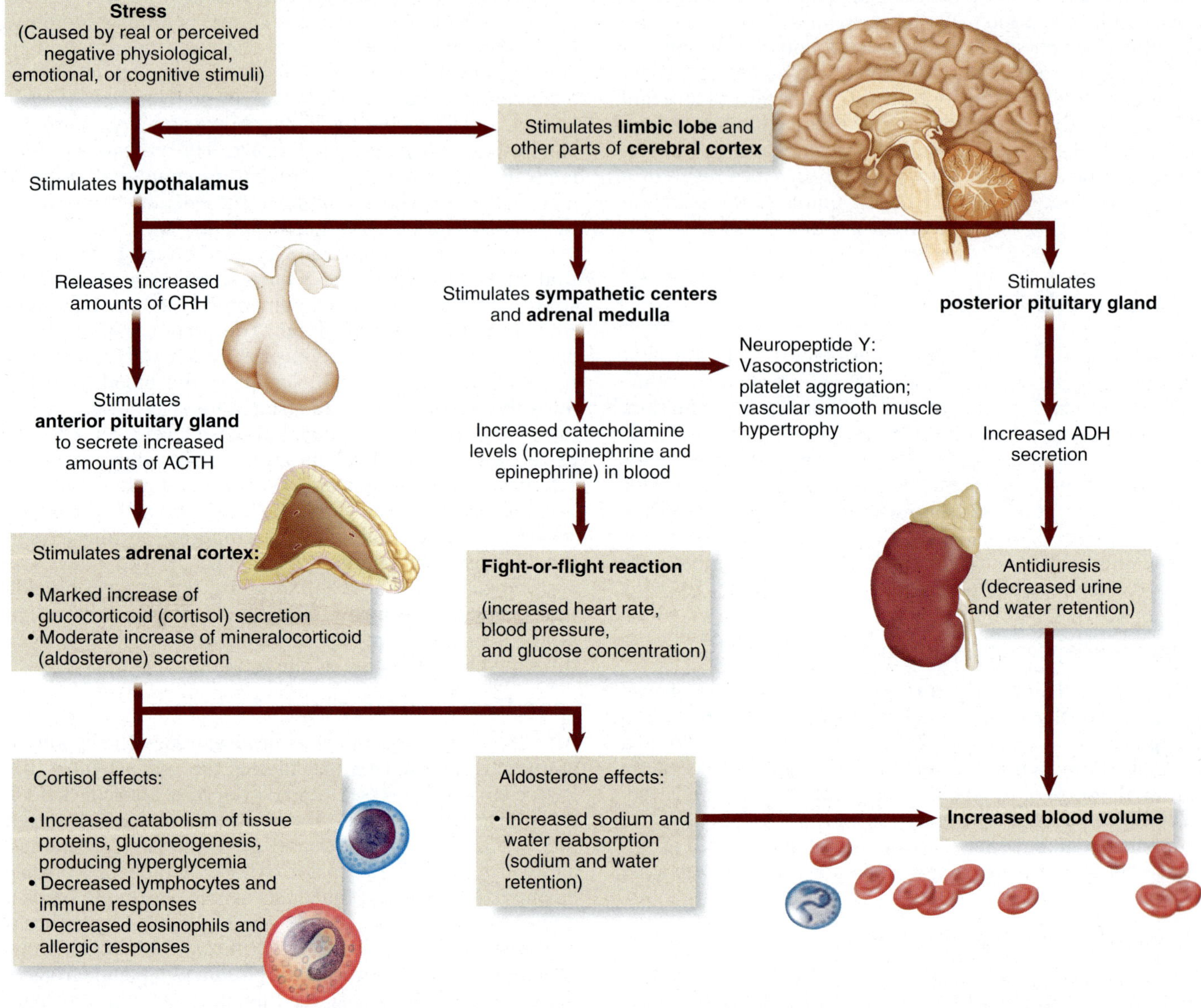

Fig. 31.1 Short-term and long-term stress response. Some effects are immediate, such as the sympathetic fight-or-flight reaction, and some effects are longer term, such as the hormonal effects. *ACTH*, adrenocorticotropic hormone; *ADH*, antidiuretic hormone; *CRH*, corticotropin-releasing hormone. (From Patton KT: *Anatomy & physiology*, ed 10, St Louis, 2019, Elsevier.)

Exhaustion From Continued Stress

The release of cortisol during the normal stress response curbs bodily functions that are nonessential in or detrimental to a fight-or-flight situation. For example, immune system responses are altered and digestive system, reproductive system, and growth processes are suppressed (Mayo Clinic, 2016). The body's stress response system is usually self-limiting. Once a perceived threat has passed, hormone levels return to normal and the body adapts physiologically. However, when stressors are always present and a person constantly feels threatened or under attack, the fight-or-flight reaction stays turned on, exhaustion develops, and serious health consequences occur (Mayo Clinic, 2016). Individuals can become more vulnerable to infection and develop anxiety, depression, heart disease, weight gain, memory and concentration impairment, and sleep problems.

Immune Response

The immune system is integrated with other physiological processes and is sensitive to changes in the central nervous system and endocrine functioning that occur during the stress response. The stress response directly influences the immune system (Huether and McCance, 2017). One effect of long-term stress is the influence of cortisol on T-lymphocyte cells, which are an essential component of cell-mediated immunity. T cells respond to molecules called interleukins by way of a signaling pathway. Cortisol blocks T cells from proliferating by preventing some T cells from recognizing the interleukin signals. It also reduces inflammation due to inhibition of histamine secretion. Continued exposure to stress thus causes prolonged changes in the immune system, which can result in increased risk for infection, as well as high blood pressure,

Table 31.1 Physical and Psychological Manifestations of Stress

System	Assessment Findings
Physical	
Cardiovascular	Tightness of chest Increased heart rate Elevated blood pressure
Respiratory	Breathing shallow Tachypnea
Neuroendocrine	Headaches, migraines Fatigue, exhaustion Insomnia, sleep disturbances Feeling uncoordinated Restlessness, hyperactivity Tremors (lips, hands) Profuse sweating (palms) Dry mouth Cold hands and feet
Gastrointestinal/ genitourinary	Urinary frequency Nausea, diarrhea, vomiting Weight gain or loss of more than 10 lb Change in appetite Gastrointestinal bleeding
Diagnostic	Blood in stools/vomitus Elevated blood glucose level Elevated cortisol levels
Musculoskeletal	Backaches, muscle aches Bruxism (clenched jaw) Slumped posture
Reproductive	Amenorrhea Failure to ovulate Impotency in men Loss of libido
Immunological	Frequent or prolonged colds/flu
Psychological	
Cognitive	Forgetfulness/preoccupation Denial Poor concentration Inattention to detail Orientation to past instead of present Decreased creativity Slower thinking, problem solving, reactions Learning difficulties Apathy Confusion Decreased attention span Calculation difficulties Memory problems
Emotional	Disruption of logical thinking Blaming others Lack of motivation to get up in the morning Crying tendencies Lack of interest Irritability Isolation Diminished initiative
Behavior/lifestyle	Worrying Decreased involvement with others Withdrawal Change in interactions with others Increased or decreased food intake Increased smoking or alcohol intake Overvigilance to environment Excessive humor or silence No exercise

diabetes, and cancer (Janowski et al., 2014; Moreira et al., 2014).

Local Adaptation Syndrome

The **local adaptation syndrome** (LAS) is the term defined as a local inflammatory response and repair process that usually occurs at the injury site and in case of severe injury it proceeds to GAS. According to Selye, stress is a general response that can occur in all types of stressors, that is, physical, psychological, and social. LAS also occurs in the same three stages and is inter-related to GAS. In response to general stress or acute stress, inflammation occurs and regulators of endocrine glands are also initiated to control the inflammatory response. Stages of LAS are associated with the stages of GAS. It would be easier to understand or relate the phases of GAS, that is, alarm, resistance, and exhaustion, to those of LAS, that is, acute and chronic phases. The progression of the stages varies from individual to individual and depends on many factors such as age, gender, nutritional status, health status, and lifestyle behavior.

Acute Local Adaptation

In response to any of the body stressors such as injury, trauma, or any immediate reflex, there will be an increase in muscle tone that further leads to ischemia and retention of metabolites. This can be defined as acute local adaptation and alarm phase in GAS. If ischemia and retention of metabolites persist, then they cause fatigue and the site of injury appears sensitive to touch and signs of inflammation also occur. There will be pain, which can become worse over time because of increased muscle tone.

Chronic Local Adaptation

In case the phase of acute local adaptation lasts for longer than few weeks, the body is at continuous exposure of stressors. This exposure of local stressors for a prolonged period of time can produce collagen and bundles of fibers are reformed with the help of these collagens to maintain the hypertonic muscles of the body. Thus, it leads to chronic adaptation. Pain in this phase also starts radiating from the site of trauma to distant areas, which leads to the development of myofascial trigger points, and lack of oxygen supply along with an increased retention of metabolites is considered to be the reason for this occurrence. Local adaptation of tendons and tendon-periosteal junction commonly occur because of this increased muscle tone. When body uses all its capacity to deal with the trauma or stressor, it enters into an exhaustive phase and it can take months to years to enter into this stage. As a result of this, dysfunction or changes occur in muscles, tissues, and joints.

PHYSICAL AND PSYCHOLOGICAL MANIFESTATIONS OF STRESS

The objective findings related to stress and coping may be assessed by observing a patient's appearance and nonverbal behavior. Observe grooming and hygiene, gait, characteristics of the patient's handshake, actions of the patient while sitting, quality of speech, facial expression and eye contact, and the attitude of the patient toward you during the interview. It is also important to assess physical signs of stress; depending on the anxiety level of the patient, take basic vital signs to assess for physiological signs of stress such as elevated blood pressure, heart rate, or respiratory rate. The physical and psychological manifestations of stress have been illustrated in Table 31.1.

COPING MECHANISMS

When a person encounters a stressor, there is an immediate process of **primary appraisal** or rating of the event. If primary appraisal results in the person identifying the event or circumstance as a harm, loss, threat, or challenge, the person experiences stress. At the same time, the person is also considering possible coping strategies or resources available to help deal with the event; this process is referred to as **secondary appraisal**. If demands placed on the person exceed the ability to cope, stress continues.

No single coping strategy works for everyone or for every stressor. Coping is important to physical and psychological health because stress is associated with a range of psychological and health outcomes (Doron et al., 2014). Effective coping strategies use a person's cognitive and behavioral traits to manage a stressor (Nielson and Knardahl, 2014). A person also copes differently at different times.

In stressful situations, most people use a combination of physiological, problem-focused, and emotion-focused coping strategies. In other words, when under stress, a person learns to relax physically (physiological), obtain information, take action to change the situation (problem-focused), and regulate emotions tied to the stress (emotion-focused). In some cases, people avoid thinking about the situation or change the way they think about it without changing the actual situation itself.

Every individual experiences stress in his or her lifetime that challenges or produces a threat to ego. Conscious and unconscious ego defense/coping mechanisms are generally used by an individual to deal with the stressful situations of day-to-day life and most of the used defense mechanisms are unconscious except suppression that is used consciously.

All the defense/coping mechanisms are used by normally healthy individuals to deal with their stressors. Coping mechanisms or ego defense mechanisms are not considered as psychotic, neurotic, and immature, but can become so if they are used excessively. An adaptive or maladaptive response of a person depends on whether the use of coping mechanisms was constructive or destructive. Use of coping mechanisms generally depends on the following:

1. Availability of a support system
2. Individual's capability to use defense mechanism

Psychological Coping Mechanism

There are many ego defense mechanisms that can be used but repression is defined as a primary coping mechanism by Sigmund Freud. Furthermore, defense mechanisms are commonly divided under different categories such as neurotic, psychotic, and mature. Below-mentioned are examples of defense mechanisms under these categories:

1. **Psychotic defense mechanisms**: Regression, denial, projection, and distortion
2. **Neurotic defense mechanisms:** Conversion, dissociation, displacement, isolation, reaction formation, undoing, rationalization, intellectualization, acting out, schizoid fantasy, introjection, hypochondriasis, inhibition, compensation, and splitting
3. **Mature defense mechanisms:** Sublimation, suppression, anticipation, and humor

Defense Mechanisms Used for Coping

The commonly used defense mechanisms used for coping are discussed as follows:

1. **Compensation:** It refers to the tendency of an individual to perform extraordinarily in any one aspect of life to overcome or compensate the failure of another aspect. Example: An adult man who is a smoker also indulges into a fitness routine to maintain health and compensate for the bad habit of smoking.
2. **Denial:** It refers to an inability to accept the reality or a denial response to avoid accountability of any action. Example: Substance abusers will deny the fact that they have a problem and a person denies the death of a loved one whenever unable to accept the reality in a grief phase.
3. **Displacement:** It is defined as relocating your anger or frustration toward a less fearful object or person rather than toward the one who was the reason behind it. Example: If a person is given reprimand by his boss, then rather than arguing with the boss, the person yells at his child when he has returned home.
4. **Introjection:** It is the complete opposite of projection in which an individual projects his/her own ideas and beliefs onto others. In introjection, the values, ideas, and opinions of the other person are internalized as own and it commonly occurs in children when they internalize the views or beliefs of their parents without giving a thought over it. Example: A lady who is a victim of domestic violence begins to believe or internalize the belief of her husband and considers herself wrong and guilty. This sort of introjection with the abuser is called as Stockholm syndrome.
5. **Projection:** It is defined as projecting or attributing one's own unacceptable or anxiety-provoking ideas, beliefs, or feelings as of others. In this, a person blames others for his/her own actions or desires. Example: A daughter-in-law hates her mother-in-law but her superego suggests that such feelings are unacceptable. So, she can resolve this conflict by considering that her mother-in-law hates her.
6. **Rationalization:** It is defined as a coping mechanism in which a person gives a reason or justification for his or her unacceptable or undesirable behavior or feelings. Example: A student who had not studied well for exam and performed poorly in exams blames his teacher for not teaching properly.
7. **Reaction formation:** It is defined as an expression of completely opposite impulses or attitude to reduce anxiety. According to Freud, people behave in an opposite manner to hide their genuine feelings, attitude, or impulses. Example: A girl who eats junk food and has a binge eating habit applauds the benefits of healthy eating practices.

8. **Repression:** It refers to unconsciously pushing out the unwanted thoughts or impulses out of conscious awareness. Freud technique of free association is based on repression as it explores repressed ideas and impulses. Example: A child suffering from abusive parenting at home completely forgets his experience when he has grown up as an adult. Forgetting the painful events can be called as an example of repression.
9. **Sublimation:** It is defined as a defense mechanism that is similar to displacement except one difference that in sublimation, a person displaces his/her unacceptable desires or emotions into socially acceptable and more constructive behavior. Example: A person who is aggressive in nature uses his aggressive impulses in sports and performs extraordinarily. Many musicians and artists who had a history of problematic life express their emotions in their artworks and music.
10. **Undoing:** It is defined as a coping mechanism in which a person tries to undo or eliminate destructive or threatening ideas and actions by getting involved into contrary or opposite behavior. Example: After a fight between siblings, one of them who initiated the fight brought a gift for another. This is considered as a response to undo the previous action by becoming nice to the person instead of directly apologizing for his or her mistake.

FACTORS INFLUENCING STRESS AND COPING

Potential stressors and coping mechanisms vary across the life span (e.g., adolescence, adulthood, and old age bring different stressors). The appraisal of stressors, the amount and type of social support, and coping strategies all balance when assessing stress and depend on previous life experiences. Furthermore, situational and social stressors place people who are vulnerable at higher risk for prolonged stress.

Situational, Maturational, and Sociocultural Factors

Potential stressors and coping mechanisms vary across the life span. For example, adolescence, adulthood, and old age bring different stressors related to separating from family, establishing oneself as an adult, and making a contribution to society. Likewise, coping strategies fluctuate from an emphasis on primarily emotional coping to problem solving as our minds grow and thinking develops.

Situational Factors

Stressors in the workplace that affect nurses and other health care professionals include high-acuity patient load, job environment, constant distractions, responsibility, conflicting priorities, and intensity of care (e.g., trauma, emergency, or critical care areas) (Ianello and Balzarotti, 2014; Mealer et al., 2014; Najimi et al., 2012). In addition, changing shifts increases fatigue and work-related stress. Coping strategies vary with the individual and the situation.

Some nurses often ease coping with shift work by knowing their own circadian rhythms. People who function best in the morning have the greatest difficulty with night work and changing shifts. As people age, they tend to become more morning oriented. Morning people need to be counseled about the potentially negative effects of night work for them. In general, people doing shift work need to maintain as consistent a sleep and mealtime schedule as possible (Lin et al., 2014; Sabo, 2011).

Adjusting to chronic illness is a situational stress. The physical limitations posed by a disease state and the uncertainty associated with treatment and illness trigger stress in patients of all ages. Sometimes illness changes how people manage their stress. For example, Parelkar et al. (2015) found that cancer survivors who made active efforts to control stress changed their physical, psychosocial, and preventive health behaviors during and after cancer treatment. Having difficulty paying for treatment and limited access to health care providers also create stress. Although being a family caregiver for someone with a chronic illness such as Alzheimer disease is stressful, the actions of competent health care providers often help minimize the stress for family caregivers.

Maturational Factors

Stressors vary with life stage. Children identify stressors related to physical appearance, family dynamics, friendships, and school. Preadolescents experience stress related to self-esteem issues, hospitalizations, or changing family structure as a result of divorce or death of a parent. Adolescents experience stress as they search for identity with peer groups and separate from their families. In addition, they face stressful questions about using mind-altering substances, sex, jobs, school, and career choices. Stress for adults centers around major changes in life circumstances. These include the many milestones of beginning a family and a career, losing parents, seeing children leave home, and accepting physical aging. In old age, stressors include the loss of autonomy and mastery resulting from general frailty or health problems that limit stamina, strength, and cognition (Box 31.2).

BOX 31.2 Care of an Older Adult

Coping Strategies

Some older adults report better mental health than younger adults because older adults appraise and cope with stress differently. Coping strategies to assist in healthy aging include the following:

- Organizing objects in the environment such as canes, walkers, handrails, hearing aids, amplifiers on telephones, and magnifying glasses to enhance daily functioning.
- Using life experiences and stress management techniques to cope with family, health, or residential stressors (Rayens and Reed, 2014).
- De-emphasizing health problems by using positive comparisons with peers and finding others who are more disabled with whom they can compare themselves.
- Using dyadic coping (two people), or joint coping, to compensate for memory problems and other physical deficits. The spouse or partner anticipates the other's needs and helps as needed. Anticipatory guidance can reduce the stress on both partners (Rayens and Reed, 2014).

Sociocultural Factors

Environmental and social stressors can lead to developmental problems. Potential stressors affect any age group, but they are especially stressful for young people. These include prolonged poverty, physical handicap, and chronic illness. The vulnerability of children escalates when they lose relationships with parents and caregivers through divorce, abandonment, imprisonment, or death or when parents have mental illness or substance-abuse disorders. Furthermore, living under conditions of continuing violence, disintegrated neighborhoods, or homelessness affects people of any age, but these factors are especially stressful to young people (Pender and Murdaugh, 2015).

Cultural variations produce stress, particularly if a person's values differ from the dominant culture in aspects of gender roles, family relationships, and religious beliefs (Giger, 2016). Other aspects of cultural variations begin with language difference, geographical location, family relationships, time orientation, access to health care programs, and disparities in health care (Box 31.3). Uncertainty about immigration status and citizenship can contribute to increased stress.

BOX 31.3 Patient-Centered Care

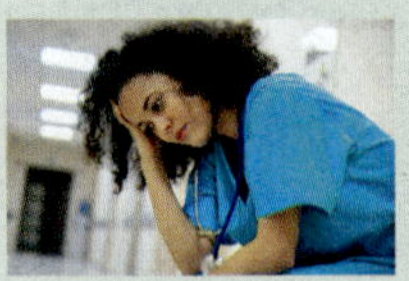

Stress and anxiety sometimes lead to insomnia, as in Rachael's case. Cultural factors influence a person's health behaviors and also influence the quality of a person's sleep (Garcia, 2016). There are significant differences in sleeping habits and routines as well as rates of insomnia among ethnic groups (Giger, 2016).

Implications for Practice

- Ask patients what their family members, especially their parents, do when they cannot sleep to learn about their cultural values associated with insomnia.
- Help patients connect their insomnia with the stress that they are experiencing by asking them what they think about while they are lying in bed awake.
- Ask patients with insomnia which coping strategies they have tried. Determine whether their coping measures include culturally specific remedies.
- If folk or culturally specific remedies are used to improve sleeping, verify that these remedies do not interact with the patient's prescribed medication.

COMPASSION FATIGUE

Compassion fatigue is a term used to describe a state of burnout and secondary traumatic stress (Potter et al., 2013). Secondary traumatic stress is the stress that health care providers experience when witnessing and caring for others who are suffering. Examples include an oncology nurse who cares for patients undergoing surgery and chemotherapy over the long term for their cancer or a spouse who witnesses his wife deteriorating over the years from Alzheimer disease. Burnout occurs when perceived demands outweigh perceived resources (Potter et al., 2013). It is a state of physical and mental fatigue and exhaustion that often affects health care providers because of the nature of their work environment. Perceived inadequate staffing, long work shifts, demands of patient acuity, and dysfunctional relationships (patients and other care providers) serve as triggers for ongoing stress. Over time, giving of oneself in often intense caring environments can result in emotional exhaustion, leaving a nurse feeling irritable, restless, and unable to focus and engage with patients. This condition may be viewed as a failure of coping because it often occurs in situations in which there is a lack of social support, organizational pressures influencing staffing, and the inability of a nurse to practice self-care.

Compassion fatigue is a condition that can overwhelm health care providers and cause physical, mental, and emotional health issues (Hunsaker et al., 2015). The feelings of hopelessness and anxiety from compassion fatigue usually result in feelings of inadequacy and lower self-esteem. These factors can lead to the health care provider lashing out in an attempt to cope with these feelings and stress. This often manifests itself as *lateral violence*, which refers to a deliberate and harmful behavior demonstrated in the workplace by one employee to another. This includes health care providers engaging in bullying and potentially assaultive behaviors toward coworkers (Christie and Jones, 2013; Embree and White, 2010).

Early recognition of the risk for compassion fatigue is essential. A supportive work environment helps guide a nursing unit in designing communication techniques to identify, prevent, and adapt to potential compassion fatigue situations (Hunsaker et al., 2015).

STRESS MANAGEMENT

There are several techniques that can be used to cope with generalized stress and arousal, with an aim to relax and soothe the body and mind. Physical relaxation aims to switch the body from sympathetic to parasympathetic dominance to restore homeostasis to the HPA axis. Other coping resources include problem-solving skills, financial status, social skills, supportive family and friends, physical attractiveness, health and energy, and personal stress management techniques such as optimism and mindfulness (O'Driscoll, 2013; van den Hurk et al., 2015). For example, physical exercise, relaxation strategies, and letting go of excess anger reduce physical and psychological tension. Exercise improves circulation and triggers the release of **endorphins**. The relaxation response, elicited by meditation or progressive muscle relaxation, restores parasympathetic function to lower blood pressure, pulse rate, and respiratory rate.

Psychological adaptive behaviors, or ego defense mechanisms, regulate emotional distress and protect a person from anxiety and stress. When you recognize that a patient is using an ego defense mechanism such as denial or displacement, do not point this out to the patient or suggest that the defense mechanism is unhealthy. Denial often helps a patient reduce stress to a manageable level until he or she can cope with it. Displacement means transferring emotions from a stressful situation to a less anxiety-producing substitute. For example, this can happen if a patient acts angrily toward a nurse when the patient is worried about his or her illness, pain, or trauma. Accept the patient's response, listen, and try to learn the specific source of his or her emotions.

Health Promotion

Intervention for relieving stress has a three-pronged approach: (1) decrease stress-producing situations, (2) increase resistance to stress, and (3) learn skills that reduce physiological response to stress (Pender, 2016; Pender and Murdaugh, 2015). First, help patients reduce the frequency of stress-inducing situations by using strategies such as instituting positive workplace habits, avoiding excessive change, and effectively managing one's personal time (Hunsaker et al., 2015). Next, increase a patient's resistance to stress by building resiliency and recommending physical and psychological conditioning, which includes enhancing self-esteem, increasing assertiveness, setting realistic goals, and building coping resources. Finally, use relaxation strategies to reduce physiological arousal (Pender and Murdaugh, 2015). As a nurse, you educate patients and families about the importance of stress reduction (Box 31.4).

BOX 31.4 Patient Teaching

Stress Reduction

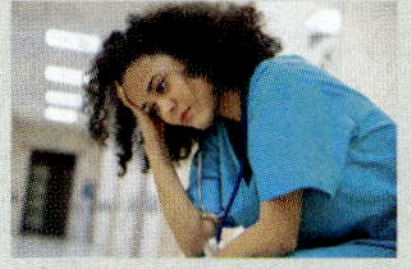

Copyright © gpointstudio/ iStock/Thinkstock.

Becky recognizes that Rachael wants to learn how to increase her resistance to stress. Becky develops the following teaching plan for Rachael.

Outcome

At the end of the teaching session, Rachael verbally identifies two methods to reduce her stress.

Teaching Strategies

- Meet with Rachael in a quiet and private setting at a time when Rachael has about 1 h to talk without interruptions.
- Schedule a follow-up hour about a week after the first session.
- Encourage Rachael to focus on two stress management strategies: regular exercise and mindfulness training.
- Ask Rachael to maintain a daily record of her physical exercise and mindfulness strategies.
- Explore with Rachael her support system, possibilities for continuing education, financial status, and her personal appearance, depending on her identified needs (Pender and Murdaugh, 2015).
- For developing insight about maintaining appropriate boundaries between work and personal space, explore with Rachael ways that she will increase awareness of her feelings of anger, pain, hurt, sadness, and joy. Discuss with her how she will recognize the limits of her responsibilities.
- Ask Rachael to keep a personal journal of her feelings for the next week.

Evaluation

- Use the principles of teach back to evaluate patient/family caregiver learning:
  - Review with Rachael her record of exercise and mindfulness activities during the week.
  - Ask Rachael to evaluate her progress toward her goal of increased resistance to stress.

Building Resiliency

Most programs aimed at improving a person's resilience recommend approaches that take a public health approach by suggesting general ways to prepare for challenges before they occur (MacLeod et al, 2016). One example is the APA's campaign to increase awareness of and provide resources for building resilience (APA, 2015). A Resilience Toolkit recommends approaches to building resilience, including maintaining strong relationships and social support, becoming active in the community, thinking positively, and maintaining hopefulness.

Regular Exercise and Rest

A regular exercise program improves muscle tone and posture, controls weight, reduces tension, improves circulation, triggers the release of endorphins, and promotes relaxation. It is important for patients to engage in exercise activities that promote stretching, improve balance, and increase conditioning. In addition, exercise reduces the risk for cardiovascular disease and improves cardiopulmonary functioning.

Regular rest and sleep help manage stress and stress-related fatigue. Encourage patients and their families to adopt regular sleep routines (see Chapter 10). People who are well rested are often able to manage stress, problem solve, and maintain control over some situations (Akerstedt et al., 2014).

Progressive Muscle Relaxation

Muscles tense during stressful thoughts and events. Physiological tension diminishes through a systematic approach to releasing tension in major muscle groups. In addition, this aids the parasympathetic nervous system to become dominant and achieve better balance. When helping a patient achieve a relaxed state, have the patient breathe deeply. Then direct the patient to relax muscles in areas that feel stiffened. Other controlled relaxation exercises such as yoga are effective in regulating stress responses and reducing blood pressure (Doron et al., 2014).

Support Systems

Patients experiencing stress benefit from a support system of family and friends who listen, offer advice, share recreation time, and provide emotional support (Doron et al., 2014). People with strong networks of friends, neighbors, and family tend to be healthier than people without support systems. Many organizations such as the American Heart Association, the American Cancer Society, local hospitals and churches, and mental health organizations offer support group services to individuals. Acceptable support systems vary by cultural group. For example, one cultural group might rely heavily on church members for support. Another cultural group values individual privacy and prefers to avoid a self-help group with "strangers."

Mindfulness-Based Stress Reduction

Mindfulness is a moment-to-moment present awareness with an attitude of nonjudgment, acceptance, and openness (Lengacher et al., 2014). Mindfulness-based stress reduction (MBSR) meditative practice is effective in reducing stressful psychological and physical symptoms or perceptions. It is an intervention that emphasizes optimism and positive emotions to enhance happiness, improve resilience, and boost well-being more effectively than reducing negative behaviors (MacLeod et al., 2016).

MBSR is effective in stress management and symptom control with certain chronic conditions including some cancers (Lengacher et al., 2015). Mindfulness training helps people learn to self-regulate awareness, identify their feelings, and implement effective changes. People use cognitive exercises and subjective experiences to process images or feelings (van den Hurk et al., 2015). These feelings are then evaluated as pleasant or unpleasant. A patient learns strategies to enhance the pleasant experiences and replace the unpleasant experiences. MBSR can be used in a variety of settings. For example, MBSR can help people control their stress response to illnesses and treatments, allow employees to manage job-related stress, and help students manage classroom stress and test anxiety.

Assertiveness Training

Assertiveness training teaches individuals to communicate effectively regarding their needs and desires. The ability to resolve conflict with others through assertiveness training reduces stress. Teaching assertiveness in a group setting increases the benefits of the experience because the participants can see how people in the group interact with one another.

Stress Management in the Workplace

Dealing with stress in the workplace as a health care provider requires a different approach for stress management. Rapid changes in health care systems and technology, organizational restructuring, ability to retain qualified staff, and changing regulatory demands place stress on nurses. Additional causes of job stress include patient acuity levels, particular job assignments, difficult schedules, shift work, fear of failure, and inadequate support services. Compassion fatigue occurs as a result of chronic stress and is associated with the human service professions (Hunsaker et al., 2015; Potter et al., 2013).

It is important that nurses participate in self-care practices. Some settings such as oncology put nurses at a higher risk for experiencing compassion fatigue because nurses see patients frequently return for care as their clinical conditions deteriorate. Recently researchers found that in other high-stress clinical settings such as critical care, trauma, and emergency departments, resilience training and clinical debriefing improved nurses' abilities to manage stress, thus reducing burnout and nursing staff turnover (Hunsaker et al., 2015; Ianello and Balzarotti, 2014; Mealer et al., 2014). Shift work and changes in schedule also contribute to work-related stress. Allowing nurses to self-schedule has been shown to provide some autonomy and choice in scheduling, which often reduces job-related stress, improves sleep quality, and improves collaboration and teamwork (Nguyen-Rodriguez et al., 2015).

If you recognize feelings of compassion fatigue, learn how to identify perceived threats that are sources of stress (e.g., angry coworker, added patient assignment, sense of not getting work done) and practice relaxation when you perceive them (Edward et al., 2014). Being able to relax at a time of perceived threat helps to switch off sympathetic dominance and allows you to think more clearly with purpose. In addition, identify the limits and scope of your responsibilities at work. Recognize what you can and cannot control and try to separate your work from your home life. Engage in an activity that is creative and active so that the stress of work will not intrude your thinking. Strengthening friendships outside of the workplace, socially finding ways for personal "recharging" of emotional energy, and spending off-duty hours in interesting activities all help reduce burnout.

Crisis Intervention

When stress overwhelms a person's usual coping mechanisms and demands mobilization of all available resources, the stress becomes a crisis. **Crisis intervention** is different from counseling. It requires excellent nurse–patient communication skills (see Chapter 4). Crisis intervention provides more direction than brief psychotherapy or counseling. It focuses on how intensely a patient views his or her problems as intolerable or how emotionally unstable a patient is. Knowledgeable members of the interdisciplinary health care team are able to initiate crisis intervention (Varcarolis, 2017).

Crisis intervention begins with defining the problem, ensuring patient safety, and providing support. First, determine that a patient is safe and not at risk for injury to self or others. Then help the patient examine alternatives, make plans, and obtain a commitment to positive action. Ideally these last three steps are completed collaboratively with a patient, but a patient in crisis may be unable to participate actively and may need a very directive approach or a crisis interventionist.

When using crisis intervention, help a person become aware of present feelings such as anger, grief, guilt, or tension. Using open-ended questions elicits feelings and responses with deeper meaning. Closed-ended questions provide important information early in the crisis intervention process. Focus on the specific problem and help a patient avoid all-encompassing, catastrophic interpretations. You may need to provide guidance and direction for obtaining resources and assistance. Provide an atmosphere of calm acceptance, yet be aware of situations that require a direct approach to ensure the safety of the patient. Capitalize on a patient's strengths when helping patients identify coping strategies, such as previous hobbies, an interest in music or sports, or religious faith (Krägeloh et al., 2015).

RECREATIONAL DIVERSION THERAPIES

Recreation includes a form of activities that are usually performed in free or leisure time for pleasure and satisfaction of personal needs. Recreation therapies are also considered as therapeutic activities where recreation-based interventions or activities are performed to promote physical, psychological, mental, social, and overall well-being of an individual. Although recreation activities are required for every individual, they play an important role in the life of people who are experiencing stress, depression, and other chronic disabilities.

Objectives of Recreational Therapies

1. To enhance the full potential of an individual including physical, mental, social, and emotional aspects
2. To minimize suffering and disability
3. To ventilate emotions and feelings
4. To improve the overall quality of life

Types of Recreational Therapies

It is difficult to define recreational therapies under particular headings because any type of activity that diverts an individual's mind and gives pleasure can be defined as a recreational therapy. It is broadly divided into indoor activities and outdoor activities and it is also considered that there are different forms of recreational activities based on the type of individual efforts they require.

1. **Indoor recreation activities:** These include those types of activities that can be performed inside closed places or in a room/unit. Examples: Reading; writing; playing indoor games such as chess, Ludo, cards, and musical games; and dancing.
2. **Outdoor recreation activities:** These include those types of activities that can be enjoyed outside or in an open place. Examples: Outdoor games such as cricket, running, swimming, camping, and hiking.
3. **Others:** There are many activities that can be considered as recreational or diversional therapies. These include yoga, meditation, and pet therapy. The list can be endless but there is only one fundamental principle: the activity should be of interest to the client.

Steps of Recreational Therapies

Recreational therapy is performed by many as a daily routine for relaxation. But in case of specific problems or stressful conditions, it is important to consult a qualified recreational therapist for an advice on the type of suitable activities. Following are the steps while conducting recreational therapies:

Assessment → Planning → Intervention → Evaluation

Disease-Specific Recreational Activities

1. **Anxiety:** Activities such as running, walking, and jogging can be helpful to deal with fear.
2. **Depression:** Any type of activity that is not competitive in nature can be suggested to clients who are depressed and sad. These clients have low self-esteem and less confidence and that's why they should be involved in group activities to improve social contact, but the activities must be noncompetitive such as running, painting, and art and craft works.
3. **Mania:** People with mania are always in an elated mood, so it is important to refrain them from huge gathering and group of people. They should be encouraged to participate in individual activities such as sports and running so that they can use their energy.
4. **Dementia:** People with dementia should be allowed to participate in activities that can cut their boredom, but such activities should be simple and interesting because most of the people are elderly. They can be involved in activities such as painting, filling the colors, and listening music to improve their quality of life.
5. **Childhood disorders:** It is important to understand and comprehend the individual interest and needs of the child before planning any activities. Motor activities such as sports and games are commonly preferred for children.
6. **Mental retardation:** People with intellectual disability are considered as slow learners compared with others, so it is important to involve them in simple activities. Their activities of leisure time can later on become their vocational training. Activities such as envelope making, candle making, dancing, and singing can be taught to them for a productive life.

Role of Nurse in Recreational Therapies

- Properly assess the client before planning activity for him or her.
- Provide a nonjudgmental and no-threatening approach toward the client.
- Motivate the client to ventilate and share his/her feelings or emotions.
- Do not be rigid with the activity routine and guidelines.
- Use a structured process to trace the continuous progress of the client.
- Encourage the patient to learn new skills and explore his/her own ability.
- Be a keen observer and understand a client's lacking to guide him/her for further steps.
- Plan such activities that can be enjoyed by clients and lead to satisfaction.

KEY POINTS

- The general adaptation syndrome (GAS), an immediate physiological response to stress, involves the autonomic nervous system and the endocrine system.
- When stress is perceived by the sensory system, impulses to the hypothalamus activate one of the following two systems: the hypothalamic-pituitary-adrenal (HPA) axis and the sympathetic nervous system (SNS).
- Physiological responses to stress also include immunological changes.
- Stress makes people ill as a result of both increased levels of powerful hormones such as cortisol that change bodily processes and coping choices that are unhealthy such as not getting enough rest or a proper diet or use of tobacco, alcohol, or caffeine.
- Post-traumatic stress disorder (PTSD) begins when a person experiences, witnesses, or is confronted with a traumatic event and responds with intense fear or helplessness. There are four types of symptoms of PTSD: reliving the event, avoiding situations that remind the person of the event, having more negative beliefs and feelings about oneself or the world, and hyperarousal.
- Compassion fatigue is a state of burnout and secondary traumatic stress that can overwhelm health care providers and result in feelings of hopelessness, inadequacy, and anxiety.
- A person experiences psychological stress only if he or she evaluates the event or circumstance as a personal threat; this is called *primary appraisal*.

- Stress includes work stress, family stress, chronic stress, acute stress, daily hassles, trauma, and crisis.
- Potential stressors and coping mechanisms vary across the life span, from childhood to adolescence, adulthood, and old age and from one culture to another.
- Coping, a process that constantly changes to manage demands on a person's resources, means making an effort to manage psychological stress.
- Resiliency is an important coping resource that you can promote in patients by suggesting general ways for them to prepare for challenges before they occur.
- Unmanaged workplace stress affects nurses' job satisfaction and patient satisfaction.

REFERENCES

Akerstedt T, Axelsson J, Lekander M, Orsini N, Kecklund G. Do sleep, stress, and illness explain daily variations in fatigue? A prospective study. J Psychosom Res 2014;76:280.

Alschuler L. The HPA axis. Integrative Therapeutics; 2016. Available from: http://www.integrativepro.com/Resources/Integrative-Blog/2016/The-HPA-Axis.

American Psychological Association (APA). The road to resilience. 2015. Available from: http://www.apa.org/helpcenter/road-resilience.aspx.

Christie W, Jones S. Lateral violence in nursing and the theory of the nurse as wounded healer. Online J Issues Nurs 2013;19(1):5.

Doron J, Trouillet R, Maneveau A, Ninot G, Neveu D. Coping profiles, perceived stress and health-related behaviors: a cluster analysis approach. Health Promot Int 2014;30:88.

Edward KL, Ousey K, Warelow P, Lui S. Nursing and aggression in the workplace: a systematic review. Br J Nurs 2014;23(12):653.

Embree JL, White AH. Concept analysis nurse-to-nurse lateral violence. Nurs Forum 2010;45(3):1266.

Garcia DS. Evaluation of 3 Behavioral Theories for Application in Health Promotion Strategies for Hispanic Women. ANS Adv Nurs Sci. 2016 Apr-Jun;39(2):165–80. doi: 10.1097/ANS.0000000000000116. PMID: 27149229.

Giger J. Transcultural nursing. 7th ed. St. Louis: Mosby; 2016.

Gillespie GL, Gates DM. Using proactive coping to manage the stress of trauma patient care. J Trauma Nurs 2013;20:44.

Harvard Medical School. Understanding the stress response. Harvard Health Publications; 2016. Available from: http://www.health.harvard.edu/staying-healthy/understanding-the-stress-response.

Huether SE, McCance KL. Understanding pathophysiology. 6th ed. St. Louis: Mosby; 2017.

Hunsaker S, Chen HC, Maughan D, Heaston S. Factors that influence the development of compassion fatigue, burnout, and compassion satisfaction in emergency department nurses. J Nurs Scholarsh 2015;47(2):186.

Ianello P, Balzarotti S. Stress and coping strategies in the emergency room. Emerg Care J 2014;10:72.

Janowski K, Kurpas D, Kusz J, Mroczek B, Jedynak T. Emotional control, styles of coping with stress and acceptance of illness among patients suffering from chronic somatic disease. Stress Health 2014;30:34.

Krägeloh CU, Billington DR, Henning MA, Chai PP. Spiritual quality of life and spiritual coping: evidence for a two-factor structure of the WHOQOL spirituality, religiousness, and personal beliefs module. Health Qual Life Outcomes 2015;13:26.

Lengacher CA, Shelton MM, Reich RR, Barta MK, Johnson-Mallard V, Moscoso MS, et al. Mindfulness based stress reduction (MBSR(BC)) in breast cancer: evaluating fear of recurrence (FOR) as a mediator of psychological and physical symptoms in a randomized control trial (RCT). J Behav Med 2014;37:185.

Lengacher CA, Reich RR, Paterson CL, Jim HS, Ramesar S, Alinat CB, Budhrani PH, Farias JR, Shelton MM, Moscoso MS, Park JY, Kip KE. The effects of mindfulness-based stress reduction on objective and subjective sleep parameters in women with breast cancer: a randomized controlled trial. Psychooncology. 2015 Apr;24(4):424–32. doi: 10.1002/pon.3603. Epub 2014 Jun 18.

Lin SH, Liao WC, Chen MY, Fan JY. The impact of shift work on nurses' job stress, sleep quality and self-perceived health status. J Nurs Manag 2014;22:604.

MacLeod S, Musich S, Hawkins K, Alsgaard K, Wicker ER. The impact of resilience among older adults. Geriatr Nurs 2016;37(4):266.

Mayo Clinic. Chronic stress puts your health at risk. 2016. Available from: http://www.mayoclinic.org/healthy-lifestyle/stress-management/in-depth/stress/art-20046037.

Mealer M, Jones J, Moss M. A qualitative study of resilience and posttraumatic stress disorder in United States ICU nurses. Intensive Care Med 2014;38:1445.

Miller DB, O'Callaghan JP. Neuroendocrine aspects of the response to stress. Metabolism 2002;51(6 Suppl. 1):5.

Moreira SR, Lima RM, Silva KE, Simões HG. Combined exercise circuit session acutely attenuates stress-induced blood pressure reactivity in healthy adults. Braz J Phys Ther 2014;18:38.

Najimi A, Goudarzi AM, Sharifirad G. Causes of job stress in nurses: a cross-sectional study. Iran J Nurs Midwifery Res 2012;17(4):301.

Nguyen-Rodriguez ST, Lisha NE, Spruijt-Metz D, Sun P, Rohrbach LA, Sussman S. Coping mediates the effects of depressive symptoms on sleep problems. Am J Health Behav 2015;39(2):183.

Nielson MB, Knardahl S. Coping strategies: a prospective study of patterns, stability, and relationships with physiological distress. Scand J Psychol 2014;55:142.

O'Driscoll MP. Coping with stress: a challenge for theory, research, and practice. Stress Health 2013;29:89.

Parelkar P, Thompson NJ, Kaw CK, Miner KR, Stein KD. Stress coping and changes in health behavior among cancer survivors: a report from the American Cancer Society's study of cancer survivors-II (SCS-II). J Psychosoc Oncol 2015;31:136.

Pender N. Health promotion model. 2016. Available from: http://www.nursing-theory.org/theories-and-models/pender-health-promotion-model.php.

Pender N, Murdaugh CL. Health promotion in nursing practice. 7th ed. Upper Saddle River, NJ: Pearson; 2015.

Potter P, Deshields T, Berger JA, Clarke M, Olsen S, Chen L. Evaluation of a compassion fatigue resiliency program for oncology nurses. Oncol Nurs Forum 2013;40(2):180.

Rayens MK, Reed DB. Predictors of depressive symptoms in older rural couples: the impact of work, stress, and health. J Rural Health 2014;30:59.

Sabo B. Reflecting on the concept of compassion fatigue. Online J Issues Nurs 2011;16(1):1.

Selye H. History of the stress concept. In: Goldberger L, Breznitz S, editors. Handbook of stress: theoretical and clinical aspects. 2nd ed. New York: Free Press; 1993.

Smith SM, Vale WW. The role of the hypothalamic-pituitary-adrenal axis in neuroendocrine response to stress. Dialogues Clin Neurosci 2006;8(4):383.

Stevens D, Wilcox HC, MacKinnon DF, Mondimore FM, Schweizer B, Jancic D, et al. Posttraumatic stress disorder increases risk for suicide attempt in adults with recurrent major depression. Depress Anxiety 2013;30:940.

van den Hurk DG, Schellekens MP, Molema J, Speckens AE, van der Drift MA. Mindfulness-based stress reduction for lung cancer patients and their partners: results of a mixed methods pilot study. Palliat Med 2015;29:652.

Varcarolis EM. Essentials of psychiatric mental health nursing. 3rd ed. St. Louis: Elsevier; 2017.

Waude A. General adaptation syndrome. Psychologist World. 2016. Available from: https://www.psychologistworld.com/stress/general-adaptation-syndrome.

32 Spiritual Health

OBJECTIVES

After reading this chapter, the student should be able to:

- Discuss the concept of spirituality and spiritual well-being.
- Describe the relationship among faith, hope, and spiritual well-being.
- Compare and contrast the concepts of religion and spirituality.
- Discuss the impact of illness on spirituality.
- Assess a patient's spirituality and spiritual health.
- Discuss nursing interventions designed to promote spiritual health.
- Establish presence with patients.
- Apply the nursing process to deal with spiritual distress.

KEY TERMS

agnostic, p. 777
atheist, p. 777
connectedness, p. 780
faith, p. 775
holistic, p. 775
hope, p. 776
self-transcendence, p. 777
spiritual distress, p. 778
spiritual well-being, p. 778
spirituality, p. 775
transcendence, p. 777

INTRODUCTION

The word *spirituality* comes from the Latin word *spiritus*, which refers to breath or wind. The spirit gives life to a person. It signifies whatever is at the center of all aspects of a person's life. **Spirituality** is an awareness of one's inner self and a sense of connection to a Supreme Being, nature, or some purpose greater than oneself. It includes personal beliefs that help a person maintain hope and get through difficult situations (March and Caple, 2016). A person's health depends on a balance of physical, psychological, sociological, cultural, emotional, developmental, and spiritual variables. This **holistic** view of health is the focus and heart of nursing practice. Spiritual care is often an overlooked part of nursing; however, the spiritual dimension does not exist in isolation from our physical and psychological being (Collins-McNeil et al., 2015). Spirituality is an important factor that helps people achieve the balance needed to maintain health and well-being and to cope with illness. Current evidence shows that spirituality positively affects health, quality of life, health promotion behaviors, and disease prevention activities (Conway-Phillips and Janusek, 2014; Jones et al., 2015).

Nurses and other health care providers often fail to recognize the spiritual dimension of human nature. In addition, some health care providers do not believe in God or a Supreme Being or believe that they do not have time to address spiritual needs. Frequently people think of the concepts of spirituality and religion interchangeably, but spirituality is a much broader and more unifying concept than religion (Carson, 2017; Dahlkemper, 2016). Florence Nightingale believed that spirituality is a force that provides energy needed in a healthy hospital environment. She also believed that caring for a person's spiritual needs is just as important as caring for his or her physical needs (O'Brien, 2014). The human spirit is powerful, and spirituality has different meanings for different people. Your personal spiritual health is important to your values and beliefs and can influence your attitudes toward spiritual care, professional commitment, and caring (Chiang et al., 2016). Therefore, you need to understand your own spirituality to integrate spirituality into your patients' care. Nursing care involves helping patients use their spiritual resources as they identify and explore what is meaningful in their lives and find ways to cope with illness and stressors of life (Ramezani et al., 2014).

CONCEPT OF SPIRITUALITY

Faith

In addition to being a part of the definition of spirituality, the concept of **faith** has other common definitions. Faith allows a person to have firm beliefs about something despite the lack of physical evidence. Although many associate faith with religious beliefs, faith can exist without them (O'Brien, 2014). Faith is a cultural or institutional religion such as Buddhism, Christianity, or Islam. It also is a relationship with a divinity, higher power, authority, or spirit that incorporates a reasoning faith (belief) and a trusting faith (action). Reasoning faith is a person's belief and confidence in something for which there is no proof. It is an acceptance of what our reasoning cannot explain. Sometimes, it involves a belief in a higher power, spirit guide, God, or Allah. Faith also is how a person chooses to live life. In this sense, it enables action. Patients who are ill frequently have a positive outlook on life and continue to participate in daily activities rather than resigning themselves to the symptoms of their disease. In these cases, a patient's faith often becomes stronger because illness is viewed as an opportunity for personal growth (Granero-Molina et al., 2014).

Religion

Religion is associated with the "state of doing," or a specific system of practices associated with a particular denomination, sect, or form of worship. It refers to the system of organized beliefs and worship that a person practices to outwardly express spirituality. Many people practice a faith or belief in a specific religion such as Hinduism is the predominant religion in India and other religions are Islam, Sikhism, Christianity, Jainism, and Buddhism. People from different religions view spirituality differently. For example, a Hindu believes in theory of Karma and a Buddhist believes in Four Noble Truths: life is suffering, suffering is caused by clinging, suffering can be eliminated by eliminating clinging, and to eliminate clinging and suffering one follows an eightfold path. The path includes the right understanding, intention, speech, action, livelihood, effort, mindfulness, and concentration. This path promotes wisdom, moral behavior, and meditation. A Hindu and a Buddhist turn inward, valuing self-control, whereas a Christian looks to the love of God to provide enlightenment and direction in life.

When providing spiritual care to patients, you need to know the differences between religion and spirituality. Although closely related, these terms are not synonymous. Religious care helps patients follow their belief systems and worship practices. Spiritual care helps people maintain personal relationships and a relationship with a Supreme Being or life force to identify meaning and purpose in life.

Hope

Spirituality and faith bring hope. When a person has the attitude of living for and looking forward to something, hope is present. **Hope** is multidimensional and gives comfort while a person endures hardship and personal challenges. It usually refers to a source of energy that helps a person plan and achieve goals (Griggs and Walker, 2016) and is used by patients to sustain themselves during illness (Dunn, 2016). It is closely associated with faith. It is energizing, giving individuals a motivation to achieve and the resources to use toward that achievement. People express hope in all aspects of their lives as a force that helps them deal with life stressors. It is a valuable personal resource and brings comfort when people face a loss (see Chapter 28) or a challenge that seems difficult to achieve (Griggs and Walker, 2016).

Spiritual Health

People gain spiritual health by finding a balance between their life values, goals, and belief systems and their relationships within themselves and with others. Throughout life, a person sometimes grows more spiritual, becoming increasingly aware of the meaning, purpose, and values of life. In times of stress, illness, loss, or recovery, a person often turns to previous ways of responding or adjusting to a situation. Often these coping styles lie within the person's spiritual beliefs.

Spiritual beliefs change as people grow and develop (Table 32.1). Spirituality begins as children learn about themselves and their relationships with others. When you

Table 32.1 Relationship Between Developmental Stage and Spiritual Beliefs

Erickson's Developmental Stage	Spiritual Beliefs
Trust versus mistrust—birth to 18 months	Spiritual well-being provided by parents Trust provides basis for hope Love, affection, security, and a stimulating environment promote spirituality
Autonomy versus shame and doubt—18–36 months	Fascination with magic and mystery Often believes that illness is related to bad behavior Begins to learn difference between right and wrong Imitates parents' spiritual or religious actions; recites prayers and sings simple religious songs, but does not understand their meanings Interprets meanings literally
Initiative versus guilt—3–6 years	Feels guilty when not acting responsibly Influenced by spiritual and religious stories, examples, moods, and actions Models moral behaviors of parents Begins to ask about God or Supreme Being
Industry versus inferiority—6–12 years	Wants to learn about spirituality Has a clear picture of God or Supreme Being, morality, and difference between right and wrong Sorts fantasy from fact Demands proof of reality and believes literal meanings of spiritual stories
Identity versus identity confusion—adolescence (12–18 years of age)	Reflects on inconsistencies in stories Begins to question spiritual practices, forms own opinions, and occasionally discards parents' beliefs Abstract reasoning leads to exploration of moral issues Spirituality comes from connectedness with family, nature, and God or Supreme Being
Intimacy versus isolation and loneliness—young adulthood (18–35 years of age)	Establishes self-identity and world view Forms independent beliefs, attitudes, and lifestyles Uses principles to solve problems when individual's and society's rules conflict

Table 32.1 Relationship Between Developmental Stage and Spiritual Beliefs—cont'd

Erickson's Developmental Stage	Spiritual Beliefs
Generativity versus stagnation—middle-age adulthood (35–65 years of age)	Develops appreciation of past spiritual experiences Embraces people from different faiths and religions Reviews value system during crisis Values others
Ego identity versus despair and disgust—older adulthood (65 years of age and older)	Values love and interactions with others Focuses on overcoming oppression and violence Beliefs vary based on many factors such as gender, past experiences, religion, economic status, and ethnic background

Data from Edelman CL, Mandle CL: *Health promotion throughout the life span,* ed 8, St Louis, 2014, Elsevier; and Hockenberry MJ, Wilson D: *Wong's nursing care of infants and children*, ed 10, St Louis, 2015, Elsevier.

understand a child's spiritual beliefs, it is easier to care for and comfort the child (Darby et al., 2014; Taylor et al., 2015). As children mature into adulthood, they experience spiritual growth by entering into lifelong relationships. An ability to care meaningfully for others and self is evidence of a healthy spirituality. A majority of older adults describe themselves as spiritual and often turn to important relationships and give themselves to others (Touhy and Jett, 2018).

SPIRITUALITY AND SPIRITUAL WELL-BEING

Spirituality

Definitions of spirituality differ. However, experts agree that it is complex and diverse (March and Caple, 2016; Timmins et al., 2014). It is unique for each individual and exists in everyone, regardless of religious beliefs. Our culture, development, life experiences, beliefs, and ideas about life influence our definition of spirituality. Spirituality exists in all people, regardless of their religious beliefs; it gives people the *energy* needed to maintain health and cope with difficult situations. Current definitions of spirituality include five distinct but overlapping constructs (Fig. 32.1).

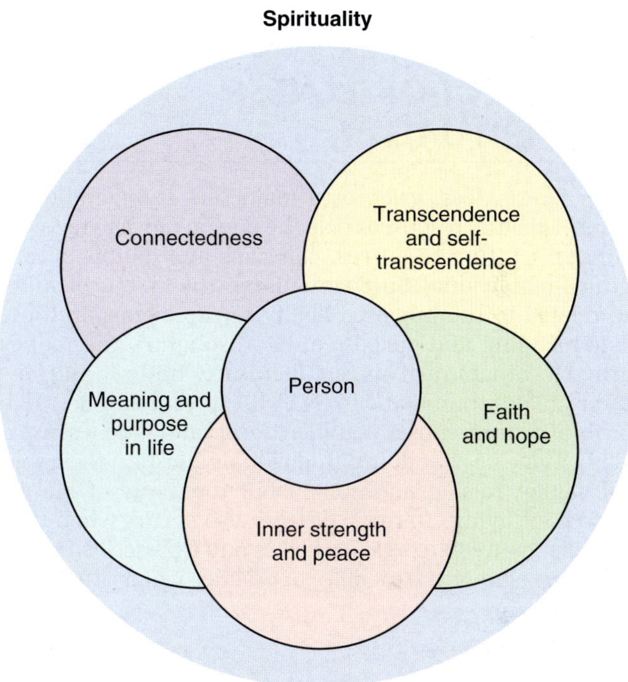

Fig. 32.1 The concept of spirituality has five distinct but overlapping constructs.

Self-transcendence refers to connecting to your inner self, which allows one to go beyond oneself to understand the meanings of experiences. For example, people with a high level of self-transcendence feel a connectedness to other living beings and the environment. In contrast, **transcendence** is the belief that there is a positive force outside of and greater than oneself that allows one to develop new perspectives that are beyond physical boundaries (Hatamipour et al., 2015). Examples of transcendent moments include the feeling of awe when holding a new baby or watching the sun rise over the mountains. Spirituality offers a sense of *connectedness* intrapersonally (connected with oneself), interpersonally (connected with others and the environment), and transpersonally (connected with God, the unseen, or a higher power). Through connectedness, patients are able to move beyond the stressors of everyday life and find comfort, faith, hope, peace, and empowerment (Hakanson and Ohlen, 2016). *Inner strength* is an energy source that instills hope, provides motivation, and promotes a positive outlook on life even during difficult times. *Inner peace* fosters calm and positive feelings despite life experiences of chaos, fear, and uncertainty (Viglund et al., 2014). These feelings help people feel comforted and find peace even in times of great distress (Hatamipour et al., 2015). Finally, spirituality helps people find *meaning and purpose in life* in both negative and positive life events (Dobratz, 2016).

Spirituality is an important concept for individuals who either do not believe in the existence of God **(atheist)** or who believe that any ultimate reality is unknown or unknowable **(agnostic)**. Atheists search for meaning in life through their work and relationships with others. It is important for agnostics to discover meaning in what they do or how they live because they find no ultimate meaning for the way things are. They believe that we, as people, bring meaning to what we do.

Spirituality is an integrating theme in life. A person's concept of spirituality begins in childhood and continues to grow throughout adulthood (Taylor et al., 2015). Spirituality represents the totality of one's being, serving as the overriding perspective that unifies the various aspects of an individual. It spreads throughout the physiological, psychological, and sociocultural dimensions of a person's life, whether or not the individual acknowledges or develops it.

Spiritual Well-Being

There are four dimensions of **spiritual well-being** as defined by Rowold (2011). The personal dimension refers to how you relate with yourself in finding meaning and purpose in life. The communal dimension relates to the quality of your interpersonal relationships. The environmental dimension describes how you interact in the world, including your sense of awe with the environment. The transcendental dimension refers to the relationship between you and some higher power (e.g., God, Buddha). Spiritual well-being has a positive effect on health and leads to spiritual health. If you are spiritually healthy, you experience joy, forgive yourself and others, accept hardship and mortality, experience enhanced quality of life, and have a positive sense of physical and emotional well-being (Cottrell, 2016; Rowold, 2011).

THE EFFECT OF ILLNESS ON SPIRITUALITY

When illness, loss, grief, or a major life change affects a person, spiritual resources help the person move to recovery. Without spiritual resources, concerns and doubts develop within an individual. **Spiritual distress** is "a state of suffering related to the impaired ability to experience and integrate meaning and purpose in life through connectedness with self, others, art, music, literature, nature, and/or a power greater than oneself" (NANDA International, 2014). Spiritual distress causes doubt, a loss of faith, and a sense of feeling alone or abandoned. Individuals question their spiritual values, raising questions about their way of life and purpose for living. Spiritual distress also occurs when there is conflict between a person's beliefs and a prescribed health treatment plan or the inability to practice usual rituals.

BOX 32.1 Evidence-Based Practice

PICO Question: Does the use of spiritual care interventions improve patient outcomes?

Summary of Evidence

Nursing care for patients needs to focus on mind, body, and spirit. It is important to include spiritual interventions in a patient's plan of care that will help to relieve spiritual distress and enhance spiritual well-being (Abuatiq, 2015). Providing spiritual care to patients helps a patient cope with illness and therapies (Trevino and McConnell, 2015). Researchers have found that spiritual interventions help decrease anxiety and reduce depression in patients with cancer (Pantuso, 2015). Spiritual interventions have also been found to contribute to spiritual well-being, improved psychological adaptation, and improved satisfaction for patients (Ramezani et al., 2014). Spiritual counseling, which includes praying with a patient, religious-specific rituals, and visits from pastoral care, had a positive effect on quality of life in patients with heart failure (Tadwalkar et al., 2014). Before providing spiritual care to patients, it is important for nurses to assess for patients' cues to respect patient beliefs and autonomy (Taylor et al., 2014).

Application to Nursing Practice

- Use active listening and therapeutic communication to develop rapport with your patients (Ramezani et al., 2014).
- Offer to pray or read scripture with patients (Tadwalkar et al., 2014).
- Turn on the patient's favorite religious music station or television channel (Abuatiq, 2015).
- Conduct a spiritual assessment or history for each of your patients (Pantuso, 2015).
- Be nonjudgmental in your assessment and care of patients, showing respect for each patient's spiritual beliefs (Ramezani et al., 2014).
- Offer to contact pastoral care or the chaplain for the patient (Abuatiq, 2015).

Acute Illness

Sudden, unexpected illness that threatens a patient's life, health, and/or well-being creates significant spiritual distress. For example, both an older man who has a heart attack and a young adult who is injured in a motor vehicle accident face crises that threaten their spiritual health. The illness or injury creates an unanticipated scramble to integrate and cope with new realities (e.g., disability). People look for ways to remain faithful to their beliefs and value systems through the use of spiritual resources. Often conflicts develop around a person's beliefs and the meaning of life. Anger is common; sometimes patients express it against God, their families, themselves, and their nurses or other health care providers. The strength of patients' spirituality influences their ability to cope with and recover from sudden illness. Having a better understanding of your patients' illnesses and conditions helps you spiritually support them (Sweat, 2015). You play a key role in helping patients resolve feelings of spiritual distress. You create a healing environment and maximize recovery by enhancing their spiritual well-being (Estores and Frye, 2015).

Chronic Illness

Patients with chronic illnesses often experience debilitating symptoms that permanently change their lifestyles. The uncertain and long-term nature of chronic illness and the potential for outcomes such as pain, changes in body image, and the need to confront death all lead to spiritual distress. Patients struggle with questions about the meaning and purpose of their lives because their independence is threatened, which often causes fear, anxiety, and powerlessness. The nursing diagnosis *Spiritual Distress* is appropriate to use for patients who experience these symptoms. A person's spirituality is a significant factor in how he or she adapts to the changes resulting from chronic illness. Successfully adapting to these changes strengthens a person spiritually, but it sometimes takes a long-term plan to help a patient with a chronic illness achieve spiritual well-being. As a nurse, you are in a unique position to help patients reevaluate their lives and achieve spiritual health (Box 32.1). Patients who have a sense of spiritual well-being are often better able to cope with their illnesses and experience enhanced quality of life (Carron, 2016). Exploring the meaning of pain and suffering with patients allows you to spiritually support them during their illnesses (Sweat, 2015).

Terminal Illness

Terminal illness commonly causes fears of physical pain, isolation, the unknown, and dying. When patients feel uncertain about what death means, they are susceptible to spiritual distress. Spirituality helps patients and families find resolution and peace by helping them prepare for and accept death (Petersen, 2014). Individuals experiencing a terminal illness often find themselves reviewing their life and questioning its meaning. Common questions they ask may include, "Why is this happening to me?" or "What have I done?" Terminal illness affects family and friends just as much as the patient. It causes members of the family to ask important questions about the meaning of life and how the illness will affect their relationship with the patient (see Chapter 28).

When caring for dying patients, help them gain a greater sense of control over their illness, whether they are in a health care setting (e.g., the hospital) or at home. Dying is a holistic process encompassing the patient's physical, social, psychological, and spiritual health (Finocchiaro, 2016; Petersen, 2014).

Near-Death Experience

You may care for a patient or have a family member who has had a near-death experience (NDE). NDE is a psychological phenomenon in which people have either been close to clinical death or recovered after being declared dead. It is not associated with a mental disorder. Experts agree that NDE describes a powerfully close brush with physical, emotional, and spiritual death. For example, people who have an NDE after cardiopulmonary arrest often tell the same story of feeling themselves rising above their bodies and watching caregivers initiate lifesaving measures. Commonly patients who experience an NDE describe feeling totally at peace, having an out-of-body experience, being pulled into a dark tunnel, seeing bright light, and encountering people who preceded them in death. Instead of moving toward the light, they learn that it is not time for them to die, and they return to life (Johnson, 2015; Rawlings and Devery, 2015).

Patients who have an NDE are often reluctant to discuss it, thinking family or caregivers will not understand. Isolation and depression often occur. NDEs can be either positive or negative experiences (Johnson, 2015). However, individuals experiencing an NDE who discuss it openly with family or caregivers find acceptance and meaning from this powerful experience. They are often no longer afraid of death, and they have a decreased desire to achieve material wealth. They also report increased sensitivity to different chemicals such as alcohol and medications. After patients have survived an NDE, promote spiritual well-being by remaining open, giving patients a chance to explore what happened, and supporting them as they share the experience with significant others (Rawlings and Devery, 2015).

DEALING WITH SPIRITUAL DISTRESS

Understanding your own spirituality is essential when you complete a spiritual assessment and provide spiritual care to your patients (Pullen et al., 2015). Remember that spirituality is very subjective and has different meanings for different people. You gather an accurate assessment of your patients' spirituality when you take time to build therapeutic relationships with them. Conduct an ongoing spiritual assessment the entire time you care for a patient. Talking about spirituality with a patient helps build a trusting relationship that often leads to conversations about spirituality and health outcomes (Carson, 2017). Focus your assessment on aspects of spirituality most likely to be influenced by life experiences, events, and questions in the case of illness and hospitalization (Table 32.2). Conducting an assessment is therapeutic for you and your patient because it conveys a level of caring and support.

One way to assess your patient's spiritual health is to ask the patient direct questions. This approach requires you to feel comfortable asking others about their spirituality. You start with a brief assessment and later follow with a more in-depth assessment (Hodge, 2015). Some health care agencies and researchers have created assessment tools to clarify values and assess spirituality. For example, the Spiritual Well-Being (SWB) scale has 20 questions that assess a patient's relationship with God and his or her sense of life purpose and life satisfaction (Life Advance, 2009). The FICA assessment tool (Borneman et al., 2010) evaluates spirituality and is closely correlated with quality of life. *FICA* is an acronym that stands for the following:

F—**Faith** or belief
I—**Importance** of spirituality
C—Individual's spiritual **Community**
A—Interventions to **Address** spiritual needs

Effective assessment tools such as the SWB and FICA help you remember important areas to assess. Patient responses to the assessment items on the tools indicate areas that you need to investigate further.

Faith

Although individual definitions vary, faith helps people find meaning in their life experiences. When assessing a

Table 32.2 Focused Patient Assessment

Factors to Assess	Questions	Physical Assessment
Past experiences with loss	How would you describe the ways you cope spiritually when faced with difficult times?	Observe the patient's facial expressions and mannerisms during the discussion.
Fear of the unknown resulting from a terminal illness	Describe the people who mean the most to you. In what way do you look to them for support? Do you consider yourself a spiritual person? If so, what gives you comfort? If not, what provides you a sense of peace?	Fear is associated with anxiety. Be alert for changes in vital signs. Observe the patient's mood, willingness to initiate conversation, and interest in surroundings.

patient's faith, first determine his or her beliefs, especially beliefs that influence hope. For example, ask how a patient believes that a treatment will affect a newly diagnosed serious illness. Determine which of your patient's beliefs serve as a guide and help the patient find meaning in life events. Ask your patient whether he or she is able to live according to his or her beliefs. Finally assess to what extent your patient interrelates with self, others, and a source of authority. Faith in an authority provides a sense of confidence that guides a person in exercising beliefs and experiencing growth. Assess a person's faith in an authority by asking, "To whom do you look to for guidance in life?" The patient's response to an open-ended question such as this will likely open the door for a meaningful discussion. Listen carefully and explore what is meaningful to the patient.

Determine whether patients have a religious source of guidance that conflicts with their medical treatment plans. This seriously affects the treatment options that nurses and other health care providers are able to offer patients. For example, if a patient is a Jehovah's Witness, blood products are not an acceptable form of treatment. Christian Scientists often refuse any medical intervention, believing that their faith will heal them.

It is also important to understand a patient's philosophy of life. Asking a patient, "Describe for me what is most important in your life," or "Tell me what gives your life meaning or purpose," helps to assess the basis of his or her spiritual belief system. This information often reveals how illness, loss, or disability affects a person's life. A patient's religious practices, views about health, and response to illness influence how you will provide support.

Life and Self-Responsibility

Assessing spiritual well-being includes looking at your patient's life and self-responsibility. People who accept change, make decisions about their lives, and are able to forgive themselves and others in times of difficulty have a higher level of spiritual well-being. During illness, patients often are unable to accept limitations or know what to do to regain a functional and meaningful life. Their sense of helplessness reflects spiritual distress. However, if a patient is able to adapt to changes and seek solutions for how to deal with any limitations, they are more responsible, and their spiritual well-being reflects an important coping resource. Assess the extent to which a patient understands any limitations or threats posed by an illness and the way the patient chooses to adjust to them. Ask, "Tell me how you feel about the changes caused by your illness," and "How do these changes affect what you now need to do?"

Connectedness

Connectedness is a dimension of spirituality that is related to the human need of belonging. Patients who are connected to themselves, others, nature, God, or another Supreme Being usually report higher levels of physical and emotional health (Hakanson and Ohlen, 2016). Patients who pray use this form of personal communication to remain connected with God (Fig. 32.2). Praying provides a sense of hope, strength, and security and is woven into one's faith. Patients often use prayer when other treatments are ineffective (O'Brien, 2014). You help patients become or remain connected by respecting each patient's unique sense of spirituality. Assess whether a patient loses the ability to express a sense of relatedness to something greater than self. You assess a patient's connectedness by asking open-ended questions, "Is prayer something helpful to you? What feelings do you have after you pray?" or "Who do you believe is the most important person in your life?"

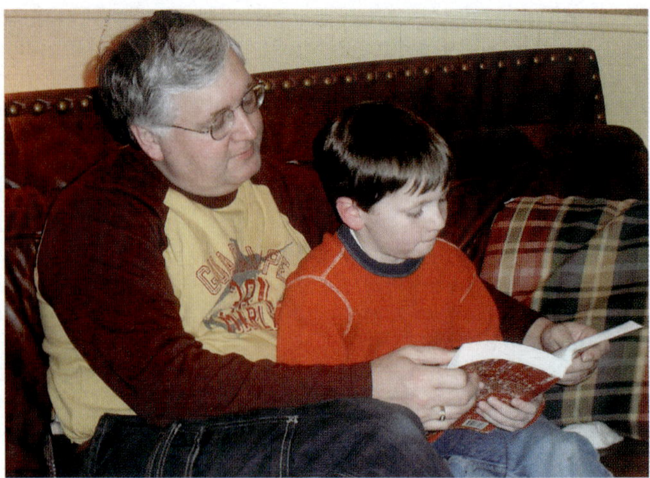

Fig. 32.2 Praying or reading a religious text together enhances connectedness between parents and their children.

Life Satisfaction

Spiritual well-being is tied to a person's satisfaction with life and what the person has accomplished (Dobratz, 2016). When people are satisfied with life and how they are using their abilities, more energy is available to deal with new difficulties and resolve problems. You assess a patient's satisfaction with life by asking, "How happy or satisfied are you with your life?" or "Tell me to what extent you feel satisfied with what you have accomplished in life."

Fellowship and Community

Fellowship is one kind of relationship that an individual has with other people, including immediate family, close friends, associates at work or school, fellow members of a church, and neighbors. More specifically, this includes the extent of the community of shared faith between people and their support networks. Many times, social support from faith-based groups helps patients cope with illness and participate in health promotion behaviors (Plunkett et al., 2015). To assess a patient's supportive community, ask questions such as, "With whom do you bond or connect with?" "Who do you find to be the greatest source of support in times of difficulty?" or "When you've faced difficult times in the past, who has been your greatest resource?"

Explore the extent and nature of a person's support networks and their relationship with the patient. Do not assume that a given network offers the kind of support that a patient desires. For example, calling a patient's pastor to request a visit is inappropriate if the patient finds little fellowship with the pastor or the pastor's faith community. Does the patient have one significant fellowship or several? What level of support does the community give? Do they visit, say prayers, or support the patient's immediate family? Learn whether openness exists between a patient and the people with whom a fellowship has formed.

Ritual and Practice

The use of rituals and practice is easy to assess and helps you understand a patient's spirituality. Rituals include participation in a religious group or private worship, prayer, participating in sacraments such as baptism or communion, fasting, singing, meditating, scripture reading, making offerings or sacrifices, or enjoying nature. Different religions have different rituals for life events. For example, Buddhists practice baptism later in life and find burial or cremation acceptable at death. Muslims wash the body of a dead family member and wrap it in white cloth with the head turned toward the right shoulder. Orthodox and Conservative Jews have their newborn sons circumcised 8 days after birth. Determine whether illness or hospitalization has interrupted a patient's usual rituals or practices. A ritual provides a patient with structure and support during challenging times. If rituals are important to a patient, use them as part of your nursing intervention.

Vocation

Individuals express their spirituality daily in their work, play, and relationships. Spirituality is often a part of a person's identity and vocation in life. Determine whether illness or hospitalization alters the ability to express some aspect of spirituality because it relates to a person's work or daily activities. Expression of spirituality is highly individual and includes showing an appreciation for life in the variety of things people do, living in the moment and not worrying about tomorrow, appreciating nature, expressing love toward others, and being productive. Assess how patients routinely express spirituality. Questions to ask include, "How has your illness affected the way you live your life spiritually at home or where you work?" or "How has your illness affected your ability to express what's important in life for you?"

Establishing Presence

You contribute to a sense of well-being and provide hope for recovery when you spend quality time with your patients. Behaviors that establish your presence include giving attention, answering questions, listening, and having a positive and encouraging (but realistic) attitude. Presence is part of the art of nursing (Carson, 2017). Benner (1984) explains that presence involves "being with" a patient versus "doing for" a patient. Presence is being able to offer closeness with a patient physically, psychologically, and spiritually. It helps to prevent emotional and environmental isolation (see Chapter 34).

When health promotion is the focus of care, your presence becomes important in instilling confidence in patients' abilities to take the steps necessary to remain healthy. You convey a caring presence by listening to patients' concerns, willingly involving family in discussions about a patient's health, showing self-confidence when providing health instruction, and supporting your patients when they make decisions about their health.

Trust is fundamental to any relationship. The attitude you convey when first interacting with a patient sets the tone for all conversations (see Chapter 4). Actively listening to the meaning of what a patient says is most important. It involves paying attention to the person's words and tone of voice and entering his or her frame of reference. By observing the patient's expressions and body language, you find cues to help him or her explore ways to achieve inner peace, take action, or manage pain. Your role as a nurse is not to solve patients' spiritual problems or impart your opinions but to provide an environment in which the patient can express spirituality.

Supporting a Healing Relationship

When giving spiritual care, look beyond isolated patient problems and recognize the broader picture of a patient's holistic needs. This is especially important when caring for older adults (Box 32.2). For example, do not look at a patient's back pain as just a problem to solve with quick remedies but rather look at how the pain influences his or her ability to function and achieve goals established in life. A holistic view enables you to assume a helping role so that you can establish a healing relationship (Benner, 1984). Three steps are evident when you establish healing relationships with your patients:

1. Mobilizing hope for you and for your patients
2. Finding an interpretation or understanding of the illness, pain, anxiety, or other stressful emotion that is acceptable to patients
3. Helping patients use social, emotional, or spiritual resources (Benner, 1984)

BOX 32.2 Care of an Older Adult

Supporting Older Adults' Spirituality

- There is an association between an older adult's spirituality and his or her ability to adjust or cope with illness and other life stressors (Manning, 2014).
- Older adults achieve spiritual resilience through frequent expressions of gratitude (e.g., via prayer, meditation, or discussions with friends) and finding ways to maintain purpose in life (e.g., helping family, volunteering) (Manning, 2014).
- Religious activities, attitudes, and spiritual experiences are very common among older adults. Older adults who experience spiritual well-being have better emotional health, experience a sense of peace that helps them accept life transitions, and experience to some extent improved physical health (Dahlkemper, 2016).
- Respecting privacy and dignity is an essential part of nursing care, especially when meeting spiritual needs of older adults (Rykkje and Raholm, 2014).
- Feelings of connectedness are important for older adults. Enhance connectedness by helping the older patient find meaning and purpose in life, listening actively to concerns, and being present (Dahlkemper, 2016).
- Beliefs in the afterlife increase as adults grow older. Make visits from clergy, social workers, lawyers, and even financial advisors available so that patients feel as though they have completed all unfinished business. Leaving a legacy to loved ones prepares the older adult to leave the world with a sense of meaning (Touhy and Jett, 2018). Legacies include oral histories, works of art, publications, photographs, or other objects of significance.

Mobilizing a patient's hope is central to a healing relationship. Hope helps people to face challenges in life (Broadhurst and Harrington, 2015). You help patients find realistic things for which to hope. For example, a patient newly diagnosed with diabetes becomes hopeful when you help him learn how to manage the disease so as to continue a productive and satisfying way of life. Your focus on controlling the pain and other symptoms a terminally ill patient is experiencing raises hope that the patient will be able to attend her daughter's graduation and live each day to the fullest.

Hope has both short-term and long-term implications. From a long-term perspective, it gives individuals a determination to endure and carry on with life responsibilities. In the short term, hope provides an incentive for constructive coping with obstacles and finding ways to realize the object of hope. Hope is future oriented and helps a patient work toward goals (Yarcheski and Mahon, 2016). You help patients achieve hope by working with them to find explanations for their situations that are mutually acceptable. Then help each patient realistically exercise hope. This includes supporting a patient's positive attitude toward life or a desire to be informed and make decisions.

To further support a healing relationship, know a patient's spiritual resources and needs. It is always important for patients to be able to express and exercise their beliefs and find spiritual comfort. When illness or treatment creates confusion or uncertainty for a patient, recognize the possible effect that this can have on the patient's well-being. How can spiritual resources be used and strengthened? Having a clear sense of what illness will be like helps a patient apply all resources toward recovery.

Support Systems

Use of support systems is important in any health care setting. They serve as a human link connecting the patient, the nurse, and the patient's lifestyle before an illness. In today's society, support comes from many areas, including family, friends, and support groups. Families often influence how patients perceive their illness. You enhance a patient's support network when you include a patient's family and friends in planning care. A patient's support system often is a source of coping, faith, and hope.

When a patient depends on family, friends, spiritual advisors, and members of the clergy for support, encourage these individuals to visit the patient regularly. Make all the patient's visitors welcome on nursing units and ensure privacy during visits to provide spiritual comfort. If the patient desires, ask the pastoral care department or hospital chaplain to notify the patient's clergy of the patient's admission. Often illness and the hospital environment produce uncertainty that frightens family members and friends. Help the family feel welcome and use their support and presence to promote the patient's healing. For example, including family members in prayer is a thoughtful gesture if it is appropriate to the patient's religion and if family members are comfortable participating. Encouraging the family to bring meaningful religious symbols to the patient's bedside and facilitating the administration of sacraments, rites, and rituals offers significant spiritual support. Do not forget to also support the family. When you support the family's spirituality and faith practices, you decrease their anxiety and feelings of uncertainty (Dobratz, 2016).

Diet Therapies

Food and nutrition are important aspects of nursing care. Food is also a significant component of some religious observances. For example, people in some Hindu and Islamic sects are vegetarian. Muslims are not allowed to eat pork, and they fast during the month of Ramadan. Orthodox Jewish patients observe kosher dietary restrictions. Native Americans have food practices influenced by individual tribal beliefs. Similar to many aspects of a particular culture or religion, food and the rituals surrounding the preparation and serving of food are important to a patient's spirituality. Integrate a patient's dietary preferences into daily care when possible, and consult with the dietitian in the health care institution. If a hospital or other health care agency cannot prepare food in the preferred way, ask the family to bring meals that are appropriate for dietary restrictions posed by the patient's condition.

Supporting Rituals

You become active in your patients' spiritual care by supporting their participation in spiritual rituals and activities. Plan care to allow time for religious readings, spiritual visitations, or attendance at religious services. Some churches and synagogues offer audiotapes of religious services. Allow family members to plan a prayer session or an organized reading when appropriate. Taped meditations, religious music, televised religious services, and some internet sites provide other effective options. Be respectful of icons, medals, prayer rugs, or crosses that patients bring to a health care setting, and make sure that they are not lost or misplaced.

Prayer and Meditation

The act of prayer gives an individual the opportunity to renew personal faith and belief in a Supreme Being in a specific, focused way that is either highly ritualized and formal or spontaneous and informal. Prayer is an effective coping resource for physical and psychological symptoms (O'Brien, 2014). Patients pray in private or pursue opportunities for group prayer with family, friends, or clergy. Some patients pray while listening to music. Be supportive of prayer by giving the patient privacy if desired, learning whether the patient wishes to have you participate, and suggesting prayer when you know that it is a coping resource for the patient. Delgado (2015) found that nurses often pray for patients rather than with patients; sharing the fact that prayer has been offered gives patients support and comfort. If prayer is not suitable for a patient, alternatives include listening to calming music or reading a book, poetry, or inspirational texts selected by the patient.

Meditation is effective in creating a relaxation response that reduces daily stress. Patients who meditate often state that they have an increased awareness of their spirituality and of the presence of God or a Supreme Being (Box 32.3). Meditation exercises give patients relief from pain, insomnia, anxiety, and depression and increase coping and the ability to relax (Starkweather, 2017). Meditation involves sitting quietly in a comfortable position with eyes closed and repeating a sound, phrase, or sacred word in rhythm with breathing while disregarding intrusive thoughts.

BOX 32.3 Patient Teaching

Meditation

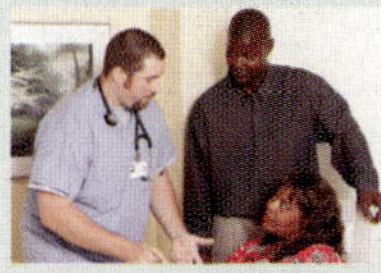

At one of her clinic visits, Victoria tells Jeff, "My friend told me yesterday that when she had cancer, she used meditation to help her cope with the side effects of her chemotherapy. I was thinking that I might try meditating to see if it would help me, but I don't know how to meditate. Can you help me?" Jeff develops the following teaching plan for Victoria:

Outcome

Victoria verbalizes feelings of relaxation and self-transcendence after meditation.

Teaching Strategies

- Provide a brief description of what will be taught.
- Give Victoria a patient-teaching sheet that describes how to meditate.
- Help Victoria identify at least one quiet place in her home that has minimal interruptions.
- Encourage her to use soft background noise such as a fan or soft music during meditation to block out distractions.
- Teach Victoria the steps of meditation—sit in a comfortable position with the back straight; breathe slowly; and focus on a sound, a prayer, or an image.
- Encourage Victoria to meditate for 10–20 min two times a day.
- Answer any questions.
- Reinforce information as needed.

Evaluation

- Use the principles of teach back to evaluate patient learning:
  - "What did you learn about yourself?"
  - "How did you feel after meditating?"

Individuals who meditate regularly (twice a day for 10 or 20 minutes) experience decreased metabolism and heart rate, easier breathing, and slower brain waves. Chapter 11 addresses relaxation approaches.

KEY POINTS

- Attending to a patient's spirituality ensures a holistic focus to nursing practice.
- Frequently the concepts of spirituality and religion are interchanged, but spirituality is a much broader and more unifying concept than religion.
- An individual's beliefs and spiritual well-being influence physical health status.
- Faith and hope are closely linked to a person's spiritual well-being, providing an inner strength for dealing with illness and disability.
- Research suggests that there is a link between a patient's spirituality and potential for healing.
- Acute and chronic illness, terminal illness, and NDEs pose spiritual problems for individuals.
- Providing appropriate spiritual care requires you to critically apply knowledge from principles related to caring, cultural care, loss and grief, and therapeutic communication.
- Avoid biases when assessing and planning spiritual care.
- Learning to practice caring and compassion helps you discover a patient's life values and meaning.
- Connectedness and fellowship with other people are a source of hope for a patient.
- Patients often have spiritual strengths that you use as resources to help them live healthier lives.
- Interruptions in or changes to customary religious practices affect the support that religion contributes to a person's well-being.
- Common religious rituals include private worship, prayer, singing, use of a rosary, and scripture reading.
- The personal nature of spirituality requires open communication and the establishment of trust between you and a patient.
- Establishing presence involves giving attention, answering questions, having an encouraging attitude, and conveying a sense of trust.
- Part of a patient's caregiving environment is the regular presence of family, friends, and spiritual advisors.

REFERENCES

Abuatiq A. Spiritual care for critical care patients. Int J Nurs Clin Pract 2015;2:128.

Benner P. From novice to expert. Menlo Park, CA: Addison-Wesley; 1984.

Borneman T, Ferrell B, Puchalski CM. Evaluation of the FICA tool for spiritual assessment. J Pain Symptom Manage 2010;40(2):163.

Broadhurst K, Harrington A. A mixed method thematic review: the importance of hope to the dying patient. J Adv Nurs 2015;72(1):18.

Carron R. Spirituality. In: Larsen PD, editor. Lubkin's chronic illness: impact and interventions. 9th ed. Burlington, MA: Jones & Bartlett; 2016.

Carson VB. Spirituality. In: Giddens JF, editor. Concepts for nursing practice. 2nd ed. St. Louis: Elsevier; 2017.

Chiang YC, Lee HC, Chu TL, Han CY, Hsiao YC. The impact of nurses' spiritual health on their attitudes toward spiritual care, professional commitment, and caring. Nurs Outlook 2016;64(3):215.

Collins-McNeil J, McCabe M, Sharp D, Hawkins T, Edwards CL. Spirituality: opportunities for advanced practice nursing and primary care. J Christ Nurs 2015;32(2):75.

Conway-Phillips R, Janusek L. Influence of sense of coherence, spirituality, social support and health perception on breast cancer screening motivation and behavior in African American women. ABNF J 2014; 25(3):72.

Cottrell L. Joy and happiness: a simultaneous and evolutionary concept analysis. J Adv Nurs 2016;72(7):1506.

Dahlkemper TR. Anderson's caring for older adults holistically. 6th ed. Philadelphia: FA Davis; 2016.

Darby K, Nash P, Nash S. Understanding and responding to spiritual and religious needs of young people with cancer. Cancer Nurs Pract 2014;13(2):32.

Delgado C. Nurses' spiritual care practices: becoming less. J Christ Nurs 2015;32(2):116.

Dobratz MC. Building a middle-range theory of adaptive spirituality. Nurs Sci Q 2016;29(2):146.

Dunn SL. Identifying and promoting hope in patients. West J Nurs Res 2016;38(3):267.

Estores IM, Frye J. Healing environments: integrative medicine and palliative care in acute care settings. Crit Care Nurs Clin North Am 2015;27:369.

Finocchiaro DN. Supporting the patient's spiritual needs at the end of life. Nursing 2016;46(5):57.

Granero-Molina J, Díaz Cortés MM, Márquez Membrive J, Castro-Sánchez AM, López Entrambasaguas OM, Fernández-Sola C. Religious faith in coping with terminal cancer: what is the nursing experience? Eur J Cancer Care (Engl) 2014;23(3):300.

Griggs S, Walker RK. The role of hope for adolescents with a chronic illness: an integrative review. J Pediatr Nurs 2016;31:404.

Hakanson C, Ohlen J. Connectedness at the end of life among people admitted to inpatient palliative care. Am J Hosp Palliat Care 2016; 33(1):47.

Hatamipour K, Rassouli M, Yaghmaie F, Zendedel K, Majd HA. Spiritual needs of cancer patients: a qualitative study. Indian J Palliat Care 2015;21(1):61.
Hodge DR. Administering a two-stage spiritual assessment in healthcare settings: a necessary component of ethical and effective care. J Nurs Manag 2015;23:27.
Johnson S. Near-death experience in patients on hemodialysis. Nephrol Nurs J 2015;42(4):331.
Jones A, Cohen D, Johnstone B, Yoon DP, Schopp LH, McCormack G, et al. Relationships between negative spiritual beliefs and health outcomes for individuals with heterogeneous medical conditions. J Spiritual Ment Health 2015;17:135.
Life Advance. The spiritual well-being scale. 2009. Available from: http://www.lifeadvance.com/spiritual-well-being-scale.html.
Manning LK. Enduring as lived experience: exploring the essence of spiritual resilience for women in later life. J Relig Health 2014;53(2):352.
March P, Caple C. Spiritual needs of hospitalized patients. In: *CINAHL Nursing Guide.* April 29, 2016.
NANDA International. Nursing diagnoses: definitions and classification, 2015–2017. 10th ed. Oxford: Wiley-Blackwell; 2014.
O'Brien ME. Spirituality in nursing: standing on Holy ground. 5th ed. Washington, DC: Jones & Bartlett; 2014.
Pantuso T. Spiritual interventions for patients with cancer. Integr Med Alert 2015;18(7):79.
Petersen CL. Spiritual care of the child with cancer at the end of life: a concept analysis. J Adv Nurs 2014;70(6):1243.
Plunkett R, Leipert B, Ray SL, Olson JK. Healthy spaces in meaningful places: the rural church and women's health promotion. J Holist Nurs 2015;33(2):122.
Pullen L, Mcguire S, Farmer L, Dodd D. The relevance of spirituality to nursing practice and education. Mental Health Pract 2015;18(5):14.
Ramezani M, Ahmadi F, Mohammadi E, Kazemnejad A. Spiritual care in nursing: a concept analysis. Int Nurs Rev 2014;61:211.
Rawlings D, Devery K. Near death experience and nursing practice: lessons from the palliative care literature. Aust Nurs Midwifery J 2015;22(8):26.
Rowold J. Effects of spiritual well-being on subsequent happiness, psychological well-being, and stress. J Relig Health 2011;50(4):950.
Rykkje L, Raholm MB. Understanding older people's experiences of dignity and its significance in caring—a hermeneutical study. Int J Hum Caring 2014;18(1):17.
Starkweather A. Pain. In: Giddens JF, editor. Concepts for nursing practice. 2nd ed. St. Louis: Elsevier; 2017.
Sweat MT. How do I spiritually support those who are suffering and in pain? J Christ Nurs 2015;32(2):123.
Tadwalkar R, Udeoji DU, Weiner RJ, Avestruz FL, LaChance D, Phan A, et al. The beneficial role of spiritual counseling in heart failure patients. J Relig Health 2014;53:1575.
Taylor EJ, Park CG, Pfeiffer JB. Nurse religiosity and spiritual care. J Adv Nurs 2014;70(11):2612.
Taylor EJ, Petersen C, Oyedele O, Haase J. Spirituality and spiritual care of adolescents and young adults with cancer. Semin Oncol Nurs 2015;31(3):227.
Timmins F, Neill F, Griffin MQ, Kelly J, De La Cruz E. Spiritual dimensions of care: developing an educational package for hospital nurses in the Republic of Ireland. Holist Nurs Pract 2014;28(2):106.
Touhy TA, Jett KF. Ebersole and Hess' gerontological nursing & healthy aging. 5th ed. St. Louis: Elsevier; 2018.
Trevino KM, McConnell TR. Religiosity and spirituality during cardiac rehabilitation. J Cardiopulm Rehabil Prev 2015;35:246.
Viglund K, Jonsén E, Strandberg G, Lundman B, Nygren B. Inner strength as a mediator of the relationship between disease and self-rated health among old people. J Adv Nurs 2014;70(1):44.
Yarcheski A, Mahon NE. Meta-analyses of predictors of hope in adolescents. West J Nurs Res 2016;38(3):345.

33 Cultural Competence

OBJECTIVES

- To describe cultural influences on health and illness.
- To explain how the many facets of culture affect a health care provider's ability to provide culturally congruent care.
- To describe health disparities and social determinants of health.
- To describe steps toward developing cultural competence.
- To describe the relationship between cultural competence and patient-centered care.
- To use cultural assessment to plan culturally competent care.
- To discuss research findings applicable to culturally competent care.
- To discuss research finding applicable to equity-focused quality improvement.

KEY TERMS

core measures, p. 794	cultural encounter, p. 787	explanatory model, p. 790
cultural assessment, p. 789	cultural knowledge, p. 787	intersectionality, p. 785
cultural awareness, p. 787	cultural skill, p. 787	linguistic competence, p. 792
cultural competence, p. 785	culturally congruent, p. 786	oppression, p. 785
cultural desire, p. 787	culture, p. 785	world view, p. 788

INTRODUCTION

Culture, in its broadest sense, reflects the whole of human behavior including ideas, beliefs, and values; ways of relating to one another; language and manners of speaking; and work and lifestyle practices. Every one of us has some type of bias that is culturally driven. A bias is an inclination or the holding of a partial perspective, often accompanied by a refusal to consider a different point of view. One might have a bias toward or against an individual based on his or her culture such as a bias toward an ethnic group, a race, gender, a nation, a religion, a social class, or a political party. When you as a nurse hold a bias toward an individual patient or group of patients, it is very difficult to provide patient-centered care. A patient-centered approach to providing care requires you to be respectful of and responsive to individual patient preferences, needs, and values and to ensure that patient values guide all clinical care decisions (Institute of Medicine [IOM], 2001). This chapter explains the importance of cultural competence and its relationship with patient-centered care. Cultural beliefs, values, and practices are learned from birth, first in the home, then in the church or other places where people congregate, and then in educational and other social settings (Purnell, 2013). This cultural learning applies to both you and your patients. The process of **cultural competence** in delivering health care services is "a culturally conscious model of care in which a healthcare professional continually strives to achieve the ability and availability to effectively work within the cultural context of a client" (family, individual, or community) (Transcultural C.A.R.E. Associates, 2015). It is a process of becoming culturally competent, not being culturally competent (Transcultural C.A.R.E. Associates, 2015).

CULTURE

Culture is associated with norms, values, and traditions passed down through generations. It also has been perceived to be the same as ethnicity, race, nationality, and language (Kleinman and Benson, 2006). A more contemporary view of culture acknowledges its many other facets such as gender, sexual orientation, location, class, and immigration status. This more dynamic perspective recognizes that we all belong simultaneously to multiple social groups within changing social and political contexts, a framework often referred to as **intersectionality** (Box 33.1). According to this framework, our memberships in social groups are not neutral. **Oppression** is a formal and informal system of advantages and disadvantages tied to our membership in social groups, such as those at work, at school, and in families (Adams et al., 2007). It impacts an individual's access to resources such as health care, housing, education, employment, and legal services. Whether we live in a disadvantaged

BOX 33.1 Key Concepts of Intersectionality

Intersectionality refers to the notion that intersecting categories such as race, ethnicity, gender, socioeconomic status, sexual orientation, and other axes of identity contribute to systemic injustice and social inequality (Cho et al., 2013).

- Social inequality: Groups have unequal access to resources, services, and positions.
- Overinclusion and underinclusion: Many groups have been overlooked in research and the design of interventions. For example, much of what is currently known about racial and ethnic disparities is drawn from national information sources and combines both sexes, despite the large body of evidence of sex and gender differences in the prevalence of health conditions and the use of health services (James et al., 2009).
- Marginalization: Groups are left out (e.g., limited access or exclusion from facets of the society such as political system, labor market, positions of power).
- Social location: One's place in society is based on membership in a social group (e.g., gender, race, class, sexual orientation) that determines access to resources. Social location is not based on biology but on the meaning that society constructs and gives to one's social group.
- Matrix of domination: Instead of thinking about race, gender, immigration status, class, and other axes of identity as descriptive categories only, it is important to understand them within the context of the larger system of power and privilege that permeates society.

Adapted from Murphy Y et al: Incorporating intersectionality in social work practice, research, policy, and education, Washington, DC, 2009, NASW Press.

community or in a community with access to social power and resources, we are all affected by the system of oppression. Understanding the dynamics of oppression that operate on various levels while simultaneously affecting you and your patients helps you engage in the process of becoming more culturally competent.

The many categories that comprise culture are not isolated from each other—they stand alone, interact, and are interdependent and mutually reinforcing. Although both groups and individuals within cultural groups may share commonalties in their experiences of oppression(s), there are also differences in these experiences. Including oppression in our definition of culture helps us recognize the profound effect it has on the individual and group experiences of all of us.

To better understand this more dynamic and complex way of thinking about culture, consider this example. As a nurse, think about how a 27-year-old homeless woman with diabetes, an 85-year-old African American retired nurse from rural Alabama, a 32-year-old Latina lesbian executive in San Francisco who is Catholic, and an undocumented immigrant woman from Eastern Europe who has a 3-year-old child with a developmental disability experience their womanhood. How may their experiences compare with the experiences of others as they live in America? How do their experiences compare with regard to using a health care system, managing their diabetes, or perceiving the presence or absence of opportunities to live a happy, safe, and productive life? How could age affect their perspective? How would these answers change if one looked at their lives 15 or 35 years ago? How would the experiences change if these individuals were men or transgender? These scenarios are likely to draw a wide range of responses.

Understanding culture requires you to adopt an intersectional perspective like the one in the example. This allows you to consider the multitude of different experiences of your patients so that you can provide effective, evidence-based, culturally competent care.

TRANSCULTURAL NURSING

Leininger (2002) defines **transcultural nursing** as a comparative study of cultures to understand their similarities (culture that is universal) and the differences among them (culture that is specific to particular groups). The goal of transcultural nursing is to provide **culturally congruent care**, or care that fits a person's life patterns, values, and system of meaning. Patterns and meaning are generated by people themselves rather than from predetermined criteria. For example, rather than instructing all patients to always take their medications at the same set times during a day, you learn their lifestyle patterns, eating habits, sleep habits, and beliefs about medications and then try to plan a dosage schedule that fits each patient's needs. Culturally congruent care is sometimes different from the values and meanings of the professional health care system. Discovering patients' cultural values, beliefs, and practices as they relate to nursing and health care requires you to assume the role of learner and to partner with your patients and their families to determine what is needed to provide meaningful and beneficial nursing care (Leininger and McFarland, 2002). Effective nursing care integrates the cultural values and beliefs of individuals, families, and communities with the perspectives of a multidisciplinary team of health care providers.

When you provide culturally congruent care, you bridge cultural gaps to provide meaningful and supportive care for all patients. For example, during nursing school, you are assigned to care for a female patient who observes Muslim beliefs. You notice the woman's discomfort with several of the male health care providers. You wonder whether this discomfort is related to your patient's religious beliefs. While preparing for clinical, you learn that Muslims differ in their adherence to tradition but that modesty is the "overarching Islamic ethic" pertaining to interaction between the sexes (Rabin, 2010). Thus, you say to the patient, "I know that for many of our Muslim patients, modesty is very important. Is there some way I can make you more comfortable?" You do not assume that the information will automatically apply to this patient. Instead, you combine your knowledge about a cultural group with an attitude of helpfulness and flexibility to provide quality, patient-centered, culturally congruent care.

CULTURAL COMPETENCE

Cultural competence is the ongoing process in which a health care professional tries to achieve the ability and availability to effectively work within the cultural context of a

BOX 33.2 National Standards for Culturally and Linguistically Appropriate Services (CLAS) in Health and Health Care

The National CLAS Standards are intended to advance health equity, improve quality, and help eliminate health care disparities by establishing a blueprint for health and health care organizations to:

Principal Standard

1 Provide effective, equitable, understandable, and respectful quality care and services that are responsive to diverse cultural health beliefs and practices, preferred languages, health literacy, and other communication needs.

Governance, Leadership, and Workforce

2. Advance and sustain organizational governance and leadership that promotes CLAS and health equity through policy, practices, and allocated resources.
3. Recruit, promote, and support a culturally and linguistically diverse governance, leadership, and workforce that are responsive to the population in the service area.
4. Educate and train governance, leadership, and workforce in culturally and linguistically appropriate policies and practices on an ongoing basis.

Communication and Language Assistance

5. Offer language assistance to individuals who have limited English proficiency and/or other communication needs, at no cost to them, to facilitate timely access to all health care and services.
6. Inform all individuals of the availability of language assistance services clearly and in their preferred language, verbally and in writing.
7. Ensure the competence of individuals providing language assistance, recognizing that the use of untrained individuals and/or minors as interpreters should be avoided.
8. Provide easy-to-understand print and multimedia materials and signage in the languages commonly used by the populations in the service area.

Engagement, Continuous Improvement, and Accountability

9. Establish culturally and linguistically appropriate goals, policies, and management accountability, and infuse them throughout the organization's planning and operations.
10. Conduct ongoing assessments of the organization's CLAS-related activities and integrate CLAS-related measures into assessment measurement and continuous quality improvement activities.
11. Collect and maintain accurate and reliable demographic data to monitor and evaluate the impact of CLAS on health equity and outcomes and to inform service delivery.
12. Conduct regular assessments of community health assets and needs and use the results to plan and implement services that respond to the cultural and linguistic diversity of populations in the service area.
13. Partner with the community to design, implement, and evaluate policies, practices, and services to ensure cultural and linguistic appropriateness.
14. Create conflict and grievance resolution processes that are culturally and linguistically appropriate to identify, prevent, and resolve conflicts or complaints.
15. Communicate the organization's progress in implementing and sustaining CLAS to all stakeholders, constituents, and the general public.

From the United States Department of Health and Human Services (USDHHS): *National standards for culturally and linguistically appropriate services (CLAS) in health and health care*, Washington, D.C., 2013. USDHHS Office of Minority Health.

patient (individual, family, or community) (Transcultural C.A.R.E. Associates, 2015). It is a developmental process that evolves over a lifetime as individuals engage with others and learn from their experiences. Campinha-Bacote's model of cultural competency has five interrelated constructs (Transcultural C.A.R.E. Associates, 2015): cultural awareness, cultural knowledge, cultural skill, cultural encounters, and cultural desire. The five constructs provide a framework for you to practice in a culturally competent manner.

- **Cultural awareness** is the process of conducting a self-examination of one's own biases toward other cultures and the in-depth exploration of one's cultural and professional background. It also involves being aware of the existence of documented racism and other "isms" in health care delivery.
- **Cultural knowledge** is the process in which a health care professional seeks and obtains a sound educational base about culturally diverse groups. In acquiring this knowledge, health care professionals must focus on the integration of three specific issues: health-related beliefs and cultural values, care practices, and disease incidence and prevalence.
- **Cultural skill** is the ability to conduct a cultural assessment of a patient to collect relevant cultural data about a patient's presenting problem as well as accurately conduct a culturally based physical assessment.
- **Cultural encounter** is a process that encourages health care professionals to directly engage in face-to-face cultural interactions and other types of encounters with patients from culturally diverse backgrounds. A cultural encounter aims to modify a health care provider's existing beliefs about a cultural group and to prevent possible stereotyping.
- **Cultural desire** is the motivation of a health care professional to "want to" (and not "have to") engage in the process of becoming culturally aware, culturally knowledgeable, and culturally skillful and seeking cultural encounters.

In 2000, the Office of Minority Health (OMH) developed the Culturally and Linguistically Appropriate Standards (CLAS). In 2013, after 10 years of successful implementation, the OMH updated the standards to reflect the tremendous growth in the field and the increasing diversity of the nation (Box 33.2).

PROVIDING CULTURALLY RESPONSIVE CARE

Two landmark reports from the Institute of Medicine (IOM)—*Crossing the Quality Chasm* (IOM, 2001) and *Unequal Treatment* (Smedley et al., 2003)—highlight the importance of patient-centered care and cultural competence. *Crossing*

BOX 33.3 Patient-Centered Care for LGBT Patients

- Create a welcoming environment that is inclusive of LGBT patients. A health care organization should have a prominently posted nondiscrimination policy or patient bill of rights that explicitly mentions sexual orientation and gender identity. Any displayed art and health materials should include images and topics relevant to LGBT patients.
- Health care organizations should create or designate unisex or single-stall restrooms because patients whose appearance may not conform to traditional gender expressions may feel less comfortable using traditional male- and female-designated restrooms.
- Ensure that visitation policies are fair and implemented in a nondiscriminatory manner. Any denial of access should have a clear medical explanation.
- Avoid assumptions about sexual orientation and gender identity, remembering that any patient can be LGBT, regardless of his or her age, appearance, and other axis of identification.
- Include LGBT-inclusive language on forms and assessments to facilitate disclosure, knowing that disclosure is a choice impacted by many factors. For example, provide options such as "partnered" under relationship status. For parents, use parent/guardian, instead of mother/father.
- Use neutral and inclusive language when talking with patients (e.g., partner or significant other), listening and reflecting the patient's choice. Remember that some LGBT patients are also legally married.

LGBT, lesbian, gay, bisexual, and transgender.
Data from Gay and Lesbian Medical Association (GLMA): *Guidelines for care of lesbian, gay, bisexual, and transgender patients*, 2006, http://www.clark.wa.gov/public-health/hiv/documents/GLMA%20Welcoming.pdf. Accessed August 2015.

the Quality Chasm identifies patient-centered care as one of six "aims" for high-quality health care, and *Unequal Treatment* stresses the importance of developing cultural competence among health care providers to eliminate racial/ethnic health care disparities (Box 33.3). The differences between cultural competence and patient-centered care are not always clear. However, Beach and colleagues (2006) succinctly summarize the differences and similarities between these two concepts.

Both patient-centeredness and cultural competence aim to improve health care quality, but each emphasizes different aspects of quality. The primary goal of the patient-centeredness movement has been to provide individualized care and restore an emphasis on personal relationships. It aims to elevate quality for all patients. Alternatively, the primary aim of the cultural competence movement has been to increase health equity and reduce disparities by concentrating on people of color and other disadvantaged populations.

Campinha-Bacote (2011) views cultural competency as an expansion of patient-centered care. More specifically, cultural competence can be seen as a necessary set of skills for nurses to attain to render effective patient-centered care. It is important for nurses to see themselves as becoming culturally competent. Your ability to exercise cultural competence by applying the components of Campinha-Bacote's (2002) model of cultural competency will allow you to deliver patient-centered care.

Cultural Awareness

Curiosity about other ways of being in the world is an important attitude for cultural competence; however, it is also important for you to understand the forces that influence your own world view. Everyone holds biases about human behavior. A bias is a predisposition to see people or things in a certain light, either positive or negative. Becoming more self-aware of your biases and attitudes about human behavior is the first step in providing patient-centered care. You should spend time reflecting on what you learned, formally and informally, throughout your life about health, illness (physical and mental), health care system, gender roles, sexual orientation, race, ability, age, family, and many other issues as a part of your commitment to becoming a culturally competent nurse. It is helpful to think about cultural competence as a lifelong process of learning about others and also about yourself.

Cultural Knowledge—World Views

Historical and social realities shape an individual's or group's **world view**, which determines how people perceive others, how they interact and relate to reality, and how they process information (Walker et al., 2010). World view refers to "the way people tend to look out upon the world or their universe to form a picture or value stance about life or the world around them" (Leininger, 2006). The cycle of socialization is the lifetime process of interacting with family, peers, communities, organizations, media, and institutions through which we develop our world view. As a nurse, it is important that you advocate for patients by gaining knowledge about their world view. When you assess a patient's cultural background and needs, you take into account each patient's world view, and then you plan and provide nursing care in partnership with each patient to ensure that it is safe, effective, and culturally sensitive (McFarland and Eipperle, 2008).

In any intercultural encounter, there is an insider perspective (emic world view) and an outsider perspective (etic world view). For example, a Korean woman requests seaweed soup for her first meal after giving birth. This request puzzles her nurse. The nurse has an insider's view of professional postpartum care but is an outsider to the Korean culture. As such, the nurse is not aware of the significance of the meal to the patient. Conversely, the Korean patient has an outsider's view of American professional postpartum care and assumes that seaweed soup is available in the hospital because, according to her cultural beliefs, the soup cleanses the blood and promotes healing and lactation (Edelstein, 2011).

It is easy for nurses to stereotype various cultural groups after reading general information about ethnic practices and beliefs (Kleinman, 2013). Avoid stereotypes or unwarranted generalizations about any particular group that prevent an accurate assessment of an individual's unique characteristics and world view. Instead, approach each person individually and ask questions to gain a better understanding of his or her perspective and needs.

Health care has its own culture of hierarchies, power dynamics, values, beliefs, and practices. Research supports the idea that group membership such as membership in a professional group shapes one's world view (Sue, 2006). Most health care providers educated in Western traditions are immersed in the culture of science and biomedicine through their course work and professional experience. Consequently, they often have a world view that differs from that of their patients (Kleinman, 2013). As a nurse, it is best to see every patient encounter as being cross-cultural.

Even when a patient and a health care provider are similar in age or have the same gender or ethnicity, two different perspectives are present each time they interact. When patients access the health care system, they want to: (1) see their health care provider, and (2) feel better. In return, the health care providers expect patients to: (1) make and keep appointments; (2) give a medication history; (3) give informed consent; (4) follow (discharge) instructions; (5) read, understand, and use health education materials; (6) correctly complete insurance forms; (7) pay their bills; and (8) go home and manage their care by taking their medication the right way, eating the right foods, and stopping/starting/changing a variety of behaviors (AMA, 2007). This list shows how complex each patient interaction is even before the interaction begins. The complexity increases as you consider the interactive effect between a health care provider's and a patient's multiple social group identities and unique life experiences.

Nurses, patients, and all other health care providers bring each of their world views into the care process. The Iceberg Analogy is a tool that helps you to visualize the visible and invisible aspects of your world view and recognize that the same applies to your patients. Just as most of an iceberg lies beneath the surface of the water, most aspects of a person's world view lie outside of his or her awareness and are invisible to those around the person. For example, a young female patient who has willingly agreed to be admitted to the hospital for a serious medical condition requiring surgery may refuse the surgery for religious reasons. In the patient's view, she came to the hospital for help to eliminate the pain and infection from her illness. At the same time, she believes that she needs to seek God's will for a decision that entails removing a body part. The patient's health care provider assumes that the patient is in the hospital to receive care for a serious illness and is willing to accept any and all treatments to cure the illness. The patient's deeply held religious beliefs about removing a body part are not obvious by assessing for a religious preference. Thus, you would need to conduct a comprehensive **cultural assessment** (Box 33.4) to understand the patient's world view, including how her religious

BOX 33.4 Nursing Assessment Questions

Open-Ended

- What do you think caused your illness?
- How do you want us to help you with your problem?
- Tell me how your beliefs affect your views on medical treatment choices and your willingness to receive care.

Focused

- Did you have this problem before?
- Is there someone with whom you want us to talk about your care?

Contrast

- How different is this problem from the one you had previously?
- What is the difference between what we are doing and what you think we should be doing for you?

Ethnohistory

- What is your ethnic background or ancestry?
- For patients who are first- or second-generation immigrants:
  - How long have you/your parents resided in this country?
  - Tell me why you/your family left your homeland.
  - How different is your life here from back home?

Sexual Orientation and Gender Identity

- What is your legal name?
- How do you prefer to be addressed?
- What is your preferred pronoun (he, she, they, or something else)?
- What is your gender?
- Are your current sexual partners men, women, or both?
- In the past, have your sexual partners been men, women, or both?
- What is your current relationship status?

Social Organization

- Who lives with you?
- Whom do you consider members of your family?
- Where do other members of your family live?
- Who makes the decisions for you or your family?
- To whom do you go outside of your family for support?
- What expectations do you have of your family members and support people? Are there different expectations for family members and support people of different ages and genders?

Socioeconomic Status

- What is your main source of income?
- If employed: What do you do for a living?

Bicultural Ecology and Health Risks

- What caused your problem?
- How does this problem affect or how has it affected your life and your family?
- How do you treat this problem at home?
- What other problems do you have?

Language and Communication

- What language(s) do you speak at home?
- What language(s) do you use to read and write?
- How should we address you or what should we call you?
- Which kinds of communication upset or offend you?

Caring Beliefs and Practices

- What do you do to keep yourself well?
- What do you do to show someone you care?
- How do you take care of sick family members?
- Which caregivers do you seek when you are sick?
- How different is what we do from what your family does for you when you are sick?

values affected her willingness to receive care. These deeply held values reside underneath the iceberg. The observed behavior (in this case, coming to the hospital) is a visible sign of a person's world view, but the beliefs, attitudes, knowledge, and experiences that guide the behavior are not visible to others; they lie under the surface. Conflict arises when health care providers interpret the behaviors of patients through their own world view lens instead of trying to uncover the world view that guides this behavior.

Because of differences in age, gender, political preferences, class, religion, or other variables, cultural values frequently differ within a single social group such as a family or a group of nurses. For patients, family members, and members of the health care team alike, culture is a process through which ordinary activities such as greeting another person or selecting a doctor take on an emotional tone and moral meaning beyond that which appears on the surface (Kleinman, 2013). Think about the complexity of culture and world views. Realize the need to develop your assessment skills and cultural interventions that will allow you to successfully negotiate the various world views present in encounters with patients and families (and frequently other team members). Most important, remember that the core of this negotiation is compassionate care. Perhaps it may be helpful to think about these encounters as gift exchanges between individuals whose relationship with one another really matters (Kleinman, 2013). During these encounters, participants exchange not only information but also acknowledgment, presence, and affirmation (Kleinman, 2013).

Skills and Interventions

You need to develop assessment skills and be able to provide culturally congruent interventions to become culturally competent. To provide patient-centered culturally competent care, you must know how to collect relevant cultural data about a patient's presenting health problem(s) and how to then use them (Campinha-Bacote, 2011). Critical to success is your ability to conduct a systematic cultural assessment, communicate effectively, and have the skills to successfully manage world view differences with others.

Cultural Assessment

The goal of a cultural assessment is to obtain accurate information from a patient that allows you to formulate a mutually acceptable and culturally relevant plan of care for each health problem of a patient (Campinha-Bacote, 2011). Nurses need skills to perform a systematic cultural assessment of individuals, groups, and communities as to their cultural beliefs, values, and practices. Numerous models and assessment tools exist to facilitate cultural assessment, including Leininger's Sunrise Model (2002), Giger and Davidhizar's Transcultural Assessment Model (2002), and the Purnell Model for Cultural Competence (Purnell, 2002). Regardless of which one you select, using a cultural assessment model will help you focus on the information that is most relevant to your patient's problems. It will also help you better understand the complex factors that influence your patient's cultural world view. You need to assess and interpret a patient's perspective during your assessment. Use open-ended, focused, and contrasted questions. Encourage your patients to describe the values, beliefs, and practices that are significant to their care. Culturally oriented questions are by nature broad and require learning more about the patient's personal narratives (see Box 33.3).

One effective approach to assessment is to ask questions that will help you understand a patient's **explanatory model**—his or her views about health and illness and its treatment. There are five questions in most explanatory models: etiology, time and mode of onset of symptoms, pathophysiology, course of illness (including severity and type of sick role), and treatment for an illness episode. Understanding a patient's perceptions of these concepts and the relationship among them helps you provide patient-centered care that combines a patient's values and beliefs with your perspectives. Using a cultural model during your assessment (such as the one in that integrates Kleinman's explanatory model with the previously discussed Iceberg Analogy) will help you develop open-ended questions that effectively reveal your patient's views on illness (Kleinman and Benson, 2006). Table 33.1 summarizes and contrasts a patient's explanatory model of illness with the biomedical explanatory model of illness (Lynch and Medin, 2006).

In contrast to standard approaches for health assessment, cultural assessment is intrusive and may take more time to conduct because it requires building a trusting relationship between participants. Miscommunication commonly occurs in intercultural transactions. This occurs because of differences in verbal communication between participants and differences in interpreting one another's behaviors. You can use transcultural communication skills to better understand a patient's behavior and to behave in a culturally congruent way. Effective communication is a critical skill in providing quality and safe care.

A number of authors have developed mnemonic cultural assessment and planning tools. Mnemonics, or memory aids, offer you a different option that makes it easier to perform assessments and communicate effectively with patients about their plan of care (Box 33.5). They help you remember the steps of each communication technique. For example, if you use the LEARN mnemonic, your first step is to ***l****isten* to the patient's explanation or story of the presenting problem. Then you ***e****xplain* your perception of the patient's problem,

Table 33.1 Explanatory Model Comparison

Patient's Explanatory Model	Biomedical Explanatory Model
What do you call your problem? What name does it have?	Etiology
What do you think has caused your problem? Why do you think it started when it did?	Time and mode of onset
What do you think your sickness does to you? How does this illness work inside your body?	Pathophysiology
What will happen to you? What do you fear most about your sickness? What are the chief problems your sickness has caused for you?	Course of illness (including symptom severity and trajectory: acute, chronic, impaired)
How should your sickness be treated?	Recommended treatment

Adapted from Lynch E, Medin D: Explanatory models of illness: study of within-culture variation, *Cogn Psychol* 53(4):285, 2006.

BOX 33.5 Communication Techniques Using Mnemonics

Communication Technique	Process
LEARN	
Berlin EA, Fowkes WC Jr: A teaching framework for cross-cultural health care, *West J Med* 139(6):934, 1982.	*L*isten with empathy and understanding to the patient's perception of problem. *E*xplain your perceptions of the problem (physiological, psychological, spiritual, and/or cultural). *A*cknowledge and discuss cultural differences and similarities between you and your patient. *R*ecommend treatment (involving the patient). *N*egotiate agreement (incorporate selected aspects of the patient's culture into patient-centered plan)
RESPECT	
Bigby JA, editor: *Cross-cultural medicine*, Philadelphia, 2003, American College of Physicians, p. 20.	*R*apport ▪ Connect on a social level. ▪ Seek the patient's point of view. ▪ Consciously attempt to suspend judgment. ▪ Recognize and avoid making assumptions. *E*mpathy ▪ Remember that the patient has come to you for help. ▪ Seek out and understand the patient's rationale for his or her behaviors or illness. ▪ Verbally acknowledge and legitimize the patient's feelings. *S*upport ▪ Ask about and try to understand barriers to care and adherence. ▪ Help the patient overcome barriers by providing resources. ▪ Involve family members if appropriate. ▪ Reassure the patient that you are and will be available to help. *P*artnership ▪ Be flexible with regard to issues of control. ▪ Negotiate roles when necessary. ▪ Stress that you will be working together to address medical problems. *E*xplanations ▪ Check often for understanding. ▪ Use verbal clarification techniques. *C*ultural competence ▪ Respect the patient and his or her culture and beliefs. ▪ Understand that the patient's view of you may be influenced by stereotypes. ▪ Be aware of your own biases and preconceptions. ▪ Know your limitations in addressing medical issues across cultures. ▪ Understand your personal style and recognize when it may not be working with a given patient. *T*rust ▪ Self-disclosure may be difficult for some patients. ▪ Do not assume trust; instead, take necessary time and consciously work to earn trust.
ETHNIC	
Levin S, Like, R, Gottlieb J: *ETHNIC: a framework for culturally competent clinical practice.* New Brunswick, NJ, 2000, Department of Family Medicine, UMDNJ-Robert Wood Johnson Medical School.	*E*xplanation: The patient explains his or her perception of problem, or you ask what most concerns the patient. *T*reatment: Which types of treatments have the patient tried for the problem? *H*ealers: Has the patient sought advice from alternative health practitioners? *N*egotiate: Try to find an option that is mutually acceptable. *I*ntervention: Agree on an appropriate intervention, which may incorporate alternate treatments. *C*ollaboration: Include the patient, family members, and other health care professionals, healers, and community resources.
C-LARA	
C-LARA was developed by the organization Love Makes a Family; *C* (check your pulse) addition has been contributed by the organization Nonviolent Peaceforce.	*C*alm yourself down. Take a deep breath. Check your pulse. *L*isten to the patient's and family's perspective. *A*ffirm: Express connection with something that was shared: a feeling, perspective, principle. *R*espond: Respond to what was said. Answer the question. *A*dd: Share additional information for the patient and family to consider. In this step, you can educate.

whether it is physiological, psychological, or cultural. Then you ***a***cknowledge the similarities and differences between the two perceptions. It is important to recognize differences but build on the similarities (Campinha-Bacote, 2011). The fourth step involves ***r***ecommendations that require you to involve the patient and family when appropriate. The last step is to then ***n***egotiate a mutually agreeable, culturally oriented, patient-centered plan. Remember, cultural assessment and care planning requires a level of negotiation. Leininger (2006) describes cultural care negotiation as assistive, accommodating, facilitative, or enabling creative provider care actions or decisions that help people with different backgrounds adapt to or negotiate with others for culturally congruent care.

Linguistic Competence

Linguistic competence is the ability of an organization and its staff to communicate effectively and convey information in a manner that is easily understood by diverse audiences. These audiences include people of limited English proficiency (LEP), those who have low literacy skills or are not literate, individuals with disabilities, and those who are deaf or hard of hearing. Linguistic competency requires organizational resources (e.g., instructional resources designed at a 6th-grade reading level or lower, interpreters) and providers who are able to respond effectively to the health and mental health literacy needs of the populations served. One important service that health care organizations must provide is an interpretive service.

Most health care providers and virtually all health care organizations nationwide are subject to federal civil rights laws. These laws outline requirements for the provision of language access services. They also help ensure meaningful access to health care for people with LEP and offer effective communication services for those who are deaf or hard-of-hearing (TJC, 2013). As a nurse, it is critical for you to know that these laws require health care organizations to do the following:

- Provide language assistance services free of charge at all points of contact to all patients who speak limited English or are deaf.
- Notify patients, both verbally and in writing, of their right to receive language assistance services.
- Take steps to provide auxiliary aids and services, including qualified interpreters, note takers, computer-aided transcription services, and written materials.
- Ensure that interpreters are competent in medical terminology and understand issues of confidentiality and impartiality.

Do not use a patient's family members to interpret for you or other health care providers. Cultural dynamics, lack of interpreting skills, low health literacy, and bias could lead to inaccurate interpretation. Box 33.6 provides guidelines for effectively working with an interpreter.

Health Literacy

The concept of linguistic competence encompasses both health literacy and LEP. Choosing a healthy lifestyle, knowing how to seek medical care, and taking advantage of preventive health care measures require people to understand and use health information. Health literacy is the ability to obtain, process, and understand health information needed to make informed health decisions (Office of Disease Prevention and Health Promotion, n.d.). Studies show that health literacy has direct effects on health outcomes, linking poor health outcomes to limited health literacy (Berkman et al., 2011; Cho et al., 2008; DeWalt et al., 2004). More specifically, lower health literacy has been associated with higher risk of mortality for seniors, poorer ability to demonstrate taking medications appropriately, poorer ability to interpret labels and health messages, and poorer overall health status among seniors (Berkman et al., 2011). Approximately 9 out of 10 people in the United States experience challenges in using health care information (NCES, 2006). Patients who are especially vulnerable are the elderly (age more than 65), immigrants, people with low incomes, people who do not have a high-school diploma or GED (The GED is a high school equivalency diploma), and people with chronic mental and/or physical health conditions (AMA, 2007).

Commonly used measures of health literacy include literacy measures such as the Rapid Estimate of Adult Literacy in

BOX 33.6 Working With Interpreters

If a patient needs an interpreter, do not ask the patient's family members and friends or other health care providers not trained as medical interpreters to help with communication. Instead, request a medically trained interpreter. The interpreter could be available in person or via technology such as speakerphone or video. During each encounter:

- Introduce yourself to the interpreter and briefly describe the purpose of the meeting.
- Determine the interpreter's qualifications.
- Make sure that the interpreter can speak the patient's dialect or has an appropriate level of certification in case of American Sign Language (ASL).
- Consider the possible impact of differences in educational and socioeconomic status between the patient and the interpreter.
- Make sure that both the patient and the interpreter are compatible and that both understand the expectations of the interpreter role.
- Introduce the interpreter to the patient.
- Do not expect the interpreter to interpret your statements word for word. Although the interpreter must ensure that everything that was said is interpreted, he or she may need to use more or fewer words to convey the meaning of your conversation with a patient.
- If you sense that the interpretation is not going well, stop and address the situation directly with the interpreter.
- Pace your speech by using short sentences but do not break your sentences. Allow time for the patient's response to be interpreted.
- Direct your questions to the patient. Look at the patient instead of at the interpreter.
- Ask the patient for feedback and clarification at regular intervals.
- Observe the patient's nonverbal and verbal behaviors.
- Thank both the patient and the interpreter.

Medicine (REALM), which is a word recognition test; and the Test of Functional Health Literacy in Adults (TOFHLA), which measures reading skills and numeracy. No gold standard instrument is currently available to assess adequately the more global concept of health literacy, including the interactions of reading ability, numeracy, and oral literacy (Berkman et al., 2011). However, researchers are beginning to develop instruments more specifically for health literacy (e.g., Newest Vital Sign, Diabetes Numeracy Test) that are framed in specific health contexts and assess condition-related skills (Berkman et al., 2011). Interestingly, in a study involving patients in the Veterans Administration (VA) system, the single question, "How confident are you filling out medical forms for yourself," showed a high correlation with being able to detect inadequate health literacy (Chew et al., 2008).

Teach Back

Evidence suggests that health care providers who attend to both health literacy and cultural differences help reduce medical errors and improve adherence, patient–provider–family communication, and outcomes of care at both individual and population levels (Lie et al., 2012). Clear communication is essential for effective delivery of quality and safe health care, but most patients experience significant challenges when communicating with their health care providers. The teach back method is an intervention that helps you to confirm that you have explained what a patient needs to know in a manner that the patient understands. The teach back technique is an ongoing process of asking patients for feedback through explanation or demonstration and presenting information in a new way until you feel confident that you communicated clearly and that your patient has a full understanding of the information presented (Fig. 33.1). You also use teach back to help you identify explanations and communication strategies that your patients most commonly understand (AHRQ, 2013b).

When using the teach back technique, do not ask a patient, "Do you understand?" or "Do you have any questions?" Instead, ask open-ended questions to verify his or her understanding. You can ask the question in the following ways:

- "I've given you a lot of information to remember. Please explain it back to me so I can be sure that I gave you the information you need to take good care of yourself."
- "What will you tell your wife (or husband/partner/child) about the changes we made to your medications today?"
- "We've gone over a lot of information today about how you might change your diet, and I want to make sure that I explained everything clearly. In your own words, please review what we talked about. How will you make it work at home?"

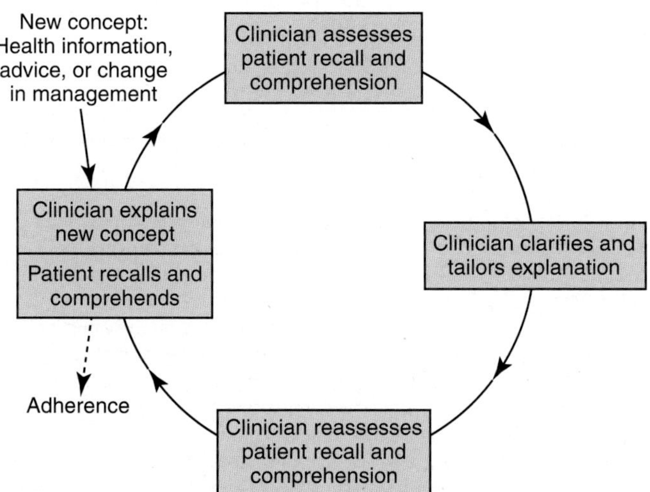

Fig. 33.1 Using teach back technique to close the loop. (From the U.S. Health Resources and Services Administration.)

It is important to understand that teach back is not intended to test a patient but rather to confirm the clarity of your communication (AHRQ, 2013b). Many patients are embarrassed by their inability to sort out health information or instructions. By regarding teach back as a test of your communication skills, you take responsibility for the success or failure of the interaction and create a shame-free environment for your patients.

Helpful hints to consider when trying the teach back method are as follows:

- *Plan your approach.* Think about how you will ask your patient to teach back in a shame-free way. Keep in mind that some situations are not appropriate for teach back (AHRQ, 2013b).
- *Use handouts, pictures,* and *models* to reinforce your teaching (AHRQ, 2013b).
- *Clarify.* If a patient cannot remember or accurately repeat your instructions, clarify your information and allow him or her to teach it back again. Do this until the patient is able to teach back in his or her own words without parroting back what you said (AHRQ, 2013b). Understand teach back as a process of "closing the loop" (see Fig. 33.1).
- *Practice.* Although it takes time to get used to teach back, studies show that it doesn't take longer to perform once it becomes a part of your routine (AHRQ, 2013b).

Cultural Encounters

A cultural encounter is an intervention that involves a nurse directly interacting with patients from culturally diverse backgrounds (Campinha-Bacote, 2011). The use of a caring, therapeutic, and culturally congruent relationship will lessen the likelihood of conflict when you engage in such encounters. A cultural encounter enables new forms of community and collective identity between you and your patients. Campinha-Bacote (2011) describes two goals of a cultural encounter: (1) to generate a wide variety of responses and to send and receive both verbal and nonverbal communication accurately and appropriately, and (2) to continuously interact with patients from culturally diverse backgrounds to validate, refine, or modify existing values, beliefs, and practices and to develop cultural desire, awareness, skill, and knowledge. The challenge is being able to show compassion, especially if cross-cultural conflict develops. However, conflict gives you an excellent opportunity for developing compassion and sharing one's suffering to achieve better health outcomes for your patients. A patient-centered and culturally competent encounter must be viewed as a "win-and-lose" situation for a patient and a "win-and-lose" situation for a nurse. Such an encounter effectively resolves cultural conflict by avoiding a "win-or-lose" situation for either the patient or the nurse and instead results in a "win–lose/win–lose" situation in which the values of both the patient and the nurse are respected (Campinha-Bacote, 2011).

Cultural Desire

It is easy to avoid cultural encounters with patients. Time, our personal discomfort in communicating with others who are "different," and a focus on physical care priorities are just some of the factors that may limit encounters with patients. Cultural desire is the motivation of a health care professional to "want to"—not "have to"—engage in the process of becoming culturally competent (Campinha-Bacote, 2011). It involves a natural inclination to engage in the cultural competence process that is characterized by passion, commitment, and caring. An ethically responsible professional nurse must embrace the importance of cultural competency and apply principles in daily patient encounters.

Within health care organizations nowadays, more changes are occurring to integrate cultural competence principles into everyday organizational processes and practices. Health care regulatory agencies, national think tanks, and government agencies expect health care organizations to incorporate cultural competence into policies and practices to ensure effective communication, patient safety and quality, and patient-centered care. Examples of such organizational policies and practices include the following:

- Instituting a requirement for all staff to be trained in cultural competence
- Embedding a broad description of family in written policies
- Expanding visitation policies and practices to include a patient's preferences
- Requiring nursing staff to conduct and document a cultural assessment on all patients within the clinical documentation system
- Ensuring that people who are deaf or speak limited English have access to an interpreter
- Embedding health literacy principles in written and verbal communication
- Collecting race, ethnicity, and language information from patients on admission and stratifying outcome data by these and other demographic indicators to identify disparities in care
- Using stratified outcome data to improve the health of populations

Core Measures

The Joint Commission (TJC) and the Centers for Medicare and Medicaid Services (CMS) are two of the many regulatory bodies that hold health care providers accountable for considering patients' unique cultural perspectives to provide safe and quality care. To improve health outcomes, TJC and the CMS developed a set of evidence-based, scientifically researched standards of care called *core measures* (TJC, 2013). The **core measures** are key quality indicators that help health care institutions improve performance, increase accountability, and reduce costs. All of the core measures such as screening for depression and controlling high blood pressure are consistent with national health priorities. They represent clinical conditions such as heart failure, acute myocardial infarction, pneumonia, and surgical-site infections. Following these standards of care on a nationwide scale is expected to reduce mortality, complications, and inpatient readmissions (Chassin et al., 2010; VanSuch et al., 2006).

In addition, core measures are intended to reduce health disparities. According to the 2013 National Health Care Disparities Report, Black people and Hispanics people received worse care than White people for about 40% of quality measures, American Indians and Alaska Natives received worse care than White people for about 30% of core measures, Asians received worse care than White people for about 25% of core measures, and poor people received worse care than high-income people for about 60% of core measures (AHRQ, 2013a).

Although most disparities in quality are significantly worse for some populations compared with White patients, there are some improvements in these outcomes as more and more effort is focused on addressing these disparities. Box 33.7 provides an example of a successful equity-focused quality improvement (QI) effort and an evidence-based process for

BOX 33.7 Evidence-Based Practice

PICO Question: What is the most effective quality improvement (QI) process that nurses can use to eliminate disparities in patient outcomes on their unit?

Evidence Summary

Health care disparities persist and indicate a clear inequity in care quality on the basis of race, ethnicity, sexual orientation, socioeconomic status, and other accesses of social identity. However, evidence for QI interventions that successfully decreased disparities is limited because of many challenges in developing, implementing, and studying QI with vulnerable populations or in under-resourced settings (Lion and Raphael, 2015). In addition, general QI interventions designed to improve overall quality (as opposed to targeting the specific needs of the population experiencing disparities) may not improve disparities and in some cases may increase them if there is greater uptake or effectiveness of the intervention among the population with better outcomes at baseline (Lion and Raphael, 2015). Designing equity-centered QI efforts is key to eliminating health care disparities.

In a recent study, the investigators used an information technology (IT) surveillance for identifying and tracking patients overdue for colorectal cancer (CRC) screening to reduce socioeconomic disparities in their screening (Berkowitz et al., 2015). CRC is the third leading cause of cancer mortality for men and women and can be effectively prevented through different screening strategies (Berkowitz et al., 2015). The investigators implemented this effort in 18 primary care practice sites, including 4 community health centers within a practice-based research network in and around Boston. After the investigators discovered that CRC screening completion was lower for patients who had not finished high school than for patients who did, they contacted identified patients via letter or a telephone call. In addition, high-risk patients received patient navigation. The

BOX 33.7 Evidence-Based Practice—cont'd

intervention resulted in a 3% increase in CRC screening overall and modestly reduced screening disparity among those with a lower level of educational attainment. Although the investigators achieved only a modest reduction in disparities, the intervention demonstrated overall screening improvement from a population health standpoint (Paluri, 2015). This study serves as an example that equity-centered QI efforts can address quality and equity.

Finding Answers, a national program office of the Robert Wood Johnson Foundation (RWJF), has been researching strategies and interventions to eliminate disparities in health outcomes. After conducting 12 systematic literature reviews and funding 33 innovative research projects, Finding Answers recommended a road map for organizations looking to implement equity-focused QI efforts and eliminate disparities in health outcomes (Clarke et al., n.d.).

Application to Nursing Practice

Emerging evidence-based strategies can help health care organizations working to reduce disparities in health outcomes. The road map offers a comprehensive approach to achieving equity. Use the following six steps described in *A Roadmap and Best Practices for Organizations to Reduce Racial and Ethnic Disparities in Health Care* (Chin et al., 2012) to implement equity-focused QI in your practice:

1. *Recognize disparities and commit to reducing them.* The Affordable Care Act makes the collection of a health care organization's performance data stratified by race, ethnicity, and language (REL) a priority. Cultural competency will improve your ability to assess for patient disparities.
2. *Implement a basic quality improvement structure and process.* An ongoing process is needed for a health care organization to build interventions. Nursing staff play a role in identifying opportunities to improve practice approaches for vulnerable patient groups.
3. *Make equity an integral component of quality improvement efforts.* It is necessary for health care organizations to think about the needs of vulnerable patients served as they design interventions to improve patient care.
4. *Design the intervention(s).* Interventions should be designed using evidence-based strategies; however, they must be tailored to fit the patient population and the context. They should target one or more of the appropriate levels of influence (i.e., the patient, provider, microsystem, organization, community, or policy).
5. *Implement, evaluate, and adjust the intervention(s).* Organizations should start by implementing a change on a small scale (pilot testing), learning from each test, and refining the intervention through performance improvement cycles (e.g., plan, do, study, and act) (PDSA). This process will help organizations prepare for implementation on a larger scale.
6. *Sustain the intervention(s).* Any change in practices must be continuously evaluated to ensure that recommended interventions are maintained.

conducting equity-focused QI. The 2013 National Health Care Disparities Report identified that the number of disparities that are getting smaller exceeded the number that are getting larger for Black people, Hispanics people, Asians, and individuals with lower socioeconomic status (AHRQ, 2013a).

Nurses and other health care providers need to be familiar with how policies and institutional forces enable or inhibit their ability to provide culturally competent, patient-centered, high-quality, safe care to all patients. When policies impede the delivery of effective care, you and your colleagues must advocate for policy change.

QSEN: Building Competency in Quality Improvement

You are a nurse on a cardiology floor. Some of your patients have been readmitted to the hospital within 30 days of discharge with the same predischarge diagnosis. You do not know why some patients are readmitted at a rate that seems higher than other patients. How might you identify patients with the highest readmission rate? What are some steps you could take to determine the patient's ability to self-manage postdischarge?

KEY POINTS

- Disparities in the access to quality of health care, preventive health, and health education contribute to poor population health.
- Health care systems and providers contribute to the problem of health disparities as a result of inadequate resources, poor patient–provider communication, lack of culturally competent care, fragmented delivery of care, and inadequate access to language services.
- Culturally competent health care providers and organizations can contribute to elimination of health disparities.
- Current evidence shows that addressing limited health literacy and cultural differences often reduces medical errors and improves adherence, patient–provider–family communication, and outcomes of care.
- Cultural desire involves a natural inclination to engage in the cultural competence process that is characterized by passion, commitment, and caring.
- A person's culture and life experiences shape his or her world view about health, illness, and health care.
- An effective approach to patient assessment is to use a patient's explanatory model instead of a traditional biomedical model to reveal your patient's views on illness.
- Becoming culturally competent is an ongoing long-term process for a health care provider.

REFERENCES

Adams M, Bell LA, Griffin P. Teaching for diversity and social justice. 2nd ed. New York: Routledge; 2007.

Administration on Aging. Profile of Older Americans: future growth. 2014. Available from: https://acl.gov/sites/default/files/Aging%20and%20Disability%20in%20America/2014-Profile.pdf. Accessed July 13, 2015.

Agency for Healthcare Research and Quality (AHRQ). 2013 National Healthcare Disparities Report. 2013a. Available from: http://www.ahrq.gov/research/findings/nhqrdr/nhdr12/index.html. Accessed May, 2014.

Agency for Healthcare Research and Quality (AHRQ). Health literacy universal precautions toolkit. 2013b. http://www.ahrq.gov/professionals/quality-patient-safety/quality-resources/tools/literacy-toolkit/index.html. Accessed April 5, 2015.

American Medical Association (AMA). Health literacy and patient safety: help patients understand. Chicago: American Medical Association Foundation; 2007.

Beach MC, Saha S, Cooper LA. The role and relationship of cultural competence and patient-centeredness in health care quality, Commonwealth Fund Publication No. 960. Medicine 2006;82(2):193.

Berkman ND, Sheridan SL, Donahue KE, Halpern DJ, Viera A, Crotty K, et al. Health literacy interventions and outcomes: an updated systematic review, Evidence Report/Technology Assessment No. 199. (Prepared by RTI International–University of North Carolina Evidence-based Practice Center under contract No. 290-2007-10056-I.) AHRQ Publication Number 11-E006. Rockville, MD: Agency for Healthcare Research and Quality; 2011.

Berkowitz SA, Percac-Lima S, Ashburner JM, Chang Y, Zai AH, He W, et al. Building equity improvement into quality improvement: reducing socioeconomic disparities in colorectal cancer screening as part of population health management. J Gen Intern Med 2015;30(7):942.

Campinha-Bacote J. The process of cultural competence in the delivery of healthcare services: a model of care. J Transcult Nurs 2002;13(3):181.

Campinha-Bacote J. Delivering patient-centered care in the midst of a cultural conflict: the role of cultural competence. Online J Issues Nurs 2011;16(2):5.

Cara V. James, Alina Salganicoff, Megan Thomas, Usha Ranji, Marsha Little Blanton, Roberta Wyn. Putting women's health care disparities on the map: examining racial and ethnic disparities at the state level. Menlo Park, CA: Kaiser Family Foundation; 2009. Available from: http://kff.org/disparities-policy/report/putting-womens-health-care-disparities-on-the/. Accessed July 13, 2015.

Chassin MR, Loeb JM, Schmaltz SP, Wachter RM. Accountability measures—using measurement to promote quality improvement. N Engl J Med 2010;363(7):6838.

Chew LD, Griffin JM, Partin MR, Noorbaloochi S, Grill JP, Snyder A, et al. Validation of screening questions for limited health literacy in a large VA outpatient population. J Gen Intern Med 2008;23(5):561–6.

Chin MH, Clarke AR, Nocon RS, Casey AA, Goddu AP, Keesecker NM, et al. A roadmap and best practices for organizations to reduce racial and ethnic disparities in health care. J Gen Intern Med 2012;27(8):992–1000.

Cho S, Crenshaw KW, McCall L. Toward a field of intersectionality studies: theory, applications, and praxis. Signs (Chic) 2013;38(4):785.

Cho YI, Lee SY, Arozullah AM, Crittenden KS. Effects of health literacy on health status and health service utilization amongst the elderly. Soc Sci Med 2008;66(8):1809–16.

Chin, M.H., Clarke, A.R., Nocon, R.S. et al. A Roadmap and Best Practices for Organizations to Reduce Racial and Ethnic Disparities in Health Care. J GEN INTERN MED 27, 992–1000 (2012). https://doi.org/10.1007/s11606-012-2082-9.

DeWalt DA, Berkman ND, Sheridan S, Lohr KN, Pignone MP. Literacy and health outcomes: a systematic review of the literature. J Gen Intern Med 2004;19(12):1228–39.

Edelstein S. Food, cuisine and cultural competency for culinary, hospitality and healthcare professionals. Sudbury, MA: Jones & Bartlett; 2011.

Giger JN, Davidhizar RD. The Giger and Davidhizar transcultural assessment model. J Transcult Nurs 2002;13(3):185.

Institute of Medicine (IOM). Crossing the quality chasm: a new health system for the 21st century. Washington DC: National Academy of Sciences, National Academies Press; 2001.

Kleinman A. From illness as culture to caregiving as moral experience. N Engl J Med 2013;368(15):1376.

Leininger MM, McFarland MR. Transcultural nursing: concepts, theories, research and practice. 3rd ed. New York: McGraw-Hill; 2002.

Leininger MM. Cultural care diversity and universality theory and evolution of the ethnonursing method. In: Leininger MM, McFarland MR, editors. Culture care diversity and universality: worldwide nursing theory. 2nd ed. Sudbury, MA: Jones & Bartlett Learning; 2006. p. 1.

Leininger MM. Culture care theory: a major contribution to advance transcultural nursing knowledge and practices. J Transcult Nurs 2002;13(3):189.

Lie D, Carter-Pokras O, Braun B, Coleman C. What do health literacy and cultural competence have in common? Calling for a collaborative health professional pedagogy. J Health Commun 2012;17:13.

Lion KC, Raphael JL. Partnering health disparities research with quality improvement science in pediatrics. Pediatrics 2015;135(2):354.

Lynch E, Medin D. Explanatory models of illness: a study of within-culture variation. Cogn Psychol 2006;53(4):285.

McFarland MR, Eipperle MK. Culture care theory: a proposed practice theory guide for nurse practitioners in primary care settings. Contemp Nurse 2008;28(1–2):48.

National Center for Education Statistics (NCES). The health literacy of America's adults: results from the 2003 National Assessment of Adult Literacy. Washington, DC: US Department of Education; 2006. Available from: http://nces.ed.gov/pubsearch/pubsinfo.asp?pubid=2006483. Accessed April 5, 2015.

Office of Disease Prevention and Health Promotion. Quick Guide to Health Literacy: Fact Sheet- Health Literacy and Health Outcomes. n.d. Available from: https://healthliteracycentre.eu/wp-content/uploads/2015/11/Quick-guide-to-health-literacy.pdf. Accessed July 18, 2015.

Paluri R. Capsule commentary on Berkowitz et al, Building equity improvement into quality improvement: reducing socioeconomic disparities in colorectal cancer screening as part of population health management. J Gen Intern Med 2015;30(7):1001.

Purnell L. The Purnell model for cultural competence. J Transcult Nurs 2002;13(3):193.

Rabin RC. Respecting Muslim patients' needs. *New York Times* 2010. Available from: http://www.nytimes.com/2010/11/01/health/01patients.html?_r=0. Accessed December 29, 2013.

Smedley B, Stith AY, Nelson AR. Unequal treatment: confronting racial and ethnic disparities in health care. Washington, DC: National Academies Press; 2003.

Sue DW. Multicultural social work practice. Ken, NJ: John Wiley & Sons; 2006.

The Joint Commission (TJC). Core measure sets. Chicago: TJC; 2013. Available from: http://www.jointcommission.org/core_measure_sets.aspx. Accessed April 5, 2015.

The Process of Cultural Competence in the Delivery of Healthcare Services | Transcultural C.A.R.E Associates [Internet]. Transculturalcare.net. 2015 [cited 12 February 2020]. Available from: http://transculturalcare.net/the-process-of-cultural-competence-in-the-delivery-of-healthcare-services/

VanSuch M, Naessens JM, Stroebel RJ, Huddleston JM, Williams AR. Effect of discharge instructions on readmission of hospitalized patients with heart failure: do all of the Joint Commission on Accreditation of Healthcare Organization's heart failure core measures reflect better care? Qual Saf Health Care 2006;15(6):414.

Walker RL, Alabi D, Roberts J, Obasi EM. Ethnic group differences in reasons for living and the moderating role of cultural worldview. Cultur Divers Ethnic Minor Psychol 2010;16(3):372.

34 *Theoretical Foundations of Nursing Practice*

OBJECTIVES

- To explain the influence of nursing theory on a nurse's approach to practice.
- To describe types of nursing theories.
- To describe the relationship among nursing theory, the nursing process, and patient needs.
- To review selected nursing theories.
- To review selected shared theories from other disciplines.
- To describe theory-based nursing practice.

KEY TERMS

assumptions, p. 799
conceptual framework, p. 799
concepts, p. 798
content, p. 800
descriptive theories, p. 800
domain, p. 799
environment/situation, p. 799
feedback, p. 800
grand theories, p. 799
health, p. 799
input, p. 800
middle-range theories, p. 800
nursing, p. 799
nursing metaparadigm, p. 799
nursing theory, p. 798
output, p. 800
paradigm, p. 799
person, p. 799
phenomenon, p. 798
practice theories, p. 800
prescriptive theories, p. 800
shared theory, p. 800
theory, p. 798

INTRODUCTION

Providing patient-centered nursing care is an expectation for all nurses. As you progress through your nursing classes, you will learn to apply knowledge from nursing; social, physical, and biobehavioral sciences; ethics; and health policy. Theory-based nursing practice helps you to design and implement nursing interventions that address individual and family responses to health problems. Some nurses find nursing theory difficult to understand or appreciate. However, as your knowledge about theories improves, you will find that they help to describe, explain, predict, and/or prescribe nursing care measures. Common questions nurses have about theory include: What is theory? How are nursing theories created? Why is theory important to the nursing profession? This chapter answers these questions and will help you understand how to use theory in your nursing practice.

Imagine that you are building a house. You need to complete the foundation before you start building the walls. Without a strong foundation, the house will not stand. Such is the case with nursing practice. Theory serves as the foundation for the art and science of nursing. Nurses use theory every day but are not always aware of it. For example, when a nurse ensures that a patient's room is free of clutter, excess noise, and soiled linens, she or he is using Florence Nightingale's environmental theory to promote healing and comfort. When encouraging a patient to set goals for his or her recovery, a nurse is using Imogene King's theory of goal attainment. A nurse uses Dorothea Orem's self-care deficit theory when feeding or bathing a patient until the patient is able to do this independently. Even though the term *theory* may sound intimidating, you will find that it is a standard part of everyday nursing practice.

The scientific work used to develop theories expands the scientific knowledge of the profession. Theories offer well-grounded rationales for how and why nurses perform specific interventions and for predicting patient behaviors and outcomes. Expertise in nursing is a result of knowledge and clinical experience. Nursing knowledge improves nursing practice by connecting theory and research. Theory, research, and practice are bound together in a continuous interactive relationship (Fig. 34.1). Nurses develop theories to explain the relationship among variables by testing the theory through research and applying it in practice. Throughout this process, new information often comes to light that indicates the need to revise a theory, and the cycle repeats (McEwen and Wills, 2014). Throughout your nursing career, you need to reflect and learn from your experiences to grow professionally and use well-developed theories as a basis for your approach to patient care.

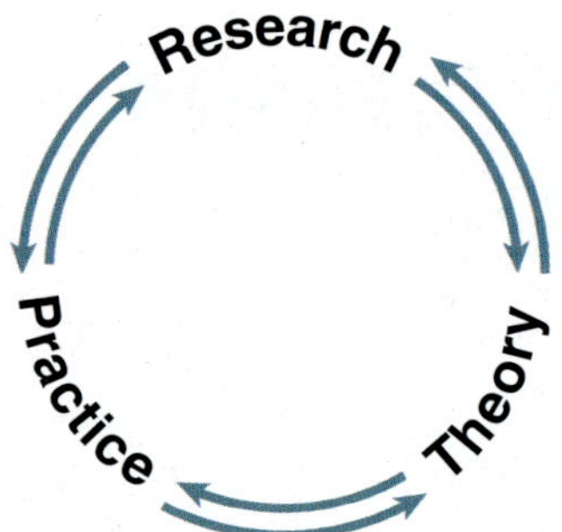

Fig. 34.1 Cyclical relationship among theory, research, and practice. (Adapted from McEwen M, Wills EM: *Theoretical basis for nursing*, ed 4, Philadelphia, 2014, Wolters Kluwer Health.)

THEORY

What is theory? A **theory** helps explain an event by defining ideas or concepts, explaining relationships among the concepts, and predicting outcomes (McEwen and Wills, 2014). In the case of nursing, theories are designed to explain a phenomenon such as self-care or caring.

A **nursing theory** conceptualizes an aspect of nursing to describe, explain, predict, or prescribe nursing care (Meleis, 2012). Theories offer a perspective for assessing your patients' situations. They also help you organize, analyze, and interpret data. For example, if you use Orem's theory in practice, you assess and interpret data to determine patients' self-care needs, deficits, and abilities in the management of their disease. Orem's theory then guides your development of patient-centered nursing interventions.

Nursing is both a science and an art. The *science* of nursing is based on data obtained from current research, whereas the *art* of nursing stems from a nurse's experience and the unique caring relationship that a nurse develops with a patient (McEwen and Wills, 2014). A nursing theory helps to identify the focus, means, and goals of practice. Nursing theories enhance communication and accountability for patient care (Meleis, 2012).

DEFINITION OF THEORY

Theories as a set of interrelated concepts that give a systematic view of a phenomenon (an observable fact or event) that is explanatory and predictive in nature.

—**Kerlinger**

A theory is a set of interrelated concept, definition, and prepositions that describes, explains, or predicts a phenomenon of interest.

PURPOSES OF THEORY

"The primary use of theory is to provide insights about nursing practice situations and guide research" and to provide a guideline or explanation of why nurses do what they do (Meleis, 2012, p. 35). Theories also have some other purposes:

- To describe, predict, and explain the phenomenon of an interest related to nursing (Chinn and Jacobs, 1978).
- To help determine what we know and what we are required to know).
- To provide the base of nursing practice, help to develop further knowledge, and indicate in which direction nursing should develop in the future.
- To distinguish what should form the basis of practice by explicitly describing nursing.
- To provide the guidelines for the nursing profession to know and maintain its professional limitation or boundaries.

COMPONENTS OF A THEORY

A theory contains a set of concepts, definitions, and assumptions or propositions that explain a phenomenon. It explains how these elements are uniquely related in the phenomenon (Fig. 34.2). These components provide a foundation of knowledge for nurses to direct and deliver caring nursing practices. Researchers test theories, and as a result they gain a clearer perspective and understanding of all parts of a phenomenon.

Phenomenon

Nursing theories focus on the phenomena of nursing and nursing care. A **phenomenon** is the term, description, or label given to describe an idea or responses about an event, a situation, a process, a group of events, or a group of situations (Meleis, 2012). Phenomena may be temporary or permanent. Examples of phenomena of nursing include caring, self-care, and patient responses to stress.

Concepts

A theory also consists of interrelated concepts that help describe or label phenomena. "Concepts are the words or phrases that identify, define, and establish structure and boundaries for ideas generated about a particular phenomenon" (Johnson and Webber, 2014, p. 18). Think of **concepts** as ideas and mental images. They can be abstract such as emotions or concrete such as physical objects (McEwen and Wills, 2014). For example, in Watson's transpersonal theory of caring, concepts include meeting human needs and instilling faith-hope (Watson, 2010). Theories use concepts to communicate meaning.

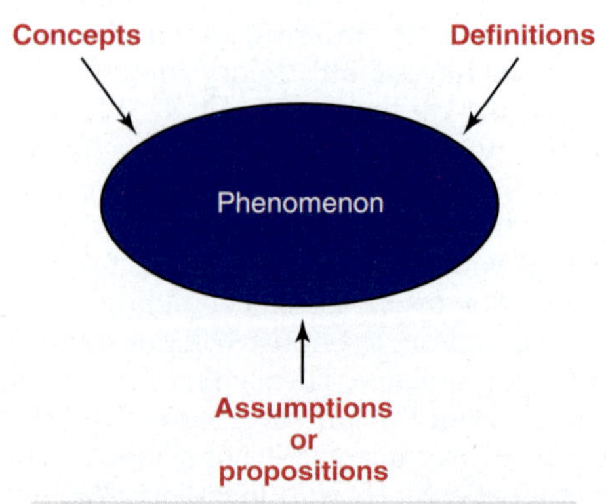

Fig. 34.2 Components of a nursing theory.

Definitions

Theorists use definitions to communicate the general meaning of the concepts of a theory. Definitions may be *theoretical/conceptual* or *operational*. Theoretical or conceptual definitions simply define a particular concept, much like what can be found in a dictionary, based on the theorist's perspective (McEwen and Wills, 2014; Meleis, 2012). Operational definitions state how concepts are measured (Johnson and Webber, 2014). For example, a nursing concept defines pain *conceptually* as physical discomfort and *operationally* as a patient reporting a score of 3 or more on a pain scale of 0–10.

Assumptions

Assumptions are the "taken-for-granted" statements that explain the nature of the concepts, definitions, purpose, relationships, and structure of a theory. They are accepted as *truths* and are based on values and beliefs (Masters, 2015; Meleis, 2012). For example, Watson's transpersonal caring theory has the assumption that a conscious intention to care promotes healing and wholeness (Watson, 2010).

THE DOMAIN OF NURSING

The **domain** is the perspective or territory of a profession or discipline (Meleis, 2012). It provides the subject, central concepts, values and beliefs, phenomena of interest, and central problems of a discipline. The domain of nursing provides both a practical and a theoretical aspect of the discipline. It is the knowledge of nursing practice and nursing history, nursing theory, education, and research. The domain of nursing gives nurses a comprehensive perspective that allows you to identify and treat patients' health care needs in all health care settings.

A **paradigm** is a pattern of beliefs used to describe the domain of a discipline. It links the concepts, theories, beliefs, values, and assumptions accepted and applied by the discipline (McEwen and Wills, 2014). Often used synonymously with paradigm is the term **conceptual framework**. A conceptual framework provides a way to organize major concepts and visualize the relationship among phenomena. Different frameworks provide alternative ways to view the subject matter of a discipline and represent the perspective of the author. For example, the grand theorists all address similar concepts in their respective theories, but each theorist defines and describes the concepts in a different way on the basis of the theorist's own ideas and experiences (Fawcett and DeSanto-Mayeda, 2013).

The **nursing metaparadigm** allows nurses to understand and explain what nursing *is*, what nursing *does*, and *why* nurses do what they do (Fawcett and DeSanto-Mayeda, 2013). It includes the four concepts of person (or human beings), health, environment/situation, and nursing. **Person** is the recipient of nursing care, including individual patients, groups, cultures, families, and communities. The person is central to the nursing care you provide. Because each person's needs are often complex, it is important to provide individualized patient-centered care. **Health** has different meanings for each patient, the clinical setting, and the health care profession. It is a state of being that people define in relation to their own values, personality, and lifestyle. It is dynamic and continuously changing. Your challenge as a nurse is to provide the best possible care based on a patient's level of health and health care needs at the time of care delivery.

Environment/situation includes all possible conditions affecting patients and the settings where they go for their health care. There is a continuous interaction between a patient and the environment. This interaction has positive and negative effects on a person's level of health and health care needs. Factors in the home, school, workplace, or community all influence the level of these needs. For example, an adolescent girl with type 1 diabetes needs to adapt her treatment plan to adjust for physical activities of school, the demands of a part-time job, and the timing of social events such as her prom.

Nursing is the "... protection, promotion, and optimization of health and abilities, prevention of illness and injury, alleviation of suffering through the diagnosis and treatment of human response, and advocacy in the care of individuals, families, communities, and populations" (ANA, 2014). The scope of nursing is broad. For example, a nurse does not medically diagnose a patient's health condition as heart failure. However, he or she assesses a patient's response to the decrease in activity tolerance as a result of the disease and develops *nursing diagnoses* of fatigue, activity intolerance, and ineffective coping (see Chapter 19). From these nursing diagnoses, the nurse creates a patient-centered plan of care for each of the patient's health problems (see Chapter 19). Use critical thinking skills to integrate knowledge, experience, attitudes, and standards into the individualized plan of care for each of your patients (see Chapter 18).

TYPES OF THEORY

The unique theories of a discipline help to distinguish the discipline from other professions. Before the development of nursing theories, nursing was considered to be a task-oriented occupation that functioned under the direction of the medical profession (McEwen and Wills, 2014). Theories are sometimes classified by levels of abstraction (grand vs. middle-range vs. practice theories) or the goals of the theory (descriptive or prescriptive). For example, a descriptive theory describes a phenomenon such as grief or caring and also identifies conditions or factors that predict a phenomenon. A prescriptive theory details nursing interventions for a specific phenomenon and the expected outcome of the care. Box 34.1 summarizes goals of theoretical nursing models.

- **Grand theories** are abstract, broad in scope, and complex; therefore, they require further clarification through research so they can be applied to nursing practice. A grand theory does not provide guidance for *specific* nursing interventions, but it provides the structural framework for general, global ideas about nursing. Grand theories intend to answer the question "What is nursing" and focus on the *whole* of nursing rather than on a *specific* type of nursing. The grand theorists developed their works based on their own experiences and the time in which they were living, which helps to explain why

BOX 34.1 Goals of Theoretical Nursing Models

- Identify domain and goals of nursing.
- Provide knowledge to improve nursing administration, practice, education, and research.
- Guide research to expand the knowledge base of nursing.
- Identify research techniques and tools used to validate nursing interventions.
- Develop curriculum plans for nursing education.
- Establish criteria for measuring quality of nursing care, education, and research.
- Guide development of a nursing care delivery system.
- Provide systematic structure and rationale for nursing activities.

there is so much variation among the theories. Grand theories address the nursing metaparadigm components of person, nursing, health, and environment.

- **Middle-range theories** are more limited in scope and less abstract. They address a specific phenomenon and reflect practice (administration, clinical, or teaching). A middle-range theory tends to focus on a concept found in a specific field of nursing such as uncertainty, incontinence, social support, quality of life, and caring rather than reflect on a wide variety of nursing care situations as the grand theories do (Meleis, 2012). For example, Kolcaba's theory of comfort encourages nurses to meet patients' needs for comfort in physical, psychospiritual, environmental, and sociocultural realms (Krinsky et al., 2014). Like many middle-range theories, Kolcaba's theory was based on the works of a grand theorist—in this case, Nightingale. Middle-range theories are also sometimes developed from research, nursing practice, or the theories of other disciplines (McEwen and Wills, 2014; Meleis, 2012).
- **Practice theories**, also known as situation-specific theories, bring theory to the bedside. Narrow in scope and focus, these theories guide the nursing care of a *specific* patient population at a *specific* time (Meleis, 2012). An example of a practice theory is a pain management protocol for patients recovering from cardiac surgery. "Practice theories have had the benefit of trial and error through clinical practice" and are often easier to understand and apply than the grand and middle-range theories (Warelow, 2013, p. 41). Fig. 34.3 demonstrates the level of abstraction for each of the grand, middle-range, and practice theory categories.
- **Descriptive theories** are the first level of theory development. They describe phenomena and identify circumstances in which the phenomena occur (Meleis, 2012). For example, theories of growth and development describe the maturation processes of an individual at various ages. Descriptive theories do not direct specific nursing activities or attempt to produce change but rather help to explain patient assessments.
- **Prescriptive theories** address nursing interventions for a phenomenon, guide practice change, and predict the consequences. Nurses use prescriptive theories to anticipate the outcomes of nursing interventions (McEwen and Wills, 2014).

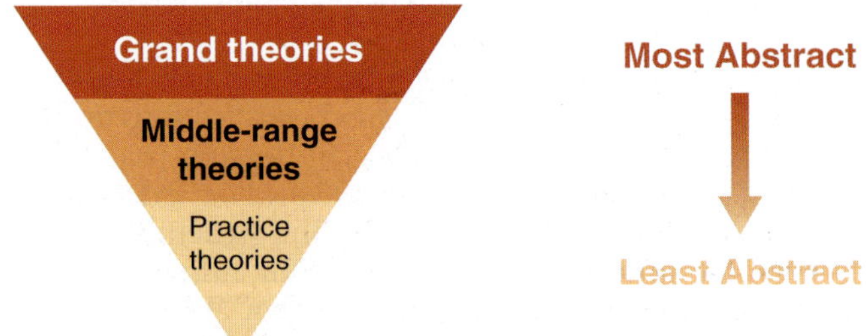

Fig. 34.3 Correlation of theory category with level of abstraction. (Adapted from McEwen M, Wills EM: *Theoretical basis for nursing*, ed 4, Philadelphia, 2014, Wolters Kluwer Health.)

Shared Theories

To practice in health care systems nowadays, nurses need a strong scientific knowledge base from nursing and other disciplines such as the biomedical, sociological, and behavioral sciences. Also known as a *borrowed* or *interdisciplinary* theory, a **shared theory** explains a phenomenon specific to the discipline that developed the theory (McEwen and Wills, 2014). For example, Piaget's theory of cognitive development helps to explain how children think, reason, and perceive the world. Knowledge and use of this theory help pediatric nurses design appropriate therapeutic play interventions for ill toddlers or school-age children. Knowles's adult learning theory helps a nurse plan and provide appropriate discharge teaching for a patient who is recovering from surgery. Several nursing theories are based on systems theory, and the nursing process is also a system (Fig. 34.4). Like all systems, the nursing process has a specific purpose or goal (see chapter 19). The goal of the nursing process is to organize and deliver patient-centered care. As a system, the nursing process has the following components: input, output, feedback, and content. **Input** for the nursing process is the data or information that comes from a patient's assessment. **Output** is the end product of a system, and in the case of the nursing process it is whether the patient's health status improves, declines, or remains stable as a result of nursing care.

Feedback serves to inform a system about how it functions. For example, in the nursing process, the outcomes reflect the patient's responses to nursing interventions. The outcomes are part of the feedback system to refine the plan of care. Other forms of feedback in the nursing process include responses from family members and consultation from other health care professionals.

The **content** is the product and information obtained from the system. For example, patients with impaired bed mobility have common skin care needs and interventions (e.g., hygiene and scheduled positioning changes) that are very successful in reducing the risk for pressure ulcers. Table 34.1 provides an overview of additional select shared theories that are often used in nursing practice.

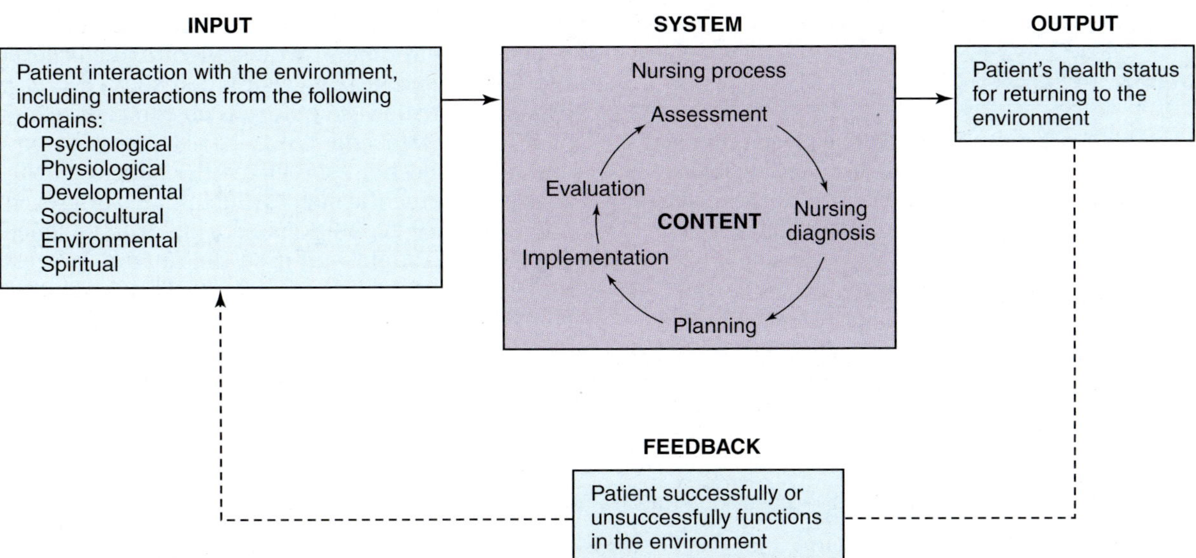

Fig. 34.4 Providing nursing services in assisted-living facilities promotes physical and psychosocial health.

Table 34.1 Overview of Select Shared Theories

Theory Categories	Focus	Application to Nursing
Human needs	Need motivates human behavior. Maslow's hierarchy of basic human needs includes five levels of priority (e.g., physiological, safety and security, love and belonging, self-esteem, and self-actualization) (see Fig 1.2, p. 3).	Basic physiological and safety needs are usually a patient's first priority, especially when he or she is severely dependent physically. When a patient has no emergent physical or safety needs, the nurse gives high priority to his or her psychological, sociocultural, developmental, or spiritual needs. Patients entering the health care system generally have unmet needs. A patient in pain after surgery (basic need) is not ready for discharge teaching (higher level need) until the pain is relieved. The hierarchy of needs is a way to plan for individualized patient care (McEwen and Wills, 2014).
Stress/adaptation	Humans respond to actual or perceived threats by adapting to maintain function and life.	Patients demonstrate a similar pattern of reacting to stress through physiological and psychological responses. Failure to adapt to stress can lead to exhaustion and decline in health. Nurses need to understand the reaction of body and mind to stress and intervene to help patients develop methods of coping/adapting to prevent or manage illness and disease (Master's, 2015).
Developmental	Humans have a common pattern of growth and development.	Human growth and development are orderly, predictive processes that begin with conception and continue through death. Varieties of well-tested theories describe and predict behavior and development at various phases of the life continuum (McEwen and Wills, 2014).
Biomedical	Theory explains causes of disease and principles related to physiology.	Nurses must have knowledge of theories from the fields of biology, medicine, public health, physiology, and pharmacology to provide holistic patient care, promote health, and prevent illness (McEwen and Wills, 2014).
Psychosocial	Theory explains and/or predicts human responses within the physiological, psychological, sociocultural, developmental, and spiritual domains.	Nursing is a diverse discipline that strives to meet holistic needs of patients. Chapter 33 discusses models for understanding cultural diversity and implementing care to meet the diverse needs of the patient. Chapter 28 discusses several models of grieving and demonstrates how to help patients through loss, death, and grief.
Educational	Theory explains the teaching–learning process by examining behavioral, cognitive, and adult learning principles.	Nurses provide education to patients, families, community groups, and members of the health care team. A basic understanding of various teaching–learning theories is critical for this aspect of the professional nursing role (Butts and Rich, 2015).
Leadership/management	Theory promotes organization, change, power/empowerment, motivation, conflict management, and decision-making.	Nurses often assume leadership positions in the health care realm and as such are expected to effectively manage individuals and groups to promote change and improve quality care and outcomes (McEwen and Wills, 2014).

OVERVIEW OF SELECTED NURSING THEORIES

Definitions and theories of nursing can help you understand the practice of nursing. The following sections describe select theories and their concepts. See Table 34.2 for a review of additional grand and middle-range nursing theories.

Nightingale's Environmental Theory

Known as the founder of modern nursing, Florence Nightingale is credited with developing the first nursing theory. The focus of Nightingale's grand theory is a patient's environment, which Nightingale believed nurses should manipulate (e.g., ventilation, light, decreased noise, hygiene, nutrition) so nature is able to restore a patient to health (McEwen and Wills, 2014). Through observation and data collection, she linked the patient's health status with environmental factors and initiated improved hygiene and sanitary conditions during the Crimean War. Nightingale taught and used the nursing process, noting that "vital observation [assessment] ... is not for the sake of piling up miscellaneous information or curious facts, but for the sake of saving life and increasing health and comfort" (Nightingale, 1860).

Table 34.2 Overview of Select Grand and Middle-Range Nursing Theories

Theory Category	Theorist	Focus	Application
Grand theory	Henderson	Principles and practice of nursing	Nurses assist patients with 14 activities (breathing, eating/drinking, elimination, movement/positioning, sleep/rest, clothing, body temperature, hygiene, safety, communication/socialization, practice of faith, learning, play/recreation, sense of accomplishment) until patients can meet these needs for themselves, or they help patients have a peaceful death (Butts and Rich, 2015; McEwen and Wills, 2014).
	Johnson	Behavioral system	Nurses perceive patients as being more important than their disease; a patient is viewed as a collection of subsystems that form an overall behavioral system focused on meeting basic drives of achievement, affiliation, aggression/protection, dependence, elimination, ingestion, sex, and restoration. The goal of nursing is to help the patient attain/maintain balance, function, and stability in each of the subsystems (Butts and Rich, 2015).
	Neuman	Systems	Nurses view a patient (physical, psychological, sociocultural, developmental, and spiritual) as being an open system that is in constant energy exchange with both internal and external environments. Nurses help a patient/client (individual, group, family, or community) cope with intrapersonal, interpersonal, and extrapersonal *stressors* that can break through the patient's line of defense and cause illness. The role of nursing is to stabilize a patient or situation, and the focus is on *wellness* and *prevention* of disease (McEwen and Wills, 2014).
	Abdellah	Patient-centered care	Nurses address 21 "nursing problems" to meet patients' physical, psychological, and social needs and should strive to *know* each patient. Nurses use knowledge constructed from previous experiences to determine a general plan of care and then personalize the plan to the patient to provide *patient-centered care*. A nurse should involve a patient's family in the plan of care (McEwen and Wills, 2014).
	Levine	Conservation	Nurses promote *balance* between nursing interventions and patient participation to help patients *conserve energy* needed for healing, *conserve structural integrity* by limiting the extent of tissue involvement/damage, *conserve personal integrity* by involving them in their care decisions, and *conserve social integrity* by facilitating patient interactions with family and loved ones (Johnson and Webber, 2014).
	King	Goal attainment	Nurses view a patient as a unique personal system that is constantly interacting/transacting with other systems (e.g., nurse, family, friends); nurses help patients become active participants in their care by working *with* them to establish goals for attaining, restoring, or maintaining health (Johnson and Webber, 2014; McEwen and Wills, 2014).
	Roy	Adaptation	Nurses help a patient cope with or adapt to changes in physiological, self-concept, role function, and interdependence domains (Masters, 2015).
	Erickson–Tomlin–Swain	Modeling/role modeling	Nurses understand a patient's *model of the world* or world view (e.g., how the patient thinks, acts, feels, communicates) and help a patient use internal and external resources to make appropriate changes *(role modeling)* to attain optimal health (McEwen and Wills, 2014).
	Watson	Caring	Nurses understand that caring is a fundamental component of professional nursing practice and is based on 10 *carative factors* (see Chapter 5). The purpose of nursing is to understand the interrelationship among health, illness, and human behavior rather than focus on the disease–cure model. Caring occurs when a nurse and a patient engage in a *transpersonal relationship* that facilitates the patient's ability for self-healing (Johnson and Webber, 2014).

Table 34.2 Overview of Select Grand and Middle-Range Nursing Theories—cont'd

Theory Category	Theorist	Focus	Application
	Rogers/Parse/ Newman	Unitary beings/ human becoming/ expanding consciousness	Nurses view a patient as a unique, dynamic energy field in constant energy exchange with the environment; nursing care focuses on helping a patient use his or her *own* potential to identify and alter personal rhythms/patterns (e.g., eating, breathing, sleeping, communicating, touching) to promote and maintain health. Nurses understand that patients are responsible for their own health and that health stems from how patients live their lives in accordance with their own values; the nurse's role is to be truly *present* with the patient and accepting of his or her view of reality while providing guidance to the patient in making health-related choices in accordance with his or her belief system (Johnson and Webber, 2014; McEwen and Wills, 2014).
Middle-range theory	Benner	Skill acquisition	Nurses progress through five stages of skill acquisition: novice, advanced beginner, competent, proficient, and expert (Butts and Rich, 2015).
	Kolcaba	Comfort	Nurses facilitate health-seeking behaviors in patients by striving to relieve physical, emotional, social, environmental, and/or spiritual distress (McEwen and Wills, 2014).
	Pender	Health promotion	Nurses understand that a patient's personal characteristics, experiences, and beliefs affect his or her motivation for adopting healthy behaviors (McEwen and Wills, 2014).
	American Association of Critical-Care Nurses	Synergy	Matching nurse competencies to patient needs in the critical care environment improves patient outcomes (McEwen and Wills, 2014).
	Mishel	Uncertainty in illness	Nurses facilitate patient coping and adaptation by performing interventions aimed at helping patients process and find meaning related to their illness (Adelstein et al., 2014).
	Eakes, Burke, and Hainsworth	Chronic sorrow	Nurses understand that the disparity between *desired* and *actual* reality often leads to continuous cycles of grief. For example, chronic sorrow sometimes occurs in parents of children with disabilities or in individuals diagnosed with a chronic illness (Vitale and Falco, 2014).

Peplau's Interpersonal Theory

Hildegard Peplau is considered to be the mother of psychiatric nursing; the focus of her middle-range theory includes interpersonal relations among a nurse, a patient, and a patient's family and developing the nurse–patient relationship (McEwen and Wills, 2014). According to Peplau, nurses help patients reduce anxiety by converting it into constructive actions (McEwen and Wills, 2014). They develop therapeutic relationships with patients that are respectful, empathetic, and nonjudgmental (Senn, 2013). The following phases characterize the nurse–patient interpersonal relationship: preorientation (data gathering), orientation (defining issue), working phase (therapeutic activity), and resolution (termination of relationship). In developing a nurse–patient relationship, the nurse serves as a resource person, counselor, and surrogate. For example, when a patient seeks help, the nurse and the patient first discuss the nature of any problems, and the nurse explains the services available. As the nurse–patient relationship develops, the nurse and the patient mutually define the problems and potential solutions. When the patient's original needs are resolved, new needs sometimes emerge. This middle-range theory is useful in establishing effective nurse–patient communication when obtaining a nursing history, providing patient education, or counseling patients and their families (see Chapter 34).

Orem's Self-Care Deficit Nursing Theory

Dorothea Orem's theory is commonly used in nursing practice (Alligood, 2014). When applying this grand theory, a nurse continually assesses a patient's ability to perform self-care and intervenes as needed to ensure that the patients meet physical, psychological, sociological, and developmental needs. According to Orem, people who participate in self-care activities are more likely to improve their health outcomes (Rustøen et al., 2014). Nursing care becomes necessary when patients are unable to fulfill biological, psychological, developmental, or social needs. Nurses continually assess and determine why patients are unable to meet these needs, identify goals to help them, intervene to help them perform self-care, and evaluate how much self-care they are able to perform. For example, a patient may need a nurse to bathe or feed him or her while acutely ill, but as his or her condition improves, the nurse encourages the patient to begin doing these activities independently.

Leininger's Culture Care Theory

As early as the 1950s, Madeleine Leininger recognized the need to focus on culture in nursing as she predicted that nursing and health care would become more global. She blended her background in anthropology with nursing to form her middle-range theory of cultural care diversity and universality (Alligood, 2014). Human caring varies among cultures in its expressions, processes, and patterns. Social structure factors such as a patient's politics, culture, and traditions are significant forces affecting care and influencing the patient's health and illness patterns. Think about the diversity of patients and their nursing care needs. The major concept of Leininger's theory is cultural diversity, and the goal of nursing care is to provide a patient with culturally specific nursing care (Alligood, 2014). To provide care to patients of unique cultures, nurses safely integrate their cultural traditions, values, and beliefs into a plan of care. Leininger's theory recognizes the importance of culture and its influence on everything that involves a patient, including health beliefs, the role of family and community, and dietary practices (Alligood, 2014). For example, some cultures believe that the leader of the community needs to be present during health care decisions. As a result, a health care team needs to reschedule when rounds occur to include the community leader. In addition, symptom expression also differs among cultures. A person with an Irish background might be stoic and not complain about pain, whereas a person from a Middle Eastern culture might be very vocal about pain. In both cases, a nurse needs to skillfully incorporate the patient's cultural practices in assessing his or her level of pain (e.g., is the pain getting worse or remaining the same?).

QSEN: Building Competency in Patient-Centered Care

You are caring for a patient from India who is visiting family in the United States. On entering this patient's room, you notice that he has not eaten any of the food on his tray. When you ask whether he was not hungry, he replies, "I am very hungry, but I cannot eat this food." How could you use *Leininger's culture care theory* to respond to this patient?

USE OF THEORIES IN NURSING PRACTICE

Theory-Based Nursing Practice

Why is theory important to the nursing profession? Nursing knowledge is derived from basic and nursing sciences, experience, aesthetics, nurses' attitudes, and standards of practice. As nursing continues to grow as a practice-oriented profession, new knowledge is needed to prescribe specific interventions to improve patient outcomes. Nursing theories and related concepts continue to evolve. Florence Nightingale spoke with firm conviction about the "nature of nursing as a profession that requires knowledge distinct from medical knowledge" (Nightingale, 1860). The overall goal of nursing knowledge is to explain the practice of nursing as different and distinct from the practice of medicine, psychology, and other health care disciplines. Theory generates nursing knowledge for use in practice, thus supporting evidence-based practice (see Chapter 34). The integration of theory into practice leads to coordinated care delivery and therefore serves as the basis for nursing (McEwen and Wills, 2014).

The nursing process is used in clinical settings to determine individual patient needs (see Chapter 19). Although the nursing process is central to nursing, it is not a theory. It provides a systematic process for the delivery of nursing care, not the knowledge component of the discipline. However, nurses use theory to provide direction in how to *use* the nursing process. For example, the theory of caring influences what nurses need to assess, how to determine patient needs, how to plan care, how to select individualized nursing interventions, and how to evaluate patient outcomes.

Link Between Theory and Knowledge Development in Nursing

Nursing has its own body of knowledge that is both theoretical and experiential. You acquire theoretical knowledge through "reading, observing, or discussing" concepts (Alligood, 2014, p. 123). Theoretical knowledge stimulates thinking and creates a broad understanding of nursing science and practice. Experiential, or clinical, knowledge, often called the *art* of nursing, is formed from nurses' clinical experience. Both types of knowledge are needed to provide safe, comprehensive nursing care.

Nursing theories guide nursing practice (McEwen and Wills, 2014). When using theory-based nursing practice, you apply the principles of a theory in delivering nursing interventions. Grand theories help shape and define your practice, middle-range theories continue to advance nursing knowledge through nursing research, and practice theories help you provide specific care for individuals and groups of diverse populations and situations (Im and Chang, 2012).

Relationship Between Nursing Theory and Nursing Research

Research validates, refutes, supports, and/or modifies theory; and theory stimulates nurse scientists to explore significant issues in nursing practice, leading to the improvement of nursing care (McEwen and Wills, 2014; Meleis, 2012). The relationship between nursing theory and nursing research builds the scientific knowledge base of nursing, which is then applied to practice. Nurses better understand the appropriate use of a theory to improve patient care as more research is conducted. The relationships between the components of a theory often help identify research questions and determine the overall design of a study. For example, nurse researchers used Peplau's interpersonal theory as the framework for a study about standardized shift report as a means of improving nurse-to-nurse communication. The results showed improved patient satisfaction with nursing care (Radtke, 2013).

Sometimes research is used to develop new theories (Meleis, 2012). *Theory-generating* research uses logic to explore relationships among phenomena (McEwen and Wills, 2014). In theory-generating research, an investigator makes observations (*without* any preconceived ideas) to view a phenomenon in a new way. Middle-range theories are often developed in this manner. For example, the middle-range theory of chronic sorrow stemmed from a researcher's initial observations of cyclic periods of sadness in parents of children with intellectual or developmental disabilities (Vitale and Falco, 2014).

Theory-testing research determines how accurately a theory describes a nursing phenomenon. Testing develops the evidence for describing or predicting patient outcomes. A researcher has *some* preconceived idea as to how patients describe or respond to a phenomenon and generates research questions or hypotheses to test the assumptions of the theory. No one study tests *all* components of a theory; researchers test the theory through a variety of research activities. For example, nurse researchers studied Kolcaba's middle-range nursing theory of comfort in relation to the pain and discomfort experienced by patients with heart

BOX 34.2 Evidence-Based Practice

PICO Question: In patients with cancer (P), how does application of Mishel's uncertainty in illness theory (I) compared with no specific theory application (C) influence physical and psychological coping abilities (O)?

Evidence Summary

Patients with cancer experience many stressors, including pain, side effects of treatment, and an uncertain future. Patients perceive this uncertainty as either a danger or an opportunity. Coping and adaptation to illness depends on reducing the uncertainty in the situation or accepting it as a sign of hope (Adelstein et al., 2014). According to Mishel's theory, people with serious illness improve their coping skills and their quality of life by helping patients "think" about their disease in a way that allows them to find meaning in their illness. This helps patients adapt to their disease and improve their quality of life. Mishel's theory provides a framework for nursing interventions to improve psychological and behavioral outcomes, especially when illness and treatment become very complex, inconsistent, random, and unpredictable (Germino et al., 2013). Although Mishel's uncertainty in illness theory can be applied to any patient experiencing a serious illness, it has been used in several research studies with patients who have cancer. For example, nursing interventions based on this theory have been found to reduce feelings of uncertainty and significantly improve coping strategies to manage uncertainty, self-efficacy, and sexual dysfunction in women with breast cancer (Germino et al., 2013; Kim et al., 2012). Research also supports the use of this theory to enhance adaptation and coping; reduce physical, psychosocial, and spiritual challenges; and achieve positive personal growth in patients who received stem cell transplants as a result of blood cancers (Adelstein et al., 2014). Finally, nursing actions based on Mishel's theory reduced anxiety and preserved quality of life in patients with incurable brain cancer (Cahill et al., 2012).

Application to Nursing Practice

- Promote meaning-making in patients with cancer or other serious illnesses.
- Help patients find meaning in their illness to improve their ability to adapt and cope.
- Implement nursing actions that reduce anxiety and preserve quality of life to balance the uncertainty that occurs when the disease is not curable.
- Recognize that a patient's sense of uncertainty often changes over the course of an illness and its treatment.

disease. The researchers explored the specific intervention of "quiet time" as a comfort measure in this patient population (Krinsky et al., 2014).

Theory-generating or theory-testing research refines the knowledge base of nursing. As a result, nurses incorporate research-based interventions into theory-based practice (Box 34.2). As research activities continue, not only does the knowledge and science of nursing increase, but also patients receive high-quality evidence-based nursing practice. As an art, nursing relies on knowledge gained from practice and reflection on past experiences. The "expert nurse" translates both the art and the science of nursing into the realm of *creative caring*, which takes the extra step of individualizing care to the specific needs of each patient. For example, a nurse provides creative caring when arranging for a hospitalized patient to visit with a beloved pet or finding a way to honor a patient's wish to die at home.

As you progress in your nursing education and practice, you will use theory in a variety of ways. Keep in mind that these theories are not only applicable to patient care but also useful in communicating with other members of the health care team. Theory is the foundation of nursing; it defines our unique profession and sets it apart from other disciplines. It provides a basis for research and practice and serves as a guide in providing safe, comprehensive, individualized care, which is the hallmark of nursing.

KEY POINTS

- A nursing theory conceptualizes an aspect of nursing to describe, explain, predict, and/or prescribe nursing care.
- Grand theories provide complex structural frameworks for broad, abstract ideas.
- Middle-range theories address specific phenomena or concepts and reflect practice. Thus, they are more limited in scope and less abstract.
- Practice or situation-specific theories bring theory to the bedside by focusing on specific types of patients in specific situations.
- The metaparadigm of nursing identifies four concepts of interest to the profession: the person, health, environment/situation, and nursing. These four components are essential to the development of nursing theory.
- Theory generates nursing knowledge used in practice. Nurses use the nursing process to apply the theory or knowledge. The integration of theory and nursing process is the basis for professional nursing.
- Theory-generating research discovers and describes relationships without imposing preconceived notions (e.g., hypotheses) of what the phenomenon under study means.
- Theory-testing research determines how accurately a theory describes nursing phenomena.

REFERENCES

Adelstein KE, Anderson JG, Taylor AG. Importance of meaning-making for patients undergoing hematopoietic stem cell transplantation. Oncol Nurs Forum. 2014 Mar 1;41(2):E172–84.

Alligood MR. Nursing theory utilization & application. 5th ed. St. Louis: Mosby; 2014.

American Nurses Association (ANA). What is nursing? American Nurses Association; 2014. http://www.nursingworld.org/EspeciallyForYou/What-is-Nursing. Accessed July 4, 2015.

Butts JB, Rich KL. Philosophies and theories for advanced nursing practice. 2nd ed. Burlington, MA: Jones & Bartlett Learning; 2015.

Cahill J, LoBiondo-Wood G, Bergstrom N, Armstrong T. Brain tumor symptoms as antecedents to uncertainty: an integrative review. J Nurs Scholarsh 2012;44(2):145.

Fawcett J, DeSanto-Mayeda S. Contemporary nursing knowledge: analysis and evaluation of nursing models and theories. 3rd ed. Philadelphia: FA Davis; 2013.

Germino BB, Mishel MH, Crandell J, Porter L, Blyler D, Jenerette C, et al. Outcomes of an uncertainty management intervention in younger African-American and Caucasian breast cancer survivors. Oncol Nurs Forum 2013;40(1):82.

Im E, Chang SJ. Current trends in nursing theories. J Nurs Sch 2012;44(2):156.

Johnson BM, Webber PB. An introduction to theory and reasoning in nursing. 4th ed. Philadelphia, PA: Lippincott Williams & Wilkins; 2014.

Kim SH, Lee R, Lee KS. Symptoms and uncertainty in breast cancer survivors in Korea: differences by treatment trajectory. J Clin Nurs 2012;21:1014.

Krinsky R, Murillo I, Johnson J. A practical application of Katharine Kolcaba's comfort theory to cardiac patients. Appl Nurs Res 2014;27:147.

Masters K. Nursing theories: a framework for professional practice. 2nd ed. Burlington, MA: Jones & Bartlett Learning; 2015.

McEwen M, Wills EM. Theoretical basis for nursing. 4th ed. Philadelphia, PA: Lippincott Williams & Wilkins; 2014.

Meleis AI. Theoretical nursing: development & progress. 5th ed. Philadelphia, PA: Lippincott Williams & Wilkins; 2012.

Nightingale F. Notes on nursing: what it is and what it is not. London: Harrison & Sons; 1860.

Radtke K. Improving patient satisfaction with nursing communication using bedside shift report. Clin Nurse Spec 2013;27(1):19.

Rustøen T, Valeberg BT, Kolstad E, Wist E, Paul S, Miaskowski C. A randomized clinical trial of the efficacy of a self-care intervention to improve cancer pain management. Cancer Nurs 2014;37(1):34.

Senn JF. Peplau's theory of interpersonal relations: application in emergency and rural nursing. Nurs Sci Q 2013;26(1):31.

Vitale SA, Falco C. Children born prematurely: risk of parental chronic sorrow. J Pediatr Nurs 2014;29:248.

Warelow PJ. Changing philosophies: a paradigmatic nursing shift from Nightingale. Aust J Adv Nurs 2013;31(1):36.

Watson J. Caring science and the next decade of holistic healing: transforming self and system from the inside out. Beginnings (American Holistic Nurses' Association), 01 Jan 2010, 30(2):14–16.

35 First Aid and Emergencies

OBJECTIVES

After reading this chapter, the student should be able to:

- Explain meaning and definition of first aid and describe the importance of first aid.
- Understand about instant action to be taken at the time of emergency.
- Describe the management of various emergencies such as poisoning, burns, and fractures.
- Demonstrate the skills to manage emergency situations strategically by analyzing the situations critically.
- Comprehend community preparedness for emergencies such as earthquakes, floods, explosions, and fire.

KEY TERMS

INTRODUCTION

First aid has been used for unwell or sick individuals since ancient time. People are seen dying because of various emergencies such as hemorrhage, burns, and poisoning, which can be prevented through simple, timely first aid interventions. First aid interventions include measures such as stabilizing body functions, for example, cardiopulmonary resuscitation (CPR), hemostasis, wound care, stabilizing the injury, and preventing further injury.

MEANING

First aid provided using available resources on site can help save the life of a person who becomes suddenly sick, sustains an injury, or is bitten by a snake. The main aim of first aid is to assess for life-threatening conditions, moving victims out of danger situations, and implementing first aid interventions to save the life or limb.

The person who volunteers to provide these services is termed a first aider. The first aider must possess the basic knowledge and skills for dos and don'ts in case of emergency life-threatening situations. There are well-recognized programs available for first aiders such as Red Cross First Aid Course; however, in emergency situations, sometimes a lay person also can provide first aid interventions, provided he or she is aware about the dos and don'ts in a particular emergency situation.

The fundamental rule in first aid is the safety of the self first and then of the victim; call for desired help and first aid must be followed by availability for advanced medical services.

DEFINITION

First aid is the assistance given to a victim or casualty in the initial period when sudden injury takes place and medical care is not available or specialized care by health care professionals cannot be met.

First aid is the instant care given to an individual who requires immediate care and medical treatment following an injury or sickness.

First aid care may be sufficient to save an individual's life and it must persist until advanced professional care arrives or the sick individual is escorted to the health care facility.

The common conditions requiring first aid management are cardiac arrest, choking, burns, bleeding, fracture, wound, shock, heat stroke, frostbite, poisoning hypoglycemia, and so on.

IMPORTANCE OF FIRST AID

- First aid treatment lessens the seriousness of the injury and sickness.
- It prevents further deterioration of the condition of the injury or illness.
- It reduces the chance of morbidity and saves a precious life.
- It enhances the chance of early recovery.

BASIC PRINCIPLES OF FIRST AID

The following are the basic principles of first aid management:

- Consider safety of self and victim as priority while providing first aid to the victim.
- Primary assessment of A, B, C, D, and E (airway, breathing, circulation, deformity, and environment) should be performed.
- Airway management should be done if the patient is suspected to have a blockage in the airway or secretions are present that may alter the respiratory pattern.
- CPR must be the priority to maintain cardiopulmonary function or to restore circulation if no pulse is felt in a victim who has suffered from a sudden cardiac arrest.
- First aid involves bleeding precautions in case the victim experienced hemorrhage as a result of head injury or trauma to the abdominal organs.
- Immediate measures need to be taken following guidelines suggesting bleeding control and applied efficiently.
- Immobilization is necessary in some circumstances to avoid further injury to the person such as immobilizing the neck or head following a spinal cord injury or stabilizing the bone following fracture.
- Assistance is required to treat severely injured persons and the caregiver must think critically to make the victim survive in emergency situations.
- Instant action is the basic principle of first aid to avoid delay in treatment and avoid complications.
- The first aid giver must be calm, confident, and physically and emotionally stable in these situations to channelize thinking in an appropriate way to resolve the danger associated with the situation.
- Raising hope and trust is mandatory side by side for the casualty and stranger gathering.
- The first aider must take all precautions to avoid any risk of cross-infection.
- Risk assessment is very necessary prior to and in every transition of the situation.

SCOPE OF FIRST AID

- Efficient skills can be attained to provide attention to the victim and first aid management promotes promptness in care.
- First aid management applies critical care thinking in analyzing the situation and acting appropriately.
- Knowledge is obtained while dealing with an emergency situation and applying necessary measures to treat victim.
- The victim can be saved following proper guidelines and those who require immediate care can be prioritized and sent for essential management in an advanced health care facility.

GENERAL RULES OF FIRST AID

- Avoid being panicked over the situation and think about measures that can be taken with the available resources.
- Prioritize care and focus on the things that must be applied first as immediate measures.
- After airway and breathing, hemorrhage control must be the priority to prevent hypovolemia and shock.
- Safely and gently handle the victim to avoid further trauma or injury.
- Make the patient comfortable and reassure the victim to reduce anxiety and fear.
- Manage the situation effectively by not allowing others at the site to avoid crowd.
- Avoid removing any object that has penetrated inside the victim's body to avoid further damage.
- Make the patient safe by creating a safe environment and removing harmful objects that surround the victim.
- Ask for help such as lifesaving equipment, for example, automated external defibrillator (AED); call for prehospital team to transport the victim to a higher health care facility.
- Carry out rapid triaging; details about the methods of triaging are illustrated in Box 35.1 and Table 35.1.

First aid management during different conditions is described in the subsequent sections.

WOUND

Wound is an injury to the skin or break in the continuity of the skin, either internal or external. An open wound is where the skin is torn, cut, or punctured, and a closed wound is a blunt force injury.

Classification of Wound

1. **Open:** A break or shattering of the skin or mucous membrane where the skin is torn, cut, or punctured

BOX 35.1 Triage

Triage stands for leveling or categorizing the degree of injury on priority basis for deciding the time limitation for professional attention from the large list of causalities for best individual benefits.

Different Color Codes According to International Guidelines

Red: Need immediate intervention without wasting any time; should be treated as urgent and if get immediate attention survival rate will be high
Orange: Need to attend within 15-min time period
Yellow: Urgency is there, still can wait for 45- to 60-min time period after first aid
Green: Not urgent, can wait for 180 min, need minor treatment
Black: Dead, should be tagged as black

Table 35.1 Field Triage Flow Chart Using International Convention Color Codes

	Red	Yellow Prime/ Orange	Yellow	Green	Black
Priority	Transfer immediately to a referral hospital with a medical escort in an equipped ambulance	Transfer only, after evacuating all Red victims, with a medical escort in an equipped ambulance	Transfer to a referral hospital in ambulance with first aid escort	Transfer to an appropriate health care facility by available vehicles without escort	Transfer to morgue
Urgency	Most urgent (fluids, intubation, fasciotomy)	Urgent (constant, intensive care)	Urgent (i.v. line, drugs, immobilize fractures)	Not urgent (splint or dressing)	Nonurgent
Condition	Shock/hypoxia present/imminent	Deep shock, needs exceed available resources	Stable for 1 h, can wait at field	Stable till end of response	No pulse or respiration No blood pressure or heartbeat
Injuries	Life-threatening	Catastrophic	Systemic effects, not yet life threatening	Localized	Fatal
Potential for survival	High after immediate care and transportation	Very poor	High after support treatment	Good	None
Examples	Intra-abdominal injury, shock status from any cause	Massive skull or chest injuries, extensive and severe burns	Heart attack, compound fractures, severe burns	Minor fractures, burns, or wounds	Dead

Source: Indian Red Cross Society.

2. **Closed:** Involves injury to a tissue that underlies the skin without a break in the skin

Types of Wound

- *Incision:* It happens with a sharp instrument such as a glass piece, knife, or blade; it can be dangerous when the cut is deep that could damage blood vessels and muscles (Fig. 35.1).
- *Abrasions:* Abrasions occur when the skin is rubbed against the hard surfaces. They cause less bleeding but can provide a good surface for a superficial skin infection (Fig. 35.2).
- *Laceration:* Laceration refers to tearing of soft tissue (Fig. 35.3), which generally occurs because of an injury with a blunt object, especially seen when mishandling of tools such as machinery.
- *Punctures:* These occur when a sharp instrument such as needles and nails is pierced into the body (Fig. 35.4).
- *Avulsion:* Avulsion occurs when tissue is partially or fully torn off, such as a body part torn out in an accident (Fig. 35.5).
- *Stab wound:* It refers to a deep incision caused by any sharp or blunt object, such as piercing injury caused by a knife or similar sharp object. A deep stab wound could

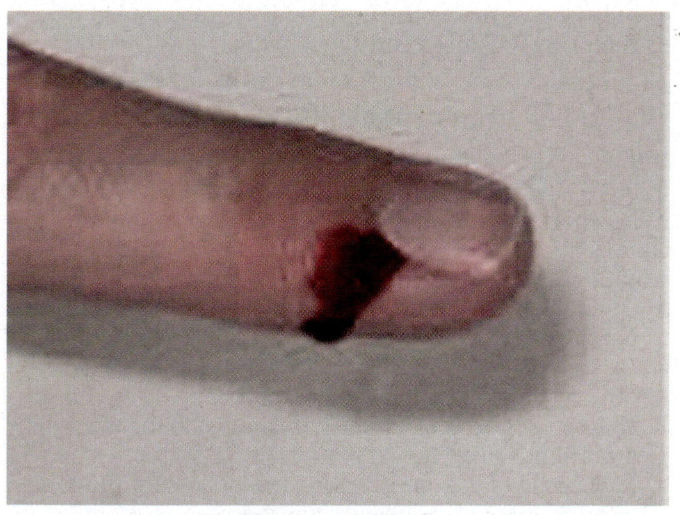

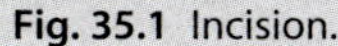

Fig. 35.1 Incision.

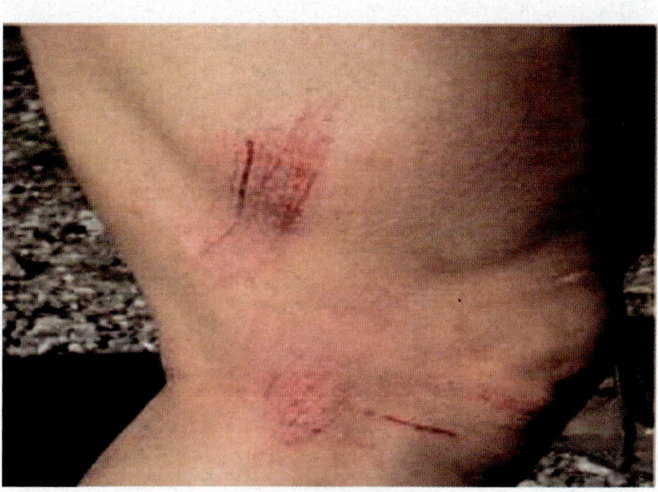

Fig. 35.2 Abrasions.

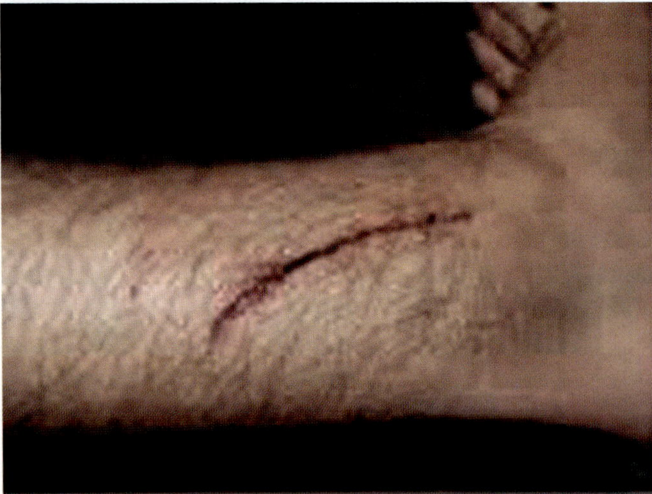

Fig. 35.3 Laceration.

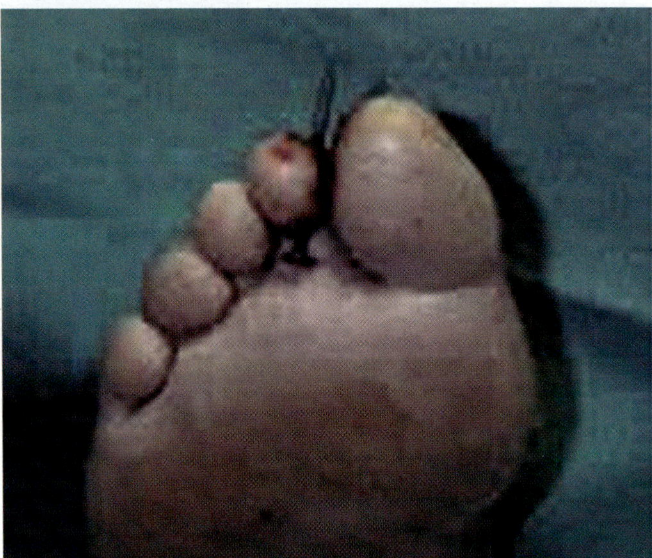

Fig. 35.4 Punctures.

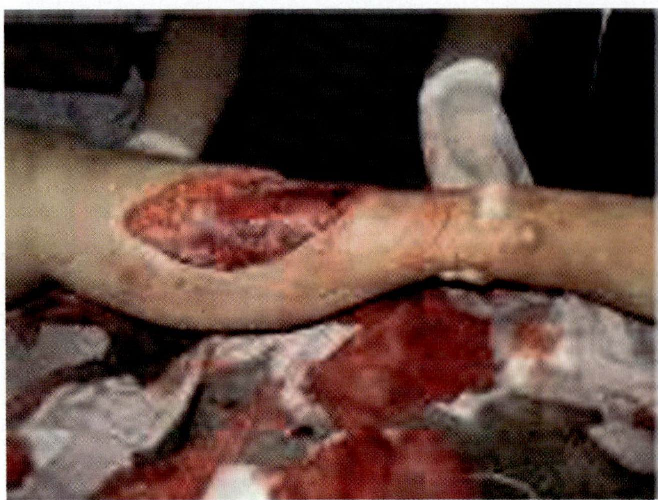

Fig. 35.5 Avulsion.

be dangerous because there may be damage to vital organs and massive internal or external bleeding.

- It should be treated very cautiously because there may be a chance of internal bleeding that can alter the function of vital organs.
- *Gunshot wound:* It refers to a deep injury caused by a bullet; although the entry of the bullet can be small, the exit can be dangerous and chances for internal bleeding are always very high.

Aims of Wound Management

- To prevent/stop the bleeding
- To avoid creating contaminated environment or prevent infection to the wound
- To treat and prevent condition of shock following excessive bleeding

First Aid Management for Open Wounds

- The first step after a cut is to stop the bleeding.
- It should be washed under running water and if the cut is small, the bleeding stops with the pressure of water. In case of a bigger cut, take a clean cloth and apply pressure.
- If dirt is present in the wound, it should be washed out to prevent infection.
- Seek immediate medical help if the cut is big or deep, or any Inidentifiable foreign body is present.
- If there is any nerve injury, the victim may experience numbness and lose sensation.
- Wound should be covered with a sterile bandage with sufficient pressure to prevent bleeding and secondary infections.

First Aid Management for Minor to Major Wound

- Wash the wound with water.
- Remove any debris if it is seen on the site.
- Apply ointments such as antibiotics if required.
- Cover the site or area with sterile bandage.
- Administer injection tetanus toxoid, if the victim is not immunized in the last 5 years.
- Take the victim to the hospital if there is major wound requiring advanced care.

First Aid Management of Infected Wound

If the wound does not start to heal after 48 hours, it can be treated as an infected wound. Mostly an open wound has more chances of getting contaminated with microorganisms. The steps of first aid management of an infected wound are listed as follows:

- After cleaning the wound, sterile gauze, pad, and bandage should be used.
- Do support the part with splint to prevent swelling.
- If any sign of infection such as fever, fatigue, swelling, or shivering is present, then immediate advanced medical attention is needed.
- Regular dressing and administration of antibiotic and tetanus toxoid are needed for the management of an infected wound.

First Aid Management of Wound With Foreign Object

If a wound is associated with any foreign object such as bullet, glass pieces, pins, or any small to large sharp pieces, then it needs to be treated little differently. The first aid management of the wound with a foreign object is listed as follows:

- If small pieces are present and embedded superficially, then they can be removed by washing under cold water or with picking through a toothed forceps. But if pieces are deeply embedded, then it is better to leave them in place because removing them may create further injury and heavy bleeding.
- Gauze, pad, and pressure bandage are required to stop bleeding.
- If tetanus toxoid injection is not administered previously, then it should be given.

First Aid Management of Wound With Severe External Bleeding

If there is a wound with severe bleeding, it can lead to shock. So, it needs immediate attention and first aid management of wounds with severe external bleeding is listed as follows:

- Expose the body to assess the wound and amount of bleeding.
- Apply adequate pressure with sterile gauze piece and apply pressure bandage.
- Check for signs of unresponsiveness of the person and open airway through head-tilt/chin-lift or jaw-thrust maneuvers.
- Check for signs of hypovolemic shock; if present, then elevate the legs, try to establish wide-bore intravenous lines, and start oxygen administration.
- Keep the person nil per oral because anesthesia administration may be required later for surgical intervention.
- Call for emergency services for safely shifting the victim to a higher health care setting.

First Aid Management of Wound With Internal Bleeding

Internal bleeding within the body cavities mainly occurs because of blunt injuries. It can be in different parts that are not visible from the outside. But it might lead to shock or can create pressure on different internal organs. The first aid management of a wound with internal bleeding is given as follows:

- Check different orifices of body parts for bleeding.
- Check signs of shock and monitor vital signs.
- Follow the treatment for shock and call for emergency services for shifting the victim to a higher health care setting.

FRACTURE

It is the break in the continuity of bone or disruption of bone tissue because of any injury or trauma such as following a fall or road traffic accident.

Symptoms

- Deformity of a limb
- Discoloration
- Severe pain at the injury site
- Swelling on the injured area
- Loss of function of the limb

Types of Fracture

- *Simple fracture:* A fracture at one site without a break in the continuity of the skin
- *Compound fracture:* Complete break of the bone that then pierces the skin
- *Greenstick fracture:* A bend-like fracture most commonly seen in children
- *Pathological fracture:* A fracture caused by underlying diseases
- *Transverse fracture:* A fracture that takes place at right angle to the axis of the bone
- *Oblique fracture:* A fracture with a curved or sloped pattern
- *Comminuted fracture*: A fracture in which the bone breaks in several pieces or fragments

Management

- Immobilize the fractured limb using bandages and splints to prevent further injury and discomfort.
- Assess and control the bleeding using sterile gauze pieces and pressure bandages. However, assess for distal pulse and warmth of the extremity.
- Assess for the patent airway, breathing, circulation, and deformity, and expose to observe any other injury or bleeding.
- Start peripheral intravenous line for fluid replacement and start oxygen administration if oxygen saturation is $<95\%$.
- Follow the "RICE" (rest, ice, compression, and elevation) strategies as a part of first aid management for a victim who has experienced fracture.
  - ***Rest*** is needed for the victim to avoid further injury.
  - ***Ice*** is applied on the site to reduce pain and avoid inflammation.
  - ***Compression*** is needed to avoid bleeding by applying pressure dressing on the site.
  - ***Elevation*** of the affected part is required to prevent edema and the extremity is elevated above the level of the heart.
- Call for ambulance to transport the victim to the higher health care setting.

DISLOCATION

It occurs when a bone partially or completely slips out of the joint or a joint is forced out of its normal position. There is a displacement of one or more bones at a joint. Shoulder, elbow, thumb, finger, and jaw are most frequently dislocated.

Causes

- Fall
- Contact sports

- Motor vehicle accident
- Sudden muscular contraction

Signs and Symptoms

- Pain at the site of dislocation
- Difficulty in moving the affected joint
- Visible deformity
- Edema or swelling at the dislocation site
- Discoloration of the dislocation site

Management

- Place the affected part in a comfortable position.
- Call for help/ambulance.
- Do not try to attempt the dislocated bone back to the place.
- Check signs of circulation below the dislocated part.
- Do not raise the dislocated part.
- First aid management is quite similar to that in fracture, for example, immobilization of the dislocated part.
- Refer the patient to a hospital as soon as possible for proper investigation and further management.

MUSCLE INJURY

It may be referred to as sprain and strain. Strain occurs because of overstretching of a muscle during exercise. Sprain occurs following a tear or twist in the ligaments such as an ankle or wrist joint. Muscle injury occurs most commonly at the back. Sprain is more severe than strain and occurs at joints, commonly at the ankle joint.

Causes

- Performing sports activity vigorously without warming up
- Heavy weight lifting

Signs and Symptoms

- Sudden pain that worsens following movement
- Tenderness at the site
- Swelling around the affected area
- Cramping of the affected area and surrounding muscles
- Loss of power
- Bruising in the initial phase
- Muscle stiffness

First Aid Treatment

- Place the victim in a proper position.
- Lift up the injured area.
- Support the injured area.
- Do not massage the area.
- Apply ice packs and cold compress to reduce inflammation at the injury site.
- Apply a crape bandage if available or a support with a cloth.
- Make sure that the bandage is not too light or too loose; check for circulation below the bandaged site.
- Refer the victim to the nearest hospital.

TRANSPORTATION OF INJURED PATIENTS

Transportation means transferring or shifting the patient from one place or location to another. The aim of transportation is to assist the victim to reach the destination without deteriorating or worsening his/her condition.

Basic Rules

- Stand as close to the victim as possible.
- Use body mechanics; bend both knees, keeping the back straight; and apply strength from legs to protect back muscles.
- Make smooth movement while holding the victim.

General Principles of Transportation

- Do not move a severely injured part.
- Do not allow the victim to sit or stand without support.
- Ask for help if it is possible and leave the victim undisturbed by promoting the safety.
- Use utmost gentleness; all movements must be slow, controlled, and careful.
- Do not try to carry a patient unless there is enough number of bearers with sufficient strength.
- Follow transportation guidelines depending on the nature and severity of the injury.

Methods of Transportation

Single-helper method of transportation:

A. *The cradle carry method:* Here, the first aider stoops by the patient's side and places one arm under the victim's knees and the other around his or her back and raises the victim using the strength from legs.

B. *Drag carry:* This is usually used for conscious patients and involves pulling the victim who is unable to stand.

C. *The human crutch method:*
   - Stand at the injured side of the victim.
   - Place his or her nearest arm around the neck.
   - Hold his or her hand with your free hands.
   - Put your other arm around the waist and grip his or her clothing at the hip.
   - A walking stick can be used for additional support.

Two-helper method of transportation:

A. *Two-hand method:*
   - The patient should be placed in a sitting position.
   - Stand on either side of the victim, maintaining a squat position.

B. *Three-handed seat:*
   - Raise the victim's legs slightly; pass the other arm under the middle of his or her thigh and grasp each other's wrist. Raise the victim together; step off with the feet outside and walk with crossover steps. Clasp hands under the thigh by a special method called the "hook grip."

C. *Four-handed seat:*
   - Stand while facing each other behind the victim.

- Grasp the left wrist of your hands and join hands to form a seat and stoop down.
- Instruct the victim to sit back on your hands and to place his or her arms around your neck to steady him or her.
- Rise up together and walk with crossover steps.

Other methods of transportation:

A. *Chair method:* It is used when a conscious victim with no serious injuries has to be moved up and down or has to be taken along a narrow passageway. The victim is placed on a steady chair and secured with broad bandages. The rescuers stand facing each other behind him or her holding the back and front legs of the chair and transport the victim.

B. *Blanket lift:* It is used when the victim is lying on a blanket or a bed sheet; fold the blanket or bed sheet on both sides and lift up the victim by holding the corners of the blanket or bed sheet; place him or her on a stretcher.

C. *Canvas or pole stretcher:* This is used to load a patient on to an ambulance trolley. A strong canvas sheet supports the casualty. Poles are inserted to move the stretcher bars and ensure that the stretcher is rigid.

FOREIGN BODY IN SKIN

A foreign body is any object that is found outside the body. Any foreign object entering the skin such as wood, stick, metal, and glass should be assessed; any superficial foreign body may be removed and the victim may also require a tetanus toxoid vaccine, if not vaccinated previously.

Steps in First Aid

- Immediately rinse the injured area with soapy solution and water.
- Use properly sterilized thumb forceps to remove the foreign object.
- Hold the foreign object with thumb forceps and pull it gently out in the same direction.
- If the object is under the skin, use a sterilized needle; lift the skin and remove the object.
- One can use a magnifying glass for visualizing the object.
- Wash it with soap and water.
- Apply antibiotic.
- Do not try to move the foreign object in different angles; if having difficulty in removing it, leave the foreign body in its place and get medical help.
- Do not remove foreign bodies if they are deep because this may cause further damage.
- Do not remove the foreign bodies near the eye.

FOREIGN BODY IN EYE

Eye is one of the sensitive parts of the body. If any foreign object enters the eye, not dealing with it carefully may cause visual impairment. Usually, dust enters the eye that can be removed by blinking continuously and washing out by water. Do not try to rub.

First Aid Management

- When a person complains of discomfort in the eye, make him or her sit comfortably on a chair with the head facing upwards.
- Tell the person not to rub the eyes.
- Use the index finger and thumb to separate eyelids.
- Ask the person to turn the eyeball up, down, left, and right for eye examination.
- In case the foreign body is present on sclera, rinse it with clean water.
- If the foreign body still remains there, use a slightly wet swab or clean cotton cloth to remove it.
- Eye irrigation can be done under the guidance of a qualified professional.
- If a foreign object or sharp instrument is found on the pupil or iris, it should not be touched; take the individual to the hospital.
- Do not remove a large object from the eye.
- Refer the victim to the nearest hospital immediately.

FOREIGN BODY IN EAR

The foreign body entering the ear could be an object or insect, which may cause temporary deafness.

First Aid Management

- Make the victim to sit down comfortably and reassure the client.
- Examine the ear under flush light. For examination of the ear, pull the earlobe backwards and downwards in case of children and backwards and upwards in case of adults.
- Remove the foreign body if it is clearly visible and hold it with forceps and gently remove it.
- Try to remove the object by gravity in case of small objects by tilting the head to the affected side.
- In case of insects, tilt the affected side of the ear upwards and try to float the insect out by pouring mineral oil into the ear; the oil should be little warm.
- Ear irrigation can be done under the guidance of a qualified professional.
- Refer the victim to a higher center for advanced care.

FOREIGN BODY IN NOSE

Younger children may unknowingly insert a small object in the nose and a sharp object may cause damage of nasal tissue.

First Aid Management

- Keep the victim calm.
- Encourage the victim to breathe through the mouth.
- Keep the unaffected nostril closed and blow slowly and gently on the affected nostril.
- Do not blow on the nose too hard.
- Do not attempt to remove the object with finger; it may enter further and cause further damage to nasal tissue.
- Do not try to search for the object with cotton swab.

- Check signs of airway obstruction.
- Transfer the victim immediately to the higher health care facility for advanced care and removal using instruments and endoscopes.

FOREIGN BODY IN THROAT

Choking or foreign body in the throat can cause obstruction in the airway and may lead to asphyxia and there is a high risk of death too because of airway obstruction. There are actions that need to be taken to prevent complications listed as follows:

Infant and younger child choking:

- Check for signs of choking such as not able to speak or breathe and signing for help.
- Never try to do blind sweep, because this may further move the foreign body deep into the respiratory tract.
- Kneel or sit with the infant in your lap.
- Hold the infant face down with the head slightly lower than the chest, resting on your forearm. Support the infant's head and jaw with your forearm on your lap or thigh to support the infant.
- Deliver up to five back slaps forcefully between the infant's shoulder blades, using the heel of your hand. Deliver each slap with sufficient force to attempt to dislodge the foreign body.
- After delivering up to five slaps, place your free hand on the infant's back, with the palm of one hand supporting the infant's face and jaw and the palm of the other hand supporting the back of the infant's head.
- Turn the infant as a unit while carefully supporting the head and neck. Hold the infant face up, with your forearm resting on your thigh. Keep the infant's head lower than the trunk.
- Provide up to five quick downward chest thrusts in the middle of the chest, over the lower half of the breastbone (same as for chest compression during CPR). Deliver chest thrush at the rate of about one per second, each with the intention of creating enough force to dislodge the foreign body.
- Repeat the sequence of up to five back slaps and up to five chest thrusts until the object is removed or the infant becomes unresponsive.
- If you fail to remove the foreign body and/or the infant becomes unresponsive, continue CPR and plan to shift the victim to a higher health care center for the expert medical help for the removal of the foreign body.

Adult and older child choking:

- Check for signs of choking such as not able to speak or breathe and signing for help by typically holding hands abound the throat.
- Never try to do blind sweep, because this may further move the foreign body deep into the respiratory tract.
- Make the victim stand in front of you by slightly leaning forward.
- Make a fist with the thumb inside and place it just above the navel, and then grab the fist with your other hand and deliver inward and upward abdominal thrusts until the foreign body is dislodged and removed. This process is called Heimlich maneuverer.
- In case the victim is pregnant or too obese, deliver chest thrush in the same manner by placing the fist just under the xiphisternum. This process is termed modified Heimlich maneuverer.
- If you fail to remove the foreign body and the victim becomes unresponsive, start CPR and plan to shift the victim to a higher health care center for the expert medical help for the removal of the foreign body.

FOREIGN BODY IN STOMACH

It is observed that a foreign body or object may accidently be ingested by children and it may enter the esophagus and stomach.

First aid management:

- Never try to let the victim to vomit; it may create further obstruction and damage.
- Take a detailed history of the victim and keep him or her under observation because most of the ingested objects pass with stool.
- Reassurance of the child and family is very important to avoid any panic among them.
- If the object is not removed and there are any signs of obstruction, the victim may be shifted to a higher health care center for the advanced medical help.

BURNS AND SCALDS

Burns are the damage caused to the skin when the body is in contact with dry heat and strong chemicals (e.g., nitric acid, sulfuric acid), electricity, and radiation. Scalds are caused when the body is in contact with moist heat such as boiling water, hot oil, hot tar, and steam.

Children are usually at more risk for burns and their related injury. It has also been observed that face is more often involved in reported burn cases of children and it can be even life threatening or challenging to treat because of its complexity.

Classification of Burn

- *First-degree burns:* Redness, swelling, pain, and blisters may develop; the area of the burn turns white while touching; and it generally takes around 3–6 days to heal.
- *Second-degree burns:* Pain, swelling, blister formation, and scars may develop, and healing depends on the extent of the injury.
- *Third-degree burns:* Numbness occurs; there is no pain, necrosis of tissues, loss of sensation, deep scar, and discoloration of the skin.

First Aid Measures

- Burn injury with fire requires immediate pouring of clean water to prevent further damage; however, ice application is not recommended because it may cause peripheral blood vessel constriction.
- A thick cloth or blanket immersed in water can be used first to cover the victim and then support the victim's head while you roll him or her on the ground.
- In case the burn occurred because of an electric source, then power off the supply as soon as possible and use a

dry rope, any wooden material, or dry cloth to take away the victim from the electric field.
- The victim should be moved quickly to a safer place to facilitate proper management.
- Clothing of the victim with burn injury should be gently removed or loosened in case removal is not possible.
- While placing the victim on his/her back for recovery, it is important to first look for effective breathing.
- If the patient is unresponsive and there no pulse and respiration, then immediately start CPR.
- It is important to assess the size and degree of the burn area for further management.
- Injection of tetanus toxoid injection is advised to the victim.
- Hospital referral should be done at the earliest possible because these victims have very high risk of developing hypovolemic shock, which could be life-threatening.

Important Points to Remember

- The victim should be refrained from using baking soda or any other sort of home remedy over the burnt area.
- Avoid frequent touching and movement of the burnt area.
- Never pull the burnt cloth on the skin; if you attempt to remove the cloth, the skin will be pulled off, causing unnecessary pain and open wound, which may predispose to infection.
- Never overcool the victim; the victim may have hypothermia.
- Do not apply ice to the burned area.
- Never bust the blisters.
- Children should be kept away from harmful items such as matchbox, flames, burning lamps, and candles.
- It is advised to keep cooking applications or other electrical appliances at a safe place or beyond children's reach.
- Avoid nylon clothing whenever working near fire or flames because it catches fire easily.
- Keep away the inflammable materials and do not come with materials such as nylon close to the fireplace.

POISONING

Ingestion of lethal substances into the body in excess can cause significant damage or problems in the body and sometimes it can be life threatening if not treated timely.

The different ways in which poison enters the body are ingestion (swallow), inhalation (breathe), absorption (by the skin), or injection.

The degree of fatality depends on different aspects such as the type of poison, total amount consumed, victim's age, and other health-related details of the individual. To deal with a poisoning case, understanding the chemical structure and toxic nature of that particular substance is necessary.

General Signs and Symptoms

- Repeated vomiting
- Pain in the abdomen
- Changes in patients' level of consciousness
- Headache and restlessness
- Change of pupillary reaction—pinpoint pupil

First Aid Management for Poisoning

1. Do not panic; be calm and act quickly.
2. Elimination of the poison:
   - Induce vomiting using syrup of ipecac or give plenty of water.
   - Immediately refer to the hospital if the victim's health deteriorates.
   - In case of kerosene poisoning, do not induce vomiting because it can be harmful.
   - Do not induce vomiting in an unconscious victim.
3. Give relevant antidote to the patient, if available.
4. Provide symptomatic management.
5. Give comfort and confidence.
6. Refer the person to a higher health care center as soon as possible.

   Special precautions:
   - Never start mouth-to-mouth resuscitation if there is a history of toxin inhalation.
   - The victim should be shifted from the actual affected area to a safe place to reduce the chance of further effect.
   - The surface of the body part where toxic substance is present should be cleaned and rinsed first before suctioning.

INSECT BITES

Bites by insects and stings are very common and they can cause minor to major symptoms such as drowsiness, dizziness, nausea, vomiting, and itching and in severe cases can lead to hives and anaphylactic shock. Sometimes insects play the role of vector and transmit diseases such as malaria, dengue, and encephalitis (tick bites). Adequate measures need to be taken to avoid any major complication in these situations.

First Aid Management

- Initial assessment is necessary to know the type of insect bite, which helps in planning for first aid interventions. For example, tick bites necessitate the removal of tick by a forceps and cleaning with antiseptic solution. Tick can be killed by using organic solvents and skin rash caused by tick bites can be treated by antibiotic administration.
- Enlist the measures to be taken according to the common insects found in that particular area.
- People may be educated about taking precautionary measures for the prevention of insect bites, for example, the use of a mosquito net, full-sleeve clothes, and mosquito replants in the areas of high mosquito prevalence.

STINGS

A sting over the body such as because of bees can cause redness, pain, itching, and swelling at the site. Bee sting can cause hives or allergies and the victim may experience nausea, vomiting, allergic reactions, anaphylactic reactions, and even anaphylactic shock. A sting on the lips can cause swelling on the lips, which may extend up to the throat, leading to breathing difficulties.

First Aid Management

- Remove stings possibly by scraping them gently but tweezers must not be used to scrape the stings because it can result in releasing venom.
- After removing the stings, wash the area with soap and water.
- Apply an ice pack over the affected site, which may reduce swelling and pain at the site caused because of the sting.
- Apply calamine lotion or if not available then baking soda and water can be applied over the site by making a paste, which may help reduce itching.

DOG BITE

The saliva from a bite or scratch of a street dog carries microorganisms that can cause infection and in severe cases can cause diseases. Rabies is a viral infection that is caused by virus of Rhabdoviridae family that gets transmitted from a bite or scratch of an infected animal. It mainly affects the nervous system and therefore leads to inflammation of the brain in humans.

Signs and Symptoms

- Difficulty in swallowing
- Lethargy and restlessness
- Hydrophobia
- Pain, itching, and numbness

First Aid Management

If the bite is superficial and received from a pet dog and the dog is immunized and healthy, then the first aid management will be as following:

- At first, clean the wound area with soapy solution and water.
- Disinfectant lotion is applied.
- Pain, pyrexia, swelling, and redness around the site of bite should be observed for signs of infection.
- The victim needs to be referred to the nearest hospital for further treatment.

If the bite is deeper and received from a strange animal:

- Wash the wound with soap and water.
- If there is bleeding from the site of bite, then apply pressure with the help of a bandage or towel to stop the bleeding.
- Clean the wound with disinfectant solution and cover it with sterile dressing.
- Take the victim to the hospital and take antirabies treatment.
- If possible, find the animal; do not kill the dog but observe it for 10–15 days.
- *If there is no history of vaccination*, then rabies immune globulin 20 IU/kg body weight should be administered around the anatomically visible wound and rest dose i.m. away from the vaccine site. Vaccines such as human diploid cell vaccine and rabies vaccine adsorbed/purified chick embryo cell vaccine should be administered in the deltoid muscles on days 0, 3, 7, 14, and 28.
- *If previously vaccinated*, then there is no need of a full regimen of rabies immune globulin. Vaccines such as human diploid cell vaccine and rabies vaccine adsorbed/purified chick embryo cell vaccine should be administered in the deltoid muscles on days 0 and 3.

SNAKE BITE

Snake bite is considered as a serious problem in many countries with both poisonous snake and nonpoisonous snake because panic kills many lives. Sometimes even wrong first aid treatment can also be fatal.

First Aid Management Guidelines for Snake Bite

- While placing the victim in recovery position, the patient is informed to avoid unnecessary movement and remain calm.
- The affected or bitten part is immobilized and kept below the level of the heart.
- Clean or wipe the bitten or sting site of the wound.
- Firm pressure or close loop with a cord can be applied above the site of bite and this should be removed within 15 minutes after antivenom has been given.

In case there is unavailability of antivenom, then perform the following measures:

- Apply firm pressure or tie a cord tightly above the bitten area.
- A cut of depth 1 cm can be made with a sterile blade or clean knife to remove the poisonous liquid.
- After removal of poison, it is advised to loosen the tightly tied area.
- Wound care should be done appropriately to avoid infection.
- Hospital referral is required for the administration of antivenom injection.

Special considerations are as follows:

- Never use suction; it is not effective, and can even worsen the condition.
- Whenever using compression in bandage, remember that it should not be too tight and too loose; see that at least one finger enters between the bandage and the skin.

FROSTBITE

Frostbite occurs when the skin and the tissues that underlie the skin freeze after an exposure to extreme cold conditions or temperatures. Most commonly, the toes, fingers, ears, exposed cheeks, and chin are affected. The area becomes numb and hard, and appears waxy. It may lead to irreversible damage of blood vessels or soft tissues. So, loss of sensation, tissue death, or even gangrene can happen. Sometimes it may be followed by hypothermia and needs immediate medical attention.

Warning Signs and Symptoms

- The skin becomes pale and a feeling of numbness occurs.
- The affected area hardens and appears waxy.
- Skin color turns white to blue.
- When gangrene occurs, the skin can turn black.
- The victim could be in a drowsy, lethargic, or unconscious state.

First Aid Management

- Hypothermia must be checked when signs such as shivering, drowsiness, lethargy, and nausea are present.
- Ask the victim to keep extremities close to the body.
- Protect the victim's skin from damage by avoiding thawing or defrosting the area immediately after frostbite.
- Provide a blanket or warm clothing to the victim.
- Remove jewelry, gloves, and shoes to continuously monitor the most affected areas and try to warm them up by rubbing.
- Warm water (temperature will be around 40°C) can be used to soak the affected areas.
- Avoid applying direct heat to the face such as by a stove, heat lamp, or heating pads.
- Offer warm beverages such as milk to the victim and avoid giving alcohol.
- Elevate the affected areas to reduce the chance of swelling.
- If numbness still persists, the victim must be referred to the higher health care facility.

HEATSTROKE

It is defined as raised body temperature in the absence of sweating, which leads to eventually loss of consciousness because of failure of the temperature regulatory mechanism of the body. It needs immediate attention because not giving significant cooling within a minute can worsen the condition.

Causes

- Cooling mechanism of the body fails because of excessive humidity and extreme heat.
- Internal body temperature rises, leading to stroke.
- It can happen because of drug use for ecstasy.

Symptoms

- Raised body temperature > 104°F
- Severe headache
- Confusion, dizziness, and disorientation
- Rapid weak pulse becoming irregular
- Rapid or shallow breaths
- Lack of sweating
- Fluctuation of blood pressure
- Alteration in consciousness or state of coma

First Aid Management

- Keep the person away from the heat and take him or her to a shady, cool place.
- Place the victim in recovery position (sitting position with a supporting pillow).
- Remove constructive clothing.
- Switch on a fan or air conditioner.
- The person should be given sponging with a wet towel to provide coolness. A wet sponge cloth can be placed under the armpit, forehead, and abdomen, or the person can be wrapped with a wet sheet and cold water poured on him or her until the temperature cools down to 38°C. Once the temperature becomes stable, dry the person using a clean and dry cloth.
- Hydration should be maintained with the help of juices, fluid, and electrolytes.
- Keep calm and confident.
- Monitor vital signs carefully.
- Contact emergency medical services immediately.

ADULT BASIC LIFE SUPPORT

A large number of people die because of cardiopulmonary arrest; therefore, basic life support (BLS) acts a lifesaving intervention. BLS involves CPR, which is a combination of chest compression, rescue breathing, and automated defibrillation. It is important to establish oxygen supply to the vital organs as soon as possible to prevent irreversible damage, which can be established through prompt initiation of BLS. The basic aim of BLS is to preserve life, promote recovery, and prevent worsening the condition.

Indications of Basic Life Support

These include cardiac arrest, pulmonary arrest, or cardiopulmonary arrest, which may have been associated with drowning, stroke, choking, smoke inhalation, drug overdose, suffocation, accident, injury, and underlying cardiac, pulmonary, endocrinal, and electrolyte morbidities.

Principles of Basic Life Support

- To restore effective circulation and ventilation
- To prevent irreversible cerebral damage because of hypoxia

Immediate Responsibilities of the Resuscitator

- To recognize the signs of cardiac arrest
- To protect the patient's brain from anoxia by immediately starting external cardiac massage and ventilation.

Chain of Survival

- Immediate recognition and prompt activation of emergency response system
- Early start of CPR (chest compression and ventilation)
- Rapid defibrillation
- Post–cardiac arrest care

Steps of CPR

- Check the scene for danger to minimize risk to yourself, bystanders, and the victim.
- Assess victim responsiveness to ascertain the level of consciousness; gently shake the victim's shoulders and ask loudly, "Are you OK?"
- If the victim is unresponsive, shout for help.
- Check breathing and carotid pulse in adults (for at least 5 seconds but not more than 10 seconds), carotid or femoral pulse in children, and brachial pulse in infants. Meanwhile, also look for the presence of breathing.
- If there is no pulse, start chest compressions and deliver 30 compressions at the rate of about 100–120 compressions/min. Position your hands and body to

perform chest compression by placing heel of one hand in the center of the victim's chest, on the lower half of the sternum, and then placing heel of the other hand on the top of the first hand. Remember to keep arms straight and position your shoulder directly over your hands.

- For children, use one or two hands for chest compression (one hand for a very small child), and for infants, use two-finger technique until the second rescuer arrives; thereafter, use the two-thumb–encircling hands technique.
- Maintain an open airway by either head-tilt/chin-lift maneuverer or if there is a suspected cervical injury, use jaw-thrust maneuver to maintain airway patency.
- For a patient not breathing, on completion of 30 compressions, deliver 2 rescues of breathing (30:2) either mouth to mouth or pocket mask or Ambu bag.
- As soon as AED arrives, switch on AED, attach pads on the chest, plug-in cord, and deliver shock if advised.
- Immediately after the delivery of shock, resume the CPR and maintain compression and respiration ratio of 30:2.
- Review the person's condition if signs of life return. If the person starts breathing by self, stop doing CPR and place the victim on his or her side with the head tilted back (recovery position).

Points to Consider

- For adults, a compression-to-ventilation ratio of 30:2 is recommended universally in case of presence of both single and more rescuers.
- A compression-to-ventilation ratio of 15:2 is maintained for children and infants if two or more rescuers are present.
- The recommended order to be followed to rescue the client is chest compression, followed by airway and breathing (CAB). The rate of compression must be at least 100–120 compressions/min.
- The depth of chest compression in adults and children is at least 5–6 cm (2–2.5 inches) and in infants it is 4–5 cm (1.5–2 inches).
- It is important to maintain high-quality CPR for a better outcome. The characteristics of high-quality CPR are as follows: (i) start chest compression within 10 seconds of recognition of cardiac arrest; (ii) push hard, push fast—compression rate of 100–120/min with a depth of about 5 cm for adults, at least one-third the depth of chest or about 5 cm for children, and at least one-third the depth of chest or about 4 cm for children; (iii) allow compete chest recoil after each compression; (iv) minimize interruptions in compression (try to limit interruptions to less than 10 seconds); (v) give effective breath that makes visible chest rise; and (vi) avoid excessive ventilation.
- Team dynamics is very important in BLS, in which clearly defined role and responsivities of every team member, constructive intervention, closed-loop communication, clear message, mutual respect, summarization, and re-evaluation are key for success.

UNCONSCIOUSNESS

A constant supply of oxygenated blood and glucose is required for the proper functioning of the brain. Interruption in the supply leads to unconsciousness within a few seconds and persistent brain damage in minutes. In this condition, the victim is unable to speak or move and cannot respond to place, people, and time.

Causes of Unconsciousness

- Brain dysfunction because of brain tumor, head injury, and vascular events such as cerebrovascular accident
- Diffuse brain dysfunction infection such as meningitis, encephalitis, and poisoning
- Metabolic and endocrine causes such as hepatic or renal failure, hypothyroidism, severe electrolyte disturbances, hypotension, or hypertensive crisis

First Aid of Unconscious Victim

Follow the sequence of A, B, C (airway, breathing, and circulation).

- Assess for any signs of bleeding.
- Place the victim in recovery position, if he or she is spontaneously breathing and progressively regaining consciousness.
- Do not offer any thing by mouth to an unconscious victim.
- Check for the pulse and breathing rate, and record any observations and initiate the level of responsiveness.
- Refer the victim to the hospital or higher health care facility as soon as possible.

HEMORRHAGE

Hemorrhage is an abnormal, severe internal or external discharge of blood that may cause hypovolemic shock and even death. In other words, it is the oozing of blood from blood vessels. Severe bleeding, if not controlled, could be life threatening; therefore, bleeding should be stopped as soon as possible.

Types of Hemorrhage

1. *External and internal hemorrhage:* External hemorrhage is visible; hence, the diagnosis is easy. In contrast, internal hemorrhage, which occurs from deep-seated vessels or following rupture of internal organs, is not seen.
2. *Arterial, venous, and capillary:* Arterial bleeding is bright red in color; venous bleeding appears to be dark red with a steady flow and capillary bleeding is blood seeping from the bed of capillaries and the blood appears to be less bright than the arterial blood.

First Aid Management

- Make the victim to lie down to assess the extent of the wound.
- Apply direct pressure on the wound by covering with sterile pressure dressing.
- If any foreign body is present, do not remove it and do not apply too much pressure.
- When bleeding stops, apply a bandage and elevate the affected limb.
- Apply tourniquet in case of severe bleeding.
- Try to establish a wide-bore intravenous cannula and start normal saline infusion.
- Do not give the victim anything to eat or drink.

- Start oxygen administration using an oxygen face mask.
- Watch for signs of hypovolemic shock and transfer the victim to the hospital

SHOCK

Shock is defined as a life-threatening medical emergency, in which the body has less blood flow (maybe fluid and/or electrolyte deficit), which in turn leads to less oxygen in the body tissues, brains, and hearts, which can lead to heart attack or organ damage. Most commonly shock occurs because of blood loss that may be visible or internal but if it exceeds more than 1.2 L, that is, one-fifth of the blood volume, the victim may start to show symptoms.

Causes

- Dehydration
- Infection
- Trauma or injuries
- Allergic reaction
- Heart failure
- Bleeding
- Burn
- Bowel obstruction

Signs and Symptoms

- Low blood pressure
- Weak or thready pulse
- Shallow breathing
- Dizziness
- Cold and clammy skin
- Weakness
- Chest pain
- Confusion
- Oliguria or anuria
- Bluish lips or fingernails
- Cyanosis: gray to blue skin color
- Restlessness associated with aggressive behavior
- Gasping
- Unresponsiveness
- Stopping of heartbeat

Types of Shock

1. *Septic shock:* It occurs when bacteria multiply in the blood and release poisonous substance.
2. *Cardiogenic shock:* It occurs when the heart is not functioning well and is unable to supply blood to vital organs.
3. *Hypovolemic shock:* It occurs because of severe blood loss or fluid and electrolyte loss
4. *Anaphylactic shock:* It occurs because of severe allergic reaction.
5. *Neurogenic shock:* It occurs because of spinal cord injury or trauma.

First Aid Management

- Lay down the victim on the back and legs should be elevated (except in case of spinal cord injury) to maintain blood supply to the vital organs.
- Maintain the patency of the airway by keeping it open and prevent tilting the head forward.
- Check for responsiveness, breathing, and pulse; in their absence, start CPR.
- Control external bleeding, if any.
- Call for help/ambulance/medical services.
- Continuously monitor vital signs.
- A blanket must be kept over the victim's body to promote warmth.
- Prevent mobilizing any fractured limb unless it has been properly splinted.
- Refer the patient to a hospital or health care facility as soon as possible.

Special Precautions

- Never ask the victim to eat or drink orally because resuscitation may be needed later on.
- If the victim is unresponsive, open the airway by head-tilt and chin-lift or jaw-thrush maneuverer and check the breathing.
- If the victim is pregnant, ask her to lie down on the left side to promote adequate blood supply to the fetus.
- Do not use any hot application that can worsen the condition.

COMMUNITY EMERGENCIES

Emergencies can happen at any time and can cause extreme damage or destruction in human life and to others. Learning and acting in these emergencies is of utmost importance to help resolve aftereffects of the disasters. There can be a hazardous or harmful impact of these emergencies such as fires, explosions, and earthquakes. The first aiders or the rescuers play an essential role in managing these life-threatening situations and promote health of the victims who experienced these disasters. Disaster preparedness prior to any nature-made or manmade disaster is mandatory to mitigate the crisis a bit. The role of a first aider is aimed to resolve various emergencies and to act as a lifesaver in the community emergency situations. The first aid management for the following common community emergency situations is discussed in this chapter: fires, explosions, floods, earthquakes, and famine.

Fire

Fire is an emergency that can spread too quickly from a minor fire to a disaster. Whenever there is an incident of fire emergency, be calm, observe, and take decisions. Keep own self safe, and try to leave and evacuate the victims as soon as possible after activating alarm or calling the emergency services.

Role of the First Aider During Fire

First of all, self-safety and the safety of those who are present at the site of incident have to be ensured while managing the situation during fire. The basic steps to be taken care are as follows:

- The first step is to rescue those who are in instant or immediate danger and one can follow **"RACE"** acronym, where **"R"** stands for rescue; **"A"** stands for being alert, shout saying "fire," and activating emergency response system; **"C"** stands for contain, which may be referred to as restraining fire by closing the doors and windows to stop spread of fire; and **"E"** stands for evacuating the building or extinguishing the fire.

- The nose and mouth must be covered to avoid inhalation of smoke while entering the premises.
- Avoid walking; instead, move forward by dragging or crawling the body or as close to the ground as possible.
- Do not use the lift in fire; do not panic and search for an exit using the stairs.
- If possible, turn off the supply of electricity.
- Sand can be used to stop the fire by throwing it on the fire.
- Water is used to stop fire. Be alert about the type of fire.
- Wait for the fire brigade and do not panic as well as prevent causing any injury to self.
- Break the *"triangle of fire"* because there are three elements responsible for a complete fire emergency, that is, a spark, the source of energy/fuel, and air or oxygen; the absence of one of them can break the chain. Therefore, allay any burning substances that can increase the energy of the fire such as paper, oil, gas, and petrol. Close the door or rap with blanket (fire blanket) to reduce the source of oxygen. Switch off or cut off the source of gas and any flame.
- If victims are stuck on any electrical source, do not touch them. Try to switch off the electrical connection. If this is not possible, then wooden material can be used to detach the victim; then move away the victim from the source of electricity. Do the initial assessment of the victim and call the emergency services for help to transfer the victim to the nearest possible hospital emergency.
- Refer first aid management of the burns and scalds given on page 814 of this chapter.

Special Considerations

- For electrical fire, switch off the source but do not use water.
- For grease fire, cover the flame with noninflammable material, switch off the source, or use a fire extinguisher but never use water.
- If a cloth catches fire, then remove it or roll over the ground.
- If trapped in a building, then close the door, come near a window, and ask for help but do not fully open the window; try to be at the ground level of the room because carbon monoxide or smoke fills the upper level of the room first.
- Never touch any electrical equipment until it is switched off.

Explosions

Explosions or blasts have a severe kind of blunt and penetrating injury consequences. They can be in an open or closed place. If they are in a closed place, there will be associated collapse of building or structure and a rescue team is needed.

Types of Explosives

High-order explosives (HE): Create huge overpressurized shock wave and are supersonic in nature, for example, dynamite and nitroglycerin.

Low-order explosives (LE): Do not create huge overpressurized shock wave and are subsonic in nature, for example, pipe bomb and gunpowder.

The classification of types of explosion injury is presented in Table 35.2.

Role of First Aider During Explosions

A victim who has experienced injury because of an explosion or blast must be rescued following the guidelines given as follows:

- Do a quick and initial assessment of the type of explosions, possible toxic substances, possible health hazards, and nearby police station and health facilities.
- The victim must be moved to safe premises or away from the site of explosion.

Table 35.2 Classification of Explosion Injury

Category	Characteristics	Body Part Injury	Types of Injury
Primary	Unique to HE, results from the impact of the overpressurization wave with body surfaces	Gas-filled structures are most susceptible—lungs, GI tract, and middle ear	Blast lung (pulmonary barotrauma) Tympanic membrane rupture and middle ear damage Abdominal hemorrhage and perforation Globe (eye) rupture Concussion (traumatic brain injury without physical signs of head injury)
Secondary	Results from flying debris and bomb fragments	Any body part may be affected	Penetrating ballistic (fragmentation) or blunt injuries Eye penetration (can be occult)
Tertiary	Results from individuals being thrown by the blast wind	Any body part may be affected	Fracture and traumatic amputation Closed and open brain injury
Quaternary	All explosion-related injuries, illnesses, or diseases not because of primary, secondary, or tertiary mechanisms–Includes exacerbation or complications of existing conditions	Any body part may be affected	Burns (flash, partial, and full thickness) Crush injuries Closed and open brain injury Asthma, COPD, or other breathing problems from dust, smoke, or toxic fumes Angina Hyperglycemia, hypertension

COPD, chronic obstructive pulmonary disease; *GI*, gastrointestinal; *HE*, high-order explosives.

- Assess the airway and injury caused following explosion such as inhalation of fervid air.
- Victims are kept safe if they experienced radiation effects and essential things must be provided.
- Do upside-down triage for priorities of the victims' needs of hospitalization and rush to the nearby hospital.
- Disposal of human excreta must be handled carefully.
- Refer the victim to the health care facility as soon as possible.
- Follow first aid management of burns (see page 814), fracture (see page 811), and hemorrhage (see page 818) given in this chapter.

Flood

Flood is one of the common natural disasters that happen frequently in the different parts of the world. This is more dangerous for the urban areas than for the rural areas because urban areas are overcrowded. If flood occurs within a few hours of heavy rainfall, it is called flash flood and it can rise above 30 m. Flood can destroy property, electricity, and road connection, and lead to prominent health hazards.

Role of First Aider During Floods

Floods can be very dangerous and water can clock people off their feet. Awareness regarding immediate management in case of floods needs to be encouraged and one must follow the following guidelines while managing victims:

- The drinking water that is to be given to the victims must be purified.
- Provision of portable toilets must be done.
- Food must be enduring or durable.
- Provide warm blankets to the victims.
- Supply of clean clothing must be kept up.
- Portable tents must be fixed at the site.
- Containers for storage of items must be present.
- Be ready with the kit for management of diarrhea, insect bites, snake bites, food poisoning, and flu.

Special Precautions During Flood

- Be alert about the position of the river, pond, dam, and manhole to avoid drowning.
- Avoid any underground area.
- Do not walk blindly without measuring the depth of the water.
- Switch off the electricity source.
- Be alert about snake bite and insect bite.
- Maintain the hygiene of the food and water to prevent food poisoning.
- Always be ready with an evacuation plan for the family during emergency.
- Store drinking water and be aware of flu outbreak.
- Be responsible for sanitation.
- Work on the drainage system.

Earthquake

Earthquake is the natural disaster resulting from the seismic waves created in the lithosphere region because of sudden release of energy. Whenever there is an event of earthquake, be aware of small-intensity earthquakes that are always known to have aftershocks.

Seven Steps to Follow During Earthquake

The public must be taught about the following guidelines for earthquake:

A. *Preparation needed before earthquake:* Whenever anyone is building his or her home, he or she should be cautious about risks associated with the structure and geographical location. Avail home earthquake insurance if applicable. Keep earthquake first aid kit ready.

B. *During earthquake:*
   - *First step:* Search for your secure space previously where you have less chances of injury from anything falling upon you. Quickly identify the potential hazardous items.
   - *Second step:* For further safety, plan beforehand how you will communicate during the time of actual emergency.
   - *Third step:* Keep aside whatever items for survival may be necessary such as first aid kit, food, and other necessary resources.
   - *Fourth step:* Keep all important documents, insurance paper, and finance-related items together and in an achievable position to avoid financial crisis.
   - *Fifth step:* When the earth is shaking, be under a safe place such as under a table; cover your head and neck and be aware of hazardous items that can create fall injury.
   - *Sixth step:* After the shakes, find out the easiest evacuation way and ask for emergency help and help others if possible.
   - *Seventh step:* Be up-to-date with the news and warning from the government and follow the recovery steps for repairing the damage after the earthquake.

Special Precautions

- Never use lift and always use stairs.
- If you are on road or in a car, search for an open place and be there. There should not be any tree, building, and electronic power supply item.
- If you are at home, search for a safe place such as under a table or bed and cover the head with a pillow and be at a safe distance from any item that can fall upon you.
- Be aware of glass windows and electronic gadgets.

Role of First Aider During Earthquakes

Earthquakes can result in loss of human lives, landslides, damage or destruction of buildings, roads, electrical equipment, and other resources. They can even be the reason for fire, flood, or dangerous tsunami. There is an essential role of the first aider in managing this disastrous situation by following these basic steps:

1. Treat injuries of the victims following the mass triage techniques and do not move or shift the victims alone in case they are trapped under any heavy object or wait for the help.
2. Relieve the anxiety of the victim by making him/her calm by assuring help.
3. Call for the helpline number and avoid any congestion in the network; use own mobile phone to report the incident.
4. Aftershocks must be expected and be aware to avoid further injury to victims.
5. Remain calm and safe while dealing with the victim.

6. Follow first aid management of fracture (see page 811) and hemorrhage (see page 818) given in this chapter.

Famine

The famine can also be called feast, which is utmost or extreme scarcity of food where there is an insufficient amount or shortage of the food. Possible causes of famine could be war, population explosion, climate changes, crop failure and food shortage, and adverse government policies.

Consequences of famine on health

- Malnutrition and starvation
- Opportunistic infection
- Epidemic diseases
- Increasing mortality rate

Preventive measures for famine

- Refocus on public health infrastructure and facilities
- Provide supplementary food for the undernourished child
- Conduct awareness program
- Implement mass immunization
- Identify vulnerable population and take remedial steps
- Arrange for needed food rations and additional fortified food
- Relief fund should be sanctioned

Role of First Aider During Famine

Some guidelines can be followed by a first aider during famine such as the following.

- Offer medical treatment including medicines of high quality and the supply that is needed on the spot for undernourished victims.
- The supply that is to be provided must be hygienic.
- Blankets and mosquito nets are provided to victims to help prevent dengue or malaria.
- Water supply must be purified as well as storage must be done.
- Distribute food to the victims following hygienic measures.

KEY POINTS

- First aid management is the technique to accomplish skills to provide prompt care to the victim in need and improves prognosis of the injured.
- It is important that the rescuer must keep safety in mind while providing first aid to the victim and avoid putting himself or herself in danger.
- First aid management needs proper assessment of the situation and application of the appropriate measures required to save the victim from danger.
- Immediate precautions need to be taken such as applying direct pressure to stop bleeding.
- The wound must be kept free of infection by avoiding unnecessary steps that can aggravate the situation.
- Three "**Ps**" to be kept in mind are the following: preserve life of the victim, prevent any further damage, and promote recovery of the victim.

REFERENCES

Austin M, Crawford R, Klaassen B. First aid mannual. 10th ed. London, New York, Munich, Melbourne, Delhi; 2014. Available from: https://www.pdfdrive.com/search?q=+first+aid+mannual&pagecount=&pubyear=&searchin=&more=true.

Chen CY, Xu W, Dai Y, Xu W, Liu C, Wu Q, et al. Household preparedness for emergency events: a cross-sectional survey on residents in four regions of China. BMJ Open. 2019;9(11):e032462.

Davis CP. First aid for floods and flash floods. On health; September 15, 2004. Available from: https://www.onhealth.com/content/1/first_aid_for_floods_and_flash_floods. Accessed March 20, 2020.

Department of Health and Human Services. Explosions and blast injuries. USA: CDC; 2003. Available from: https://www.cdc.gov/masstrauma/preparedness/primer.pdf.

Earthquake. Available from: https://en.wikipedia.org/wiki/Earthquake. Accessed March 8, 2020.

Famine. Available from: https://en.wikipedia.org/wiki/Famine. Accessed March 10, 2020.

First Aid & Personal Safety. The American National Red Cross. 1st ed. New York: Doubleday; 1978. Available from: https://www.biblio.com/standard-first-aid-and-personal-by-american-red-cross/work/777967. Accessed March 10, 2020.

First aid management and accident prevention for health extension workers. Ethiopia: Ethioipia Public Health Training Initiatives, The Carter Center; 2004. Available from: https://www.cartercenter.org/resources/pdfs/health/ephti/library/lecture_notes/health_extension_trainees/LN_HEW_First_Aid_Mgmt_final.pdf.

First Aid Manual: the step by step guide for everyone. 5th ed. United States: Dorling Kindersey Limited; 2014. Available from: https://kuiyem.ku.edu.tr/wp-content/uploads/2016/12/American-College-of-Emergency-Physicians-ACEP-First-Aid-Manual.pdf. Accessed March 9, 2020.

First aid. Available from: https://en.wikipedia.org/wiki/First_aid. Accessed March 10, 2020.

Flood preparedness. Available from: https://www.nsc.org/home-safety/safety-topics/emergency-preparedness/flood. Accessed March 8, 2020.

Florio I. First aid. G Ital Med Lav 1986;8(5–6):243–4.

Gilks JML. Principles of Emergency Treatment for Swallowed Poisons: First-Aid Treatment of Accidentally Ingested Poisons in Industry. Proceedings of the Royal Society of Medicine. 1977;70(11):770–772.

Hoque DM, Islam MI, Sharmin Salam S, Rahman QS, Agrawal P, Rahman A, et al. Impact of first aid on treatment outcomes for non-fatal injuries in rural Bangladesh: Findings from an injury and demographic census. Int J Environ Res Public Health 2017;14(7):762.

Indian First Aid Manual. 7th ed. New Delhi: 2016. Available from: https://www.indianredcross.org/publications/FA-manual.pdf. Accessed March 8, 2020.

Jouhari Z, Pirasteh A, Ghassemi GR, Bazrafkan L. The effects of educational program on health volunteers' knowledge regarding their approach to earthquake in health centers in Tehran. J Adv Med Educ Prof 2015;3(2):56.

Module 2 Emergency First Aid. Indian Red Cross Society. Available from: https://www.indianredcross.org/fmr/Module2.pdf. Accessed March 12, 2020.

Pourhosseini SS, Ardalan A, Mehrolhassani MH. Key aspects of providing healthcare services in disaster response stage. Iran J Public Health 2015;44(1):111.

Presutti JR. Prevention and treatment of dog bites. Am Fam Physician. 2001;63(8):1567–73. Available from: https://www.aafp.org/afp/2001/0415/p1567.html.

Randy DK. Blast injuries and burn care. EMS World; February 4, 2013. Available from: https://www.emsworld.com/article/10913345/blast-injuries-and-burn-care. Accessed March 7, 2020.

Seven steps to earthquake safety. Available from: https://www.earthquakeauthority.com/California-Earthquake-Risk/Personal-Preparedness/Seven-Steps-to-Earthquake-Safety. Accessed March 12, 2020.

Singletary EM, Charlton NP, Epstein JL, Ferguson JD, Jensen JL, MacPherson AI, et al. Part 15: first aid: 2015 American Heart Association and American Red Cross guidelines update for first aid. Circulation 2015;132(18 Suppl. 2):S574–89.

Triage. Available from: https://en.wikipedia.org/wiki/Triage#/media/File:13049_2012_Article_483_Fig2_HTML.jpg. Accessed March 12, 2020.

Zideman DA, De Buck ED, Singletary EM, Cassan P, Chalkias AF, Evans TR, et al. European resuscitation council guidelines for resuscitation 2015 section 9. First aid. Resuscitation 2015;95:278–87.

Index

b indicates boxes, *f* indicates illustrations, and *t* indicates tables.

N

Q

R